To borrow: send email to
library@sharp.com with your
*name, phone, email barcode
of the book or CD*. Item will
be due back in 4 weeks.

Valvular Heart Disease

A Companion to Braunwald's Heart Disease

BRAUNWALD'S HEART DISEASE COMPANIONS

BRAUNWALD'S HEART DISEASE COMPANIONS

Upcoming Titles

Theroux: Acute Coronary Syndromes, 2nd Edition
Mann: Heart Failure, 2nd Edition
Blumenthal, Foody & Wong: Prevention of Cardiovascular Disease
Kormos & Miller: Mechanical Circulatory Support and Artificial Hearts
Taylor: Atlas of Cardiac CT
Kramer & Hundley: Atlas of Cardiovascular MR
Cerqueira: Atlas of Nuclear Cardiology
Thomas: Atlas of Echocardiography

Published Titles

Ballantyne: Clinical Lipidology
Issa, Miller & Zipes: Clinical Arrhythmology and Electrophysiology
Antman: Cardiovascular Therapeutics, 3rd Edition
Black & Elliott: Hypertension
Creager, Dzau & Loscalzo: Vascular Medicine
Chien: Molecular Basis of Cardiovascular Disease, 2nd Edition
Manson: Clinical Trials in Heart Disease, 2nd Edition
St. John-Sutton & Rutherford: Clinical Cardiovascular Imaging

Valvular Heart Disease

A Companion to Braunwald's Heart Disease

Third Edition

Catherine M. Otto, MD, FACC, FAHA
J. Ward Kennedy-Hamilton Endowed Professor of Cardiology
Director, Cardiology Fellowship Programs
University of Washington School of Medicine
Seattle, Washington

Robert O. Bonow, MD, MACC, FAHA
Goldberg Distinguished Professor of Cardiology
Northwestern University Feinberg School of Medicine
Chief, Division of Cardiology
Co-Director, Bluhm Cardiovascular Institute
Northwestern Memorial Hospital
Chicago, Illinois

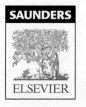

SAUNDERS

ELSEVIER

SAUNDERS
ELSEVIER

1600 John F. Kennedy Blvd.
Ste 1800
Philadelphia, PA 19103-2899

VALVULAR HEART DISEASE:
A COMPANION TO BRAUNWALD'S HEART DISEASE

978-1-4160-5892-2

Library of Congress Cataloging-in-Publication Data

Valvular heart disease : a companion to Braunwald's heart disease / [edited by] Catherine M. Otto, Robert O. Bonow. – 3rd ed.
    p. ; cm.
    Rev. ed. of: Valvular heart disease / Catherine M. Otto. c2004.
    Includes bibliographical references and index.
    ISBN 978-1-4160-5892-2
    1. Heart valves–Diseases. I. Otto, Catherine M. II. Bonow, Robert O. III. Otto, Catherine M. Valvular heart disease. IV. Braunwald's heart disease.
    [DNLM: 1. Heart Valve Diseases–therapy. 2. Heart Valve Diseases–diagnosis. 3. Heart Valve Diseases–pathology. WG 260 V2152 2009]
    RC685.V2O78 2009
    616.1'25–dc22

2008044872

Executive Publisher: Natasha Andjelkovic
Project Manager: Bryan Hayward
Design Direction: Steve Stave

Printed in China

Last digit is the print number: 9 8 7 6 5 4 3 2 1

David H. Adams, MD
Professor and Chairman
Department of Cardiothoracic Surgery
Mount Sinai Medical Center
New York, New York

Thomas M. Bashore, MD
Professor of Medicine
Vice Chief, Division of Cardiology
Duke University Medical Center
Durham, North Carolina

Helmut Baumgartner, MD
Professor of Adult Congenital Heart Disease
Adult Congenital and Valvular Heart Disease Center
University Hospital Muenster
University of Muenster
Muenster, Germany

Michael A. Beardslee, MD
Associate Professor of Medicine
Cardiovascular Division
Department of Medicine
Washington University School of Medicine
St. Louis, Missouri

Ronen Beeri, MD
Cardiovascular Research Center,
Heart Institute
Hadassah-Hebrew University Medical Center
Jerusalem, Israel

Peter C. Block, MD
Director, Clinical Trials Office
Department of Cardiology
Emory University Hospital
Atlanta, Georgia

Robert O. Bonow, MD
Goldberg Distinguished Professor of Cardiology
Northwestern University Feinberg School of Medicine
Chief, Division of Cardiology
Co-Director, Bluhm Cardiovascular Institute
Northwestern Memorial Hospital
Chicago, Illinois

Alan C. Braverman, MD
Professor of Medicine
Cardiovascular Division
Department of Medicine
Washington University School of Medicine
St. Louis, Missouri

Charles J. Bruce, MD
Associate Professor of Medicine
Mayo Clinic College of Medicine
Consultant, Division of Cardiovascular Diseases
Department of Internal Medicine, Mayo Clinic
Rochester, Minnesota

Blase A. Carabello, MD
Professor and Vice-Chair
Department of Medicine
The W.A. "Tex" and Deborah Moncrief, Jr. Baylor College
    of Medicine
Medical Care Line Executive
Department of Medicine, Veterans Affairs Medical Center
Houston, Texas

Heidi M. Connolly, MD
Professor of Medicine
Mayo Clinic College of Medicine
Division of Cardiovascular Diseases
Mayo Clinic
Rochester, Minnesota

Mario J. Garcia, MD
Professor of Medicine and Radiology
Director Cardiovascular Imaging
Mount Sinai Medical Center
New York, New York

Brian P. Griffin, MD
John and Rosemary Brown Endowed Chair in
    Cardiovascular Medicine
Department of Cardiovascular Medicine
Cleveland Clinic
Cleveland, Ohio

Bernard Iung, MD
Department of Cardiology
Bichat Hospital
Paris, France

Jong Mi Ko, BA
Research Assistant
Baylor Heart and Vascular Institute
Baylor University Medical Center
Dallas, Texas

Robert A. Levine, MD
Professor of Medicine
Harvard Medical School
Cardiac Ultrasound Laboratory
Massachussets General Hospital
Boston, Massachussets

vi **S. Chris Malaisrie, MD**
Assistant Professor of Surgery
Northwestern University Feinberg School of Medicine
Director of Thoracic Aortic Surgery
Bluhm Cardiovascular Institute
Northwestern Memorial Hospital
Chicago, Illinois

Patrick M. McCarthy, MD
Heller-Sacks Professor of Surgery
Northwestern University Feinberg School of Medicine,
Chief, Division of Cardiothoracic Surgery
Co-Director, Bluhm Cardiovascular Institute
Northwestern Memorial Hospital
Chicago, Illinois

George A. Mensah, MD
Chief Medical Officer
Associate Director for Medical Affairs
National Center for Chronic Disease Prevention and
    Health Promotion
Centers for Disease Control and Prevention
Atlanta, Georgia

L. LuAnn Minich, MD
Professor, Department of Pediatrics
University of Utah School of Medicine
Primary Children's Medical Center
Salt Lake City, Utah

Brad Munt, MD
Echocardiography Laboratory
St. Paul's Hospital and Providence Health
Vancouver, British Columbia, Canada

Rick A. Nishimura, MD
Judd and Mary Morris Leighton Professor of
    Cardiovascular Diseases
Professor of Medicine
Mayo Clinic College of Medicine
Division of Cardiovascular Diseases
Mayo Clinic
Rochester, Minnesota

Patrick T. O'Gara, MD
Associate Professor of Medicine
Harvard Medical School
Director of Clinical Cardiology
Brigham & Women's Hospital
Boston, Massachusetts

Yutaka Otsuji, MD
Second Department of Internal Medicine
University of Occupational and Environmental Health
Sangyo University of Occupational and Environmental
    Health
Kitakyushu, Japan

Catherine M. Otto, MD
J. Ward Kennedy-Hamilton Endowed Professor of Cardiology
Director, Cardiology Fellowship Programs
University of Washington School of Medicine
Seattle, Washington

Michael D. Puchalski, MD
Assistant Professor
Department of Pediatrics
University of Utah School of Medicine
Primary Children's Medical Center
Salt Lake City, Utah

Nalini Marie Rajamannan, MD
Associate Professor of Medicine
Division of Cardiology
Department of Medicine
Feinberg Cardiovascular Research Institute
Northwestern University Feinberg School of Medicine
Chicago, Illinois

William C. Roberts, MD
Executive Director
Baylor Heart and Vascular Institute
Baylor University Medical Center
Dallas, Texas

Raphael Rosenhek, MD
Associate Professor
Department of Cardiology
Medical University Vienna
Vienna, Austria

Hartzell V. Schaff, MD
Stuart W. Harrington Professor of Surgery
Mayo Clinic College of Medicine
Division of Cardiovascular Surgery
Mayo Clinic
Rochester, Minnesota

Ehud Schwammenthal, MD
Department of Cardiac Rehabilitation
Heart Institute
Sheba Medical Center
Tel Hashomer, Israel

Pravin M. Shah, MD
Chair and Medical Director
Hoag Heart Valve Center
Medical Director
Non-Invasive Cardiac Imaging
Hoag Heart and Vascular Institute
Newport Beach, California

David M. Shavelle, MD
Associate Professor of Medicine
Division of Cardiology
David Geffen School of Medicine at UCLA
Director, Interventional Cardiology Fellowship
Los Angeles County/Harbor-UCLA Medical Center
Torrance, California

Paul Stelzer, MD
Professor, Department of Cardiothoracic Surgery
Mount Sinai Medical Center
New York, New York

Karen Stout, MD
Director, Adult Congenital Heart Disease Program
Assistant Professor of Medicine
Adjunct Assistant Professor of Pediatrics
University of Washington School of Medicine
Seattle, Washington

Lloyd Y. Tani, MD
Professor, Department of Pediatrics
University of Utah School of Medicine
Primary Children's Medical Center
Salt Lake City, Utah

Pilar Tornos, MD
Servei de Cardiologia
Hospital Universitari Vall d'Hebron
Barcelona, Spain

Alec Vahanian, MD
Department of Cardiology
Bichat Hospital
Paris, France

Richard V. Williams, MD
Associate Clinical Professor
Department of Pediatrics
University of Utah School of Medicine
Primary Children's Medical Center
Salt Lake City, Utah

Worldwide, valvular heart disease remains a major cause of morbidity and mortality. In the United States, there are approximately 100,000 open-heart operations each year for valve replacement or repair, which accounts for about 20% of all cardiac surgical cases. A far greater number of patients have valve disease that is managed medically. Because the prevalence of valve disease increases as a function of age, we anticipate that even greater numbers of patients will come to medical attention with the aging of the population in this country and abroad.

Recognition of a heart murmur remains central to the practice of medicine because primary care physicians usually make the initial diagnosis of valvular heart disease followed by referral to a specialist. Noninvasive methods for diagnosis and evaluation of disease severity have greatly increased our knowledge of valvular heart disease: the ability to monitor stenosis severity with varying flow rates has broadened our understanding of the complex hemodynamics of valvular stenosis and regurgitation; serial noninvasive studies in patients with mild or moderate degrees of valve dysfunction have improved our understanding of the natural history of valvular disease; and these noninvasive methods now allow precise assessment of the changes in valvular and ventricular function after medical or surgical interventions. In addition, better options for correction of valve dysfunction, including percutaneous interventions, improved valve substitutes, and the increasing use of valve repair procedures now are available. Earlier intervention is increasingly being considered as the risk-benefit ratio improves and as the potential long-term adverse consequences of valve disease are more clearly defined.

Optimal care of the patient with valvular heart disease requires knowledgeable collaboration among several different types of health professionals. The diagnosis often is suspected by the primary care physician or nurse practitioner based on auscultation of a cardiac murmur or recognition of symptoms that might be due to valvular disease. Further evaluation by a cardiologist typically involves subspecialists in echocardiography and interventional cardiology, as well as the skilled assistance of cardiac sonographers, radiology technicians, and cardiac catheterization laboratory technologists. Cardiac surgeons expert in valve repair or replacement have made enormous advances in the past two decades that have transformed the outlook of patients with valve disease. In patients undergoing surgical or percutaneous intervention, cardiovascular anesthesiologists, cardiac perfusionists, and coronary care unit nurses are all key members of the team. Increasingly, cardiac surgeons and interventional cardiologist are working together to decide on the optimal treatment plan in each patient, with the increasing use of "hybrid" approach where a combination of surgical and nonsurgical techniques are used in an procedure suite designed for both open surgical or robotic and percutaneous procedures. In addition, optimal management of patients with valvular heart disease often depends on close collaboration with other medical specialties, for example, high-risk obstetrics in the pregnant patient with valvular heart disease, medical genetics in patients with inherited conditions, electrophysiologists when arrhythmias complicate the clinical presentation, and the heart transplant team in patients with irreversible ventricular dysfunction.

This book integrates the diverse knowledge required for optimal care of the patient with valvular heart disease by each of these health professionals. Since the publication of the second edition of Otto's *Valvular Heart Disease*, there have been substantial advances in our understanding of the disease processes and optimal treatments for valvular heart disease, with an upsurge of interest in understanding the causes of valve disease and improved diagnostic techniques. With publication of updated guidelines by the American College of Cardiology/ American Heart Association (ACC/AHA) and the European Society of Cardiology, evidence-based approaches to the treatment of valvular heart disease are becoming accepted. We anticipate more clinical outcome studies in patients with valvular heart disease in the future. This field has now matured to the point where a multi-author book, building on the material in the second edition, and inclusion as part of the Braunwald Companion Series is appropriate.

The authors for each chapter were chosen for their clinical and research expertise, although we acknowledge that there now are many other experts in valvular heart disease worldwide who could not be included in this volume due to space limitations. Each chapter provides a summary of the pathophysiology, clinical presentation, and natural history of the disease process along with a discussion of medical therapy and timing of surgical intervention, including postoperative outcome. Each chapter is extensively illustrated and the major clinical trials are summarized in tables whenever possible. Current guidelines are provided and discussed in each chapter, with an appendix providing the exact definitions of the recommendation grades and levels of evidence used in the ACC/AHA guideline documents. The reference list for each chapter emphasizes more recent studies, with only the most important earlier studies cited.

The book begins with a section on basic principles in diagnosis and management of valvular heart disease. Chapters discuss disease prevalence and anatomic pathology followed by an in-depth chapter on our rapidly expanding knowledge of the cellular and molecular mechanisms of disease initiation and progression. A chapter on the left ventricular response to pressure and/or volume overload is included as this is a key factor in the decision-making process regarding the optimal timing of surgical intervention. Next are several chapters on diagnostic evaluation of valvular heart disease by echocardiography, cardiac catheterization, and advanced cardiac imaging techniques. The chapter on basic principles of medical management in patients with valvular heart disease serves as a quick clinical reference source with tables summarizing indications for echocardiography and timing of follow-up studies, diagnosis and prevention of rheumatic fever, updated endocarditis guidelines, recommendations for physical activity in patients with valve disorders, an overview of anticoagulation recommendations, and indications for coronary angiography.

The next section of the book addresses aortic valve disease and includes chapters on aortic stenosis, aortic regurgitation, the bicuspid aortic valve, and both surgical and percutaneous approaches to treatment of aortic valve disease. The section on mitral valve disease includes separate chapters on rheumatic valve disease, myxomatous mitral valve disease, functional mitral regurgitation, timing of surgery for mitral regurgitation, mitral valve repair and replacement, and percutaneous approaches to mitral valve dysfunction. The final section of the book covers several topics, including intraoperative echocardiography, right-sided valve disease, endocarditis, prosthetic valves, valve disease in children, and management of valvular heart disease during pregnancy.

While every attempt has been made to provide accurate and up-to-date information, medicine is an ever-changing field, so readers always should check the recent literature for any changes in diagnostic approaches or therapy. The number of new publications in the area of valve disease is so large that not all could be included in the cited references in this book. It is expected that the interested reader will use electronic databases to find additional references as needed. In addition, professional organizations such as the AHA, ACC, and European Society of Cardiology periodically develop consensus guidelines for patient management and the latest update of those guidelines should be consulted. Chapters on specific diagnostic techniques and surgical and percutaneous interventions are provided as

background information. Of course, expertise in these areas requires appropriate education and experience as defined by the relevant accreditation and credentialing bodies and professional organizations.

Valvular heart disease historically has been an interest for physicians and continues to be an area of fascination for many of us, with the initial stimulus for learning often being the appreciation of a cardiac murmur on physical examination as a medical student. Now that we are on the verge of understanding the cellular and molecular mechanisms of valve disease, it is important to consolidate our current knowledge in order to focus on the possibility of preventing disease initiation and progression in the future. An improved understanding of the mechanisms of disease, combined with well-designed clinical outcomes trials, will lead to even more advances in prevention and treatment of valvular heart disease in the future.

CATHERINE M. OTTO, MD

ROBERT O. BONOW, MD

Valvular heart disease is an important clinical problem, responsible for an estimated 20,000 deaths and 100,000 hospitalizations each year in the United States alone. Although it has been recognized for centuries, in recent decades valvular disease has been caught in two important cross-currents. The first is demographic. Despite the recent decline in the prevalence of rheumatic heart disease in North America, Western Europe, and Australia, the total number of patients with valvular heart disease in these regions is rising steadily because of the increase in degenerative valvular diseases that accompanies the aging of the population. The numbers of patients with valvular heart disease in developing countries is rising particularly rapidly because the incidence of new cases of rheumatic heart disease has not (yet) fallen to the low levels observed in the developed nations, while the number of the elderly and the accompanying degenerative valve diseases are increasing.

The second important cross-current relates to the changes in the diagnosis and management of valvular heart disease. Until relatively recently, the cardiac catheterization laboratory was the site at which the diagnosis and functional assessment of valvular heart disease were obtained, while the management of advanced valvular disorders took place in the operating room. Now, noninvasive imaging techniques—echocardiography, including three-dimensional echocardiography, as well as cardiac magnetic resonance imaging and computed tomography—all provide rich anatomic and functional information. The cardiac catheterization laboratory is becoming increasingly the site of catheter-based correction of valvular disorders. This approach began 25 years ago with balloon mitral valvuloplasty and now involves growing efforts to perfect correction of severe mitral regurgitation and transcatheter insertion of prosthetic aortic valves.

The editors of *Valvular Heart Disease*, Drs. Otto and Bonow, are among the world's leaders in this field. They have selected outstanding authors, each an authority in the particular area that they cover. They cover in depth the cross-currents mentioned above, which make the understanding and management of valvular heart diseases much more dynamic than ever. They also cover systematically the pathogenesis, pathophysiology, clinical findings, imaging, natural history, and therapeutic options. We congratulate the editors and authors for their important contributions and welcome this excellent book to our growing list of *Companions to Heart Disease*. We anticipate that this text will become the standard in this important field.

EUGENE BRAUNWALD, MD

PETER LIBBY, MD

DOUGLAS L. MANN, MD

DOUGLAS P. ZIPES, MD

Acknowledgments

Sincere thanks are due to the many individuals who helped make this book a reality. In particular, we would like to thank the chapter authors for their time and efforts in providing excellent chapters. Some of the chapters in this edition include material from the second edition of *Otto's* *Valvular Heart Disease* with the full knowledge and consent of Catherine Otto, the author of the previous chapters.

Finally, as always, we would like to thank our families for their constant encouragement and support.

Contents

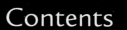

The Burden of Valvular Heart Disease

George A. Mensah

KEY POINTS

- The dramatic decline in the incidence of acute rheumatic fever has led to a corresponding reduction in rheumatic valve disease in most industrialized nations. Nevertheless, nearly 16 million people worldwide live with rheumatic heart disease, and an estimated 233,000 deaths are attributable to rheumatic fever or rheumatic heart disease each year.
- The reduction in rheumatic valve disease has not resulted in a decrease in valvular heart disease burden because increasing life expectancy in many countries and a continuing epidemic of atherosclerotic risk factors have led to an increase in age-related and degenerative valvular heart disease.
- Mild to moderate degrees of valvular heart disease are relatively common in adults, increase in prevalence with advancing age, and are associated with reduced survival.
- Sclerosis of the aortic and mitral valves, even in the absence of hemodynamic obstruction, is associated with increased cardiovascular mortality.
- Hospitalization for symptom management and valve repair or replacement constitutes the major morbidity, and heart failure is the major sequela leading to death. An estimated 20,260 deaths and 100,000 hospitalizations for valvular heart disease occur in the United States annually.
- Procedures for repair or replacement of heart valves more than doubled in the United States in the last two decades with an increasing preference for bioprosthetic over mechanical valves.
- Health disparities in access to care and quality of care for valvular heart disease exist by age, gender, race/ethnicity, and socioeconomic status. Continued investments in strategies to improve health care quality for all and eliminate these disparities are necessary.

Diseases and disorders of the heart valves constitute a major worldwide cause of disability, reduced quality of life, and premature mortality from cardiovascular diseases. Throughout most of the 19th and early 20th centuries, rheumatic fever and consequent rheumatic valvulopathy were the leading causes of valvular heart disease worldwide and remain so today in most developing countries where rheumatic fever remains the leading cause of heart disease in children and young adults.[1] In most industrialized nations, however, the dramatic decline in the incidence and sequelae of rheumatic fever coupled with significant increases in life expectancy and prevalence of persons aged 65 years and older has led to a changing etiology and an increasing burden of age-related valvular heart disease. In addition, a better understanding of valvular biology and pathophysiology, improved diagnostic imaging, and novel approaches to valve repair and replacement in most developed countries have contributed to improved patient survival and an increasing prevalence of valvular heart disease.[2,3]

In this chapter, the changing etiology of valvular heart disease is first reviewed. The overall burden of valvular heart disease, together with the incidence, prevalence, natural history, and clinical outcomes of aortic, mitral, tricuspid, and pulmonary valve diseases and their sequelae are then presented. The epidemiology of multivalvular and mixed valvular heart disease is also reviewed. Endocarditis and associated morbidity and mortality are discussed. Disease burden in women of reproductive age is then reviewed. Trends in heart valve procedures and the epidemiology of prosthetic valve dysfunction are then presented. Finally, disparities in access to quality health care in the prevention, treatment, and the control of valvular heart disease are reviewed.

A CHANGING ETIOLOGY

Valvular heart disease may be congenital, acquired, or both (as in progressive calcification of a congenitally bicuspid aortic valve or endocarditis of a congenitally malformed mitral leaflets). Acquired valvular heart disease may be of rheumatic or nonrheumatic origin. Until the mid-20th century, the predominant etiology of acquired valvular heart disease worldwide was rheumatic, a nonsuppurative cardiovascular sequela of group A streptococcal pharyngitis.[4] Although a dramatic decline in the incidence of rheumatic fever and rheumatic heart disease has been observed in industrialized nations over the past five decades, rheumatic fever and rheumatic heart disease remain major clinical and public health problems in developing countries where their most devastating effects are on children and young adults in their most productive years.[4] In developing countries, the majority of cases of rheumatic valve disease affect the mitral valve, with mitral stenosis (MS) being the most common lesion in adults, but aortic and tricuspid valve involvement may be seen as well. In children aged 5 years and younger, mitral regurgitation (MR) is the most common cardiac manifestation in developing countries, and obstructive valve disease is distinctly rare in this age group.[5]

In their recent analysis of the global burden of group A streptococcal diseases, Carapetis et al[6] estimated a worldwide rheumatic heart disease prevalence of 15.6 million people, with 470,000 new cases of rheumatic fever and 233,000 deaths attributable to rheumatic fever or rheumatic heart disease each year. Table 1-1 shows the estimated number of deaths and disability adjusted life years lost to rheumatic heart disease in 2000 by World Health Organization regions.[4] As shown in Figure 1-1, almost all of these cases and deaths occur in developing countries, with the highest calculated regional prevalence of the disease among children noted in sub-Saharan Africa (5.7 per 1000), the Pacific and indigenous populations in Australia and New Zealand (3.5 per 1000), and south central Asia (2.2 per 1000).[6] In fact, as many as half of the 2.4 million children affected by rheumatic heart disease globally reside in Africa alone.[7]

In many countries in these regions, more than 50% of patients with rheumatic heart disease are unaware of the diagnosis and, thus, do not receive secondary prophylaxis for prevention of recurrent rheumatic fever. The prevalence of diagnosed rheumatic heart disease in many countries in which echocardiographic imaging is not available may represent a significant underestimation of the true burden of disease.[8] Marijon et al[8] recently showed that systematic screening with echocardiography reveals as much as a 10-fold greater prevalence of rheumatic heart disease, compared with clinical screening in the same population.[8] Both the primary episode of rheumatic fever and the long-term valvular sequelae lead to substantial medical costs for this potentially preventable disease. Recognizing the huge burden of morbidity and mortality from rheumatic heart disease in Africa and the availability of cost-effective and relatively inexpensive

TABLE 1–1	The Global Burden of Rheumatic Heart Disease: Estimated Number of Deaths and Disability Adjusted Life Years Lost to Rheumatic Heart Disease in 2000, by World Health Organization (WHO) Region			
	Deaths		DALYs Lost	
WHO Region	n (×10³)	Rate (per 100,000 population)	n (×10³)	Rate (per 100,000 population)
Africa	29	4.5	0.77	119.8
The Americas	15	1.8	0.24	27.4
Eastern Mediterranean	21	4.4	0.59	121.6
Europe	38	4.3	0.49	56.1
Southeast Asia	117	7.6	2.66	173.4
Western Pacific	115	6.8	1.78	105.4
World	332	5.5	6.63	109.6

DALYs, disability adjusted life years.
From World Health Organization: Rheumatic fever and rheumatic heart disease. World Health Organ Tech Rep Ser 2004;923:1–122, with permission.

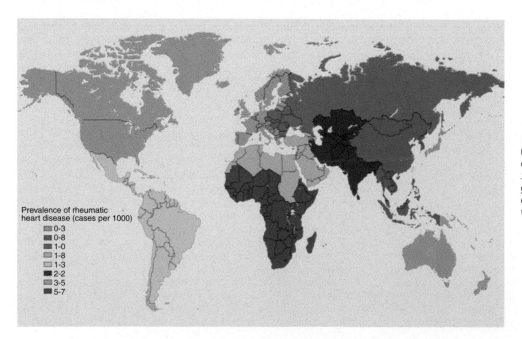

Prevalence of rheumatic heart disease (cases per 1000)

- 0-3
- 0-8
- 1-0
- 1-8
- 1-3
- 2-2
- 3-5
- 5-7

FIGURE 1–1 The worldwide prevalence (cases per 1000) of rheumatic heart disease in children aged 5-14 years. (*From Carapetis JR, Steer AC, Mulholland EK, Weber M: The global burden of group A streptococcal diseases. Lancet Infect Dis 2005;5:685-694, with permission.*)

interventions for prevention and control, a recent initiative (the Drakensberg Declaration) called for a comprehensive program using awareness, surveillance, advocacy, and prevention to eliminate rheumatic fever and rheumatic heart disease in the region.[7,9]

In sharp contrast to the picture in developing countries, the incidence of acute rheumatic fever has dramatically declined in most developed countries to less than 1 per 100,000.[4] This has resulted in a dramatic decline in the incidence of rheumatic valve disease in developed countries. The overall burden of valvular heart disease has, however, not declined because of an increase in age-related degenerative valve disease.[10-14] This pattern is expected to persist as life expectancy continues to improve and the proportion of persons aged older than 65 years increases significantly in developed nations.

For example, from 1950 to 2005, the total resident population of the United States increased from 151 to 296 million, representing an average annual growth rate of 1.2%. During that same period, however, the population aged 65 years and older grew, on average, 2.0% per year, increasing from 12 to 37 million, and the population aged 75 years and older more than quadrupled from 4 to 18 million persons. Current projections suggest that the population aged 75 years and older will continue to increase to 12% in 2050.[15] As a result of increasing life expectancy and continuing decline of rheumatic fever incidence, nonrheumatic and age-related degenerative valvular heart disease will predominate in developed countries.

In addition to the increasing life expectancy and declining incidence of acute rheumatic fever, the continuing epidemic of major cardiovascular risk factors is likely to contribute to the changing etiology of valvular heart disease. Several studies have now shown that valve calcification, typically seen in age-related valvular heart disease, is the result of an active process that is preceded by basement membrane disruption, inflammatory cell infiltration, lipid deposition, neurohormonal influence, and endothelial dysfunction.[10-20] This process is associated with diabetes, hypercholesterolemia, hypertension, and tobacco use and thus is likely to be exacerbated and adversely impact the prevalence of valvular heart disease in the setting in which these risk factors are suboptimally controlled.[16,21] In addition, adverse changes in the synthetic, morphologic, and metabolic functions of the valvular endothelial cells contribute to progressive age-related valvulopathy[22] Thus, in the setting of uncontrolled cardiovascular risk factors and a continuing epidemic of obesity and diabetes, the epidemiologic burden of valvular heart disease is likely to increase.[14,23-27]

NONRHEUMATIC VALVULAR HEART DISEASE

The worldwide burden of nonrheumatic valvular heart disease in the population has not been estimated. Two recent publications provide data on the U.S. experience at the population and community levels[28] and the European experience in a survey of clinical patients (the Euro Heart Survey).[29] In the U.S. experience, Nkomo et al[28] pooled three population-based studies to obtain data for 11,911 randomly selected adults from the general population who had been assessed prospectively with echocardiography. They also analyzed data from a community study of 16,501 adults who had been assessed using clinically indicated echocardiography.

From the population-based studies, they estimated a national prevalence of valvular heart disease, corrected for age and sex distribution from the U.S. 2000 population, to be 2.5%. The prevalence of moderate or severe valvular heart disease increased with age, from 0.7% in 18 to 44 year olds to 13.3% in the 75 years and older group. No significant sex-related differences were noted. In the community group,

valve disease was diagnosed in 1505 (1.8% adjusted) adults and disease frequency increased considerably with age, from 0.3% of the 18 to 44 year olds to 11.7% of those aged 75 years and older, but was diagnosed less often in women than in men (odds ratio 0.90, 0.81 to 1.01; $P = 0.07$).[28] Importantly, the adjusted mortality risk ratio associated with valve disease was 1.36 (1.15 to 1.62; $P = 0.0005$) in the population and 1.75 (1.61 to 1.90; $P < 0.0001$) in the community. These findings suggest that moderate or severe valvular diseases are relatively common in the United States, that their prevalence increases with age (Figure 1-2), and that they are associated with significantly reduced survival (Figure 1-3).[28]

The Euro Heart Survey on valvular heart disease prospectively included 5001 outpatients or hospitalized patients from 92 centers in 25 European countries. All patients had to have echocardiographic evidence of primary and significant valvular heart disease and, as such, the survey cannot inform us of the population burden of valve disease in Europe.[29] However, it provides very useful information on the spectrum of valve disease in this population, overall management, and survival. Native valve disease was present in 71.9% with the remaining 28.1% having undergone previous valve surgery.[29] Aortic stenosis (AS) and MR were the most common native valve disorders (34% and 25%, respectively) and were mostly caused by degenerative diseases (the mean age was 69 and 65 years, respectively). Multivalvular disease was present in 20% of the patients and at least one comorbidity was noted in 36.3% of the patients. A major contribution from this sur-

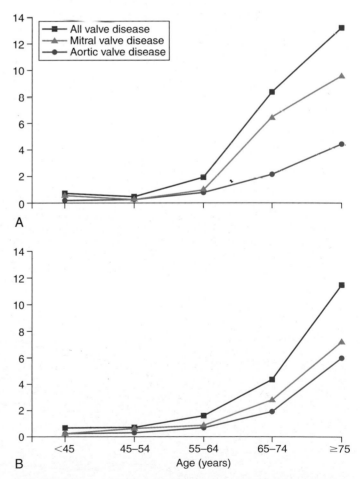

FIGURE 1–2 The prevalence of valvular heart disease in the United States. Frequency in (**A**) population–based studies and (**B**) in the Olmsted County community. (*From Nkomo VT, Gardin JM, Skelton TN, et al: Burden of valvular heart diseases: A population–based study. Lancet 2006;368:1005-1011, with permission.*)

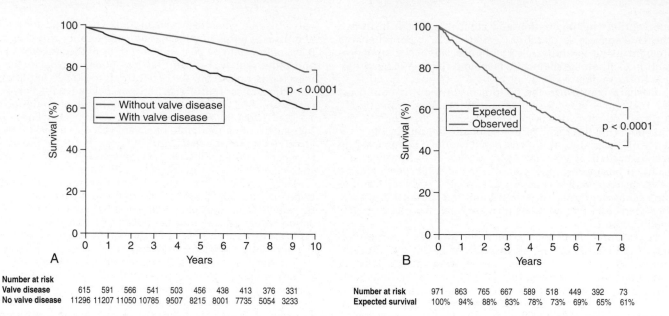

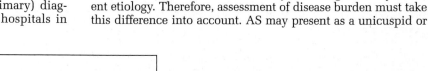

FIGURE 1–3 Survival after detection of moderate or severe valvular heart disease in the United States. (**A**) Survival in population-based studies. (**B**) Expected versus observed survival in Olmsted County. The blue line represents survival of 971 residents diagnosed with valve diseases between 1990 and 1995; the yellow line represents the expected survival in the age-matched and sex-matched population of the county. *(From Nkomo VT, Gardin JM, Skelton TN, et al: Burden of valvular heart diseases: A population-based study. Lancet 2006;368:1005-1011, with permission.)*

vey is that symptomatic patients with severe valve disease were frequently denied surgery (32.3% in AS after the age of 75 and 51.3% in MR), more on the basis of age and left ventricular function than comorbidities. Compared with symptomatic patients, asymptomatic patients were more likely to receive interventions in accordance with established practice guideline recommendations.[29]

Hospitalization for symptom management and surgical repair or replacement of heart valves constitute the major morbidity in valvular heart disease. In the United States, there were 1.5 million hospital discharges with any diagnosis of valvular heart disease in 2005, compared with 675,000 discharges 20 years earlier.[30] Mitral and aortic valve disease constitute the largest contributors to these increased hospital discharges (Figure 1-4).[30] Only 94,000 of these hospital discharges were related to surgical procedures for heart valve disease in 2005 (Figure 1-5), a number that is significantly lower than the 466,000 coronary artery bypass procedures that year. The American Heart Association reported that in 2006, there were an estimated 93,000 hospital discharges for valvular heart disease as the first-listed (primary) diagnosis for inpatients discharged from short-stay hospitals in

the United States and more than half of these (49,000) were related to aortic valve disease.[31]

Although the total-mention mortality for valvular heart disease in the United States was 43,900 in 2005, only an estimated 20,891 were primarily due to valve disease.[31] This mortality is predominantly related to aortic valve disease (more than 13,137 deaths in 2005) with the remainder related to mitral valve disease and endocarditis (valve unspecified).[31] Pulmonary and tricuspid valve disease rarely are indicated as a primary or first-listed cause of death. The mechanism of death in patients with valvular heart disease most often is congestive heart failure, either due to primary valve dysfunction or due to residual ventricular dysfunction after valve surgery. Other mechanisms of death in patients with valvular heart disease include sudden cardiac death, cardiac arrhythmias, stroke, endocarditis and surgical complications.

AORTIC STENOSIS

In children and older adults, AS may have a significantly different etiology. Therefore, assessment of disease burden must take this difference into account. AS may present as a unicuspid or

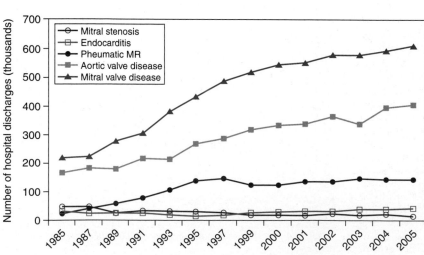

FIGURE 1–4 Number of all discharge diagnoses of valvular heart disease in the United States between 1985 and 2005 based on the National Center for Health Statistics ICD-9 discharge code data. ICM-9-CM codes used were mitral valve disease (424.0), aortic valve disease (424.1), rheumatic mitral regurgitation (396.2 + 396.3 + 394.1), mitral stenosis (394.0 + 394.2 + 396.0), and endocarditis (424.9). *(From National Center for Health Statistics: National Hospital Discharge Survey: Annual Summaries with Detailed Diagnosis and Procedure Data; Series 13. Data on Health Resources Utilization. Available at http://www.cdc.gov/nchs/products/pubs/pubd/series/ser.htm#sr13.)*

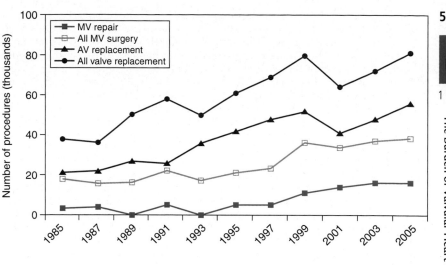

FIGURE 1–5 Number of heart valve surgery procedures performed in the United States between 1985 and 2005 based on data from the National Hospital Discharge Survey from the National Center for Health Statistics. ICD-9-CM procedure codes: all valve replacements (35.2), aortic valve (AV) replacement (35.22 + 35.21), mitral valve (MV) replacement (35.23 + 35.24), and MV repair (35.12). *(From National Center for Health Statistics: National Hospital Discharge Survey: Annual Summaries with Detailed Diagnosis and Procedure Data; Series 13. Data on Health Resources Utilization. Available at http://www.cdc.gov/nchs/products/pubs/pubd/series/ser.htm#sr13.)*

severely deformed bicuspid valve, which must be distinguished from a membranous or muscular subaortic cause of stenosis in children and young adults. In older adults, valvular AS is most commonly due to secondary calcification of a congenitally bicuspid valve or degenerative calcific changes of a trileaflet valve (Table 1-2).[32,33] In these older patients, the primary differential diagnosis is obstructive hypertrophic cardiomyopathy, although previously unrecognized subaortic stenosis may be seen.

In surgical pathologic cases in the United States, calcific AS is most commonly encountered, accounting for 51% of cases, with bicuspid and rheumatic etiologies accounting for 36% and 9% of cases, respectively.[11] In a series of meticulous surgical pathologic examinations, Roberts et al reported on the valve structure and the early and late survival in nonagenarians,[34] octogenarians,[35] septuagenarians,[36] sexagenarians,[37] and quinquagenarians[38] among 1,112 patients who underwent aortic valve replacement (AVR) with or without simultaneous coronary artery bypass surgery and without mitral valve replacement (MVR) at one medical center from 1993 to 2005. As shown in Figure 1-6, a tricuspid aortic valve was more commonly seen in stenotic valves from patients in their 8th, 9th, and 10th decades of life, whereas the bicuspid valve was predominant in younger patients.[34-38] Surprisingly however, three of the nine nonagenarians had a bicuspid valve. No unicuspid or quadricuspid valves were found in octogenarians or nonagenarians.[34,35] In general, unadjusted survival was not affected by gender, valve structure, preoperative severity of the AS, or performance of simultaneous coronary artery bypass surgery in sexagenarians.[37]

In both community and population-based studies from the United States, the prevalence of valve disease rose strikingly with age, with an odds ratio of 2.51 (2.02-3.12; $P < 0001$) for the association of AS with advancing age (per decade of life; see Figure 1-2).[28] In the clinical population from the Euro Heart Survey, the most striking observation was old age.[29] The mean age of patients with AS was 69 years, with more than half of them aged 70 years or older and 13.8% at least 80 years old.[29] Not surprisingly, the most common etiology of AS was degenerative calcification (81.9%) followed by rheumatic valvular stenosis (11.2%).[29] Rheumatic involvement of the aortic valve is characterized by fusion of the commissures between the aortic valve leaflets and is invariably accompanied by rheumatic mitral valve disease.

The annual incidence of bicuspid aortic valve is estimated to be 13.7 per 1000 live births in the United States.[31] The prevalence estimate is 1% to 2% of the general population with a three- to fourfold male predominance.[39] More recently, a lower prevalence (0.8%) was noted in nearly 21,000 young male military conscripts (mean age 18 years) who underwent screening echocardiography for the military in Italy.[40] A similarly lower prevalence between 0.5% and 0.6% was reported in two large independent databases of young athletes and clinic patients.[41] The 2009 statistical update from the American Heart Association estimated that 2 million adults and 1 million children now have a congenital bicuspid aortic valve with approximately 54,800 new cases in the United States every year.[31]

TABLE 1–2	Causes of Aortic Stenosis

Congenital
  Bicuspid valve
  Unicuspid valve
  Quadricuspid
  Other (e.g., dome–shaped diaphragm)
Calcific (degenerative)
  Trileaflet valve
  Superimposed on bicuspid valve
  Superimposed on other congenitally abnormal valve

Rheumatic valve disease

Other conditions
  Homozygous type II hyperlipoproteinemia
  Metabolic (e.g., Fabry disease)
  Systemic lupus erythematosus
  Ochronosis with alkaptonuria

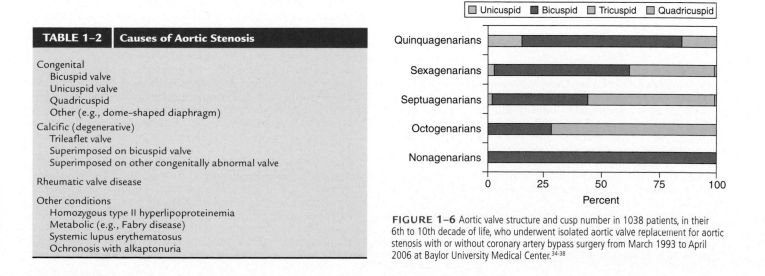

FIGURE 1–6 Aortic valve structure and cusp number in 1038 patients, in their 6th to 10th decade of life, who underwent isolated aortic valve replacement for aortic stenosis with or without coronary artery bypass surgery from March 1993 to April 2006 at Baylor University Medical Center.[34-38]

Most patients with a congenital bicuspid valve develop superimposed calcific changes, eventually requiring intervention for valve stenosis in the sixth or seventh decade of life. The cusp number of the calcified valve can be fairly predicted on the basis of the patient's age at the time of surgical intervention; in patients aged 15 to 65 years, nearly 75% are bicuspid or unicuspid, whereas in patients aged older than 75 years, 90% of stenotic aortic valves are trileaflet.[42]

Clinical outcome in adults with AS depends on symptom status and stenosis severity. Symptomatic patients, regardless of the degree of severity, have a very high risk of cardiac mortality, approaching 50% at 1 to 2 years. In patients who refuse surgical intervention for symptomatic severe AS, the major causes of death are congestive heart failure and sudden cardiac death. It is generally assumed that asymptomatic patients have clinical outcomes similar to those of normal age-matched adults. However, recent data suggest that the natural history of asymptomatic patients with severe AS (aortic valve area 0.8 cm^2 or less) is not benign[43-45] and that many asymptomatic patients may benefit from AVR.[43]

Increasingly, the presence of comorbid atherosclerotic risk factors are being recognized as important factors in the progression of AS.[46] For example, in a retrospective analysis of 105 consecutive patients with moderate AS, Briand et al[46] found that the hemodynamic progression of AS was twice as fast (-0.14 ± 0.13 cm^2/year vs. -0.08 ± 0.08 cm^2/year; $P = 0.008$) and the 3-year event-free survival was markedly lower ($44 \pm 8\%$ vs. $69 \pm 6\%$; $P = 0.002$) among patients with the metabolic syndrome (Figure 1-7). In multivariate analysis, metabolic syndrome was a strong predictor of both stenosis progression and event-free survival, independent of traditional risk factors.[46] Despite successful treatment with lipid-lowering therapy to achieve the recommended goal of the National Cholesterol Education Program-Adult Treatment Panel III in all patients with metabolic syndrome, the average rate of AS progression in patients with the metabolic syndrome was twice as fast as that in patients without metabolic syndrome (see Figure 1-7).[46] In an earlier study, the authors showed that the presence of the metabolic syndrome was independently associated with faster bioprosthetic valve degeneration.[47]

AORTIC SCLEROSIS

Aortic sclerosis is a common echocardiographic finding that manifests as varying degrees of focal thickening of the aortic valve leaflets with commissural sparing, normal leaflet mobility, and no evidence of obstruction of the left ventricular outflow (transaortic velocity ≤2.5 m/s).[48] It is seen in about one in four persons aged 65 years and older[48] and in nearly half of persons aged older than 80 years, although the presence of hypertension or end-stage renal disease requiring hemodialysis increases the prevalence.[49,50] Taylor et al[51] recently reported a lower prevalence of aortic sclerosis (8%) in African Americans in the Atherosclerosis Risk in Communities Study.

In the population-based Cardiovascular Health Study of 5176 adults aged older than 65 years, aortic sclerosis was present in 26% of subjects (Table 1-3). The prevalence of aortic sclerosis increased with age, being present in 48% of adults at least 85 years of age, and was seen in 31% of men versus 22% of women.[52] The Helsinki Aging Study of 651 adults aged older than 55 years showed an even higher prevalence of aortic sclerosis and stenosis, most likely related to a slightly different definition of the severity of valve disease in this study.[53]

The relationship between aortic sclerosis and age is nonlinear, with a sharp increase in the prevalence of disease in men aged about 65 years and women aged about 75 years.[54] Clinical factors associated with aortic sclerosis or stenosis on echocardiography included age, male sex, a history of hypertension, low-density lipoprotein cholesterol levels, lipoprotein(a) levels, height, and current smoking (Table 1-4).[52] Other studies also support the association of these clinical factors with calcific aortic valve disease with the magnitude of the association being similar to that seen in atherosclerosis. Other factors that were related to the presence of aortic valve disease in these studies include diabetes, elevated homocysteine levels, and metabolic syndrome.[16,21,22] Hereditary factors, genetic polymorphisms, and single-gene defects have also been associated with calcific aortic valve disease[55-58]; however, definitive evidence is still lacking but anticipated.[59,60]

Several population studies suggest that aortic sclerosis is not benign. It has been associated with a 50% increased risk of cardiovascular mortality, even after adjustments for age, sex, hypertension, current smoking, shorter height, elevated low-density lipoprotein cholesterol and the presence of diabetes.[61] In the LIFE study of treatment of 961 hypertensive patients, the composite clinical end point of cardiovascular death, myocardial infarction, or stroke occurred in 15% of patients with aortic sclerosis compared with 8% of those with a normal aortic valve.[49]

Although the precise pathophysiologic basis for the increased cardiovascular and all-cause mortality in aortic sclerosis is incompletely understood, it is unlikely that it directly causes myocardial infarction or death, given the normal valve hemodynamics and the absence of any evidence that thrombosis occurs on the valve leaflets.[62] Studies showing an association between valve sclerosis and atherosclerosis of the aorta support the hypothesis that valve sclerosis is a subclinical marker of vascular atherosclerosis in general.[63,64] However, the discordance between the severity of aortic valve sclerosis or stenosis and coronary artery disease seen in daily clinical practice suggests that the relation may be more nuanced than anticipated. Most patients with severe coronary artery disease never develop aortic valve stenosis. Conversely, only 50% of adults undergoing AVR for severe AS have coronary disease severe enough to warrant a concurrent coronary bypass graft.

AORTIC REGURGITATION

Regurgitation or insufficiency of the aortic valve results from incomplete closure of the valve during diastole and can be caused by a wide variety of disease processes affecting the valve cusps or commissures, aortic sinuses, aortic root, or ascending aorta (Table 1-5). Congenital or acquired deformities of the valve cusps or commissures and dilatation, distortion, or enlargement of the aortic root and ascending aorta are often the underlying causes. The extent to which these abnormalities contribute individually to aortic regurgitation (AR) depends on the age, sex, and other characteristics of the population. The spectrum of etiologies in developing countries also differs from that in the developed world.

In developing countries, a rheumatic etiology predominates, whereas in most developed nations, the most common cause is aortic root dilation or a congenitally bicuspid aortic valve. Rheumatic aortic valve disease in this setting is characterized by thickening and deformity along the valve commissures and is invariably accompanied by rheumatic mitral valve disease.

Age is also important in the etiology of AR. In patients younger than 50 years, the echocardiographic finding of more than trace AR is of concern, especially if there is no history of hypertension, so that a careful clinical history and echocardiographic examination of the valve leaflets and aortic root is indicated to determine the mechanism and severity of regurgitation. For mild AR, Singh et al[65] found a prevalence of 0.5%, 0.6%, and 2.2% in men at ages 50 to 59, 60 to 69, and

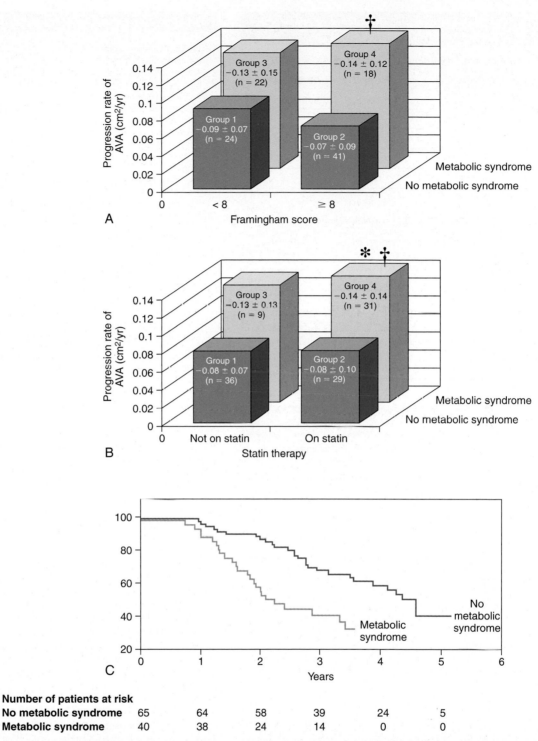

FIGURE 1–7 Impact of the presence of metabolic syndrome on overall survival and hemodynamic progression of aortic stenosis. (**A**) The rate of progression of aortic valve area (AVA) among the two groups separated according to the median value of the Framingham score in patients with (orange bars) and those without metabolic syndrome (blue bars). †Significant difference versus group 2 ($P < 0.05$). (**B**) The rate of progression of AVA among the two groups separated according to the presence or absence of statin therapy in patients with (orange bars) and those without metabolic syndrome (blue bars). *Significant difference versus group 1 ($P < 0.05$); †significant difference versus group 2 ($P < 0.05$). (**C**) Kaplan-Meier analysis of event–free survival in 40 patients with compared with 65 patients without metabolic syndrome. *(From Briand M, Lemieux I, Dumesnil JG, et al: Metabolic syndrome negatively influences disease progression and prognosis in aortic stenosis. J Am Coll Cardiol 2006;47:2229-2236, with permission.)*

70 to 83, respectively. For women in similar age groups, the prevalence of mild AR was 1.9%, 6.0%, and 14.6%. Moderate to severe AR was relatively more common with a prevalence of 3.7%, 12.1%, and 12.2% in men at ages 50 to 59, 60 to 69, and 70 to 83, respectively. The comparable values in women were 0.2%, 0.8%, and 2.3%.[65]

Moderate or severe AR is uncommon in the United States general population especially in those younger than age 50.[28,65] Moderate or severe AR was noted in only 0.1% to 0.2% in pooled population-based study subjects aged younger than 65 years, in 1% of those aged 65 to 74 years, and in 2% in those aged 75 years and older.[28] It was also infrequently diagnosed in Olmstead County in persons younger than 75 years (0.1% to 0.6%) or those older (1.7%).[28]

In the clinical population from the Euro Heart Survey on valvular heart disease, AR was more common in men than in

TABLE 1–3 | **Echocardiographic Prevalence of Aortic Valve Abnormalities**

Aortic Valve Abnormality* (Cardiovascular Health Study, n = 5201[†])

Age Group	None (%)	Sclerosis (%)	Stenosis (%)
All subjects	72	26	2
Women	76	22	1.5
Men	67	31	2
65–74 years	78	20	1.3
75–84 years	62	35	2.4
≥85 years	48	48	4

Aortic Valve Calcification and Thickening* (Helsinki Aging Study, n = 651[‡])

Age Group	None (%)	Slight (%)	Severe (%)
55–71 years	72	21	7
75–76 years	52	39	9
80–81 years	45	38	17
85–86 years	25	56	19

* Percentages of patients in each age group with the observed valve abnormality.
[†] Data from Stewart et al.[52]
[‡] Data from Lindroos et al.[53]

TABLE 1–4 | **Clinical Factors Associated with Calcific Aortic Valve Disease (Cardiovascular Health Study)**

	P Value	Odds Ratio
Age	<0.001	2.18*
Male gender	<0.001	2.03
Lipoprotein(a)	<0.001	1.23[†]
Height	0.001	0.84[‡]
History of hypertension	0.002	1.23
Present smoking	0.006	1.35
Low-density lipoprotein cholesterol (mg/day)	0.006	1.12[†]

*10-year increase.
[†]10-unit increase.
[‡]75th versus 25th percentile.
From Stewart BF, Siscovick D, Lind BK, et al: Clinical factors associated with calcific aortic valve disease: Cardiovascular Health Study. J Am Coll Cardiol 1997;29:630–634, with permission.

women.[29] The most frequent etiology was degenerative heart valve disease, except in patients younger than 50 years in whom a congenital etiology (predominantly a bicuspid aortic valve) was the most frequent finding and accounted for 15.2% of the cases, the same percentage as observed for rheumatic valve disease in this age group.[29] About 15% to 20% of patients with a congenitally bicuspid valve have incomplete valve closure owing to distorted valve anatomy and therefore present clinically with significant regurgitation. These patients typically present in the third or fourth decade of life with an asymptomatic murmur, cardiac enlargement on chest radiography, or symptoms due to AR.[13,66,67]

The finding of a bicuspid aortic valve prompts evaluation for associated abnormalities, including aortic coarctation and aortic root dilation.[68,69] Aortic root dilation in patients with a bicuspid aortic valve is unrelated to age or to the hemodynamic severity of the valvular lesion.[70] In addition, patients

TABLE 1–5 | **Causes of Aortic Regurgitation**

Valve Leaflet Abnormalities
 Congenital bicuspid
 Rheumatic fever
 Bacterial endocarditis (active or healed)
 Marantic endocarditis
 Myxomatous (floppy) valve
 Systemic lupus erythematosus
 Rheumatoid arthritis
 Ankylosing spondylitis
 Congenital fenestration
 Trauma
Aortic Root Disease
 Idiopathic aortic root dilation
 Systemic arterial hypertension
 Marfan syndrome
 Cystic medial necrosis with aortic aneurysm
 Dissecting aneurysm
 Ehlers-Danlos syndrome
 Pseudoxanthoma elasticum
 Inflammatory bowel disease
 Osteogenesis imperfecta
 Annuloaortic ectasia
 Syphilitic aortitis
 Ankylosing spondylitis
 Reiter syndrome
 Trauma

with a bicuspid valve are at increased risk for acute aortic dissection.[71,72] Thus, a patient with baseline mild-moderate valve dysfunction may present acutely with severe AR due to a superimposed aortic dissection. Other rare congenital causes of AR include congenital valve fenestrations, a unicommissural valve, or a quadricuspid valve.[66,73]

In surgical series of patients undergoing aortic valve surgery, isolated AR accounts for about 20% to 30% of cases, whereas mixed stenosis and regurgitation accounts for an additional 12% to 30% of cases.[73,74] In patients aged older than 70 years, a lower percentage of patients undergo AVR for AR and a higher percentage for AS.[74] In the Euro Heart Survey, patients undergoing surgical intervention for valvular regurgitation represent only the extreme of the disease spectrum. Less severe AR, which does not require surgical intervention, is much more common. Although accurate estimates of disease prevalence are not available, several echocardiographic studies have noted an increasing prevalence of detectable AR with age,[75-77] with up to 11% of subjects aged older than 50 years[77,78] and 29% of subjects aged older than 75 years showing AR on Doppler examination.[53] Most of these elderly patients do not have hemodynamically significant regurgitation, show no evidence of left ventricular dilation, and usually require no specific follow-up or treatment.

The presumed etiology of AR in elderly individuals is a combination of mild aortic root dilation[79] and mild fibrocalcific changes of the valve leaflets. Chronic hypertension is associated with mild aortic root dilation[80] and although an increased prevalence of AR has not been documented in asymptomatic hypertensive patients, AR is a feature of end-stage hypertensive heart disease.[81] Small congenital valve fenestrations may be another cause of a small amount of AR. Some systemic diseases result in thickening and incomplete closure of the aortic valve leaflets including irradiation, Fabry disease, mucopolysaccharidosis, and Cogan syndrome.[73] Degenerative valve disease may lead to mild AR but rarely causes a hemodynamically significant lesion unless concurrent aortic root dilation is present. Nonbacterial thrombotic endocarditis or other valve masses (such as a papillary fibroelastoma) rarely result in significant valve incompetence.

AORTIC ROOT DILATION

Aortic root dilatation and abnormal geometry of the outflow tract and sinuses play important pathophysiologic roles in AR. Congenital or genetic abnormalities may be the underlying culprit, and recent studies suggest that heredity explains a substantial proportion of the variability of aortic root size that is not accounted for by age, sex, body size, and blood pressure.[82] Examples include a perimembranous ventricular septal defect with inadequate support of the base of the aortic annulus, Tetralogy of Fallot with associated enlarged aortic root, and sinus of Valsalva aneurysms with distortion of the normal supporting structures and collagen-vascular diseases such as Ehlers-Danlos syndrome, pseudoxanthoma elasticum, and osteogenesis imperfecta, which result in aortic root dilation due to the abnormal molecular components of the aortic wall. Marfan syndrome, although rare, is important to recognize as a potential cause of AR because diagnosis and appropriate surgical therapy in patients with this genetic disease can be life-saving.

Acquired dilation of the aortic root or distortion of its normal anatomy leads to AR either through symmetric stretching of the annulus until the size of the stretched valve leaflets is inadequate to cover the cross-sectional area of the outflow tract, resulting in a central regurgitant jet, or through inadequate support of the valve commissures, resulting in a more eccentric jet origin and direction.

The most prevalent acquired abnormality of the aortic root is dilation due to hypertension and/or atherosclerotic changes of the aortic wall. Cuspidi et al[83] showed in a consecutive series of 3366 patients with untreated and treated essential hypertension (mean age, 53 years) that aortic root dilatation, defined by the sex-specific echocardiographic criterion of 40 mm in men and 38 mm in women, was present in 8.5% of men and in 3.1% of women. Compared with 3160 patients with normal aortic size, the group of 206 patients with an enlarged aortic root was older, had higher diastolic blood pressure values, and included a greater fraction of subjects receiving antihypertensive treatment, with type 2 diabetes and metabolic syndrome.[83]

Annuloaortic ectasia, also known as cystic medial necrosis, is more likely to lead to progressive root dilation and hemodynamically significant regurgitation, requiring surgical intervention.[84] Systemic diseases that are accompanied by aortic root dilation and may result in significant AR include rheumatoid arthritis,[85] psoriatic arthritis, ankylosing spondylitis,[86-88] systemic lupus erythematosus, Reiter syndrome,[89] relapsing polychondritis,[90] syphilitic aortitis, Kawasaki disease, and Takayasu aortitis.[73]

MITRAL STENOSIS

The most frequent cause of MS is chronic rheumatic carditis, a sequela of one or more prior episodes of acute rheumatic fever. The dramatic decline in the incidence of acute rheumatic fever in most developed countries has led to a corresponding decline in the incidence and prevalence of MS. In the United States, MS is the least common valve disease in adults aged 18 years and older with an overall age-adjusted prevalence of 0.1% 0.2% in population-based studies and the community.[28] The ratio of women to men presenting with MS is about 2:1; however, it may be as high as 4:1 as noted in the European experience of valvular heart disease in the community.[28,29] In both the European and American experiences, rheumatic heart disease remained the predominant cause of MS. Acquired causes of mitral valve obstruction, other than rheumatic heart disease, are rare and include left atrial myxoma, ball valve thrombus, mucopolysaccharidosis, and severe annular calcification (Table 1-6).[91]

TABLE 1–6	Causes of Mitral Stenosis

Rheumatic Fever
  Carditis with mitral valve damage (>95%)
Congenital Heart Disease
  Papillary muscle hypoplasia or fusion
  Short and thickened chordae tendineae
Metabolic
  Whipple disease
  Mucopolysaccharidosis
  Fabry disease
  Carcinoid
  Methysergide therapy
Other
  Severe mitral annular calcification
  Atrial tumor with prolapse into mitral annulus
  Active infective endocarditis with large vegetation

Isolated MS occurs in 40% of all patients presenting with rheumatic heart disease, although a history of rheumatic fever can be elicited from approximately 60% of patients presenting with pure MS.[92,93] Surgical pathologic series show rheumatic involvement in 99% of mitral valves excised for stenosis.[94,95] In about 38% of cases of MS, there is multivalve involvement. The aortic valve is affected most often (93%), with rheumatic tricuspid valve changes seen in 6% of patients with rheumatic mitral valve disease and involvement of all three valves in 1% of patients with rheumatic mitral valve disease.[96,97]

Severe mitral annular calcification (MAC) with involvement of the mitral leaflets by the degenerative process is an unusual cause of hemodynamically significant MS, accounting for less than 3% of cases of MS. These patients tend to be elderly and often have associated aortic valve calcification.[98] Rarer causes of MS include carcinoid disease,[99] Fabry disease,[100] mucopolysaccharidosis,[101,102] Whipple disease,[103,104] gout,[105] rheumatoid arthritis, or obstruction by a large valvular vegetation.[106,107]

Congenital causes of MS are seen almost exclusively in infants and children and account for less than 1% of MS.[108-110] Congenital malformations that lead to MS include shortened chordae and obliteration of interchordal spaces, a hypoplastic mitral valve associated with hypoplastic left heart syndrome, a supramitral ring, and a "parachute" mitral valve with insertion of all the chordae into a single papillary muscle. Congenital MS is often associated with other congenital abnormalities and is rarely seen in adults, given that the median age at death is only 2 months.[108]

MITRAL REGURGITATION

MR is the most commonly encountered clinically significant valvular disease in both population- and community-based studies in the United States.[28] Its overall frequency of 1.7% in population-based studies reflects an increase from 0.5% in persons aged 45 to 54 years to 9.3% in those aged 75 years and older.[28] The corresponding prevalence in the community was 7.1% overall and also increased gradually with age from 0.1% in persons aged 18 to 44 years to 7.1% in those aged 75 years and older.[28] In the Euro Heart Survey on valvular heart disease, MR was the second most frequent single native valve disease and accounted for 31.6% of patients.[29] The mean age in this European multicenter survey was 65 years, and although patients with MR were younger than the patients with AS, those with MR had more frequent comorbidities.[29]

MR may be due to a primary disorder of the valve leaflets, annulus, and/or subvalvular apparatus or may represent a secondary consequence of another cardiac disease or a systemic or genetic disease that involves the mitral valve (Table 1-7).

TABLE 1-7	Causes of Mitral Regurgitation

Primary Mitral Valve Disease
   Myxomatous mitral valve disease (mitral valve prolapse)
   Rheumatic valve disease
   Acute rheumatic fever
   Chronic rheumatic valvular disease
   Infective endocarditis
   Congenital lesions
   Cleft anterior mitral leaflet
   Leaflet fenestration
   Mitral annular calcification/degenerative leaflet changes
   Idiopathic chordal rupture
Mitral Regurgitation Secondary To Another Cardiac Disease
   Coronary artery disease (ischemic mitral regurgitation)
   Papillary muscle rupture
   Transmural myocardial infarction
   Ischemic regional dysfunction
   Global ventricular dysfunction
   Dilated cardiomyopathy
   Marfan syndrome or other inherited connective tissue disorder
   Hypertrophic cardiomyopathy
   Endomyocardial fibrosis
Mitral Valve Involvement in a Systemic Disease
   Systemic lupus erythematosus
   Hypereosinophilic syndrome
   Amyloidosis
   Rheumatoid arthritis
   Ehlers-Danlos types I and III
   Scleroderma
External Causes
   Radiation therapy
   Pharmacologic agents
   Fenfluramine-phentermine
   Methysergide
   Trauma
   Surgical
   Percutaneous valvuloplasty

The relative prevalence of the differing etiologies of MR depends on whether only patients with severe regurgitation requiring surgical intervention are considered or whether patients with milder degrees of regurgitation are included in the clinical study. In particular, estimates of disease prevalence are confounded by the observation that a small degree of physiologic MR can be detected on careful Doppler echocardiography in up to 80% of normal individuals.[65]

Table 1-7 shows the wide variety of disease processes that lead to MR. They include primary valve abnormalities, other cardiac diseases with mitral valvular involvement, systemic diseases that also affect the mitral valve, and external forces, such as radiation therapy[111] or surgical trauma. In addition to myxomatous mitral valve disease, such as mitral valve prolapse (MVP), primary disease of the valve leaflets includes endocarditis with destruction of valve tissue leading to perforation, incomplete leaflet coaptation, chordal rupture, and consequent MR. Congenital abnormalities of the leaflets include a cleft anterior mitral leaflet and mitral valve fenestrations. A cleft anterior leaflet often accompanies defects of the atrioventricular septum but also may occur as an isolated defect.

In the clinical population represented in the Euro Heart Survey, the most frequent etiology overall was degenerative heart valve disease, followed by rheumatic heart disease.[29] However, in patients aged younger than 50 years, rheumatic heart disease was just as prevalent as degenerative disease. In patients undergoing surgical intervention for severe MR, the most common etiologies are MVP (20% to 70% of cases), ischemic MR (13% to 30% of cases), rheumatic disease (3% to 40% of cases), and endocarditis (10% to 12% of cases).[94,95,112] In patients followed medically in general clinical practices, the most common underlying etiologies of MR include ischemic heart disease, MVP, dilated cardiomyopathy, and MAC.[113]

MITRAL ANNULAR CALCIFICATION

MAC is a common echocardiographic finding, especially in older adults. In the Cardiovascular Health Study, a prospective community-based observational study designed to assess cardiovascular risk factors and outcomes in elderly persons (mean age of 76 years), MAC was found in 42% of participants. Participants with MAC were older and had worse cardiovascular, renal, metabolic, and functional profiles than those without MAC.[114]. In the relatively much younger African-American participants of the Atherosclerotic Risk in Communities study, the overall prevalence of MAC was 4.6% for women and 5.6% for men.[115] In participants aged 70 years and older, the prevalence of MAC was 10% in women and 15.2% in men.[115]

MAC can be a cause of MR. The presumed mechanism of regurgitation with MAC is increased rigidity of the annulus, although calcification may involve the base of the posterior leaflet in some patients. In addition to MR, MAC has been associated with hypertension, AS, renal failure, and diabetes mellitus. Typically the degree of MR is only mild to moderate and these patients rarely need intervention for MR.

MAC, like calcific aortic valve disease, is associated with standard cardiovascular risk factors.[116] However, Kizer et al[117] recently showed that the presence of MAC but not of aortic valve sclerosis was a strong risk factor for incident stroke in a cohort of American Indians without clinical cardiovascular disease after extensive adjustment for other predictors. MAC is also associated with coronary atherosclerosis and a wide variety of clinical conditions.[115,117-120]

More recently, caseous calcification of the mitral annulus, a lesser known variant of MAC, has been described as "a round mass with a central echolucent area composed of a puttylike admixture of fatty acids, cholesterol, and calcium."[121] Of 20,468 consecutive patients referred for transthoracic echocardiography, a total of 14 patients (0.64% of all patients with MAC and 0.068% of all studied) were given the diagnosis of caseous calcification of the mitral annulus.[121] This variant of MAC carries a benign prognosis; however, it is important that it not be mistaken for a cardiac tumor.[121-123]

TRICUSPID AND PULMONARY VALVE DISEASE

Acquired primary disorders of intrinsically normal tricuspid and pulmonary valves are rare. However, congenital malformations of the right-sided heart valves and associated structural and functional disorders and complications are not uncommon. In addition, acquired disorders of intrinsically normal tricuspid and pulmonary valves due to other cardiovascular and noncardiac systemic disorders are relatively more common. For example, more than 50% of patients with carcinoid syndrome eventually develop carcinoid heart disease, which characteristically may include severe tricuspid regurgitation (TR), with or without tricuspid stenosis, and pulmonary stenosis and regurgitation.[99,124,125] In fact, in nearly 20% of patients, these cardiac manifestations may be the initial presentation of carcinoid syndrome.[99]

The major congenital abnormalities of the right-sided heart valves include congenital pulmonic stenosis, congenital pulmonary regurgitation, Ebstein anomaly of the tricuspid valve, and tricuspid atresia. Congenital valvular pulmonic stenosis is relatively common and constitutes about 13.5% of the congenital heart disease abnormalities.[31] In 2002, it had an estimated prevalence of 134,000 (about 58,000 in children and 76,000 in adults). In the United States[31] stenosis occurs in about 7% to 10% of patients with congenital heart disease. Ebstein anomaly is a rare congenital heart disorder that is seen in about 1 per 200,000 live births and accounts for less than 1% of all cases of congenital heart disease.[126] The other congenital abnormalities are significantly less frequent; however, they can be a cause of significant morbidity such as endocarditis.

Trace or minor degrees of TR can be detected in up to 90% of normal individuals and are not associated with progressive valve dysfunction or adverse clinical outcomes.[127] Although these degrees of TR are considered to be normal, mild to moderate TR may be associated with decreased survival, independent of the level of associated right or left ventricular dilatation and dysfunction or abnormal pulmonary artery pressure.[128] Severe TR is associated with a poor prognosis, independent of age, biventricular systolic function, right ventricular size, and dilation of the inferior vena cava.[128] The disorders that contribute to intrinsic valvular TR include rheumatic, congenital, and carcinoid heart disease, infective endocarditis, toxic effects of chemicals, tumors, blunt trauma, and myxomatous degeneration.[127]

Although trace or a minor degree of pulmonary regurgitation is also commonly seen and considered physiologic, isolated pulmonary regurgitation of mild to moderate degrees is rare and not benign.[129] Abnormal pulmonary regurgitation is most commonly a result of pulmonary hypertension or complications after surgical or percutaneous relief of pulmonary stenosis and after repair of tetralogy of Fallot.[129]

MULTIVALVULAR AND MIXED VALVULAR HEART DISEASE

Although many studies include only patients with regurgitation or stenosis involving only one heart valve, several scenarios in which patients present with regurgitation and/or stenosis involving two or more valves exist. The etiology of these multivalvular and mixed valvular heart diseases includes both congenital[130-133] and acquired cardiac causes[134] and noncardiac systemic diseases,[135,136] as well as adverse drug effects and complications.[137-147] Thus, the burden of multivalvular and mixed valvular heart disease in the population will depend on the prevalence of these contributing etiologies. For example, complex congenital cardiac anomalies, with or without chromosomal aberrations, may involve several valves with regurgitation and or stenosis.[131-133] Kowal-Vern et al[131] reported that 93% of patients with trisomy 18 have polyvalvular disease, and more than one-third of them have all four valves involved. In four patients with polyvalvular disease without chromosomal abnormalities, all four valves were markedly abnormal, bicuspid and unicuspid valves were seen, the chordae tendineae were generally abbreviated, and papillary muscles were hypoplastic.[131]

Among the acquired cardiac disorders that lead to multiple valve involvement, the most prevalent include recurrent acute rheumatic fever,[148] endocarditis, severe biventricular dilatation, and thoracic/mediastinal radiation therapy.[88,149,150] Noncardiac disorders that contribute to the burden of multivalvular and mixed valvular heart disease include heritable disorders of connective tissue,[151] carcinoid syndrome, and the rare condition of cardiac ochronosis with alkaptonuria.[152,153] Although AS is the most frequent cardiac manifestation of ochronosis, mitral and tricuspid involvement do occur and typically manifest as leaflet thickening with subsequent dysfunction.[152]

Adverse drug effects and complications can contribute to the burden of valvular heart disease as recently reported in some patients with Parkinson disease treated with ergot-derived dopamine agonists[137-144,154] or the reports from a decade earlier in patients prescribed anorectic medications.[145-147] For example, between 1995 and 1997, an estimated 1.2 to 4.7 million persons (mostly women and persons younger than 60 years old) in the United States were exposed

to fenfluramine (Pondimin) or its dextroisomer dexfenfluramine (Redux), alone or in combination with phentermine (Adipex, Fastin, and Ionamin) as prescription appetite suppressants.[155] In 1997, Connolly et al[156] reported 24 cases of valvular heart disease in women who had been treated with fenfluramine and phentermine. The histopathologic features were similar to those observed in carcinoid-induced valvular disease, except that MR or AR or both were always present, and about half of the women also had tricuspid valve involvement.[155,156]

One nonrandomized study suggested that valvulopathy (mild or greater degree of AR, and moderate or greater degree of MR) could be seen in up to 12.8% of persons taking dexfenfluramine alone, 22.8% of those taking a dexfenfluramine and phentermine combination, and 25.2% of those taking a fenfluramine and phentermine combination.[157] Both regression and progression of valvulopathy have been observed during follow-up, including a recent report of aortic and mitral valve disease that deteriorated and was discovered 7 years after cessation of treatment with fenfluramine.[157-159] Although the weight of the evidence supports an increased risk of multivalvular regurgitation in patients exposed to these anorectants,[145,160] the magnitude of the risk appears to be lower than the initial case reports suggested.[161]

ENDOCARDITIS

Although relatively uncommon, infective endocarditis (IE) is a serious clinical and public health problem associated with significant morbidity and mortality. Its precise worldwide burden and epidemiologic trends have been difficult to establish because of varying case definitions used in different studies, differences in risk level of populations assessed, and biases in case ascertainment and incidence estimates. Despite these challenges, the recent advances in invasive interventions, increasing numbers and types of susceptible hosts, continuing global antimicrobial resistance, and an aging population have led to a general suspicion that the incidence and prevalence of IE may be changing. Until recently, however, definitive evidence of this had been lacking.

In a rigorous systematic review that included 15 population-based studies with 2371 patients with IE from Denmark, France, Italy, the Netherlands, Sweden, United Kingdom, and United States from 1969 to 2000, Tleyjeh et al[162] showed (1) a nonsignificant decline in patients with underlying rheumatic heart disease, (2) a 7% per decade increase in the proportions of patients with IE undergoing valve surgery, and (3) a 7% per decade increase in those with underlying prosthetic valves. They observed no significant temporal trends in the causative organisms.

A recent community-based temporal trend study from Olmsted County, Minnesota, found no substantial change in the incidence of IE over the past 3 decades.[163] In this study, the age- and sex-adjusted incidence of IE ranged from 5.0 to 7.0 cases per 100,000 person-years during the study period and did not change significantly over time. However, a nonsignificant increasing temporal trend was observed in the proportions of patients with IE who have prosthetic valves and patients with MVP. There was no time trend in rates of valve surgery or 6–month mortality during the study period.[163]

In 2004, the total-mention mortality from IE was 2438 with an estimated hospital discharge burden of 30,000 instances of IE as the primary or secondary diagnosis in the United States. Advancing age is a powerful independent predictor of mortality in IE.[164] Concurrent with improved therapies for IE, there has been an increase in the age of affected individuals, with an estimated mean age of 30 years in the preantibiotic era compared with a mean age ranging from 40 to 70 years currently.[164,165]

Valvular heart disease in women of child-bearing age is an important clinical and public health burden because of the increased risk specific valve lesions pose to fetal and maternal health during pregnancy and delivery.[166,167] Recent advances in the diagnosis and treatment of congenital heart disease in infants and children have led to an increased prevalence of adults with congenital heart disease, many of whom are women in their child-bearing years.[167,168] In addition, anticoagulation often administered in the management of mechanical prosthetic valves poses an additional risk to the fetus.[168,169] Nevertheless, many women can have uneventful pregnancies as long as appropriate specialized care is provided before and during the pregnancy, labor, and perinatal periods.[91,166-170]

Valvular heart diseases in this population are usually residua of corrected congenital abnormalities, acquired lesions (such as rheumatic valvulopathy and degenerative calcification or sclerosis of a congenitally bicuspid aortic valve), and MVP due to myxomatous and floppy mitral leaflets.[170] MVP is generally considered to be the most common valvular heart lesion in women of reproductive age and is estimated to contribute about 4% of obstetric cardiac problems.[171,172] However, quantitative echocardiographic studies that are designed to be free of referral bias show a much lower prevalence (1.4% for classic MVP and 1.3% for nonclassic MVP) in women.[173]

The most common valve lesion of rheumatic origin in this population is MS, followed by MR, with AS and regurgitation accounting for the remainder. For example, in one study of pregnancies complicated by heart disease from 1970 to 1983 in Ireland, 60% of heart disease was of rheumatic origin, and MS, MR, and AR accounted for 61%, 33%, and 6% of cases, respectively.[167] Although the prevalence and incidence of rheumatic heart disease have dramatically declined in Europe and North America since that time, rheumatic valve disease still remains common in women of child-bearing age.[170,174,175] Other causes of valvular heart disease that should be considered in this population include prior endocarditis and the valvulopathy of systemic disease such as inflammatory vascular disorders, systemic lupus erythematosus, and Marfan syndrome.[170]

Definitive epidemiologic data on incidence, prevalence, case fatality, and overall burden of specific valve diseases in women of child-bearing age for most parts of the world are lacking. Nevertheless, the available data suggest that MS is the most frequent significant valvular heart disease encountered in pregnant women, and it is almost always of rheumatic origin.[166,176] MS is often poorly tolerated when the mitral valve area is less than 1.5 cm^2, even in previously asymptomatic patients.[176,177] For example, Silversides et al[178] showed that in 80 pregnancies in 74 women with rheumatic MS, the incidence of maternal complications was 67% in women with severe MS, 38% in women with moderate MS, and 26% in women with mild MS.

AS is significantly less common in women of child-bearing age and in pregnant women. The two leading causes of AS in this population are of congenital and rheumatic origin, with rheumatic AS typically seen in conjunction with mitral valve disease in an estimated 5% of pregnant women with rheumatic valvular disease.[177,179] Most patients tolerate pregnancy well when valve area exceeds 1.0 cm^2 in the absence of symptoms and close follow-up care is provided. Isolated pulmonic stenosis is most commonly a result of congenital obstruction at the valve level, and, in contrast to MS or AS, it is well tolerated in pregnancy even when severe.[166] AR in this population may be due to a congenitally bicuspid valve, dilated aortic annulus, or rheumatic valvulopathy or be a sequela of endocarditis.[166] When unaccompanied by symptoms or left ventricular systolic dysfunction, mild AR and also MR are well tolerated.[166] In general, however, maternal and fetal outcomes with mitral and aortic valvular disease in pregnancy are related to hemodynamic severity and associated symptoms.[91,176]

Functional regurgitation involving all valves except the aortic valve also occurs with pregnancy. Campos et al[180] reported that physiologic valvular regurgitation, involving only the tricuspid (38.9%) and pulmonary (22.2%) valves in early pregnancy, was similar to that in a control group of healthy nonpregnant women. However, there was a progressive and significant increase of multivalvular regurgitation that became maximal at full-term (mitral, 27.8%; tricuspid, 94.4%; and pulmonary, 94.4%; $P < 0.05$ versus early pregnancy).[180] Thus, physiologic, multivalvular regurgitation is frequent in late pregnancy, occasionally persisting in the early puerperium. As with biventricular enlargement, cardiac remodeling and valve annular dilatation resulting from chronic volume overload account for these multivalvular regurgitation.

In the presence of severe symptomatic valvular heart disease before conception, definitive treatment in accordance with established clinical guidelines often yields good clinical outcomes. For example, in 267 young women with rheumatic heart disease who underwent isolated mechanical MVR between 1975 and 2003, De Santo et al[181] reported very impressive outcomes after 3708 patient-years of follow-up. Actuarial survival at 5, 10, 20, and 25 years was 90%, 85%, 72%, and 70%, respectively.[181] Freedom from thromboembolic events at these same time points was 94%, 89%, 81%, and 75%, respectively.[181] Remarkably, when treated with warfarin, no patient undertaking pregnancy (n = 35) experienced adverse cardiac or valve-related events, and fetal complications were significantly less frequent with a daily warfarin dose less than 5 mg.[181] At the end of the 25-year study, 208 of 267 (78%) were still alive; of these survivors, 61.1% and 33.6% were in New York Heart Association functional class I and II, respectively, suggesting that mechanical prosthetic valves in the mitral position provided excellent performance, safety, and durability in women of reproductive age.[181]

HEART VALVE PROCEDURES

Summary data from the Society of Thoracic Surgeons National Database show that 17,592 aortic valve procedures and 4251 mitral valve procedures were performed by the 756 participating sites in 2007.[31] The corresponding mean postprocedure lengths of stay for aortic and mitral valve procedures were 8.1 and 10.6 days, respectively, with associated unadjusted operative mortality for the two procedures of 3% and 6%.[31] The national total number of open heart valvuloplasty without replacement, heart valve replacement, and other operations on heart valves was estimated in men and women to be 61,000 and 43,000, respectively.[31]

The costs and complications associated with therapeutic heart valve procedures represent another part of the burden of valvular heart disease. The most recent data from the Healthcare Cost and Utilization Project for the United States show that in 2006, the mean charges for heart valve procedures ($141,120) was substantially higher than those for coronary artery bypass surgery (99,743) or implantable defibrillators ($104,743). In addition, the in-hospital death rate was also higher at 5.1% compared with 1.94% and 0.64% for coronary artery bypass surgery and implantable defibrillators, respectively.[31,182]

Allareddy et al[183] analyzed the Nationwide Inpatient Sample for the years 2000 to 2003 to provide nationally representative estimates of in-hospital mortality, length of

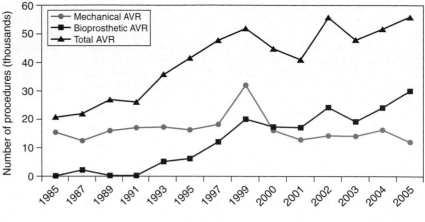

FIGURE 1–8 Number of aortic valve replacement (AVR) procedures performed in the United States between 1985 and 1999 based on the National Center for Health Statistics. ICD-9-CM procedure codes: all AVRs (35.22 + 35.21), bioprosthetic AVR (35.21), and mechanical AVR (35.22). Note the recent increase in the use of bioprosthetic aortic valve prostheses. *(From National Center for Health Statistics: National Hospital Discharge Survey: Annual Summaries With Detailed Diagnosis and Procedure Data; Series 13. Data on Health Resources Utilization. Available at http://www.cdc.gov/nchs/products/pubs/pubd/series/ser.htm#sr13.)*

stay, and hospital charges after AVR and MVR and to quantify the impact of different types of complications on in-hospital outcomes. Complications occurred in 35.2% of the 43,909 patients who underwent AVR and in 36.4% of 16,516 patients who had MVR.[183] Importantly, nearly half of these complications were cardiac complications and one-quarter involved hemorrhage, hematoma, or seroma. Thus, cardiac complications were relatively common and had a considerable impact on hospital mortality, length of stay, and hospital charges even after adjustment for patient and hospital characteristics.[183]

Important advances in diagnostic imaging, percutaneous interventions, and improvements in surgical techniques have led to increasing numbers of valve procedures in the United States. In the two decades since 1985, the number of heart valve replacements have more than doubled and mitral valve repair has increased steadily, especially since 1993 (Figure 1-8).[30] In addition, implantation of a bioprosthetic valve now exceeds that of a mechanical valve in the aortic position, although 20 years earlier, nearly all AVRs involved mechanical valves (Figure 1-8).[30] In 2006, an estimated 104,000 operations or procedures were performed on heart valves in the United States.[31] Although more than half of these procedures were performed on persons aged 65 years and older, nearly one-third of procedures were in younger patients aged 45 to 64 years.[31]

VALVE REPLACEMENT AND PROSTHETIC VALVE DYSFUNCTION

For most types of severely diseased valves, the definitive treatment is replacement with a prosthetic heart valve. Prosthetic valve replacement, however, does not restore normal cardiac function and is invariably associated with significant operative mortality. For example, risk-adjusted operative mortality for AVR is about 3% for isolated valve replacement and 6% when combined with coronary bypass grafting.[184] For mitral valve surgery, the risk adjusted operative mortality is about 2% for mitral valve repair, 8% for mitral valve repair plus coronary bypass grafting, 6% for MVR, and 12% for MVR plus bypass grafting.[184] Both short-term and long-term postoperative complications may include thromboembolism, endocarditis, hemolytic anemia, anticoagulation-related bleeding, structural deterioration, and other structural and functional dysfunction.[185]

The prevalence of prosthetic valve dysfunction and the overall death rate have traditionally been considered to depend on the specific type of valve implanted, the site of implantation, and comorbid risk factors. For example, in a meta-analysis of 5837 patients who underwent bioprosthetic AVR with a total follow-up of 31,874 patient-years, the annual rates of valve thrombosis, thromboembolism, hemorrhage, and nonstructural dysfunction were 0.03%, 0.87%, 0.38%, and 0.38%, respectively (Figure 1-9).[186] The annual

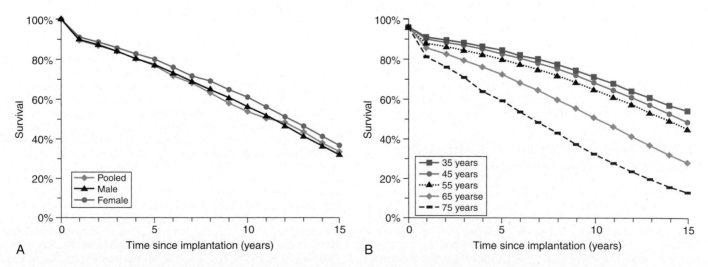

FIGURE 1–9 Survival after implantation of stented porcine bioprosthesis. (A) Pooled estimate from the literature (pooled) and predicted survival for 62-year-old men and women according to model. (B) Predicted survival for men of different ages. *(From Puvimanasinghe JP, Steyerberg EW, Takkenberg JJ, et al: Prognosis after AVR with a bioprosthesis: Predictions based on meta-analysis and microsimulation. Circulation 2001;103:1535-1541, with permission.)*

rate of endocarditis was estimated to be 0.68% for longer than 6 months of implantation and was five times as high during the first 6 months.[186]

In a long-term (19-year) follow-up study of 440 patients who received an isolated MVR with a St. Jude mechanical prosthesis, Remadi et al[187] found linearized rates (in percent patient-years) of thromboembolism, thrombosis, and hemorrhage of 0.69, 0.2, and 1, respectively.[187] Freedom from endocarditis and reoperation was 98.6% and 90%, respectively. In these studies, age, sex, New York Heart Association class, and atrial fibrillation were significantly correlated with overall mortality.[187] In a more recent meta-analysis that included 32 articles with 15 mechanical and 23 biologic valve series totaling 17,439 patients and 101,819 patient-years, Lund and Bland[188] found no difference in risk factor–corrected overall death rate between mechanical or bioprosthetic aortic valves irrespective of age. Mean age of the prosthetic valve series was directly related to the death rate with no interaction with valve type.[188]

Kulik et al[189] examined the long-term outcomes of mechanical versus bioprosthetic valves in middle-aged (50 to 65 years old) persons who had first-time AVR and/or MVR with contemporary prostheses followed prospectively for a total of 3,402 patient-years (mean ± SD 5.1 ± 4.1 years; maximum 18.3 years). The 10–year survival was 73.2 ± 4.2% after mechanical AVR, 75.1 ± 12.6% after bioprosthetic AVR, 74.1 ± 4.6% after mechanical MVR, and 77.9 ± 7.4% after bioprosthetic MVR (P=NS).[189] Reoperation rates at 10 years were 35.4% and 21.3% with aortic and mitral bioprostheses, respectively. The overall freedom from major adverse prosthesis-related events at 10 years was 70.2 + 4.1% for patients with mechanical AVR, 41.0 ± 30.3% for patients with bioprosthetic AVR, 53.3 + 8.8% for patients with mechanical MVR, and 61.2 ± 9.2% for patients with bioprosthetic MVR.

In the 15-year follow-up comparison of long-term survival and valve-related complications between bioprosthetic and mechanical heart valves in 575 patients who underwent single AVR or MVR at 13 Veterans Affairs medical centers, Hammermeister et al[190] found that all-cause mortality after AVR was lower with a mechanical valve versus a bioprosthesis (66% versus 79%; P = 0.02) but not after MVR. Primary valve failure occurred mainly in patients aged younger than 65 years (bioprosthesis versus mechanical, 26% versus 0%; P < 0.001 for AVR and 44% versus 4%; P = 0.0001 for MVR). In patients aged 65 years and older primary valve failure after AVR for bioprosthesis versus mechanical valves was 9 ± 6% versus 0%. The reoperation rate was significantly higher for bioprosthetic AVR, and bleeding occurred more frequently in patients with mechanical valves. However, there were no statistically significant differences in thromboembolism and all valve-related complications. The investigators concluded that at 15 years, patients undergoing AVR had better survival with a mechanical valve than with a bioprosthetic valve, largely because primary valve failure was virtually absent with a mechanical valve. Primary valve failure was greater with a bioprosthesis, both for AVR and MVR, and occurred at a much higher rate in patients aged younger than 65 years.

DISPARITIES IN ACCESS TO CARE AND QUALITY OF HEALTH CARE

Disparities in access to care and the quality of health care for the prevention, diagnostic evaluation, treatment, and control of cardiovascular diseases constitute an important component of the overall burden of disease.[191-193] Several publications, including an Institute of Medicine summary of the literature[194-201] and a review conducted jointly by the American College of Cardiology Foundation and Kaiser Family Foundation[202] concluded (after examining the most rigorous studies investigating racial/ethnic differences in angiography, angioplasty, coronary artery bypass graft surgery, and thrombolytic therapy) that disparities in the quality of medical care are pervasive, and they persist even after adjustment for potentially confounding factors.

The determinants of these disparities are complex and may include contributing factors at the patient, provider, and health care system levels. What is now well established is that (1) disparities are pervasive, (2) they are observed in almost all aspects of health care, and (3) are seen across all dimensions of quality of health care including effectiveness, patient safety, timeliness, and patient centeredness.[203-205] In addition, these disparities are present across many levels and types of care including preventive care, treatment of acute conditions, and overall disease management in the long-term.[203] In general, Hispanics, African Americans, American Indians, Alaska Natives, persons without health insurance, and poor people of any race or ethnicity receive poorer quality of care than whites and Asian Americans.[203,204,206] These disparities also transcend race, ethnicity, and socioeconomic status to include age, gender, and educational attainment. Until recently, however, disparities in the burden and care of patients with valvular heart disease had not been carefully evaluated.

In the general population experience from the United States, there were no gender-related differences in the frequency of moderate or severe valve disease. However, in the community setting, MR and AR were more often diagnosed in men than in women.[28] In addition, several reports in surgical series of MR or AR consistently show a 60% to 75% greater preponderance of men than women, suggesting a possible gender disparity in referral patterns and/or surgical intervention.[207,208] In the Euro Heart Survey,[209] women with severe AS presented at an older age and with more severe symptoms, whereas men had more frequent comorbidity and coronary disease. Importantly, sex had no impact on the decision to operate; however, age did.[209]

Not all sex-based differences in the epidemiology of valvular heart disease are related to disparities in access and quality of care, although the basis for the differences are often incompletely understood.[41,210] For example, as many as two-thirds of all patients with rheumatic MS are female[91]; however, rheumatic MR is more common in men, although some studies showed an equal prevalence in men and women.[41] MAC is common in both older men and women; however, MR resulting from severe MAC is more common in women than in men.[211] In addition, MVP syndrome is more prevalent in women, in whom it generally has a benign course, whereas severe myxomatous disease is more common in older men, who have a higher risk of complications, including the need for surgical mitral valve repair.[212-214]

Age-related differences are also well recognized and are often preventable. For example, in nearly one-third of patients with severe single-valve disease who did not undergo guideline-recommended intervention while in New York Heart Association class III or IV, the most frequent noncardiac reason stated for denying an intervention was old age (27.6% and as a sole reason in 1.3%).[181] This observation was again confirmed in the 2007 European experience,[29] suggesting that disparate care for patients with severe valve disease was provided solely on the basis of age rather than the established practice guideline recommendations. Analysis of the therapeutic decision in patients with severe valve diseases showed that symptomatic patients were frequently denied surgery (32.3% in AS after the age of 75 and 51.3% in MR) more on the basis of age rather than the recommendations of clinical practice guidelines.

Taylor et al[215] used the Society of Thoracic Surgeons National Cardiac Database comprising 3137 black and 46,249 white patients to examine the association between race and operative mortality after isolated AVR or MVR from 1999 through 2002. Unadjusted operative mortality for MVR only was 5.60% for blacks versus 6.18% for whites. The corresponding mortality for AVR only was 4.60% for blacks versus 3.62% for whites. In contrast with previous publications that suggested that as an independent risk factor for operative mortality after coronary artery bypass surgery, race was not a significant predictor of operative mortality after isolated AVR or MVR.

Other recent data suggest that system-level factors, such as hospital volume, provider board certification, access to subspecialty care, and hospital characteristics may play a more important role than patient-level factors in disparities in the care and outcomes for valvular heart disease. For example, Groeneveld et al[216] showed that low rates of technology utilization in hospitals with high proportions of black inpatients may be an important contributor to and a remediable cause of health care disparities. In their study of 2,348,952 elderly Medicare beneficiaries potentially eligible for tissue replacement of the aortic valve and four other emerging medical technologies from 1989 to 2000, blacks had significantly lower adjusted rates ($P < 0.001$) for tissue replacement of the aortic valve than whites.[216] Hospitals with more than 20% black inpatients were less likely to perform the procedure on both white and black patients than hospitals with less than 9% black inpatients, and the racial disparity was greater in hospitals with larger black populations.[216] They concluded that blacks may be disadvantaged in access to new procedures by receiving care at hospitals that have both lower procedure rates and greater racial disparity.[216]

More recently, Groeneveld et al[217] identified 87,536 potential candidates for bioprosthetic AVR hospitalized at Veterans Administration Medical Centers (VAMCs) between 1998 and 2003 and examined racial differences in procedure rates both across and within hospital-level classifications. They found that VAMCs with more than 30% black inpatients had greater racial differences compared with predominantly white VAMCs (adjusted black-white odds ratios of 0.45 versus 0.81 for AVR; $P = 0.07$). Thus, although VAMCs with larger black inpatient populations performed cardiac procedures at rates similar to those of predominantly white VAMCs, racial differences in procedures were greater within VAMCs with larger black populations.[217] Schelbert et al[218] also compared the use of bioprosthetic valves in 78,154 black and white Medicare beneficiaries aged 65 years or older undergoing AVR in 904 U.S. hospitals during 1999 through 2001. After adjustment for patient characteristics, bioprosthetic valve use was lower in blacks relative to whites (relative risk, 0.93; 95% CI, 0.91 to 0.95; $P < 0.001$).[218] However, black patients were more likely to undergo surgery in hospitals in the lowest quintile of bioprosthesis use overall (29% versus 20% of white patients; $P < 0.001$). In fact, after accounting for hospital-level variability in bioprosthesis use, the use of bioprostheses was somewhat higher in black patients (relative risk, 1.06; 95% CI, 1.04 to 1.09; $P < 0.001$).[218]

Lucas et al[219] used national Medicare data to identify all patients undergoing one of eight cardiovascular and cancer procedures that included AVR between 1994 and 1999 to examine relationships between race and operative mortality. Black patients had higher crude mortality rates than white patients for AVR.[219] However, patient characteristics had only modest or no effect on odds ratios of mortality by race,[219] and adjustment for hospital characteristics accounted for most of the differences. Hospitals that treated a large proportion of black patients had higher mortality rates for all eight procedures and for white as well as black patients.[219] The authors concluded that the higher operative mortality risks across a wide range of surgical procedures observed for blacks resulted in large part because of higher mortality rates at the hospitals they attend.[219]

In another study that examined the clinical presentation and surgical outcome for severe mitral valve disease in African American compared with white patients, DiGiorgi et al[220] found no significant differences in the incidences of postoperative complications or hospital mortality (2.4% African American versus 5.1% white; $P = 0.19$). However, African Americans presented for mitral valve surgery at a significantly younger age than whites and with higher prevalence of many risk factors.[220] In addition, African Americans were less likely to undergo mitral valvuloplasty than whites.[220]

SUMMARY AND CONCLUSIONS

Diseases and disorders of heart valves remain an important clinical and public health burden associated with significant morbidity and mortality. Recent evidence suggests that this burden is increasing as a result of the continuing recurrence of acute rheumatic fever and associated rheumatic valvulopathy in many developing countries and an aging population with an increasing prevalence of degenerative valve disease in developed countries. Mild to moderate degrees of valvular heart disease are relatively common in adults, increase in prevalence with aging, and result in reduced overall survival. Hospitalization for symptom management and valve repair or replacement are the major causes of morbidity and costs, whereas heart failure remains the chief cause of death. In the United States and Europe, disparities in the care of patients with valvular heart disease have been documented. However, the determinants of these disparities are complex and include contributing factors at the patient, provider, and health care systems level. Definitive epidemiologic data including the incidence, prevalence, morbidity, access to care, case fatality, overall mortality, and the determinants of survival in valvular heart disease global level remain incomplete. Renewed emphasis on the population science and clinical epidemiology of valvular heart disease is needed to better inform the prevention, treatment, and control of valvular heart disease.[221]

Acknowledgment

I am grateful to Nancy Sonnenfeld and Carol DeFrances of the U.S. National Center for Health Statistics for their support and for providing me access to unpublished data from the National Hospital Discharge Data.

REFERENCES

1. Carapetis JR: Rheumatic heart disease in developing countries. N Engl J Med 2007;357:439-441.
2. Schoen FJ: Cardiac valves and valvular pathology: Update on function, disease, repair, and replacement. Cardiovasc Pathol 2005;14:189-194.
3. Yacoub MH, Takkenberg JJ: Will heart valve tissue engineering change the world? Nat Clin Pract Cardiovasc Med 2005;22:60-61.
4. World Health Organization: Rheumatic fever and rheumatic heart disease. World Health Organ Tech Rep Ser 2004;923:1-122.
5. Chockalingam A, Prabhakar D, Dorairajan S, et al: Rheumatic heart disease occurrence, patterns and clinical correlates in children aged less than five years. J Heart Valve Dis 2004;13:11-14.
6. Carapetis JR, Steer AC, Mulholland EK, Weber M: The global burden of group A streptococcal diseases. Lancet Infect Dis 2005;5:685-694.
7. Mayosi B, Robertson K, Volmink J, et al: The Drakensberg declaration on the control of rheumatic fever and rheumatic heart disease in Africa. S Afr Med J 2006;96(3 Pt 2):246.
8. Marijon E, Ou P, Celermajer DS, et al: Prevalence of rheumatic heart disease detected by echocardiographic screening. N Engl J Med 2007;357:470-476.
9. Robertson KA, Volmink JA, Mayosi BM: Towards a uniform plan for the control of rheumatic fever and rheumatic heart disease in Africa—the Awareness Surveillance Advocacy Prevention (A.S.A.P.) Programme. S Afr Med J 2006;96(3 Pt 2):241.
10. Rajamannan NM, Bonow RO, Rahimtoola SH: Calcific aortic stenosis: An update. Nat Clin Pract Cardiovasc Med 2007;45:254-262.
11. Dare AJ, Veinot JP, Edwards WD, et al: New observations on the etiology of aortic valve disease: A surgical pathologic study of 236 cases from 1990. Hum Pathol 1993;24:1330-1338.
12. National Center for Health Statistics: Vital and Health Statistics. Series 13 ed. Hyattsville, MD, US Department of Health and Human Services, 1999.
13. Passik CS, Ackermann DM, Pluth JR, Edwards WD: Temporal changes in the causes of aortic stenosis: A surgical pathologic study of 646 cases. Mayo Clin Proc 1987;62:119-123.
14. Supino PG, Borer JS, Preibisz J, Bornstein A: The epidemiology of valvular heart disease: A growing public health problem. Heart Fail Clin 2006;24:379-393.
15. National Center for Health Statistics: Health, United States, 2007. With Chartbook on Trends in the Health of Americans. Atlanta, National Center for Health Statistics, 2007.

16. Goldbarg SH, Elmariah S, Miller MA, Fuster V: Insights into degenerative aortic valve disease. J Am Coll Cardiol 2007;50:1205-1213.
17. Osman L, Chester AH, Sarathchandra P, et al: A novel role of the sympatho-adrenergic system in regulating valve calcification. Circulation 2007;116(11 Suppl):I282-I287.
18. Caira FC, Stock SR, Gleason TG, et al: Human degenerative valve disease is associated with up-regulation of low-density lipoprotein receptor-related protein 5 receptor-mediated bone formation. J Am Coll Cardiol 2006;47:1707-1712.
19. Kaden JJ, Dempfle CE, Grobholz R, et al: Inflammatory regulation of extracellular matrix remodeling in calcific aortic valve stenosis. Cardiovasc Pathol 2005;14:80-87.
20. Borer JS, Herrold EM, Carter JN, et al: Cellular and molecular basis of remodeling in valvular heart diseases. Heart Fail Clin 2006;24:415-424.
21. Li YB, Hu CL, Liu J, et al: Calcific aortic valve disease should not be considered as a degenerative disease anymore. Med Hypotheses 2007;68:1233-1235.
22. Leask RL, Jain N, Butany J: Endothelium and valvular diseases of the heart. Microsc Res Tech 2003;60:129-137.
23. Caballero B: The global epidemic of obesity: An overview. Epidemiol Rev 2007; 29:1-5.
24. Mainous AG III, Baker R, Koopman RJ, et al: Impact of the population at risk of diabetes on projections of diabetes burden in the United States: An epidemic on the way. Diabetologia 2007;50:934-940.
25. Caterson ID, Hubbard V, Bray GA, et al: Prevention Conference VII: Obesity, a worldwide epidemic related to heart disease and stroke: Group III: Worldwide comorbidities of obesity. Circulation 2004;110:e476-e483.
26. Mensah GA, Mokdad AH, Ford E, et al: Obesity, metabolic syndrome, and type 2 diabetes: Emerging epidemics and their cardiovascular implications. Cardiol Clin 2004;22:485-504.
27. Mokdad AH, Bowman BA, Ford ES, et al: The continuing epidemics of obesity and diabetes in the United States. JAMA 2001;286:1195-1200.
28. Nkomo VT, Gardin JM, Skelton TN, et al: Burden of valvular heart diseases: A population-based study. Lancet 2006;3689:1005-1011.
29. Iung B, Baron G, Tornos P, et al: Valvular heart disease in the community: A European experience. Curr Probl Cardiol 2007;32:609-661.
30. National Center for Health Statistics: National Hospital Discharge Survey: Annual Summaries with Detailed Diagnosis and Procedure Data; Series 13. Data on Health Resources Utilization. Available at http://www.cdc.gov/nchs/products/pubs/pubd/series/ser.htm#sr13.
31. Lloyd-Jones D, Adams R, Casnethon M, et al: Heart disease and stroke statistics—2009 update: A report from the American Heart Association Statistics Committee and Stroke Statistics Subcommittee. Circulation 2009;119:e21-e181.
32. Roberts WC: Morphologic aspects of cardiac valve dysfunction. Am Heart J 1992;123:1610-1632.
33. Selzer A: Changing aspects of the natural history of valvular aortic stenosis. N Engl J Med 1987;317:91-98.
34. Roberts WC, Ko JM, Matter GJ: Aortic valve replacement for aortic stenosis in nonagenarians. Am J Cardiol 2006;989:1251-1253.
35. Roberts WC, Ko JM, Garner WL, et al: Valve structure and survival in octogenarians having aortic valve replacement for aortic stenosis (± aortic regurgitation) with versus without coronary artery bypass grafting at a single US medical center 1993 to 2005. Am J Cardiol 2007;100:489-95.
36. Roberts WC, Ko JM, Filardo G, et al: Valve structure and survival in septuagenarians having aortic valve replacement for aortic stenosis (±aortic regurgitation) with versus without coronary artery bypass grafting at a single US medical center 1993 to 2005. Am J Cardiol 2007;100:1157-6115.
37. Roberts WC, Ko JM, Filardo G et al: Valve structure and survival in sexagenarians having aortic valve replacement for aortic stenosis (±aortic regurgitation) with versus without coronary artery bypass grafting at a single US medical center 1993 to 2005. Am J Cardiol 2007;100:1286-1292.
38. Roberts WC, Ko JM, Filardo G et al: Valve structure and survival in quinquagenarians having aortic valve replacement for aortic stenosis (±aortic regurgitation) with versus without coronary artery bypass grafting at a single US medical center 1993 to 2005. Am J Cardiol 2007;100:1584-1591.
39. Roberts WC: The congenitally bicuspid aortic valve. A study of 85 autopsy cases. Am J Cardiol 1970;26:72-83.
40. Nistri S, Basso C, Marzari C, et al: Frequency of bicuspid aortic valve in young male conscripts by echocardiogram. Am J Cardiol 2005;96:718-721.
41. Movahed MR, Hepner AD, Ahmadi-Kashani M: Echocardiographic prevalence of bicuspid aortic valve in the population. Heart Lung Circ 2006;15:297-299.
42. Waller BF, Howard J, Fess S: Pathology of aortic valve stenosis and pure aortic regurgitation: A clinical morphologic assessment—part II. Clin Cardiol 1994;17:150-156.
43. Pai RG, Kapoor N, Bansal RC, Varadarajan P: Malignant natural history of asymptomatic severe aortic stenosis: Benefit of aortic valve replacement. Ann Thorac Surg 2006;826:2116-2122.
44. Varadarajan P, Kapoor N, Bansal RC, Pai RG: Clinical profile and natural history of 453 nonsurgically managed patients with severe aortic stenosis. Ann Thorac Surg 2006;82:2111-2115.
45. Rosenhek R, Klaar U, Schemper M, et al: Mild and moderate aortic stenosis: Natural history and risk stratification by echocardiography. Eur Heart J 2004;253:199-205.
46. Briand M, Lemieux I, Dumesnil JG, et al: Metabolic syndrome negatively influences disease progression and prognosis in aortic stenosis. J Am Coll Cardiol 2006;47:2229-2236.
47. Briand M, Pibarot P, Despres JP, et al: Metabolic syndrome is associated with faster degeneration of bioprosthetic valves. Circulation 2006;114(1 Suppl):I512-I517.
48. Freeman RV, Otto CM: Spectrum of calcific aortic valve disease: Pathogenesis, disease progression, and treatment strategies. Circulation 2005;111:3316-3326.
49. Olsen MH, Wachtell K, Bella JN, et al: Aortic valve sclerosis relates to cardiovascular events in patients with hypertension (a LIFE substudy). Am J Cardiol 2005;95: 132-136.
50. Turkmen F, Emre A, Ozdemir A, et al: Relationship between aortic valve sclerosis and left ventricular hypertrophy in chronic haemodialysis patients. Int Urol Nephrol 2008:40:497-502.
51. Taylor HA Jr, Clark BL, Garrison RJ, et al: Relation of aortic valve sclerosis to risk of coronary heart disease in African-Americans. Am J Cardiol 2005;95:401-404.
52. Stewart BF, Siscovick D, Lind BK, et al: Clinical factors associated with calcific aortic valve disease. Cardiovascular Health Study. J Am Coll Cardiol 1997;29:630-634.
53. Lindroos M, Kupari M, Heikkila J, Tilvis R: Prevalence of aortic valve abnormalities in the elderly: An echocardiographic study of a random population sample. J Am Coll Cardiol 1993;21:1220-1225.
54. Agmon Y, Khandheria BK, Meissner I, et al: Aortic valve sclerosis and aortic atherosclerosis: Different manifestations of the same disease? Insights from a population-based study. J Am Coll Cardiol 2001;38:827-834.
55. Garg V: Molecular genetics of aortic valve disease. Curr Opin Cardiol 2006213:180-184.
56. Probst V, Le SS, Legendre A, et al: Familial aggregation of calcific aortic valve stenosis in the western part of France. Circulation 2006;113:856-860.
57. Le GG, Bertault V, Bezon E, et al: Heterogeneous geographic distribution of patients with aortic valve stenosis: Arguments for new aetiological hypothesis. Heart 2005;91:247-249.
58. O'Brien KD: Epidemiology and genetics of calcific aortic valve disease. J Investig Med 2007;55:284-291.
59. Ortlepp JR, Pillich M, Mevissen V, et al: APOE alleles are not associated with calcific aortic stenosis. Heart 2006;92:1463-1466.
60. Bosse Y, Mathieu P, Pibarot P: Genomics: The next step to elucidate the etiology of calcific aortic valve stenosis. J Am Coll Cardiol 2008;51:1327-1336.
61. Otto CM, Lind BK, Kitzman DW, et al: Association of aortic-valve sclerosis with cardiovascular mortality and morbidity in the elderly. N Engl J Med 1999;341:142-147.
62. Otto CM: Why is aortic sclerosis associated with adverse clinical outcomes? J Am Coll Cardiol 2004;43:176-178.
63. Agmon Y, Khandheria BK, Jamil TA, et al: Inflammation, infection, and aortic valve sclerosis; insights from the Olmsted County (Minnesota) population. Atherosclerosis 2004;174:337-342.
64. Adler Y, Shemesh J, Tenenbaum A, et al: Aortic valve calcium on spiral computed tomography (dual slice mode) is associated with advanced coronary calcium in hypertensive patients. Coron Artery Dis 2002;13:209-213.
65. Singh JP, Evans JC, Levy D, et al: Prevalence and clinical determinants of mitral, tricuspid, and aortic regurgitation (the Framingham Heart Study). Am J Cardiol 1999;83:897-902.
66. Olson LJ, Subramanian R, Edwards WD: Surgical pathology of pure aortic insufficiency: A study of 225 cases. Mayo Clin Proc 1984;59:835-841.
67. Subramanian R, Olson LJ, Edwards WD: Surgical pathology of pure aortic stenosis: A study of 374 cases. Mayo Clin Proc 1984;59:683-690.
68. Becker AE, Becker MJ, Edwards JE: Anomalies associated with coarctation of aorta: Particular reference to infancy. Circulation 1970;41:1067-1075.
69. Edwards JE: The congenital bicuspid aortic valve. Circulation 1961;23:485-488.
70. Hahn RT, Roman MJ, Mogtader AH, Devereux RB: Association of aortic dilation with regurgitant, stenotic and functionally normal bicuspid aortic valves. J Am Coll Cardiol 1992;19:283-288.
71. Larson EW, Edwards WD: Risk factors for aortic dissection: A necropsy study of 161 cases. Am J Cardiol 1984;53:849-855.
72. Edwards WD, Leaf DS, Edwards JE: Dissecting aortic aneurysm associated with congenital bicuspid aortic valve. Circulation 1978;57:1022-1025.
73. Edwards WD: Surgical pathology of the aortic valve. In Pathology of the Heart and Great Vessels. New York, Churchill Livingstone, 1988, pp. 43-100.
74. Fremes SE, Goldman BS, Ivanov J, et al: Valvular surgery in the elderly. Circulation 1989;80(Suppl I):I77-I90.
75. Aronow WS, Kronzon I: Correlation of prevalence and severity of aortic regurgitation detected by pulsed Doppler echocardiography with the murmur of aortic regurgitation in elderly patients in a long-term health care facility. Am J Cardiol 1989;63:128-129.
76. Akasaka T, Yoshikawa J, Yoshida K, et al: Age-related valvular regurgitation: A study by pulsed Doppler echocardiography. Circulation 1987;76:262-265.
77. Klein AL, Burstow DJ, Tajik AJ, et al: Age-related prevalence of valvular regurgitation in normal subjects: A comprehensive color flow examination of 118 volunteers. J Am Soc Echocardiogr 1990;3:54-63.
78. Lebowitz NE, Bella JN, Roman MJ, et al: Prevalence and correlates of aortic regurgitation in American Indians: The Strong Heart Study. J Am Coll Cardiol 2000;362:461-467.
79. Seder JD, Burke JF, Pauletto FJ: Prevalence of aortic regurgitation by color flow Doppler in relation to aortic root size. J Am Soc Echocardiogr 1990;3:316-319.
80. Kim M, Roman MJ, Cavallini MC, et al: Effect of hypertension on aortic root size and prevalence of aortic regurgitation. Hypertension 1996;28:47-52.
81. Waller BF, Zoltick JM, Rosen JH, et al: Severe aortic regurgitation from systemic hypertension (without aortic dissection) requiring aortic valve replacement: Analysis of four patients. Am J Cardiol 1982;49:473-477.
82. Bella JN, MacCluer JW, Roman MJ, et al: Genetic influences on aortic root size in American Indians: The Strong Heart Study. Arterioscler Thromb Vasc Biol 2002;22:1008-1011.
83. Cuspidi C, Meani S, Fusi V, et al: Prevalence and correlates of aortic root dilatation in patients with essential hypertension: Relationship with cardiac and extracardiac target organ damage. J Hypertens 2006;24:573-580.
84. Carlson RG, Lillehei CW, Edwards JE: Cystic medial necrosis of the ascending aorta in relation to age and hypertension. Am J Cardiol 1970;25:411-415.
85. Robinowitz M, Virmani R, McAllister JHA: Rheumatoid heart disease: A clinical and morphologic analysis of 34 autopsy patients. Lab Invest 1980;42:145.
86. Roberts WC, Hollingsworth JF, Bulkley BH, et al: Combined mitral and aortic regurgitation in ankylosing spondylitis: Angiographic and anatomic features. Am J Med 1974;56:237-243.

87. Bulkley BH, Roberts WC: Ankylosing spondylitis and aortic regurgitation: Description of the characteristic cardiovascular lesion from study of eight necropsy patients. Circulation 1973;48:1014-1027.
88. Roberts WC, Dangel JC, Bulkley BH: Nonrheumatic valvular cardiac disease: A clinicopathologic survey of 27 different conditions causing valvular dysfunction. Cardiovasc Clin 1973;5:333-446.
89. Paulus HE, Pearson CM, Pitts W Jr: Aortic insufficiency in five patients with Reiter's syndrome: A detailed clinical and pathologic study. Am J Med 1972;53:464-472.
90. Pearson CM, Kroening R, Verity MA, Getzen JH: Aortic insufficiency and aortic aneurysm in relapsing polychondritis. Trans Assoc Am Physicians 1967;80:P71-90.
91. Bonow RO, Carabello BA, Chatterjee K, et al: ACC/AHA 2006 guidelines for the management of patients with valvular heart disease: A report of the American College of Cardiology/American Heart Association Task Force on Practice Guidelines (Writing Committee to revise the 1998 guidelines for the management of patients with valvular heart disease) developed in collaboration with the Society of Cardiovascular Anesthesiologists endorsed by the Society for Cardiovascular Angiography and Interventions and the Society of Thoracic Surgeons. J Am Coll Cardiol 2006;48:e1-e148.
92. Horstkotte D, Niehues R, Strauer BE: Pathomorphological aspects, aetiology and natural history of acquired mitral valve stenosis. Eur Heart J 1991;12(Suppl):BP55-60.
93. Multicenter experience with balloon mitral commissurotomy. NHLBI Balloon Valvuloplasty Registry Report on immediate and 30–day follow-up results. The National Heart, Lung, and Blood Institute Balloon Valvuloplasty Registry Participants. Circulation 1992;85:448-461.
94. Hanson TP, Edwards BS, Edwards JE: Pathology of surgically excised mitral valves: One hundred consecutive cases. Arch Pathol Lab Med 1985;109:823-828.
95. Olson LJ, Subramanian R, Ackermann DM, et al: Surgical pathology of the mitral valve: A study of 712 cases spanning 21 years. Mayo Clin Proc 1987;62:22-34.
96. Olson LJ, Subramanian R, Ackermann DM, et al: Surgical pathology of the mitral valve: A study of 712 cases spanning 21 years. Mayo Clin Proc 1987;62:22-34.
97. Waller BF: Morphological aspects of valvular heart disease: Part I. Curr Probl Cardiol 1984;9:1-66.
98. Hammer WJ, Roberts WC, deLeon AC: "Mitral stenosis" secondary to combined "massive" mitral anular calcific deposits and small, hypertrophied left ventricles: Hemodynamic documentation in four patients. Am J Med 1978;64:371-376.
99. Pellikka PA, Tajik AJ, Khandheria BK, et al: Carcinoid heart disease: Clinical and echocardiographic spectrum in 74 patients. Circulation 1993;87:1188-1196.
100. Leder AA, Bosworth WC: Angiokeratoma corporis diffusum universale (Fabry's disease) with mitral stenosis. Am J Med 1965;38:814-819.
101. John RM, Hunter D, Swanton RH: Echocardiographic abnormalities in type IV mucopolysaccharidosis. Arch Dis Child 1990;65:746-749.
102. Roberts WC: Morphologic features of the normal and abnormal mitral valve. Am J Cardiol 1983;51:1005-1028.
103. McAllister HA Jr, Fenoglio JJ Jr: Cardiac involvement in Whipple's disease. Circulation 1975;52:152-156.
104. Rose AG: Mitral stenosis in Whipple's disease. Thorax 1978;33:500-503.
105. Scalapino JN, Edwards WD, Steckelberg JM, et al: Mitral stenosis associated with valvular tophi. Mayo Clin Proc 1984;59:509-512.
106. Waller BF, McManus BM, Roberts WC: Mitral valve stenosis produced by or worsened by active bacterial endocarditis. Chest 1982;82:498-500.
107. Matula G, Karpman LS, Frank S, Stinson E: Mitral obstruction from staphylococcal endocarditis, corrected surgically. JAMA 1975;233:58-59.
108. Ruckman RN, Van Praagh R: Anatomic types of congenital mitral stenosis: Report of 49 autopsy cases with consideration of diagnosis and surgical implications. Am J Cardiol 1978;42:592-601.
109. McElhinney DB, Sherwood MC, Keane JF, et al: Current management of severe congenital mitral stenosis: Outcomes of transcatheter and surgical therapy in 108 infants and children. Circulation 2005;112:707-714.
110. Moore P, Adatia I, Spevak PJ, et al: Severe congenital mitral stenosis in infants. Circulation 1994;89:2099-2106.
111. Jones RA, Hall RJ, Fraser AG: Severe mitral regurgitation caused by immobile posterior leaflet after radiotherapy. J Am Soc Echocardiogr 1995;8:207-210.
112. Turri M, Thiene G, Bortolotti U, et al: Surgical pathology of disease of the mitral valve, with special reference to lesions promoting valvar incompetence. Int J Cardiol 1989;22:213-219.
113. Boudoulas H, Sparks EE, Wooley CF: Mitral valvular regurgitation: Etiology, pathophysiologic mechanisms, clinical manifestations. Herz 2006;31:6-13.
114. Barasch E, Gottdiener JS, Larsen EK, et al: Clinical significance of calcification of the fibrous skeleton of the heart and aortosclerosis in community dwelling elderly. The Cardiovascular Health Study (CHS). Am Heart J 2006;151:39-47.
115. Fox E, Harkins D, Taylor H, et al: Epidemiology of mitral annular calcification and its predictive value for coronary events in African Americans: The Jackson Cohort of the Atherosclerotic Risk in Communities Study. Am Heart J 2004;148:979-984.
116. Boon A, Cheriex E, Lodder J, Kessels F: Cardiac valve calcification: Characteristics of patients with calcification of the mitral annulus or aortic valve. Heart 1997;78:472-474.
117. Kizer JR, Wiebers DO, Whisnant JP, et al: Mitral annular calcification, aortic valve sclerosis, and incident stroke in adults free of clinical cardiovascular disease: The Strong Heart Study. Stroke 2005;36:2533-2537.
118. Sharma R, Pellerin D, Gaze DC, et al: Mitral annular calcification predicts mortality and coronary artery disease in end stage renal disease. Atherosclerosis 2007;191: 348-354.
119. Davutoglu V, Yilmaz M, Soydinc S, et al: Mitral annular calcification is associated with osteoporosis in women. Am Heart J 2004;147:1113-1116.
120. Fox CS, Parise H, Vasan RS, et al: Mitral annular calcification is a predictor for incident atrial fibrillation. Atherosclerosis 2004;173:291-294.
121. Deluca G, Correale M, Ieva R, et al: The incidence and clinical course of caseous calcification of the mitral annulus: A prospective echocardiographic study. J Am Soc Echocardiogr 2008;21:828-833.
122. Fernandes RM, Branco LM, Galrinho A et al: Caseous calcification of the mitral annulus: A review of six cases. Rev Port Cardiol 2007;26:1059-1070.
123. Marcu CB, Ghantous AE, Prokop EK: Caseous calcification of the mitral valve ring. Heart Lung Circ 2006;153:187-188.
124. Bhattacharyya S, Toumpanakis C, Caplin ME, Davar J: Analysis of 150 patients with carcinoid syndrome seen in a single year at one institution in the first decade of the twenty-first century. Am J Cardiol 2008;101:378-381.
125. Bernheim AM, Connolly HM, Hobday TJ, et al: Carcinoid heart disease. Prog Cardiovasc Dis 2007;49:439-451.
126. Attenhofer Jost CH, Connolly HM, et al: Ebstein's anomaly. Circulation 2007;115:277-285.
127. Shah PM, Raney AA: Tricuspid valve disease. Curr Probl Cardiol 2008;33:47-84.
128. Nath J, Foster E, Heidenreich PA: Impact of tricuspid regurgitation on long-term survival. J Am Coll Cardiol 2004;43:405-409.
129. Bouzas B, Kilner PJ, Gatzoulis MA: Pulmonary regurgitation: Not a benign lesion. Eur Heart J 2005;26:433-439.
130. Bartram U, Bartelings MM, Kramer HH, et al: Congenital polyvalvular disease: A review. Pediatr Cardiol 2001;22:93-101.
131. Kowal-Vern A, Bharati S, Melnyk A, Husain AN: Congenital polyvalvular cardiac disease without chromosomal abnormalities. Pediatr Pathol Lab Med 1995;15:299-308.
132. Matsuoka R, Misugi K, Goto A, et al: Congenital heart anomalies in the trisomy 18 syndrome, with reference to congenital polyvalvular disease. Am J Med Genet 1983;14:657-668.
133. Bharati S, Lev M: Congenital polyvalvular disease. Circulation 1973;47:575-586.
134. Krake PR, Zaman F, Tandon N: Native quadruple-valve endocarditis caused by Enterococcus faecalis. Tex Heart Inst J 2004;31:90-92.
135. Straumann E, Meyer B, Misteli M, et al: Aortic and mitral valve disease in patients with end stage renal failure on long-term haemodialysis. Br Heart J 1992;67:236-239.
136. Castillo JG, Filsoufi F, Rahmanian PB, Adams DH: Quadruple valve surgery in carcinoid heart disease. J Card Surg 2008;23:523-525.
137. Yamashiro K, Komine-Kobayashi M, Hatano T, et al: The frequency of cardiac valvular regurgitation in Parkinson's disease. Mov Disord 2008;23:935-941.
138. Antonini A, Poewe W: Fibrotic heart-valve reactions to dopamine-agonist treatment in Parkinson's disease. Lancet Neurol 2007;6:826-829.
139. Zanettini R, Antonini A, Gatto G, et al: Valvular heart disease and the use of dopamine agonists for Parkinson's disease. N Engl J Med 2007;356:39-40.
140. Kast RE, Altschuler EL: Dopamine agonists and valvular heart disease. N Engl J Med 2007;356:1677-1680.
141. Schade R, Andersohn F, Suissa S, et al: Dopamine agonists and the risk of cardiac-valve regurgitation. N Engl J Med 2007;356:29-38.
142. Kim JY, Chung EJ, Park SW, Lee WY: Valvular heart disease in Parkinson's disease treated with ergot derivative dopamine agonists. Mov Disord 2006;21:1261-1264.
143. Waller EA, Kaplan J: Pergolide-associated valvular heart disease. Compr Ther 2006;32:94-101.
144. Horvath J, Fross RD, Kleiner-Fisman G, et al: Severe multivalvular heart disease: A new complication of the ergot derivative dopamine agonists. Mov Disord 2004;19: 656-662.
145. Palmieri V, Arnett DK, Roman MJ, et al: Appetite suppressants and valvular heart disease in a population-based sample: The HyperGEN study. Am J Med 2002;112:710-715.
146. Weissman NJ: Appetite suppressants and valvular heart disease. Am J Med Sci 2001;321:285-291.
147. Jick H, Vasilakis C, Weinrauch LA, et al: A population-based study of appetite-suppressant drugs and the risk of cardiac-valve regurgitation. N Engl J Med 1998;339:719-724.
148. Sani MU, Karaye KM, Borodo MM: Prevalence and pattern of rheumatic heart disease in the Nigerian Savannah: An echocardiographic study. Cardiovasc J Afr 2007;18:295-299.
149. Tamura A, Takahara Y, Mogi K, Katsumata M: Radiation-induced valvular disease is the logical consequence of irradiation. Gen Thorac Cardiovasc Surg 2007;55:53-56.
150. Carlson RG, Mayfield WR, Normann S, Alexander JA: Radiation-associated valvular disease. Chest 1991;99:538-545.
151. Boudoulas H: Etiology of valvular heart disease. Expert Rev Cardiovasc Ther 2003;1:523-532.
152. Erek E, Casselman FR, Vanermen H: Cardiac ochronosis: Valvular heart disease with dark green discoloration of the leaflets. Tex Heart Inst J 2004;31:445-447.
153. Gaines JJ Jr, Pai GM: Cardiovascular ochronosis. Arch Pathol Lab Med 1987;111:991-994.
154. Rasmussen VG, Poulsen SH, Dupont E, et al: Heart valve disease associated with treatment with ergot-derived dopamine agonists: A clinical and echocardiographic study of patients with Parkinson's disease. J Intern Med 2008;263:90-98.
155. Cardiac valvulopathy associated with exposure to fenfluramine or dexfenfluramine: U.S. Department of Health and Human Services interim public health recommendations, November 1997. MMWR Morb Mortal Wkly Rep 1997;46:1061-1066.
156. Connolly HM, Crary JL, McGoon MD, et al: Valvular heart disease associated with fenfluramine-phentermine. N Engl J Med 1997;337:581-588.
157. Khan MA, Herzog CA, St Peter JV, et al: The prevalence of cardiac valvular insufficiency assessed by transthoracic echocardiography in obese patients treated with appetite- suppressant drugs [see comments]. N Engl J Med 1998;339:713-718.
158. Dahl CF, Allen MR: Regression and progression of valvulopathy associated with fenfluramine and phentermine. Ann Intern Med 2002;136:489.
159. Greffe G, Chalabreysse L, Mouly-Bertin C, et al: Valvular heart disease associated with fenfluramine detected 7 years after discontinuation of treatment. Ann Thorac Surg 2007;83:1541-1543.
160. Hopkins PN, Polukoff GI: Risk of valvular heart disease associated with use of fenfluramine. BMC Cardiovasc Disord 2003;3:5.
161. Loke YK, Derry S, Pritchard-Copley A: Appetite suppressants and valvular heart disease—a systematic review. BMC Clin Pharmacol 2002;2:6.

18

162. Tleyjeh IM, Abdel-Latif A, Rahbi H, et al: A systematic review of population-based studies of infective endocarditis. Chest 2007;132:1025-1035.

163. Tleyjeh IM, Steckelberg JM, Murad HS, et al: Temporal trends in infective endocarditis: A population-based study in Olmsted County, Minnesota. JAMA 2005;293:3022-3028.

164. Hill EE, Herijgers P, Claus P, et al: Infective endocarditis: Changing epidemiology and predictors of 6-month mortality: A prospective cohort study. Eur Heart J 2007;28:196-203.

165. Werner GS, Schulz R, Fuchs JB et al: Infective endocarditis in the elderly in the era of transesophageal echocardiography: Clinical features and prognosis compared with younger patients. Am J Med 1996;100:90-97.

166. Elkayam U, Bitar F: Valvular heart disease and pregnancy: Part I: Native valves. J Am Coll Cardiol 2005;46:223-230.

167. McFaul PB, Dornan JC, Lamki H, Boyle D: Pregnancy complicated by maternal heart disease: A review of 519 women. Br J Obstet Gynaecol 1988;95:861-867.

168. Elkayam U, Bitar F: Valvular heart disease and pregnancy: Part II: Prosthetic valves. J Am Coll Cardiol 2005;46:403-410.

169. Elkayam U, Singh H, Irani A, Akhter MW: Anticoagulation in pregnant women with prosthetic heart valves. J Cardiovasc Pharmacol Ther 2004;9:107-115.

170. Stout KK, Otto CM: Pregnancy in women with valvular heart disease. Heart 2007;93:552-558.

171. Chia YT, Yeoh SC, Lim MC, et al: Pregnancy outcome and mitral valve prolapse. Asia Oceania J Obstet Gynaecol 1994;20:383-388.

172. Jana N, Vasishta K, Khunnu B, et al: Pregnancy in association with mitral valve prolapse. Asia Oceania J Obstet Gynaecol 1993;19:61-65.

173. Freed LA, Levy D, Levine RA, et al: Prevalence and clinical outcome of mitral-valve prolapse. N Engl J Med 1999;341:1-7.

174. Davies GA, Herbert WN: Acquired heart disease in pregnancy. J Obstet Gynaecol Can 2007;29:507-509.

175. Soler-Soler J, Galve E: Worldwide perspective of valve disease. Heart 2000;83:721-725.

176. Vahanian A, Baumgartner H, Bax J, et al: Guidelines on the management of valvular heart disease: The Task Force on the Management of Valvular Heart Disease of the European Society of Cardiology. Eur Heart J 2007;28:230-268.

177. Hameed A, Karaalp IS, Tummala PP, et al: The effect of valvular heart disease on maternal and fetal outcome of pregnancy. J Am Coll Cardiol 2001;37:893-899.

178. Silversides CK, Colman JM, Sermer M, Siu SC: Cardiac risk in pregnant women with rheumatic mitral stenosis. Am J Cardiol 2003;91:1382-1385.

179. Bhatla N, Lal S, Behera G, et al: Cardiac disease in pregnancy. Int J Gynaecol Obstet 2003;82:153-159.

180. Campos O, Andrade JL, Bocanegra J, et al: Physiologic multivalvular regurgitation during pregnancy: A longitudinal Doppler echocardiographic study. Int J Cardiol 1993;403:265-272.

181. De Santo LS, Romano G, Della CA, et al: Mitral mechanical replacement in young rheumatic women: Analysis of long-term survival, valve-related complications, and pregnancy outcomes over a 3707-patient-year follow-up. J Thorac Cardiovasc Surg 2005;130:13-19.

182. Agency for Healthcare Research and Quality. Healthcare Cost and utilization project HCUPnet. Available at http://www.hcup.ahrq.gov/HCUPnet.jsp Accessed February 2, 2009.

183. Allareddy V, Ward MM, Ely JW, et al: Impact of complications on outcomes following aortic and mitral valve replacements in the United States. J Cardiovasc Surg (Torino) 2007;48:349-357.

184. Society of Thoracic Surgeons: STS National Database: Spring 2002 Executive Summary. Available at http://www.ctsnet.org/file/2002ExecutiveReport_Rev.pdf.

185. Vesey JM, Otto CM: Complications of prosthetic heart valves. Curr Cardiol Rep 2004;6:106-111.

186. Puvimanasinghe JP, Steyerberg EW, Takkenberg JJ, et al: Prognosis after aortic valve replacement with a bioprosthesis: Predictions based on meta-analysis and microsimulation. Circulation 2001;103:1535-1541.

187. Remadi JP, Baron O, Roussel C, et al: Isolated mitral valve replacement with St. Jude medical prosthesis: Long-term results: A follow-up of 19 years. Circulation 2001;103:1542-1545.

188. Lund O, Bland M: Risk-corrected impact of mechanical versus bioprosthetic valves on long-term mortality after aortic valve replacement. J Thorac Cardiovasc Surg 2006;132:20-26.

189. Kulik A, Bédard P, Lam BK, et al: Mechanical versus bioprosthetic valve replacement in middle-aged patients. Eur J Cardiothorac Surg 2006;30:485-491.

190. Hammermeister K, Sethi GK, Henderson WG, et al: Outcomes 15 years after valve replacement with a mechanical versus a bioprosthetic valve: Final report of the Veterans Affairs randomized trial. J Am Coll Cardiol 2000;36:1152-1158.

191. Bonow RO, Grant AO, Jacobs AK: The cardiovascular state of the union: Confronting healthcare disparities. Circulation 2005;111:1205-1207.

192. Mensah GA, Brown DW: An overview of cardiovascular disease burden in the United States. Health Aff (Millwood) 2007;26:38-48.

193. Mensah GA, Mokdad AH, Ford ES, et al: State of disparities in cardiovascular health in the United States. Circulation 2005;111:1233-1241.

194. Gordon HS, Paterniti DA, Wray NP: Race and patient refusal of invasive cardiac procedures. J Gen Intern Med 2004;19:962-966.

195. Martin R, Lemos C, Rothrock N, et al: Gender disparities in common sense models of illness among myocardial infarction victims. Health Psychol 2004;23:345-353.

196. Rothenberg BM, Pearson T, Zwanziger J, Mukamel D: Explaining disparities in access to high-quality cardiac surgeons. Ann Thorac Surg 2004;78:18-24.

197. Walker DR, Stern PM, Landis DL: Examining healthcare disparities in a disease management population. Am J Manag Care 2004;10(2 Pt 1):81-88.

198. Grace SL, Abbey SE, Bisaillon S, et al: Presentation, delay, and contraindication to thrombolytic treatment in females and males with myocardial infarction. Womens Health Issues 2003;13:214-221.

199. O'Connell L, Brown SL: Do nonprofit HMOs eliminate racial disparities in cardiac care? J Health Care Finance 2003;30:84-94.

200. Litaker D, Koroukian SM: Racial differences in lipid-lowering agent use in medicaid patients with cardiovascular disease. Med Care 2004;42:1009-1018.

201. Institute of Medicine: Unequal Treatment: Confronting Racial and Ethnic Disparities in Health Care. Washington, DC, National Academies Press, 2003.

202. Lillie-Blanton M, Maddox TM, Rushing O, Mensah GA: Disparities in cardiac care: Rising to the challenge of Healthy People 2010. J Am Coll Cardiol 2004;44:503-508.

203. U.S. Department of Health and Human Services: 2005 National Healthcare Disparities Report. Available at http://www.ahrq.gov/qual/nhdr05/nhdr05.pdf.

204. U.S. Department of Health and Human Services: 2006 National Healthcare Disparities Report. Available at http://www.ahrq.gov/qual/nhdr06/nhdr06report.pdf.

205. U.S. Department of Health and Human Services: 2006 National Healthcare Quality Report. Available at http://www.ahrq.gov/qual/nhqr06/nhqr06report.pdf.

206. Agency for Healthcare Research and Quality: 2007 National Healthcare Disparities Report (AHRQ Publication No. 08-0041). Rockville, MD. U.S. Department of Health and Human Services, Agency for Healthcare Research and Quality, 2008.

207. Klodas E, Enriquez-Sarano M, Tajik AJ, et al: Surgery for aortic regurgitation in women. Contrasting indications and outcomes compared with men. Circulation 1996;94:2472-2478.

208. Mohty D, Orszulak TA, Schaff HV, et al: Very long-term survival and durability of mitral valve repair for mitral valve prolapse. Circulation 2001;104(Suppl 1):I1-I7.

209. Iung B, Baron G, Butchart EG, et al: A prospective survey of patients with valvular heart disease in Europe: The Euro Heart Survey on Valvular Heart Disease. Eur Heart J 2003;24:1231-1243.

210. Douglas PS: Rheumatic heart disease and other valvular disorders in women. Cardiovasc Clin 1989;19:259-265.

211. Carabello BA: Progress in mitral and aortic regurgitation. Prog Cardiovasc Dis 2001;43:457-475.

212. Angella FR, Lewis JF: Mitral valve prolapse: Gender differences in evaluation and management. Cardiol Rev 1999;73:161-168.

213. Devereux RB, Jones EC, Roman MJ, et al: Prevalence and correlates of mitral valve prolapse in a population-based sample of American Indians: The Strong Heart Study. Am J Med 2001;1119:679-685.

214. Devereux RB, Kramer Fox R, Kligfield P: Mitral valve prolapse: Causes, clinical manifestations, and management. Ann Intern Med 1989;111:305-317.

215. Taylor NE, O'Brien S, Edwards FH, et al: Relationship between race and mortality and morbidity after valve replacement surgery. Circulation 2005;111:1305-1312.

216. Groeneveld PW, Laufer SB, Garber AM: Technology diffusion, hospital variation, and racial disparities among elderly Medicare beneficiaries: 1989-2000. Med Care 2005;43:320-329.

217. Groeneveld PW, Kruse GB, Chen Z, Asch DA: Variation in cardiac procedure use and racial disparity among Veterans Affairs Hospitals. Am Heart J 2007;15:320-327.

218. Schelbert EB, Rosenthal GE, Welke KF, Vaughan-Sarrazin MS: Treatment variation in older black and white patients undergoing aortic valve replacement. Circulation 2005;112:2347-2353.

219. Lucas FL, Stukel TA, Morris AM, et al: Race and surgical mortality in the United States. Ann Surg 2006;243:281-286.

220. DiGiorgi PL, Baumann FG, O'Leary AM, et al: Mitral valve disease presentation and surgical outcome in African-American patients compared with white patients. Ann Thorac Surg 2008;85:89-93.

221. Takkenberg JJ, Rajamannan NM, Rosenhek R, et al: The need for a global perspective on heart valve disease epidemiology: The SHVD Working Group on Epidemiology of Heart Valve Disease founding statement. J Heart Valve Dis 2008;17:135-139.

CHAPTER 2

Clinical Pathology of Valvular Heart Disease

William C. Roberts and Jong Mi Ko

KEY POINTS

- The frequency of various valvular disorders has changed considerably in the Western world in the last 30 years.
- Aortic stenosis (with or without aortic regurgitation) is now the most common valvular disorder requiring operative treatment, and if systemic hypertension were not considered, it would be the second most common potentially fatal cardiac disease.
- Among patients with aortic stenosis (with or without aortic regurgitation) that is not associated with mitral stenosis or severe mitral regurgitation, the congenitally malformed aortic valve (unicuspid or bicuspid) is more common than is the tricuspid aortic valve.
- The average age of death in patients with aortic stenosis (with or without aortic regurgitation) that is not associated with mitral stenosis or severe mitral regurgitation is 61 years in men and 71 years in women, the same mean ages as in patients with coronary heart disease not receiving coronary artery bypass grafting.
- The weight of operatively excised stenotic aortic valves correlates well with the peak systolic pressure gradient across the valve but not well with valve area.
- Among patients with isolated aortic stenosis (with or without aortic regurgitation), unicuspid and bicuspid valves contain more calcific deposits than do stenotic tricuspid valves and, as a consequence, they weigh more.
- Pure aortic regurgitation (no element of stenosis) is much less common than is aortic stenosis and the etiologies are far more varied. There are two basic causes: 1) disease of the ascending aorta and 2) disease of the aortic valve.
- Mitral stenosis remains very common in the non-Western world and is essentially always the consequence of rheumatic heart disease. As societies gain in wealth, the prevalence of rheumatic fever and rheumatic heart disease wanes.
- Pure mitral regurgitation (no element of stenosis) is the second most common major valvular disorder in the Western world. Although its causes are varied, in contrast with mitral stenosis, mitral valve prolapse is the most common mitral disorder leading to valvular operations in the Western world today.
- Although mitral valve prolapse is more common in women than in men, the latter more commonly develop sufficient regurgitation to require operative repair or replacement.

SOURCES FOR MORPHOLOGIC STUDIES

Before 1960, the only source to study the heart itself was the autopsy. The early years of cardiac valve replacement provided a rich source of necropsy "material" until valve techniques and artificial heart valves became more refined. During the 1960s and 1970s many thousands of patients with rheumatic heart disease underwent replacement of one or more cardiac valves. By the 1980s most of this rheumatic heart disease pool of patients had undergone operations, and in addition, the frequency of rheumatic fever and subsequently rheumatic heart disease had dropped dramatically. Also, in the 1950s and 1960s most physicians attributed valvular heart disease in adults at that time to rheumatic heart disease. By the 1970s, the congenitally malformed aortic valve that was found frequently in adults with aortic stenosis (AS), and mitral valve prolapse (MVP) was being recognized as a common cause of pure (no associated stenosis) mitral regurgitation (MR). Also, by the 1990s, the frequency of autopsies in hospitals in the United States had dropped enormously compared with that in the 1950s, and operatively excised cardiac valves were becoming the major source of anatomic study. Although established by the 1980s, cardiac transplantation was rarely performed because of valvular heart disease.

FREQUENCY OF VARIOUS VALVULAR DISORDERS IN NECROPSY STUDIES

Roberts[1] personally studied 1010 hearts at necropsy in patients with fatal valvular heart disease (Table 2-1). All had died between 1955 and 1980, and the specimens were retrieved from a number of different hospitals, most of which were located in the Washington, DC, area. As shown in Table 2-1, these cases were given both a functional (valve stenosis with or without regurgitation or pure regurgitation [no element of stenosis]) and an anatomic classification. A number of these patients had only one dysfunctional valve but, in addition, had one or more anatomically abnormal valves (normal function). (A valve may be anatomically abnormal yet function normally.) AS was the most common functional disorder (29%); in 35 (12%) of these 292 patients, the mitral leaflets were diffusely thickened (rheumatic heart disease), but there was no clinical evidence of mitral dysfunction. Most of the 256 patients with AS and anatomically normal mitral valves had congenitally unicuspid or bicuspid aortic valves. Mitral stenosis (MS) was the next most common functional valve disease, but 72 (38%) of these 189 patients also had anatomic involvement of one or more other cardiac valves. All patients with MS, whether isolated or associated with a functional disorder of another cardiac valve, had the valvular disease attributed to rheumatic heart disease. Combined MS and AS was the third most common functional valvular disease (15%), and 32 (21%) of these 152 patients also had anatomic disease of the tricuspid valve leaflets. The purely regurgitant lesions (aortic regurgitation [AR], MR, or both) were less common. Tricuspid stenosis of rheumatic etiology occurred in only 3% of the 1010 patients, and all had associated MS with or without associated AS. No other large series of patients with valvular heart disease studied at necropsy has been reported in the last 25 years, and it is unlikely that such a large series, all studied by the same physician (namely, WCR) will be accumulated in the future because of the low autopsy rates in most hospitals today and also because few specimens are retained indefinitely after autopsy.

CHANGING FREQUENCY OF VARIOUS VALVULAR DISORDERS IN RECENT DECADES

Today the most frequently studied operatively excised valve is the stenotic aortic valve followed by excision of a portion of the posterior mitral leaflet in patients with MR due to MVP (Table 2-2). Operatively excised purely regurgitant aortic valves with or without excision of portions of the ascending aorta are also common. Purely regurgitant mitral valves that are replaced usually yield only anterior mitral leaflets as specimens; the posterior leaflet usually is not excised. Operative excision of a tricuspid valve is rare today.

SPECIFIC VALVULAR DISORDERS

Aortic Stenosis (with or without Regurgitation)

Frequency and Causes

If systemic hypertension is not considered, AS is the second most common potentially fatal or fatal heart disease after coronary heart disease. There are three major causes of AS: atherosclerosis (formerly called degenerative); congenitally malformed valves, and rheumatic heart disease.

That atherosclerosis is a cause of AS is derived primarily from five pieces of evidence: 1) patients with familial homozygous hyperlipidemia usually develop calcific deposits on the aortic aspects of their aortic valve cusps at a very young age, usually by the teenage years (these individuals have serum total cholesterol levels >800 mg/dl from the time of birth)[2]; 2) progression of AS can be slowed by lowering total and low-density lipoprotein cholesterol levels with statins[3]; 3) patients older than 65 years of age with AS involving a three-cusp aortic valve (unassociated with mitral valve disease) usually have extensive atherosclerosis involving the major epicardial coronary arteries and usually other systemic arterial systems[4]; 4) serum total cholesterol levels

TABLE 2–1	Functional and Anatomic Classification of Valvular Heart Disease in 1010 Necropsy Patients Age ≥ 15 Years*					
		Anatomic Class (%)				
Functional Class	No. of Patients (%)	AV	MV	MV-AV	TV-MV	TV-MV-AV
1. AS	292 (29)	256 (88)	0	35 (12)	0	1 (0.3)
2. MS	189 (19)	0	117 (62)	40 (21)	13 (7)	19 (10)
3. MS + AS	152 (15)	0	0	120 (79)	0	32 (21)
4. AR†	119 (12)	107 (90)	0	10 (8)	0	2 (2)
5. MR	97 (10)	0	85 (88)	8 (8)	1 (1)	3 (3)
6. MS + AR	65 (6)	0	52 (80)	0	0	13 (20)
7. MR + AR	45 (4)	0	0	39 (87)	0	6 (13)
8. AS + MR	23 (2)	0	0	21 (91)	0	2 (9)
9. Tricuspid stenosis + MS ± AS	28 (3)	0	0	0	4 (14)	24 (86)
Totals	1010 (100)‡	363 (36)	254 (25)	273 (27)	18 (2)	102 (10)

*Excludes patients with MR due to coronary heart disease (papillary muscle dysfunction), carcinoid heart disease, or hypertrophic cardiomyopathy and those with infective endocarditis limited to one or both right-sided cardiac valves. TV regurgitation was present in many patients in most of the nine functional groups. All patients were in functional class III or IV (New York Heart Association), and more than half had had one or more cardiac operations.

†In many patients, the aortic valve cusps were normal or nearly normal, and the regurgitation was the result of disease of the aorta (Marfan and Marfan-like syndrome, syphilis, systemic hypertension, or healed aortic dissection).

‡The hearts in all 1010 patients were examined and classified by WCR.

AR, aortic regurgitation; AS, aortic stenosis; AV, aortic valve; MR, mitral regurgitation; MS, mitral stenosis; MV, mitral valve; TV, tricuspid valve.

From Roberts WC: Morphologic features of the normal and abnormal mitral valve. Am J Cardiol 1983;51:1005-1028, with permission.

TABLE 2–2	Type of Valvular Dysfunction in Patients* Having Aortic Valve Replacement and/or Mitral Valve Replacement or Repair at Baylor University Medical Center (Dallas), 1993-2006
Valve Dysfunction	Number of Patients (%)
1. AS	985 (53)
2. MS	129 (7)
3. MS + AS	54 (3)
4. AR†	326 (17)
5. MR	313 (17)
6. MS + AR	10 (<1)
7. MR + AR	28 (1)
8. AS + MR	27 (1)
9. Tricuspid stenosis + MS + AS	0
TOTALS	1872 (100)‡

*Excludes patients with MR due to coronary heart disease (papillary muscle dysfunction), carcinoid heart disease, or hypertrophic cardiomyopathy and those with infective endocarditis limited to one or both right-sided cardiac valves. Tricuspid regurgitation was present in many patients in most of the nine functional groups.

†In many patients, the aortic valve cusps were normal or nearly normal, and the regurgitation was the result of disease of the aorta (Marfan and Marfan-like syndrome, syphilis, systemic hypertension, or healed aortic dissection).

‡The operatively excised valves in all 1872 patients were examined and classified by WCR.

AR, aortic regurgitation; AS, aortic stenosis; MR, mitral regurgitation; MS, mitral stenosis.

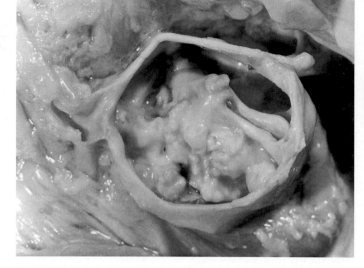

FIGURE 2–1 Aortic stenosis. Congenitally unicuspid unicommisured aortic valve in a 18-year-old man. The heart weighed 750 g. *(From Falcone MW, Roberts WC, Morrow AG, Perloff JK: Congenital aortic stenosis resulting from unicommissural valve: Clinical and anatomic features in twenty-one adult patients. Circulation 1971;44:272-280, with permission.)*

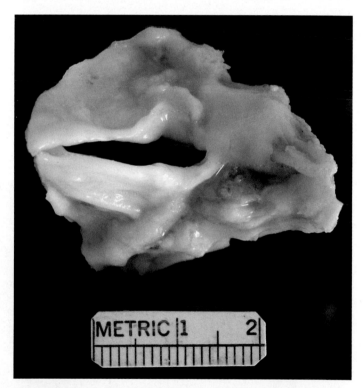

FIGURE 2–2 Aortic stenosis. Operatively excised unicuspid unicommissural aortic valve in a 41-year old man. The valve weighed 5.42 g. The mean transvalvular pressure gradient was 51 mm Hg.

and concomitant coronary bypass grafting tend to be higher in patients with AS involving three-cuspid aortic valves than in patients of similar age and sex without AS or with congenitally bicuspid aortic valves[5], and 5) histologic study of three-cuspid stenotic aortic valve demonstrates features similar to those in atherosclerotic plaques.[2]

The unicuspid aortic valve appears to be stenotic from the time of birth.[6,7] The congenitally bicuspid valve, however, infrequently is stenotic at birth but becomes stenotic as calcific deposits form on the aortic aspects of the cusps.[8] Rheumatic heart disease never involves the aortic valve anatomically without also involving the mitral valve.[9] Although the mitral valve may be diffusely abnormal anatomically, its function can be normal and consequently a patient with rheumatic heart disease can present initially with only aortic valve dysfunction, and therefore rheumatic heart disease has to be considered a cause of functionally isolated AS (with or without AR) or pure AR.[9]

Valve Structure

In patients with isolated AS (with or without AR) (only cardiac valve anatomically abnormal), the aortic valve may be unicuspid, bicuspid, tricuspid, or quadricuspid. The congenitally unicuspid valve is of two types: acommissural and unicommissural.[7,10] The acommissural valve, which represents less than 10% of the unicuspid valves, has a central orifice and no distinct commissures. The unicommissural valve, which constitutes most of the unicuspid valves, has one commissure and usually two other rudimentary commissures and a vertical orifice extending out from the only true commissure (Figures 2-1 and 2-2).[9]

The congenitally bicuspid valve (Figures 2-3 and 2-4) has two cusps, and they are usually of slightly unequal size in both cuspal surface area and weight. Usually one of the two cusps contains a raphe (rudimentary commissure) in its central portion. Often the raphe cusp has free margins that are V-shaped with the apex of the V pointing to the raphe

producing a concave configuration. The nonraphe cusp in this circumstance commonly has a convex configuration that fits nicely into the concave shape of the raphe cusp such that associated regurgitation is absent or minimal. These bicuspid valves with a concave configuration of the raphe cusp and a convex appearance of free margin of the nonraphe cusp are often confused with tricuspid valves with fusion of one of three commissures. In other bicuspid valves the free margins of both cusps are relatively straight.

The tricuspid aortic valve is common in older patients with AS (atherosclerotic origin) and in patients in whom the AS

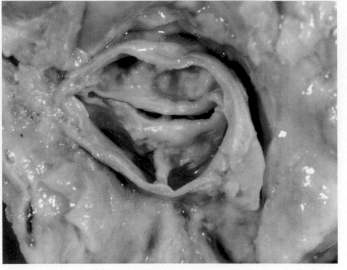

FIGURE 2–3 Aortic stenosis. Congenitally bicuspid aortic valve in a 61-year-old man. At catheterization 2 years before his death, the peak systolic transvalvular pressure gradient was 45 mm Hg when the cardiac index was 2.6 L/min/m². He had complete heart block due to destruction of the atrioventricular bundle by calcium. The heart weighed 700 g.

is of rheumatic etiology. (These latter patients always have mitral leaflets that are diffusely fibrotic [with or without focal calcific deposits] or at least the margins of both leaflets are everywhere thickened by fibrous tissue.). In patients with AS of rheumatic etiology, one or more of the three commissures are often fused, and the cusps may be either diffusely or focally fibrotic with or without commissural fusion or calcific deposits. The stenotic tricuspid aortic valve in older persons contains calcific deposits on the aortic surfaces, usually involving the sites of cuspal attachments, and the

commissures characteristically are not fused (Figure 2-5). Thus, operative excision produces three cusps, none of which are attached to another (Figure 2-6). Older patients with AS often also have a calcified mitral anomaly. Figure 2-7 shows how calcium might develop in both the aortic valve and in the mitral anulus.

The quadricuspid aortic valve is rare.[11] When present and if dysfunctional, the dysfunction is usually pure AR. AS with a quadricuspid valve is exceedingly rare, seen by Roberts and coworkers[12] in 1 of 1112 operatively excised stenotic aortic valves.

Necropsy Studies of Patients with Isolated Aortic Stenosis (with or without Aortic Regurgitation) and Never a Cardiac Operation—Natural History

During a 32-year-period at the National Institutes of Health, Roberts collected (mainly from hospitals in the Washington, DC, area) the hearts of 192 adults (aged 16 to 99 years) with isolated AS, and none of them had ever had a cardiac operation (unpublished data). Of the 192 patients, 139 (72%) were men and 53 (28%) women (Table 2-3). The average age of the men was 61 years and that of the women was 71 years, the same average ages of death as in coronary heart disease. The weight of the hearts was 610 ± 135 g (normal <400 g) in the men and 486 ± 111 g (normal <350 g) in the women. The aortic valve was congenitally unicuspid in 17 patients (9%), congenitally bicuspid in 89 patients (46%), and tricuspid in 86 patients (45%) (Table 2-4). Other observations in these 192 patients are shown in Tables 2-3 and 2-4.

Weights of Operatively Excised Stenotic Aortic Valves

The weight of operatively excised stenotic aortic valves is useful in quantitating the severity of stenosis because the weight is determined primarily by the quantity of calcific deposits, and the larger the calcific deposits are, the greater the transvalvular pressure gradient is.[12-23] Roberts and colleagues[21] reported weights for 1849 operatively excised stenotic valves

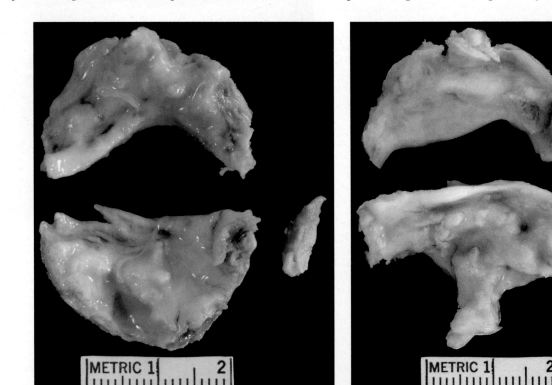

FIGURE 2–4 Aortic stenosis. Two operatively excised congenitally bicuspid aortic valves. **A**, Valve in a 60-year-old man. The valve weighed 4.65 g. The patient had severe heart failure. **B**, Valve in a 66-year-old man. The valve weighed 4.79 g, and the peak systolic transvalvular gradient was 84 mm Hg.

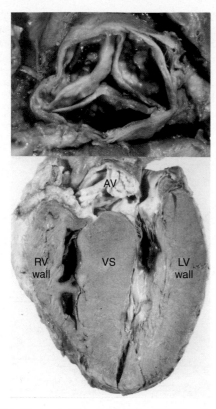

FIGURE 2–5 Aortic stenosis. Three-cuspid aortic valve (*top*) and longitudinal section of heart in an 89-year-old man whose heart weighed 440 g. None of the three aortic valve commissures are fused. The mitral annulus contains calcific deposits. *(From Roberts WC, Perloff JK, Costantino T: Severe valvular aortic stenosis in patients over 65 years of age: A clinicopathologic study. Am J Cardiol 1971;27:497-506, with permission.)*

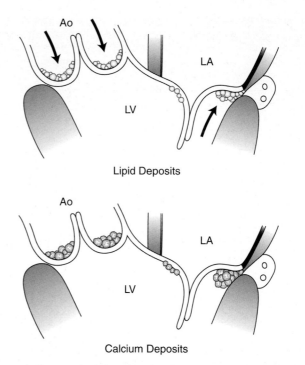

FIGURE 2–7 Aortic valve and mitral annular calcium. Commonly calcific deposits are present in the aortic valve cusps, mitral annulus, and epicardial coronary arteries (also referred to as the "senile cardiac calcification syndrome." The cause of the calcific deposits in these locations is speculative, but atherosclerosis seems to be the most reasonable. In younger individuals lipid deposits are usually present on the aortic aspects of the aortic valve cusps and on the ventricular aspects of the posterior mitral leaflet and to a much less extent on the ventricular aspect of the anterior mitral leaflet. The lipid in these locations is usually both intracellular and extracellular. Degeneration of the lipid probably leads to the calcific deposits in these locations. AO, aorta; LA, left atrium; LV, left ventricle.

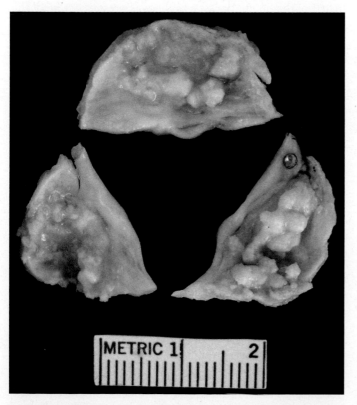

FIGURE 2–6 Aortic stenosis. Operatively excised aortic valve in a 70-year old man. The valve weighed 1.69 g, the peak systolic transvalvular gradient was 55 mm Hg, and left ventricular function was normal (ejection fraction = 60%).

TABLE 2–3	Findings at Necropsy in Isolated Aortic Valve Stenosis in Men Versus Women	
Variable	**Men**	**Women**
No. of patients (%)	139 (72%)	53 (28%)
Age (years), range (mean)	16-99 (61)	32-90 (71)
Symptomatic	103/129 (80%)	41/49 (84%)
Total cholesterol (mg/dl)	206 ± 63	161 ± 26
Severity of stenosis		
1+	24 (17%)	7 (13%)
2+	22 (16%)	9 (17%)
3+	93 (67%)	37 (70%)
Coronary narrowing		
absent	73 (53%)	20 (38%)
present	66 (47%)	33 (62%)
Mitral annular calcium		
0	101 (73%)	23 (43%)
1+-3+	38 (27%)	30 (57%)
Heart weight (g)	610 ± 135	486 ± 111
Aortic valve		
Unicuspid	16 (12%)	1 (2%)
Bicuspid	66 (47%)	23 (43%)
Total unicuspid and bicuspid	82 (59%)	24 (45%)
Tricuspid	57 (41%)	29 (55%)
Left ventricular		
Fibrosis	57 (41%)	13 (25%)
Necrosis	13 (9%)	5 (9%)

TABLE 2–4	Underlying Structure of the Aortic Valve in Patients Studied at Necropsy with Isolated Aortic Valve Stenosis with or without Associated Aortic Regurgitation		
Variable	Unicuspid	Bicuspid	Tricuspid
No. of patients (%)	17 (9%)	89 (46%)	86 (45%)
Ages (years), range (mean)	25-73 (46)	16-87 (62)	36-99 (64)
Male sex	16 (94%)	66 (74%)	57 (66%)
Symptomatic	15 (88%)	73/84 (87%)	57/78 (73%)
Total cholesterol (mg/dl)	216	203	173
Mode of death			
Sudden (outside hospital)	1 (6%)	15 (17%)	11 (13%)
Sudden (inside hospital)	1 (6%)	13 (15%)	6 (7%)
Nonsudden (cardiac)	14 (82%)	47 (53%)	45 (52%)
Vascular	0	2 (2%)	4 (5%)
Noncardiovascular	1 (6%)	12 (14%)	20 (23%)
Severity of stenosis			
1+	1 (6%)	11 (12%)	19 (22%)
2+	0	14 (16%)	17 (20%)
3+	16 (94%)	64 (72%)	50 (58%)
Coronary narrowing			
0	15 (88%)	57 (64%)	41 (48%)
≥1	2 (12%)	32 (36%)	45 (52%)
Mitral annular calcium			
0	12 (71%)	72 (81%)	40 (47%)
1+-3+	5 (29%)	17 (19%)	46 (53%)
Heart weight (g) (mean)	617	578	573
Left ventricular			
Fibrosis	8/15 (53%)	34/88 (39%)	28/85 (33%)
Necrosis	1/16 (6%)	8/87 (9%)	9/85 (11%)

in patients aged 21 to 91 years without concomitant mitral valve replacement or MS. These authors found that the weight of the stenotic valves varied inversely with the number of aortic valve cusps.[13] The unicuspid valves were the heaviest, the bicuspid valves were the next heaviest, and the tricuspid aortic valves were the lightest. The men had heavier valves than did the women (Figure 2-8), and the younger patients had heavier valves than did the older patients. The mean weights of the valves were similar in patients whose body mass index was less than 25, 25 to 30, and more than 30 kg/m². Mean valve weights also were heavier in the patients who did not undergo simultaneous coronary artery bypass grafting versus those who did.

Table 2-5 shows various clinical findings in the 1849 patients whose stenotic aortic valves were studied by Roberts and colleagues.[21] The patients underwent aortic valve replacement at three different institutions: the National Institutes of Health (NIH) from 1963 to 1989; Georgetown University Medical Center (GUMC) from 1969 to 1992, and Baylor University Medical Center (BUMC) from 1993 to 2004. All 1849 operatively excised stenotic valves were examined and classified by WCR. Patients having simultaneous mitral valve replacement or MS were excluded. The valves excised at NIH and at GUMC from 1963 to 1992 were heavier than the valves excised at BUMC from 1993 to 2004: men 4.05 ± 1.91 g (NIH), 4.36 ±1.83 g (GUMC), and 3.11 ± 1.51 g (BUMC); women 2.80 ± 1.26 g (NIH), 3.02 ± 1.26 g (GUMC), and 1.89 ±0.87 g (BUMC).

Not only did the valve weights vary according to valve structure (unicuspid > bicuspid > tricuspid), but also there was often variation in individual cusps among patients with bicuspid valves and among patients with tricuspid valves.[14,15] Of 200 operatively excised stenotic congenitally bicuspid valves, the two cusps in 152 patients (76%) differed in weight by more than 0.2 g, and in 48 patients

(24%) the cusps were of similar weight (≤0.2 g difference).[14] In 161 of the 200 patients, a raphe was present in one of the two cusps: the raphe and nonraphe cusps differed in weight in 120 patients (74%) with the raphe cusps being heavier in 89 patients (55%), lighter in 31 patients (19%), and of similar weight in 41 patients (26%). Of the 39 patients without a raphe in one cusp, in 32 patients (82%) the two cusps were of different (>0.2 g) weight and in 7 patients (18%) were of similar weight (≤0.2 g).

Of 260 operatively excised stenotic three-cuspid aortic valves, all three cusps differed (by >0.1 g) in weight in 71 patients (27%). All three cusps were similar (≤0.1 g difference) in weight in 33 patients (13%), and in 156 patients (60%) one cusp differed from both of the other two cusps, which were similar in weight.[15]

Why might cusps of operatively excised stenotic valves differ in weight? The most likely explanation seems to be that the cusps differ in size, that is, in surface area, from the time of birth. The cusp with the largest surface area has a larger area on which calcium can be deposited, and the weight of a cusp is determined primarily by the amount of calcium deposited on its aortic surface.

Relation of Aortic Valve Weight to Transvalvular Peak Systolic Pressure Gradient

The best determinant of the magnitude of obstruction in patients with AS has been a topic of debate. Determinants considered have been aortic valve area or index, mean transvalvular systolic gradient, and peak transvalvular systolic gradients. Roberts and Ko[16] compared the weights of operatively excised stenotic aortic valves to peak transvalvular systolic pressure gradient and to aortic valve area. The results of these studies in 201 men and in 123 women with isolated AS are shown in Table 2-6. In both men and women the weights

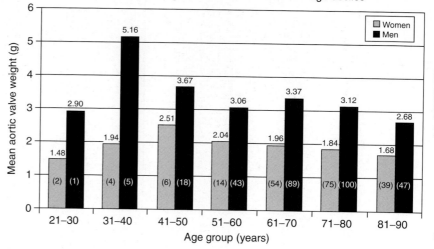

Mean aortic valve weights of women and men in 7 age deciles

FIGURE 2–8 Bar graph showing aortic valve weights in men and women in each of seven decades. All had aortic stenosis. *(From Roberts WC, Ko JM: Weights of operatively excised stenotic unicuspid, bicuspid, and tricuspid aortic valves and their relation to age, sex, body mass index, and presence or absence of concomitant coronary artery bypass grafting. Am J Cardiol 2003;92:1057-1065, with permission.)*

2

Clinical Pathology of Valvular Heart Disease

TABLE 2–5	Data in Patients Having Isolated Aortic Valve Replacement for Aortic Stenosis (with or without ± Aortic Regurgitation) at Three Different Medical Centers		
Variable	**NIH (1963-1989)**	**GUMC (1969-1992)**	**BUMC (1993-2004)**
Valve structure			
Unicuspid			
Men	84/342 (25%)	56/255 (22%)	36/601 (6%)
Women	14/110 (13%)	24/145 (17%)	12/356 (4%)
Bicuspid			
Men	158/342 (46%)	129/255 (50%)	316/601 (53%)
Women	53/110 (48%)	68/145 (47%)	153/356 (43%)
Tricuspid			
Men	47/342 (14%)	63/255 (25%)	242/601 (40%)
Women	28/110 (25%)	48/145 (33%)	186/356 (52%)
Indeterminate			
Men	53/342 (15%)	7/255 (3%)	7/601 (1%)
Women	15/110 (14%)	5/145 (3%)	5/356 (1%)
Ages (years), range (mean ± SD)			
Men	21-82 (54 ± 12)	24-88 (64 ± 11)	25-91 (69 ± 12)
Men ≥65	62/331 (19%)	124/251 (49%)	424/601 (71%)
Women	33-86 (57 ± 11)	22-89 (67 ± 12)	27-91 (70 ± 11)
Women ≥65	27/104 (26%)	94/142 (66%)	273/356 (77%)
Sex			
Men	342/452 (76%)	255/400 (64%)	601/957 (63%)
Women	110/452 (24%)	145/400 (36%)	356/957 (37%)
Aortic valve weight (g)			
Men	0.70-10.2 (4.05 ± 1.91)	1.20-11.0 (4.36 ± 1.83)	0.89-11.30 (3.11 ± 1.51)
Women	0.55-5.50 (2.80 ± 1.26)	0.40-6.70 (3.02 ± 1.26)	0.45-4.97 (1.89 ± 0.87)
Left ventricular to aortic peak systolic gradient (mm Hg)			
Men	10-145 (69 ± 30)	10-160 (69 ± 25)	10-141 (52 ± 23)
Women	10-165 (76 ± 34)	30-170 (81 ± 32)	10-133 (54 ± 28)
Aortic valve area (cm²)			
Men	0.20-1.90 (0.66 ± 0.32)	0.27-1.97 (0.75 ± 0.31)	0.20-1.90 (0.78 ± 0.26)
Women	0.23-1.10 (0.53 ± 0.21)	0.20-1.30 (0.57 ± 0.21)	0.18-1.49 (0.67 ± 0.22)
Cardial index (L/min/m²)			
Men	1.10-5.00 (2.58 ± 0.72)	1.00-7.30 (2.87 ± 0.93)	—
Women	1.60-4.50 (2.68 ± 0.69)	1.60-6.20 (2.79 ± 0.81)	—
Simultaneous coronary bypass			
Men	21/238 (9%)	77/198 (39%)	332/601 (55%)
Women	6/74 (8%)	29/118 (25%)	167/356 (47%)

AV, aortic valve; BUMC, Baylor University Medical Center; GUMC, Georgetown University Medical Center; NIH, National Institutes of Health.
From Roberts WC, Ko JM, Hamilton C: Comparison of valve structure, valve weight, and severity of the valve obstruction in 1849 patients having isolated aortic valve replacement for aortic valve stenosis (with or without associated aortic regurgitation) studied at 3 different medical centers in 2 different time periods. Circulation 2005;112:3919-3929, with permission.

TABLE 2-6 Ages, Body Mass Index, and Concomitant Coronary Artery Bypass, Left Ventricular to Aortic Peak Systolic Gradients, and Aortic Valve Areas in Seven Aortic Valve Weight Groups in Men and in Women

AV Weight (g)	No. of Patients	Ages (years), Range (Average)	BMI (kg/m²), Range (Average)	AV Weights (g), Range (Average)	LV-Aorta PSG (mm Hg), Range (Average)	AV, Range (Mean)	Coronary Bypass	UAV or BAV	Ejection Fraction No.	Range (mean)	No. (%) ≤40	No. (%) >40
Men												
≤1	0	—	—	—	—	—	—	—	—	—	—	—
>1-2	41	47-90 (72)	19-37 (27)	1.16-2.00 (1.64)	11-81 (36)	0.27-1.43 (0.86)	27 (66%)	11 (27%)	37	15-78 (48)	13 (35%)	24 (65%)
>2-3	60	29-87 (69)	20-43 (29)	2.01-3.00 (2.58)	15-97 (45)	0.42-2.25 (0.89)	32 (53%)	24 (40%)	52	10-85 (51)	14 (27%)	38 (73%)
>3-4	50	37-84 (69)	17-40 (27)	3.03-4.00 (3.40)	20-100 (56)	0.20-1.63 (0.75)	26 (52%)	30 (60%)	44	15-80 (53)	7 (16%)	37 (84%)
>4-5	29	42-87 (69)	18-45 (28)	4.01-4.84 (4.40)	20-108 (64)	0.32-1.06 (0.67)	11 (38%)	25 (86%)	26	15-70 (53)	5 (19%)	21 (81%)
>5-6	12	49-90 (70)	24-36 (28)	5.03-5.93 (5.60)	50-116 (71)	0.40-0.88 (0.60)	3 (25%)	10 (83%)	10	20-65 (43)	4 (40%)	6 (60%)
>6	9	38-84 (58)	21-38 (28)	6.24-11.30 (7.92)	35-141 (87)	0.39-1.23 (0.71)	2 (22%)	8 (89%)	8	15-70 (51)	2 (25%)	6 (75%)
Women												
≤1	10	55-85 (74)	21-44 (30)	0.69-0.95 (0.83)	15-62 (28)	0.34-1.28 (0.83)	7 (70%)	2 (20%)	9	30-70 (47)	4 (44%)	5 (56%)
>1-2	73	19-88 (71)	17-51 (29)	1.02-1.99 (1.46)	10-119 (49)	0.18-1.49 (0.72)	40 (55%)	14 (19%)	66	15-80 (56)	9 (14%)	57 (86%)
>2-3	29	30-87 (70)	18-50 (28)	2.04-3.00 (2.42)	26-113 (63)	0.27-1.09 (0.58)	15 (52%)	12 (41%)	23	30-80 (54)	4 (17%)	19 (83%)
>3-4	10	47-85 (73)	17-35 (26)	3.14-4.00 (3.42)	53-131 (85)	0.23-0.78 (0.51)	3 (30%)	9 (90%)	9	45-75 (53)	0	9 (100%)
>4-5	1	83	29	4.27	53	0.75	0	1 (100%)	1	50	0	1 (100%)
>5-6	0	—	—	—	—	—	—	—	—	—	—	—
>6	0	—	—	—	—	—	—	—	—	—	—	—

AV, aortic valve; BAV, bicuspid aortic valve; BMI, body mass index; LV, left ventricular; PSG, peak systolic gradient; UAV, unicuspid aortic valve.

From Roberts WC, Ko JM: Relation of weights of operatively excised stenotic aortic valves to preoperative transvalvular peak systolic pressure gradients and to calculated aortic valve areas. J Am Coll Cardiol 2004;44:1847-1855, with permission.

of the stenotic aortic valves increased significantly as the peak left ventricular-to-aortic systolic gradient increased but valve weight had essentially no relation to aortic valve area. Women had significantly lower valve weights with peak gradients similar to those in men. In men with valve weights from 1 to 2 g the peak transvalvular gradient averaged 36 mm Hg, and the valve area averaged 0.86 cm^2; in the men with valve weights more than 6 g the peak gradient averaged 87 mm Hg, whereas the valve area averaged 0.71 cm^2. In women with valve weights ≤1 g the peak gradient averaged 28 mm Hg and valve area averaged 0.83 cm^2; in women whose valve weighed from more than 3 to 4 g the peak gradient averaged 85 mm Hg, and the valve area averaged 0.51 cm^2 (see Table 2-6).

Relatively few operatively excised aortic valves in adults with AS are ≥5 g, and those that are are usually congenitally malformed. Of unicuspid valves, 37 (30%) of 124 valves in men and 5 (11%) of 44 in women reached this weight; of bicuspid valves, 96 (18%) of 521 valves in men and 4 (2%) of 236 valves in women reached this weight (unpublished data). In contrast, only 15 (4%) of 361 tricuspid valves in men and only 2 (0.72%) of 281 valves in women reached this weight. Of 1038 operatively excised stenotic aortic valves in men, 161 (16%) weighed >5 g, and of 571 valves in women, only 13 (2%) reached this weight. Seven operatively excised stenotic valves weighed ≥10 g; all were in men, and all seven were either unicuspid or bicuspid and the peak pressure gradient across them ranged from 80 to 143 mm Hg (average 101 mm Hg) (unpublished data).

Associated Coronary Arterial Narrowing

Patients with operatively excised congenitally unicuspid and bicuspid valves have significantly less epicardial coronary arterial narrowing than do patients with tricuspid aortic valves (Table 2-7). Concomitant coronary artery bypass grafting also varies according to the era during which the AVR was done and on the institution in which it was done. Also, the criteria for performing coronary artery bypass grafting in patients having AVR have changed with time.

Relation to Left Bundle Branch Block and/or Complete Heart Block

At one time, patients with AS and left bundle branch block or complete heart block were believed to have conduction disturbance because of associated severe coronary arterial narrowing from atherosclerosis. Study at necropsy of many patients with combined AS and left bundle branch block or complete heart block, however, has indicated that the conduction disturbance was due not to associated coronary narrowing but to destruction of the left bundle branches or the atrioventricular bundle by calcific deposits that had extended caudally from the aortic valve (WC Roberts, unpublished data). Most of these patients had congenitally malformed aortic valves, not tricuspid valves, and severe degrees of hemodynamic obstruction as a result of the heavy calcific deposits.

TABLE 2–7	Frequency of Concomitant Coronary Artery Bypass Grafting Among Patients Having Isolated Aortic Valve Replacement for Aortic Stenosis at Three Different Institutions*		
Valve Structure	NIH (1963-1989)	GUMC (1969-1992)	BUMC (1993-2007)
No. of patients	259	308	1351
Unicuspid	2/61 (3%)	13/55 (24%)	13/83 (16%)
Bicuspid	13/140 (9%)	42/162 (26%)	280/646 (43%)
Tricuspid	10/58 (17%)	47/91 (52%)	390/622 (63%)

*Excludes cases in which the number of valve cusps was unclear (indeterminate).
BUMC, Baylor University Medical Center; GUMC, Georgetown University Medical Center; NIH, National Institutes of Health.

Pure Aortic Regurgitation

There are two major causes of pure (no element of stenosis) AR: 1) conditions affecting primarily the valve and 2) conditions affecting the aorta and only secondarily causing the valve to be incompetent. Roberts and Ko[24] recently reviewed the cause of pure AR in 268 patients having isolated AVR at BUMC from 1993 to 2005. As shown in Table 2-8, conditions affecting primarily the valve were the cause of the AR in 122 patients (46%), and nonvalve conditions was the cause in 146 patients (54%). Among the former, the congenitally bicuspid valve unassociated with infective endocarditis was the problem in 59 patients, 22 (37%) of whom had resection of portions of the dilated ascending aorta. Eleven of the 22 patients with resected aortas had severe loss of medial elastic fibers. Infective endocarditis was the cause in 46 patients, 15 (33%) of whom had congenitally bicuspid aortic valves. Thus, of the 122 with valve conditions causing the AR, 74 (61%) had congenitally bicuspid aortic valves. Why one congenitally bicuspid aortic valve becomes stenotic,[8,25] another shows purely regurgitation without superimposed infective endocarditis,[26] another becomes severely dysfunctional only when infective endocarditis appears,[27] and some function normally an entire lifetime is unclear.[8] Of 85 patients, aged 15 to 79 years, with congenitally bicuspid aortic valves studied at autopsy by Roberts,[8] 61 (72%) valves were stenotic, 2 (2%) were purely regurgitation without superimposed infective endocarditis, 9 (11%) had AR because of infective endocarditis, and 13 (15%) functioned normally during the patients' 23 to 59 years of life (mean 45 years).

Rheumatic heart disease is a relatively infrequent cause of pure AR in patients with normally functioning mitral valves.[9] All such patients (by our definition of rheumatic heart disease) have diffuse fibrosis of the mitral leaflets or at least diffuse thickening of the margins of these leaflets. In this circumstance mitral valve function would be normal despite the anatomic abnormality.

Infective endocarditis more commonly involves a three-cuspid aortic valve than a two-cuspid valve because the tricuspid valve is much more common than the bicuspid valve.[27]

Rheumatoid arthritis is a rare cause of AR. The anatomic abnormality is specific for this condition and consists of rheumatoid nodules within the aortic valve cusps.[28,29]

Conditions affecting the ascending aorta and causing it to dilate produce AR more commonly than conditions affecting primarily the aortic valve. Of 146 patients having pure AR and isolated AVR, the cause of the AR was not determined after examination of the operatively excised aorta and aortic valve.[24] Many of these patients had systemic hypertension but only mild dilation of the aorta, and all had normal or nearly normal three-cuspid aortic valves. It is likely that systemic hypertension in some way played a role in the AR.[30,31]

Aortic dissection usually produces acute AR due to splitting of the aortic media behind the aortic valve commissures that results in prolapse of one or more cusps toward the left ventricular cavity.[32]

Diffuse thickening of the tubular portion of the central ascending aorta with sparing of the wall of aorta behind the sinuses is characteristic of cardiovascular syphilis.[33] These patients generally undergo a cardiovascular operation because of diffuse aneurysmal dilatation of the tubular portion of ascending aorta, not usually because of severe AR. Granulomatous (giant cell) aortitis grossly mimics cardiovascular syphilis but is far less common. During the past 10 years, 15 patients have had resection of aneurysmally dilated syphilitic aortas with or without simultaneous aortic valve replacement at BUMC (unpublished data). The characteristic histologic feature of cardiovascular syphilis is extensive thickening of the aortic wall due to fibrous thickening of the

TABLE 2-8 | Causes of Aortic Regurgitation in Patients Having Isolated Aortic Valve Replacement at Baylor University Medical Center (1993-2005)

Causes of Aortic Regurgitation	Total	Ages (years) at Operation, Range (Mean)	M	F	Acute	Chronic	SH	CABG	Portions of Ascending Aorta Excised	Examined Histologically	CMN (3+,4+)*	BAV	Calcium Deposits on AV Cusps	Aortic Valve Weight (g), Range (Mean) Men	Women
Valve: 122 (46%)															
Congenital malformation without infective endocarditis															
Bicuspid	59 (22%)	22-77 (55)	49	10	0	59	39 (66%)	18 (31%)	22	22	11	59	31	0.52-2.99 (1.42)	0.68-1.80 (1.24)
Quadricuspid	2 (1%)	53, 79 (66)	0	2	0	2	0	1 (50%)	0	0	0	0	0	—	0.57, 1.13 (.85)
Tricuspid	5 (2%)	33-48 (40)	3	2	0	5	2 (40%)	0	1	1	0	0	0	1.11-1.40 (1.23)	0.34, 0.66 (.050)
Infective endocarditis	46 (17%)	21-82 (45)	31	15	27	19	29 (63%)	7 (15%)	6	4	0	15	8	0.77-2.31 (1.53)	0.44-2.50 (0.98)
Rheumatic?	8 (3%)	25-63 (47)	6	2	0	8	6 (75%)	2 (25%)	0	0	0	0	3	1.10-2.45 (1.81)	1.31, 1.83 (1.57)
Miscellaneous	2 (1%)	24, 42 (33)	1	1	0	2	2 (100%)	1 (50%)	0	0	0	0	0	0.55	—
Nonvalve: 146 (54%)															
Aortic dissection	28 (10%)	25-78 (58)	20	8	21	7	22 (79%)	5† (17%)	28	20	5	3	4	0.51-1.19 (0.81)	0.37-0.90 (0.59)
Marfan or forme fruste	15 (6%)	21-71 (47)	9	6	0	15	10 (67%)	1‡ (7%)	15	13	13	0	2	0.73-1.01 (0.94)	0.35-0.85 (0.66)
Aortitis	12 (4%)	35-82 (66)	5	7	0	12	10 (83%)	5 (42%)	12	12	12	0	2	0.63-0.79 (0.70)	0.35-0.70 (0.54)
Etiology unclear	91 (34%)	50-84 (66)	58	33	0	91	83 (91%)	46 (51%)	7	7	0	0	26	0.48-2.13 (1.08)	0.31-1.74 (0.73)
Total	268 (100%)	21-84 (57)	182 (68%)	86 (32%)	48 (18%)	220 (82%)	203 (76%)	86 (32%)	91 (34%)	76	41	77 (29%)	76/263 (29%)	0.48-2.99 (1.22) 151§	0.31-2.50 (0.81) 75§

AV, aortic valve; BAV, bicuspid aortic valve; CABG, coronary artery bypass grafting; CMN, cystic medial necrosis; F, female; M, male; SH, systemic hypertension.

*Cystic medial necrosis is used here to refer to the magnitude of loss of elastic fibers in the media of the aorta.

†Four other patients had CABG due to extension of the aortic dissection into a coronary artery.

‡One additional patient had CABG due to extension of the aortic dissection into a coronary artery.

§Number of cases with aortic valve weight.

From Roberts WC, Ko JM, Moore TR, Jones WH III. Causes of pure aortic regurgitation in patients having isolated aortic valve replacement at a single US tertiary hospital (1993-2005). Circulation 2006;114:422-429, with permission.

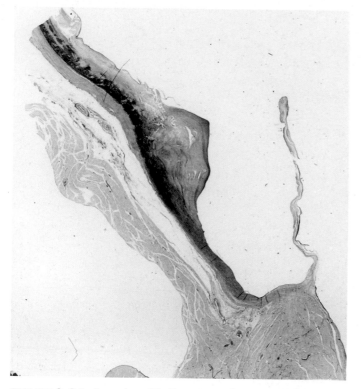

FIGURE 2–9 Cardiovascular syphilis. Photomicrographs of an aortic valve cusp, sinus portion of aorta (behind the cusp) and proximal tubular portion of ascending aorta which is thickened by intimal and adventitial fibrous tissue. Many medial elastic fibers have been destroyed. The location of the process in the tubular portion of the aorta with sparing of the sinus portion of aorta is characteristic of cardiovascular syphilis. Elastic tissue stain, ×4.5.

intima and of the adventitia (Figure 2-9). The medial elastic fibers and smooth muscle cells are also replaced focally by scars due to narrowings in the vasa vasora. Focal collections of plasma cells and lymphocytes are present in the adventitia. Giant-cell aortitis is similar to syphilitic aortitis except for the presence of multinucleated giant cells.

The AR in patients with Marfan syndrome and forme fruste varieties of it is the result of severe dilatation of the sinus portion and proximal tubular portion of the aorta.[34] The consequence of the "aortic root" dilatation is stretching of the aortic valve cusps in roughly a straight line between the commissures, leading to a wide-open central regurgitant stream. In contrast to cardiovascular syphilis, the aortic wall in the Marfan syndrome is thinner than normal because of the massive loss of medial elastic fibers and lack of thickening of either the intima or the adventitia.

There is one condition that causes AR by involving both the valve cusp and the portion of the aorta behind and adjacent to the lateral attachments of the aortic valve cusps. That condition is ankylosing spondylitis.[35,36] About 5% of patients with this form of arthritis develop AR. The bases of the aortic valve cusps become densely thickened by fibrous tissue, which is also present on the ventricular aspect of anterior mitral leaflet and on the left ventricular aspect of the membranous ventricular septum. Varying degrees of heart block may be a consequence of this subaortic deposit of dense fibrous tissue. The AR associated with ankylosing spondylitis is usually severe with diastolic pressures in both aorta and left ventricle often being similar. The histologic appearance of the aorta in ankylosing spondylitis is similar to that in syphilis but the syphilitic process never extends onto the aortic valve cusps or subvalvularly and rarely involves the wall of aorta behind the sinuses.

Mitral Stenosis

Of the 1010 patients aged 15 years or older with functionally severe valvular cardiac disease studied at necropsy by Roberts up to 1980, 434 (44%) had MS.[1] MS occurred alone in 189 (44%) patients and in combination with other functional valve lesions in the other 245 (56%) patients. MS was of rheumatic etiology in all 434 patients.

Rheumatic heart disease may be viewed as a disease of the mitral valve; other valves also may be involved both anatomically and functionally, but anatomically the mitral valve is always involved[37,38] (Figure 2-11). Aschoff bodies have never been reported in hearts without anatomic disease of the mitral valve.[38] Of the first 543 patients with severe valvular heart disease that Roberts and Virmani[39] studied at necropsy, 11 (2.7%) had Aschoff bodies, and all had anatomic mitral valve disease. The 11 patients ranged in age from 18 to 68 years (mean 38 years) and 9 had a history of acute rheumatic fever, 9 had MS with or without dysfunction of one or more other cardiac valves, 1 had isolated AR, and 1 had both AR and MR. All 11 had diffuse fibrous thickening of the mitral leaflets, and all but 1 had diffuse anatomic lesions of at least two other cardiac valves. Thus, among patients with chronic valve disease, Aschoff bodies, the only anatomic lesions pathognomic of rheumatic heart disease, usually indicate diffuse anatomic lesions of more than one cardiac valve, and the most common hemodynamic lesion is MS with or without MR.

Although rare at necropsy in patients with fatal chronic valve disease, Aschoff bodies are fairly common in the hearts of patients having mitral commissurotomy for MS. Among 481 patients having various valve operations, Aschoff bodies were found by Virmani and Roberts[40] in 40 (21%) of 191 operatively excised left atrial appendages, in 4 (2%) of 273 operatively excised left ventricular papillary muscles, and in 1 (6%) of 17 patients in whom both appendage and papillary muscle were excised. Of these 45 patients with Aschoff bodies, 44 had MS (Figure 2-12) and only 1, a 10-year-old boy, had pure MR. Sinus rhythm was present preoperatively in 38 (84%), and atrial fibrillation in 7 (16%).

Not only is rheumatic heart disease a disorder of the cardiac valves, but it may also affect mural endocardium, epicardium, and myocardium. The atrial walls virtually always have increased amounts of fibrous tissue in both myocardial interstitium and in the mural endocardium, atrophy of some myocardial cells and hypertrophy of others, and hypertrophy of smooth muscles in the mural endocardium. In all patients with rheumatic MS, the leaflets are diffusely thickened either by fibrous tissue or calcific deposits or both, the two commissures are usually fixed, and the chordae tendineae are usually (but not always) thickened and fused (Figures 2-13 and 2-14).

The amount of calcium in the leaflets of stenotic mitral valves varies considerably (Figure 2-15). Generally, the calcific deposits are more frequent and in larger quantities in men than in women, in older than in younger patients, and in those with higher than in those with lower pressure gradients between left atrium and left ventricle (see Figure 2-14). The rapidity with which calcium develops also varies considerably: it is present at a younger age in men than in women. Lachman and Roberts[41] determined the presence or absence and the extent of calcific deposits in operatively excised stenotic mitral valves in 164 patients aged 26 to 72 years. The amount of calcific deposits in the stenotic mitral valves correlated with sex and with the mean transvalvular pressure gradient (Figure 2-16), but it did not correlate with the patients' age (after 25 years), cardiac rhythm, pulmo-

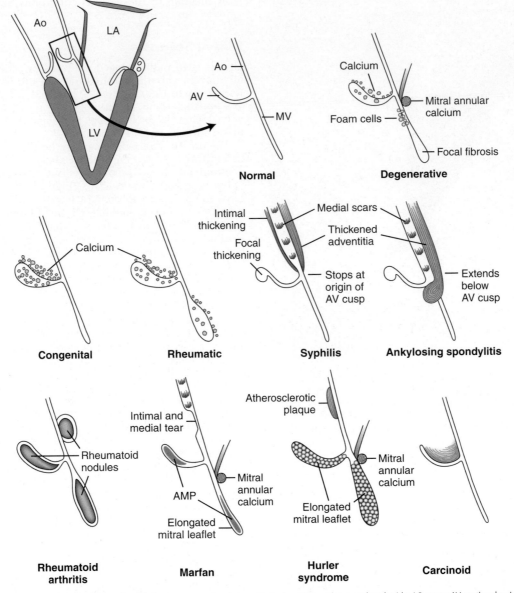

FIGURE 2–10 Diagram of some of the conditions affecting the aorta or aortic valve or mitral valve. AMP, acid mucopolysacharide; AO, aorta; AV, aortic valve; LA, left atrium; LV, left ventricle; MV, mitral valve. *(From Roberts WC, Perloff JK: Mitral valvular disease: A clinicopathologic survey of the conditions causing the mitral valve to function abnormally. Ann Intern Med 1972;77: 939-975, with permission.)*

nary arterial or pulmonary arterial wedge pressure, previous mitral commissurotomy, presence of thrombus in the body or appendage of the left ventricle, or presence of disease in one or more other cardiac valves. Of the 164 patients, radiographs of the operatively excised valve showed no calcific deposits in 14 of them, and only minimal deposits in 43 of them. Of the 57 patients, however, 37 had moderate or severe MR. The remaining 20 in an earlier era would have been ideal or near-ideal candidates for mitral commissurotomy.[42]

A major complication of MS is thrombus formation in the left atrial cavity. The thrombus may be limited to the atrial appendage (by far most common) or be located in both the appendage and body of the left atrium. Left atrial "body" thrombus was observed in 5% of the 1010 patients with fatal valvular heart disease studied at necropsy by Roberts, and all had severe MS (unpublished data). Left atrial body thrombus was not found in any of the 165 patients with pure MR. All patients with left atrial body thrombus had atrial fibrillation. In contrast, of 46 patients with MS having a cardiotomy at the National Heart, Lung, and Blood Institute and thrombus in the left atrial body, 42 (91%) had atrial fibrillation and 4 (9%) had sinus rhythm.

Thrombus appears to occur in the body of the left atrium only in patients with MS, and atrial fibrillation in the absence of MS is incapable of forming thrombus in the left atrial body.

Calcific deposits on the mural endocardium of left atrium almost certainly are indicative of previous organization of left atrial thrombi.[43] Histologically, the "calcific thrombi" also contain cholesterol clefts and are identical to atherosclerotic plaques. The observation that left atrial thrombi can organize into lesions identical to atherosclerotic plaques supports the view that atherosclerotic plaques may in part be the result of organization of thrombi.

Nonrheumatic causes of MS include congenital anomalies,[37,38] large mitral annular calcific deposits associated with left ventricular outflow obstruction[44,45] (Figure 2-17), neoplasms (particularly myxoma) protruding through the mitral orifice,[46] large vegetations from active infective endocarditis,[47] and a mechanical prosthesis or bioprosthesis used to replace a native mitral valve.[48]

Histologic examination of sections of stenotic mitral valves when stained for elastic fibers show the mitral leaflet to have lost most or all of its spongiosa element such that the leaflet

Rheumatic Heart Disease —
Mitral valve involved anatomically in
one of two ways — diffuse or margins only

I. Diffuse

Leaflets

Posterior   Anterior   Posterior

Chordae
tendineae

Papillary
muscle

LA

LV

II. Margins

☐ Portion of leaflets abormal structurally

FIGURE 2–11 Rheumatic heart disease. Diagram showing the two types of anatomic involvement of the mitral valve in rheumatic heart disease.

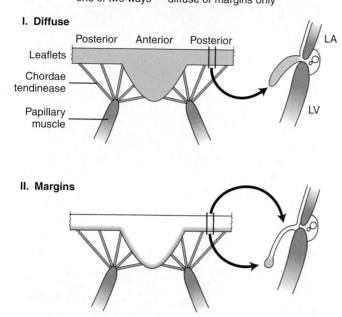

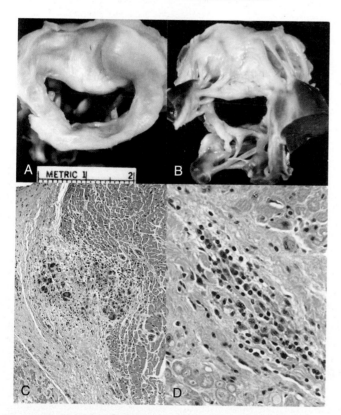

FIGURE 2–12 Acute rheumatic fever and mitral stenosis. Excised mitral valve in a 23-year-old Indian woman with mitral stenosis (13 mm Hg mean diastolic pressure gradient between pulmonary artery wedge and left ventricle) and regurgitation. She had had acute rheumatic fever initially at age 7 and recurrence of migratory polyarthritis at age 22 years. During the early postoperative course after mitral valve replacement, she had swelling and pain in one knee and one ankle and erythema around two joints. Shown are the excised valves viewed from the left atrium (**a**) and from the left ventricle (**b**) and Aschoff bodies (**c** and **d**), which were numerous in both excised left ventricular papillary muscles. Hematoxylin and eosin: ×110 (**c**), ×400 (**d**). *(From Virmani R, Roberts WC: Aschoff bodies in operatively excised atrial appendages and in papillary muscles: Frequency and clinical significance. Circulation 1977;55:559-556, with permission.)*

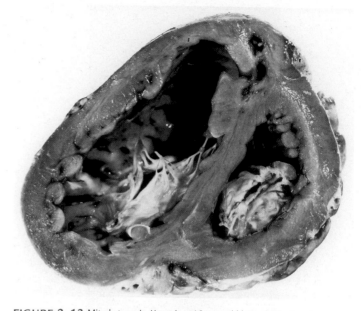

FIGURE 2–13 Mitral stenosis. Heart in a 16-year-old boy who had acute rheumatic fever at age 6 and chronic heart failure beginning at age 10. He had severe mitral stenosis and tricuspid valve regurgitation. At cardiac catheterization 10 hours before death, the right ventricular pressure was 100/20 and the left ventricular pressure was 100/10 mm Hg. By a left ventricular angiogram, the left ventricular cavity was of normal size, and there was no mitral regurgitation. At necropsy, the heart weighed 450 g (the patient weight 43 kg). The right ventricular cavity was greatly dilated and both ventricular walls were of similar thickness. Both mitral and tricuspid valve leaflets were diffusely thickened and free of calcific deposits. No Aschoff bodies were found. *(From Roberts WC: Morphologic features of the normal and abnormal mitral valve. Am J Cardiol 1983;51:1005-1028, with permission.)*

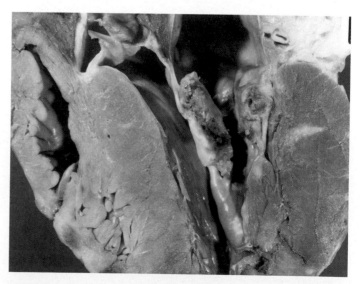

FIGURE 2–14 Mitral stenosis. Longitudinal view of a very narrow and thickened mitral valve in a 55-year-old man with equal peak systolic pressures in the right and left ventricles and no associated mitral regurgitation during cannulation of the aorta for planned mitral valve replacement. Both anterior and posterior mitral leaflets are heavily calcified. *(From Roberts WC: Morphologic features of the normal and abnormal mitral valve. Am J Cardiol 1983;51:1005-1028, with permission.)*

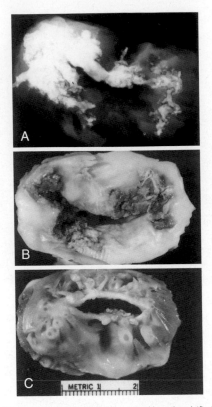

FIGURE 2–15 Mitral stenosis. Operatively excised heavily calcified stenotic mitral valve in a 57-year-old man with combined mitral stenosis (12 mm Hg mean transvalvular diastolic gradient) and aortic stenosis. **a,** Radiograph of the excised valve. **b,** View of valve from the left atrial aspect. Thrombi are present near and at the commissures. **c,** View from the left ventricular aspect. The orifice is severely narrowed.

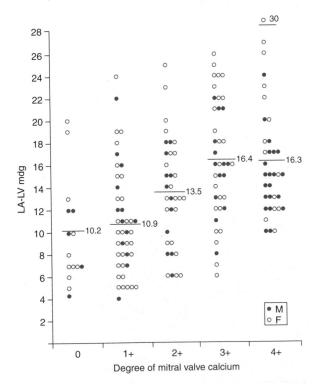

FIGURE 2–16 Mitral stenosis. Diagram comparing the relation of the mean left atrial (LA)-left ventricular (LV) mean diastolic gradient to the quantity of mitral valve calcium graded by radiograph of the operatively excised mitral valve. The greater the quantity of mitral calcium is, the greater the transvalvular gradient. *(From Lachman AS, Roberts WC: Calcific deposits in stenotic mitral valves: Extent and relation to age, sex, degree of stenosis, cardiac rhythm, previous commissurotomy and left atrial body thrombus from study of 164 operatively excised valves. Circulation 1978;57:808-815, with permission.)*

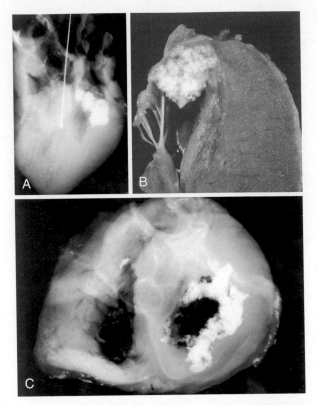

FIGURE 2–17 Mitral annular calcium. Heavily calcified mitral annulus in a 71-year-old woman with previous second-degree heart block and a pacemaker for 23 months. She died of acute myocardial infarction complicated by rupture of the left ventricular free wall. **a,** Radiograph of the heart at necropsy showing mitral annular calcium and the pacemaker leads. **b,** Longitudinal section showing heavy calcific deposits behind the posterior mitral leaflet. **c,** Radiograph of the base of the heart after removal of its apical one-half, showing the circumferential extent of the mitral annular calcific deposits. *(From Roberts WC, Dangel JC, Bulkley BH: Nonrheumatic cardiac disease: A clinicopathologic survey of 27 different conditions causing valvular dysfunction. Cardiovasc Clin 1973;5:333-446, with permission.)*

itself consists entirely or nearly entirely of the fibrosa element. The leaflet (as are the chordae) is outlined by an elastic fibril (which stains black by an elastic tissue stain) and covering it on both atrial and ventricular aspects is dense fibrous tissue containing focally some vascular channels. Similar dense fibrous tissue surrounds the chordae and the chordae themselves appear normal.

Patients with MS usually have distinct pulmonary vascular changes due to the pulmonary venous and arterial hypertension. These anatomic changes consist of thickening of the media of the muscular and elastic pulmonary arteries and focal intimal fibrous plaques. Plexiform lesions never occur in the lungs as a result of MS. The alveolar septa also thicken due to dilatation of the capillaries, proliferation of lining alveolar cells, and some increase of alveolar septal fibrous tissue.

Pure Mitral Regurgitation

Pure MR (no element of MS) is the most common dysfunctional cardiac valve disorder, and, in contrast to MS, it has many different causes. If patients with MR due to left ventricular dilatation from any cause (e.g., ischemic cardiomyopathy, idiopathic dilated cardiomyopathy, or anemia) are excluded, the most common cause of MR treated operatively in the Western world today is MVP (Figures 2-18 and 2-19). This condition, which was described initially in the 1960s by Barlow and colleagues[49] and by Criley and colleagues,[50] is now recognized to occur in approximately 5% of the adult population, and, if this condition is considered a congenital

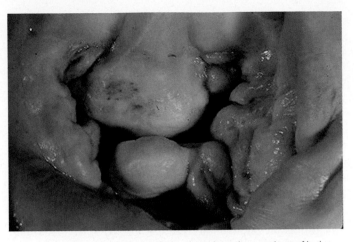

FIGURE 2–18 Mitral valve prolapse. View from above shows prolapse of both anterior and posterior cusps in a man who died from consequences of an acute myocardial infarction.

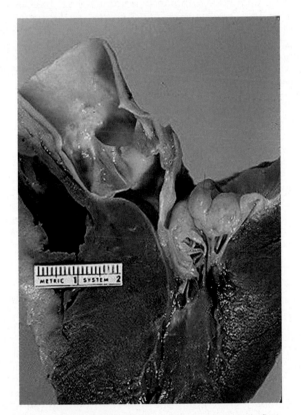

METRIC 1 SYSTEM 2

FIGURE 2–19 Mitral valve prolapse. View of prolapsed posterior leaflet in a 74-year-old woman who during life was found to have a precordial murmur but never had symptoms of cardiac dysfunction.

deficiency of mitral tissues, as we do, it is the most common congenital cardiovascular disease. Among 97 patients having mitral valve replacement for pure MR from 1968 to 1981 at the National Heart, Lung, and Blood Institute, MVP was responsible in 60 patients (62%), papillary muscle dysfunction from coronary heart disease in 29 (30%), infective endocarditis in 5 (5%), and possibly rheumatic disease in 3 (3%).[51]

Although several authors have attempted to do so, defining MVP has not been easy.[1] The following criteria have proved useful in separating the valve affected by MVP from other conditions affecting the mitral valve:

1. Focal lengthening of the posterior and/or anterior mitral leaflets from their site of attachment to their distal margins. Normally, the length of the posterior leaflet from its attachment to distal margin is about 1 cm. In MVP, this leaflet focally often is as long as the anterior leaflet.[51]
2. Elongation and thinning of chordae tendineae.
3. Focal thickening of the posterior and/or anterior leaflet. This finding is particularly prominent on the portion of leaflet that prolapses toward or into the left atrium during ventricular systole. The atrial surface is uniformly smooth. The thickening of the leaflet produces a spongy feel.
4. The mitral leaflet is increased in area, either focally or diffusely.[51]
5. Loss of chordae tendineae on the ventricular aspect of posterior mitral leaflet. It is rare to actually see a ruptured chorda, but what is seen are areas where chordae should be attached but none are there. They presumably ruptured in the past and with time were matted down on the ventricular aspect of the leaflets, giving this surface a "bumpy" appearance and feel. Chordae are nearly uniformly missing (previously ruptured) in portions of posterior mitral leaflet excised during mitral valve repair or during replacement. Indeed, MVP appears to be by far the most common cause of ruptured chordae tendineae. Infective endocarditis is the next most frequent cause.[52]
6. Dilatation of the mitral annulus. Annular dilatation probably is the major cause of development of severe MR in the presence of MVP.[51,53] (The other cause is rupture of the chordae tendineae.) Normally, the mitral annulus in adults averages about 9 cm in circumference. In patients with left ventricular dilatation from any cause, with or without MR, the mitral circumference usually dilates slightly, usually to about 11 cm or less than 25% above normal.[54] Among patients with MVP associated with severe MR, this annular circumference generally increases more than 50% to 12 to 18 cm. Acute rupture of chordae tendineae may occur in patients with MVP in the absence of mitral annular dilatation.
7. An increase in the transverse dimension of the mitral leaflets such that the length of the mitral circumference measured on a line corresponding to the distal margin of the posterior leaflet is much larger than the circumference measured at the level of the mitral annulus.[51] In the normal mitral valve, the two are the same. This feature is analogous to a skirt gathered at the waist. The leaflets of the opened normal mitral valve are flat or smooth on the atrial aspect (such as the mucosa of the ileum), whereas those of the opened floppy mitral valve are undulating (such as those of the duodenum or jejunum).
8. Focal thickening of mural endocardium of left ventricle behind the posterior mitral leaflet. Salazar and Edwards[55] called these fibrous thickenings "friction lesions" to indicate that they are believed to be the result from friction between the overlying leaflets and chordae and the underlying left ventricular wall. Lucas and Edwards[56] observed these friction lesions in 77 (75%) of 102 necropsy cases of MVP, and Dollar and Roberts[57] found them in 23 (68%) of 34 necropsy cases of MVP.
9. Fibrinous deposits on the atrial surface of the prolapsed portion of mitral leaflet and particularly at the angle formed between prolapsed leaflet and left atrial wall (mitral valve to left atrial angle). These fibrin deposits may be a source of emboli.

Histologically, the MVP valve is distinctive. With the use of elastic tissue stains, the mitral leaflet and chordae are surrounded by a single thick elastic fibril. The underlying leaflet generally, but not always, contains an excess amount of the spongiosa element, and this causes the leaflet itself to be a bit thicker than normal. Most of the leaflet thickening, however, is due to superimposed fibrous tissue on both its atrial and ventricular aspects. The covering on the atrial side of the leaflet contains numerous elastic fibers, whereas that on the

2

ventricular aspect contains few or no elastic fibrils. Often on the ventricular aspect previously ruptured and now "matted" chordae tendineae are covered by fibrous tissue. The spongiosa element within the leaflet itself appears normal, just increased in amount, and therefore the phrase "mucoid degeneration" seems to be inappropriate.

Ultrastructural studies of mitral valves grossly characteristic of MVP have disclosed alterations of the collagen fibers in the leaflets and in the chordae tendineae.[58] These changes have included fragmentation, splitting, swelling, and course granularity of the individual collagen fibers and also spiraling and twisting of the fibers. These alterations in the structure of the collagen are probably far more important than the excess acid mucopolysaccharide material in the leaflet in that they lead to focal weakness of the leaflets and chordae and their subsequent elongation. The left ventricular systolic pressure exerted against these weakened areas may account for the prolapse.

Just as the frequency of MVP varies clinically depending on the age and sex group being examined and the clinical criteria used for diagnosis (auscultatory, echocardiographic, or angiographic), its frequency at necropsy is quite variable, and the variation is determined by several factors: 1) age and sex group of the population being examined; 2) type of institution in which necropsy is performed (general hospital, referral hospital for cardiovascular disease, or medical examiner's [coroner's] office); 3) expertise in cardiovascular disease of the physician performing the necropsy or reporting the findings; 4) percentage of total deaths having autopsies at the particular hospital; 5) presence or absence of evidence of cardiac disease before death; 6) presence or absence of mitral valve replacement or repair; and 7) prevalence of Marfan syndrome, infective endocarditis, atrial septal defect, and so on.

No study shows better how bias alters the finding in necropsy studies than the one performed by Lucas and Edwards[56] (Table 2-9). These investigators, in one portion of their study, determined the frequency and complications of floppy mitral valves observed at necropsy in one community (nonreferral) hospital for adults. Of 1376 autopsies performed, 102 patients (7%) had morphologically floppy mitral valves at necropsy. Their mean age at death was 69 ± 12 years; 62 (61%) were men and 40 (39%) were women. Of the 102 patients, MVP was the cause of death in only 4. One leaflet had prolapsed in 34 patients and two leaflets in 68. Only 18 had anatomic evidence of previous MR, 7 had infective endocarditis, 7 had ruptured chordae tendineae (without infection), 1 had Marfan syndrome, and 3 had secundum atrial septal defect. No patient died suddenly. In contrast, in the other portion of their study, these authors described complications in 69 patients at necropsy whose hearts had been sent to Edwards for his opinion and interest. Among these 69 patients, 16 (23%) had died suddenly and unexpectedly, 19 (28%) had ruptured chordae tendineae (without infection), 7 (10%) had infective endocarditis, 20 (29%) had Marfan syndrome, and 9 (13%) had a secundum-type atrial septal defect. Thus, in contrast to their infrequency in their community hospital series, most patients submitted to their cardiovascular registry from other institutions had ruptured chordae, infective endocarditis, sudden unexpected and unexplained death, or Marfan syndrome.

The earlier studies by Pomerance[59] and by Davies and colleagues[60] can also be compared to the community hospital series of Lucas and Edwards[56] (see Table 2-9). The study by Dollar and Roberts[57] (see Table 2-9) is comparable to the study of Lucas and Edwards and their selected cases. These authors studied at necropsy 56 patients, aged 16 to 70 years (mean 48 years), and they compared findings in the 15 who died suddenly and unexpectedly with those for the other 41 who did not. Compared with the 34 patients without associated congenital heart disease and with non-MVP conditions

capable in themselves of being fatal, the 15 patients who died suddenly with isolated MVP were younger (mean age 39 years versus 52 years), were more often women (67% versus 26%), had a lower frequency of MR (7% versus 38%), and were less likely to have ruptured chordae tendineae (29% versus 67%).

The frequency of atrial fibrillation is different in patients with MVP and those with MS immediately before a mitral valve replacement or "repair." Among 246 patients aged 21 to 84 years (mean 61 years) (66% men) who had mitral valve repair or replacement for MR due to MVP, Berbarie and Roberts[61] found only 37 patients (15%) (mean 60) with atrial fibrillation and 209 patients (88%) with sinus rhythm. In contrast, of 104 patients, aged 33 to 80 years (12% men), with rheumatic MS severe enough or symptomatic enough to warrant MVP, Sims and Roberts[62] found atrial fibrillation by electrocardiogram immediately preoperatively in 47 (45%) and sinus rhythm in 57 (55%).

Another cause of pure MR is cleft anterior mitral leaflet. Partial atrioventricular "defect" includes a spectrum of five anatomic anomalies.[63] Some patients have all five and others have only one or two. The five are the following: 1) a defect in the lower portion of the atrial septum, the so-called primum atrial septal defect; 2) a defect in or absence of the posterobasal portion of the ventricular septum; 3) a cleft, anterior mitral leaflet; 4) an anomalous chordae tendineae from the anterior mitral leaflet to the crest of the ventricular septum; and 5) partial or complete absence of the septal tricuspid valve leaflet. There are at least four potential functional consequences of these five anatomic anomalies: 1) shunt at the atrial level, 2) shunt at the ventricular level, 3) MR, and 4) obstruction to left ventricular outflow. Well over 95% of patients with a partial atrioventricular defect have a primum-type atrial septal defect, and most of those without a primum defect have a shunt at the ventricular level. The occurrence of MR from a cleft in the anterior mitral leaflet unassociated with a defect in either the atrial or ventricular septa is rare, but this has been the case in several reported patients.[64]

Left-Sided Atrioventricular Valve Regurgitation Associated with Corrected Transposition of the Great Arteries

Corrected transposition is an entity that has produced much confusion.[65,66] Corrected transposition and complete transposition are quite different; the only thing they have in common is the word "transposition." Complete transposition is essentially one defect: The great arteries are transposed, so that the aorta arises from the right ventricle and the pulmonary trunk from the left ventricle. In corrected transposition, the great arteries also are transposed, but, in addition, the ventricles, atrioventricular valves, epicardial coronary arteries, and conduction system are inverted. Patients with complete transposition die because they have inadequate communications between the two circuits. Patients with corrected transposition theoretically should be able to live a full lifespan but usually this is not the case because associated defects, namely, ventricular septal defect or regurgitation of the left-sided atrioventricular valve or both, cause the heart to function abnormally. The left-sided valve anatomically is a tricuspid valve (in the case of the situs solitus heart) and its most frequent abnormality is the Ebstein-type abnormality (Figure 2-20). Although most patients with corrected transposition present with excessive pulmonary blood flow because of the left-to-right shunt via the ventricular septal defect, an occasional patient with corrected transposition has no defect in the cardiac septa and has evidence of pure "MR," occasionally mistaken for other causes of MR.[67]

TABLE 2–9 | **Reported Necropsy Cases of Mitral Valve Prolapse**

Authors	Year of Publication	No. with MVP	Ages (Years)	Male/Female	MVP Cause of Death	No. of Mitral Leaflets Prolapsed ½	MR	RCT	IE	SD	MS	ASD*	MAC	HW Increased	DMA
Pomerance	1969	35†	51-98 (mean 74)	23/12	4	12/23	8	2‡	2	1	0	1	9	13	—§
Davies et al.	1978	90¶	<40-100	44/46	6	69/21	23	—	9	13	0	0	3	8¶	6
Lucas and Edwards	1982	102**	69 ± 12	62/40	4	34/68	18	7‡	7	0	1	3	—	—	—
Lucas and Edwards	1982	69††	—	—	—	—	—	19‡	7	16	20	9	—	—	—
Dollar and Roberts	1991	56‡‡	16-70 (mean 48)	33/23	29	50/6	32	18‡	0	15	2	4	12	30‡‡	40

ASD, atrial septal defect; DMA, dilated mitral annulus; HW, heart weight; IE, infective endocarditis; MAC, mitral annular calcium; MR, mitral regurgitation; MS, Marfan syndrome; MVP, mitral valve prolapse; RCT, ruptured chordae tendineae; SD, sudden death.

*Secundum-type atrial septal defect.

†Thirty cases from a single hospital (1% of autopsies).

‡Unassociated with infective endocarditis.

§—, no information available.

¶Cases acquired from four different hospitals (4.5% of autopsies).

¶Heart weight >300 g.

**Cases seen in a single community hospital (7% of autopsies).

††Cases "whose hearts had been sent to Edwards or Roberts for his opinion and interest."

‡‡Heart weight >350 g in women and >400 g in men.

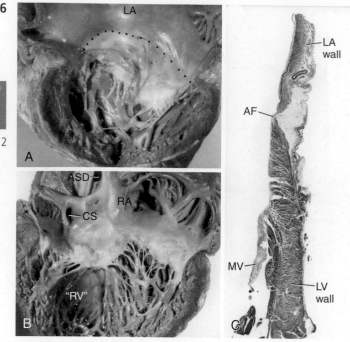

FIGURE 2–20 Corrected transposition of the great arteries and Ebstein's anomaly of the left-sided atrioventricular valve in a 38-year-old woman who was cyanotic from birth and in heart failure periodically all of her life. She also had severe pulmonic valve stenosis and ventricular septal defect. She died shortly after operative insertion of a conduit between the left subclavian and left main pulmonary arteries. **a**, Opened left atrium (LA) and anatomic right ventricle (RV). The normal annulus is shown by the dotted line. **b**, Opened right atrium (RA) and anatomic left ventricle (RV). ASD, atrial septal defect; CS, ostium of coronary sinus. **c**, Histologic section of left atrial (LA) and left ventricular (LV) walls showing the normal annulus fibrosis (AF) and insertion of the mitral valve (MV) considerably caudal to the annulus and directly from the ventricular wall. Verhoeff-von Gieson stain: ×4. *(From Berry WB, Roberts WC, Morrow AG, Braunwald E: Corrected transposition of the aorta and pulmonary trunk: Clinical, hemodynamic and pathologic findings. Am J Med 1964;36:35-53, with permission.)*

Infective Endocarditis

The most common cardiac valve affected by infective endocarditis is the aortic valve, and the mitral valve is most commonly affected by vegetations growing down the anterior mitral leaflet from the regurgitant aortic valve causing mitral leaflet damage and chordal rupture.[68,69] Infection isolated to the mitral valve is far less common, and when this situation occurs the vegetations are on the atrial aspects of the mitral leaflets.[70]

Coronary Heart Disease

MR in patients with coronary heart disease is due to myocardial infarction, which may acutely cause necrosis of one or more left ventricular papillary muscles (usually the posteromedial one) with or without rupture of the entire muscle or, far more commonly, rupture of a portion of the "tip" of the papillary muscle[37,71-72] (Figure 2-21). Rupture, either partial or complete, of a papillary muscle during acute myocardial infarction is far less common a cause of acute MR than is necrosis of a papillary muscle and the free wall beneath it. When it occurs late after acute myocardial infarction, the MR is usually the result of dilatation of the left ventricular cavity and severe scarring of a papillary muscle, which tends to pull the mitral leaflets laterally, preventing proper coaptation of the two mitral leaflets during ventricular systole.

Cardiomyopathy

Most patients with idiopathic dilated cardiomyopathy,[73] ischemic cardiomyopathy,[74,75] and hypertrophic cardiomyopathy[76] have MR at some time in the course of their condition. The first two conditions are associated with dilatation of the left ventricular cavity primarily in a lateral or right-to-left direction, not a caudal-cephalad direction, and the consequence is abnormal papillary muscle "pull" on the

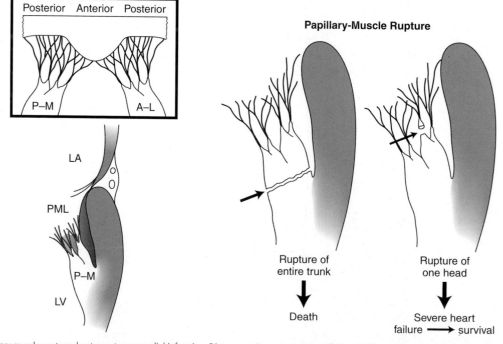

FIGURE 2–21 Papillary muscle rupture due to acute myocardial infarction. Diagrammatic representation of the possible consequences of papillary muscle rupture during acute myocardial infarction. Rupture of the entire trunk is incompatible with survival (*left*). With rupture of an apical "head" (*right*), survival depends on the extent to which function of the left ventricle has been impaired by the infarct. With severely impaired left ventricular function, the additional burden of even modest mitral regurgitation may be intolerable. If the left ventricle is less severely compromised, survival is possible for weeks or months, but heart failure will almost invariably develop. *(From Morrow AG, Cohen LS, Roberts WS, et al: Severe mitral regurgitation following acute myocardial infarction and ruptured papillary muscle: Hemodynamic findings and results of operative treatment in four patients. Circulation 1968;37:II-124-II-132, with permission.)*

mitral leaflets during ventricular systole with resulting incomplete coaptation of the mitral leaflets. Evidence that mitral annulus dilation is the prime cause of MR in patients with dilated cardiomyopathy is lacking.[54] The cause of MR in patients with hypertrophic cardiomyopathy is entirely different from that in patients with dilated cardiomyopathy and results at least in part in anterior movement of the anterior mitral leaflet toward the ventricular septum during ventricular systole.[76] Patients with chronic anemia, e.g., sickle cell anemia, usually also have MR from papillary muscle fibrosis and left ventricular cavity dilatation.[77]

Tricuspid Valve Disease

Tricuspid Regurgitation

The most common cause of pure tricuspid regurgitation (TR) is dilation of the right ventricular cavity from any cause, with the most common being left ventricular dilatation followed by parenchymal lung disease. In contrast with mitral annular dilatation, which is severe only in patients with MVP, tricuspid annular dilatation is by far the most common cause of TR. The tricuspid valve is the only cardiac valve with a true annulus bordering its entire circumference, whereas the mitral valve has a true annulus only for its posterior leaflet and its anterior leaflet is braced, so to speak, by its connection to ascending aorta. Usually patients with functional TR also have functional MR because both ventricular cavities are so commonly dilated together.

Infective endocarditis on the right side of the heart usually (90%) attacks the tricuspid valve and TR may be the consequence.[78] Operative treatment of active infective endocarditis involving the tricuspid valve has initially been total tricuspid valve excision (to remove the source of infective pulmonary emboli) with later valve replacement.[79]

Tricuspid Valve Stenosis

This hemodynamic lesion is rare and probably still is most commonly the result of rheumatic heart disease. If the tricuspid valve is made stenotic on the basis of rheumatic heart disease, the mitral valve is always stenotic also and never purely regurgitant.[1] Carcinoid heart disease affects the right side of the heart by producing pulmonic stenosis and usually pure TR (although some degree of tricuspid stenosis may occur as well).[80,81] The combination of pulmonic stenosis and tricuspid regurgitation usually results in considerable heart failure, and, indeed, a good experimental method to produce right-sided heart failure is to place a tight band on the pulmonary trunk ("pulmonic stenosis") and partially destroy the tricuspid valve by a surgical instrument ("tricuspid regurgitation"). This combination is seen in carcinoid heart disease.[80,81] On rare occasions a tumor or vegetation has produced tricuspid valve obstruction.[46]

Pulmonic Valve

Pulmonic stenosis is usually the result of congenital heart disease, either isolated or associated with one or more other major cardiovascular congenital defects.[33] In isolated pulmonic stenosis the valve is usually acommissural unicuspid with a central very stenotic orifice. These valves by adulthood collect calcific deposits on their ventricular aspect rather than on the arterial aspect as occurs with the left-sided semilunar valve. In a rare patient with rheumatic heart disease, pulmonic stenosis has occurred. In this circumstance all four cardiac valves have been affected. Tumors in the right ventricular outflow tract or pulmonary trunk also have produced "pulmonic stenosis."[82] Pulmonic regurgitation is usually of iatrogenic origin.

1. Roberts WC: Congenital cardiovascular abnormalities usually silent until adulthood. In Roberts WC (ed): Adult Congenital Heart Disease. Philadelphia, FA Davis, 1987, pp 631–691.
2. Sprecher DL, Schaefer EJ, Kent KM, et al: Cardiovascular features of homozygous familial hypercholesterolemia: analysis of 16 patients. Am J Cardiol 1984; 54:20-30.
3. Moura LM, Ramos SF, Zamorano JL: Rosuvastati affecting aortic valve endothelium to slow the progression of aortic stenosis. J Am Coll Cardiol 2007; 49:554-561.
4. Roberts WC, Perloff JK, Costantino T: Severe valvular aortic stenosis in patients over 65 years of age: A clinicopathologic study. Am J Cardiol 1971; 27:497-506.
5. Stephan PJ, Henry AC III, Hebeler RF Jr: Comparison of age, gender, number of aortic valve cusps, concomitant coronary artery bypass grafting, and magnitude of left ventricular-systemic arterial peak systolic gradient in adults having aortic valve replacement for isolated aortic valve stenosis. Am J Cardiol 1997; 79:166-172.
6. Roberts WC, Morrow AG: Congenital aortic stenosis produced by a unicommissural valve. Br Heart J 1965; 27:505-510.
7. Falcone MW, Roberts WC, Morrow AG, Perloff JK: Congenital aortic stenosis resulting from unicommissural valve: Clinical and anatomic features in twenty-one adult patients. Circulation 1971; 44:272-280.
8. Roberts WC: The congenitally bicuspid aortic valve: A study of 85 autopsy cases. Am J Cardiol 1970; 26:72-83.
9. Roberts WC: Anatomically isolated aortic valvular disease. The case against its being of rheumatic etiology. Am J Med 1970; 49:151-159.
10. Roberts WC, Ko JM: Clinical and morphologic features of the congenitally unicuspid acommissural stenotic and regurgitant aortic valve. Cardiology 2007; 108:79-81.
11. Hurwitz LE, Roberts WC: Quadricuspid semilunar valve. Am J Cardiol 1973; 31: 623-626.
12. Roberts WC, Ko JM, Filardo C, et al: Valve structure and survival in sexagenarians having aortic valve replacement for aortic stenosis (±aortic regurgitation) with versus without coronary artery bypass grafting at a single US medical center (1993 to 2005). Am J Cardiol 2007; 100:1287-1292.
13. Roberts WC, Ko JM: Weights of operatively-excised stenotic unicuspid, bicuspid, and tricuspid aortic valves and their relation to age, sex, body mass index, and presence or absence of concomitant coronary artery bypass grafting. Am J Cardiol 2003; 92:1057-1065.
14. Roberts WC, Ko JM: Weights of individual cusps in operatively-excised stenotic congenitally bicuspid aortic valves. Am J Cardiol 2004; 94:678-681.
15. Roberts WC, Ko JM: Weights of individual cusps in operatively-excised stenotic congenitally three-cuspid aortic valves. Am J Cardiol 2004; 94:681-684.
16. Roberts WC, Ko JM: Relation of weights of operatively excised stenotic aortic valves to preoperative transvalvular peak systolic pressure gradients and to calculated aortic valve areas. J Am Coll Cardiol 2004; 44:1847-1855.
17. Roberts WC, Ko JM: Frequency by decade of unicuspid, bicuspid, and tricuspid aortic valves in adults having isolated aortic valve replacement for aortic stenosis, with or without associated aortic regurgitation. Circulation 2005; 111:920-925.
18. Roberts WC, Ko JM, Matter GJ: Isolated aortic valve replacement without coronary bypass for aortic valve stenosis involving a congenitally bicuspid aortic valve in a nonagenarian. Am J Geriatr Cardiol 2006; 15:389-391.
19. Roberts WC, Ko JM, Garner WL, et al: Valve structure and survival in octogenarians having aortic valve replacement for aortic stenosis (±aortic regurgitation) with versus without coronary artery bypass grafting at a single US medical center (1993-2005). Am J Cardiol 2007; 100:489-498.
20. Roberts WC, Ko JM, Filardo G, et al: Valve structure and survival in septuagenarians having aortic valve replacement for aortic stenosis (±aortic regurgitation) with versus without coronary artery bypass grafting at a single US medical center (1993-2005). Am J Cardiol 2007; 100:1157-1165.
21. Roberts WC, Ko JM, Hamilton C: Comparison of valve structure, valve weight, and severity of the valve obstruction in 1849 patients having isolated aortic valve replacement for aortic valve stenosis (with or without aortic regurgitation) studied at 3 different medical centers in 2 different time periods. Circulation 2005; 112:3919-3929.
22. Roberts WC, Ko JM, Filardo G, et al: Valve structure and survival in quinquagenarians having aortic valve replacement for aortic stenosis (±aortic regurgitation) with versus without coronary artery bypass grafting at a single US medical center (1993 to 2005). Am J Cardiol 2007; 100:1584-1591.
23. Roberts WC, Ko JM, Filardo G, et al: Valve structure and survival in quadragenarians having aortic valve replacement for aortic stenosis (±aortic regurgitation) with versus without coronary artery bypass grafting at a single US medical center (1993 to 2005). Am J Cardiol 2007; 100:1683-1690.
24. Roberts WC, Ko JM, Moore TR, Jones WH III: Causes of pure aortic regurgitation in patients having isolated aortic valve replacement at a single US tertiary hospital (1993-2005). Circulation 2006; 114:422-429.
25. Roberts WC: The structure of the aortic valve in clinically-isolated aortic stenosis: An autopsy study of 162 patients over 15 years of age. Circulation 1970; 42:91-97.
26. Roberts WC, Morrow AG, McIntosh CL, et al: Congenitally bicuspid aortic valve causing severe, pure aortic regurgitation without superimposed infective endocarditis: Analysis of 13 patients requiring aortic valve replacement. Am J Cardiol 1981; 47:206-209.
27. Roberts WC, Oluwole BO, Fernicola DJ: Comparison of active infective endocarditis involving a previously stenotic versus a previously nonstenotic aortic valve. Am J Cardiol 1993; 71:1082-1088.
28. Carpenter DF, Golden A, Roberts WC: Quadrivalvular rheumatoid heart disease associated with left bundle branch block. Am J Med 1967; 43:922-929.
29. Roberts WC, Kehoe JA, Carpenter DF, Golden A: Cardiac valvular lesions in rheumatoid arthritis. Arch Intern Med 1968; 122:141-146.
30. Waller BF, Zoltick JM, Rosen JH, et al: Severe aortic regurgitation from systemic hypertension (without aortic dissection) requiring aortic valve replacement: Analysis of four patients. Am J Cardiol 1982; 49:473-477.

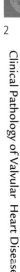

31. Waller BF, Kishel JC, Roberts WC: Severe aortic regurgitation from systemic hypertension. Chest 1982; 82:365-368.

32. Roberts WC: Aortic dissection: anatomy, consequences, and causes. Am Heart J 1981; 101:195-214.

33. Roberts WC, Dangel JC, Bulkley BH: Non-rheumatic valvular cardiac disease: A clinicopathologic survey of 27 different conditions causing valvular dysfunction. Cardiovasc Clin 1973; 5:333-446.

34. Roberts WC, Honig HS: The spectrum of cardiovascular disease in the Marfan syndrome: A clinico-morphologic study of 18 necropsy patients and comparison to 151 previously reported necropsy patients. Am Heart J 1982; 104:115-135.

35. Bulkley BH, Roberts WC: Ankylosing spondylitis and aortic regurgitation: Description of the characteristic cardiovascular lesion from study of eight necropsy patients. Circulation 1973; 48:1014-1027.

36. Roberts WC, Hollingsworth JF, Bulkley BH, et al: Combined mitral and aortic regurgitation in ankylosing spondylitis: Angiographic and anatomic features. Am J Med 1974; 56:237-243.

37. Roberts WC, Perloff JK: Mitral valvular disease: A clinicopathologic survey of the conditions causing the mitral valve to function abnormally. Ann Intern Med 1972; 77:939-975.

38. Roberts WC: Morphologic features of the normal and abnormal mitral valve. Am J Cardiol 1983; 51:1005-1028.

39. Roberts WC, Virmani R: Aschoff bodies at necropsy in valvular heart disease: Evidence from an analysis of 543 patients over 14 years of age that rheumatic heart disease at least anatomically, is a disease of the mitral valve. Circulation 1978; 57:803-807.

40. Virmani R, Roberts WC: Aschoff bodies in operatively excised atrial appendages and in papillary muscles: Frequency and clinical significance. Circulation 1977; 55:559-563.

41. Lachman AS, Roberts WC: Calcific deposits in stenotic mitral valves: Extent and relation to age, sex, degree of stenosis, cardiac rhythm, previous commissurotomy and left atrial body thrombus from study of 164 operatively-excised valves. Circulation 1978; 57:808-815.

42. Roberts WC, Lachman AS: Mitral valve commissurotomy versus replacement: Considerations based on examination of operatively excised stenotic mitral valves. Am Heart J 1979; 98:56-62.

43. Roberts WC, Humphries JO, Morrow AG: Giant right atrium in rheumatic mitral stenosis: Atrial enlargement restricted by mural calcification. Am Heart J 1970; 79:28-35.

44. Hammer WJ, Roberts WC, de Leon AC Jr: "Mitral stenosis" secondary to combined "massive" mitral annular calcific deposits and small, hypertrophied left ventricles. Am J Med 1978; 64:371-376.

45. Theleman KP, Grayburn PA, Roberts WC: Mitral "annular" calcium forming a complete circle "O" causing mitral stenosis in association with a stenotic congenitally bicuspid aortic valve and severe coronary artery disease. Am J Geriatr Cardiol 2006; 15:58-61.

46. Roberts WC: Neoplasms involving the heart, their simulators, and adverse consequences of their therapy. Proc (Bayl Univ Med Cent) 2001; 14:358-376.

47. Roberts WC, Ewy GA, Glancy DL, Marcus FI: Valvular stenosis produced by active infective endocarditis. Circulation 1967; 36:449-451.

48. Roberts WC, Bulkley BH, Morrow AG: Pathologic anatomy of cardiac valve replacement: A study of 224 necropsy patients. *Prog Cardiovasc Dis* 1973; 15:539-587.

49. Barlow JB, Pocock WA, Marchand P, Denny M: The significance of late systolic murmurs: Am Heart J 1963; 66:443-452.

50. Criley JM, Lewis KB, Humphries JO, Ross RS: Prolapse of the mitral valve: Clinical and cine-angiocardiographic finding. *Br Heart J* 1966; 28:488-496.

51. Waller BJ, Morrow AG, Maron BJ, et al: Etiology of clinically isolated, severe, chronic, pure mitral regurgitation: Analysis of 97 patients over 30 years of age having mitral valve replacement. Am Heart J 1982; 104:276-288.

52. Roberts WC, Braunwald E, Morrow AG: Acute severe mitral regurgitation secondary to ruptured chordae tendineae: Clinical, hemodynamic, and pathologic considerations. Circulation 1966; 33:58-70.

53. Roberts WC, McIntosh CL, Wallace RB: Mechanisms of severe mitral regurgitation in mitral valve prolapse determined from analysis of operatively excised valves. Am Heart J 1987; 113:1316-1323.

54. Bulkley BH, Roberts WC: Dilatation of the mitral anulus: A rare cause of mitral regurgitation. Am J Med 1975; 59:457-463.

55. Salazar AE, Edwards JE: Friction lesions of ventricular endocardium: Relation to chordae tendineae of mitral valve. Arch Pathol 1970; 90:364-376.

56. Lucas RV Jr, Edwards JE: The floppy mitral valve. Curr Probl Cardiol 1982; 7(4):1-48.

57. Dollar AL, Roberts WC: Morphologic comparison of patients with mitral valve prolapse who died suddenly with patients who died from severe valvular dysfunction or other conditions. J Am Coll Cardiol 1991; 17:921-931.

58. Renteria VG, Ferrans VJ, Jones M, Roberts WC: Intracellular collagen fibrils in prolapsed ("floppy") human atrioventricular valves. Lab Invest 1976; 35:439-443.

59. Pomerance A: Ballooning deformity (mucoid degeneration) of atrioventricular valves. Br Heart J 1969; 31:343-351.

60. Davies MJ, Moore BP, Braimbridge MV: The floppy mitral valve: Study of incidence, pathology and complications in surgical, necropsy, and forensic material. Br Heart J 1978; 40:468-481.

61. Berbarie RF, Roberts WC: Frequency of atrial fibrillation in patients having mitral valve repair or replacement for pure mitral regurgitation secondary to mitral valve prolapse. Am J Cardiol 2006; 97:1039-1044.

62. Sims JB, Roberts WC: Comparison of findings in patients with vs. without atrial fibrillation just before isolated mitral valve replacement for rheumatic mitral stenosis (with or without associated mitral regurgitation). Am J Cardiol 2006; 97:1035-1038.

63. Braunwald E, Ross RS, Morrow AG, Roberts WC: Differential diagnosis of mitral regurgitation in childhood: Clinical pathological conference at the National Institutes of Health. Ann Intern Med 1961; 54:223-1242.

64. Barth CW III, Dibdin JD, Roberts WC: Mitral valve cleft without cardiac septal defect causing severe mitral regurgitation but allowing long survival. Am J Cardiol 1985; 55:1129-1231.

65. Schiebler GL, Edwards JE, Burchell HB, et al Congenital corrected transposition of the great vessels: A study of 33 cases. Pediatrics 1961; 27(Suppl):851-888.

66. Berry WB, Roberts WC, Morrow AG, Braunwald E: Corrected transposition of the aorta and pulmonary trunk: Clinical, hemodynamic and pathologic findings. Am J Med 1964; 36:35-53.

67. Roberts WC, Ross RS, Davis FW Jr: Congenital corrected transposition of the great vessels in adulthood simulating rheumatic valvular disease. Bull Johns Hopkins Hosp 1964; 114:157-172.

68. Buchbinder NA, Roberts WC: Left-sided valvular active infective endocarditis: A study of forty-five necropsy patients. Am J Med 1972; 53:20-35.

69. Arnett EN, Roberts WC: Active infective endocarditis: A clinicopathology analysis of 137 necropsy patients. Curr Probl Cardiol 1976; 1:1-76.

70. Fernicola DJ, Roberts WC: Clinicopathologic features of active infective endocarditis isolated to the mitral valve. Am J Cardiol 1993; 71:1186-1197.

71. Morrow AG, Cohen LS, Roberts WC, et al:. Severe mitral regurgitation following acute myocardial infarction and ruptured papillary muscle: Hemodynamic findings and results of operative treatment in four patients. Circulation 1968; 37(Suppl II):124-132.

72. Barbour DJ, Roberts WC: Rupture of a left ventricular papillary muscle during acute myocardial infarction: analysis of 22 necropsy patients. J Am Coll Cardiol 1986; 8:558-565.

73. Roberts WC, Siegel RJ, McManus BM: Idiopathic dilated cardiomyopathy: Analysis of 152 necropsy patients. Am J Cardiol 1987; 60:1340-1355.

74. Virmani R, Roberts WC: Quantification of coronary arterial narrowing and of left ventricular myocardial scarring in healed myocardial infarction with chronic eventually fatal, congestive cardiac failure. Am J Med 1980; 68:831-838.

75. Ross EM, Roberts WC: Severe atherosclerotic coronary arterial narrowing and chronic congestive heart failure without myocardial infarction: analysis of 18 patients studied at necropsy. Am J Cardiol 1986; 57:51-56.

76. Klues HG, Maron BJ, Dollar AL, Roberts WC: Diversity of structural mitral valve alterations in hypertrophic cardiomyopathy. Circulation 1992; 85:1651-1660.

77. Berezowski K, Roberts WC: Scarring of the left ventricular papillary muscles in sickle-cell disease. Am J Cardiol 1992; 70:1368-1370.

78. Roberts WC, Buchbinder NA: Right-sided valvular infective endocarditis: A clinicopathologic study of twelve necropsy patients. Am J Med 1972; 53:7-19.

79. Barbour DJ, Roberts WC: Valve excision only versus valve excision plus replacement for active infective endocarditis involving the tricuspid valve. Am J Cardiol 1986; 57:475-481.

80. Roberts WC, Sjoerdsma A: The cardiac disease associated with the carcinoid syndrome (carcinoid heart disease). Am J Med 1964; 36:5-34.

81. Ross EM, Roberts WC: The carcinoid syndrome: comparison of 21 necropsy subjects with carcinoid heart disease to 15 necropsy subjects without carcinoid heart disease. Am J Med 1985; 79:339-354.

82. Shmookler BM, Marsh HB, Roberts WC: Primary sarcoma of the pulmonary trunk and/or right or left main pulmonary artery: A rare cause of obstruction to right ventricular outflow. Report on two patients and analysis of 35 previously described patients. Am J Med 1977; 63:263-272.

Cellular, Molecular, and Genetic Mechanisms of Valvular Heart Disease

Nalini Marie Rajamannan

KEY POINTS

- Recent studies have shown that myxomatous mitral valve disease has an associated cartilage phenotype.
- Rheumatic valve disease is characterized by an inflammatory cellular process that has an associated osteoblast phenotype.
- Aortic valve calcification develops due to an active cellular biologic process with an osteoblast-like calcification process.
- Epidemiologic studies have demonstrated parallel clinical risk factors for aortic valve disease that are similar to those for vascular atherosclerosis.
- Experimental hypercholesterolemia in vivo models have elucidated a number of cellular processes important in the development of calcific valve disease.

In the last decade, a number of studies have transformed our understanding of the cellular biology of diseases affecting the heart valve. Several studies demonstrated a correlation between atherosclerosis risk factors and degenerative aortic valve and mitral valve disease. Although a unifying hypothesis for the role of atherosclerotic risk factors in the mechanism of vascular and aortic valve disease is emerging, progress in studying the cell biology of this disease has been limited in the past because of the paucity of experimental models available. This chapter reviews the cellular pathways and emerging experimental models important in the understanding of the most common valvular heart disorders: myxomatous mitral valve disease, rheumatic heart valve disease, and calcific aortic stenosis. Bicuspid aortic valve disease is discussed in Chapter 11.

MYXOMATOUS MITRAL VALVE DISEASE

Myxomatous "degenerative" mitral valve disease is associated with abnormal movement of the leaflets into the left atrium during systole due to inadequate chordal support (elongation or rupture) and excessive valvular tissue.

There is a spectrum of pathologic changes ranging from mild leaflet thickening and redundancy to a marked increase in valve area and length with secondary rupture of chordae (Figure 3-1). Annular myxomatous changes may lead to dilation and calcification of the annulus. The valve leaflets appear thickened with a white appearance along the atrial surface. This lesion has various clinical presentations including prolapse, retraction, and redundancy of the leaflet. Over the past decade, there have been many descriptions of mitral valve disease: myxomatous mitral valve disease, Barlow's syndrome, and fibroelastic deficiency. The reported differences between these various types of valve lesions are the degree of leaflet redundancy and matrix composition of each leaflet. Over time progressive regurgitation commonly develops, suggesting that these types of mitral valve disease represent a continuum of the same underlying cellular disorder with variable clinical presentations, depending on the associated factors in each individual patient. Most patients present with slow and gradual progression of the disease process resulting from slow thickening of the valve leaflets. Chordal rupture develops in a subset of patients, leading to a more rapid increase in the severity of mitral regurgitation. Further understanding of cellular biology of myxomatous mitral valve disease will provide insight into its different presentations.

Histologic Findings

The basic microscopic feature of primary mitral valve prolapse is marked proliferation of the interstitial cells and deposition of mucopolysaccharides and glycosaminoglycans in the spongiosa, the delicate connective tissue between the atrialis (a thick layer of collagen and elastic tissue forming the atrial aspect of the leaflet) and the fibrosis, or ventricularis, which is composed of dense layers of collagen and forms the basic support of the leaflet.[1] In primary mitral valve prolapse, an increase in the synthesis of acid mucopolysaccharides and glycosaminoglycans containing spongiosa tissue causes focal interruption of the fibrosa. In Figure 3-2, the cells present

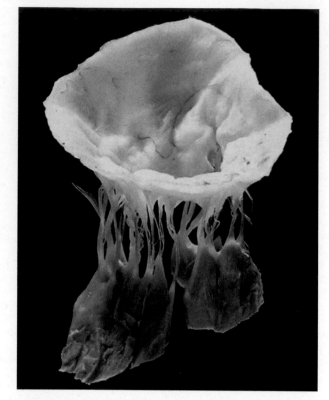

FIGURE 3–1 Photograph of myxomatous mitral valve and chordae tendineae, demonstrating the redundant thickened mitral valve leaflets and cartilaginous thickening along the atrial surface of the mitral valve. *(From Willerson JT, Cohn JN, McAllister HA, et al (Eds): Atlas of Valvular Heart Disease: Clinical and Pathologic Aspects. New York, Churchill Livingstone, 1998, with permission.)*

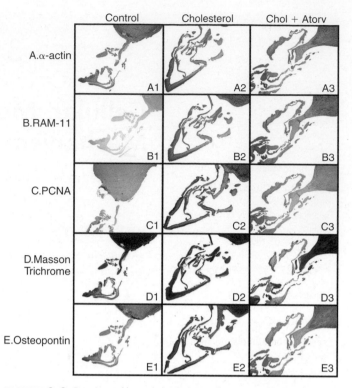

FIGURE 3–3 Experimental hypercholesterolemia effects on the mitral valve of New Zealand rabbits showing control versus cholesterol versus atorvastatin effects on the mitral valve. **A,** α-Actin. **B,** Ram-11 (macrophage stain). **C,** Proliferating cell nuclear antigen (PCNA). **D,** Masson trichrome stain. **E,** Osteopontin. *(From Makkena B, Salti H, Subramaniam M, et al: Atorvastatin decreases cellular proliferation and bone matrix expression in the hypercholesterolemic mitral valve. J Am Coll Cardiol 2005;45:631-633, with permission.)*

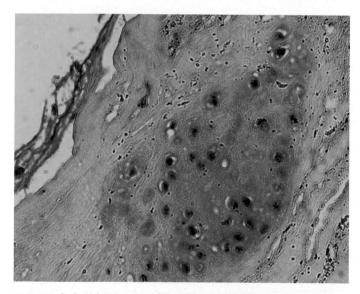

FIGURE 3–2 Light microscopy of Alcian blue stain demonstrating hypertrophic chondrocytes in myxomatous mitral valve. Alcian blue stain is specific for cartilaginous tissue. The stain is a phthalocyanine dye that contains copper and stains acid mucopolysaccharides and glycosaminoglycans.

Experimental Models of Mitral Valve Disease

Experimental models[5,6] of mitral valve disease show an active, complex process that can be triggered by hypercholesterolemia. These models demonstrate parallel mechanisms in the aortic and mitral valves involving endothelial abnormalities, macrophage infiltration, myofibroblast cell proliferation, and osteopontin expression due to hypercholesterolemia. Moreover, this process may be modified by atorvastatin (Figure 3-3) in the mitral as well as the aortic valve.[5] Osteopontin is found in active skeletal metabolism and is present in the differentiation process that results in valvular heart disease[7] with upregulation of both gene expression and synthesis of these skeletal bone matrix proteins. Osteopontin is an extracellular matrix protein that has multiple functions. It is important in cellular adhesion and matrix binding. Further studies are necessary to determine the cellular mechanisms important in the development of mitral valve disease. These early findings raise the intriguing question of whether cholesterol levels are a clinical risk factor for development of mitral valve disease and whether medical treatment might slow disease progression.

RHEUMATIC VALVE DISEASE

Rheumatic disease is the most common cause of valvular heart disease in developing countries. Improvement in living standards and the aggressive treatment of penicillin-sensitive group A β-hemolytic *Streptococcus* are changing the epidemiology of rheumatic valve disease throughout the world. In 1924, Dr. Carey Coombs wrote the first textbook on rheumatic heart disease, describing the inflammatory lesion in the rheumatic valve leaflet and the presence of new vessels within the

in the center of the mitral valve leaflet are consistent with hypertrophic chondrocyte cells; these differentiated cells are responsible for the synthesis of glycosaminoglycans.[2,3] Over time the myofibroblast cells differentiate into chondrocytes. In addition, several studies have demonstrated that cartilage is present in this tissue and that cartilaginous thickening contributes to the disease process.[1,2,4]

cellular architecture of the valve leaflet.[8] The Jones criteria, which were developed in the 1940s to help characterize the disease process, have been revised over time and are still being used today (see Table 8-2). Acute rheumatic fever is characterized by exudative and proliferative inflammatory lesions of the connective tissue, primarily in the heart, joints, and subcutaneous tissue. When carditis ensues, all layers of the heart are involved. Pericarditis is common, and fibrinous pericarditis is occasionally present. The pericardial inflammation usually resolves over time with no clinically significant sequelae, and tamponade is rare. In fatal cases, myocardial involvement leads to enlargement involving all four chambers of the heart. In the myocardium, initially there is fragmentation of collagen fibers, lymphocytic infiltration, and fibrinoid degeneration. These are followed by the appearance of Aschoff nodules, which are considered pathognomic of acute rheumatic fever.

Endocardial involvement is responsible for chronic rheumatic valvulitis. Small, fibrinous vegetations (1 to 2 mm in diameter) are found on the atrial surface at sites of valve coaptation and on the chordae tendineae. Over time, thickening and fibrosis develop in the valve leaflet and fusion of the chordae results in stenosis and/or regurgitation. The valvulitis that develops results in mitral regurgitation with a blowing holosystolic murmur best heard at the apex and radiating to the axilla and occasionally to the base of the heart or the back. Over time, mitral stenosis can develop, and the classic diastolic rumble is heard across the mitral valve. In the aortic valve position, a diastolic murmur develops across the regurgitant aortic valve.

The histopathologic lesions of the valve are specified for rheumatic carditis, with Aschoff bodies, nonspecific edema, and leukocyte infiltration.[9] More recently, studies have demonstrated that superimposed calcification and fibrosis are associated with a bone formation process.[10] In addition, there is prominent neo-vascularization. The mechanism for new vessel formation or angiogenesis is expression of vascular endothelial growth factor. Vascular endothelial growth factor is localized to inflammatory cells in the regions of the valve fibrosis, specifically the macrophages and myofibroblasts (Figure 3-4).[10] At the cellular level, there is a more intense inflammatory infiltrate found in rheumatic valves compared with degenerative aortic stenosis or degenerative mitral valve disease. However, the fundamental bone-like phenotype is present in both calcific and rheumatic aortic valve disease. These findings suggest that rheumatic valve disease is also an active biologic process or, more likely, that calcific valve disease is superimposed on chronic rheumatic valve disease.

CALCIFIC AORTIC STENOSIS

The most common causes of aortic valve stenosis are rheumatic disease, calcification of a congenital bicuspid valve, and calcific changes of a normal trileaflet valve. Rare causes of aortic stenosis include Paget's disease, renal failure, drugs (including methysergide[11] and fenfluramine-phentermine)[12], familial hypercholesterolemia, systemic lupus erythematosus, radiation, and ochronosis.[13]

Epidemiologic and experimental data support the hypothesis that calcific aortic stenosis is not a passive phenomena but an active cellular biologic process that develops within the valve leaflet. Vascular atherosclerosis was also once thought to be a degenerative process but is now recognized to be an active biologic process that can be targeted with medical therapy. A similar phenomenon has occurred in our understanding of aortic valve disease. Growing evidence points toward a "response to injury" mechanism for the etiology of degenerative calcific aortic valve disease, similar to what has been described for vascular atherosclerosis. The hallmark of end-stage aortic stenosis is calcification (Figure 3-5),[14] which occurs predominantly on the aortic surface of the valve.

Aortic Valve Histology

Histologically, the normal aortic valve is composed of three layers—the fibrosa, the spongiosa, and the ventricularis—and both sides of the valve are covered with an endothelial surface.[15] The interstitial myofibroblast cells,[16] which reside below the endothelial surface, are important in maintaining the physical architecture of the valve tissue.

Genetics of Aortic Valve Disease

Several studies have provided evidence for a genetic predisposition for aortic valve disease (Table 3-1). Some of these studies have used a case-control approach to study genetic polymorphisms in candidate genes including apolipoproteins[17,18] and the vitamin D receptor.[19,20] One case-control study showed that the B allele of the vitamin D receptor is more common in patients with calcific aortic valve stenosis.[19] The frequency of allele penetrance was compared in 100 adults with aortic stenosis and 100 adults without aortic stenosis who were undergoing coronary angiography. In the aortic stenosis group, the frequency for the B allele was 0.54, and for the b allele frequency was 0.46: 24 patients were homozygous for the B allele, 15 patients were homozygous for the b allele, and 61 patients were heterozygous. Compared to the control group, the B allele frequency was 27% higher in the case group. Interestingly, the B allele also predisposes carriers to a decrease in calcium absorption and therefore an increase in bone loss. Therefore, the association of the Vitamin D receptor B allele with calcific aortic stenosis suggests a link between abnormal regulation of vitamin D metabolism, abnormalities in bone metabolism and an increased occurrence of calcific aortic stenosis.

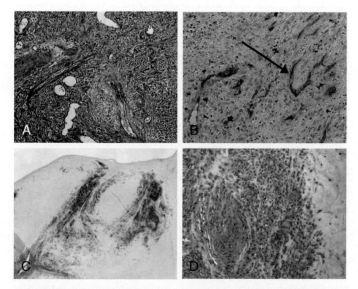

FIGURE 3–4 Immunohistochemistry vascular endothelial growth factor and bone markers staining in rheumatic calcified heart valves. **A,** Masson trichrome stain. **B,** Vascular endothelial growth factor (VEGF). **C,** Alizarin red stain. **D,** osteocalcin. *(From Rajamannan NM, Nealis TB, Subramaniam M, et al: Calcified rheumatic valve neoangiogenesis is associated with vascular endothelial growth factor expression and osteoblast-like bone formation. Circulation 2005;111:3296-3301, with permission.)*

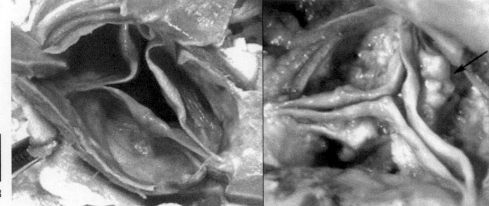

FIGURE 3–5 Photograph of normal (*left*) versus diseased (*right*) aortic valve, demonstrating marked calcification along the aortic surface of the aortic valve. (*From Freeman RV, Otto CM: Spectrum of calcific aortic valve disease: pathogenesis, disease progression, and treatment strategies. Circulation 2005;111:3316-3326, with permission.*)

TABLE 3–1	Genetic Studies of Calcific Aortic Stenosis	
Gene	**First Author (Year)**	**Reference**
Vitamin D receptor	Ortlepp (2001)	19
Apolipoproteins AI, B, and E	Avakian (2001)	17
Estrogen receptor alpha	Nordstrom (2003)	20
Apolipoprotein E	Novaro (2003)	18
Interleukin 10, connective tissue growth factor, CR5	Ortlepp (2001)	21
Notch1	Garg (2005)	22

Another genetic study identified *Pvull* polymorphisms in the estrogen receptor α gene.[21] These investigators found a correlation between polymorphism in the estrogen receptor and an increased prevalence of aortic stenosis in postmenopausal woman. They also demonstrated that the polymorphism is associated with elevated lipid levels in adolescent patients. The increased prevalence of the disease in postmenopausal women with this polymorphism in the estrogen receptor and the physiologic lack of estrogen is a novel finding that parallels the hypothesis that postmenopausal women have an increased incidence of vascular atherosclerosis. This discovery defines the importance of gender and hormonal effects in conjunction with the lipid risk factor playing a role in the development of calcific aortic stenosis.

In family studies of large kindreds with inherited valve and congenital disease, a mutation in the *Notch1* receptor was associated with bicuspid aortic valve disease, calcific aortic stenosis,[22] and other congenital heart conditions. *Notch1* plays a roll in cellular differentiation and, in it serves as an inhibitor of osteoblast differentiation.[23,24] The results from the genetic study suggest that mutations in *Notch1* result in a lack of inhibition of calcification, which may play a role in the rapid progression of calcification. The *Notch1* signaling pathway also is critical in embryonic development explaining why this mutation leads to development of congenital heart defects. Four Notch receptors have been identified in mammals (Notch1 to 4), and five Notch ligands (δ-like [DII]-1, DII3, DII4, Jagged1, and Jagged2) have been identified. Abnormal *Notch1* regulation has been implicated in a number of cardiovascular diseases. Abnormalities in the receptor and mutations in the *Jagged* ligands have demonstrated congenital heart abnormalities in mutant mice.[25] Genes that are downstream to Notch receptor activation such as *HRT2/HEY2*, have also been implicated in cardiovascular development.[26] In addition, Notch receptors and their ligands have been localized to the vasculature and are present on the endocardial cells important in endocardial cushion formation.[27,28]

These experimental results provide the foundation for the discovery of mutations in the *Notch1* receptor that play a role in congenital heart abnormalities and also in the accelerated calcification found in this patient population. The findings from this important genetic study have provided a valuable clue in the cell signaling pathways involved in the development of bicuspid aortic valve disease. Further experimental studies are necessary for full understanding of this pathway.

Using another approach to studying potential genetic factors, the geographic distribution of calcific valve disease was evaluated in 2527 consecutive patients operated on for calcific aortic stenosis at one institution in the western part of France between 1992 and 2002.[29] These investigators found that the geographic distribution of calcific aortic valve disease is heterogeneous, with an average frequency of operations for calcific aortic valve disease of 1.13 per 1000 inhabitants but up to 9.38 per 1000. Screening of the population from the parishes with the highest rate of operations for calcific aortic valve disease identified five families with three or more siblings affected by this disease. A large genealogic analysis performed in one of these families linked 48 patients in 34 families with a single common ancestor within 13 generations.

These genetic studies confirm experimental studies demonstrating that the cellular pathways important in the development of aortic stenosis are similar to those of osteoblast differentiation. Important factors include the vitamin D and Notch1 signaling pathways. The finding of the role of estrogen parallels the studies in vascular disease, which have shown that postmenopausal woman develop accelerated vascular disease. Finally, the increased prevalence in families with aortic valve disease provides further evidence that aortic valve disease is not a random process or simple "wear-and-tear:" degeneration of the valve. Future studies are needed to understand whether screening of families for the development of calcific aortic valve disease would be helpful.

Cardiovascular Risk Factors

A number of epidemiologic studies have shown that the risk factors for calcific valve disease are similar to those for vascular atherosclerosis. These epidemiologic studies defined aortic sclerosis as focal leaflet thickening or calcification with normal valve function and then compared subjects with sclerosis with those with normal valve leaflets. In the Cardiovascular Health Study, the independent risk factors for aortic valve sclerosis were age, male gender, serum lipoprotein(a) levels, height, a history of hypertension, smoking, and elevated low-density lipoprotein (LDL) cholesterol levels.[25] Several subsequent studies supported these findings and suggested other clinical factors associated with aortic sclerosis,[30-40] which are similar to those that promote the development of vascular atherosclerosis.[41-43] Surgical pathologic studies have demonstrated the presence of LDL[44] and atherosclerosis in calcified human aortic valves. These studies demonstrate similarities between the genesis of valvular and vascular disease and suggest a common cellular mechanism of atherosclerosis.[45]

The role of lipids and other cardiovascular risk factors as risk factors for vascular atherosclerosis is well known. Atherosclerosis is a complex multifactorial process that produces a lesion composed of lipids and[46,47] macrophages,[48] with proliferation of smooth muscle cells[49] and areas of apoptosis.[50] Published studies have shown that the endothelial surface of the artery and the aortic surface of the valve express endothelial nitric oxide synthase.[51-55] Cholesterol-rich LDL has a critical role in the onset and further progression of the atherosclerotic lesion via inactivation of endothelial nitric-oxide synthase,[50,56-58] contributing to an abnormal oxidation state within the vessel. Experimental hypercholesterolemia studies demonstrate that mechanisms of the development of aortic valve disease are similar to those seen with vascular atherosclerosis. However, unlike atherosclerosis, a cause-effect relationship has not been definitively established between clinical factors and calcific aortic valve disease. The literature to date supports a statistical association; convincing evidence for a cause-effect relationship requires demonstrating that removing or altering the "risk factor" prevents the disease process.

Molecular and Cellular Events

Lipids

Surgical pathologic studies have shown the presence of oxidized LDL in calcified valves (Figure 3-6).[44,45] Patients with homozygous familial hypercholesterolemia provide an opportunity to test the hypothesis that lipids play a role in the development of calcific aortic stenosis because these patients have extremely elevated levels of LDL cholesterol without other traditional risk factors for coronary artery disease. Before the advent of lipid-lowering therapy, patients with familial hypercholesterolemia developed aggressive peripheral vascular disease, coronary artery disease, and aortic valve lesions that calcified with age.[59-61] The first index case of an early atherosclerotic lesion in the aortic valve in this patient population was found in a 7-year-old boy who died of the

disease in 1956 (Figure 3-7).[62] Autopsy studies of these patients demonstrate a severe form of aortic stenosis associated with supravalvar narrowing in these patients.[60]

Lipids also play a role in the cell signaling of vascular calcification.[63] Studies in the field of vascular calcification have played an important role in the recent experimental studies in valvular heart disease. In vitro and in vivo models have shown that treatment of vascular smooth muscle cells is important in the development of extracellular matrix production and mineralization.[64-66] The in vivo models of vascular calcification have shown that lipids play an important role in the expression of extracellular bone matrix proteins and progressive calcification.[66] Parallel studies in the field of vascular calcification have tested the effect of lipids in the development of osteoporosis.[65,67,68] These studies point in the direction of a paradox between osteoporosis and atherosclerosis. The findings from these studies suggest that as osteoporosis develops, bone formation decreases in the skeleton but calcification and bone formation increase in the vasculature.

Renin-Angiotensin Signaling Pathway

Angiotensin-converting enzyme is expressed and colocalizes with LDL in calcified aortic valves.[69] Histologic studies of diseased aortic valves show the presence of angiotensin-converting enzyme (Figure 3-8).[69] Furthermore, there is colocalization of LDL in the areas of increased staining for angiotensin-converting enzyme.[69] A retrospective clinical study showed a lower rate of progression of aortic valve

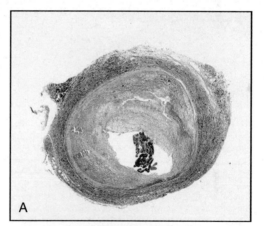

Left Circumflex Artery

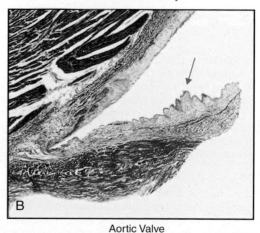

Aortic Valve

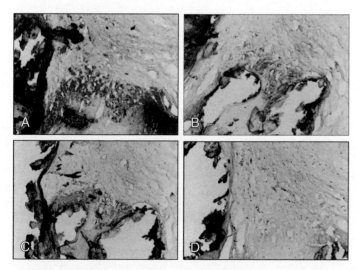

FIGURE 3–6 Lipids and inflammatory cells in a stenotic valve. Colocalization of lipid (**A,** oil red O), apolipoprotein B (**B,** ApoB immunostaining), oxidized low-density lipoproteins (**C,** NA59 immunostaining), and T lymphocytes (**D,** CD6 immunostaining) close to a calcium deposit in a stenotic valve. Original magnification, ×20. *(From Olsson M, Thyberg J, Nilsson J: Presence of oxidized low density lipoprotein in nonrheumatic stenotic aortic valves. Arterioscler Thromb Vasc Biol 1999;19:1218-1222, with permission.)*

FIGURE 3–7 Light microscopy of cardiac pathologic lesions from a patient with familial hypercholesterolemia. **A,** Atherosclerosis of the left circumflex artery. **B,** Cross-section of the aortic valve attachment to the aorta. *(From Rajamannan NM, Edwards WD, Spelsberg TC: Hypercholesterolemic aortic-valve disease. N Engl J Med 2003;349:717-718, with permission.)*

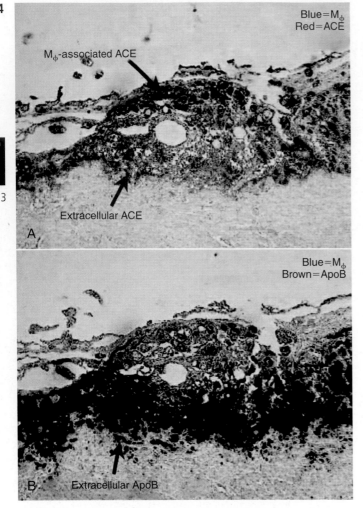

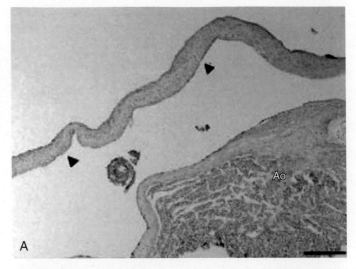

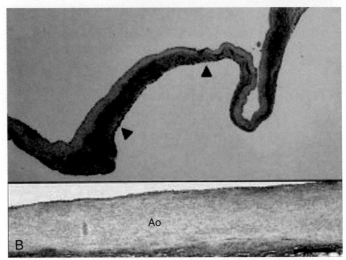

FIGURE 3–8 Angiotensin-converting enzyme (ACE) in a human aortic valve lesion. **A,** Double immunostaining for macrophages (blue stain) and ACE (red stain) demonstrate that the majority of macrophages are blue, indicating the absence of ACE protein. A minority of macrophages contain ACE protein, identified by their purple stain. In contrast, the vast majority of red ACE staining is extracellular. **B,** Double immunostaining for macrophages (blue stain) and apolipoprotein B (ApoB), the primary protein of low-density lipoprotein cholesterol particles (brown stain), demonstrates the presence of extensive extracellular ApoB staining, which colocalizes with extracellular ACE. Original magnification, ×400. *(From O'Brien KD, Shavelle DM, Caulfield MT, et al: Association of angiotensin-converting enzyme with low-density lipoprotein in aortic valvular lesions and in human plasma. Circulation 2002;106:2224-2230, with permission.)*

disease in patients taking angiotensin-converting enzyme inhibitors compared with those not receiving this therapy.[70] Another study demonstrated that angiotensin receptor-1 blocker inhibits atherosclerotic changes and endothelial disruption of the aortic valve in hypercholesterolemic rabbits (Figure 3-9).[71] The potential for blocking this pathway with angiotensin-converting enzyme inhibitors and angiotensin receptor blockers may be one approach to targeting of this disease process.

Calcification

Calcification in the aortic valve is responsible for hemodynamic progression of aortic valve stenosis. Recent descriptive studies from patient specimens have demonstrated the critical features of aortic valve calcification, including osteoblast expression, cell proliferation, and atherosclerosis.[7,72-74] Furthermore, these studies have also shown that specific bone cell phenotypes are present in calcifying valve tissue from human specimens[2,75] and demonstrate the potential for vascular cells to differentiate into calcifying phenotypes.[3,64,65]

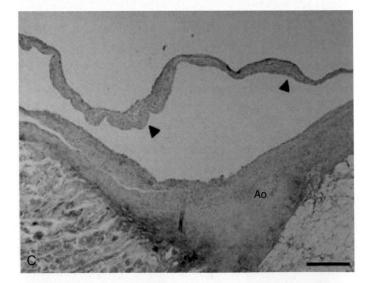

FIGURE 3–9 Treatment effects of angiotensin receptor blocker (olmesartan) on experimental hypercholesterolemia in the aortic valve. Angiotensin-converting enzyme (ACE) immunostaining (black) in sections of aortic valve from control (**A**), hypercholesterolemic (**B**), and hypercholesterolemic olmesartan-treated (**C**) rabbits. Sections are counterstained with methyl green. *Inset* in **B** shows the aorta from the same section. *Arrowheads* indicate the aortic side of the valve leaflet. *(From Arishiro K, Hoshiga M, Negoro N, et al: Angiotensin receptor-1 blocker inhibits atherosclerotic changes and endothelial disruption of the aortic valve in hypercholesterolemic rabbits. J Am Coll Cardiol 2007;49:1482-1489, with permission.)*

Recent intriguing observations in an ex vivo human tissue analysis provide new insights in our understanding of the basic mechanisms involved in the initiation and progression of vascular and valvular calcification. Because an osteoblast phenotype is present, factors important in the regulation of bone development and regeneration must be considered in the understanding of calcification of the aortic valve. Cardiovascular calcification is composed of hydroxyapatite deposited on a bone-like matrix of collagen, osteopontin, and other minor bone matrix proteins.[73,76,77] Calcified aortic valves removed during surgical valve replacement show osteoblast bone formation.[2,73,74]

Immunohistochemical staining of calcified bicuspid aortic valves shows the expression of osteopontin (Figure 3-10).[74] In addition, osteopontin expression has been demonstrated in the mineralization zones of heavily calcified aortic valves obtained at autopsy and surgery.[2,72,73] Examination of calcified aortic valves, removed at the time of valve replacement, confirms the presence of an osteogenic bone gene program demonstrated by semiquantitative reverse transcriptase-polymerase chain reaction analysis, histomorphometry, and micro-computed tomography. In addition, an osteoblast-like cellular phenotype is present.[74]

Extraction of messenger RNA from calcified versus normal aortic valves confirms upregulation of osteoblast bone markers in calcified aortic valves including osteopontin, bone sialoprotein, osteocalcin, alkaline phosphatase, and the osteoblast-specific transcription factor Cbfa-1. There is evidence at the RNA level for the activation of the osteoblast gene program in calcified human aortic valves removed at the time of surgical valve replacement compared with valves removed at the time of heart transplantation (Figure 3-11).[74] Gene expression of osteopontin, bone sialoprotein, and Cbfa-1 were all increased in the calcified aortic valves compared with the control valves, obtained from explanted hearts at the time of heart transplantation. These results demonstrate that this bone phenotype is regulated both at the protein production level and at the RNA gene transcription level. These data provide the first molecular evidence that a parallel osteoblast gene program is important in the mineralizing phenotype found in calcified human aortic valves.

The cell responsible for the development of calcification is the myofibroblast cell. This important cell is resident in the aortic valve and normally has a phenotype that was characterized initially as a subendothelial or interstial cell.[16] Nomenclature for this specific cell type and a classification scheme provide a framework to conceptualize the different phases of plasticity that describe this cell's potential to differentiate from one phenotype to another. Five functional phenotypes have been proposed for the transitions this cell can go through while it becomes a calcifying cell.[78]

The classification includes the following. (1) Embryonic progenitor endothelial/mesenchymal cells give rise to resident quiescent valve interstitial cells (VICs), which are the normal heart valve leaflet cells as described by Johnson et al.[10] (2) Quiescent VICs maintain physiologic valve structure and function and inhibit angiogenesis in the normal leaflets. (3) Progenitor VICs are the bone marrow, circulation, and/or the heart valve leaflet cells. These cells have the ability to enter the valve or are resident in the valve to provide

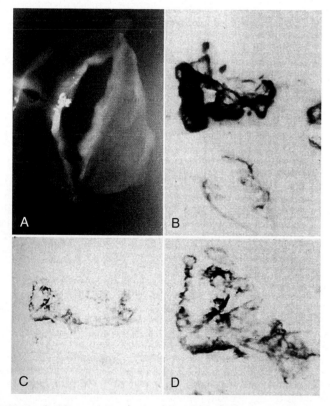

FIGURE 3–10 Association of osteopontin and calcification with minimal valvular calcification. **A,** Radiograph, using mammography, of a congenital bicuspid aortic valve replaced owing to severe regurgitation. Calcific deposits are seen as bright white regions at the midportion of the tip and base of the left leaflet. **B,** Photomicrograph of a section of the calcified tip of the left leaflet that was stained with alizarin red S. **C** and **D,** Low- and high-power photomicrographs, respectively, of a section of the calcified tip of the left leaflet, using anti-osteopontin antibody to identify osteopontin. These findings indicate that osteopontin is present in aortic valves that have minimal calcification. *(From Mohler ER 3rd, Adam LP, McClelland P, et al: Detection of osteopontin in calcified human aortic valves. Arterioscler Thromb Vasc Biol 1997;17:547-552, with permission.)*

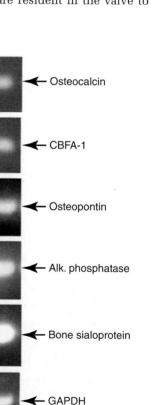

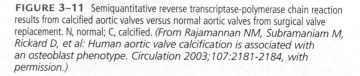

FIGURE 3–11 Semiquantitative reverse transcriptase-polymerase chain reaction results from calcified aortic valves versus normal aortic valves from surgical valve replacement. N, normal; C, calcified. *(From Rajamannan NM, Subramaniam M, Rickard D, et al: Human aortic valve calcification is associated with an osteoblast phenotype. Circulation 2003;107:2181-2184, with permission.)*

activator VICs to repair the heart valve and may be CD34-, CD133-, and/or S100-positive. (4) Activator VICs are the heart valve leaflet cells that are activated to undergo the initial stage of differentiation. These are α-smooth muscle actin–containing VICs with activated cellular repair processes including proliferation, migration, and matrix remodeling. These cells respond to valve injury attributable to pathologic conditions and abnormal hemodynamic/mechanical forces. (5) VICs that undergo osteoblastic degeneration are also of heart valve leaflet origin. These cells have the ability to undergo calcification, chondrogenesis, and osteogenesis in the heart valve. This classification demonstrates the stepwise stages of the transformation process in the valve myofibroblast cells as shown in Table 3-2. Several in vitro experimental studies demonstrate the growth factors/cytokines and signaling pathways important in the differentiation pathway of the evolution of this type of cell into a calcifying phenotype.[79-82]

The ontogeny of osteoblast cell differentiation is illustrated in Figure 3-12. Osteoblast cells originally derived from the mesoderm in embryo development. These cells are given the

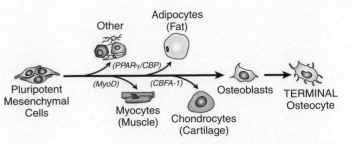

FIGURE 3–12 The ontogeny pathway for differentiation of the valve myofibroblast to a calcifying phenotype. This figure demonstrates the different regulator pathways important in the mesenchymal stem cell derivation of osteoblast cells.

name *mesenchymal stem cell*, which is derived from their mesoderm origin. These cells have a pluripotential ability to differentiate into different cell types, depending on the path that is chosen for the cells. The pathway fate of these cells is dictated by which transcription factor is activated in the nucleus. The potential pathways for the mesenchymal precursor cell include (1) adipocyte differentiation regulated by peroxisome proliferator-activated receptor-γ/cAMP response element–binding protein–binding protein; (2) myocyte differentiation regulated by MyoD; and (3) chondrocyte and osteoblast differentiation regulated by Cbfa-1. Therefore, the final common pathway for each of these cells is regulated by a master switch transcription factor that is specified by a specific transcription factor for a potential path for the life of these cells. Osteoblast bone formation is a complex process involving multiple growth and differentiation cellular mechanisms. The presence of osteoblast bone formation in the aortic valve has provided the foundation for the hypothesis that the cells residing in the aortic valve have the potentiality to differentiate into a bone-forming cell, which over time mineralizes and expresses an ossification phenotype. These studies have further defined not only the phenotype important in the understanding of how calcification develops in the aortic valve but also have identified the specific gene pathways important to the understanding of the molecular regulation of the calcification process.

Cell Signaling Pathways

Numerous studies have identified the signaling pathways critical in the development of calcific aortic stenosis. A number of these signaling factors are similar to those found in vascular atherosclerosis and bone formation. Matrix metalloproteinases,[75,83] interleukin-1,[84] transforming growth factor-β,[85] purine nucleotides,[80,81] receptor activator of nuclear factor κB (RANK),[86] osteoprotegrin (OPG),[86] and tumor necrosis factor-α[87] have all been identified as signaling pathways important in the development of this disease process.

In human tissue removed at the time of surgical valve replacement, increased expression of elastolytic cathepsins S, K, and V and their inhibitor cystatin C has been noted.[88] This study was the first to suggest a potential involvement of cathepsins S, K, and V in the pathogenesis of aortic stenosis (Figure 3-13).[88] The increased levels of these elastolytic cathepsins in stenotic aortic valves and their ability to degrade aortic valvular elastin suggest that they may disturb the balance between matrix synthesis and degradation in the diseased valves. The degree of cathepsin-mediated matrix degradation is regulated by their natural inhibitor, cystatin C, and, these investigators found that its expression was increased in the stenotic aortic valves. The factors that stimulate cystatin C expression in the stenotic valves are unknown, and these investigators proposed that the mechanism by which this effect takes place may be through the transforming growth factor-β pathway.

The tumor necrosis factor superfamily that is involved in the regulation of bone resorption and vascular calcification

TABLE 3–2	Classification of the Valvular Interstitial Cell (VIC) Markers and Function into Five Phenotypes	
Cell Type	**Location**	**Function**
Embryonic progenitor endothelial/ mesenchymal cells	Embryonic cardiac cushions	Give rise to resident quiescent VICs, possibly through an activated stage. Endothelial-mesenchymal transition can be detected by the loss of endothelial and the gain of mesenchymal markers
Quiescent VICs	Heart valve leaflet	Maintain physiologic valve structure and function and inhibit angiogenesis in the leaflets
Progenitor VICs	Bone marrow, circulation, and/or heart valve leaflet	Enter valve or are resident in valve to provide activator VICs to repair the heart valve, may be CD34-, CD133-, and/or S100-positive
Activator VICs	Heart valve leaflet	α-Smooth muscle actin-containing VICs with activated cellular repair processes including proliferation, migration, and matrix remodeling. Respond to valve injury attributable to pathologic conditions and abnormal hemodynamic/ mechanical forces
VICs that undergo osteoblastic degeneration	Heart valve leaflet	Calcification, chondrogenesis, and osteogenesis in the heart valve. Secrete alkaline phosphatase, osteocalcin, osteopontin, bone sialoprotein

From Liu AC, Joag VR, Gotlieb AI: The emerging role of valve interstitial cell phenotypes in regulating heart valve pathobiology. Am J Pathol 2007;171:1407-1418, with permission.

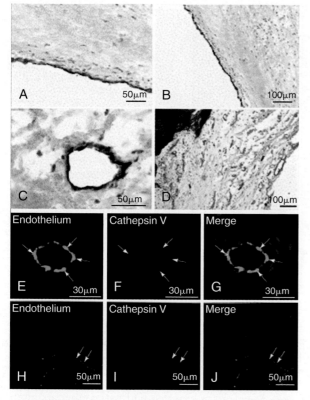

FIGURE 3–13 Immunohistochemistry to test for cathepsin S and cystatin C expression. **A,** In the control aortic valves, cathepsin S protein was detected only in the aortic lining endothelium. **B,** In the stenotic valves, positive staining of cathepsin S was found in the aortic endothelium lining the valves and also in the deeper areas of the subendothelial space in the valve and rich with inflammatory cells. **C-E,** Double immunofluorescence staining demonstrated that cathepsin S colocalized with macrophages in the inflammatory areas of the stenotic valves, and large regional differences in the amount of cathepsin S–positive macrophages between the different valvular regions. **F-H,** Cathepsin S protein was detected in the ossified areas of the valves, where it appeared as a perinuclear rim in the majority of the S100-positive chondroblast-like cells, suggesting active cathepsin S synthesis by these cells. **I-J,** Colocalization of cathepsin S and cystatin C was detected in the superficial endothelium lining the valves as well as in a fraction of macrophages in the stenotic valves. *(From Helske S, Syvaranta S, Lindstedt KA, et al: Increased expression of elastolytic cathepsins S, K, and V and their inhibitor cystatin C in stenotic aortic valves. Arterioscler Thromb Vasc Biol 2006;26: 1791-1798, with permission.)*

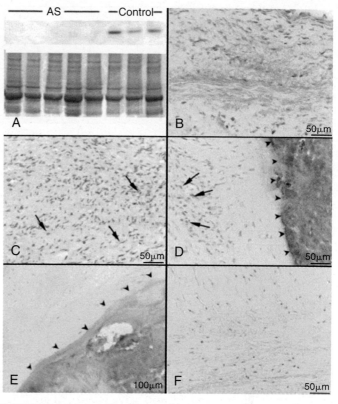

FIGURE 3–14 Immunohistochemistry of osteoprotegerin (OPG) in calcified aortic valves. Western blotting of native protein extracts for OPG demonstrated bands at 40 kDa in control valves and no detectable bands in stenotic valves. **A,** Immunohistochemistry showed a high proportion of OPG-positive cells in control valves. **B,** Staining of thickened, but not calcified, areas of stenotic valves demonstrated an increased total cell count but a reduced percentage of OPG-positive cells. **C,** Regions from stenotic valves containing focal calcification showed scattered cells weakly positive for OPG. **D,** The calcium deposits in these sections were stained intensely by the OPG antibody. **E,** However, calcium deposits were also stained in a comparable fashion by an isotype-matched IgG control antibody. **F,** Noncalcified tissue demonstrated no staining. *(From Kaden JJ, Bickelhaupt S, Grobholz R, et al: Receptor activator of nuclear factor κB ligand and osteoprotegerin regulate aortic valve calcification. J Mol Cell Cardiol 2004;36:57-66, with permission.)*

has also been discovered in calcific valve disease. This cytokine system consists of the transmembrane protein RANK, its ligand (RANKL), and the soluble receptor OPG. Mouse studies have shown that the RANKL-RANK pathway is the gatekeeper of osteoclast differentiation and activation[89] and that RANKL is a key regulator of osteoclastogenesis and lymphocyte development. OPG is a soluble decoy receptor that binds to RANKL, thereby inhibiting the interaction of RANKL and RANK. OPG is expressed at high concentrations by a variety of tissues and cell types including arterial smooth muscle cells and endothelial cells, whereas RANKL and RANK are not expressed in vascular tissue under physiologic conditions.[89]

Elegant studies have demonstrated[86] the expression and localization of OPG as assessed by Western blotting and immunohistochemistry in calcified valves (Figure 3-14). The staining of calcium deposits by the OPG antibody probably represents nonspecific binding. More studies demonstrated[90] the potential mechanism for OPG in aortic valve calcification, and the phenotypic diversity between the endothelium aortic surface and the ventricular surface of the aortic valve was explored. These studies demonstrated the upregulation of OPG along the ventricular surface of the aortic valve, which is most likely one of the key factors responsible for the lack of calcification found along the ventricular surface of the aortic valve. The conclusions from these studies are that the aortic valve has specific osteoblast differentiation signaling pathways, implicating active cellular biologic pathways instead of a passive degenerative process.

Wnt/Lrp5 Signaling Pathway

The LDL receptor-related protein 5 (Lrp5), a coreceptor of the LDL receptor family, has been discovered as an important receptor in the activation of skeletal bone formation via binding to the secreted glycoprotein wingless (Wnt), which activates β-catenin to induce bone formation. The canonical Wnt/Lrp5 pathway is a highly conserved pathway that has evolved as one of the leading signaling mechanisms in early embryologic development.[91,92] It is a highly conserved pathway across species.[93] The Wnt pathway is a critical pathway in the development of bone formation. When Wnt binds to the Lrp5/Frizzled receptor, calcification develops within the myofibroblast cell in the aortic valve[53] and in the vasculature.[66]

Specific mutations in Lrp5 result in a high bone mass phenotype versus an osteoporosis phenotype, implicating this coreceptor and the canonical Wnt signaling pathway in bone formation and bone mass regulation.[94,95] Recent studies

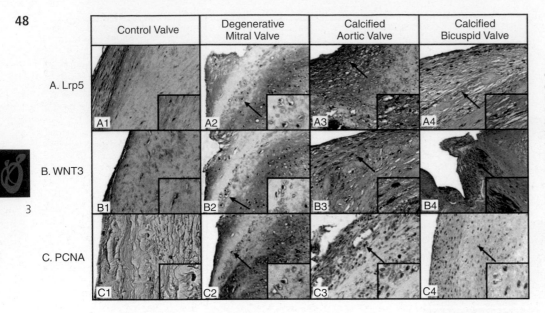

| Control Valve | Degenerative Mitral Valve | Calcified Aortic Valve | Calcified Bicuspid Valve |

A. Lrp5 — A1, A2, A3, A4

B. WNT3 — B1, B2, B3, B4

C. PCNA — C1, C2, C3, C4

FIGURE 3-15 Immunohistochemistry for control, myxomatous, bicuspid, and tricuspid diseased aortic valves demonstrating an increase in low-density lipoprotein receptor-related protein 5 (Lrp5), wingless 3a (Wnt3a), and proliferating cell nuclear antigen (PCNA) in the diseased valves compared with the control valve tissue. **A,** Lrp5 immunohistochemistry. **B,** Wnt3a immunohistochemistry. **C,** PCNA immunohistochemistry. *(From Caira FC, Stock SR, Gleason TG, et al: Human degenerative valve disease is associated with up-regulation of low-density lipoprotein receptor-related protein 5 receptor-mediated bone formation. J Am Coll Cardiol 2006;47:1707-1712, with permission.)*

have shown regulation by the Lrp5 pathway in both experimental animal models[66,82] and human vascular disease. In addition, a study in adults with valve disease demonstrated the upregulation of Lrp5 diseased valves removed at the time of surgical valve replacement and valve repair (Figure 3-15).[2] The results provide the first evidence of a mechanistic pathway for the initiation of bone differentiation in degenerative valve lesions, which is expressed in the mitral valve as a cartilage phenotype and in the calcified aortic valve as a bone phenotype. In normal adult skeleton formation the initiation of bone formation occurs with the development of a cartilaginous template, which eventually mineralizes and forms calcified bone. Therefore, the mitral valve expresses early cartilage formation, and the aortic valve demonstrates the mineralized osteoblast phenotype, which follows the spectrum of normal skeletal bone formation. These findings implicate an osteoblast differentiation process that is mediated by the Lrp5/Wnt3 pathway with an active endochondral bone formation mechanism central in the development of heart valve disease.

EXPERIMENTAL MODELS OF VALVULAR HEART DISEASE

In Vivo Rabbit Model

If atherosclerotic risk factors are important in the development of valvular heart disease, then experimental models of atherosclerosis are the next step toward understanding this disease process. Experimental models in mice and rabbits have confirmed that hypercholesterolemia results in both atherosclerosis and calcification in the aortic valves.[7,96-100]

In vivo studies have demonstrated that experimental cholesterol[96,101] and vitamin D[97] induce early stenosis in the valve (Table 3-3).[97] A preliminary study[101] tested experimental cholesterol in rabbits and demonstrated early endothelial abnormalities in the aortic valves. This rabbit model was further analyzed for multiple markers of the atherosclerotic process within the valve, which are critical steps toward the development of valvular calcification process.[7] This initial study of the cholesterol versus the normal control aortic valve (Figure 3-16) shows that atherosclerosis, cell proliferation, and apoptosis are early markers and hallmark features in the development of valve atherosclerosis (Figure 3-17).[96] Atorvastatin

attenuates bone gene expression, macrophage infiltration, and cellular proliferation.[7] The next step was to increase the duration of the cholesterol diet to determine the early mineralization process within the valve leaflet. The cholesterol diet was tested for 3 months, and early mineralization was found by micro-computed tomography, which was attenuated by atorvastatin.[53] This study also demonstrated that endothelial nitric-oxide synthase was regulated in the valves from the different treatment groups.

To determine whether the chronicity of the diet allows calcification to develop, many investigators have tested the long-term effects of lipids. One study tested the effects of a 6-month cholesterol diet with and without atorvastatin on the aortic valves and showed that it contributed to the formation of a calcified atherosclerotic lesion (see Figure 3-17).[82] The marked thickening of the rabbit aortic valve leaflets and complex calcification within the valve leaflet with attenuation of the calcification was demonstrated by micro-computed tomographic analysis.[82] This study also showed Lrp5 receptor regulation in rabbit aortic valves in the in vivo as well as the in vitro cell culture model. It was also the first study to use echocardiography in rabbits treated with cholesterol and vitamin D. A pulsed-wave echocardiogram demonstrating early stenosis is shown in Figure 3-18. This pulsed-wave Doppler tracing indicates the presence of early stenosis across the vitamin D– and cholesterol-treated aortic valve leaflet.

In Vivo Mouse Models

In vivo mouse models have emerged as a powerful approach to study aortic valve disease. A recent study[98] demonstrated the first evidence that elevated cholesterol in a genetic mouse model causes severe aortic stenosis by echocardiographic measurements and hemodynamic catheterization studies. This study tested elderly mice with a genetic knockout for the LDL receptor (LDLr) and expression of only the receptor for the human apolipoprotein (Apo) B100 (LDLr$^{-/-}$ApoB$^{100/100}$). This model induces mineralization as confirmed by Von Kossa staining, which stains for calcium and phosphate mineral. The study also demonstrated an abnormal oxidation state in the diseased aortic valves as shown in Figure 3-19, showing increase in superoxide dismutase in the aortic valve leaflets from the high cholesterol mouse model.

TABLE 3–3	**In Vivo Models of Experimental Hypercholesterolemia and Aortic Valve Disease**				
Author	**Journal, Year**	**Model**	**Diet**	**Medical Therapy**	**Experimental Results**
Rabbit species					
Sarphie	Atherosclerosis, 1985	New Zealand White rabbit	Cholesterol	None	Endothelial structural changes along aortic surface of the aortic valve
Sarphie	American Journal of Anatomy, 1985	New Zealand White rabbit	Cholesterol	None	Anionic surface properties of the endothelium
Sarphie	Experimental Molecular Pathology, 1986	New Zealand White rabbit	Cholesterol	None	Cytochemical surface properties
Sarphie	Atherosclerosis, 1985	New Zealand White rabbit	Cholesterol	None	Interactions of IgG and β-VLDL
Rajamannan	Journal of Heart Valve Disease, 2001	New Zealand White rabbit	Cholesterol	None	Apoptosis
Rajamannan	Circulation, 2002	New Zealand White rabbit	Cholesterol	Atorvastatin	Cell proliferation, extracellular matrix production, foam cell formation, Cbfa-1 expression, statin inhibits cell proliferation and matrix
Rajamannan	Heart, 2005	New Zealand White rabbit	Cholesterol	Atorvastatin	eNOS expression and regulation in the aortic valve, calcification
Rajamannan	Circulation, 2005	Watanabe rabbit/LDLr+	Cholesterol	Atorvastatin	Lrp5/Wnt/Cbfa-1 regulation in severely calcified aortic valves and regulation of cell proliferation in myofibroblast cell culture
Drolet	Journal of the American College of Cardiology, 2003	New Zealand White rabbit	Cholesterol and vitamin D	None	Hemodynamic evidence of early stenosis
Cimini	Journal of Heart Valve Disease, 2001	New Zealand White rabbit	Cholesterol	None	Early aortic valve sclerosis and atherosclerosis
Arishiro	Journal of the American College of Cardiology, 2007	Japanese rabbit	Cholesterol	Olmesartan	ARB1 inhibits endothelial disruption and atherosclerosis
Mouse species					
Shao	Journal of Clinical Investigation, 2005	LDLr+	Cholesterol	None	Valvular fibrosis via Wnt-Msx2 regulation
Drolet	Journal of the American College of Cardiology, 2006	LDLR+	Cholesterol	None	Hemodynamic evidence of early stenosis and metabolic syndrome
Weiss	Circulation, 2006	LDLr+/ApoB$^{100/100}$	Cholesterol	None	Hemodynamic evidence of severe stenosis, mineralization, and abnormal oxidative stress
Aikawa	Circulation, 2007	ApoE+	Cholesterol	None	Multimodality imaging in atherosclerotic aortic valves; measuring osteogenic activities

ARB, angiotensin receptor blocker; Apo, apolipoprotein; eNOS, endothelial nitric-oxide synthase; LDLR, low-density lipoprotein receptor; Lrp5, low-density lipoprotein receptor-related protein 5; VLDL, very low-density lipoprotein; Wnt, wingless.

From Rajamannan NM: Low-density lipoprotein and aortic stenosis. Heart 2008;94:1111-1112, with permission.

From Rajamannan NM: Calcific Aortic Stenosis: Lessons Learned from Experimental and Clinical Studies. ATVB 2008; Nov 20, Epub ahead of print, with permission.

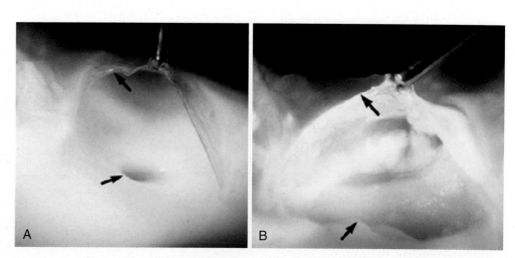

FIGURE 3–16 Rabbit aortic valve leaflet attached to the aorta. The control aortic valve on the left demonstrates a clear glistening aortic valve leaflet with the normal coronary ostia and aorta. The experimental hypercholesterolemia aortic valve shows an atherosclerotic lesion that develops along the aortic surface of the valve and extends out to along the proximal aortic surface. **A,** Control diet with normal-appearing clear glistening aortic valve leaflet. **B,** Cholesterol diet treatment with atherosclerotic leaflet with macrophages and lipid infiltration. *(From Rajamannan NM: Role of statins in aortic valve disease. Heart Fail Clin 2006;2: 395-413, with permission.)*

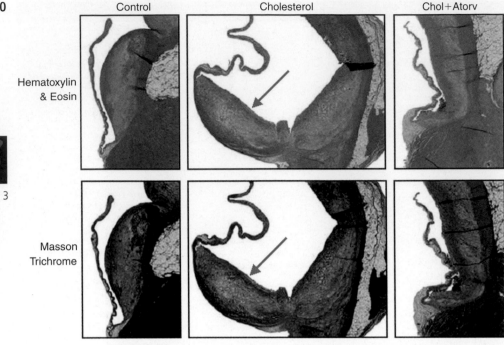

| | Control | Cholesterol | Chol+Atorv |

Hematoxylin & Eosin

Masson Trichrome

FIGURE 3–17 Six-month hypercholesterolemic rabbit aortic valve study. Light microscopy of rabbit aortic valves and aorta. *Left column,* control diet; *middle column,* cholesterol diet; *right column,* cholesterol diet plus atorvastatin. In each panel, the aortic valve leaflet is positioned on the left, with the aorta on the right. *Arrow* points to aortic valve in each figure. All frames ×12.5 magnification. **A,** Hematoxylin and eosin stain. **B,** Masson trichrome stain. *(From Rajamannan NM, Subramaniam M, Caira F, et al: Atorvastatin inhibits hypercholesterolemia-induced calcification in the aortic valves via the Lrp5 receptor pathway. Circulation 2005;112:I229-I234, with permission.)*

Another elegant mechanistic study[103] demonstrated that 10% of cells within the atherosclerotic lesion in native aortic valves of hypercholesterolemic mice are bone marrow–derived cells (Figure 3-20). In this study, the investigators demonstrated that aortic valve flow velocity increases with aging in wild-type mice as well as in ApoE$^{-/-}$ mice.

However, a marked increase in aortic valve flow velocity was detected only in ApoE$^{-/-}$ mice. The investigators hypothesized that probably both altered lipid metabolism and aging are essential for the development of murine aortic sclerosis, which potentially causes functional stenosis and regurgitation. Their findings suggest that some of the smooth muscle–like and osteoblast-like cells in degenerative valves might derive from bone marrow. Bone marrow–derived cells were also integrated to the endothelium of the aortic valve. The molecular mechanism by which bone marrow cells are mobilized and recruited to the site of valvular degeneration remains to be elucidated. It is likely that growth factors expressed in the endothelium with abnormal oxidative stress may play a role, at least in part, in the recruitment and homing of bone marrow–derived cells to the site of valvular remodeling.

The next step in the translation of these scientific findings was using multimodality imaging in the ApoE-null mice with valve disease (Figure 3-21).[99] Endothelial cell activation occurs in the commissures of diseased aortic valves. The authors determined that the flexion area of the aortic leaflets near the attachment of the aortic root (commissure) encounters the highest mechanical forces, which might induce endothelial cell activation/injury and expression of adhesion molecules such as vascular cell adhesion molecule-1, intracellular adhesion molecule-1, and E-selectin. These results suggest that endothelial cell activation/damage occurs at the regions of high flexure and increased mechanical forces. The data also suggest that inflammatory cells probably enter the leaflets via the circulation in response to endothelial cell activation or injury.

Conventional structural imaging modalities can identify prominent late-stage calcification, but before these studies no current imaging methods could detect in vivo early mineralization and osteogenesis in cardiac valves. The imaging techniques in this article demonstrated the presence of calcium-hydroxyapatite complexes formed by smooth muscle actin-positive cells. The data are consistent with previous studies showing the association of valvular lesions with features typical of atherosclerotic plaques, including endothelial activation, inflammation, proteolytic activity, and osteogenesis. Therefore, modification of atherogenic factors and pharmacologic therapies that target proinflammatory pathways may retard the progression of aortic valve calcification. Molecular

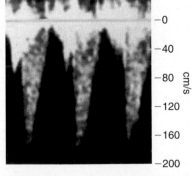

Control

Chol+Vit D$_2$

FIGURE 3–18 Transvalvular aortic gradients in control (*top*) and cholesterol plus vitamin D$_2$ rabbits (*bottom*) by continuous-wave Doppler imaging. *(From Drolet MC, Arsenault M, Couet J: Experimental aortic valve stenosis in rabbits. J Am Coll Cardiol 2003;41:1211-1217, with permission.)*

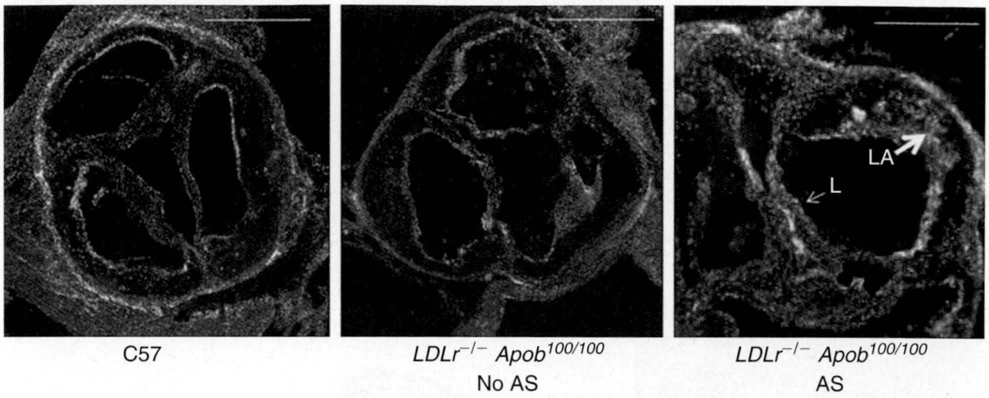

FIGURE 3–19 Superoxide dismutase stain in the control (C57BL/6) versus LDLr⁻/⁻apoB$^{100/100}$ control versus cholesterol diet. Images depict oxyethidium fluorescence, a reporter for tissue superoxide, as discrete bright white pixels. L, leaflet; LA, leaflet attachment. In the image on the *far right,* there appears to be fusion of the attachment surfaces of adjacent valve leaflets (*larger white arrow*). Bar, 0.3 mm. *(From Weiss RM, Ohashi M, Miller JD, et al: Calcific aortic valve stenosis in old hypercholesterolemic mice. Circulation 2006;114:2065-2069, with permission.)*

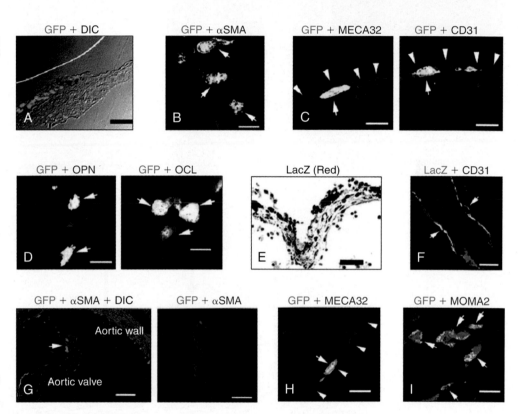

FIGURE 3–20 Bone marrow transplant experiment to determine percentage of transplanted cells into hypercholesterolemic aortic valve. **A,** Bone marrow transplantation (BMT) was performed from green fluorescent protein (GFP) mice to 59-week-old apolipoprotein E–deficient (ApoE⁻/⁻) mice. **B-D,** Studies to show adjacent sections with double immunofluorescence technology; nuclei were counterstained with Hoechst 33258 (blue). **B,** GFP-positive cells (green) that expressed α-smooth muscle actin (SMA) (red). *Arrows* indicate double-positive cells. **C,** GFP-positive endothelial-like cells (green) that expressed MECA32 or CD31 (red). *Arrowheads* indicate the surface of the aortic valves. *Arrows* indicate double-positive cells (yellow). **D,** GFP-positive cells (green) that expressed osteopontin (OPN) or osteocalcin (OCL) (red). *Arrows* indicate double-positive cells (yellow). **E,** Aortic valves of 80-week-old BMT$^{LacZ→ApoE}$ mice. BMT was performed from LacZ mice to ApoE⁻/⁻ mice. **F,** LacZ-positive cells (green) that expressed CD31 (red). *Arrows* indicate double-positive cells (yellow). **G,** BMT was performed from GFP mice to C57BL/6 mice (BMT$^{GFP→wild-type}$ mice). **H,** Bone marrow–derived endothelial-like cell or macrophages. **I,** Aortic valve of BMT$^{GFP→wild-type}$ mice. *Arrows* indicate the double-positive cells (yellow). *(From Tanaka K, Sata M, Fukuda D, et al: Age-associated aortic stenosis in apolipoprotein E-deficient mice. J Am Coll Cardiol 2005;46:134-141, with permission.)*

imaging of the earliest stages of calcification may identify high-risk valves while disease is silent and may enable the monitoring of valvular osteogenic activity during therapeutic interventions such as lipid lowering.

SUMMARY

Data from the experimental studies outlined in this chapter provide a foundation for our understanding of the molecular mechanisms of aortic valve calcification. Figure 3-22 shows the importance of the initial studies in the field of population science, demonstrating the risk factors important in calcific aortic stenosis. Furthermore, these risk factors are similar to those important in the development of vascular atherosclerosis. In the presence of the different atherogenic risk factors, the initiating events important in the development of valve calcification are activated.[104]

Low-density lipoproteins are important in initial oxidative stress and increased expression of superoxide dismutase.[105] Once the oxidative environment is present, numerous pathways similar to those present in vascular atherosclerosis are activated. Angiotensin II levels are increased, which in turn activates bradykinin and increases cell proliferation. Decreases in normal endothelial nitric-oxide synthase enzyme function occurs, which causes further increases in cellular proliferation via growth factor and cytokine activation of the mitogen-activated protein kinase pathways.

Over time the myofibroblast cell activates extracellular matrix production via the Wnt/Lrp5, transforming growth factor-β pathways. Osteopontin, bone sialoprotein, osteocalcin, and alkaline phosphatase matrix proteins are increased. As the synthesis of these matrix proteins is occurring, these matrix proteins increase cellular adhesion and binding of hydroxyapatite proteins. Over time, this mineralization process causes calcification and formation of ectopic bone.

3

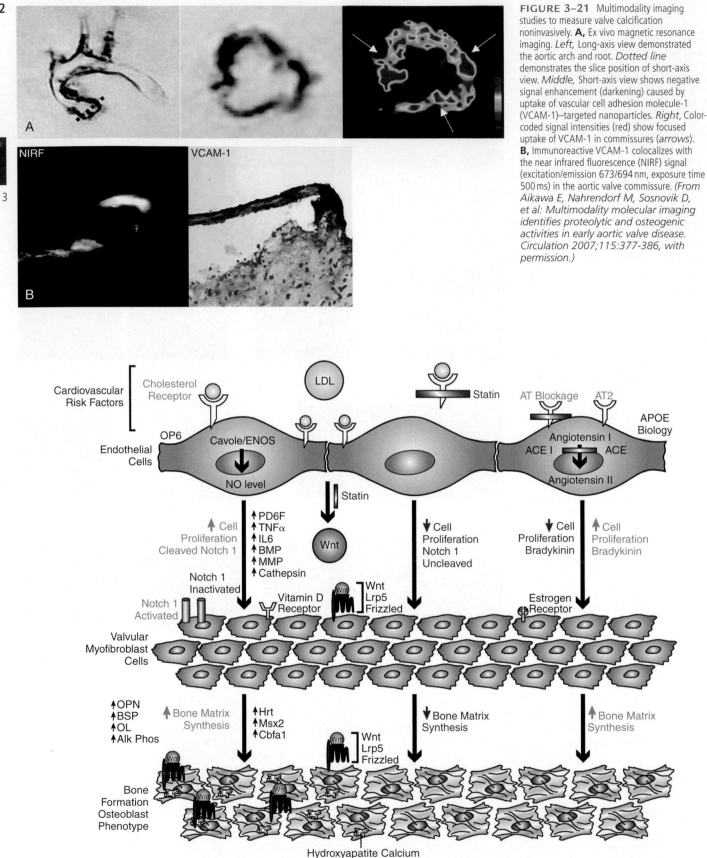

FIGURE 3–21 Multimodality imaging studies to measure valve calcification noninvasively. **A,** Ex vivo magnetic resonance imaging. *Left,* Long-axis view demonstrated the aortic arch and root. *Dotted line* demonstrates the slice position of short-axis view. *Middle,* Short-axis view shows negative signal enhancement (darkening) caused by uptake of vascular cell adhesion molecule-1 (VCAM-1)–targeted nanoparticles. *Right,* Color-coded signal intensities (red) show focused uptake of VCAM-1 in commissures (*arrows*). **B,** Immunoreactive VCAM-1 colocalizes with the near infrared fluorescence (NIRF) signal (excitation/emission 673/694 nm, exposure time 500 ms) in the aortic valve commissure. *(From Aikawa E, Nahrendorf M, Sosnovik D, et al: Multimodality molecular imaging identifies proteolytic and osteogenic activities in early aortic valve disease. Circulation 2007;115:377-386, with permission.)*

FIGURE 3–22 Overview of the signaling pathways involved in aortic valve calcification. The cell layers as indicated are the endothelial cell layer along the aortic surface and the myofibroblast cell that resides below the endothelial cell. The myofibroblast cell is the cell that is activated to differentiate to a bone-synthesizing phenotype in response to different signaling proteins as indicated in the diagram. Medications such as statins, angiotensin-converting enzyme inhibitors, and angiotensin receptor blockers have the potential to target receptors and enzyme pathways to slow the progression of this disease. *(From Rajamannan NM: Calcific Aortic Stenosis: Lessons Learned from Experimental and Clinical Studies. ATVB;2008, Nov 20, Epub ahead of print, with permission.)*

The experimental models recapitulate the process found in vascular atherosclerosis, with an early, soft, lipid-laden lesion.[106] The longer the duration of the atherogenic diet, the longer the opportunity the mineral has to bind and form bone. Echocardiographic measurements further confirm the progressive disease process that leads to eventual stenosis. If the disease process is recognized early enough, then there is a potential for medical therapy to target this disease. Statins have the potential to modify the disease process by inhibiting the 3-hydroxy-3-methylglutaryl-coenzyme A reductase pathway, increasing endothelial nitric-oxide synthase functional activity and inhibiting the Wnt/Lrp5 pathway. However, if treatment is too late, the window has closed, and the calcification process progresses. The timing of the initial events in the disease, which is an atherosclerotic process, will be critical in development of medical therapies for calcific aortic stenosis.

Acknowledgments

This work was completed with the support of an American Heart Association Grant-in-Aid (0350564Z) and a grant from the US National Institutes of Health (1K08HL073927-01) and (1R01HL085591-01A1). The author is the inventor on a patent for methods to slow progression of valvular heart disease. This patent is owned by the Mayo Clinic, and the author does not receive any royalties from this patent.

REFERENCES

1. Grande-Allen KJ, Calabro A, Gupta V, et al: Glycosaminoglycans and proteoglycans in normal mitral valve leaflets and chordae: association with regions of tensile and compressive loading. Glycobiology 2004;14:621-633.
2. Caira FC, Stock SR, Gleason TG, et al: Human degenerative valve disease is associated with up-regulation of low-density lipoprotein receptor-related protein 5 receptor-mediated bone formation. J Am Coll Cardiol 2006;47:1707-1712.
3. Tintut Y, Alfonso Z, Saini T, et al.: Multilineage potential of cells from the artery wall. Circulation 2003;108:2505-2510.
4. Grande-Allen, KJ, Borowski AG, Troughton RW, et al: Apparently normal mitral valves in patients with heart failure demonstrate biochemical and structural derangements: an extracellular matrix and echocardiographic study [see comment]. J Am Coll Cardiol 2005;45:54-61.
5. Makkena B, Salti H, Subramaniam M, et al: Atorvastatin decreases cellular proliferation and bone matrix expression in the hypercholesterolemic mitral valve. J Am Coll Cardiol 2005;45:631-633.
6. Sarphie TG: A cytochemical study of the surface properties of aortic and mitral valve endothelium from hypercholesterolemic rabbits. Exp Mol Pathol 1986;44:281-282.
7. Rajamannan NM, Subramaniam M, Springett M, et al: Atorvastatin inhibits hypercholesterolemia-induced cellular proliferation and bone matrix production in the rabbit aortic valve. Circulation 2002;105:2260-2265.
8. Coombs C: Rheumatic Heart Disease. New York, William Wood and Co, 1924.
9. Edwards WD, Peterson K, Edwards JE: Active valvulitis associated with chronic rheumatic valvular disease and active myocarditis. Circulation 1978;57:181-185.
10. Rajamannan NM, Nealis TB, Subramaniam M, et al: Calcified rheumatic valve neoangiogenesis is associated with vascular endothelial growth factor expression and osteoblast-like bone formation. Circulation 2005;111:3296-3301.
11. Mason JW, Billingham ME, Friedman JP: Methysergide-induced heart disease: a case of multivalvular and myocardial fibrosis. Circulation 1977;56:889-990.
12. Connolly HM, Crary JL, McGoon MD, et al: Valvular heart disease associated with fenfluramine-phentermine. N Engl J Med 1997;337:581-588.
13. Rajamannan, NM, Gersh B, Bonow RO: Calcific aortic stenosis: from bench to the bedside—emerging clinical and cellular concepts. Heart 2003;89:801-805.
14. Freeman RV, Otto CM: Spectrum of calcific aortic valve disease: pathogenesis, disease progression, and treatment strategies. Circulation 2005;111:3316-3326.
15. Johnson CM, Helgeson SC: Platelet adherence to cardiac and noncardiac endothelial cells in culture: lack of a prostacyclin effect. J Lab Clin Med 1988;112:372-379.
16. Johnson CM, Hanson MN, Helgeson SC: Porcine cardiac valvular subendothelial cells in culture: cell isolation and growth characteristics. J Mol Cell Cardiol 1987;19:1185-1193.
17. Avakian SD, Annicchino-Bizzacchi JM, Grinberg M, et al: Apolipoproteins AI, B, and E polymorphisms in severe aortic valve stenosis. Clin Genet 2001;60:381-384.
18. Novaro GM, Sachar R, Pearce GL: Association between apolipoprotein E alleles and calcific valvular heart disease. Circulation 2003;108:1804-1808.
19. Ortlepp JR, Hoffmann R, Ohme F, et al: The vitamin D receptor genotype predisposes to the development of calcific aortic valve stenosis. Heart 2001;85:635-638.
20. Ortlepp JR Schmitz F, Mevissen V, et al: The amount of calcium-deficient hexagonal hydroxyapatite in aortic valves is influenced by gender and associated with genetic polymorphisms in patients with severe calcific aortic stenosis. Eur Heart J. 2004;25:514-522.
21. Nordstrom P, Glader CA, Dahlen G, et al: Oestrogen receptor alpha gene polymorphism is related to aortic valve sclerosis in postmenopausal women. J Intern Med 2003;254:140-146.
22. Garg V, Muth AN, Ransom JF, et al: Mutations in NOTCH1 cause aortic valve disease. Nature 2005;437:270-274.
23. Sciaudone M, Gazzerro E, Priest L, et al: Notch 1 impairs osteoblastic cell differentiation. Endocrinology 2003;144:5631-5639.
24. Deregowski V, Gazzerro E, Priest L, et al: Notch 1 overexpression inhibits osteoblastogenesis by suppressing Wnt/β-catenin but not bone morphogenetic protein signaling. J Biol Chem 2006;281:6203-6210.
25. Le Caignec C, Lefevre M, Schott JJ, et al: Familial deafness, congenital heart defects, and posterior embryotoxon caused by cysteine substitution in the first epidermal-growth-factor–like domain of Jagged 1. Am J Hum Genet 2002;71:180-186.
26. Rutenberg JB, Fischer A, Jia H, et al: Developmental patterning of the cardiac atrioventricular canal by Notch and Hairy-related transcription factors. Development 2006;133:4381-4390.
27. Watanabe Y, Kokubo H, Miyagawa-Tomita S, et al: Activation of Notch1 signaling in cardiogenic mesoderm induces abnormal heart morphogenesis in mouse. Development 2006;133:1625-1634.
28. Noseda M, McLean G, Niessen K, et al: Notch activation results in phenotypic and functional changes consistent with endothelial-to-mesenchymal transformation. Circ Res 2004;94:910-917.
29. Probst V, Le Scouarnec S, Legendre A, et al: Familial aggregation of calcific aortic valve stenosis in the western part of France. Circulation 2006;113:856-860.
30. Deutscher S, Rockette HE, and V. Krishnaswami, Diabetes and hypercholesterolemia among patients with calcific aortic stenosis. J Chronic Dis 1984;37:407-15.
31. Aronow WS, Schwartz KS, Koenigsberg M: Correlation of serum lipids, calcium, and phosphorus, diabetes mellitus and history of systemic hypertension with presence or absence of calcified or thickened aortic cusps or root in elderly patients. Am J Cardiol 1987;59:998-999.
32. Mohler ER, Sheridan MJ, Nichols R, et al: Development and progression of aortic valve stenosis: atherosclerosis risk factors—a causal relationship? A clinical morphologic study. Clin Cardiol 1991;14:995-999.
33. Lindroos M, Kupari M, Valvanne J, et al: Factors associated with calcific aortic valve degeneration in the elderly. Eur Heart J 1994;15:865-870.
34. Boon A, Cheriex E, Lodder J, Kessels F: Cardiac valve calcification: characteristics of patients with calcification of the mitral annulus or aortic valve. Heart 1997;78:472-474.
35. Stewart BF, Siscovick D, Lind BK, et al: Clinical factors associated with calcific aortic valve disease. Cardiovascular Health Study. J Am Coll Cardiol 1997;29:630-634.
36. Wilmshurst PT, Stevenson RN, Griffiths H, Lord JR: A case-control investigation of the relation between hyperlipidaemia and calcific aortic valve stenosis. Heart 1997;78:475-479.
37. Chan KL, Ghani M, Woodend K, Burwash IG: Case-controlled study to assess risk factors for aortic stenosis in congenitally bicuspid aortic valve. Am J Cardiol 2001;88:690-693.
38. Aronow WS, Ahn C, Kronzon I, Goldman ME: Association of coronary risk factors and use of statins with progression of mild valvular aortic stenosis in older persons. Am J Cardiol 2001;88:693-695.
39. Chui MC, Newby DE, Panarelli M, et al: Association between calcific aortic stenosis and hypercholesterolemia: is there a need for a randomized controlled trial of cholesterol-lowering therapy? Clin Cardiol 2001;24:52-55.
40. Peltier M, Trojette F, Sarano ME, et al: Relation between cardiovascular risk factors and nonrheumatic severe calcific aortic stenosis among patients with a three-cuspid aortic valve. Am J Cardiol 2003;91:97-99.
41. Whyte HM: The relative importance of the major risk factors in atherosclerotic and other diseases. Aust N Z J Med 1976;6:387-393.
42. Wilson PW, Castelli WP, Kannel WB: Coronary risk prediction in adults (the Framingham Heart Study). Am J Cardiol 1987;59:91G-94G.
43. D'Agostino RB, Kannel WB, Belanger AJ, Sytkowski PA: Trends in CHD and risk factors at age 55-64 in the Framingham Study. Int J Epidemiol 1989;18(3 Suppl 1): S67-S72.
44. Olsson M, Thyberg J, Nilsson J: Presence of oxidized low density lipoprotein in nonrheumatic stenotic aortic valves. Arterioscler Thromb Vasc Biol 1999;19:1218-1222.
45. O'Brien KD, Reichenbach DD, Marcovina SM, et al: Apolipoproteins B, (a), and E accumulate in the morphologically early lesion of 'degenerative' valvular aortic stenosis. Arterioscler Thromb Vasc Biol 1996;16:523-532.
46. Desai MY, Rodriguez A, Wasserman BA, et al: Association of cholesterol subfractions and carotid lipid core measured by MRI. Arterioscler Thromb Vasc Biol 2005;25:e110-e111.
47. Subbaiah PV, Gesquiere LR, Wang K: Regulation of the selective uptake of cholesteryl esters from high density lipoproteins by sphingomyelin. J Lipid Res 2005;46:2699-2705.
48. Kim WJ, Chereshnev I, Gazdoiu M, et al: MCP-1 deficiency is associated with reduced intimal hyperplasia after arterial injury. Biochem Biophys Res Commun 2003;310:936-942.
49. Tanner FC, Boehm M, Akyurek LM, et al: Differential effects of the cyclin-dependent kinase inhibitors p27(Kip1), p21(Cip1), and p16(Ink4) on vascular smooth muscle cell proliferation. Circulation 2000;101:2022-2025.
50. Zhang R, Luo D, Miao R, et al: Hsp90-Akt phosphorylates ASK1 and inhibits ASK1-mediated apoptosis. Oncogene 2005;24:3954-3963.
51. Laufs U, Liao JK: Post-transcriptional regulation of endothelial nitric oxide synthase mRNA stability by Rho GTPase. J Biol Chem 1998;273:24266-24271.
52. Venema RC, Sayegh HS, Kent JD, Harrison DG: Identification, characterization, and comparison of the calmodulin-binding domains of the endothelial and inducible nitric oxide synthases. J Biol Chem 1996;271:6435-6440.
53. Rajamannan NM, Subramaniam M, Stock SR, et al: Atorvastatin inhibits calcification and enhances nitric oxide synthase production in the hypercholesterolaemic aortic valve. Heart 2005;91:806-810.
54. Charest A, Pépin A, Shetty R, et al: Distribution of SPARC during neovascularization of degenerative aortic stenosis. Heart 2006;92:1844-1849.
55. Ngo DT, Hereztyn T, Mishra K, et al: Aortic stenosis is associated with elevated plasma levels of asymmetric dimethylarginine (ADMA). Nitric Oxide 2007;16:197-201.
56. Blair A, Shaul PW, Yuhanna IS, et al: Oxidized low density lipoprotein displaces endothelial nitric-oxide synthase (eNOS) from plasmalemmal caveolae and impairs eNOS activation. J Biol Chem 1999;274:32512-32519.

54

57. Smart EJ, Anderson RG: Alterations in membrane cholesterol that affect structure and function of caveolae. Methods Enzymol 2002;353:131-139.
58. Pritchard KA, Ackerman AW, Ou J, et al: Native low-density lipoprotein induces endothelial nitric oxide synthase dysfunction: role of heat shock protein 90 and caveolin-1. Free Radic Biol Med 2002;33:52-62.
59. Goldstein JL, Brown MS, Familial hypercholesterolemia: identification of a defect in the regulation of 3-hydroxy-3-methylglutaryl coenzyme A reductase activity associated with overproduction of cholesterol. Proc Natl Acad Sci U S A 1973;70:2804-2808.
60. Sprecher DL, Schaefer EJ, Kent KM, et al: Cardiovascular features of homozygous familial hypercholesterolemia: analysis of 16 patients. Am J Cardiol 1984;54:20-30.
61. Kawaguchi A, Miyatake K, Yutani C, et al: Characteristic cardiovascular manifestation in homozygous and heterozygous familial hypercholesterolemia. Am Heart J 1999;137:410-418.
62. Rajamannan NM, Edwards WD, Spelsberg TC: Hypercholesterolemic aortic-valve disease. N Engl J Med 2003;349:717-718.
63. Demer LL: Cholesterol in vascular and valvular calcification. Circulation 2001;104:1881-1883.
64. Parhami F, Basseri B, Hwang J, et al: High-density lipoprotein regulates calcification of vascular cells. Circ Res 2002;91:570-576.
65. Parhami F, Morrow AD, Balucan J, et al: Lipid oxidation products have opposite effects on calcifying vascular cell and bone cell differentiation: a possible explanation for the paradox of arterial calcification in osteoporotic patients. Arterioscler Thromb Vasc Biol 1997;17:680-687.
66. Shao JS, Cheng SL, Pingsterhaus JM, et al: Msx2 promotes cardiovascular calcification by activating paracrine Wnt signals. J Clin Invest 2005;115:1210-1220.
67. Parhami F, Jackson SM, Tintut Y, et al: Atherogenic diet and minimally oxidized low density lipoprotein inhibit osteogenic and promote adipogenic differentiation of marrow stromal cells. J Bone Miner Res 1999;14:2067-2078.
68. Tintut Y, Abedin M, Cho J, et al: Regulation of RANKL-induced osteoclastic differentiation by vascular cells. J Mol Cell Cardiol 2005;39:389-393.
69. O'Brien KD, Shavelle DM, Caulfield MT, et al: Association of angiotensin-converting enzyme with low-density lipoprotein in aortic valvular lesions and in human plasma. Circulation 2002;106:2224-2230.
70. Shavelle DM, Takasu J, Budoff MJ, et al: HCoA reductase inhibitor (statin) and aortic valve calcium. Lancet 2002;359:1125-1126.
71. Arishiro K, Hoshiga M, Negoro N, et al: Angiotensin receptor-1 blocker inhibits atherosclerotic changes and endothelial disruption of the aortic valve in hypercholesterolemic rabbits. J Am Coll Cardiol 2007;49:1482-1489.
72. O'Brien KD, Kuusisto J, Reichenbach DD, et al: Osteopontin is expressed in human aortic valvular lesions [see comment]. Circulation 1995;92:2163-2168.
73. Mohler ER 3rd, Gannon F, Reynolds C, et al Bone formation and inflammation in cardiac valves. Circulation 2001;103:1522-1528.
74. Rajamannan NM, Subramaniam M, Rickard D, et al: Human aortic valve calcification is associated with an osteoblast phenotype. Circulation 2003;107:2181-2184.
75. Jian B, Jones PL, Li Q, et al: Matrix metalloproteinase-2 is associated with tenascin-C in calcific aortic stenosis. Am J Pathol 2001;159:321-327.
76. Mohler ER 3rd, Adam LP, McClelland P, et al: Detection of osteopontin in calcified human aortic valves. Arterioscler Thromb Vasc Biol 1997;17:547-552.
77. O'Brien KD, Kuusisto J, Reichenbach DD, et al: Osteopontin is expressed in human aortic valvular lesions. Circulation 1995;92:2163-2168.
78. Liu AC, Joag VR, Gotlieb AI: The emerging role of valve interstitial cell phenotypes in regulating heart valve pathobiology. Am J Pathol 2007;171:1407-1418.
79. Osman L, Yacoub MH, Latif N, et al: Role of human valve interstitial cells in valve calcification and their response to atorvastatin. Circulation 2006;114(1 Suppl):I547-I552.
80. Osman L, Chester AH, Amrani M, et al: A novel role of extracellular nucleotides in valve calcification: a potential target for atorvastatin. Circulation 2006;114(1 Suppl):I566-I572.
81. Osman L, Amrani M, Isley C, et al: Stimulatory effects of atorvastatin on extracellular nucleotide degradation in human endothelial cells. Nucleosides Nucleotides Nucleic Acids 2006;25:1125-1128.

82. Rajamannan NM, Subramaniam M, Caira F, et al: Atorvastatin inhibits hypercholesterolemia-induced calcification in the aortic valves via the Lrp5 receptor pathway. Circulation 2005;112(9 Suppl):I229-I234.
83. Kaden JJ, Vocke DC, Fischer CS, et al: Expression and activity of matrix metalloproteinase-2 in calcific aortic stenosis. Z Kardiol 2004;93:124-130.
84. Kaden JJ, Dempfle CE, Grobholz R, et al: Interleukin-1β promotes matrix metalloproteinase expression and cell proliferation in calcific aortic valve stenosis. Atherosclerosis 2003;170:205-211.
85. Jian B, Narula N, Li QY, et al: Progression of aortic valve stenosis: TGF-β1 is present in calcified aortic valve cusps and promotes aortic valve interstitial cell calcification via apoptosis. Ann Thorac Surg 2003;75:457-465; discussion 465-466.
86. Kaden JJ, Bickelhaupt S, Grobholz R, et al: Receptor activator of nuclear factor κB ligand and osteoprotegerin regulate aortic valve calcification. J Mol Cell Cardiol 2004;36:57-66.
87. Kaden JJ, Kilic R, Sarikoc A, et al: Tumor necrosis factor α promotes an osteoblast-like phenotype in human aortic valve myofibroblasts: a potential regulatory mechanism of valvular calcification. Int J Mol Med 2005;16:869-872.
88. Helske S, Syvaranta S, Lindstedt KA, et al: Increased expression of elastolytic cathepsins S, K, and V and their inhibitor cystatin C in stenotic aortic valves. Arterioscler Thromb Vasc Biol 2006;26:1791-1798.
89. Simonet WS, Lacey DL, Dunstan CR, et al: Osteoprotegerin: a novel secreted protein involved in the regulation of bone density. Cell 1997;89:309-319.
90. Davies PF, Passerini AG, Simmons CA: Aortic valve: turning over a new leaf(let) in endothelial phenotypic heterogeneity. Arterioscler Thromb Vasc Biol 2004;24:1331-1333.
91. Nusse R: Wnt signaling in disease and in development. Cell Res 2005;15:28-32.
92. Johnson ML, Rajamannan N: Diseases of Wnt signaling. Rev Endocr Metab Disord 2006;7(1-2):41-49.
93. Nusse R: Developmental biology: making head or tail of Dickkopf [see comment]. Nature 2001;411:255-256.
94. Gong Y, Slee RB, Fukai N, et al: LDL receptor-related protein 5 (LRP5) affects bone accrual and eye development. Cell 2001;107:513-523.
95. Little RD, Carulli JP, Del Mastro RG, et al: A mutation in the LDL receptor-related protein 5 gene results in the autosomal dominant high-bone-mass trait. Am J Hum Genet 2002;70:11-19.
96. Rajamannan NM, Sangiorgi G, Springett M, et al: Experimental hypercholesterolemia induces apoptosis in the aortic valve. J Heart Valve Dis 2001;10:371-374.
97. Drolet MC, Arsenault M, Couet J: Experimental aortic valve stenosis in rabbits. J Am Coll Cardiol 2003;41:1211-1217.
98. Weiss RM, Ohashi M, Miller JD, et al: Calcific aortic valve stenosis in old hypercholesterolemic mice. Circulation 2006;114:2065-2069.
99. Aikawa E, Nahrendorf M, Sosnovik D, et al Multimodality molecular imaging identifies proteolytic and osteogenic activities in early aortic valve disease. Circulation 2007;115:377-386.
100. Drolet MC, Roussel E, Deshaies Y, et al: A high fat/high carbohydrate diet induces aortic valve disease in C57BL/6J mice. J Am Coll Cardiol 2006;47:850-855.
101. Sarphie TG: Surface responses of aortic valve endothelia from diet-induced, hypercholesterolemic rabbits. Atherosclerosis 1985;54:283-299.
102. Ortlepp JR, Pillich M, Schmitz F, et al: Lower serum calcium levels are associated with greater calcium hydroxyapatite deposition in native aortic valves of male patients with severe calcific aortic stenosis. J Heart Valve Dis 2006;15:502-508.
103. Tanaka K, Sata M, Fukuda D, et al: Age-associated aortic stenosis in apolipoprotein E-deficient mice. J Am Coll Cardiol 2005;46:134-141.
104. Otto CM, Calcific aortic stenosis—time to look more closely at the valve. N Engl J Med. 2008;359:1395-1398.
105. Miller JD, Chu, Y, Brooks RM, et al: Dysregulation of antioxidant mechanisms contributes to increased oxidative stress in calcific aortic valvular stenosis in humans. J Am Coll Cardiol. 2008;52:843-850.
106. Rajamannan NM: Calcifc Aortic Stenosis: Lessons Learned from Experimental and Clinical Studies. ATVB; 2008, Nov 20, Epub ahead of print.

CHAPTER **4**

Left Ventricular Adaptation to Pressure and/or Volume Overload

Blase A. Carabello

KEY POINTS

- Each valve lesion imparts a unique hemodynamic load on the left ventricle wherein aortic stenosis creates a pure pressure overload, mitral regurgitation presents a pure volume overload, aortic regurgitation causes combined pressure and volume overload, and mitral stenosis leads to volume underload and potentially increased afterload. In turn, each lesion causes its own type of hypertrophy and remodeling.
- Individuals respond to similar load in very different ways, presumably based on their genetic makeup.
- Hypertrophy can accrue not just from increased protein synthesis but also from reduced protein degradation.
- The terms *remodeling* and *hypertrophy* are not synonymous.
- In almost all cases hypertrophy is both adaptive and maladaptive.
- The transition from hypertrophy to heart failure is not a simplistic change in a single system but represents a complex biologic cascade not yet completely defined.

Each form of valvular heart disease places a unique hemodynamic load on the left ventricle. Although the left ventricle is an amazingly complex sea of biologic processes, in fact, it can respond to these overloads using only three basic mechanisms. These are (1) activation of the Frank-Starling mechanism, (2) use of the adrenergic (and other) neurohumoral systems, and (3) chamber remodeling. In this chapter, I attempt to summarize the response of the left ventricle to the load it faces in each of the four major left-sided valve lesions: aortic stenosis (AS), mitral regurgitation (MR), aortic regurgitation (AR), and mitral stenosis (MS).

BACKGROUND

In 1973, Grossman et al.[1] proposed the schema shown in Figure 4-1 as the foundation on which the left ventricle responds to valvular heart disease.[1] In this concept, the increased systolic stress (s) caused by pressure overload induces sarcomere production in parallel, increasing myocyte width, and in turn increasing left ventricular (LV) wall thickness. Because $s = p \times r/2h$ where p = LV pressure, r = LV radius, and h = thickness, increased pressure in the numerator is offset by increased thickness in the denominator so that stress remains normal. Systolic wall stress is a reasonable surrogate for LV afterload. Because the ejection fraction varies inversely with afterload, the concentric hypertrophy and remodeling that occur through this process are thought of as initially compensatory because they help maintain LV function.

In the same hypothesis, volume overload increases diastolic stress that causes sarcomeres to be laid down in series, lengthening each myocyte, and in turn increasing LV volume. Increased volume then allows total stroke volume to increase, helping to compensate for the wasted volume lost to regurgitation. Because this mechanism is a requisite to normalizing forward stroke volume, it too is considered compensatory, at least in part. Table 4-1 demonstrates the patterns of remodeling found in the left-sided overloading valve lesions.[2] AS, the classic pressure overload lesion produces typical concentric LV hypertrophy (LVH) with the highest mass-to-volume ratio and the lowest radius-to-thickness ratio. MR is the prototypical volume overload lesion leading to the lowest mass to volume ratio and the highest radius-to-thickness ratio. AR, a combined pressure and volume LV overload causes the greatest amount of LVH with hybrid geometry between that of AS and MR.

Hypertrophy versus Remodeling

It has become fashionable to use the term *remodeling* when changes in ventricular size and geometry are discussed, and most remodeling is associated with LVH. However, the two terms are not synonymous. Hypertrophy means an increase in mass whereas remodeling indicates a change in geometry and/or volume. Thus, a situation in which increased wall thickness is accompainied by increased LV mass should be considered concentric hypertrophy, whereas one in which increased thickness is accompanied by a reduction in volume leading to no change in LV mass[3] should be

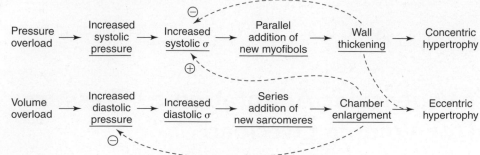

FIGURE 4–1 The diagram shown is a framework for how mechanical stress (σ) is transduced into pressure versus volume overload hypertrophy. *(From Grossman W, Jones D, McLaurin LP: Wall stress and patterns of hypertrophy in the human left ventricle. J Clin Invest 1975; 53:332-341, with permission.)*

4

TABLE 4–1	Hypertrophy in Human Left-Sided Overload Valve Lesions		
	Mass Index (g/m²)	r/h	m/v
NL	86 (259)*	3.05 (88)	1.25 (225)
MR	158 (146)	4.03 (64)	0.87 (117)
AR	230 (148)	3.52 (31)	1.00 (141)
AS	178 (302)	2.35 (93)	1.55 (296)

*Numbers in parentheses indicate numbers of subjects analyzed.
AR, aortic regurgitation; AS, aortic stenosis; MR, mitral regurgitation; *m/v*, ratio of left ventricular mass to volume; NL, normal subject; *r/h*, ratio of left ventricular radius to thickness.
From Carabello BA: The relationship of left ventricular geometry and hypertrophy to left ventricular function in valvular heart disease. J Heart Valve Dis 1995 (Suppl 2):S132-S138, with permission.

termed *concentric remodeling*. Whereas the term remodeling is most often used in the context of LV dilatation, a distinction should also be made between ventricles that enlarge with concomitant wall thinning where LV mass could remain the same (pure remodeling) versus those left ventricles that also increase their mass (eccentric hypertrophy) (Figure 4-2).

AORTIC STENOSIS

The normal aortic valve opens, slightly through not entirely understood mechanisms before pressure in the left ventricle exceeds aortic pressure[4,5] and then offers almost no resistance to LV outflow. As the valve becomes diseased it stiffens and the orifice area diminishes. Even when aortic valve area is reduced by half, the LV pressure only exceeds that of the aorta by 5 to 10 mm Hg. However, further reductions in aortic valve area cause progressively greater pressure gradients across the valve. The transvalvular gradient represents the additional pressure that the left ventricle must generate to drive blood past the obstruction to outflow. It is generally agreed that this mechanical stress is transduced into a biologic response, leading to hypertrophy and/or remodeling.

As noted above, because the development of hypertrophy helps normalize afterload, thereby normalizing ejection performance, such hypertrophy has been viewed as compensatory. According to the paradigm raised in Figure 4-1, just enough hypertrophy should develop to return wall stress to normal. Indeed, in some cases this expected course is borne out. However, such perfect compensation often fails to occur (Figures 4-3 and 4-4). Figure 4-3 demonstrates that frequently in patients with LV dysfunction, such dysfunction is due to afterload excess, indicating that not enough hypertrophy developed to normalize stress.[6] In fact, the majority of patients with AS have some element of afterload excess, indicating a lack of fully compensatory hypertrophy.[7]

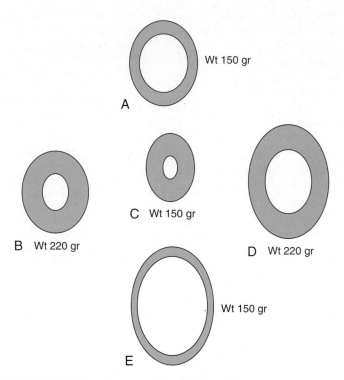

FIGURE 4–2 A schematic representation of the types of hypertrophy and remodeling that occur in valvular heart disease is shown. **A**, Normal. **B**, Concentric left ventricular hypertrophy (LVH). **C**, Concentric remodeling. **D**, Eccentric LVH. **E**, Eccentric remodeling.

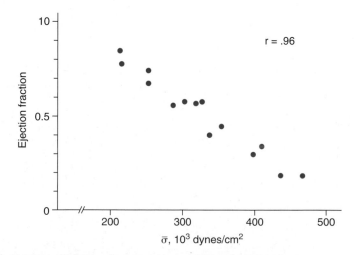

FIGURE 4–3 Ejection fraction is plotted against mean systolic wall stress (afterload) for patients with aortic stenosis. As afterload increases from inadequate left ventricular hypertrophy, ejection fraction falls. *(From Gunther S, Grossman W: Determinants of ventricular function in pressure-overload hypertrophy in man. Circulation 1979;59:679-688, with permission.)*

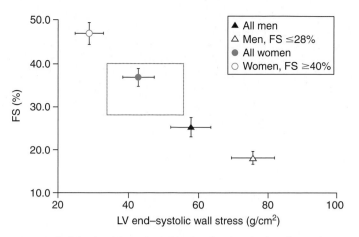

FIGURE 4–4 Fractional shortening (FS) is plotted against systolic wall stress for patients with aortic stenosis. Some patients, especially women, have abnormally low stress and very high shortening fractions suggesting that more left ventricular (LV) hypertrophy is present than that needed simply to normalize stress. *(From Carroll JD, Carroll EP, Feldman T, et al: Sex-associated differences in left ventricular function in aortic stenosis of the elderly. Circulation 1992;86:1099-1107, with permission.)*

The opposite end of the spectrum is shown in Figure 4-4.[8] In some patients, especially elderly women and children born with congenital AS,[9] there appears to be excessive hypertrophy. In such patients afterload is actually subnormal, leading to higher than expected ejection performance, at least at the endocardial level. It should be noted that assessment of LV function at the endocardial level often overestimates contractility. Ejection of blood from the LV cavity during systole is primarily a function of wall thickening. The more sarcomeres present in parallel, the more thickening occurs with shortening of the sarcomeres. Thus, in concentric remodeling and hypertrophy, subnormal shortening can still produce a normal ejection fraction.[10] Therefore, for accurate assessment of LV function in concentrically altered ventricles, midwall shortening should be evaluated and when done, it may reveal diminished LV function, although this is not always the case.

In still other patients yet another response—concentric remodeling—develops to AS. In these patients there is no increase in LV mass.[3] Rather there is a reduction in LV volume together with an increase in LV wall thickness, acting to normalize stress without actual hypertrophy.

Variability in the Response to Pressure Overload

The question arises, why is there such inhomogeneity in the hypertrophic response to pressure overload? Is the differing LV geometry that occurs a response to different disease characteristics, i.e., valve area, rate of progression, body habitus, or others? Or is there an inherent difference in response to a similar pressure overload? Koide et al[11] addressed this question by creating a model of AS in which a gradually imposed gradient was identical in dogs of similar size and weight. The hypertrophy that subsequently developed recapitulated that seen in humans. Some animals developed modest concentric hypertrophy, whereas others developed severe hypertrophy. Of interest, the group with modest hypertrophy had persistently higher wall stress yet far less myocardial mass despite this greater stimulus for hypertrophy (Figure 4-5). These data suggest a different set point for response to the overload for which the stimulus was greater and the response less. It is likely that these inherent differences also explain the difference in the hypertrophic response in humans noted above.

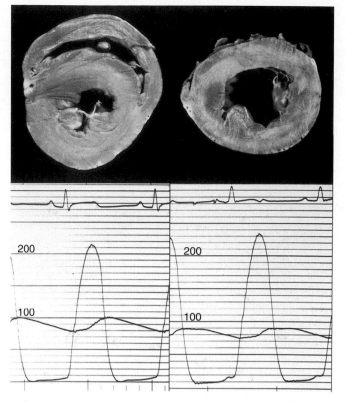

FIGURE 4–5 The heterogeneous response of the left ventricle to pressure overload is demonstrated in ventricles from two dogs with identical pressure gradients. *(From Koide M, Nagatsu M, Zile MR, et al: Premorbid determinants of left ventricular dysfunction in a novel mode of gradually induced pressure overload in the adult canine. Circulation 1997;95:1349-1351, with permission.)*

Concentric Hypertrophy and Left Ventricular Function

LV ejection is controlled by preload, afterload, and contractility. The reduction in the ejection fraction in AS stems from increased afterload, decreased contractility, or both.[7,12] Increased afterload occurs when remodeling fails to offset the increased systolic pressure required of the left ventricle. Whereas concentric LVH has long been considered a compensatory mechanism, this issue is not clear-cut. In studies of hypertrophy in general, LVH has led to increased cardiac mortality, especially in the presence of coronary artery disease.[13] Genetic maneuvers in mice that prevent or diminish the hypertrophic response have led to both increased mortality[14,15] and, conversely, beneficial effects,[16,17] leaving the question of the compensatory role of LVH in doubt. In the canine model cited above, contractility was preserved at both the sarcomere and LV chamber level in the animals with extreme hypertrophy in which wall stress was normalized. In dogs with high afterload, contractility was depressed, at least in part due to microtubular hyperpolymerization, acting as an internal stent inhibiting sarcomere shortening.[18] Conversely, in a recent human study of AS, the best outcome was in patients without LVH who underwent concentric remodeling.[3] LV mass was not increased, but increased relative wall thickness normalized afterload, allowing for compensated systolic function.

When contractile dysfunction does occur, its mechanism is probably multifactorial. Concentric LVH clearly results in abnormal coronary blood flow and blood flow reserve.[19-21] Normally the subendocardium receives about 20% more blood flow than the epicardium, but this ratio is reversed in LVH.[22]

Thus, the myocardial layer with the highest oxygen demand receives the least oxygen supply. Further coronary reserve is limited in concentric LVH. Whereas in normal individuals, coronary flow can increase by 5- to 8-fold in response to increased myocardial energy demands, flow reserve in AS is limited to 2- to 3-fold.[19] Abnormal flow reserve and flow distribution lead to subendocardial ischemia and contractile dysfunction during periods of stress.[22] It is also possible, but unproven, that this chronic imbalance could cause myocardial hibernation or stunning. The cytoskeletal abnormalities noted above as well as disordered calcium handling and apoptosis also probably play a role.[23-25] Finally, there is the general belief that LVH transitions from a compensatory phase to a pathologic one.[26] Although certainly plausible, this concept, too, has been questioned. Animals destined to develop contractile dysfunction demonstrated gene expression different from that in those who maintained normal function early in the course of pressure overload, suggesting that two separate patterns of hypertrophy exist rather than one transitioning into another,[27] consistent with the Koide dog model.

It is well recognized that diastolic function is abnormal in concentric LVH. Dysfunction accrues from delayed relaxation, increased wall thickness, and changes in myocardial structure with an increase in stiffness mediated by increased collagen content.[28,29]

In summary, the body of evidence supports the concept that concentric LVH is compensatory in the pressure overload of AS. However, concentric LVH is also associated with adverse outcomes, and the differences between compensatory and pathologic LVH have yet to be clearly delineated but are not explained by magnitude alone.

MITRAL REGURGITATION

Whereas a variety of cardiac lesions are classified as volume overload lesions, most are actually combined pressure and volume overload lesions.[30,31] In conditions such as AR, anemia, complete heart block, and others, the additional volume pumped by the left ventricle is ejected into the aorta where it increases stroke volume, widening pulse pressure and causing an element of systolic hypertension. Conversely, MR is a pure volume overload lesion. The extra volume pumped by the left ventricle in MR is ejected into the relatively low pressure zone of the left atrium and systemic systolic pressure tends to be reduced. Thus, MR is an ideal lesion in which to examine volume overload. As noted above, the remodeling in MR is eccentric, with a large increase in LV radius and little, if any, increase in LV thickness. In fact, LV thickness in MR may even be less than normal.

This type of remodeling is beneficial for diastolic filling of the left ventricle but may impair systolic emptying. MR is one of the few cardiac diseases in which diastolic function is supernormal (Figure 4-6).[32,33] The thin-walled left ventricle in MR requires less filling pressure to fill it to any given filling volume. Thus, the ventricle is equipped to fill rapidly to accept the large blood volume stored in the left atrium during systole that helps compensate for the volume wasted to regurgitation.

However, the large r/h ratio found in this type of remodeling (see Table 4-1) does not facilitate and may even impede LV ejection. The misconception that MR unloads the left ventricle by way of the low impedance pathway for ejection into the left atrium is common. Although to some extent this concept must be valid, afterload is reduced only in acute MR. Thereafter, as the radius term in the Laplace equation increases, afterload returns to normal. As remodeling progresses, the enlarging r/h ratio actually causes afterload to become abnormally high, impeding rather than unloading the left ventricle during ejection.[34] In reexamining Grossman's

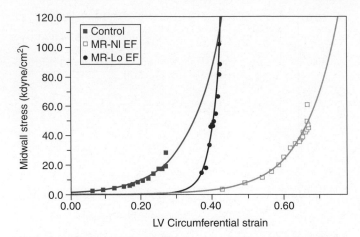

FIGURE 4–6 Stress-strain plots (stiffness) for normal subjects, for patients with mitral regurgitation (MR) with normal left ventricular (LV) function (MR-Nl EF), and for patients with MR with reduced LV function (MR Lo EF) are demonstrated. Patients with MR with a normal ejection fraction have reduced myocardial stiffness with their curves falling down and to the right of normal. *(From Corin WJ, Murakami T, Monrad ES, et al: Left ventricular passive diastolic properties in chronic mitral regurgitation. Circulation 1991;83:797-807, with permission.)*

hypothesis, it appears that the pressure term in the Laplace equation is more effective than the radius term in causing LV thickening, because increased systolic stress from pressure overload but not from volume overload induces wall thickening. Alternatively it may be the lack of isovolumic pressure generation that causes this type of remodeling. In MR and ventricular septal defect, ejection from the left ventricle begins almost immediately, lacking the isovolumic period before the aortic valve opens, and in both cases the relative lack of LV muscle mass seems connected with reduced LV function.[2,31,34,35]

Left Ventricular Function in Mitral Regurgitation

Increased preload together with normal afterload work in concert with initially normal contractility to maintain the LV ejection fraction at higher than normal levels. A "normal" ejection fraction in MR is about 70%. However, contractility eventually becomes impaired in severe prolonged MR so that by the time ejection fraction falls to less than 60%, prognosis is impaired.[36,37]

Coronary blood flow is normal in MR and thus is not responsible for impaired contractile function.[38] Reduced contractility stems from loss of sarcomeric contractile elements (Figure 4-7) and impaired calcium handling.[39,40] The former can be reversed by correction of the volume overload or institution of β-blockade, implying sympathetic overdrive as a cause for the abnormal contractile function.[41,42]

The force frequency response in MR is impaired, with peak force occurring at relatively low heart rates followed by an early descending limb. These data indicate impaired calcium handling. Forskolin also reverses contractile dysfunction, indicating that abnormal cyclic AMP generation is also involved in abnormal contractility.[40]

MECHANISMS OF HYPERTROPHY IN AORTIC STENOSIS VERSUS MITRAL REGURGITATION

The contractile proteins of the myocardium are in constant flux, turning over every 10 days or so. For hypertrophy to occur, the rate of protein synthesis (K_s) must exceed the rate

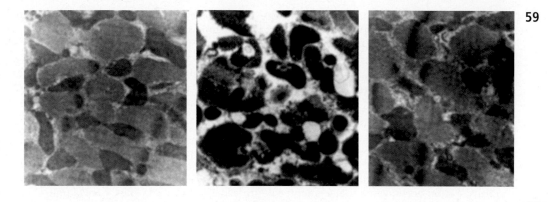

FIGURE 4–7 Myocardial ultrastructure of normal dogs (*left*), dogs with severe mitral regurgitation (MR) (*center*), and dogs that had severe MR corrected surgically (*right*) is shown. During severe MR there is a loss of contractile elements that is restored after surgery. *(From Spinale FG, Ishihara K, Zile M, et al: Structural basis for changes in left ventricular function and geometry because of chronic mitral regurgitation and after correction of volume overload. J Thorac Cardiovasc Surg 1993;106: 1147-1157, with permission.)*

of protein degradation (K_d). Obviously, the only way for this to occur is for K_s to increase or for K_d to decrease. By infusing an experimental animal with a tritiated amino acid such as leucine, the rate of incorporation of new protein (K_s) can be determined. When a pressure overload is imposed on the canine left ventricle, K_s increases by 35% within 6 hours of the onset of the overload (Figure 4-8).[43] K_s then remains elevated for several days and returns to normal once afterload is normalized, strongly supporting Grossman's hypothesis.[44] Increased protein synthesis does not accrue from increased DNA transcription in this model but rather by enhanced message translation as there is no increase in myosin message but rather an increase in ribosomal number and in polysome formation.

Conversely, even when severe MR was imposed on the canine left ventricle, no increase in K_s could be detected acutely nor at 2 weeks, 1 month, or 3 months after creation of MR (Figure 4-9).[43,45] Because eccentric LVH did occur, the lack of an increase in K_s implies that hypertrophy ensued by a decrease in K_d, an opposite mechanism for hypertrophy development from that of pressure overload. A rabbit model of MR produced similar findings.[46] In an isolated myocyte study in which load was imposed either during systole as it would be in pressure overload versus in diastole as it would occur in volume overload, different signaling pathways were activated, again speaking to potentially differing mechanisms for generating pressure versus volume overload hypertrophy.[47]

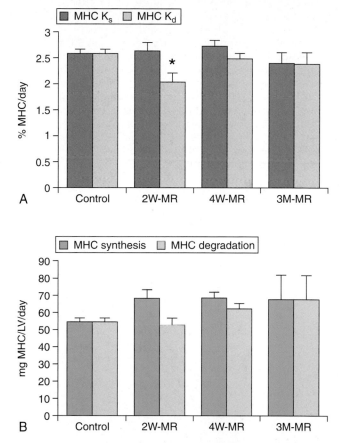

A

B

FIGURE 4–9 Myosin heavy chain (MHC) synthesis rate (K_s) and calculated degradation rate (K_d) are shown for controls and for dogs with mitral regurgitation (MR) at 2 weeks (2w-MR), 4 weeks (4w-MR), and 3 months (3m-MR) after creation of MR. An increase in K_s was not seen during the course of the lesion. *(From Matsuo T, Carabello BA, Nagatomo Y, et al: Mechanisms of cardiac hypertrophy in canine volume overload. Am J Physiol 1998;275:H65-H74, with permission.)*

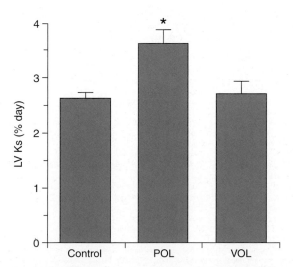

FIGURE 4–8 Myosin heavy chain synthesis rate (K_s) is demonstrated for controls, for acute pressure overload (POL), and for acute volume overload (VOL). Whereas K_s increased substantially in POL, no increase could be detected in VOL. LV, left ventricular. *(From Imamura T, McDermott PJ, Kent RL, et al: Acute changes in myosin heavy chain synthesis rate in pressure versus volume overload. Circ Res 1994;75:418-425.)*

AORTIC REGURGITATION, A HYBRID DISEASE

Long lumped together with MR as a volume overload lesion, it is clear that aortic AR is really a combined pressure and volume overload.[30] Here the relatively high systolic pressure generated by the high total stroke volume ejected into the aorta combined with a large LV radius produces afterload that may be as high as that seen in AS, the traditional pressure overload. Not surprisingly then, both types of hypertrophy develop in AR. LV volume is increased and to a lesser extent so is LV wall thickness.[48] Thus, LV mass in AR is the highest of all valve lesions. Of interest, the mechanism of hypertrophy in AR also appears to be a hybrid of AS and MR, established by an increase in K_s but maintained by a decrease in K_d.[49]

Left Ventricular Function in Aortic Regurgitation

LV function in even severe AR may remain normal for years and the rate of progression to LV dysfunction or symptom onset in asymptomatic patients is slow, probably less than 4% per year.[50] As with AS, when LV dysfunction does occur, it appears to be due both to excess afterload as well as to diminished contractility.[51] After aortic valve replacement, a depressed ejection fraction may improve dramatically especially if the duration of dysfunction has been short (Figure 4-10).[52] Recovery is primarily due to a postoperative reduction in afterload.[53] If the ejection fraction is only mildly depressed preoperatively, it is likely to return to normal postoperatively. Even if the preoperative ejection fraction is severely reduced, significant improvement postoperatively is the rule because of the fall in afterload. The mechanisms of depressed contractility have been studied in a rabbit model,[54,55] in which there is an abundant growth of the noncollagen interstitial matrix, especially fibronectin. This abundant overgrowth appears to "choke" existing contractile elements, often replacing them. To what extent this process is reversible after correction of the volume overload is unknown, as is the degree of its role in human AR.

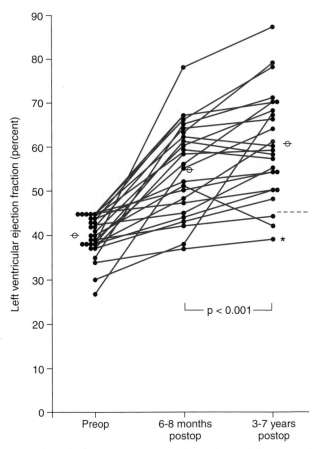

Early increase in LV ejection fraction

p < 0.001

FIGURE 4–10 Left ventricular (LV) ejection fraction before (pre-op) and after (post-op) aortic valve replacement for patients with aortic regurgitation is demonstrated. *(From Bonow RO, Dodd JT, Maron BJ, et al: Long-term serial changes in left ventricular function and reversal of ventricular dilatation after valve replacement for chronic aortic regurgitation. Circulation 1988;78:1108-1120, with permission.)*

MITRAL STENOSIS: THE UNDERLOADED LEFT VENTRICLE

Approximately one third of patients with MS have reduced LV ejection performance, perhaps surprising because this lesion "protects" the left ventricle from the consequences of MS.[56,57] Although the issue of whether the rheumatic process causes a contractile or "myocardial factor" leading to impaired myocardial function remains controversial, it does not appear to be operative in developed countries where the consequences of rheumatic fever seem milder than in the developing world. Why then should LV ejection performance be reduced in MS? It appears that increased afterload is partly to blame. Although MS is not usually thought of as an afterloading lesion, systolic wall stress is increased in many patients with MS.[56] Increased afterload seems predicated on reduced wall thickness and reflexively increased systemic vascular resistance. At the same time, impaired LV filling prevents the use of the preload reserve to compensate for the afterload excess. These abnormalities are reversed after balloon mitral valvotomy.[58] It is plausible, although far from being proven, that reduced filling also impairs the ventricle from receiving the mechanical signals necessary for maintaining the mass and geometry needed for normalizing wall stress.

CONCLUSION

Each valve lesion creates its own unique set of loading conditions that lead to LV remodeling and/or hypertrophy. These changes in many cases provide compensation for the load presented by the lesion, but remarkable differences exist among patients with similar types and severities of lesions, suggesting a great deal of modulation downstream from the initial mechanical signal. Although hypertrophy and remodeling may be compensatory, this often is not the case as they may also lead to negative consequences including heart failure and death. Future efforts to understand when and why these processes become pathologic are almost certain to augment our current armamentarium for deciding when to intervene in valvular heart disease.

REFERENCES

1. Grossman W, Jones D, McLaurin LP: Wall stress and patterns of hypertrophy in the human left ventricle. J Clin Invest 1975;53:332-341.
2. Carabello BA: The relationship of left ventricular geometry and hypertrophy to left ventricular function in valvular heart disease. J Heart Valve Dis 1995;4 (Suppl 2): S132-S138; discussion S138-S139.
3. Kupari M, Tutro H, Lommi J: Left ventricular hypertrophy in aortic valve stenosis—preventive or promotive of systolic dysfunction and heart failure? Eur Heart J 2005; 26:1790-1796.
4. Rodriguez F, Green GR, Dagum P, et al: Left ventricular volume shifts and aortic root expansion during isovolumic contraction. J Heart Valve Dis 2006;15:465-473.
5. Pang DC, Choo SJ, Luo HH, et al: Significant increase of aortic root volume and commissural area occurs prior to aortic valve opening. J Heart Valve Dis 2000;9:9-15.
6. Gunther S, Grossman W: Determinants of ventricular function in pressure-overload hypertrophy in man. Circulation 1979;59:679-688.
7. Huber D, Grimm J, Koch R, Krayenbuehl HP: Determinants of ejection performance in aortic stenosis. Circulation 1981;64:126-134.
8. Carroll JD, Carroll EP, Feldman T, et al: Sex-associated differences in left ventricular function in aortic stenosis of the elderly. Circulation 1992;86:1099-1107.
9. Donner R, Carabello BA, Black I, Spann JF: Left ventricular wall stress in compensated aortic stenosis in children. Am J Cardiol 1983;51:946-951.
10. deSimone G, Devereux RB, Celentano A, et al: Left ventricular chamber and wall mechanics in the presence of concentric geometry. J Hypertens 1999;17:1001-1006.
11. Koide M, Nagatsu M, Zile MR, et al: Premorbid determinants of left ventricular dysfunction in a novel mode of gradually induced pressure overload in the adult canine. Circulation 1997;95:1349-1351.
12. Carabello BA, Green LH, Grossman W, et al: Hemodynamic determinants of prognosis of aortic valve replacement in critical aortic stenosis and advanced congestive heart failure. Circulation 1980;62:42-48.
13. Levy D, Garrison RJ, Savage DD, et al: Prognostic implications of echocardiographically determined left ventricular mass in the Framingham Heart Study. N Engl J Med 1990;322:1561-1566.

14. Meguro T, Hong C, Asai K, et al: Cyclosporine attenuates pressure-overload hypertrophy in mice while enhancing susceptibility to decompensation and heart failure. Circ Res 1999;84:735-740.

15. Rogers JH, Tamirisa P, Kovacs A, et al: RGS4 causes increased mortality and reduced cardiac hypertrophy in response to overload. J Clin Invest 1999;104:567-576.

16. Esposito G, Rapacciuolo A, Naga Prasad SV, et al: Genetic alterations that inhibit in vivo pressure-overload hypertrophy prevent cardiac dysfunction despite increased wall stress. Circulation 2002;105:85-92.

17. Hill JA, Karimi M, Kutschke W, et al: Cardiac hypertrophy is not a required compensation response to short-term pressure overload. Circulation 2000;101:2863-2869.

18. Koide M, Hamawaki M, Narishige T, et al: Microtubule depolymerization normalizes in vivo myocardial contractile function in dogs with pressure-overload left ventricular hypertrophy. Circulation 2000;102:1045-1052.

19. Marcus ML, Doty DB, Hiratzka LF, et al: Decreased coronary reserve: a mechanism for angina pectoris in patients with aortic stenosis and normal coronary arteries. N Engl J Med. 1982;307:1362-1366.

20. Julius BK, Spillman M, Vassali G, et al: Angina pectoris in patients with aortic stenosis and normal coronary arteries: mechanisms and pathophysiological concepts. Circulation 1997;95:892-898.

21. Rajappan K, Rimoldi OE, Dutka DP, et al: Mechanisms of coronary microcirculatory dysfunction in patients with aortic stenosis and angiographically normal coronary arteries. Circulation 2002;105:470-476.

22. Nakano K, Corin WJ, Spann JF, et al: Abnormal subendocardial blood flow in pressure overload hypertrophy is associated with pacing-induced subendocardial dysfunction. Circ Res 1989;65:1555-1564.

23. Tsutsui H, Oshihara K, Cooper GT: Cytoskeletal role in the contractile dysfunction of hypertrophied myocardium. Science 1993;260:682-687.

24. Ito K, Yan X, Feng X, et al: Transgenic expression of sarcoplasmic reticulum Ca^{2+} ATPase modifies the transition from hypertrophy to early heart failure. Circ Res 2001;89:422-9.

25. Olivetti G, Abbi R, Quaini F, et al: Apoptosis in the failing human heart. N Engl J Med 1997;336:1131-1141.

26. Hein S, Arnon E, Kostin S, et al: Progression from compensated hypertrophy to failure in the pressure-overloaded human heart: structural deterioration and compensatory mechanisms. Circulation 200325;107:984-989.

27. Buermans HPJ, Redout EM, Schiol AE, et al: Micro-array analysis reveals pivotal divergent mRNA expression profiles early in the development of either compensated ventricular hypertrophy or heart failure. Physiol Genomics 2005;21:314-323.

28. Zile MR, Brutsaert DL: New concepts in diastolic dysfunction and diastolic heart failure: part II-causal mechanisms and treatment. Circulation 2002;105:1503-1508.

29. Hess OM, Ritter M, Schneider J, et al: Diastolic stiffness and myocardial structure in aortic valve disease before and after valve replacement. Circulation 1984; 69:855-865.

30. Wisenbaugh T, Spann JF, Carabello BA: Differences in myocardial performance and load between patients with similar amounts of chronic aortic versus chronic mitral regurgitation. J Am Coll Cardiol 1984;3:916-923.

31. Carabello BA: Mitral regurgitation. Part I: Basic pathophysiological principles. Mod Concepts Cardiovasc Dis 1988;57:53-58.

32. Zile Mr, Tomita M, Nakano K, et al: Effects of left ventricular volume overload produced by mitral regurgitation on diastolic function. Am J Physiol 1991;261:II1471-H1480.

33. Corin WJ, Murakami T, Monrad ES, et al: Left ventricular passive diastolic properties in chronic mitral regurgitation. Circulation 1991;83:797-807.

34. Corin WJ, Monrad ES, Murakami T, et al: The relationship of afterload to ejection performance in chronic mitral regurgitation. Circulation 1987;76:59-67.

35. Corin WJ, Swindle MM, Spann JF Jr, et al: Mechanisms of decreased forward stroke volume in children and swine with ventricular septal defect and failure to thrive. J Clin Invest 1988;82:544-551.

36. Enriquez-Sarano M, Tajik AJ, Schaff HV, et al: Echocardiographic prediction of survival after surgical correction of organic mitral regurgitation. Circulation 1994;90:830-837.

37. Schuler G, Peterson KL, Johnson A, et al: Temporal response of left ventricular performance to mitral valve surgery. Circulation 1979;59:1218-1231.

38. Carabello BA, Nakano K, Ishihara K, et al: Coronary blood flow in dogs with contractile dysfunction due to experimental volume overload. Circulation 1991;83:1063-1075.

39. Spinale FG, Ishihara K, Zile M, et al: Structural basis for changes in left ventricular function and geometry because of chronic mitral regurgitation and after correction of volume overload. J Thorac Cardiovasc Surg 1993;106:1147-1157.

40. Mulieri LA, Leavitt BJ, Martin BJ, et al: Myocardial force-frequency defect in mitral regurgitation heart failure is reversed by forskolin. Circulation 1993;88:2700-2704.

41. Nakano K, Swindle MM, Spinale F, et al: Depressed contractile function due to canine mitral regurgitation improves after correction of the volume overload. J Clin Invest 1991;87:2077-2086.

42. Tsutsui H, Spinale FG, Nagatsu M, et al: Effects of chronic β-adrenergic blockade on the left ventricular and cardiocyte abnormalities of chronic canine mitral regurgitation. J Clin Invest 1994;93:2639-2648.

43. Imamura T, McDermott PJ, Kent RL, et al: Acute changes in myosin heavy chain synthesis rate in pressure versus volume overload. Circ Res 1994;75:418-425.

44. Nagatomo Y, Carabello BA, Hamawaki M, et al: Translational mechanisms accelerate the rate of protein synthesis during canine pressure-overload hypertrophy. Am J Physiol 1999;277:H2176-H2184.

45. Matsuo T, Carabello BA, Nagatomo Y, et al: Mechanisms of cardiac hypertrophy in canine volume overload. Am J Physiol 1998;275:H65-H74.

46. Borer JS, Carter JN, Jacobson MH, et al: Myofibrillar protein synthesis rates in mitral regurgitation. Circulation 1997;96(Suppl 1):I-469.

47. Yamamoto K, Dang Q, Maeda Y, et al: Regulation of cardiomyocyte mechanotransduction by the cardiac cycle. Circulation 2001;103:1459-1464.

48. Feiring AJ, Rumberger JA: Ultrafast computed tomography analysis of regional radius-to-wall thickness ratios in normal and volume-overloaded human left ventricle. Circulation 1992;85:1423-1432.

49. Magid NM, Wallerson DC, Borer JS: Myofibrillar protein turnover in cardiac hypertrophy due to aortic regurgitation. Cardiology 1993;82:20-29.

50. Bonow RO, Lakatos E, Maron BJ, Epstein SE: Serial long-term assessment of the natural history of asymptomatic patients with chronic aortic regurgitation and normal left ventricular systolic function. Circulation 1991;84:1625-1635.

51. Sutton M, Plappert T, Spegel A, et al: Early postoperative changes in left ventricular chamber size, architecture, and function in aortic stenosis and aortic regurgitation and their relation to intraoperative changes in afterload: a prospective two-dimensional echocardiographic study. Circulation 1987;76:77-89.

52. Bonow RO, Dodd JT, Maron BJ, et al: Long-term serial changes in left ventricular function and reversal of ventricular dilatation after valve replacement for chronic aortic regurgitation. Circulation 1988;78:1108-1120.

53. Taniguchi K, Nakano S, Kawashima Y, et al: Left ventricular ejection performance, wall stress, and contractile state in aortic regurgitation before and after aortic valve replacement. Circulation 1990;82:798-807.

54. Borer JS, Truter S, Herrold EM, et al: Myocardial fibrosis in chronic aortic regurgitation: molecular and cellular responses to volume overload. Circulation 2002;105:1837-1842.

55. Borer JS, Herrold EM, Carter JN, et al: Cellular and molecular basis of remodeling in valvular heart diseases. Heart Fail Clin 2006;2:415-424.

56. Gash AK, Carabello BA, Cepin D, et al: Left ventricular ejection performance and systolic muscle function in patients with mitral stenosis. Circulation 1983;67:148-154.

57. Horwitz LD, Mullins CB, Payne PM, Curry CG: Left ventricular function in mitral stenosis. Chest 1973;64:609-614.

58. Fawzy ME, Choi WB, Mimish L, et al: Immediate and long-term effect of mitral balloon valvotomy on left ventricular volume and systolic function in severe mitral stenosis. Am Heart J 1996;132:356-360.

Left Ventricular Adaptation to Pressure and/or Volume Overload

Evaluation of Valvular Heart Disease by Echocardiography

Catherine M. Otto

KEY POINTS

- Echocardiography provides an accurate diagnosis of the presence and cause of valve disease.
- Quantitative echocardiographic evaluation of left ventricular size and systolic function is a key factor in clinical decision making in adults with valvular heart disease.
- Aortic stenosis severity is defined by maximum aortic jet velocity, mean gradient, and continuity equation valve area.
- Mitral stenosis severity is defined by mean gradient and valve area, determined by two-dimensional planimetry and the pressure half-time method.
- Color Doppler flow mapping provides information on regurgitant jet origin and direction but is no longer recommended for evaluation of regurgitant severity.
- Regurgitant severity is defined by vena contracta width, the continuous wave Doppler velocity signal, and the presence of distal flow reversals. In selected cases, calculation of regurgitant volume and regurgitant orifice area is recommended.
- Other key echocardiographic data includes left ventricular diastolic function, left atrial enlargement and thrombus formation, pulmonary pressure estimates, and evaluation of right heart function.
- Aortic dilation associated with aortic valve disease can be diagnosed by echocardiography but other imaging modalities may be needed for complete evaluation.
- Primary indications for transesophageal imaging include detection of left atrial thrombus, evaluation of prosthetic mitral valves, mitral valve repair, aortic dilation, and nondiagnostic transthoracic data.

Echocardiography provides detailed, non-invasive information about the anatomy and etiology of valve disease, the severity of valve stenosis and/or regurgitation, the impact of the valvulars lesion on left ventricular (LV) size and function, and any associated cardiac abnormalities. Thus, echocardiographic evaluation now is the standard diagnostic approach to the patient with suspected or known valvular heart disease. This chapter provides a concise overview of the echocardiographic evaluation of the patient with valvular heart disease; more detailed discussions are available in standard echocardiography texts.[1-3]

ANATOMIC IMAGING

The first step in evaluation of the patient with valvular heart disease is assessment of valvular anatomy on two-dimensional (2D) imaging (Table 5-1). Although in many patients the specific valve involved is known from previous evaluation or on the basis of clinical history and physical examination; in other patients, the exact diagnosis may be unknown or may have been incorrectly inferred from clinical data. Thus, a careful examination of all four valves and screening for other lesions that might be mistaken for valvular disease are important aspects of the examination (Figure 5-1). For example, in a patient with a systolic murmur referred for suspected valvular aortic stenosis, other diagnostic possibilities that might account for the systolic murmur include a subaortic membrane, mitral regurgitation, ventricular septal defect, or hypertrophic obstructive cardiomyopathy. An appropriate examination includes exclusion (or confirmation) of each differential diagnosis as well as evaluation of the aortic valve itself. Normal echocardiographic values for imaging and Doppler flows are shown in Tables 5-2 and 5-3.

Echocardiographic Valve Anatomy

2D imaging allows identification of the involved valve and often allows precise definition of the etiology of the valvular lesion, based on the typical anatomic features of each disease process. Mitral stenosis most often is due to rheumatic valvular disease with pathognomonic features of commissural fusion, thickening of the leaflet tips, and chordal thickening, fusion, and

TABLE 5–1	Echocardiographic Evaluation of the Patient with Valvular Heart Disease

2D imaging
Valve anatomy and etiology of disease
2D echocardiographic valve area (in mitral stenosis)
Qualitative evaluation of global and regional LV function
Quantitative LV dimensions, volumes, ejection fraction, and mass
Qualitative evaluation of global and regional LV function
Quantitative LV dimensions, volumes, ejection fraction and mass
Associated chamber enlargement (e.g., left atrium)
Right heart structure and function
Complications of valve disease (i.e., left atrial thrombus)
Aortic root anatomy and dimensions

Doppler evaluation of severity of valve disease
Valve stenosis
   Maximum velocity
   Mean pressure gradient
   Valve area (continuity equation and/or pressure half-time)
   Other measures of stenosis severity, if needed
Valve regurgitation
   Vena contracta width
   Continuous-wave Doppler signal
   Distal flow reversals
   Regurgitant volume and orifice area

Other Doppler echocardiographic data
LV diastolic function
Pulmonary pressures at rest and with exercise

2D, two-dimensional; LV, left ventricular.

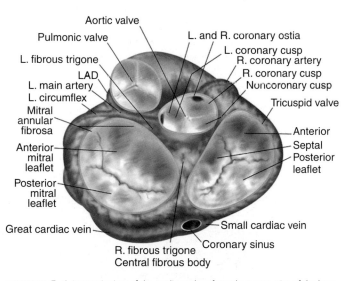

FIGURE 5–1 Anatomic view of the cardiac valves from the perspective of the base of the heart with the left and right atrium cut away and the great vessels transected. Note the close anatomic relationships of all four cardiac valves. In particular, the aortic valve is adjacent to the mitral valve along the midsegment of the anterior mitral valve leaflet. The pulmonic valve is slightly superior to the aortic valve and the aortic and pulmonic valve planes are nearly perpendicular to each other. L., left; LAD, left anterior descending coronary artery; R., right. (*Drawing by Starr Kaplan.*)

shortening, all of which are easily recognized on 2D imaging.[4-6] In contrast, the occasional elderly patient with functional mitral stenosis due to extension of mitral annular calcification onto the valve leaflets, has thin, mobile leaflet tips, with calcification and thickening at the leaflet bases (Figure 5-2). In addition, the specific anatomic features of the rheumatic mitral valve apparatus, as seen on 2D imaging, are important factors in predicting prognosis and in clinical decision making, particularly with regard to mitral commissurotomy as discussed in Chapter 14.

While aortic valve stenosis of any cause is characterized by thickened, stiff leaflets with reduced systolic opening, calcific aortic stenosis (most commonly seen) is typified by increased echogenicity and thickness in the body of the leaflets without evidence of commissural fusion, resulting in a stellate-shaped orifice in systole (Figure 5-3).[7,8] It may be difficult to separate calcific changes superimposed on a bicuspid aortic valve from calcification of a trileaflet valve by 2D imaging alone. However, the different age distribution of symptom onset in patients with stenosis due to a bicuspid (age 50 to 70 years) versus a trileaflet valve (age 70 to 90 years) allows a reasonable guess as to disease etiology.[9] Rheumatic aortic valve disease is characterized by a commissural fusion with increased thickening and echogenicity along the leaflet closure lines and invariably is associated with rheumatic mitral valve disease.[10] Congenital aortic stenosis, seen in young adults, is characterized by a deformed (often unicuspid) valve, which "domes" in systole with a restrictive orifice.

Evaluation of the etiology of a regurgitant lesion by echocardiography is more challenging, given the wide range of abnormalities that can lead to valvular incompetence. Mitral regurgitation may be due to abnormalities of the mitral apparatus including the annulus, leaflets, subvalvular apparatus, or papillary muscle, or may be due to LV dysfunction, either global or regional. (Figures 5-4 and 5-5) Echocardiographic imaging allows assessment of each of these components of the valve apparatus, so that the etiology of the regurgitant lesion can be discerned in many patients, as discussed in detail in Chapters 15 and 16. This evaluation is critical is selecting patients for mitral valve repair procedures as discussed in Chapter 18. However, in some patients, multiple abnormalities of the valve apparatus may make determination of the mechanism of regurgitation difficult. For example, in a patient with a dilated, hypokinetic left ventricle and irregular thickening of the valve leaflets, it may be unclear whether mitral regurgitation is due to the abnormal leaflets, annular dilation, malalignment or dysfunction of the papillary muscles, or a combination of these factors. In the future, three-dimensional (3D) reconstruction of echocardiographic images, in combination with computer modeling of normal valve anatomy and function, may provide a more precise definition of the mechanism of regurgitation in individual patients.[11-13] Quantitation evaluation of regurgitant severity, as described below, also may be helpful in determining whether mitral regurgitation is the cause or consequence of ventricular dysfunction.

Aortic regurgitation may be due to abnormalities of the valve leaflets (such as a bicuspid valve or endocarditis), inadequate support of the valve structures (e.g., a subaortic ventricular septal defect), or aortic root dilation (such as Marfan syndrome or annuloaortic ectasia) (Figures 5-5 and 5-6).[14-16] Echocardiographic imaging provides accurate measurements of aortic root dimensions and allows detailed evaluation of valve anatomy and dynamics. A bicuspid valve is diagnosed on the basis of the typical appearance in systole of two open leaflets; the closed valve in diastole may mimic a trileaflet valve if there is a raphe in one leaflet. Other recognized abnormalities of the valve leaflets that correspond to a specific etiology include valvular vegetations in endocarditis, redundant leaflets in myxomatous disease, and commissural thickening and associated mitral valve involvement in rheumatic disease, all of which can be recognized on 2D imaging.

With aortic root disease, the specific pattern of root dilation and associated features may indicate a specific etiology, such as the "water balloon" appearance of the root in Marfan syndrome with loss of the normal tapering at the sinotubular junction and associated mitral valve abnormalities.[17,18] In other cases, the pattern of root dilation is nonspecific so that incorporation of other clinical information is needed to

TABLE 5–2 | **Reference Values for Echocardiographic Chamber Quantification**

Chamber	Measurement	Normal Range (Women)	Normal Range (Men)	Units
Left ventricle	Diastolic diameter	3.9-5.3	4.2-4.9	cm
	(indexed to BSA)	2.4-3.2	2.2-3.1	cm/m²
	(indexed to height)	2.5-3.2	2.4-3.3	cm/m
	Diastolic volume	56-104	67-155	mL
	(indexed to BSA)	35-75	35-37	mL/m²
	Systolic volume	19-49	22-58	mL
	(indexed to BSA)	12-30	12-30	mL/m²
	Ejection fraction	≥55	≥55	%
	Septal wall thickness	0.6-0.9	0.6-1.0	cm
	Posterior wall thickness	0.6-0.9	0.6-1.0	cm
	LV mass (2D method)	66-150	96-200	g
	(indexed to BSA)	44-88	50-102	g/m²
	Relative wall thickness	0.22-0.42	0.24-0.42	cm
Left atrium	AP diameter	2.7-3.8	3.0-4.0	cm
	(indexed to BSA)	1.5-2.3	1.5-2.3	cm/m²
	LA area	≤20	≤20	cm²
	LA volume	22-52	18-52	mL
	(indexed to BSA)	22±6	22±6	mL/m²
		Normal Range		
Right ventricle	Mid-RV diastolic diameter	2.7-3.3		cm
	RV diastolic area (A4C)	11-28		cm²
	RV systolic area (A4C)	7.5-16		cm²
	Fractional area change	32-60		%
	Tricuspid annular excursion	>1.5		cm
Right atrium	RA dimension (A4C)	2. 9-4.5		cm
	(indexed to BSA)	1.7-2.5		cm/m²

2D, two-dimensional; A4C, apical four-chamber view; AP, anterior-posterior diameter in long-axis view; BSA, body surface area; LA, left atrium; RA, right atrium.
From Otto CM, Schwaegler RG: Echocardiography Review Guide: Companion to the Textbook of Clinical Echocardiography. Philadelphia, Saunders, 2007, with permission.

TABLE 5–3 | **Normal Antegrade Doppler Flow Velocities**

	Normal range
Ascending aorta	1.0-1.7 m/s
LV outflow tract	0.7-1.1 m/s
LV inflow	
E-velocity	0.6-1.3 (0.72 ± 0.14)
Deceleration slope	5.0 ± 1.4 m/s
A-velocity	0.2-0.7 (0.47-0.4)
Pulmonary artery	0.5-1.3
RV inflow	
E-velocity	0.3-0.7
RV filling (SVC, HV)	
Systole	0.32-0.69 (0.46 ± 0.08) m/s
Diastole	0.06-0.45 (0.27 ± 0.08) m/s
LA filling (pulmonary vein)	
Systole	0.56 ± 0.13 m/s
Diastole	0.44 ± 0.16 m/s
Atrial reversal	0.32 ± 0.07 m/s

A, late (atrial) diastolic peak; E, early diastolic peak; HV, hepatic vein; LA, left atrial; LV, left ventricular; RA, right atrial; RV, right ventricular; SVC, superior vena cava.
Data from Wilson et al: Br Heart J 1985;53:451; Hatle and Angelsen: Doppler Ultrasound in Cardiology, 2nd ed. Lea & Febiger, 1985; Van Dam et al: Eur Heart J 1987;8:1221, 1988;9:165; Jaffe et al: Am J Cardiol 1991;68:550; Appleton et al: J Am Coll Cardiol 1987;10:1032.
From Otto CM: Textbook of Clinical Echocardiography, 3rd ed. Philadelphia, Saunders, 2004, with permission.

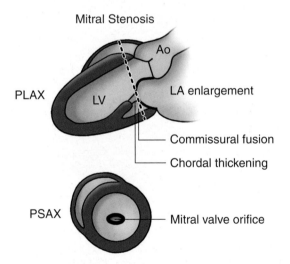

FIGURE 5–2 Schematic diagram of the two-dimensional echo findings in mitral stenosis. In the parasternal long-axis view (PLAX), commissural fusion with diastolic doming of the mitral leaflets is seen, as well as chordal thickening and fusion. In a parasternal short-axis view (PSAX), at the mitral valve orifice, the area of opening can be planimetered. The plane of the short-axis view is indicated by a dashed line on the long-axis image. Ao, aorta; LV, left ventricle. *(From Otto CM: Textbook of Clinical Echocardiography, 3rd ed. Philadelphia, Saunders, 2004, with permission.)*

determine the etiology of disease. For example, aortic root dilation in a patient with a systemic immune-mediated process (such as rheumatoid arthritis) is probably due to this systemic disease process.[19] In contrast, dilation of the ascending aorta in a patient with a bicuspid aortic valve probably is related to bicuspid aortic valve disease.[20,21]

Right-sided valve abnormalities in adults are most likely due to residual congenital heart disease (e.g., congenital pulmonic stenosis or Ebstein anomaly of the tricuspid valve) or are secondary to left-sided heart disease (e.g., tricuspid annular dilation due to pulmonary hypertension in a patient with mitral stenosis). Again, 2D imaging usually allows determination of the valve anatomy and etiology of the valvular lesion, particularly when other aspects of the examination and clinical features are incorporated in the echocardiographic interpretation.

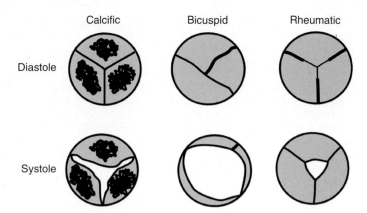

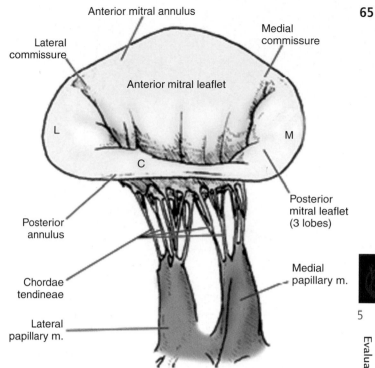

FIGURE 5–3 Schematic diagram of the three most common causes of valvular aortic stenosis. Calcific aortic stenosis is characterized by fibrocalcific masses on the aortic side of the leaflet that result in increased leaflet stiffness, without commissural fusion. A congenital bicuspid valve undergoes secondary degenerative changes. The diagnostic features of rheumatic stenosis are commissural fusion and mitral valve involvement. *(From Otto CM: Textbook of Clinical Echocardiography, 2nd ed. Philadelphia, Saunders, 2000, with permission.)*

FIGURE 5–5 The mitral valve apparatus consists of the mitral annulus, anterior and posterior leaflets, chordae tendineae, and the papillary muscles. Abnormal function of any one these components results in mitral regurgitation. The posterior leaflet has three scallops: lateral (L or P1), central (C or P2) and medial (M or P3). *(Drawing by Starr Kaplan.)*

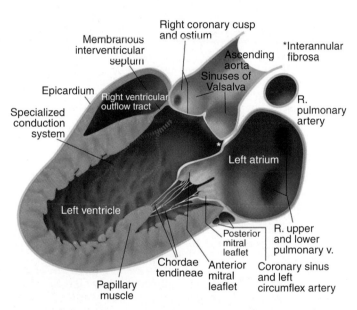

FIGURE 5–4 Anatomic drawing in a long-axis orientation illustrating the close relationship between the aortic root and anterior mitral valve leaflet. Note that the mitral valve apparatus includes the left atrial wall, the annulus, the anterior and posterior mitral leaflets, the mitral chordae and the papillary muscles. R., right. *(Drawing by Starr Kaplan.)*

Transthoracic versus Transesophageal Imaging

Transthoracic imaging provides diagnostic images in the vast majority of patients with valvular heart disease and is the standard approach both for the initial evaluation and for follow-up studies. Transesophageal imaging is reserved for patients for whom transthoracic images are nondiagnostic or when higher resolution images are needed for clinical decision making. With trained and experienced sonographers, diagnostic images can be obtained on transthoracic imaging in most patients; exceptions include patients with poor ultrasound access due to body habitus, hyperexpanded lungs, or the postoperative state. In these patients, transesophageal imaging may be necessary. In addition, the improved image quality, particularly of posterior structures (such as the mitral valve), may provide critical anatomic information in specific clinical situations, such as determining the likelihood of mitral valve repair in a patient with myxomatous mitral valve disease or excluding left atrial thrombus in a candidate for mitral balloon commissurotomy.

Other indications for transesophageal echocardiography in patients with valvular disease include assessment of regurgitant severity when transthoracic images are nondiagnostic or when a prosthetic mitral valve is present, intraoperative monitoring of valve repair procedures, and determining the exact level of obstruction in a patient with a differential diagnosis of valvular versus subvalvular obstruction. Rarely, transesophageal imaging is needed for evaluation of stenosis severity, when transthoracic data are not diagnostic.

Three-Dimensional Echocardiography

Anatomic images in a 3D gray-scale format derived from real-time 3D imaging probes or alignment of multiple tomographic images provide intuitive images of valve anatomy and motion.[22,23] The exact role of 3D echocardiography is evaluation of patients with valvular heart disease is in evolution, but this approach appears to be most valuable for 3D transesophageal imaging of the myxomatous mitral valve. These 3D cine images provide a "surgical" view of the mitral valve from the perspective of the left atrium which allows evaluation of the presence, location, and severity of prolapse; chordal rupture; and the anatomy of the valve commissures (Figure 5-7). 3D echocardiography has been less useful for evaluation of the aortic valve because signal drop-out due to the nonperpendicular angle of the ultrasound signal results in artifactual "holes" in the valve leaflets.

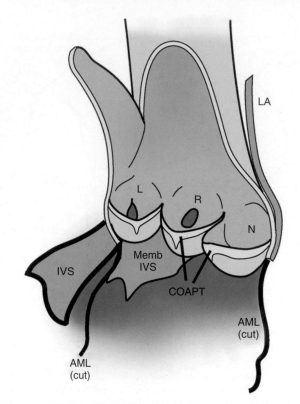

FIGURE 5–6 Detailed view of the aortic valve with the aorta opened to show the valve leaflets and the anterior leaflet bisected. The aortic valve consists of three leaflets and associated sinuses of Valsalva; the left (L), right (R) and non (N) coronary leaflets and sinuses. Each leaflet-sinus pair forms a cup-shaped unit when the valve is closed. The load-bearing section of the leaflet appears linear when viewed in long-axis (see Figure 5-4) but curved in cross-section consistent with a hemicylindrical shape. The coaptation (COAPT) surfaces of the leaflets thicken toward the center of each leaflet with areas of prominent thickening termed the nodes of Arantius. Lambl's excrescences, filamentous attachments on the ventricular side of the nodules of Arantius, are common in older subjects. AML, anterior mitral leaflet; IVS, interventricular septum; LA, left atrium *(From Otto CM: Textbook of Clinical Echocardiography, 3rd ed. Philadelphia, Elsevier Saunders, 2004, with permission.)*

EVALUATION OF LEFT VENTRICULAR SYSTOLIC FUNCTION

Evaluation of the LV response to pressure and/or volume overload is a critical step in echocardiographic examination of the patient with left-sided valvular heart disease. The degree of LV dilation and evidence of impaired contractility is particularly important in patients with chronic valvular regurgitation as discussed in Chapter 4.

Left Ventricular Volumes and Ejection Fraction

2D echocardiography allows both qualitative and quantitative evaluation of LV size and systolic function.[1,24] Images of the left ventricle are acquired from the parasternal window in a long axis view and in sequential short axis views at the basal, midventricular, and, when possible, apical levels. From an apical approach, images are acquired in four-chamber, two-chamber and long-axis views. Additional subcostal views in four-chamber and short-axis orientations can be used to supplement the parasternal and apical windows, particularly if image quality is suboptimal from parasternal and apical windows. Tissue harmonic imaging provides excellent endocardial definition in most patients. If endocardial definition is suboptimal even with tissue harmonic imaging, intravenous contrast agents for opacification of the left ventricle may be helpful.

Qualitative Evaluation

When quantitative evaluation of LV systolic function is not possible, qualitative evaluation of global and regional systolic function by an experienced observer has great clinical utility. Classification of overall LV systolic function as normal or mildly, moderately or severely reduced is of prognostic value in patients with valvular heart disease, for example, in patients with symptomatic aortic stenosis.[25] Evaluation of overall systolic function by an experienced observer correlates well with quantitative measures of systolic function. Individual echocardiographers can "calibrate" themselves and improve the accuracy of qualitative assessment by ongoing comparison with other measures of LV function, whenever possible.

Regional wall motion is assessed as normal, hypokinetic, akinetic, or dyskinetic for each region of the left ventricle using the standard 17-segment nomenclature.[26] The ventricle is divided into thirds from base to apex (basal, midventricular, and apex) with evaluation (clockwise in a short-axis view) of anterior septum, anterior wall, lateral wall, posterior wall, inferior wall, and inferior septum at the basal and midventricular levels with four segments (anterior, lateral, posterior, and inferior) at the apical level and an additional segment for the tip of the LV apex (see Figure 5-6). Although regional wall motion abnormalities are not a feature of valvular heart disease per se, their presence may alert the clinician to the probability of coexisting coronary artery disease. Because wall motion may be normal at rest even when significant coronary disease is present, if there is a high clinical suspicion of coronary disease, coronary angiography may be indicated.

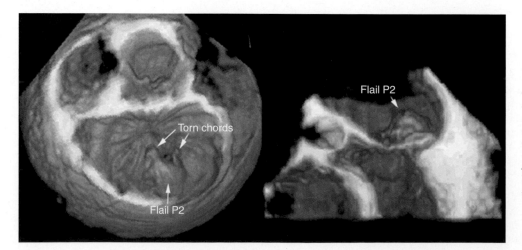

FIGURE 5–7 Three-dimensional reconstructed images from a rotational transesophageal echocardiographic scan are oriented to show the mitral valve from the left atrial aspect (*left*) and in a long-axis orientation (*right*) The torn chords and flail central scallop of the posterior mitral leaflet (P2) are clearly seen. (*From Oxorn D, Otto CM: Atlas of Intraoperative Transesophageal Echocardiography. Philadelphia, Elsevier Saunders, 2007, with permission.*)

The simplest quantitative measures of LV size are 2D-guided M-mode recordings at the midventricular level (see Table 5-2) for end-diastolic dimensions and end-systolic dimensions. The American College of Cardiology/American Heart Association practice guidelines rely on precise values of ventricular dimension for clinical decision making so use of a careful measurement technique is critical.[27] By using both long- and short-axis views from a parasternal window, the 2D image is used to ensure that the M-mode beam is centered in the LV chamber and is perpendicular to the long axis of the left ventricle. The advantages of M-mode measurements, compared with measurements from 2D images, are that they are based on the axial resolution of the ultrasound system (rather than the less accurate lateral resolution) and there is a much higher temporal resolution allowing better identification of endocardial borders. 2D guided measurements are reasonably reproducible when performed by experienced laboratories using careful recording and measurement techniques. On serial studies, side-by-side comparisons of the image planes and measurement sites are needed to ensure consistency in recording and measurement techniques between the two examinations.

The disadvantages of M-mode data are that an oblique orientation of the M-mode beam or incorrect identification of endocardial borders lead to measurement errors. Of course, when only an oblique M-mode alignment is possible, 2D measurements should be used instead. With either measurement approach, end-diastolic dimensions change with changes in preload, as a result of volume status or medications. End-systolic dimensions are less dependent on preload but may be affected by afterload (see Chapter 4).

Quantitative 2D measurements of LV size and function include LV end-diastolic volume (EDV) and end-systolic volume (ESV) with calculation of the ejection fraction (EF):

$$EF = (EDV - ESV)/EDV$$

Several methods for calculation of LV volumes from tomographic 2D images have been described,[28-31] some of which are shown in Figure 5-8. The consensus of the American Society of Echocardiography is that the preferred method is the apical biplane approach,[24]

$$V = (\pi / 4) \sum_{i=1}^{20} a_i b_i \times (L / 20)$$

where *a* and *b* represent the minor axis dimensions in two image planes at each of 20 intervals perpendicular to the long axis of the ventricle, from apex to the base, with a length (*L*). For the apical biplane method, images of the left ventricle are acquired in apical four-chamber and two-chamber views for tracing of endocardial borders at end-diastole and end-systole.

Accurate LV volume measurements on 2D imaging depend on correct image plane orientation and inclusion of the true long axis of the ventricle in the image (see Table 5-2). Use of a cut-out in the bed to allow positioning of the transducer on the apex with the patient in a steep left lateral decubitus position helps avoid inadvertent foreshortening of the apex. Accuracy also depends on accurate identification of endocardial borders. Manual tracing of borders by an experienced observer remains the most accurate method for calculation of volumes from 2D images. Approaches to automated border detection remain experimental and alternate approaches, including 3D echocardiography, require further validation. During image acquisition, care is taken to optimize endocardial definition based on patient positioning, transducer frequency and focusing, subtle adjustments in transducer position and orientation, pre- and postprocessing curves, gray scale, and gain settings. Harmonic imaging markedly improves endocardial definition

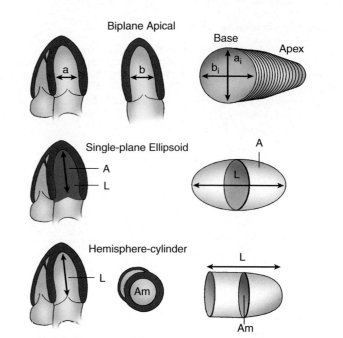

FIGURE 5–8 Examples of three formulas for left ventricular volume calculations showing the two-dimensional echocardiographic views and measurements on the left and the geometric model on the right. For the biplane apical method, endocardial borders are traced in apical four-chamber and two-chamber views, which are used to define a series of orthogonal diameters (a and b). A Simpson rule assumption based on stacked discs is used to calculate volume. The single plane ellipsoid method uses the two-dimensional area (A) and length (L) in a single (usually apical four-chamber) view. The hemisphere-cylinder method uses a short-axis endocardial area at the midventricular level (Am) and a long-axis length (L). For each method, both end-diastolic and end-systolic measurements are needed for calculation of end-diastolic and end-systolic volumes, respectively, and for ejection fraction determination. *(From Otto CM: Textbook of Clinical Echocardiography, 3rd ed. Philadelphia, Saunders, 2004, with permission.)*

in most patients and should be used whenever possible for assessment of ventricular function.

The quality of image acquisition is improved if the LV borders are traced by the sonographer performing the examination. Systems that allow evaluation of the motion of the endocardium during the tracing process (i.e., using a cine-loop feature) facilitate correct border identification. Even so, the views most suited to quantitative measurement (the apical views) use the lateral (rather than axial) resolution of the ultrasound system, limiting the overall precision with which the endocardial border can be identified.

In a experienced laboratory the accuracy and reproducibility of 2D echocardiographic LV volumes and ejection fractions is high, with 95% confidence intervals for LV end-diastolic volume of ±15%, for end-systolic volume of ±25%, and for ejection fraction of ±10%.[32] These values are similar to the reported variability for ventricular volumes or ejection fraction determined by contrast or radionuclide ventriculography.[33] Because many of the factors leading to measurement variability are constant in an individual patient, when serial studies are evaluated a change in end-systolic volume of greater than 5% and a change in ejection fraction of greater than 2% is clinically significant.[32]

LV mass can be determined by 2D echocardiography using a mean end-diastolic wall thickness, calculated from traced endocardial and epicardial borders in a parasternal short-axis view at the mid-ventricular level.[24,34] The mean wall thickness allows calculation of the volume of myocardium as the difference between the epicardial (V_{epi}) and endocardial volume (V_{endo}), which then is multiplied by the mass density of myocardium to yield LV mass:

$$LV\ mass = 1.05 \times (V_{epi} - V_{endo})$$

Evaluation of Valvular Heart Disease by Echocardiography

LV wall stress can be calculated from 2D echocardiographic data in combination with measurement of ventricular systolic pressure. Wall stress calculations provide a relatively load-independent measure of LV systolic function. Meridional wall stress (σ_m) is calculated as the ratio of total myocardial area (A_m) to ventricular cavity area (A_c) in a short-axis view at the midventricular level times LV pressure[35-37]:

$$\sigma_m = 1.33P \, (A_m/A_c) \times 103 \text{ dyne/cm}^2$$

Circumferential stress (σ_c) requires a measurement of ventricular length (L) from an apical four-chamber view, in addition to the above variables[36,38,39]:

$$\sigma_c = \frac{1.33P\sqrt{A_c}}{\sqrt{A_m}+A_c-\sqrt{A_c}} \times \left(\frac{\left(4A_c\sqrt{A_c}\right)3/2/\pi L^2}{\sqrt{A_m}+A_c-\sqrt{A_c}} \right) \text{kdyn/cm}^2$$

Wall stress can be calculated at any point in the cardiac cycle at which these measurements can be made, but end-systolic wall stress provides the most useful information.

Doppler Cardiac Output

Another clinically useful measure of LV systolic function is stroke volume or cardiac output (Figure 5-9). Stroke volume (SV) can be measured using 2D and Doppler echocardiography at any intracardiac site where flow is undisturbed by multiplying the cross-sectional area (CSA) of flow, by flow velocity (v) and duration of flow (t):

$$SV \text{ (cm}^3\text{)} = CSA \text{ (cm}^2\text{)} \times v \text{ (cm/sec)} \times t \text{ (sec)}$$

Because the Doppler spectral output displays the instantaneous velocity on the y-axis versus time on the x-axis, the velocity-time integral (VTI in cm) represents the mean velocity during the period of flow so that (see Figure 5-8):

$$SV = CSA \times VTI$$

Cardiac output (CO) then is stroke volume times heart rate (HR):

$$CO = SV \times HR$$

The cross-sectional area typically is calculated from a 2D echocardiographic measurement of diameter (D) as the area of a circle:

$$CSA = (D/2)^2$$

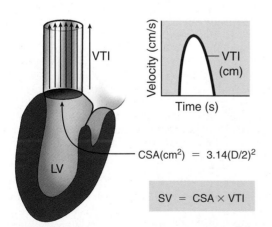

$$CSA(cm^2) = 3.14(D/2)^2$$

$$SV = CSA \times VTI$$

FIGURE 5–9 Doppler stroke volume calculation. The cross-sectional area (CSA) of flow is calculated as a circle based on a two-dimensional echo diameter (D) measurement. The length of the cylinder of blood ejected through this cross-sectional area on a single beat is the velocity-time integral (VTI) of the Doppler curve. Stroke volume (SV) is then calculated as CSA × VTI. LV, left ventricle. *(From Otto CM: Textbook of Clinical Echocardiography, 3rd ed. Philadelphia, Saunders, 2004, with permission.)*

with the assumption that flow fills the anatomic cross-sectional area. Several other assumptions factor into this equation. First, flow velocity and cross-sectional area must be measured at the same anatomic site; this factor becomes important when diameter and flow must be measured nonsimultaneously in different views. Second, the pattern of flow is assumed to be laminar with an undisturbed pattern of flow in parallel streamlines at uniform velocities. In addition, measurement of a centerline velocity assumes that the spatial flow profile is "flat" with the same velocity at the edges and center of the flow stream. Finally, the ultrasound beam is assumed to be oriented parallel to the direction of flow for accurate velocity measurement.

Despite potential theoretical concerns as to whether these assumptions are strictly met, there have been numerous studies demonstrating the accuracy and reproducibility of Doppler stroke volume measurements.[40-43] The most useful sites for stroke volume measurement in patients with valvular disease are the LV outflow tract proximal to the aortic valve, the mitral annulus, and the pulmonary artery. In normal individuals, volume flow rates are equal at these sites; however, when valvular regurgitation is present, differences in volume flow rates can be used to quantify regurgitant severity. In addition, accurate quantitation of stenosis severity depends on measurement of the antegrade volume flow rate across the affected valve.

For the LV outflow tract (LVOT), diameter is averaged from three to five measurements in midsystole, parallel to the valve plane and adjacent to the aortic valve leaflet insertions, from the endocardium of the septum to the leading edge of the anterior mitral valve leaflet (Figure 5-10). A parasternal long-axis image is used to facilitate identification of the correct site of measurement and to use the axial resolution of the ultrasound system. The flow velocity curve is recorded from an apical approach (anteriorly angulated four-chamber or long-axis view) with sample volume (2 to 5 mm in length) positioned on the ventricular side of the aortic valve. Care is taken to obtain a parallel intercept angle between the direction of flow and the ultrasound beam by careful patient positioning and transducer angulation. The region of flow acceleration proximal to the jet (recognized by spectral broadening in midsystole) must be avoided while a position immediately adjacent to the valve is maintained for correspondence with the site of diameter measurement. Optimal sample volume positioning results in a smooth velocity curve with a well-defined peak velocity and an aortic valve closing click. Wall filters are adjusted to a low setting and the sweep speed of the recording device is maximized to allow precise identification of the onset and end of flow. Transaortic stroke volume (SV_{Ao}) then is calculated as

$$SV_{Ao} = CSA_{LVOT} \times VTI_{LVOT}$$

This approach results in an accurate calculation of transaortic stroke volume even when stroke volume across the aortic valve is increased (as with aortic regurgitation) or when there is downstream flow obstruction (as with aortic stenosis) because the upstream flow pattern remains laminar[42] and flow in the outflow tract continues to equal transaortic flow even when aortic stenosis or regurgitation is present.

Transmitral stroke volume (SV_{MV}) is calculated as the product of the annular cross-sectional area (CSA_{MA}) and the velocity time integral of flow at the mitral annulus (VTI_{MA}):

$$SV_{MV} = CSA_{MA} \times VTI_{MA}$$

Measurement of stroke volume at the annulus assumes that flow is laminar at this site with a spatially flat velocity profile, assumptions that are likely to be valid in patients with a normal mitral valve or with mitral regurgitation but may not be appropriate in patients with mitral stenosis given proximal flow acceleration on the left atrial side of the stenotic valve in diastole.

Mitral annular cross-sectional area is best described as the area of an ellipse with the major axis measured from the four-chamber

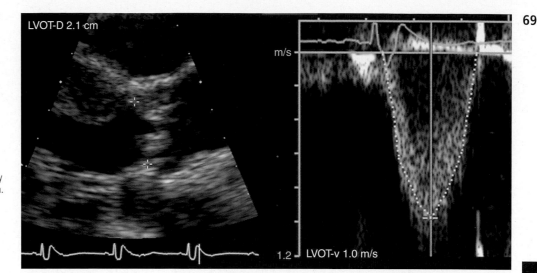

FIGURE 5–10 Example showing the data needed to calculate stroke volume in the left ventricular outflow tract (LVOT). Outflow tract diameter is measured in a parasternal long-axis view (*left*) to take advantage of the axial resolution of the ultrasound system. The flow velocity at this site is measured from an apical approach using pulsed Doppler echocardiography (*right*). LV, left ventricle; LA, left atrium; Ao, aorta.

view and the minor axis measured from an apical or parasternal long axis view; however, a simplified approach using a single diameter measurement with calculation of a circular cross-sectional area provides acceptable results. Transmitral flow velocity is recorded from an apical approach with the sample volume positioned at the level of the mitral annulus in diastole. A sample volume length of 2 to 5 mm with low wall filters and a fast sweep speed on the spectral display is used to improve the accuracy of tracing the velocity time integral. The major potential source of error in calculating stroke volume across the mitral annulus is measurement of annulus diameter because the annulus is at a substantial depth in the image from the apical view, resulting in beam width artifact superimposed on the lateral resolution of the imaging system.

Stroke volume in the pulmonary artery is calculated from 2D measurement of pulmonary artery diameter in a parasternal short axis or right ventricular outflow view, assuming a circular cross-sectional area (CSA_{PA}) and the velocity time integral of flow at that site (VTI_{PA}):

$$SV_{PA} = CSA_{PA} \times VTI_{PA}$$

As for the mitral annulus approach, the major potential source of error, particularly in adults, is accurate diameter measurement because it often is difficult to clearly define the lateral wall of the pulmonary artery. Alternatively, diameter and flow can be measured in the right ventricular outflow tract, just proximal to the pulmonary valve, although it may be difficult to obtain a parallel intercept angle between the Doppler beam and flow direction at this site.

EVALUATION OF STENOSIS SEVERITY

Velocity Data and Pressure Gradients

The fluid dynamics of a stenotic valve are characterized by a high-velocity jet in the narrowed orifice; laminar, normal-velocity flow proximal to the stenosis; and a flow disturbance distal to the obstruction (Figure 5-11).[44,45] The pressure gradient across the valve (ΔP) is related to the high-velocity jet (V_{max}) in the stenosis, the proximal velocity (V_{prox}), and the mass density of blood (ρ), as stated in the Bernoulli equation, which includes terms for conversion of potential to kinetic energy (convective acceleration), the effects of local acceleration, and viscous (v) losses:

$$\Delta P = \frac{1}{2}\rho(V^2_{max} - V^2_{prox}) + \rho(dv/dt)dx + R(v)$$
$$\text{Convective} \quad \text{Local} \quad \text{Viscous}$$
$$\text{acceleration} \quad \text{acceleration} \quad \text{losses}$$

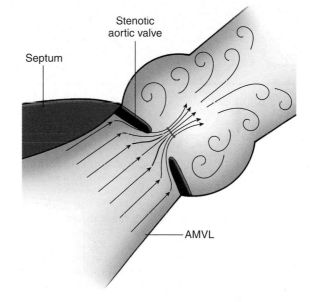

FIGURE 5–11 Schematic illustration of the fluid dynamics of the stenotic aortic valve in systole. The left ventricular outflow tract (LVOT) is bounded by the septum and anterior mitral valve leaflet (AMVL). As LVOT flow accelerates and converges, a relatively flat velocity profile occurs proximal to the stenotic valve, as indicated by the *arrows*. Flow accelerates in a spatially small zone adjacent to the valve as blood enters the narrowed orifice. In the stenotic orifice, a high-velocity laminar jet is formed with the narrowest flow stream (vena contracta, indicated by the dots) occurring downstream from the orifice. Beyond the jet, flow is disturbed with blood cells moving in multiple directions and velocities. *(From Otto CM: Textbook of Clinical Echocardiography, 3rd ed. Philadelphia, Saunders, 2004, with permission.)*

In clinical practice, the terms for acceleration and viscous losses are ignored, so that

$$\Delta P = 4\ (V^2_{max} - V^2_{prox})$$

where the constant 4 accounts for the mass density of blood and conversion factors for measurement of pressure in mmHg and velocity in m/s. When the proximal velocity is low (<1.5 m/s) and the jet velocity is high ($v1^2 << v2^2$) this equation can be further simplified as[46,47]

$$\Delta P = 4V^2_{max}$$

Maximum instantaneous gradient is calculated from the maximum transvalvular velocity, whereas mean gradient is calculated by averaging the instantaneous gradients over the flow period (Figure 5-12).

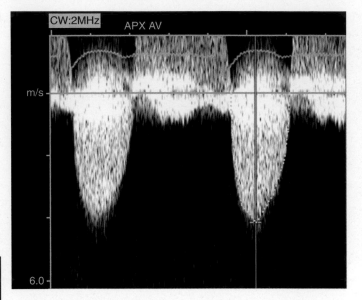

FIGURE 5–12 Doppler aortic velocity curve recorded with continuous wave Doppler from an apical window. The maximum instantaneous pressure gradient (*arrow*) corresponds to the maximum instantaneous velocity across the valve. Mean transaortic gradient is calculated by integrating the instantaneous gradients over the systolic ejection period.

sources of error include beat-to-beat variability with irregular rhythms, and interim changes in volume flow rates, leading to changes in velocity and pressure gradient.

In many clinical situations, the velocity itself across the stenotic valve provides important diagnostic and prognostic information. As stated in the Bernoulli equation, there is a consistent relationship between maximum velocity and maximum pressure gradient. In addition, there is a consistent relationship between maximum velocity and mean gradient in native aortic valve stenosis so that maximum velocity, maximum gradient, and mean gradient all convey the same information about the degree of valve narrowing. Increasingly, clinicians rely on velocity data alone in clinical decision making, without the intermediate step of converting velocities to pressure gradients.

Valve Area

Pressure gradients and velocities depend on the volume flow rate across the valve as well as the degree of valve narrowing. Both in theory and in practice, valve area (or the 2D size of the stenotic orifice) is a robust measure of stenosis severity that more closely reflects valve anatomy independently of the flow rate across the valve. Valve area can be calculated from invasive data as discussed in Chapter 6 or noninvasively from 2D and Doppler data as described below.

Whereas the concept of valve area is simple, the actual extent of valve opening in a patient with valvular disease is more elusive. The fluid dynamics of a stenotic valve are complex so that there may be no simple descriptor of stenosis severity that is constant for a given valve anatomy. In addition, there is a difference between anatomic and functional valve area, related to the coefficients of orifice contraction and velocity, which in turn depend on the specific shape and eccentricity of the valve orifice and on the geometry and tapering of proximal flow.[52,53] Finally, several studies have demonstrated that valve area is flow dependent to some extent, at least in valvular aortic stenosis (see Chapter 9).[54-61] Despite these concerns, valve area determination remains a standard clinical approach for evaluation of patients with valvular disease.

The accuracy of the simplified Bernoulli equation in measuring transvalvular pressure gradients has been shown in in vitro studies, animal models, and clinical studies of patients with valvular disease (Table 5-4).[46-51] However, accuracy depends on optimal data acquisition as detailed in textbooks of echocardiography.[1-3] Specifically, care is needed to obtain a parallel intercept angle between the continuous wave Doppler beam and direction of blood flow to avoid underestimation of the velocity and hence of the pressure gradient across the valve. The high velocities encountered in aortic and pulmonic stenosis mandate the use of continuous wave Doppler to avoid signal aliasing. A dedicated small dual-crystal continuous wave Doppler transducer is recommended. Pulsed or high pulse repetition frequency Doppler can be used for evaluation of the lower velocities seen in mitral and tricuspid stenosis with the advantage of a better signal-to-noise ratio and clearer definition of the diastolic deceleration slope than with continuous wave Doppler. Other potential technical sources of error in measuring transvalvular velocities include poor acoustic access with an inadequate flow signal, incorrect identification of the flow signal (e.g., mistaking the mitral regurgitation signal for aortic stenosis), respiratory motion, and measurement variability. In addition, physiologic

Two-Dimensional Imaging

The valve orifice in rheumatic mitral stenosis is a relatively planar structure with a constant shape and size throughout diastole (Figure 5-13). From a parasternal short-axis view, the orifice can be imaged, taking care to identify the minimum orifice area by scanning from the apex toward the base, using low gain settings, and tracing the inner border of the black-white interface.[62] Measurement of 2D mitral valve area has been well validated compared with direct measurement at surgery[4,63] and with invasive valve area calculations.[64]

TABLE 5–4	Selected Studies Validating Doppler Pressure Gradients in Valvular Aortic Stenosis				
First Author (Year)	**N**	**Study Group/Model**	**R**	**Range (mm Hg)**	**SEE (mm Hg)**
Callahan (1985)	120	Supravalvular constriction (canines)	0.99 (ΔP_{max})	7-179	5.2
			0.98 (ΔP_{mean})	N/A	4.3
Smith (1985)	88	Supravalvular constriction (canines)	0.98 (ΔP_{max})	5-166	5.3
			0.98 (ΔP_{mean})	5-116	3.3
Currie (1985)	100	Adults with valvular aortic stenosis	0.92 (ΔP_{max})	2-180	15
			0.92 (ΔP_{mean})	0-112	10
Smith (1986)	33	Adults with valvular aortic stenosis	0.85 (ΔP_{max})	27-138	N/A
Simpson (1985)	24	Adults with valvular aortic stenosis	0.98 (ΔP_{max})	0-120	N/A
Burwash (1993)	98	Chronic valvular aortic stenosis (canines)	0.95 (ΔP_{max})	10-128	8.4
			0.91 (ΔP_{mean})	5-77	5.3

Data from Callahan et al: Am J Cardiol 1985;56:989-993; Smith et al: J Am Coll Cardiol 1985;6:1306-1314; Currie PJ et al: Circulation 1985;71:1162-1169; Smith MD et al: Am Heart J 1986;111:245-252; Simpson et al: Br Heart J 1985;53:636-639; Burwash et al: Am J Physiol 1993;265:H1734-1743.

From Otto CM: Textbook of Clinical Echocardiography, 3rd ed. Philadelphia, Saunders, 2004, with permission.

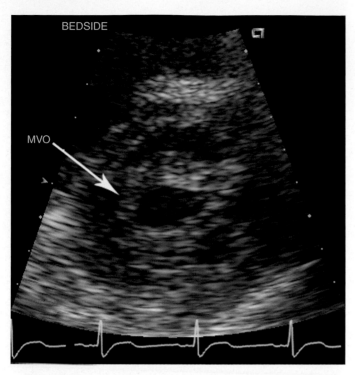

FIGURE 5–13 Two-dimensional echocardiographic short-axis views at the level of the mitral valve orifice in mid-diastole in a patient with moderate mitral stenosis. The mitral valve orifice (MVO) is identified by scanning slowly from the apex toward the base with valve area calculated directly by planimetry of the white-black interface.

The anatomy of valvular aortic stenosis is variable and more complex than that of mitral stenosis. A congenitally unicuspid valve may have a relatively symmetric orifice that can be imaged in a single tomographic plane. Although the opening of a bicuspid valve often is clearly seen early in the disease course, superimposed calcific changes result in shadowing

and reverberations, making planimetry of the stenotic valve orifice problematic. The orifice of a calcified trileaflet valve may be quite complex with a nonplanar stellate shape, further complicating direct planimetry of valve area. Some of these limitations are minimized on transesophageal imaging, and accurate measurement of aortic valve area has been reported using this approach in comparison with continuity equation valve area and invasive valve area calculations.[65-68] However, this approach is rarely needed as aortic valve area can be calculated on transthoracic echocardiography using the continuity equation in nearly all patients.[42,49,69,70] Planimetry of aortic valve area on transesophageal imaging is most useful in the operating room when unexpected aortic valve disease is encountered, i.e., when no transthoracic study is available.

Continuity Equation

Valve area is calculated using the continuity equation based on the principle of conservation of mass, specifically that the stroke volumes proximal to and in the stenotic orifice are equal:

$$SV_{Proximal} = SV_{Stenotic\ orifice}$$

Because stroke volume is the product of cross-sectional area and velocity time integral of flow:

$$CSA_{Proximal} \times VTI_{Proximal} = Area_{Stenotic\ orifice} \times VTI_{Stenotic\ orifice}$$

This equation then is solved for stenotic orifice area:

$$Area_{Stenotic\ orifice} = (CSA_{Proximal} \times VTI_{Proximal})/VTI_{Stenotic\ orifice}$$

The continuity equation is used routinely for evaluation of aortic stenosis severity.[71-73,74] For calculation of aortic valve area, transaortic stroke volume is measured in the LV outflow tract just proximal to the stenotic valve. The high-velocity aortic jet signal is recorded with continuous wave Doppler from whichever window yields the highest velocity signal.

Continuity equation valve area calculations depend both on accurate measurement of transaortic stroke volume and on optimal recording of the high-velocity flow in the stenotic orifice (Figure 5-14). The underlying assumptions of these

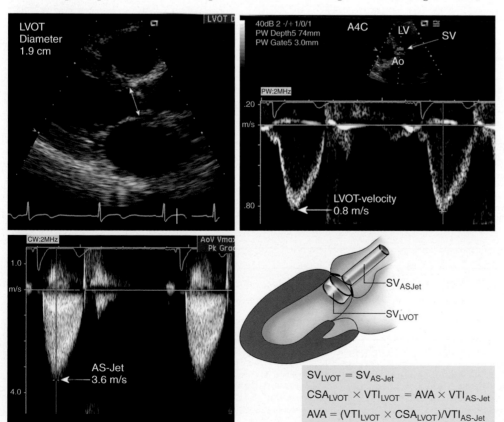

FIGURE 5–14 Continuity equation aortic valve area (AVA) calculations require measurement of left ventricular outflow tract (LVOT) diameter in a parasternal long-axis view for circular cross-sectional area (CSA) calculation (*top, left*), pulsed Doppler recording of the left ventricular outflow tract velocity-time integral (VTI) from an apical approach (*top, right*), and continuous wave Doppler recording of the aortic stenosis velocity-time integral (VTI AS-jet) from whichever window gives the highest velocity signal (bottom, *left*). (*From Otto CM: Textbook of Clinical Echocardiography, 3rd ed. Philadelphia, Saunders, 2004, with permission.*)

$$SV_{LVOT} = SV_{AS\text{-}Jet}$$

$$CSA_{LVOT} \times VTI_{LVOT} = AVA \times VTI_{AS\text{-}Jet}$$

$$AVA = (VTI_{LVOT} \times CSA_{LVOT})/VTI_{AS\text{-}Jet}$$

methods and potential sources of error are described in the sections on cardiac output and velocity measurement above (Table 5-5). Continuity equation valve area calculations have been validated in comparison with invasive measures of valve area both in animal models and in clinical studies, and the utility of this measurement is patient management is clear (Table 5-6).[42,69] In an experienced laboratory, with meticulous attention to technical details, the reproducibility of continuity equation valve area measurements is 5% to 8% so that an interim change greater than 0.15 cm² is clinically significant.[75]

Pressure Half-Time

In contrast to stenosis of a semilunar valve, in which ventricular ejection drives blood across the narrowed orifice resulting in the characteristic ejection type velocity curve, the time course of the decline in velocity (or pressure gradient) across a narrowed atrioventricular valve is a passive process, largely dependent on the area of the stenotic valve. This rate of pressure decline across the stenotic valve is independent of heart rate and volume flow rate and is inversely related to valve area.[76] The rate of pressure decline typically is measured as the pressure half-time ($T\frac{1}{2}$) defined as the time interval between the maximum initial gradient and the point where this gradient has declined to ½ the initial value (Figure 5-15). Although this method was initially described using invasive pressure measurement,[76] it now is used noninvasively with the pressure half-time measured

TABLE 5–5	Potential Sources of Error in Echocardiographic Valve Area Calculations

Two-dimensional valve area
  Tomographic plane not a minimum valve orifice
  Image plane oblique
  Image quality
  Gain settings
  Measurement error
  Complex, nonplanar, valve anatomy
  Shadowing and reverberations

Continuity equation valve area
  Proximal flow diameter measurement
  Position of proximal sample volume
  Proximal spatial flow profile
  Intercept angle between proximal flow and ultrasound beam
  Identification of stenotic jet velocity
  Intercept angle between stenotic jet and ultrasound beam
  Measurement and calculation error

Pressure half-time valve area
  Definition of maximum early diastolic velocity
  Definition of early diastolic deceleration slope
  Nonlinear diastolic deceleration slope
  Use of empiric constant for prosthetic valves
  Short early diastolic filling period (rapid heart rate, prolonged PR in sinus rhythm)
  Changing left ventricular and left atrial compliances

TABLE 5–6	Selected Studies of Aortic Valve Area Determination					
First Author (Year)	Comparison	N	Study Group	R*	Range (cm2)	SEE (cm2)*
Hakki (1981)	Simplified vs original Gorlin formula	60	Aortic stenosis	0.96	0.2-2.0	0.10
Skjaerpe (1985)	Cont eq vs Gorlin	30	Aortic stenosis	0.89	0.4-2.4	0.12
Zoghbi (1986)	Cont eq vs Gorlin	39	Aortic stenosis	0.95	0.4-2.0	0.15
Otto (1988)	Cont eq vs Gorlin	103	Aortic stenosis	0.87	0.2-3.7	0.34
Teirstein (1986)	Cont eq vs Gorlin	30	Aortic stenosis	0.88	0.3-1.6	0.17
Oh (1988)	Cont eq vs Gorlin	100	Aortic stenosis	0.83	0.2-1.8	0.19
Danielson (1989)	Cont eq vs Gorlin	100	Aortic stenosis	0.96	0.4-2.0	—
Cannon (1985)	Gorlin vs videotape of valve opening	42	Porcine valves in pulsatile flow model	0.87	0.6-2.5	0.28
	New formula vs actual orifice area	42	Porcine valves in pulsatile flow model	0.98	0.6-2.5	0.11
Segal (1987)	Cont eq vs actual valve area		In vitro pulsatile flow with orifice plates	0.99	0.05-0.5	0.016
	Gorlin formula vs actual valve area			0.87		0.047
Cannon (1988)	Gorlin vs known valve area	135	Prosthetic aortic valves	0.39	0.6-2.3	—
Nishimura (1988)	Cont eq vs Gorlin	55	Pre-BAV Post-BAV	0.72 0.61	0.2-0.9 0.5-1.3	0.10 0.17
Desnoyers (1988)	Cont eq vs Gorlin	42	Pre-BAV	0.74	0.3-1.3	—
Tribouilloy (1994)	TEE vs cont eq TEE vs Gorlin	54	Aortic stenosis	0.96 0.90	0.3-2.0	0.11 0.12
Cormier (1996)	TEE vs Gorlin	45	Aortic stenosis	0.74	0.5-1.4	—
Kim (1997)	TEE vs Gorlin	81	Aortic stenosis	0.89	0.4-2.0	0.04

*If not stated in the publication, statistics were calculated from the raw data provided in tables. A blank indicates that data for this calculation were not available. AS, aortic stenosis; BAV, balloon aortic valvuloplasty; Cont eq, continuity equation; Gorlin, Gorlin formula for valve area; TEE, planimetered two-dimensional valve area on transesophageal echocardiography.

Data from Hakki et al: Circulation 1981;63:1050-1055; Skjaerpe et al: Circulation 1985;72:810-818; Zoghbi et al: Circulation 1986;73:452-459; Otto et al: Arch Intern Med 1988;148:2553-2560; Teirstein et al: J Am Coll Cardiol 1986;8:1059-1065; Oh et al: J Am Coll Cardiol 1988;11:1227-1234; Danielson et al: Am J Cardiol 1989;63:1107-1111; Cannon et al: Circulation 1985;71:1170-1178; Segal et al: J Am Coll Cardiol 1987;9:1294-1305; Cannon et al: Am J Cardiol 1988;62:113-116; Nishimura et al: Circulation 1988;78:791-799; Desnoyers et al: Am J Cardiol 1988;62:1078-1084; Tribouilloy et al. Am Heart J 1994;128:526-532; Cormier et al: Am J Cardiol 1996;77: 882-885; Kim KS et al: Am J Cardiol 1997;79:436-441.

From Otto CM: Textbook of Clinical Echocardiography, 3rd ed. Philadelphia, Saunders, 2004, with permission.

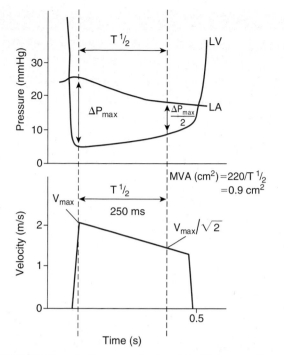

FIGURE 5 15 Schematic diagram showing the relationship between left ventricular (LV) and left atrial (LA) pressures (*top*) and the transmitral velocity curve (*bottom*) recorded with Doppler ultrasound. The shape of the pressure gradient is reflected in the Doppler velocity curve. The pressure half-time ($T\frac{1}{2}$) is the same whether measured from the pressure data or from the velocity data. Mitral valve area (MVA) is calculated using an empiric constant as $220/T\frac{1}{2}$, where valve area is in cm² and $T\frac{1}{2}$ is in ms. *(From Otto CM: Textbook of Clinical Echocardiography, 3rd ed. Philadelphia, Saunders, 2004, with permission.)*

from the Doppler velocity curve as the time from maximum velocity to the maximum velocity divided by the square root of 2 (given the quadratic relationship between velocity and pressure).[47,77-79] A normal pressure half-time is 40 to 60 ms with progressively longer half-times indicating more severe stenosis. For the stenotic native mitral valve an empiric constant of 220 is used to convert the half-time (in ms) to mitral valve area (MVA in cm²):

$$MVA = 220/T\frac{1}{2}$$

The pressure half-time concept also can be applied to the stenotic tricuspid valve and to prosthetic valves, although it is preferable to report only the half-time itself as the empiric constant has not been as well validated in these situations.

A major assumption of the pressure half-time method is that valve area is the predominant factor affecting ventricular diastolic filling. Whereas this assumption is appropriate in clinically stable patients with severe mitral stenosis, caution in needed in other clinical situations. For example, when mitral stenosis is not severe, the time course of the pressure decline between the left atrium and left ventricle in diastole is determined by the diastolic compliance of the two chambers, the initial (or opening) gradient across the valve, and atrial contractile function, in addition to the effect of the restrictive mitral orifice. Similarly, in the patient undergoing percutaneous mitral commissurotomy, changing ventricular and atrial compliances in the immediate postprocedure period can lead to inaccuracies.[80,81] Another potential concern is coexisting aortic regurgitation, because LV diastolic filling is due to both antegrade transmitral and retrograde transaortic flow, although this theoretic concern does not appear to significantly affect the accuracy of the pressure half-time in the clinical setting.[82]

Despite these limitations, the mitral pressure half-time is an established clinical technique that provides accurate results, particularly in patients with evidence of significant mitral stenosis on 2D echocardiography (Table 5-7). As for other methods of evaluation of stenosis severity, careful attention to technical details and an awareness of potential pitfalls are essential to the accuracy of the techniques.

Other Measures of Stenosis Severity

Several other echocardiographic measures of stenosis severity have been proposed for aortic stenosis including the valve resistance, stroke work loss, and valve impedance. These proposed measures have not gained wide acceptance, although studies are ongoing to determine if any might provide better prediction of symptom onset and long-term clinical outcome compared with standard measures of maximum velocity, mean gradient, and valve area.

A simplified version of the continuity equation is the velocity ratio—the dimensionless ratio of the maximum velocity proximal to a stenosis (LV outflow velocity) to the maximum velocity in the stenotic aortic orifice (V_{max}):

$$\text{Velocity ratio} = V_{LVOT}/V_{max}$$

A normal velocity ratio is slightly less than 1, with smaller ratios indicating more severe stenosis. For example, a velocity ratio of 0.25 implies that valve opening is reduced to one-fourth (25%) its normal size. In one sense, the velocity ratio is a simplification of the continuity equation, with elimination of the term for cross-sectional area of the proximal flow stream. In another sense, the velocity ratio is a more robust descriptor of stenosis severity. Normal valve area is a function of body size so that stenotic valve areas need to be interpreted in the context of patient size, specifically by indexing valve area to body surface area. The velocity ratio has the advantage that it is already "indexed" to body size. Normal intracardiac velocities are similar in people of all ages and sizes; differences in stroke volume relate to differences in the cross-sectional area of flow rather than to flow velocities. By looking at velocities alone, the velocity ratio assumes that the proximal cross-sectional area is "normal" for that patient and thus the resulting descriptor of stenosis severity is already indexed for body size. The velocity ratio has proven to be most useful in patients with native aortic stenosis when outflow tract diameter is difficult to visualize and in patients with prosthetic valves in the aortic and pulmonic positions.[83,84]

Stenosis Severity with Changes in Flow Rate

Valve area is relatively constant for a rheumatic mitral valve so that increases in flow rate result in increases in pressure gradient, with little change in valve area due to the anatomic effects of commisural fusion. In contrast, a calcified aortic valve is "stiff," and the degree of leaflet opening depends on the applied force, or volume flow rate in the clinical setting. Given the recognition that clinical measures of stenosis severity are flow dependent, there has been increasing interest in using the degree of change in stenosis severity relative to a change in volume flow rate as an index of disease severity. This concept has been applied predominantly to valvular aortic stenosis in an effort to separate those patients with a small valve area due to LV systolic dysfunction from those with severe aortic stenosis resulting in LV dysfunction. This evaluation typically is performed with a low-dose dobutamine stress test, measuring the maximum velocity, mean gradient, stroke volume, and valve area at each stage of the protocol (see Chapter 9).

EVALUATION OF VALVULAR REGURGITATION

Echocardiographic assessment of valvular regurgitation includes integration of data from 2D imaging of the valve and

TABLE 5–7 | **Selected Studies of Mitral Valve Area Determination**

First Author (Year)	Comparison	N	Study Group	R	Range (cm²)	SEE (cm²)
Gorlin (1951)	MVA by Gorlin formula vs direct at autopsy or surgery	11	MS	0.89	0.5-1.5	0.15
Libanoff (1968)	T½ at rest vs exercise	20	Mitral valve disease	0.98	20-340 ms	21 ms
Henry (1975)	2D echo vs direct measurement at surgery	20	MS pts undergoing surgery	0.92	0.5-3.5	—
Holen (1977)	MVA by Doppler vs Gorlin	10	MS	0.98	0.6-3.4	0.18
Hatle (1979)	T½ vs Gorlin MVA	32	MS	-0.74	0.4-3.5	—
Smith (1986)	2D echo vs Gorlin	37	MS alone	0.83	0.4-2.3	0.26
	T½ MVA vs Gorlin	35	Prior commissurotomy	0.58		0.28
		(37)	MS alone	0.85		0.22
		(35)	Prior commissurotomy	0.90		0.14
Come (1988)	T½ MVA vs Gorlin	37	Pre-MBC	0.51	0.6-1.3	—
	Gorlin vs Gorlin		Post-MBC	0.47	1.2-3.8	—
			Repeat cath	0.74	0.4-1.4	—
Thomas (1988)	Predicted vs actual T½	18	Pre-MBC	0.93-0.96		
			Post-MBC	0.52-0.66		
Chen (1989)	T½ MVA vs Gorlin	18	Pre-MBC	0.81	0.4-1.2	0.11
			Immediately post-MBC	0.84	1.3-2.6	0.20
			24-48 h post-MBC	0.72	1.3-2.6	0.49
Faletra (1996)	2D echo vs direct measurement	30	MS undergoing surgical mitral valve replacement	0.95	0.6-2.0	0.06
	T½ vs direct measurement	30		0.80		0.09
	Continuity equation vs direct measurement	30		0.87		0.09
	Flow area vs direct measurement	30		0.54		0.10

2D, two-dimensional; Gorlin, Gorlin formula valve area; MBC, mitral balloon commissurotomy; MS, mitral stenosis; MVA, mitral valve area; pts, patients; T½, pressure half-time.
Data from Gorlin et al: Am Heart J 1951;41:1-29; Libanoff et al: Circulation 1968;38:144-150; Henry et al: Circulation 1975;51:827-831; Holen et al: Acta Med Scand 1977;201:83-88; Hatle et al: Circulation 1979;60:1096-1104; Smith et al: Circulation 1986;73:100-107; Come et al: Am J Cardiol 1988;61:817-825; Thomas et al: Circulation 1988;78:980-993; Chen et al: J Am Coll Cardiol 1989;13:1309-1313; Faletra et al: J Am Coll Cardiol 1996;28:1190-1197.
From Otto CM: Textbook of Clinical Echocardiography, 3rd Edition. Philadelphia, Saunders, 2004, with permission.

ventricle as well as Doppler measures of regurgitant severity. No single Doppler method provides a definitive measure of regurgitant severity nor can the Doppler findings be interpreted in the absence of qualitative and quantitative imaging data. The standard examination in a patient with valvular disease includes vena contracta measurement on color flow imaging, continuous wave Doppler velocity curves, evaluation for distal flow reversals, and transvalvular volume flow data (Table 5-8). Quantitative measures of regurgitant severity, including regurgitant orifice area and regurgitant volume, are increasingly used, particularly when regurgitation is moderate on qualitative evaluation or when the cause of ventricular dilation is not clear.[85,86]

Color Flow Mapping

Color flow imaging provides a 2D display of blood flow direction and velocity superimposed on the 2D image. Although the physics of color Doppler imaging are complex and numerous factors affect the final display, the color flow image provides an intuitive and appealing real-time display of blood flow patterns in the heart.[87-90] Color flow Doppler has a high sensitivity (nearly 100%) and specificity (nearly 100%) for identification of valvular regurgitation based on identification of the flow disturbance in the receiving chamber, exceeding the detection rates for auscultation or angiography.[91] With a meticulous examination, a small degree of valvular regurgitation is seen in

TABLE 5–8 | **Doppler Evaluation of Valvular Regurgitation**

Method	Doppler parameters	Limitations	Invasive Analog
Color flow imaging	Jet origin Jet direction Jet size	Variation with technical and physiologic factors	Angiography
Continuous wave Doppler	Signal intensity Shape of velocity curve	Qualitative	Hemodynamics
Vena contracta width	Width of regurgitant jet at origin	Small values, careful measurement needed	None
PISA	Calculation of RV and ROA	Less accurate with eccentric jets Peak values only	None
Volume flow at two sites	Calculation of RV and ROA	Tedious	Invasive RV and RF
Distal flow reversals	Pulmonary vein (MR) or aorta (AR)	Qualitative, affected by LA pressure, AF (MR)	None

AR, aortic regurgitation; MR, mitral regurgitation; PISA, Proximal isovelocity surface area (RV, regurgitant volume; ROA, regurgitant orifice area; RF, regurgitant fraction).
From Otto CM: Textbook of Clinical Echocardiography, 3rd ed. Philadelphia, Saunders, 2004, with permission.

many normal individuals; tricuspid regurgitation is detectable in 80% to 90% of normal individuals, pulmonic regurgitation in 70% to 80%, mitral regurgitation in 70% to 80%, and aortic regurgitation in 5% to 10% with an increasing frequency of detectable regurgitation with age.[92] Physiologic or normal regurgitation is characterized by a small volume of backflow with only a small area of flow disturbance seen on color flow and a weak continuous wave Doppler signal.

Pathologic regurgitation is associated with a larger area of flow disturbance on color flow imaging. Although it is tempting to interpret the size of the flow disturbance as synonymous with the severity of regurgitation, the color flow display is affected by numerous factors other than regurgitant severity and is not recommended as a measure of regurgitant severity. However, the origin and direction of the regurgitant jet may be helpful in determining the anatomic mechanism of regurgitation, as discussed in subsequent chapters.

Vena Contracta

Color Doppler evaluation of regurgitant severity focuses on the geometry of the regurgitant signal as it passes through the narrowed orifice (Figure 5-16). The narrowest segment of the regurgitant flow stream, the vena contracta, typically occurs just beyond the regurgitant orifice. The vena contracta is not dependent on flow rate or pressure and is less sensitive to instrument settings than conventional color flow mapping. For example, the size of the aortic regurgitant jet often is overestimated in the apical views owing to beam width artifact and depth of interrogation from this window. However, the parasternal long- and short-axis views just on the LV side of the aortic valve provide clear images of jet width relative to the diameter of the outflow tract.[93-95]

For aortic regurgitation, the vena contracta width is measured as the smallest flow diameter, immediately beyond the flow convergence region, in the parasternal long-axis view. An aortic regurgitant vena contracta jet width more than 6 mm indicates severe aortic regurgitation and less than 3 mm indicates mild regurgitation.[86,96] For mitral regurgitation, the vena contracta also is best imaged in the parasternal long-axis view, taking advantage of the axial resolution at this depth. However, identification of the vena contracta is most reliable when both the proximal convergence zone and distal expansion of the jet can be seen, with the vena contracta as the narrow segment joining these two regions. Thus, a mitral regurgitant vena contracta often is better visualized in an apical four-chamber or long-axis view. Vena contracta width should

not be measured in a two-chamber view as this is a tangential plane through the flow signal. A mitral regurgitant vena contracta jet width more than 7 mm indicates severe regurgitation and less than 3 mm indicates mild regurgitation.[86]

Proximal Flow Convergence

Blood flow accelerates on the upstream side of a regurgitant valve resulting in successively higher velocities as flow approaches the regurgitant orifice, which can be seen on color Doppler imaging (see Figure 5-16).[97-101] Color flow imaging uses pulsed Doppler technology so that signal aliasing occurs when velocity exceeds a value determined by instrument settings and depth. Aliasing is displayed as a change in color from blue to red (or vice versa) with the color change occurring at the specific aliasing velocity, which can be adjusted to some extent. Thus, visualization of the hemisphere of flow acceleration proximal to a regurgitant orifice represents an isovelocity surface area where flow is equal to the aliasing velocity (v) on the color flow image. By definition, the instantaneous flow rate (Q) at this site (e.g. regurgitant flow rate) is the cross-sectional area of flow times velocity. The area of flow can be calculated as the area of a hemisphere (with radius r), so that

$$Q = 2\pi r^2 v$$

With the continuity equation principle, this flow rate then can be used to calculate an instantaneous regurgitant orifice area (ROA), in conjunction with the maximal continuous wave Doppler velocity (V) through the regurgitant orifice, as[102]

$$ROA = Q/V$$

In the clinical setting this approach has proven most useful for evaluation of mitral regurgitation, as imaging of proximal acceleration is more difficult for aortic regurgitation.[85] The proximal isovelocity surface area (PISA) method also can be used to estimate regurgitant volume and orifice area over the cardiac cycle, as discussed below (Figure 5-17).

Continuous Wave Doppler Data

Two types of data are inherent in the continuous wave Doppler spectral recording of a regurgitant jet velocity curve. First, the signal strength, especially relative to antegrade flow, is directly related to the volume of regurgitation.[103] Although acoustic attenuation and instrumentation variability make quantitation of signal strength problematic, qualitative assessment is a simple and useful clinical measure.

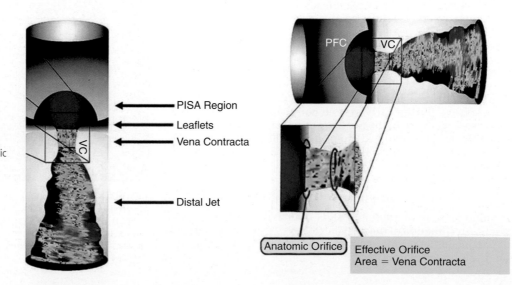

FIGURE 5–16 *Left panel:* The three components of a regurgitant jet: The proximal isovelocity surface area region also referred to as proximal flow convergence region, vena contracta (VC) and distal jet. *Right panel:* The effective regurgitant orifice area is the orifice area defined by the narrowest regurgitant flow stream and typically occurs distal to the anatomic orifice defined by the valve leaflets. *(Adapted from Roberts BJ, Grayburn P: Color flow imaging of the vena contracta in mitral regurgitation: Technical considerations. J Am Soc Electrocardiogr 2003;16: 1002-1006, with permission.)*

PISA Region

Leaflets

Vena Contracta

Distal Jet

PFC

VC

Anatomic Orifice

Effective Orifice Area = Vena Contracta

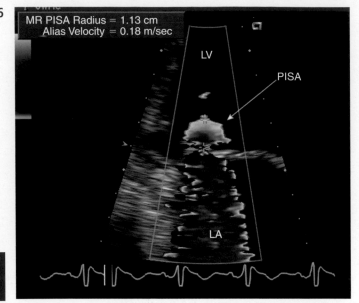

FIGURE 5–17 Proximal isovelocity surface area (PISA) in a patient with a dilated cardiomyopathy. The PISA has been optimized by decreasing the depth, narrowing the sector, and using the zoom mode. In addition, the velocity color scale (no variance) has been adjusted to an aliasing velocity away from the transducer that maximizes the size of the PISA. The PISA radius of 1.1 cm (surface area = $2\pi r^2$ = 7.6 cm²) at an aliasing velocity of 18 cm/s indicates an instantaneous regurgitant flow rate of 137 ml/s. The maximum mitral regurgitant jet velocity was 4.3 m/s, so that regurgitant orifice area is 0.32 cm², consistent with moderate mitral regurgitation. *(From Otto CM: Textbook of Clinical Echocardiography, 3rd ed. Philadelphia, Saunders, 2004, with permission.)*

Second, the time-velocity curve reflects the time course of the instantaneous pressure difference across the regurgitant valve. For each instantaneous velocity, the pressure difference across the valve is $4v^2$ (as stated in the Bernoulli equation) so that inferences about intracardiac pressures and the time course of pressure changes can be derived from the Doppler data.

For aortic regurgitation, the rate of pressure decline between the aorta and left ventricle in diastole relates to chronicity of disease and LV compensation as illustrated in Figure 5-18.[82,104-106] In addition, the end-diastolic velocity across the regurgitant aortic valve corresponds to the end-diastolic pressure gradient which, when subtracted from the cuff diastolic blood pressure, provides an approximation of LV end-diastolic pressure, although wide measurement variability limits the clinical utility of this estimate.[107]

The mitral regurgitant signal is characterized by a high maximum velocity, reflecting the high LV systolic pressure and low left atrial pressure in compensated disease. Typically, this high velocity persists through most of systole. However, when left atrial pressure rises in late systole (e.g., a v-wave) due to severe and/or acute mitral regurgitation, the velocity curve shows a steep decline in velocity in late systole, the Doppler "v-wave." In addition, the rate of pressure rise in the left ventricle during early systole correlates with the rate of increase in velocity in the regurgitant jet (Figure 5-19). In fact, LV dP/dt can be calculated from the Doppler mitral regurgitant jet as the time interval (in ms) between the points on the curve corresponding to 1 and 3 m/s divided by the pressure difference between these two points:

$$dP/dt = time/[4(3)^2 - 4(1)^2] = time/32$$

A value more than 1000 mm Hg/s indicates significant contractile dysfunction of the left ventricle.[108-110] Similarly, the rate of decline in the mitral regurgitant jet velocity corresponds to LV diastolic relaxation.[109]

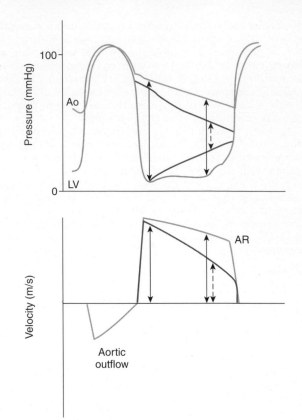

FIGURE 5–18 Left ventricular (LV) and central aortic (Ao) pressures and the corresponding Doppler velocity curve are shown for chronic (*green lines*) and acute (*blue lines*) aortic regurgitation (AR). The shape of the velocity curve is related to the instantaneous pressure differences across the valve, as stated in the Bernoulli equation. With acute aortic regurgitation, aortic pressure falls more rapidly and ventricular diastolic pressure rises more rapidly, resulting in a steeper deceleration slope on the Doppler curve. *(From Otto CM: Textbook of Clinical Echocardiography, 3rd ed. Philadelphia, Saunders, 2004, with permission.)*

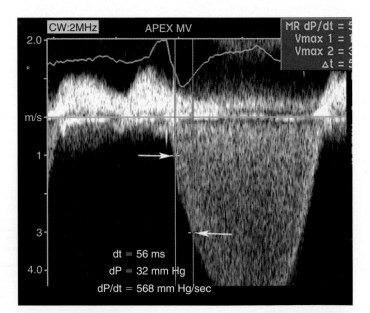

FIGURE 5–19 An enlarged view of a continuous wave Doppler recording of mitral regurgitation shows the measurements for calculation of left ventricular *dP/dt* by placing markers on the Doppler signal at 1 and 3 m/s and measuring the time interval between these markers. The change in pressure gradient (32 mm Hg) then is divided by the time interval in seconds. The value of 568 mm Hg/s in this case is consistent with severely decreased contractility.

On the right side of the heart, the tricuspid regurgitant jet velocity corresponds to the right ventricular to right atrial pressure difference in systole, so that right ventricular (and pulmonary systolic pressures) can be calculated from the maximum tricuspid regurgitant jet, based on the Bernoulli equation as discussed below. As for mitral regurgitation, severe or acute tricuspid regurgitation may result in a right atrial v-wave, seen as a late systolic rapid decline in the velocity curve.

The pulmonic regurgitant jet velocity is related to the diastolic pressure difference between the pulmonary artery and right ventricle and, given that the normal pressure difference is low, typically is low in velocity. When pulmonary hypertension is present, pulmonic regurgitant velocities are increased and the end-diastolic velocity, in combination with an estimate of right ventricular diastolic pressure, allows calculation of diastolic pulmonary pressure.

Distal Flow Reversals

When atrioventricular valve regurgitation is severe, the backflow across the valve not only fills the atrium but extends into the veins, resulting in reversal of the normal flow pattern in systole. Severe tricuspid regurgitation results in retrograde systolic flow in the vena cavae and hepatic veins, which can be demonstrated from the subcostal view using pulsed Doppler recordings. Severe mitral regurgitation results in systolic flow reversal in the pulmonary veins. On transthoracic echocardiography, the flow pattern in the right inferior pulmonary vein can be recorded from the apical four-chamber view in most patients, although the signal-to-noise ratio may be suboptimal at this depth in some adult patients. On transesophageal echocardiography, the flow pattern in the pulmonary veins can be recorded at high resolution. Examination of all four pulmonary veins is especially helpful with an eccentric regurgitant jet, as the pattern of systolic flow reversal may not be uniform.

Other physiologic factors also affect the atrial inflow patterns, including respiratory phase, cardiac rhythm, atrial and venous compliance, ventricular diastolic filling, and age.[111-115] Thus, although the presence and severity of venous systolic flow reversal is a useful adjunct in evaluation of atrioventricular valve regurgitant severity, it certainly is not a pathognomonic finding and should not be relied on when the patient is not in normal sinus rhythm.

For the semilunar valves (aortic and pulmonic), severe regurgitation results in diastolic flow reversal in the associated great vessels as blood flows back into the ventricular chamber across the incompetent valve. A quantitative aortic regurgitant fraction can be derived from the extent of diastolic flow reversal in the descending aorta, when systolic and diastolic aortic diameters and velocity time integrals are used to calculated antegrade versus retrograde volume flow rates.[116,117] Because the distance that holodiastolic flow reversal extends down the aorta correlates with regurgitant severity, the presence of holodiastolic flow reversal in the proximal abdominal aorta provides a simple indicator of severe aortic regurgitation (Figure 5-20).[118] Holodiastolic flow reversal in the descending thoracic aorta is a more sensitive, but less specific, indicator of significant regurgitant because both patients with severe and those with moderate aortic regurgitation will be detected. When performed carefully, with an adequate signal-to-noise ratio and low wall filters, this approach is a simple and reliable method for qualitative evaluation of regurgitant severity. False-negative results are due to poor examination technique or limited acoustic access. False-positive results are due to other sources of diastolic run-off in the aorta, such as a patent ductus arteriosus,

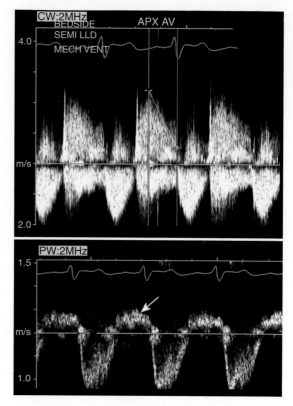

FIGURE 5–20 Severe acute aortic regurgitation with a dense continuous wave Doppler signal with a steep deceleration slope (*top*) and holodiastolic flow reversal in the descending thoracic aorta recorded from a suprasternal notch window (*bottom*). (From Otto CM: Textbook of Clinical Echocardiography, 3rd ed. Philadelphia, Saunders, 2004, with permission.)

or misinterpretation of the normal early diastolic flow reversal for holodiastolic reversal.

Regurgitant Volume and Orifice Area

Regurgitant volume (the amount of backflow across the valve) and regurgitant orifice area (the cross-sectional area of the flow stream) both can be calculated from Doppler data based on the PISA approach (Table 5-9). Measurements based on a single still-frame image provide only an instantaneous regurgitant flow rate and orifice area. This may suffice when the orifice is relatively uniform during systole. However, many causes of mitral regurgitation are associated with a dynamic orifice area, for example mitral prolapse with only late systolic mitral regurgitation. In this situation, PISA-based calculations overestimate regurgitant severity. With holosystolic regurgitation and a continuous wave Doppler signal showing similar density over the regurgitant flow period, quantitation of regurgitant severity using the PISA approach can be helpful when disease severity is uncertain. For mitral regurgitation a regurgitant orifice area greater than 0.4 cm^2 corresponds to severe regurgitation and less than 0.2 cm^2 indicates mild regurgitation.[86]

Another approach to calculation of regurgitant stroke volume (RSV) is 2D and pulsed Doppler echocardiographic measurement of cardiac output at two intracardiac sites. Regurgitant stroke volume is total stroke volume (TSV) antegrade across the regurgitant valve minus the forward stroke volume (the amount of blood delivered to the body) across a normal valve (Figure 5-21). For aortic regurgitation

TABLE 5–9 | **Validation of Quantitative Evaluation of Regurgitant Severity Using Doppler Echocardiography**

First Author (Year)	Method	Standard of Reference	N	R	SEE
Color jet area					
Spain (1989)	Color jet area	Angio LV, TD-CO	15 MR pts	0.62 (RF)	—
Tribouilloy (1992)	Regurgitant jet width at origin	Angio LV, TD-CO	31 MR pts	0.85 (RSV)	—
Enriquez-Sarano (1993)	Color jet area	Doppler SV at two sites	80 MR pts	0.69 (RF)	4.4 cm²
Vena contracta					
Tribouilloy (2000)	Vena contracta width	Doppler EROA and RV	79 AR pts	0.89 (EROA) 0.90 (RV)	0.08 cm² 18 mL
Hall (1997)	Vena contracta width	Doppler EROA and RV	80 MR pts	0.86 0.85 (RV)	0.15 cm² 20 mL
PISA					
Recusani (1991)	PISA (hemispherical)	Rotometer	In vitro, constant flow	0.94-0.99 (flow rate)	1-1.6 L/min
Utsunomiya (1991)	PISA (hemispherical)	Actual flow rate stopwatch and cylinder	In vitro, pulsatile flow	0.99 (flow rate)	0.53 L/min
Vandervoort (1993)	PISA	Actual flow rate	In vitro, steady flow	0.98-0.99 (flow rate)	—
Giesler (1993)	PISA	LV angio, Fick CO	16 MR pts	0.88 (RSV)	17 mL
Chen (1993)	PISA	Doppler SV at two sites	46 MR pts	0.94 (RSV)	18 mL
Continuous wave Doppler					
Teague (1986)	AR half-time	Angio LV, Fick CO	32 AR pts	−0.88 (RF)	11%
Masuyama (1986)	AR half-time	Angio LV, ID-CO	20 AR pts	−0.89 (RF)	—
Volume flow at two sites					
Ascah (1985)	Transmitral vs transaortic SV	EM-flow	30 flow rates in canine model	0.83 (RF)	—
Kitabatake (1985)	Transaortic vs transpulmonic SV	Angio LV, TD-CO	20 AR pts	0.94 (RF)	—
Rokey (1986)	Transmitral vs transaortic SV	Angio LV, TD-CO	19 MR and 6 AR pts	0.91 (RF)	7%
Distal flow reversals					
Boughner (1975)	Diastolic flow reversal in descending Ao	Angio LV, Fick CO	15 AR pts	0.91 (RF)	—
Touche (1985)	Diastolic flow reversal in descending Ao	Angio LV, TD-CO	30 AR pts	0.92 (RF)	8.8%

Ao, aortic; AR, aortic regurgitation; CO, cardiac output; EM-flow, volume flow rate measured by electromagnetic flowmeter; EROA, effective regurgitant orifice area; ID, indicator dilation; LV, left ventricle; MR, mitral regurgitation; PISA, proximal isovelocity surface area method; pts, patients; RF, regurgitant fraction; RSV, regurgitant stroke volume; RV, right ventricle; SV, stroke volume; TD, thermodilution.

Data from Boughher et al: Circulation 1975;52:874-879; Touche et al: Circulation 1985;72:819-824; Ascah et al: Circulation 1985;72:377-383; Kitabatake et al: Circulation 1985;72:523-529; Rokey et al: J Am Coll Cardiol 1986;7:1273-1278; Teague et al: J Am Coll Cardiol 1986;8:592-599; Masuyama et al: Circulation 1986;73:460-466; Jenni et al: Circulation 1989;79:1294-1299; Spain et al: J Am Coll Cardiol 1989;13:585-590; Tribouilloy et al: Circulation 1992;85:1248-1253; Enriquez-Sarano et al: J Am Coll Cardiol 1993;21:1211-1219; Rescusani et al: Circulation 1991;83:594-604; Utsunomiya et al: J Am Soc Echocardiogr 1991;4:338-348; Vandervoort et al: J Am Coll Cardiol 1993;22:535-541; Giesler et al: Am J Cardiol 1993;71:217-224; Chen et al: J Am Coll Cardiol 1993;21:374-383; Tribouilloy CM et al. Circulation 2000;102:558-564; Hall SA et al. Circulation 1997;95: 636-642.

From Otto CM: Textbook of Clinical Echocardiography, 3rd Edition. Philadelphia, Saunders, 2004, with permission.

(AR), total stroke volume is measured in the left ventricular outflow tract (LVOT) and forward stroke volume across the mitral or pulmonic (PA) valve:

$$RSV_{AR} = (CSA_{LVOT} \times VTI_{LVOT}) - (CSA_{PA} \times VTI_{PA})$$

For mitral regurgitation (MR), total stroke volume is measured across the mitral annulus (MA) and forward stroke volume across the LVOT or pulmonic valve:

$$RSV_{MR} = (CSA_{MA} \times VTI_{MA}) - (CSA_{LVOT} \times VTI_{LVOT}).$$

Regurgitant fraction (RF) then is the ratio of regurgitant stroke volume to total stroke volume:

$$RF = RSV/TSV$$

The validity of this method has been demonstrated in animal and clinical studies of valvular regurgitation.[119-121] However, the accuracy of this method for calculation of regurgitant fraction depends on the caveats described above for measurement of cardiac output by Doppler echocardiography. Given the potential error with this approach, particularly if there are errors in diameter measurement, and the complexity of data acquisition and measurement, most laboratories perform these calculation only in selected patients.

A simpler approach to quantitation of mitral regurgitation used at many centers is to use the 2D biplane LV stroke volume, instead of transmitral flow, for total stroke volume. Then, regurgitant volume and orifice area are calculated

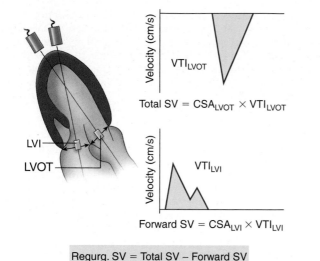

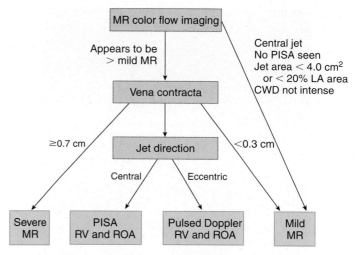

FIGURE 5–21 Calculation of aortic regurgitant stroke volume (SV) by measurement of transvalvular volume flow rate at two intracardiac sites is illustrated. Transaortic flow, representing total SV, is calculated from the cross-sectional area (CSA) and velocity-time integral (VTI) of the left ventricular outflow tract (LVOT). Transmitral flow, representing forward SV, is calculated from the CSA and VTI of LV inflow (LVI) across the mitral annulus. Regurgitant stroke volume is the difference between total and forward SV. *(From Otto CM: Textbook of Clinical Echocardiography, 3rd ed. Philadelphia, Saunders, 2004, with permission.)*

FIGURE 5–22 Approach to quantitation of mitral regurgitant severity. Other quantitative measures may be needed in some patients with a vena contracta width of 0.7 cm or greater. Evaluation of systolic flow reversal in the pulmonary veins provides useful additional information in patients with sinus rhythm. Transesophageal imaging often is needed for complete evaluation of mitral regurgitant severity in patients with moderate to severe disease. CWD, continuous wave Doppler; LV, left ventricle; MR, mitral regurgitation; PISA, proximal isovelocity surface area; RV, right ventricle; ROA, regurgitant orifice area. *(From Otto CM: Textbook of Clinical Echocardiography, 3rd ed. Philadelphia, Saunders, 2004, with permission.)*

using the forward stroke volume measured by pulsed Doppler in the LV outflow tract. This approach uses measurements performed as part of a routine examination and avoids the measurement variability inherent in determination of mitral annulus diameter.

Integration of Regurgitant Parameters

A step-wise approach to use of Doppler measures of regurgitant severity is recommended by the American Society of Echocardiography.[86] For both mitral and aortic regurgitation, the initial step is measurement of the vena contracta diameter. With mitral regurgitation and a small (<0.3 cm) or very large (>0.7 cm) vena contracta diameter, further evaluation is not typically needed (Figure 5-22). For a vena contracta diameter of 0.3 to 0.7 cm, regurgitant severity is quantitated by the PISA method for central holosystolic jets or by the volume flow method in other cases. With aortic regurgitation, the combination of vena contracta diameter, continuous wave Doppler signal strength and diastolic pressure half-time and distal flow reversal in the aorta usually are adequate, with further quantitation only if regurgitant severity remains uncertain (Figure 5-23).

OTHER ECHOCARDIOGRAPHIC DATA

Echocardiographic evaluation of the patient with valvular heart disease also includes assessment of other parameters, depending on the specific valve involved and the severity of valve disease. For example, in a patient with mitral stenosis, measurement of left atrial size and estimation of pulmonary pressures are important components of the examination. In a patient with severe aortic stenosis and heart failure symptoms despite normal LV systolic function, evaluation of diastolic ventricular function may be needed.

Left Ventricular Diastolic Function

Left ventricular diastolic function is reflected in the Doppler velocity patterns of ventricular inflow and atrial filling

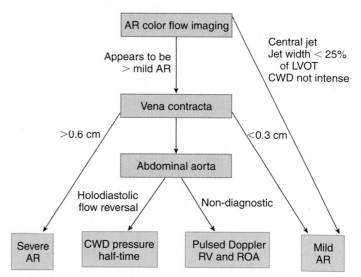

FIGURE 5–23 Approach to echocardiographic quantitation of aortic regurgitant severity. In some patients quantitation using pulsed and continuous wave Doppler techniques may be helpful when vena contracta width is greater than 0.6 cm. AR, atrial regurgitation; CWD, continuous wave Doppler; LV, left ventricle; LVOT, left ventricular outflow tract; PISA, proximal isovelocity surface area; RV, right ventricle; ROA, regurgitant orifice area. *(From Otto CM: Textbook of Clinical Echocardiography, 3rd ed. Philadelphia, Saunders, 2004, with permission.)*

(Figure 5-24).[122-125] LV diastolic inflow is recorded from the transthoracic approach in the apical four-chamber view with the sample volume positioned at the mitral leaflet tips in diastole. The normal pattern of LV diastolic filling in young healthy individuals is a short isovolumic relaxation time, a high early diastolic filling velocity (E-velocity), a steep early diastolic deceleration slope, and a smaller late diastolic filling velocity after atrial contraction (A-velocity) with a high ratio of early to late diastolic filling velocities (E/A ratio).

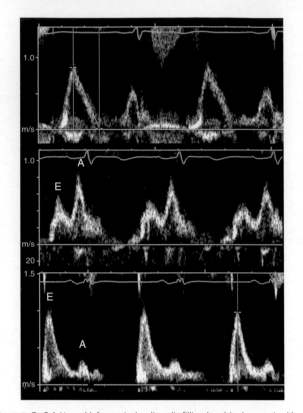

FIGURE 5–24 Normal left ventricular diastolic filling (*top*) is characterized by rapid early diastolic filling (E) with a normal deceleration slope and a small atrial contribution to ventricular filling (A). With impaired ventricular relaxation (*middle*), as is seen in patients with concentric hypertrophy, the early diastolic filling velocity is diminished, the deceleration slope is prolonged, and the atrial contribution to filling is more prominent. With decreased compliance (*bottom*), there is prominent early diastolic filling with a steep deceleration slope and a very small A-velocity.

Pulmonary vein flow is recorded from the apical four-chamber view on transthoracic echocardiography with the sample volume positioned in the right inferior pulmonary vein using color Doppler to aid in positioning the Doppler beam. Higher quality pulmonary vein flow signals can be obtained from the transesophageal approach with the sample volume positioned in the left superior pulmonary vein. Normal pulmonary vein flow patterns show systolic and diastolic flow into the atrium with diastolic flow (D) exceeding systolic flow (S) in young normal individuals. A small flow reversal after atrial contraction (a-reversal) also is seen.

With diastolic dysfunction due to impaired LV relaxation, the E-velocity is reduced and the A-velocity is increased, resulting in a low E/A ratio. In addition, the isovolumic relaxation time is prolonged, and the deceleration slope is reduced. Pulmonary vein flow shows a reduced diastolic filling velocity, prominent systolic filling velocity, and increased atrial reversal.

With diastolic dysfunction due to decreased compliance of the left ventricle, the pattern of LV diastolic filling is characterized by an increased E-velocity and reduced A-velocity resulting in a high E/A ratio in conjunction with an increased early diastolic deceleration slope and a reduced isovolumic relaxation time. A reduced systolic filling and increased diastolic filling curve is seen on the pulmonary venous flow curve with an increase in the velocity and duration of the atrial reversal velocity curve. Between these two extremes, diastolic dysfunction may present with a "pseudo-normal" pattern in which the LV filling curve appears normal yet the pulmonary vein flow pattern shows reduced diastolic filling and an increased atrial reversal velocity.

Unfortunately, although the Doppler velocity curves accurately portray LV diastolic filling, evaluation of LV diastolic function by echocardiography is limited by the numerous technical and physiologic factors other than the diastolic properties of the ventricle that affect diastolic filling. LV diastolic filling is affected by technical factors such as sample volume position and intercept angle; normal physiological variation including respiration, heart rate, age and PR interval; and other physiologic variables such as preload, coexisting mitral regurgitation, LV systolic function, and atrial contractile function.[112,113,126-129] Pulmonary vein flow is affected by age, left atrial size, left atrial pressure, atrial contractile function, and cardiac rhythm in addition to LV and left atrial compliance, LV diastolic relaxation, and the pressure gradient from the pulmonary veins to the left ventricle. Thus, evaluation of diastolic function in an individual patient, must take into consideration whether technical or physiologic factors may affect the findings. With knowledge of these potential limitation, clinically useful information about LV diastolic function can be derived from the Doppler patterns of LV inflow and pulmonary vein flow in patients with valvular heart disease.

Left Atrial Enlargement and Thrombus Formation

Left atrial size can be assessed with 2D transthoracic imaging from parasternal, apical, and subcostal views. Although methods for calculation of left atrial volume based on planimetry of atrial area in two views have been validated and provide a quantitative measure of atrial size, in most clinical situations a single anterior-posterior diameter, in conjunction with 2D visual estimates of atrial size, provides adequate information for patient management.

The specificity of identification of a left atrial thrombus on transthoracic imaging is high (95% to 99%); however, sensitivity is low (about 60%) because of poor image quality at the depth of the left atrium and difficulty in visualizing the atrial appendage.[130-132] Transesophageal imaging provides high-quality images of the left atrium and atrial appendage, resulting in a very high sensitivity (nearly 100%) and specificity (nearly 100%) for detection of atrial thrombus.[133,134] Thus, when atrial thrombus is suspected clinically, transesophageal imaging is necessary for reliable exclusion of this potential diagnosis.

Determination of Pulmonary Pressures

Pulmonary pressure is estimated on the basis of measurement of tricuspid regurgitant jet velocity, in combination with an estimate of right atrial pressure (Figure 5-25).[49,135,136] A small degree of tricuspid regurgitation is present in most normal individuals with an even higher prevalence in patients with valvular disease. Because the velocity of the regurgitant jet relates to the pressure difference across the valve and not to the volume of regurgitation, this degree of tricuspid regurgitation, although not hemodynamically significant, allows recording of jet velocity and calculation of pulmonary pressures.

The velocity in the tricuspid regurgitant jet (TR$_{jet}$) reflects the right ventricular to right atrial systolic pressure difference, as stated in the Bernoulli equation. Addition of right atrial pressure (RAP) to this pressure difference yields right ventricular systolic pressure, which, in the absence of pulmonic stenosis, equals pulmonary artery systolic pressure (PA$_{systolic}$):

$$PA_{systolic} = 4(TR_{jet})^2 + RAP$$

Right atrial pressure is estimated from the appearance of the inferior vena cava at its entrance into the right

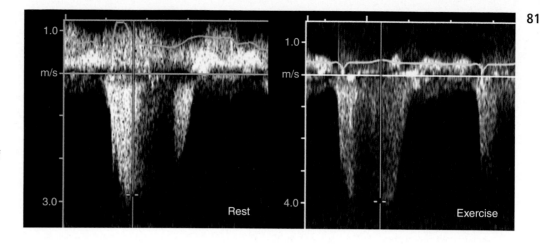

FIGURE 5–25 In a patient with mitral regurgitation, the pulmonary artery pressure at rest is 36 mm Hg (based on the tricuspid regurgitant jet velocity of 2.8 m/s and an estimated right atrial pressure of 5 mm Hg). Immediately after symptom-limited treadmill exercise, the tricuspid regurgitant jet is 3.9 m/s, consistent with a pulmonary systolic pressure of 66 mm Hg.

atrium as imaged from a subcostal view during normal respiration.[137,138] Because this method depends on normal intrathoracic pressure changes with respiration, it is not applicable in the mechanically ventilated patient. Examination of the tricuspid regurgitant jet from parasternal and apical windows with careful transducer angulation to record the highest velocity signal is essential to avoid underestimation of jet velocity (and hence pulmonary artery pressures). When a clear maximum regurgitant jet velocity cannot be identified or only an incomplete waveform is obtained, pulmonary pressures cannot be reliably determined with this method. Instead, indirect evidence for pulmonary hypertension (e.g., midsystolic notching and short time to peak velocity in the pulmonary artery velocity wave, abnormal septal motion, and other) or another method must be used. In patients with mitral stenosis, assessment of the rise in pulmonary pressures with exercise provides insight into the relationship between hemodynamic severity and clinical symptoms. Exercise Doppler data also may be useful in determining the optimal timing of intervention in patients with mitral stenosis to prevent the development of irreversible pulmonary hypertension (see Chapter 14).

Right Heart Structure and Function

Qualitative evaluation of right ventricular size and systolic function on 2D echocardiography is an important component of the examination in patients with valvular heart disease. The right ventricle is imaged in the parasternal short axis and right ventricular inflow views and in apical and subcostal four-chamber views. Right ventricular size is described as normal or mildly, moderately, or severely enlarged on the basis of integration of data from these views. Similarly, right ventricular systolic function is graded on a normal to severely reduced scale. The pattern of ventricular septal motion also is helpful in diagnosis of right ventricular pressure or volume overload. Although quantitative evaluation of right ventricular size and function has been described using 3D echocardiography, these techniques are complex and have not been widely used clinically. When right-sided valve disease is present and quantitative evaluation of right ventricular function is needed, cardiac magnetic resonance imaging may be considered.

Aortic Anatomy and Dilation

Aortic dilation often accompanies aortic valve disease (See Chapter 11). On echocardiography, the aortic annulus, sinuses, and proximal ascending aorta are well visualized in parasternal views. Additional views of the ascending aorta often can be obtained from a higher intercostal space, the aortic arch can be imaged from a suprasternal notch approach, and portions of the descending thoracic and proximal abdominal aorta are seen on apical and subcostal views, respectively.

Basic measurements on echocardiography include the maximum end-diastolic diameter of the aortic root, typically at the sinus level, measured from a 2D long-axis image. If this measurement is abnormal or if there is effacement of the sinotubular junction, measurements are taken at multiple sites in the aortic root. The American Society of Echocardiography recommends calculation of an expected aortic root size, on the basis of age and body size.[139,140] Additional imaging with chest computed tomography or cardiac magnetic resonance imaging may be helpful when the aortic involvement is suspected or known.

REFERENCES

1. Otto CM: Textbook of Clinical Echocardiography, 3rd ed. Philadelphia, Saunders, 2004.
2. Oh JK, Seward JB, Tajik AJ: The Echo Manual, 3rd ed. Baltimore, Lippincott Williams & Wilkins, 2006.
3. Feigenbaum H, Armstrong WF, Ryan T: Echocardiography, 6th ed. Baltimore, Lippincott Williams & Wilkins, 2004.
4. Henry WL, Griffith JM, Michaelis LL, et al: Measurement of mitral orifice area in patients with mitral valve disease by real-time, two-dimensional echocardiography. Circulation 1975;51:827-831.
5. Abascal VM, Wilkins GT, Choong CY, et al: Echocardiographic evaluation of mitral valve structure and function in patients followed for at least 6 months after percutaneous balloon mitral valvuloplasty. J Am Coll Cardiol 1988;12:606-615.
6. Reid CL, Otto CM, Davis KB, et al: Influence of mitral valve morphology on mitral balloon commissurotomy: immediate and six-month results from the NHLBI Balloon Valvuloplasty Registry. Am Heart J 1992;124:657-665.
7. Roberts WC: Morphologic aspects of cardiac valve dysfunction. Am Heart J 1992;123:1610-1632.
8. Selzer A: Changing aspects of the natural history of valvular aortic stenosis. N Engl J Med 1987;317:91-98.
9. Beppu S, Suzuki S, Matsuda H, et al: Rapidity of progression of aortic stenosis in patients with congenital bicuspid aortic valves. Am J Cardiol 1993;71:322-327.
10. Roberts WC: Anatomically isolated aortic valvular disease: the case against its being of rheumatic etiology. Am J Med 1970;49:151-159.
11. He S, Fontaine AA, Schwammenthal E, et al: Integrated mechanism for functional mitral regurgitation-leaflet restriction versus coapting force: In vitro studies. Circulation 1997;96:1826-1834.
12. Otsuji Y, Handschumacher MD, Schwammenthal E, et al: Insights from three-dimensional echocardiography into the mechanism of functional mitral regurgitation: direct in vivo demonstration of altered leaflet tethering geometry. Circulation 1997;96:1999-2008.
13. Levine RA: Dynamic mitral regurgitation—more than meets the eye. N Engl J Med 2004;351:1681-1684.
14. Subramanian R, Olson LJ, Edwards WD: Surgical pathology of combined aortic stenosis and insufficiency: a study of 213 cases. Mayo Clin Proc 1985;60:247-254.
15. Olson LJ, Subramanian R, Edwards WD: Surgical pathology of pure aortic insufficiency: a study of 225 cases. Mayo Clin Proc 1984;59:835-841.

82

16. Maurer G: Aortic regurgitation. Heart 2006;92:994-1000.
17. Pyeritz RE, McKusick VA: The Marfan syndrome: diagnosis and management. N Engl J Med 1979;300:772-777.
18. Marsalese DL, Moodie DS, Vacante M, et al: Marfan's syndrome: natural history and long-term follow-up of cardiovascular involvement. J Am Coll Cardiol 1989;14:422-428.
19. Roldan CA, Shively BK, Crawford MH: An echocardiographic study of valvular heart disease associated with systemic lupus erythematosus. N Engl J Med 1996;335:1424-1430.
20. Schaefer BM, Lewin MB, Stout KK, et al: Usefulness of bicuspid aortic valve phenotype to predict elastic properties of the ascending aorta. Am J Cardiol 2007;99:686-690.
21. Fedak PW, Verma S, David TE, et al: Clinical and pathophysiological implications of a bicuspid aortic valve. Circulation 2002;106:900-904.
22. Picard MH: Three dimensional echocardiography. In Otto CM (ed): The Practice of Clinical Echocardiography, 3rd ed. Philadelphia, Saunders, 2007, pp 86-114.
23. Hung J, Lang R, Flachskampf F, et al: 3D echocardiography: a review of the current status and future directions. J Am Soc Echocardiogr 2007;20:213-233.
24. Schiller NB, Shah PM, Crawford M, et al: Recommendations for quantitation of the left ventricle by two-dimensional echocardiography. American Society of Echocardiography Committee on Standards, Subcommittee on Quantitation of Two-Dimensional Echocardiograms. J Am Soc Echocardiogr 1989;2:358-367.
25. Otto CM, Mickel MC, Kennedy JW, et al: Three-year outcome after balloon aortic valvuloplasty: insights into prognosis of valvular aortic stenosis. Circulation 1994;89:642-650.
26. Cerqueira MD, Weissman NJ, Dilsizian V, et al: Standardized myocardial segmentation and nomenclature for tomographic imaging of the heart: a statement for healthcare professionals from the Cardiac Imaging Committee of the Council on Clinical Cardiology of the American Heart Association. Circulation 2002;105:539-542.
27. Bonow RO, Carabello BA, Chatterjee K, et al: ACC/AHA 2006 guidelines for the management of patients with valvular heart disease: a report of the American College of Cardiology/American Heart Association Task Force on Practice Guidelines (writing Committee to Revise the 1998 guidelines for the management of patients with valvular heart disease) developed in collaboration with the Society of Cardiovascular Anesthesiologists endorsed by the Society for Cardiovascular Angiography and Interventions and the Society of Thoracic Surgeons. J Am Coll Cardiol 2006;48:e1-e148.
28. Folland ED, Parisi AF, Moynihan PF, et al: Assessment of left ventricular ejection fraction and volumes by real-time two-dimensional echocardiography: a comparison of cineangiographic and radionuclide techniques. Circulation 1979;60:760-766.
29. Zile MR, Tanaka R, Lindrith JR, et al: Left ventricular volume determined echocardiographically by assuming a constant left ventricular epicardial long-axis/short-axis dimension ratio throughout the cardiac cycle. J Am Coll Cardiol 1992;20:986-993.
30. Zoghbi WA, Buckey JC, Massey MA, Blomqvist CG, Determination of left ventricular volumes with use of a new nongeometric echocardiographic method: clinical validation and potential application. J Am Coll Cardiol 1990;15:610-617.
31. Smith MD, MacPhail B, Harrison MR, et al: Value and limitations of transesophageal echocardiography in determination of left ventricular volumes and ejection fraction. J Am Coll Cardiol 1992;19:1213-1222.
32. Gordon EP, Schnittger I, Fitzgerald PJ, et al: Reproducibility of left ventricular volumes by two-dimensional echocardiography. J Am Coll Cardiol 1983;2:506-513.
33. Nessly ML, Bashein G, Detmer PR, et al: Left ventricular ejection fraction: single-plane and multiplanar transesophageal echocardiography versus equilibrium gated-pool scintigraphy. J Cardiothorac Vasc Anesth 1991;5:40-45.
34. Reichek N, Helak J, Plappert T, et al: Anatomic validation of left ventricular mass estimates from clinical two-dimensional echocardiography: initial results. Circulation 1983;67:348-352.
35. Mirsky I, Cohn PF, Levine JA, et al: Assessment of left ventricular stiffness in primary myocardial disease and coronary artery disease. Circulation 1974;50:128-136.
36. Gaasch WH, Zile MR, Hoshino PK, et al: Stress-shortening relations and myocardial blood flow in compensated and failing canine hearts with pressure-overload hypertrophy. Circulation 1989;79:872-883.
37. Reichek N, Wilson J, St-John SM, et al: Noninvasive determination of left ventricular end-systolic stress: validation of the method and initial application. Circulation 1982;65:99-108.
38. Douglas PS, Reichek N, Plappert T, et al: Comparison of echocardiographic methods for assessment of left ventricular shortening and wall stress. J Am Coll Cardiol 1987;9:945-951.
39. St-John-Sutton MG, Plappert TA, Hirshfeld JW, Reichek N: Assessment of left ventricular mechanics in patients with asymptomatic aortic regurgitation: a two-dimensional echocardiographic study. Circulation 1984;69:259-268.
40. Lewis JF, Kuo LC, Nelson JG, et al: Pulsed Doppler echocardiographic determination of stroke volume and cardiac output: clinical validation of two methods using the apical window. Circulation 1984;70:425-431.
41. Bouchard A, Blumlein S, Schiller NB, et al: Measurement of left ventricular stroke volume using continuous wave Doppler echocardiography of the ascending aorta and M-mode echocardiography of the aortic valve. J Am Coll Cardiol 1987;9:75-83.
42. Otto CM, Pearlman AS, Gardner CL, et al: Experimental validation of Doppler echocardiographic measurement of volume flow through the stenotic aortic valve. Circulation 1988;78:435-441.
43. Burwash IG, Forbes AD, Sadahiro M, et al: Echocardiographic volume flow and stenosis severity measures with changing flow rate in aortic stenosis. Am J Physiol 1993;265:H1734-H1743.
44. Baumgartner H, Hung J, Bermejo J, Chambers JB, Evangelista A, Griffin BP, Iung B, Otto CM, Pellikka PA, Quiñones M. Echocardiographic assessment of valve stenosis:

EAE/ASE recommendations for clinical practice. Eur J Echocardiogr. 2008 Dec 8. [Epub ahead of print]
45. Yoganathan AP: Fluid mechanics of aortic stenosis. Eur Heart J 1988;9(Supple E):13-17.
46. Holen J, Aaslid R, Landmark K, Simonsen S: Determination of pressure gradient in mitral stenosis with a non-invasive ultrasound Doppler technique. Acta Med Scand 1976;199:455-460.
47. Hatle L, Angelsen B, Tromsdal A: Noninvasive assessment of atrioventricular pressure half-time by Doppler ultrasound. Circulation 1979;60:1096-1104.
48. Hatle L, Angelsen A, Tromsdal A: Non-invasive assessment of aortic stenosis by Doppler ultrasound. Br Heart J 1980;43:284-292.
49. Currie PJ, Seward JB, Reeder GS, et al: Continuous-wave Doppler echocardiographic assessment of severity of calcific aortic stenosis: a simultaneous Doppler-catheter correlative study in 100 adult patients. Circulation 1985;71:1162-1169.
50. Smith MD, Dawson PL, Elion JL, et al: Correlation of continuous wave Doppler velocities with cardiac catheterization gradients: an experimental model of aortic stenosis. J Am Coll Cardiol 1985;6:1306-1314.
51. Nishimura RA, Tajik AJ: Quantitative hemodynamics by Doppler echocardiography: a noninvasive alternative to cardiac catheterization. Prog Cardiovasc Dis 1994;36:309-342.
52. Flachskampf FA, Weyman AE, Guerrero JL, Thomas JD: Influence of orifice geometry and flow rate on effective valve area: an in vitro study. J Am Coll Cardiol 1990;15:1173-1180.
53. Segal J, Lerner DJ, Miller DC, et al: When should Doppler-determined valve area be better than the Gorlin formula? Variation in hydraulic constants in low flow states. J Am Coll Cardiol 1987;9:1294-1305.
54. Burwash IG, Thomas DD, Sadahiro M, et al: Dependence of Gorlin formula and continuity equation valve areas on transvalvular volume flow rate in valvular aortic stenosis. Circulation 1994;89:827-835.
55. Burwash IG, Pearlman AS, Kraft CD, et al: Flow dependence of measures of aortic stenosis severity during exercise. J Am Coll Cardiol 1994;24:1342-1350.
56. Casale PN, Palacios IF, Abascal VM, et al: Effects of dobutamine on Gorlin and continuity equation valve areas and valve resistance in valvular aortic stenosis. Am J Cardiol 1992;70:1175-1179.
57. Cochrane T, Kenyon CJ, Lawford PV, et al: Validation of the orifice formula for estimating effective heart valve opening area. Clin Phys Physiol Meas 1991;12:21-37.
58. Montarello JK, Perakis AC, Rosenthal E, et al: Normal and stenotic human aortic valve opening: vitro assessment of orifice area changes with flow. Eur Heart J 1990;11:484-491.
59. Tardif JC, Rodrigues AG, Hardy JF, et al: Simultaneous determination of aortic valve area by the Gorlin formula and by transesophageal echocardiography under different transvalvular flow conditions. Evidence that anatomic aortic valve area does not change with variations in flow in aortic stenosis. J Am Coll Cardiol 1997;29:1296-1302.
60. Badano L, Cassottano P, Bertoli D, et al: Changes in effective aortic valve area during ejection in adults with aortic stenosis. Am J Cardiol 1996;78:1023-1028.
61. Bermejo J, García Fernández MA, Torrecilla EG, et al: Effects of dobutamine on Doppler echocardiographic indexes of aortic stenosis. J Am Coll Cardiol 1996;28:1206-1213.
62. Iung B, Vahanian A: Echocardiography in patients undergoing balloon mitral valvuloplasty. In Otto CM (ed): The Practice of Clinical Echocardiography, 3rd ed. Philadelphia, Saunders, 2007, pp 481-501.
63. Smith MD, Handshoe R, Handshoe S, et al: Comparative accuracy of two-dimensional echocardiography and Doppler pressure half-time methods in assessing severity of mitral stenosis in patients with and without prior commissurotomy. Circulation 1986;73:100-107.
64. Smith MD, Kwan OL, DeMaria AN: Value and limitations of continuous-wave Doppler echocardiography in estimating severity of valvular stenosis. JAMA 1986;255:3145-3151.
65. Kim KS, Maxted W, Nanda NC, et al: Comparison of multiplane and biplane transesophageal echocardiography in the assessment of aortic stenosis. Am J Cardiol 1997;79:436-441.
66. Cormier B, Iung B, Porte JM, et al: Value of multiplane transesophageal echocardiography in determining aortic valve area in aortic stenosis. Am J Cardiol 1996;77:882-885.
67. Tribouilloy C, Shen WF, Peltier M, et al: Quantitation of aortic valve area in aortic stenosis with multiplane transesophageal echocardiography: comparison with monoplane transesophageal approach. Am Heart J 1994;128:526-532.
68. Stoddard MF, Hammons RT, Longaker RA: Doppler transesophageal echocardiographic determination of aortic valve area in adults with aortic stenosis. Am Heart J 1996;132:337-342.
69. Galan A, Zoghbi WA, Quinones MA: Determination of severity of valvular aortic stenosis by Doppler echocardiography and relation of findings to clinical outcome and agreement with hemodynamic measurements determined at cardiac catheterization. Am J Cardiol 1991;67:1007-1012.
70. Otto CM, Nishimura RA, Davis KB, et al: Doppler echocardiographic findings in adults with severe symptomatic valvular aortic stenosis. Am J Cardiol 1991;68:1477-1484.
71. Otto CM, Pearlman AS, Gardner CL: Hemodynamic progression of aortic stenosis in adults assessed by Doppler echocardiography. J Am Coll Cardiol 1989;13:545-550.
72. Roger VL, Tajik AJ, Bailey KR, et al: Progression of aortic stenosis in adults: new appraisal using Doppler echocardiography. Am Heart J 1990;119:331-338.
73. Oh JK, Taliercio CP, Holmes DRJ, et al: Prediction of the severity of aortic stenosis by Doppler aortic valve area determination: prospective Doppler-catheterization correlation in 100 patients. J Am Coll Cardiol 1988;11:1227-1234.
74. Rosenhek R: Aortic stenosis: role of echocardiography in evaluation of disease severity, disease progression, and the role of echocardiography in clinical decision making.

In Otto CM (ed): The Practice of Clinical Echocardiography, 3rd ed. Philadelphia, Saunders, 2007, pp 516-551.

75. Otto CM: Valvular aortic stenosis: disease severity and timing of intervention. J Am Coll Cardiol 2006;47:2141-2151.

76. Libanoff AJ, Rodbard S: Atrioventricular pressure half-time: measure of mitral valve orifice area. Circulation 1968;38:144-150.

77. Thomas JD, Weyman AE: Doppler mitral pressure half-time: a clinical tool in search of theoretical justification. J Am Coll Cardiol 1987;10:923-929.

78. Holen J, Aaslid R, Landmark K, et al: Determination of effective orifice area in mitral stenosis from non-invasive ultrasound Doppler data and mitral flow rate. Acta Med Scand 1977;201:83-88.

79. Knutsen KM, Bae EA, Sivertssen E, Grendahl H: Doppler ultrasound in mitral stenosis: assessment of pressure gradient and atrioventricular pressure half-time. Acta Med Scand 1982;211:433-436.

80. Thomas JD, Wilkins GT, Choong CY, et al: Inaccuracy of mitral pressure half-time immediately after percutaneous mitral valvotomy: dependence on transmitral gradient and left atrial and ventricular compliance. Circulation 1988;78:980-993.

81. Braverman AC, Thomas JD, Lee RT: Doppler echocardiographic estimation of mitral valve area during changing hemodynamic conditions. Am J Cardiol 1991;68:1485-1490.

82. Grayburn PA, Handshoe R, Smith MD, et al: Quantitative assessment of the hemodynamic consequences of aortic regurgitation by means of continuous wave Doppler recordings. J Am Coll Cardiol 1987;10:135-141.

83. Otto CM, Pearlman AS, Gardner CL, et al: Simplification of the Doppler continuity equation for calculating stenotic aortic valve area. J Am Soc Echocardiogr 1988;1:155-157.

84. Zoghbi WA, Galan A, Quinones MA: Accurate assessment of aortic stenosis severity by Doppler echocardiography independent of aortic jet velocity. Am Heart J 1988;116:855-863.

85. Hung J: Quantitation of valvular regurgitation. In Otto CM (ed): The Practice of Clinical Echocardiography, 3rd ed. Philadelphia, Saunders, 2007, pp 405-429.

86. Zoghbi WA, Enriquez-Sarano M, Foster E, et al: Recommendations for evaluation of the severity of native valvular regurgitation with two-dimensional and Doppler echocardiography. J Am Soc Echocardiogr 2003;16:777-802.

87. Bolger AF, Eigler NL, Pfaff JM, et al: Computer analysis of Doppler color flow mapping images for quantitative assessment of in vitro fluid jets. J Am Coll Cardiol 1988;12:450-457.

88. Krabill KA, Sung HW, Tamura T, et al: Factors influencing the structure and shape of stenotic and regurgitant jets: an in vitro investigation using Doppler color flow mapping and optical flow visualization. J Am Coll Cardiol 1989;13:1672-1681.

89. Simpson IA, Valdes-Cruz LM, Sahn DJ, et al: Doppler color flow mapping of simulated in vitro regurgitant jets: evaluation of the effects of orifice size and hemodynamic variables. J Am Coll Cardiol 1989;13:1195-1207.

90. Stevenson JG: Comparison of several noninvasive methods for estimation of pulmonary artery pressure. J Am Soc Echocardiogr 1989;2:157-171.

91. Spain MG, Smith MD, Grayburn PA, et al: Quantitative assessment of mitral regurgitation by Doppler color flow imaging: angiographic and hemodynamic correlations. J Am Coll Cardiol 1989;13:585-590.

92. Klein AL, Burstow DJ, Tajik AJ, et al: Age-related prevalence of valvular regurgitation in normal subjects: a comprehensive color flow examination of 118 volunteers. J Am Soc Echocardiogr 1990;3:54-63.

93. Taylor AL, Eichhorn EJ, Brickner ME, et al: Aortic valve morphology: an important in vitro determinant of proximal regurgitant jet width by Doppler color flow mapping. J Am Coll Cardiol 1990;16:405-412.

94. Enriquez-Sarano M, Tajik AJ, Bailey KR, Seward JB: Color flow imaging compared with quantitative Doppler assessment of severity of mitral regurgitation: influence of eccentricity of jet and mechanism of regurgitation [published erratum appears in J Am Coll Cardiol 1993;22:342]. J Am Coll Cardiol 1993;21:1211-1219.

95. Veyrat C, Lessana A, Abitbol G, et al: New indexes for assessing aortic regurgitation with two-dimensional Doppler echocardiographic measurement of the regurgitant aortic valvular area. Circulation 1983;68:998-1005.

96. Tribouilloy CM, Enriquez-Sarano M, Bailey KR, et al: Quantification of tricuspid regurgitation by measuring the width of the vena contracta with Doppler color flow imaging: a clinical study. J Am Coll Cardiol 2000;36:472-478.

97. Recusani F, Bargiggia GS, Yoganathan AP, et al: A new method for quantification of regurgitant flow rate using color Doppler flow imaging of the flow convergence region proximal to a discrete orifice: an in vitro study. Circulation 1991;83:594-604.

98. Utsunomiya T, Ogawa T, Doshi R, et al: Doppler color flow "proximal isovelocity surface area" method for estimating volume flow rate: effects of orifice shape and machine factors [published erratum appears in J Am Coll Cardiol 1993;21:1537]. J Am Coll Cardiol 1991;17:1103-1111.

99. Vandervoort PM, Rivera JM, Mele D, et al: Application of color Doppler flow mapping to calculate effective regurgitant orifice area: an in vitro study and initial clinical observations. Circulation 1993;88:1150-1156.

100. Giesler M, Grossmann G, Schmidt A, et al: Color Doppler echocardiographic determination of mitral regurgitant flow from the proximal velocity profile of the flow convergence region. Am J Cardiol 1993;71:217-224.

101. Chen C, Koschyk D, Brockhoff C, et al: Noninvasive estimation of regurgitant flow rate and volume in patients with mitral regurgitation by Doppler color mapping of accelerating flow field. J Am Coll Cardiol 1993;21:374-383.

102. Reimold SC, Byrne JG, Caguioa ES, et al: Load dependence of the effective regurgitant orifice area in a sheep model of aortic regurgitation. J Am Coll Cardiol 1991;18:1085-1090.

103. Jenni R, Ritter M, Eberli F, Grimm J, Krayenbuehl HP: Quantification of mitral regurgitation with amplitude-weighted mean velocity from continuous wave Doppler spectra. Circulation 1989;79:1294-1299.

104. Labovitz AJ, Ferrara RP, Kern MJ, et al: Quantitative evaluation of aortic insufficiency by continuous wave Doppler echocardiography. J Am Coll Cardiol 1986;8:1341-1347.

105. Teague SM, Heinsimer JA, Anderson JL, et al: Quantification of aortic regurgitation utilizing continuous wave Doppler ultrasound. J Am Coll Cardiol 1986;8:592-599.

106. Masuyama T, Kodama K, Kitabatake A, et al: Noninvasive evaluation of aortic regurgitation by continuous-wave Doppler echocardiography. Circulation 1986;73:460-466.

107. Mulvagh S, Quinones MA, Kleiman NS, et al: Estimation of left ventricular end-diastolic pressure from Doppler transmitral flow velocity in cardiac patients independent of systolic performance. J Am Coll Cardiol 1992;20:112-119.

108. Pai RG, Bansal RC, Shah PM: Doppler-derived rate of left ventricular pressure rise: its correlation with the postoperative left ventricular function in mitral regurgitation. Circulation 1990;82:514-520.

109. Chen C, Rodriguez L, Lethor JP, et al: Continuous wave Doppler echocardiography for non-invasive assessment of left ventricular dP/dt and relaxation time constant from mitral regurgitant spectra in patients. J Am Coll Cardiol 1994;23:970-976.

110. Chen C, Rodriguez L, Levine RA, et al: Noninvasive measurement of the time constant of left ventricular relaxation using the continuous-wave Doppler velocity profile of mitral regurgitation. Circulation 1992;86:272-278.

111. Gardin JM, Drayer JI, Weber M, et al: Doppler echocardiographic assessment of left ventricular systolic and diastolic function in mild hypertension. Hypertension 1987;9:II90-II96.

112. Harrison MR, Clifton GD, Pennell AT, DeMaria AN: Effect of heart rate on left ventricular diastolic transmitral flow velocity patterns assessed by Doppler echocardiography in normal subjects. Am J Cardiol 1991;67:622-627.

113. Berk MR, Xie G, Kwan OL, et al: Reduction of left ventricular preload by lower body negative pressure alters Doppler transmitral filling patterns. J Am Coll Cardiol 1990;16:1387-1392.

114. Choong CY, Abascal VM, Thomas JD, et al: Combined influence of ventricular loading and relaxation on the transmitral flow velocity profile in dogs measured by Doppler echocardiography. Circulation 1988;78:672-683.

115. Dabestani A, Takenaka K, Allen B, et al: Effects of spontaneous respiration on diastolic left ventricular filling assessed by pulsed Doppler echocardiography. Am J Cardiol 1988;61:1356-1358.

116. Touche T, Prasquier R, Nitenberg A, et al: Assessment and follow-up of patients with aortic regurgitation by an updated Doppler echocardiographic measurement of the regurgitant fraction in the aortic arch. Circulation 1985;72:819-824.

117. Boughner DR: Assessment of aortic insufficiency by transcutaneous Doppler ultrasound. Circulation 1975;52:874-879.

118. Takenaka K, Dabestani A, Gardin JM, et al: A simple Doppler echocardiographic method for estimating severity of aortic regurgitation. Am J Cardiol 1986;57:1340-1343.

119. Rokey R, Sterling LL, Zoghbi WA, et al: Determination of regurgitant fraction in isolated mitral or aortic regurgitation by pulsed Doppler two-dimensional echocardiography. J Am Coll Cardiol 1986;7:1273-1278.

120. Ascah KJ, Stewart WJ, Jiang L, et al: A Doppler two-dimensional echocardiographic method for quantitation of mitral regurgitation. Circulation 1985;72:377-383.

121. Kitabatake A, Ito H, Inoue M, et al: A new approach to noninvasive evaluation of aortic regurgitant fraction by two-dimensional Doppler echocardiography. Circulation 1985;72:523-529.

122. Desai MY, Klein AL: Assessment of diastolic function by echocardiography. In Otto CM (ed): The Practice of Clinical Echocardiography, 3rd ed. Philadelphia, Saunders, 2007, pp 237-261.

123. Redfield MM, Jacobsen SJ, Burnett JC Jr, et al: Burden of systolic and diastolic ventricular dysfunction in the community: appreciating the scope of the heart failure epidemic. JAMA 2003;289:194-202.

124. Thomas JD, Popovic ZB: Assessment of left ventricular function by cardiac ultrasound. J Am Coll Cardiol 2006;48:2012-2025.

125. Gilman G, Nelson TA, Hansen WH, et al: Diastolic function: a sonographer's approach to the essential echocardiographic measurements of left ventricular diastolic function. J Am Soc Echocardiogr 2007;20:199-209.

126. Stoddard MF, Pearson AC, Kern MJ, et al: Influence of alteration in preload on the pattern of left ventricular diastolic filling as assessed by Doppler echocardiography in humans. Circulation 1989;79:1226-1236.

127. Thomas JD, Choong CYP, Flachskampf FA, Weyman AE: Analysis of the early transmitral Doppler velocity curve: effect of primary physiologic changes and compensatory preload adjustment. J Am Coll Cardiol 1990;16:644-655.

128. Appleton CP: Influence of incremental changes in heart rate on mitral flow velocity: assessment in lightly sedated, conscious dogs. J Am Coll Cardiol 1991;17:227-236.

129. Zoghbi WA, Bolli R: The increasing complexity of assessing diastolic function from ventricular filling dynamics. J Am Coll Cardiol 1991;17:238-248.

130. Shrestha NK, Moreno FL, Narciso FV, et al: Two-dimensional echocardiographic diagnosis of left-atrial thrombus in rheumatic heart disease: a clinicopathologic study. Circulation 1983;67:341-347.

131. Chiang CW, Pang SC, Lin FC, et al: Diagnostic accuracy of two-dimensional echocardiography for detection of left atrial thrombus in patients with mitral stenosis. J Ultrasound Med 1987;6:525-529.

132. Bansal RC, Heywood JT, Applegate PM, Jutzy KR: Detection of left atrial thrombi by two-dimensional echocardiography and surgical correlation in 148 patients with mitral valve disease. Am J Cardiol 1989;64:243-246.

84

133. Aschenberg W, Schluter M, Kremer P, et al: Transesophageal two-dimensional echocardiography for the detection of left atrial appendage thrombus. J Am Coll Cardiol 1986;7:163-166.

134. Olson JD, Goldenberg IF, Pedersen W, et al: Exclusion of atrial thrombus by transesophageal echocardiography. J Am Soc Echocardiogr 1992;5:52-56.

135. Yock PG, Popp RL: Noninvasive estimation of right ventricular systolic pressure by Doppler ultrasound in patients with tricuspid regurgitation. Circulation 1984;70:657-662.

136. Berger M, Haimowitz A, Van TA, et al: Quantitative assessment of pulmonary hypertension in patients with tricuspid regurgitation using continuous wave Doppler ultrasound. J Am Coll Cardiol 1985;6:359-365.

137. Simonson JS, Schiller NB: Sonospirometry: a new method for noninvasive estimation of mean right atrial pressure based on two-dimensional echocardiographic measurements of the inferior vena cava during measured inspiration. J Am Coll Cardiol 1988;11:557-664.

138. Kircher BJ, Himelman RB, Schiller NB: Noninvasive estimation of right atrial pressure from the inspiratory collapse of the inferior vena cava. Am J Cardiol 1990;66:493-496.

139. Lang RM, Bierig M, Devereux RB, et al: Recommendations for chamber quantification: a report from the American Society of Echocardiography's Guidelines and Standards Committee and the Chamber Quantification Writing Group, developed in conjunction with the European Association of Echocardiography, a branch of the European Society of Cardiology. J Am Soc Echocardiogr 2005;18:1440-1463.

140. Roman MJ, Devereux RB, Kramer-Fox R, O'Loughlin J: Two-dimensional echocardiographic aortic root dimensions in normal children and adults. Am J Cardiol 1989;64:507-512.

5

CHAPTER **6**

Evaluation of Valvular Heart Disease by Cardiac Catheterization and Angiocardiography

David M. Shavelle

KEY POINTS

- Cardiac Catheterization and angiocardiography is useful in patients:
  - whom require coronary angiography prior to surgical intervention,
  - with complex multivalve disease when data from echocardiography and cardiac catheterization must be integrated,
  - with suboptimal echocardiographic imaging (large body habitus, obese, chronic lung disease),
  - when discrepancies exist between the clinical information and findings from echocardiography,
  - when the diagnosis remains uncertain despite echocardiography and additional non-invasive imaging studies, and
  - with low gradient aortic stenosis when the administration of dobutamine can differentiate between true and 'pseudo' aortic stenosis.
- Accurate and detailed measurements are essential in patients with valvular heart disease so that the subsequently derived data remain accurate.
- Evaluation of left ventricular systolic function includes ventriculography, measurement of cardiac output and measurement of left ventricular pressures throughout the cardiac cycle.
- The principles to evaluate the severity of stenosis of each of the cardiac valves are similar and involve:
  - measurement of the pressure gradient,
  - analysis of the pressure waveforms,
  - measurement of cardiac output,
  - calculation of the valve area and occasionally,
  - angiocardiography of the chamber upstream to the site of stenosis.
- The pressure gradient between the left ventricle and the aorta in aortic stenosis is described by three invasive measurements: the mean gradient, the peak-to-peak gradient, and the maximum gradient.
- Adults with true severe aortic stenosis and a low gradient due to left ventricular dysfunction can be differentiated from pseudo-stenosis based on hemodynamics after dobutamine infusions showing:
  - a mean aortic valve gradient > 30 mm Hg and
  - an aortic valve area that remains ≤ 1.2 cm².
- Angiographic evaluation of regurgitant severity is based on injection of a contrast agent into the chamber downstream to the affected valve with imaging of contrast agent reflux into the chamber receiving the regurgitant volume.

In the majority of patients with valvular heart disease, information obtained from the history, physical examination, and noninvasive imaging studies (electrocardiogram, chest radiograph, and echocardiogram) is sufficient to establish the correct diagnosis and allow appropriate clinical decision making, including referral for percutaneous or surgical intervention. However, cardiac catheterization and angiocardiography continue to play an important role in selected patients with valvular heart disease.[1] These include those 1) who require coronary angiography before surgical intervention, 2) who have complex multivalve disease when data from echocardiography and cardiac catheterization must be integrated, 3) who have suboptimal echocardiographic imaging (e.g., large body habitus, obesity, or chronic lung disease), 4) for whom discrepancies exist between the clinical information and findings from echocardiography, 5) for whom the diagnosis remains uncertain despite echocardiography and additional non-invasive imaging studies, and 6) who have low-gradient aortic stenosis when the administration of dobutamine can differentiate between true and "pseudo" aortic stenosis.

A variety of approaches can be used in the cardiac catheterization laboratory to evaluate patients with valvular heart disease (Table 6-1). The fundamental basis of each approach relies on the premise that obtaining accurate and detailed measurements during the procedure is essential, so that the subsequently derived data remain accurate.

TABLE 6–1	Protocol for Evaluation of Valvular Heart Disease at Cardiac Catheterization

Pressure measurements
Right heart (including pulmonary capillary wedge pressure)
Left ventricle
Left atrium (for mitral stenosis evaluation)
Aorta
Transvalvular gradients: simultaneous pressure recordings on both sides of stenotic valve

Cardiac output
Thermodilution or Fick method (simultaneous with transvalvular gradient)

Angiocardiography
Left ventricle: end-diastolic volume, end-systolic volume, stroke volume, ejection fraction, evaluation of mitral regurgitation
Ascending aortography: for evaluation of aortic regurgitation
Coronary: for assessment of coexisting coronary artery disease

Calculated values
Valve area: Gorlin and Gorlin formula, Hakki formula
Valve resistance
Pulmonary vascular resistance: baseline and after vasodilator challenge
Systemic vascular resistance
Regurgitant volume and fraction

TABLE 6–2	Potential Sources of Error in Evaluation of Valvular Heart Disease at Catheterization

Pressure data
Frequency response
Side-hole versus end-hole catheters
Catheter whip and impact artifacts
Signal damping
Calibration and zero
Recorder sweep speed and scale
Peripheral amplification

Cardiac output
Fick: measurement of O_2 consumption
  Timing of arterial and venous O_2 samples
  Site of arterial and venous sampling
Thermodilution: uneven mixing of injectate within right atrium (tricuspid regurgitation)
  Poor accuracy at low outputs (extrapolation of curve)

Angiography
Geometric assumptions
Endocardial border identification
Catheter positioning
Cardiac rhythm

Valve area calculations
Transvalvular volume flow rate
Pressure measurements
Empiric constant

A number of potential sources of error can be present during the cardiac catheterization laboratory procedure (Table 6-2). The specific methods and techniques used during a cardiac catheterization procedure are selected to provide answers to specific clinical questions. The significance of the hemodynamic findings must be integrated with the complete set of clinical data, including information from the history, physical examination, electrocardiogram, chest radiograph, and echocardiogram.

EVALUATION OF LEFT VENTRICULAR SYSTOLIC FUNCTION

Evaluation of left ventricular systolic function includes ventriculography, measurement of cardiac output, and measurement of left ventricular pressures throughout the cardiac cycle. Contractility is defined as the intrinsic ability of the myocardium to shorten independent of loading conditions. However, measurement of left ventricular contractility in the clinical setting is problematic because most conventional measures of left ventricular systolic function depend on both ventricular preload and afterload as well as on myocardial contractility. Increased preload, defined as left ventricular end-diastolic volume or pressure, increases myocardial shortening as described by the Frank-Starling relationship. In contrast, afterload, defined as the resistance or impedance to left ventricular ejection, is inversely related to myocardial shortening. Loading conditions are frequently altered in patients with valvular heart disease. For example, with aortic stenosis, afterload is increased, and with aortic regurgitation, preload is increased. These alterations complicate the assessment of left ventricular systolic function.

Angiocardiography

Left ventricular end-diastolic volume (EDV) and end-systolic volume (ESV) can be calculated by tracing the respective endocardial boundaries on angiographic images and applying a validated geometric formula for volume calculation. Stroke volume (SV) is calculated as

$$SV = EDV - ESV$$

and ejection fraction (EF) as

$$EF = SV/EDV$$

The stroke volume (cardiac output divided by heart rate) calculated by angiocardiography represents the total amount of blood ejected by the ventricle, whether that blood is ejected forward into the aorta or backward into the left atrium across an incompetent mitral valve. Thus, angiographic stroke volume is termed *total* stroke volume.

The geometric formulas for angiographic calculation of volume (V) typically assume a prolate ellipsoid shape of the left ventricle. Endocardial border tracings from two orthogonal views of the ventricle (right and left anterior oblique projections) are used to measure the area (A) and length (L) of the ventricle with the minor axis diameter (D) calculated for each view as

$$D = (4A)/\pi L$$

Calculated ventricular volume (V_c) then is

$$V_c = (\pi/6)(L \times D_a \times D_b)$$

where D_a and D_b are the minor axis dimensions in the two orthogonal views. In the clinical setting, a single plane right anterior oblique angiogram using the modified formula of Dodge and Sandler also provides acceptable results[2]:

$$V_c = (8A^2)/(3\pi L) \text{ or } V_c = (\pi/6)(LD^2)$$

Whereas both angiography and echocardiography depend on manual border tracing, a slight, but consistent, overestimation of left ventricular volumes by angiography is due to contrast agent filling the ventricular trabeculations so that the traced endocardial border represents the outer edge of the myocardial trabeculations, in contrast to echocardiography in which ultrasound is reflected from the inner edge of the myocardial trabeculations so that volume tends to be underestimated slightly.[3-5] In addition, the volume occupied by the papillary muscles (which are excluded from the endocardial border tracing) needs to be taken into account. Regression equations have been derived in an attempt to correct for the overestimation of volume on angiography resulting from these two factors[2,6,7]

$$V = 0.81 V_c + 1.9$$

where V_c is the calculated volume and V is the corrected volume.

With careful angiographic technique, tracing of endocardial borders by an experienced observer, and use of appropriate correction factors, ventricular volumes derived from angiography correlate well with directly measured volumes and with echocardiographic volumes.[4,6,8,9] A biplane imaging approach[3,5] using borders traced from both the right and left anterior oblique radiographic projections provides accurate results with a mean difference for measurement variability of 6 to 10 mL for end-systolic and 7 to 20 mL for end-diastolic volumes.[10]

Technical factors important in performing ventricular angiography include the need for complete opacification of the ventricle with clear definition of the endocardial borders both at end-diastole and end-systole. This can be achieved with a 6-French side-hole pigtail catheter and a power contrast agent injector using an injection rate and volume appropriate to the type of catheter, ventricular size, and hemodynamics. A nonionic contrast agent is optimal in patients with valvular disease to avoid myocardial depression or hemodynamic changes. Correct positioning of the catheter in the mid-ventricle is needed to provide complete opacification of the chamber, to prevent movement of the catheter during the contract agent injection, and to minimize the risk of arrhythmias. Optimal catheter positioning also avoids artifactual mitral regurgitation due to entrapment of the catheter in the mitral valve apparatus. In addition, a correction factor for the effect of magnification must be determined by filming a calibrated grid at the estimated level of the ventricle. Other factors that affect the accuracy and reproducibility of angiographic volumes include image quality, the experience of the individual tracing the endocardial borders, heart rate and rhythm, and the potential cardiodepressant effect of the contrast agent.

Methods for determining left ventricular mass by angiographic techniques have been described, with left ventricular (LV) mass calculated on the basis of the thickness (h) of the anterior wall (assuming a symmetric thickness around the ventricle), ventricular diameter in anterior-posterior (D_{AP}) and lateral views (D_{lat}), long-axis length (L), and ventricular volume (V) as

$$\text{LV mass (g)} = \left(\frac{4}{3}\right)\pi\left[\frac{D_{AP}}{3}+h\right]\left[\frac{D_{lat}}{2}+h\right]\left[\frac{L}{2}+h\right]-V \times 1.05$$

However, ventricular mass calculations are limited by the inaccuracy in measuring left ventricular wall thickness from the angiographic image and, thus, are not widely used clinically.[11,12]

Left ventricular angiography also allows qualitative and quantitative assessment of wall motion in patients with valvular heart disease with concurrent coronary artery disease.[13,14]

Cardiac Output

Cardiac output can be calculated in the cardiac catheterization by the dilution of a known concentration of an indicator (e.g., dye, oxygen, or cold saline) as it passes through the vascular bed. This concept is illustrated by the injection of a known volume and concentration of dye (typically indocyanine green) into the venous circulation. From the rate at which this dye appears in the arterial circulation, the volume of blood the dye was diluted in (i.e., the cardiac output) can be calculated. Although indicator dilution dye curves provide accurate measurement of cardiac output, the procedure is time consuming and depends on meticulous technique such that other methods are now used more commonly.

Fick Technique

Oxygen serves as the indicator for cardiac output calculations in the Fick method. The Fick principle states that the uptake or release of oxygen by a tissue is the product of the amount of oxygen delivered to the tissue times the difference in oxygen content between the blood entering and leaving the tissue.[15] Thus, for the uptake of oxygen by the lungs:

$$\text{Oxygen uptake} = \text{Pulmonary blood flow}/(\text{O}_2 \text{ content}_{PV} - \text{O}_2 \text{ content}_{PA})$$

If the amount of oxygen consumed by the patient (oxygen uptake) and the oxygen content of pulmonary arterial (PA) and pulmonary venous (PV) blood are measured, this equation can be solved for pulmonary blood flow:

$$\text{Pulmonary blood flow} = \text{O}_2 \text{ consumption}/(\text{O}_2 \text{ content}_{PV} - \text{O}_2 \text{ content}_{PA})$$

In the absence of an intracardiac shunt, pulmonary and systemic blood flows are equal so that this method provides a measure of systemic (or forward) cardiac output, which can be calculated as

$$\text{Cardiac output} = \text{O}_2 \text{ consumption}/[(\text{O}_2 \text{ content})_{arterial} - (\text{O}_2 \text{ content})_{venous}]$$

where O_2 consumption is measured in mL O_2/min and O_2 content as mL O_2/100 mL blood (often referred to as volume percent).

To ensure that the sample of venous blood represents total venous return with adequate mixing of the sample, a pulmonary artery blood sample is used for mixed systemic venous oxygen content in this equation (in the absence of an intracardiac shunt). Whereas pulmonary venous blood provides the most accurate sample of oxygenated blood, the arterial sample is obtained from a systemic artery or the left ventricle. When an intracardiac shunt is present, separate calculations for systemic and pulmonary blood flow (using the appropriate arterial and venous oxygen contents) allow determination of the shunt ratio.

In clinical practice, oxygen consumption is usually measured by the polarographic O_2 method or by the paramagnetic method. Collection of expired air with the Douglas bag method is rarely used. The polarographic method uses a hood or face mask with the rate of air flow through the servo unit controlled by an oxygen sensor cell to maintain a constant fractional content of oxygen. Oxygen consumption (VO_2) then is calculated from the fractional content of oxygen and flow rates of air entering and exiting the patient mask, assuming a respiratory quotient of 1.0. The paramagnetic method measures both oxygen and carbon dioxide in expired air, which allows calculation of the respiratory quotient for each patient.

The arteriovenous oxygen difference is calculated from measurement of oxygen content in simultaneously drawn samples of arterial and mixed venous blood collected midway during the oxygen consumption measurement. Oxygen content typically is calculated as oxygen saturation times the theoretic oxygen capacity, which is estimated from the patient's hemoglobin (Hgb) level:

$$\text{O}_2 \text{ content} = \text{Hgb (g/dL)} \times 1.36 \text{ (mL O}_2\text{/g Hgb)} \times 10 \times \% \text{ saturation}$$

For accurate cardiac output calculations it is important that the arterial and venous oxygen samples are collected from the correct sites with prompt processing of the samples and that oxygen consumption and content measurements are simultaneous. Even with careful technique, the average error in measuring oxygen consumption is approximately 6%,[16] and the error in measurement of the arteriovenous oxygen difference is approximately 5%,[17] resulting in an error in cardiac output measurement of about 10% by the Fick method.[18] Measurements are more inaccurate if physiologic changes that affect cardiac output, such as heart rate or loading conditions, occur during the analysis period. Use of an assumed, rather than measured, oxygen consumption also leads to significant error as there is wide variation in the normal rate of oxygen consumption in adults.[19,20] Fick cardiac outputs tend to be more accurate for low outputs, and thermodilution outputs are more accurate at high flow rates.

Thermodilution

Measurement of cardiac output by the thermodilution method is widely used in the evaluation of patients with valvular heart disease. With the thermodilution method, a known volume of cold saline is injected into the right atrium while a thermistor in the pulmonary artery continuously records temperature. Cardiac output then is calculated from the known temperature (T) and volume (V) of the injectate, and the integral of temperature over time (T/dt) in the pulmonary artery,[21,22]

$$\text{Cardiac output} = \text{Constant } [V_{\text{injectate}} \times (T_{\text{blood}} - T_{\text{injectate}})]/(\Delta T/dt)$$

where the constant incorporates factors for the specific gravity and specific heat of blood and the injectate (1.08 if the injectate is 5% dextrose). In addition, an empiric correction factor (multiplication by 0.825) for the effect of warming of the injectate as it passes through the catheter also is needed.[23,24]

As with the Fick technique, the thermodilution method measures the "forward" cardiac output in patients with left sided valve disease, specifically the output of the right heart. Advantages of the thermodilution method include ease and repeatability of use, thus allowing multiple measurements over short time intervals with reasonable accuracy (a reproducibility of about 5% to 10% with proper technique).[24] Disadvantages include relatively poor accuracy at low cardiac outputs[25] and dependence on careful attention to technique, particularly avoidance of warming of the injectate. Because this method depends on even mixing of the injectate with the right atrial blood, thermodilution output measurements may be inaccurate when tricuspid regurgitation is present.

Pressure-Volume Loops

Direct measurement of left ventricular pressures throughout the entire cardiac cycle provides valuable data on left ventricular systolic function, although the effect of concurrent valvular disease must also be taken into account. The rate of rise of left ventricular pressure (dP/dt) during isovolumic contraction provides a relatively load-independent measure of left ventricular systolic function, which is particularly useful in patients with altered loading conditions due to valvular disease.

The relationship between left ventricular pressure and volume throughout the cardiac cycle can be examined in detail by graphing instantaneous pressure (on the vertical axis) versus volume (on the horizontal axis). Left ventricular stroke volume is the distance on the horizontal axis between end-diastole and end-systole, whereas left ventricular stroke work (the integral of pressure times volume over the cardiac cycle) is the area enclosed by the pressure-volume loop. When pressure-volume loops are recorded under different loading conditions, the slope of the end-systolic pressure-volume relationship, termed elastance or E_{max}, provides a load-independent measure of left ventricular systolic function.[26,27]

Valvular heart disease characterized by pressure overload of the left ventricle results in a taller pressure-volume loop that is shifted upward, reflecting the higher ventricular systolic pressures and greater left ventricular stoke work. Volume overload of the left ventricle also increases stroke work with a larger loop that is shifted upward and to the right. However, despite these shifts in the pressure-volume loop, the slope of the end-systolic pressure-volume relationship remains normal in patients with valvular disease and compensated ventricular systolic function. A reduced slope indicates impaired

contractility superimposed on the pressure and/or volume overload state.

In practice, measurement of pressure-volume loops is technically demanding. Ventricular pressures must be recorded with high-fidelity catheters and volumes must be determined at multiple points in the cardiac cycle either using contrast or radionuclide angiography or experimental approaches such as a conductance catheter.[28] Thus, although this approach provides insight into the pathophysiology of disease and provides essential information in research studies, it rarely is used in the routine clinical management of patients with valvular heart disease.[29]

EVALUATION OF STENOSIS SEVERITY

Normal cardiac valves offer little to no resistance to blood flow when the valve is open in either systole (semilunar valves—aortic and pulmonic) or diastole (atrioventricular valves—tricuspid and mitral). In the setting of disease, restriction to leaflet opening (stenosis) occurs and blood flow across the valve is hindered. Resistance to blood flow results in a pressure drop or gradient across the valve. The principles to evaluate the severity of stenosis of each of the cardiac valves are similar and involve (1) measurement of the pressure gradient, (2) analysis of the pressure waveforms, (3) measurement of cardiac output, (4) calculation of the valve area, and, occasionally, (5) angiocardiography of the chamber upstream to the site of stenosis.

Pressure Gradients

Pressure gradients are most accurately measured using two transducers that allow for simultaneous measurement of the upstream and downstream pressures. A systematic approach to the review of pressure waveforms includes optimization of the pressure scale and recording speed (i.e., sweep paper), with assessment of (1) cardiac rhythm, (2) the pressure measurements on both sides of the valve across the valve, (3) pressures in all adjacent cardiac chambers (Table 6-3), (4) the rate and shape of the upslope and downslope of pressure waveforms, and (5) recording artifacts. Both technical and physiologic factors can affect the measured pressure gradients (see Table 6-2).

Technical Factors

Technical factors can significantly affect the accuracy of the reported transvalvular gradients. The frequency response of the pressure measurement system significantly affects the recorded pressure waveform. Although micromanometer-tipped catheters have an optimal frequency response (at least 20 cycles/sec) for intracardiac pressure recording, these catheters are expensive and require meticulous technique. In the clinical setting, fluid-filled catheters and strain-gauge external transducers that are commonly used have a frequency response of only 10 to 20 cycles/sec. The frequency response can be optimized by use of stiff wide-bore catheters, a short length of connecting tubing, and a low-density liquid.

External pressure transducers are subject to a phenomenon called "ring-down," resulting from the conversion of pressure energy to an electrical signal, similar to the sound resulting from striking a bell. The use of a fluid-filled catheter between the chamber of interest and the transducer amplifies this phenomenon, leading to apparent fluctuations in the recorded pressure signal. This phenomenon, called underdamping, is characterized by a waveform consisting of diminishing harmonic oscillations of the underlying pressure signal. To counter this effect, the recording system is damped just enough to avoid excessive oscillations while maintaining the frequency response of the system. Overdamping must also be avoided as it can lead to underestimation of pressure gradients.

TABLE 6–3	Normal Values at Cardiac Catheterization (Supine, Resting Adults)		
Angiographic left ventricular volumes	**Mean ± 1 SD**		
End-diastolic volume	70 ± 20 mL/m²		
End-systolic volume	24 ± 0 mL/m²		
Ejection fraction	0.67 ± 0.08		
LV mass	92 ± 16 g/m²		
Cardiac output			
Rest	3.0 L/min/m²		
Exercise	18.0 L/min/m²		
O₂ consumption (resting)	126 ± 26 mL/min/m²		
Arterial O₂ saturation	95%		
Venous O₂ saturation	75%		
AV oxygen difference	40 mL/L (volume %)		
Pressures (mm Hg)	**Systolic/ Diastolic**	**Mean**	
Right atrium	a3-6, v1-4	1-5	
Right ventricle	20-30/2-7		
Pulmonary artery	16-30/4-13	9-18	
Pulmonary wedge	5-12		
Left atrial	a4-14, v6-16	6-11	
Left ventricular	90-140/6-12		
Aorta	90-140/70-90	70-110	
Vascular resistance	**Mean ± 1 SD**	**Indexed to BSA**	
Pulmonary resistance	67 ± 30	123 ± 54 dynes-second cm⁻⁵m²	
Wood units (mm Hg-L⁻¹-min)	0.8-1.1 ± 0.3-0.5		
Systemic resistance	1170 ± 270	2130 ± 450	
Valve areas (cm²)	**Overall**	**Male**	**Female**
Aortic	4.6 ± 1.1	4.8 ± 1.3	3.7 ± 1.0
Mitral	7.8 ± 1.9	8.3 ± 2.0	6.7 ± 1.3
Tricuspid	10.6 ± 2.6	11.5 ± 2.5	8.8 ± 1.7
Pulmonic	4.7 ± 1.2	4.9 ± 1.3	4.3 ± 1.0

AV, arteriovenous; BSA, body surface area; LV, left ventricular.

Damping typically can be optimized by using short, stiff tubing to connect the catheter to the pressure transducer, minimizing the number of connections in the system, and using contrast agent (instead of saline) to fill the catheter.

Pressure recording systems must be zeroed and calibrated both before and after data collection. Calibration is optimally performed using a known input pressure, such as with a mercury manometer, but many systems now include electronic calibration, which is usually adequate. The zero and the reference standard need to be rechecked periodically during and at completion of the study to avoid erroneous data interpretations. When two catheters are used to measure pressures simultaneously on both sides of a stenotic valve, the calibrations are checked together and, if possible, data are

re-recorded after switching the transducers to the other catheters to avoid any systematic bias.

Pressures are recorded at a fast sweep speed to allow accurate time measurements and to display the waveform in enough detail to allow analysis of the degree of damping and the subtleties of the pressure waveform. The vertical axis is adjusted, depending on the pressures being recorded, to use the full height of the recording while including the pressure waveforms of interest on the scale. For example, left atrial and left ventricular pressures across a stenotic mitral valve might be recorded on a 0 to 25 mm Hg scale, whereas severe aortic stenosis might require a 0 to 200 mm Hg scale.

Physiologic Factors

The exact location of the pressures recorded on the upstream and downstream sides of a stenotic valve can significantly affect the measured transvalvular gradient. This occurs for several reasons. First, the timing of the pressure waveform is different closer to the valve than at a greater distance from the valve so that realignment of the waveforms may be needed for accurate gradient calculations. For example, the femoral artery pressure upstroke is delayed compared with the central aortic pressure as predicted by the velocity of pressure propagation between these two sites. If a femoral artery waveform is used in place of central aortic pressure for calculating the aortic transvalvular gradient, this timing difference needs to be taken into account. Similarly, if the diastolic pressure curve uses the pulmonary capillary wedge pressure in place of directly measured left atrial pressure in a patient with mitral stenosis, failure to consider timing differences may lead to erroneous mitral gradient calculations.

Second, the shape of the waveform adjacent to the valve versus more distally may affect the apparent transvalvular gradient. This is most evident when central aortic and peripheral arterial (e.g., femoral artery) pressures are compared. Because of summation of the transmitted and reflected pressure waveforms, the femoral artery pressure curve is narrower with a higher peak compared with central aortic pressure, a phenomenon known as peripheral amplification (Figure 6-1). Whereas simultaneously measured central aortic and left ventricular pressures are used whenever possible for calculation of transaortic pressure gradients, if only a femoral pressure is

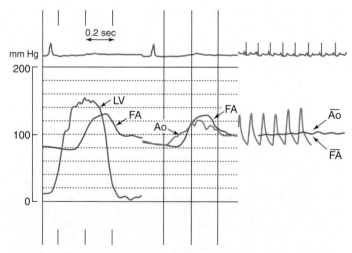

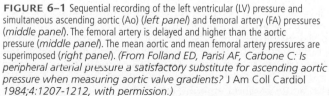

FIGURE 6–1 Sequential recording of the left ventricular (LV) pressure and simultaneous ascending aortic (Ao) (*left panel*) and femoral artery (FA) pressures (*middle panel*). The femoral artery is delayed and higher than the aortic pressure (*middle panel*). The mean aortic and mean femoral artery pressures are superimposed (*right panel*). (*From Folland ED, Parisi AF, Carbone C: Is peripheral arterial pressure a satisfactory substitute for ascending aortic pressure when measuring aortic valve gradients?* J Am Coll Cardiol 1984;4:1207-1212, with permission.)

available, realignment of timing and correction of the peripheral amplification are needed.

The third physiologic issue that may affect the measured transvalvular gradient is the phenomenon of pressure recovery that occurs distal to a site of stenosis. Pressure recovery is especially important with aortic stenosis.[30-32] As the high-velocity jet flows through the stenotic orifice, it decelerates and expands distal to the valve. The associated turbulence results in an increase in aortic pressure ("pressure recovery") such that the pressure difference between the left ventricle and the distal ascending aorta is less than the difference between the left ventricle and the pressure in the stenotic orifice itself. Whereas pressure recovery may account for some of the observed discrepancies between Doppler- and catheter-based data and conceivably could lead to underestimation of stenosis severity, the magnitude of this effect in the clinical setting appears to be small (approximately 5 to 10 mm Hg) and is unlikely to affect clinical decision making. Pressure recovery is greatest when stenosis severity is mild and aortic root dimension is small and least with severe stenosis and poststenotic dilation. Potential underestimation of stenosis severity due to pressure recovery can be avoided by recording pressures immediately adjacent to the valve on the downstream side of the stenosis.

Several other factors also may affect recorded pressure gradients. The transaortic pressure gradient may be affected by the presence of the catheter itself in the stenotic orifice. The catheter may increase the transvalvular pressure gradient either by further decreasing the cross-sectional flow area or by inducing aortic regurgitation.[33] Other physiologic variables that may affect the pressure gradient include the effect of atrial contraction, cardiac arrhythmias, and the compliance of the receiving chamber when regurgitation is present. Irregular heart rhythms affect measured pressure gradients in valvular stenosis because of the varying volume flow rates across the valve, necessitating averaging of several beats for clinical interpretation.

Aortic Valve

The most commonly encountered valvular heart disease condition in the cardiac catheterization laboratory in recent years is aortic stenosis. With the widespread use of echocardiography, the diagnosis and severity of aortic stenosis are frequently known before referral to the cardiac catheterization laboratory. The cardiac catheterization procedure therefore usually involves confirming the findings of echocardiography. Occasionally, however, the diagnosis and/or severity of stenosis remain in question, and cardiac catheterization is requested to further clarify the situation; in this setting, it is essential to obtain complete, accurate, and reliable data during the procedure.

Pressure Gradients

All pressures should be measured before contrast ventriculography. A variety of catheters and techniques can be used to cross the aortic valve in a retrograde manner to measure the pressure gradient. A 0.038-inch straight wire in combination with a pigtail, Judkins right, or Amplatz left coronary catheter is commonly used.[34] Occasionally, a catheter specifically designed to cross the aortic valve called a Feldman catheter may be required.[35] When the straight wire cannot be passed across the valve, supravalvular angiography may be useful to localize the position of the valve orifice. Although the risk of retrograde passage of catheters across a narrowed and diseased aortic valve is small, a recent study showed that 3% of patients experienced a clinically significant neurologic event and 22% had magnetic resonance imaging evidence of an acute cerebral embolic event.[36] In the setting of severe

aortic valve calcification, critical aortic stenosis, or the presence of coexisting mitral stenosis, transseptal puncture should be considered.

The pressure gradient between the left ventricle and the aorta can be described by three invasive measurements: (1) the mean gradient, (2) the peak-to-peak gradient, and (3) the maximum gradient (Figure 6-2). The mean gradient represents the area under the left ventricular-aortic pressure curve and corresponds to the mean gradient measured by echocardiography. The peak-to-peak gradient has no true physiologic meaning and represents the difference between maximum aortic and the maximum left ventricular pressures. Note that these maximum pressures do not occur at the same time and the peak-to-peak gradient is not the same as the maximum gradient. The maximum gradient represents the maximum difference that can be measured between the left ventricle and aorta during systole and corresponds to the maximum instantaneous gradient measured by echocardiography. The maximum gradient occurs early during ventricular ejection, before the peak left ventricular pressure.

In the absence of aortic stenosis, there may occasionally be a small, early gradient between the left ventricle and aorta that is referred to as an "impulse" gradient (Figure 6-3).[37] This gradient can only be detected using high-fidelity micromanometer-tipped catheters and may be present during high-flow states such as exercise.[38]

There are five invasive methods that can be used to measure pressure gradients between the left ventricle and the aorta. The single catheter pullback technique is not recommended because spontaneous changes in cardiac cycle length, especially in the setting of atrial and or ventricular arrhythmias, result in significant variations in the measured gradient.[39] Simultaneous measurement of the proximal aortic and the left ventricular pressure using two transducers yields the most accurate data. The most common approach uses a single arterial puncture with placement of a 6-French sheath within the femoral artery and advancement of a 6-French double lumen catheter (Langston dual lumen catheter; Vascular Solutions, Minneapolis, MN) into the left ventricle. This catheter provides simultaneous measurement of the aortic and left ventricular pressures through ports within these locations.[40] After measurement

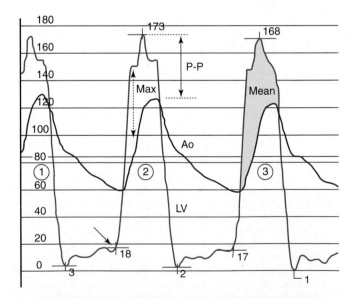

FIGURE 6–2 The gradient between the left ventricle and the aorta in aortic stenosis can be described by three invasive measures. The mean gradient (beat 3) represents the area under the left ventricular-aortic pressure curve. The peak-to-peak gradient (beat 2) is the difference between the maximum aortic and the maximum left ventricular systolic pressure. The maximum gradient (beat 2) is the maximum difference that can be measured between the left ventricle and aorta during systole.

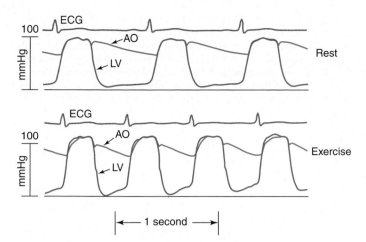

FIGURE 6–3 Simultaneous aortic (AO) and left ventricular (LV) pressure measured at rest (*top*) and at exercise (*bottom*). A small early systolic gradient is present during exercise and is referred to as an impulse gradient. *(From Pasipoularides A: Clinical assessment of ventricular ejection dynamics with and without outflow obstruction.* J Am Coll Cardiol *1990;15:859-882, with permission.)*

of the gradient, a contrast agent can be injected through the left ventricular port of the catheter to perform a left ventriculogram. The second approach requires two arterial punctures with one catheter positioned within the left ventricle and a second catheter (from the second arterial puncture site) located within the ascending aorta. The third method uses femoral venous access to allow a transseptal puncture with subsequent positioning of a catheter into the left ventricle and a second catheter (from an arterial puncture) positioned into the ascending aorta. The fourth method uses a single arterial puncture with placement of a standard, short 6-French sheath within the femoral artery and advancement of a 4- or 5-French pigtail catheter (through the 6-French sheath) into the left ventricle. The femoral artery pressure is measured via the side arm of the sheath and is used as a surrogate to the central aortic pressure. By nature of its peripheral location, the femoral artery pressure is delayed and higher than the central aortic pressure (see Figure 6-1). When this delay is accounted for by realignment of the pressures, the mean left ventricular to aortic gradient is underestimated by approximately 10 mm Hg. Without realignment, the mean gradient is overestimated by approximately 9 mm Hg.[41] Therefore, to obtain accurate data, the central aortic pressure should be measured. The fifth method uses a single arterial puncture with placement of a long (55 cm) 6-French sheath into the ascending aorta with a smaller 4- or 5-French sheath advanced through the long sheath into the left ventricle.[42]

Recently, a novel method was introduced to simultaneously measure both aortic and left ventricular pressures. Bertog et al[43] described performing a single arterial puncture with placement of a 4-French catheter into the ascending aorta. Left ventricular pressure is measured using a 0.014-inch pressure wire (placed through the 4-French catheter), which is the same wire used to assess fractional flow reserve. In a small series of four patients, correlation with traditional methods to measure the aortic valve gradient was excellent. In a larger series of 18 patients with aortic stenosis, Bae et al[44] also found high correlation with traditional methods for measuring the aortic valve gradient and an average procedure time of 36 minutes.[44]

In the setting of critical aortic stenosis, the presence of a catheter positioned across the aortic valve can influence the pressure gradient. This phenomenon was initially described by Carabello in 1987.[45] In the setting of an aortic valve area less than 0.6 cm², Carabello observed an increase in 10 mm Hg in the peripheral arterial pressure when the catheter

was withdrawn from the left ventricle across the aortic valve. This was thought to be related to the catheter further narrowing the orifice of a severely narrowed valve.

Pressure Waveform Analysis

In the absence of aortic stenosis, the slope and magnitude of the aortic and left ventricular systolic pressures are similar and rise together to a mid-systolic peak. With aortic stenosis, the pressure in the aorta rises slowly and achieves a late systolic peak. In an attempt to reduce wall stress, the left ventricle responds to the pressure overload of aortic stenosis by developing hypertrophy. Left ventricular hypertrophy limits the ability of the left ventricle to fill at a normal pressure, which results in a higher end-diastolic pressure.

Valve Area

General Concepts In 1951 Gorlin and Gorlin[46] published their classic manuscript describing data derived from hydraulic systems that was used to determine the orifice of various cardiac valves. The calculated valve area from the formula was validated by directly measuring the valve orifice from autopsy or surgical specimens in 11 patients. The formula states that the area of a valve (cm²) is equal to the flow across the valve (mL/sec) divided by the product of two constants and the square root of the pressure difference (mm Hg) across the valve. The first constant (C) is an empirical constant that accounts for energy loss and issues related to orifice contraction. For the aortic, pulmonic, and tricuspid valves, C is assumed to be 1.0. For the mitral valve, C was initially assumed to be 0.7 by Gorlin and Gorlin; this value was later revised in 1972 to be 0.85.[47] The second constant is equal to the square root of twice the gravity acceleration factor (980 cm/sec/sec) and is 44.3:

$$\text{Valve area} = \frac{\text{Flow across valve}}{44.3C\sqrt{\Delta P}}$$

$$\text{Valve area} = \frac{\text{CO/(SEP)(HR)}}{44.3C\sqrt{\Delta P}}$$

where P is the mean pressure gradient, CO is the cardiac output, SEP is the systolic ejection period, and HR is heart rate. For mitral stenosis, the diastolic filling period is used instead of the systolic ejection period in the equation.

A simplified formula for calculating valve areas was later proposed in 1981 by Hakki et al.[48] The Hakki equation for valve area uses the cardiac output (L/min) divided by the square root of the pressure difference across the valve:

$$\text{Valve area} = \frac{\text{CO}}{\sqrt{P_{\text{mean}}}}$$

For the aortic valve, either the mean or the peak pressure gradient can be used; for the mitral valve, the mean pressure gradient should be used. In a series of 100 patients with mitral and aortic stenosis, the correlation coefficients for the simplified Hakki equation compared with those for the Gorlin formula were 0.94 and 0.96, respectively.

Measurement of Aortic Valve Area Worksheets can be useful to organize the measured and derived data when the aortic valve area is determined (Table 6-4). Simultaneous aortic and left ventricular pressures are measured using one of the techniques discussed above. Traditionally, gradients were measured using hand-held planimeter devices. Currently, however, computer-based monitoring systems can accurately determine the mean, maximum, and peak-to-peak gradients. Manual confirmation of the computer-measured gradients can be performed using a grid-based system (Figure 6-4). If sinus rhythm is present, 5 cardiac beats should be used to determine the gradients. If atrial fibrillation or other arrhythmias

TABLE 6–4	Valve Area Calculation Worksheet for the Aortic and Mitral Valves

Aortic valve area (valve constant = 1)

Step 1. Determine the average gradients for 5 cardiac beats if in sinus rhythm and 10 cardiac beats if in atrial fibrillation

Step 2. Determine the mean systolic ejection period for 5 cardiac beats

Step 3. Heart rate = _____ beats/min

Step 4. Cardiac output = _____ mL/min

Step 5. Valve area = $\dfrac{\text{Cardiac output}/(\text{heart rate} \times \text{systolic ejection period})}{44.3 \times \text{Valve constant}\sqrt{\text{mean gradient}}}$

Mitral valve area (valve constant = 0.85)

Step 1. Determine the average gradients for 5 cardiac beats if in sinus rhythm and 10 cardiac beats if in atrial fibrillation

Step 2. Determine the mean diastolic filling period for 5 cardiac beats

Step 3. Heart rate = _____ beats/min

Step 4. Cardiac output = _____ ml/min

Step 5. Valve area = $\dfrac{\text{Cardiac output}/(\text{heart rate} \times \text{diastolic filling period})}{44.3 \times \text{Valve constant}\sqrt{\text{mean gradient}}}$

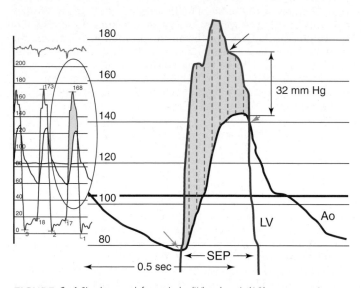

FIGURE 6–4 Simultaneous left ventricular (LV) and aortic (AO) pressure tracings in a patient with severe aortic stenosis. The systolic ejection period (SEP) begins with opening of the aortic valve (*orange arrow*) and ends with closure of the aortic valve (*orange arrowhead*). The shaded area represents the mean systolic gradient. To confirm the computer-measured pressure gradients, a grid-based system can be used. Ten vertical lines are drawn at equal spaces throughout systole. Each line is measured to determine the gradient at that time period. For example, the 7th line from the left (*black arrow*) shows a gradient of 32. Summing all of the values together and dividing by 10 (10 lines were drawn), yields manual confirmation of the mean gradient.

are present, 10 cardiac beats should be required for accurate results. The cardiac output is measured by both the methods of thermodilution and Fick. The systolic ejection period (SEP) is measured from the opening of the aortic valve (left ventricular pressure exceeds aortic pressure) to the closing of the aortic valve (left ventricular pressures falls below aortic pressure) in units of seconds per beat. The SEP should also be measured for 5 beats and an average taken. The aortic valve area is reported using the cardiac output as measured by both the Fick and thermodilution methods. The severity of aortic stenosis is classified on the basis on the valve area as mild (>1.5 cm²), moderate (1.0 to 1.5 cm²), severe (<1.0 cm²), and critical (<0.5 cm²). The valve area index is calculated as the aortic valve area divided by the body surface area.

There are often discrepancies between the aortic valve area and transvalvular gradients measured by cardiac catheterization and Doppler echocardiography. When systematically evaluated, the aortic valve area tends to be higher when measured by cardiac catheterization than with Doppler echocardiography.[49-51] These discrepancies are due to the pressure recovery phenomenon,[52,53] changes in hemodynamics (transaortic flow rate and heart rate) between the time of the studies,[54] and suboptimal echocardiographic recording of the aortic jet velocity. In the setting of coexisting aortic regurgitation, the valve area by the Gorlin equation can only provide a minimum value for the valve area.

Angiocardiography

Left ventriculography should be routinely performed in patients with aortic stenosis as it provides assessment of left ventricular systolic function, the anatomy of the aortic valve, and coexisting mitral regurgitation. The aortic valve should be assessed for calcification, leaflet morphology (bicuspid), and leaflet mobility. A bicuspid aortic valve may show systolic doming of the leaflets.

Low-Output, Low-Gradient Aortic Stenosis

A small proportion of patients evaluated in the cardiac catheterization laboratory for aortic stenosis will be found to have a low transvalvular gradient in the setting of a low cardiac output. The Gorlin equation is flow dependent, and this is particularly true when the cardiac output is less than 4 L/min. Differentiating true, severe aortic stenosis from mild aortic stenosis with a coexisting cardiomyopathy (so-called "pseudo" aortic stenosis) is clinically important as the former group of patients derive benefit from aortic valve replacement.[55]

A widely accepted definition of low-gradient aortic stenosis is a mean aortic valve gradient less than 40 mm Hg in the setting of an ejection fraction less than 40%.[56] For patients with pseudo aortic stenosis, medications that increase cardiac output will usually increase the calculated aortic valve area. In contrast, for patients with true, severe aortic stenosis, an increase in cardiac output will not result in a significant increase in the calculated aortic valve area. Intravenous dobutamine can be used in the cardiac catheterization laboratory to differentiate true from pseudo aortic stenosis (Figure 6-5). A standard protocol involves obtaining baseline measurements of cardiac output, heart rate, and simultaneous left ventricular and aortic pressures and initiating dobutamine by continuous infusion at 5 µg/kg/min.[57] The dose is then increased by 3 to 10 µg/kg/min every 5 minutes until a maximum dose of 40 µg/kg/min is achieved, the mean gradient increases to greater than 40 mm Hg, cardiac output increases by 50%, heart rate increases to less than 140 beats/min, or intolerable symptoms or side effects occur. Patients with true, severe aortic stenosis can be identified after dobutamine infusion as those with (1) a mean aortic valve gradient greater than 30 mm Hg and (2) an aortic valve area that remains 1.2 cm or less.[2,57]

Aortic Valve Resistance

Aortic valve resistance has been proposed as another measure to assess the severity of aortic stenosis.[58,59] Aortic valve resistance is calculated as the mean pressure gradient divided by the flow rate ratio and is expressed in units of dyne-seconds cm⁻⁵:

$$\text{Aortic valve resistance} = \frac{1.33\sqrt{\Delta P_{\text{mean}}}}{(\text{CO/HR}) \times \text{SEP}}$$

A cutoff value of greater than 300 dyne-seconds cm⁻⁵ is commonly used to identify patients with severe aortic stenosis.[59] It was previously felt that aortic valve resistance was less flow dependent than the Gorlin formula–derived aortic valve area. However, recent in vitro and clinical studies

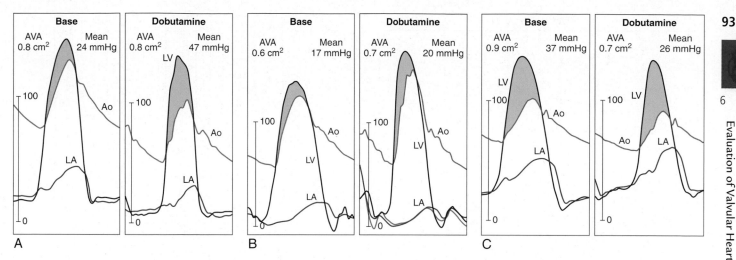

FIGURE 6–5 Hemodynamic tracings from three patients with aortic stenosis receiving intravenous dobutamine. **A**, Cardiac output and aortic valve gradient increase in response to dobutamine and the aortic valve area remained 0.8 cm². This patient had severe aortic stenosis at the time of valve surgery. **B**, Dobutamine infusion resulted in an increase in cardiac output and aortic valve gradient. Final aortic valve area was 0.7 cm². The patient was found to only have mild aortic stenosis at valve surgery. **C**, Dobutamine infusion did not change cardiac output and the mean aortic valve gradient decreased from 37 to 26 mm Hg. Dobutamine was stopped because of hypotension. This patient was found to have severe aortic stenosis at the time of surgery. *(From Nishimura RA, Grantham JA, Connolly HM, et al. Low-output, low-gradient aortic stenosis in patients with depressed left ventricular systolic function: the clinical utility of the dobutamine challenge in the catheterization laboratory. Circulation 2002;106:809-813, with permission.)*

suggest that aortic valve resistance is flow dependent and not superior to calculated aortic valve area for the assessment of aortic stenosis.[60,61]

Pulmonic Valve

Most cases of valvular pulmonic stenosis are congenital in origin. Adults commonly present with dyspnea and exertional fatigue due to the inability to increase cardiac output sufficiently during exercise. Stenosis is frequently diagnosed by Doppler echocardiography, and cardiac catheterization is usually only performed before balloon valvotomy.

Pressure Gradients

The severity of valvular pulmonic stenosis is evaluated on the basis of the peak-to-peak gradient between the right ventricle and pulmonary artery. A peak-to-peak gradient of greater than 30 mm Hg is considered hemodynamically significant and warrants consideration for balloon valvotomy. As opposed to the assessment of aortic stenosis, the gradient between the right ventricle and pulmonary artery can be measured by the pullback technique using an end-hole catheter. By using the peak-to-peak gradient, the severity of pulmonic stenosis is classified as mild (25 to 49 mm Hg), moderate (50 to 79 mm Hg), and severe (≥80 mm Hg).[62]

Pressure Waveform Analysis

Pressure waveform analysis in valvular pulmonic stenosis is notable for an elevated right ventricular systolic pressure, a gradient (described above) across the pulmonic valve, and a pulmonary artery pressure that rises slowly to achieve a late systolic peak.

Valve Area

The normal pulmonary valve orifice is 2.0 cm²/m² and in the absence of disease, there is no gradient across the valve.[63] However, the concept of valve area is not used in the evaluation of pulmonic stenosis, and decisions regarding therapy are based on the peak-to-peak gradient.

Angiocardiography

Right ventriculography in a left lateral projection displays the pulmonic valve, the right ventricle, and the proximal portion

of the main pulmonary artery in a relatively straight line. With valvular pulmonic stenosis, the valve appears thickened and domes during systole. Right ventricular function and the presence and severity of tricuspid regurgitation should also be assessed. A right anterior oblique projection with 25 to 30° of cranial angulation allows visualization of the right ventricle and also profiles the pulmonic valve.

Mitral Valve

Patients with mitral stenosis are currently referred to the cardiac catheterization laboratory for evaluation of disease severity before percutaneous mitral balloon valvuloplasty or mitral valve replacement. Complete assessment includes right and left heart catheterization, simultaneous measurement of left atrial (or pulmonary capillary wedge) and left ventricular pressures, and measurement of cardiac output.

Pressure Gradients

A transseptal puncture is required for accurate assessment of left atrial pressure. A transseptal sheath is placed into the left atrium, and simultaneous measurement of left atrial and left ventricular pressure is performed. The mean and maximum pressure gradients should be recorded at various sweep speeds and pressure scales. The optimal sweep speed and pressure scale are usually 100 mm/sec and 0 to 40 mm Hg, respectively. Mean gradients are measured by averaging the instantaneous gradients over the flow period using carefully recorded and correctly aligned tracings of the left atrial and left ventricular pressure curves.

In clinical practice, the pulmonary capillary wedge pressure is often used as a surrogate of the left atrial pressure to assess the severity of mitral stenosis (Figure 6-6). To ensure that an accurate pulmonary capillary wedge pressure is obtained, the mean pulmonary capillary wedge pressure should be less than the mean pulmonary artery pressure and the saturation of blood should be greater than 95%. In a systematic study, Lange et al[64] found that the pulmonary capillary wedge pressure exceeded estimated left atrial pressure by 1.7+/−0.6 mm Hg.

Pressure Waveform Analysis

Atrial fibrillation may be present in patients with long-standing mitral stenosis and results in loss of the a wave in the

PCWP and LV

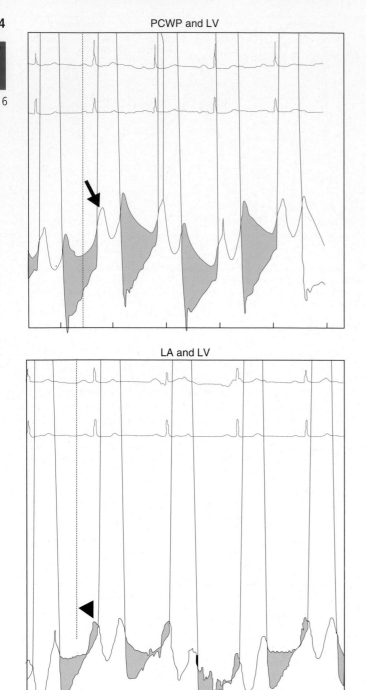

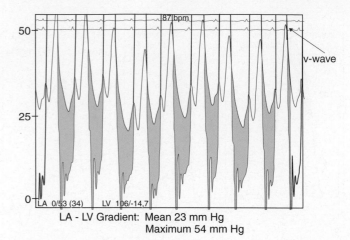

LA - LV Gradient: Mean 23 mm Hg
Maximum 54 mm Hg

FIGURE 6–7 Simultaneous left atrial (LA) (from transseptal puncture) and left ventricular (LV) pressures in a patient with critical mitral stenosis. The mean gradient is 23 mm Hg, and the maximum gradient is 54 mm Hg. The v waves (*arrow*) are prominent and approach 52 mm Hg.

LA and LV

FIGURE 6–6 An example of a good quality pulmonary capillary wedge pressure tracing that mirrors the left atrial pressure tracing in a patient with severe mitral stenosis. *Top,* Simultaneous pulmonary capillary wedge pressure (PCWP) and left ventricular (LV) pressure tracing. The vertical dotted line marks the beginning of the p wave in the electrocardiogram. The a wave in the pulmonary capillary wedge pressure tracing (*arrow*) occurs approximately 120 msec after the p wave. *Bottom,* Simultaneous left atrial (LA) and left ventricular (LV) pressure tracing in the same patient with severe mitral stenosis. Note that the gradient is higher when the pulmonary capillary wedge pressure tracing is used, instead of the left atrial pressure. The a wave in the left atrial pressure tracing (*arrowhead*) occurs 80 ms after the p wave.

left atrial (and pulmonary capillary wedge) pressure tracing; v waves are frequently prominent and thought to be the result of low compliance of the left atrium (Figure 6-7). The presence of v waves may also be present because of coexisting mitral regurgitation.

Valve Area

The normal mitral valve area is 4.0 to 6.0 cm². When the mitral valve area is reduced to 1.0 cm², a significant diastolic gradient at rest will be present. At this severity of mitral stenosis, increases in cardiac output will result in a significant elevation in left atrial pressure and pulmonary edema. Increases in heart rate preferentially shorten diastole more than systole and therefore limit the time available for flow across the mitral valve.

The Gorlin equation for the mitral valve area is

$$\text{Valve area} = \frac{\text{CO/(DFP)(HR)}}{44.3 C \sqrt{\Delta P_{\text{mean}}}}$$

where P_{mean} is the mean pressure gradient, CO is the cardiac output, DFP is the diastolic filling period, HR is heart rate, and C is an empirical constant that is 0.85. A worksheet to determine the mitral valve area is shown in Table 6-4. Simultaneous left atrial (or pulmonary capillary wedge) and left ventricular pressures are measured. Manual confirmation of the computer-measured gradients can be performed using the grid-based system as discussed in the assessment of aortic stenosis. If sinus rhythm is present, 5 cardiac beats should be used to determine the mean gradient. If atrial fibrillation is present, 10 cardiac beats are required for accurate results. The cardiac output is measured by both the thermodilution and Fick methods. The diastolic filling period (DFP) is measured from the opening of the mitral valve (left atrial pressure exceeds left ventricular pressure) to the closing of the mitral valve (left atrial pressure falls below left ventricular pressure) in units of seconds per beat. The diastolic filling period should also be measured for 5 beats and an average taken. Mitral valve area is reported using both the cardiac output as measured by the Fick and thermodilution methods. The severity of mitral stenosis is classified on the basis of the valve area as mild (>1.5 cm²), moderate (1.0-1.5 cm²), and severe (<1.0 cm²).

Tricuspid Valve

Before technologic advances in echocardiography, cardiac catheterization was used to confirm the presence and severity of tricuspid stenosis. Simultaneous recordings of the right atrial and right ventricular diastolic pressures were needed for accurate assessment because the pressure gradients are small, and there are considerable respiratory variations in the pressure waveforms.

Pressure Gradients

The gradient between the right atrium and right ventricle should be measured simultaneously with two catheters. This can be accomplished with a long 6-French sheath advanced into the right atrium and an end-hole catheter (multipurpose) placed through the sheath and into the right ventricle. A mean gradient of 2 mm Hg or greater that is present throughout diastole is the hallmark of tricuspid stenosis.[65]

Pressure Waveform Analysis

Characteristic findings in tricuspid stenosis include a prominent a wave and a blunted or absent y descent in the right atrial pressure waveform.

Valve Area

The Gorlin formula can be used to determine the tricuspid valve area using a constant of 1.0. Significant tricuspid stenosis is present when the valve area is less than 1.3 cm².

Angiocardiography

Right ventriculography may be useful in the evaluation of tricuspid stenosis. The tricuspid valve may be calcified with decreased mobility and associated tricuspid regurgitation is frequently present.[65]

EVALUATION OF VALVULAR REGURGITATION

Valvular regurgitation is evaluated by cardiac catheterization with direct measurement of intracardiac pressures and evaluation of pressure waveforms, semiquantitative evaluation of regurgitant severity by angiocardiography and calculation of the regurgitant fraction. Evaluation of the pressure waveforms on both sides of the regurgitant valve allows evaluation of the severity and chronicity of the regurgitant lesion and left ventricular systolic function. Angiographic evaluation of regurgitant severity is based on injection of contrast into the chamber downstream to the affected valve with imaging of contrast reflux into the chamber receiving the regurgitant volume. The regurgitant fraction is calculated as the difference between the angiographic (total) and forward (Fick or thermodilution method) stroke volume.

Aortic Regurgitation

Pressure Waveform Analysis

Aortic regurgitation results in a systolic pressure gradient across the aortic valve (even in the absence of coexisting stenosis) because of the high volume flow rate. This pressure gradient occurs predominantly in early systole. Although the magnitude of the systolic pressure gradient is related to volume flow rate, pressure gradients in isolated severe aortic regurgitation are small, with mean gradients ranging from 5 to 20 mmHg. Higher pressure gradients indicate associated aortic stenosis or another cause of left ventricular outflow obstruction.

In diastole, central aortic pressure falls more rapidly than normal, because of the diastolic run-off into the left ventricle, so that end-diastolic aortic pressure is lower than normal (Figure 6-8). Conversely, left ventricular diastolic pressure rises more rapidly than normal because of rapid ventricular filling retrograde across the incompetent aortic valve as well as antegrade across the mitral valve. With acute severe aortic regurgitation, this fall in aortic pressure and rise in ventricular diastolic pressure result in equalization of aortic and ventricular pressures at end-diastole. Thus, the rate of equalization of aortic and left ventricular diastolic pressures relates to regurgitant severity. This concept serves as the basis for using the diastolic slope of the Doppler velocity curve as a measure of regurgitant severity (see Chapter 5). However, this approach is limited because chronic aortic regurgitation results in compensatory changes in left ventricular diastolic compliance such that the left ventric-

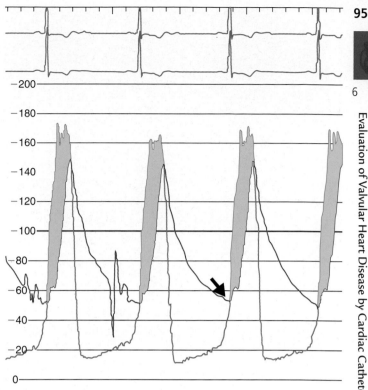

FIGURE 6–8 Simultaneous aortic and left ventricular pressures in a patient with mild aortic stenosis and severe aortic regurgitation. Note that the pulse pressure is wide (approximately 100 mm Hg) and the aortic diastolic pressure (*arrow*) is low.

ular end-diastolic pressure may remain low, even with severe regurgitation. Thus, interpretation of the pressure waveforms must take disease chronicity as well as severity into account.

This combination of systolic and diastolic pressure abnormalities leads to the most characteristic hemodynamic feature of chronic aortic regurgitation, that is, an increased pulse pressure. Because systolic pressure is increased and end-diastolic pressure is decreased, the pulse pressure is increased. However, the magnitude of the increase in pulse pressure only modestly correlates with regurgitation severity.[66] Even so, this simple measure of regurgitant severity should be integrated with other imaging and hemodynamic data in patient evaluation.

Angiocardiography

A contrast agent is injected into the aortic root and regurgitation is graded on a semiquantitative 0 to 4+ scale as shown in Table 6-4[67,68] (Figure 6-9). Angiographic grading of regurgitation severity has several limitations.[69] First, interobserver variability in grading regurgitant severity can be considerable unless there is strict adherence to the definitions outlined in Table 6-4. Although mild regurgitation is distinct from severe regurgitation, intermediate grades are often difficult to estimate. Second, technical factors may lead to an erroneous interpretation. The volume and rate of contrast agent injection must provide complete opacification of the upstream chamber. The catheter should be positioned close to the valve but should not interfere with valve closing. The angiocardiogram should be recorded from an angle and with an image size that includes both the upstream and downstream chambers without overlapping structures. For aortic regurgitation, a 45° left anterior oblique view with 10% to 15% of cranial angulation results in a image perpendicular to the valve plane and allows accurate assessment of the degree of reflux from the aortic root into the left ventricle. Third, physiologic factors including heart rate, cardiac rhythm, and preload and afterload affect the severity of regurgitation so that images recorded under

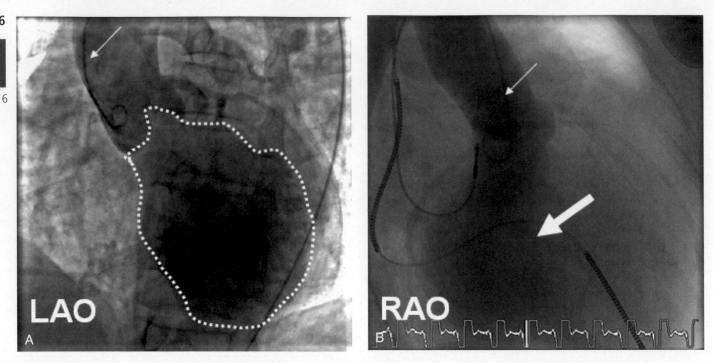

FIGURE 6–9 A, Pigtail catheter (*arrow*) is positioned in the ascending aorta in a left anterior oblique (LAO) projection to perform angiography in a patient with severe aortic regurgitation. Note that in a LAO projection, the left ventricle (*dotted white line*) is superimposed on the spine and the severity of aortic regurgitation (4+ in this patient) is difficult to evaluate. **B**. Pigtail catheter (arrow) is positioned in the ascending aorta in a right anterior oblique (RAO) projection in another patient with severe aortic regurgitation. In the ROA projection, the left ventricle is no longer superimposed on the spine. Radiographic density of contrast within the left ventricle (large white arrow) is similar to the aortic root, consistent with 4+ aortic regurgitation.

conditions disparate from the patient's baseline hemodynamic state may not accurately reflect disease severity.

Regurgitant Fraction

Regurgitant volume and fraction can be calculated at cardiac catheterization on the basis of measurement of the amount of blood ejected by the left ventricle (total stroke volume [SV]) and the amount of blood delivered to the body (forward stroke volume). Total stroke volume is calculated from the left ventriculogram as the difference between the end-diastolic and end-systolic left ventricular volumes. The forward stroke volume is calculated by dividing the measured cardiac output (either Fick or thermodilution technique) by the heart rate. The regurgitant stroke volume is calculated as

$$\text{Regurgitant SV} = \text{Total SV} - \text{Forward SV}$$

The regurgitation fraction is the regurgitant stroke volume divided by the total stroke volume. A regurgitation fraction less than 20% indicates mild, 20% to 40% moderate, 40% to 60% moderately severe, and greater than 60% severe regurgitation. Although this method has the potential to provide a quantitative measure of regurgitant severity, it is rarely used in clinical practice now that reliable noninvasive measures of regurgitant severity are available.

The regurgitant volume index is calculated by dividing the regurgitant volume by the body surface area and is another measure of regurgitation severity. A regurgitation volume index of greater than 700 mL/min/m² indicates mild, 700 to 1700 mL/min/m² moderate, 1700 to 3000 mL/min/m² severe, and greater than 3000 mL/min/m² very severe regurgitation.

Mitral Regurgitation

Pressure Waveform Analysis

Mitral regurgitation results in an increase in left atrial pressure, which peaks in late systole and is represented by the v wave. The height of the v wave relates to regurgitation

severity, although other factors, such as left atrial size and compliance, also play a role. The left atrial pressure curve is variably transmitted to the pulmonary capillary wedge pressure tracing, again related to the modulating effects of the size and compliance of the pulmonary vascular bed. For example, a patient with a prosthetic mitral valve with mild mitral regurgitation may show a prominent v wave due to a noncompliant pulmonary vascular bed. In contrast, a patient with chronic severe mitral regurgitation may have no v wave because of compensatory changes in the left atrium and pulmonary vasculature. Thus, although a v wave is often considered the hallmark of mitral regurgitation, this finding is not sensitive for the diagnosis nor is the absolute value a reliable predictor of regurgitation severity.[70]

Left atrial pressure is not routinely measured in patients with mitral regurgitation and information from the pulmonary artery and pulmonary capillary wedge pressure tracings should be used. The large v wave may result in a bifed appearance to the pulmonary artery pressure tracing. A large v wave in the pulmonary capillary wedge pressure tracing may occasionally give the appearance of a pulmonary artery pressure tracing (Figure 6-10).[71]

The rate of rise of left ventricular pressure during "isovolumic" contraction (*dP/dt*) provides a measure of left ventricular systolic function in patients with mitral regurgitation. Normally *dP/dt* is greater than 1000 mm Hg/sec, and lower values reflect progressively more severe impairment of left ventricular contractility. Peak left ventricular systolic pressure typically is normal in patients with mitral regurgitation although severe regurgitation associated with decreased forward cardiac output may lead to decreased left ventricular systolic pressure and subsequent hypotension.

Angiocardiography

A 30° right anterior oblique view separates the left ventricle and the left atrium in a plane perpendicular to the mitral valve annulus. The descending aortic shadow is superimposed on the left atrium in this view so that contrast agent in the descending

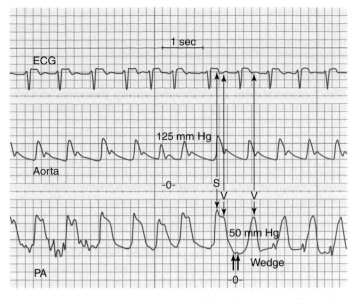

FIGURE 6–10 ECG, aortic, pulmonary artery (PA), and pulmonary capillary wedge pressure tracings in a patient with acute severe mitral regurgitation. The bottom tracing shows the change in the waveform between the PA pressure and the wedge pressure (double arrows). A prominent v wave is present in both the pulmonary artery and wedge pressure tracing. The pulmonary artery pressure is bifed because of the presence of both the pulmonary artery systolic wave and the v wave. The right-hand side of the figures shows the pulmonary capillary wedge pressure tracing (double arrow indicates inflation of pulmonary wedge balloon). The large v wave can cause the wedge tracing to be confused for a pulmonary artery tracing. *(From Sharkey SW: Beyond the wedge: clinical physiology and the Swan-Ganz catheter. Am J Med 1987;83:111-122, with permission.)*

aorta may be mistaken for mitral regurgitation. A left ventriculogram is performed with a sufficient amount of contrast agent to completely opacify the left ventricle. Mitral regurgitation is graded on the same semiquantitative scale (0 to 4+) as that used for aortic regurgitation (Table 6-5 and Figure 6-11).

Regurgitant Fraction

The regurgitant fraction for mitral regurgitation is calculated in the same manner as that used for aortic regurgitation.

Tricuspid Regurgitation

Pressure Waveform Analysis

Severe tricuspid regurgitation results in elevation in right atrial pressure, a prominent right atrial v wave (or c-v wave), and a prominent and sharp y descent (Figure 6-12). The prominent

v or c-v wave causes "ventricularization" of the right atrial pressure waveform. The right ventricular end-diastolic pressure is elevated. The Kussmaul sign, a lack of a decrease or even a small rise in mean right atrial pressure with inspiration, may be present.[72] Elevated pulmonary artery pressures (>60 mm Hg) suggest that the cause of tricuspid regurgitation is secondary (i.e., right ventricular dilation resulting from pulmonary hypertension).

Angiocardiography

As with mitral regurgitation, a 30° right anterior oblique view separates the right ventricle and the right atrium in a plane perpendicular to the tricuspid valve annulus. The presence of a catheter across the tricuspid valve may cause a small amount (usually negligible) of tricuspid regurgitation. The presence of ventricular tachycardia during right ventriculography precludes assessment of tricuspid regurgitation. An angled pigtail catheter placed into the body of the right ventricle usually provides adequate imaging. Tricuspid regurgitation is graded on the same semiquantitative scale (0 to 4+) as discussed above (see Table 6-5).

TABLE 6–5	Angiographic Grading of Regurgitant Severity	
Severity	**Aortic Regurgitation**	**Mitral Regurgitation**
1+	Contrast refluxes from the aortic root into the LV but clears on each beat	Contrast refluxes into the left atrium but clears on each beat
2+	Contrast refluxes into the LV with a gradually increasing density of contrast in the LV that never equals contrast intensity in the aortic root	Left atrial contrast density gradually increases but never equals LV density
3+	Contrast refluxes into the LV with a gradually increasing density such that left ventricular and aortic root density are equal after several beats	The density of contrast in the atrium and ventricle equalize after several beats
4+	Contrast fills the LV rapidly resulting in an equivalent radiographic density in the LV and aortic root on the first beat	The left atrium becomes as dense as the LV on the first beat and contrast agent is seen refluxing into the pulmonary veins

LV, left ventricle.

From Sellers RD, Levy MJ, Aplatz K, et al: Left retrograde cardioangiography in acquired cardiac disease: technique, indications and interpretations in 700 cases. Am J Cardiol 1964;14:437-447.

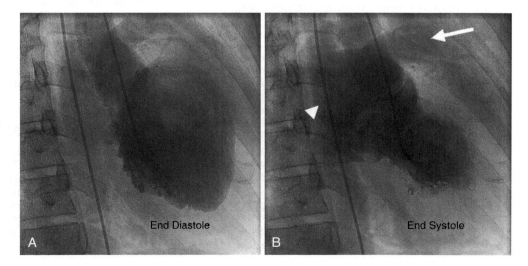

FIGURE 6–11 **A**, End-diastolic image in the right anterior oblique projection in a patient with severe (4+) mitral regurgitation. The left ventricle is dilated. **B**, End-systolic image showing complete opacification of a dilated left atrium (*arrowhead*) with a density of contrast that is equal to the left ventricle, 4+ mitral regurgitation. Contrast agent also fills the left atrial appendage (*arrow*).

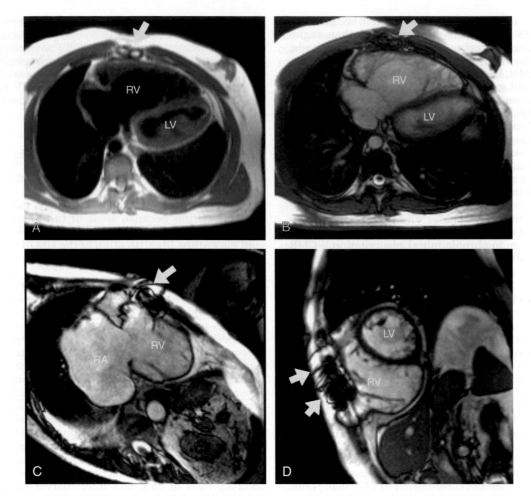

FIGURE 7–1 "Black-blood" horizontal (**A**), cine horizontal (**B**), cine longitudinal (**C**), and cine short-axis (**D**), right ventricular end-diastolic projections obtained from a patient with severe tricuspid regurgitation. CMR permits visualization of the complex geometry of the right ventricle and obtaining of accurate volume determinations. The *arrows* indicate sternal wire artifacts. LV, left ventricle; RV, right ventricle.

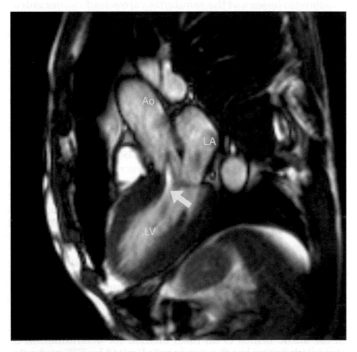

FIGURE 7–2 Cine CMR mid-systolic frame obtained in the long-axis left ventricular (LV) projection demonstrating flow acceleration (*arrow*) in the LV outflow tract in a patient with hypertrophic obstructive cardiomyopathy.

In a recent study, 40 consecutive patients underwent cardiac catheterization, TEE, and CMR.[35] AVA was determined by direct planimetry on CMR and TEE and calculated indirectly from catheterization using the Gorlin formula. Pressure gradients from cardiac catheterization and Doppler echocardiography were also compared. Mean AVA was $0.91 \pm 0.25\,cm^2$ by CMR, $0.89 \pm 0.28\,cm^2$ by TEE, and $0.64 \pm 0.26\,cm^2$ by catheterization. The correlation between CMR-derived and TEE-derived AVA was $r = 0.96$, significantly higher than the correlations between TEE and catheterization or between CMR and catheterization.

Degenerative aortic stenosis is invariably accompanied by calcification. Severe calcification is associated with a faster rate of stenosis progression and increased cardiac event rates. Echocardiography may detect the presence of calcification but has limited ability to quantify its severity. Aortic valve calcification can be accurately quantified with excellent interscan reproducibility (>90%) using CCT.[36-38] The amount of calcification is directly correlated with stenosis severity, although the relationship is nonlinear. The incremental value of the information derived from the aortic valve calcium score may be particularly useful to evaluate stenosis severity in patients with low cardiac output and reduced transvalvular gradients.

Contrast-enhanced CCT can precisely evaluate valve morphology and accurately differentiate trileaflet from bicuspid valves. Planimetric determinations of the aortic valve area have shown excellent correlation with echocardiographic measurements.[39,40]

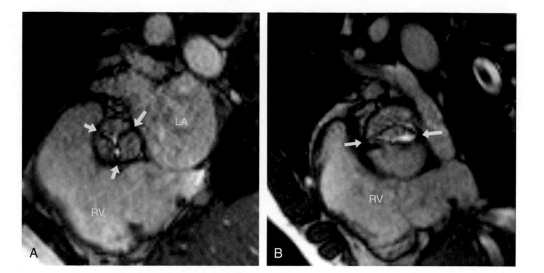

FIGURE 7–3 Cine CMR images obtained at mid-systole in a patient with tricuspid (**A**) and bicuspid (**B**) aortic valve stenosis. *Arrows* indicate the valve commissures.

TABLE 7–2	CCT and CMR methods for evaluating stenotic and regurgitant lesions	
Valvular Lesion	**Modality**	**Method**
Stenosis	CCT	Calcium scoring
	CCT	Stenotic orifice planimetry
	CMR	Stenotic orifice planimetry
	CMR	PC-VENC pressure gradients
	CMR	PC-VENC continuity valve area
	CMR	PC-VENC pressure half-time (mitral)
Regurgitation	CCT	Regurgitant orifice planimetry
	CCT	Regurgitant volume (LV-RV stroke volume difference)
	CMR	PC-VENC aortic regurgitant volume
	CMR	Regurgitant volume (LV-RV stroke volume difference)
	CMR	Regurgitant volume (Ao-Pa stroke volume difference)
	CMR	Regurgitant volume (Ao-mitral inflow stroke volume difference)
	CMR	Vena contracta
	CMR	Flow acceleration radius
	CMR	Signal void area

Ao, aortic; CCT, cardiac computed tomography; CMR, cardiac magnetic resonance; LV, left ventricular; RV, right ventricular; Pa, pulmonary artery; PC-VENC, phase-contrast velocity-encoding.

Mitral Stenosis

CMR can easily demonstrate the thickened leaflets and reduced diastolic opening of the valve in patients with mitral stenosis. The maximal extent of leaflet opening determined by CMR correlates with stenosis severity.[41]

In-plane as well as through-plane velocity mapping by CMR has been used to measure the transmitral peak velocity in mitral stenosis. Compared with Doppler echocardiography, an accuracy rate of 87% has been reported, with an interobserver reproducibility rate of 96%.[42,43] CMR-determined peak early filling ($r = 0.99$) and atrial contraction ($r = 0.99$) velocities and

estimated mitral valve area by the pressure half time ($r = 0.94$) method have been validated against those obtained with Doppler echocardiography.[44]

The presence of calcium in the mitral annulus is associated with systemic atherosclerosis and has negative prognostic implications. The amount of mitral annular calcium can also be quantified with CCT, although reproducibility appears to be somewhat lower than that for the aortic valve. In rheumatic mitral stenosis calcification can extend to the leaflets, commissures, subvalvular apparatus or even the left atrial wall (Figure 7-4). CCT has been reported to be useful in evaluating mitral valve morphology in patients undergoing balloon mitral commissurotomy.[45]

Mitral stenosis is often accompanied by marked atrial enlargement involving the appendage. The presence or absence of thrombus can be determined after contrast agent administration

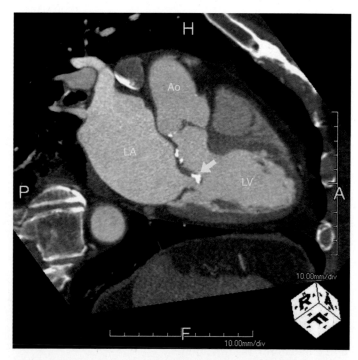

FIGURE 7–4 CCT long-axis view from a patient with rheumatic mitral stenosis showing thickened and mildly calcified leaflets.

with very high sensitivity although lower specificity, as slow flow may often impair contrast agent opacification in the left atrial appendage. Planimetry of the mitral opening by CCT provides accurate assessment of stenosis severity.[46]

PULMONARY AND TRICUSPID VALVE STENOSIS

7

Thickened tricuspid valve leaflets in patients with rheumatic or carcinoid heart disease can be recognized on both MRI and CT imaging.[47] CMR can assess three-dimensional morphology in patients with pulmonary stenosis and congenital heart disease without exposure to X-rays. The morphology of the RV outflow tract may vary significantly in these patients.[48] CMR has been proposed as a method to determine which patients may be suitable for percutaneous pulmonary valve replacement. Moreover, pulmonary valve valvuloplasty and pulmonary valve replacement may be performed under CMR guidance, reducing the need for radiation exposure.

ASSESSMENT OF VALVULAR REGURGITATION

CMR evaluation of patients with regurgitant valve disease includes (1) anatomic assessment of valves, great vessels, and the cardiac chamber, (2) estimation of ventricular volumes and function, and (3) quantification of valvular regurgitant volume and fraction. Numerous studies have documented the accuracy and reliability of these methods.[49-53]

Regurgitant jets may be visualized in cine bright-blood images as a region of signal void. This is produced by dephasing of the spins caused by turbulence. The presence of a signal void provides accurate identification of the presence of aortic or mitral regurgitation with a sensitivity greater than 93% and a specificity greater than 89% compared with Doppler flow imaging or angiography.[54] Further, as with color Doppler flow imaging, the three-dimensional spatial distribution of the signal void is related to regurgitant severity, allowing separation of mild from severe degrees of regurgitation.[55] However, the magnitude of signal void depends on multiple imaging parameters such as echo time and flip angle used on the acquisition sequence. Moreover, turbulence may actually decrease in the presence of severe regurgitation, when the flow becomes laminar. Thus, direct semiquantitative assessment of regurgitant lesion severity is limited on the basis of jet visualization alone.

In many patients, the acceleration of flow proximal to the regurgitant orifice may be visualized by CMR as an area of signal loss (Figure 7-5). As with the Doppler proximal isovelocity surface area method, the diameter and persistence of the detected proximal convergence zone is a marker of regurgitant flow severity.[56,57]

CMR ventricular volumes may be used for quantification of valvular regurgitation. In the absence of valvular regurgitation, the difference between LV and RV stroke volumes is less than 5%.[58,59] In the presence of single valvular regurgitation, regurgitant volume may be calculated as the difference between left and right ventricular stroke volumes and regurgitant fraction as the ratio of regurgitant volume to LV (for left sided valve regurgitation) or RV (for right sided regurgitation) volume. The use of CMR for calculation of regurgitant volume using the latter approach has been demonstrated for isolated mitral and aortic regurgitation.[60]

Most commonly, regurgitant volumes are measured as the difference between ventricular stroke volume and forward

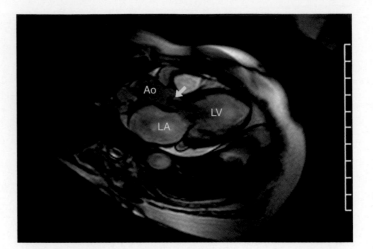

FIGURE 7–5 Cine CMR mid-diastolic image obtained in a patient with moderate-to-severe aortic regurgitation. Notice the proximal acceleration zone and the vena contracta at the regurgitant orifice (*arrow*). Ao, aorta, LA, left atrium; LV, left ventricle.

transvalvular flow determined from phase contrast velocity data. CMR has been shown to measure regurgitant fractions with 90% accuracy compared with radionuclide ventriculography[61] and echocardiography.[62] Alternatively, the difference in phase-contrast velocity flow between the aorta and pulmonary artery can be used to quantify the severity of either aortic or mitral regurgitation (Figure 7-6).[63]

The evaluation of regurgitant lesions by CCT is limited by the fact that its acquisition is not dynamic; therefore, regurgitant flow cannot be visualized or quantified. However, in isolated regurgitant lesions, the regurgitant volume (and fraction) can be derived from the difference between the left and right stroke volumes.[64] Significant regurgitation of any valve eventually causes ipsilateral ventricular dilatation, often accompanied by eccentric hypertrophy. With EBCT, regurgitant volume can be calculated as the difference between left ventricular stroke volume determined from cine images and forward stroke volume determined using the indicator dilution method in the ascending aorta.[65]

Aortic Regurgitation

Aortic regurgitant volume is usually determined from the phase-contrast velocity–encoded diastolic regurgitant flow velocities at the aortic root. Phase-contrast velocity–encoded CMR imaging of the ascending and descending aorta has been used to identify patients with severe aortic regurgitation. Similar to the Doppler method, CMR identifies severe aortic regurgitation as the presence of holodiastolic flow reversal (Figure 7-7).[66] However, this method has several limitations. Normally, 3% to 15% of the forward aortic flow is reversed during diastole into the coronary arteries.[67] In addition, the normal movement of the imaging plane from a position between the aortic valve and the coronary ostia to a position 2 cm distal to the sinotubular junction may lead to a 30% to 70% underestimation in regurgitant volume.[68] Nevertheless this method has been validated in several studies, revealing accuracy of 90%, interstudy reproducibility rate of 95%, and interobserver reproducibility rate of 94%.[69] This technique has been used to demonstrate beneficial effects of vasodilator therapy in chronic aortic regurgitation.[70]

CCT may be useful in evaluating the mechanism leading to aortic regurgitation. In degenerative valve disease there is increased leaflet thickness and calcification, and the area

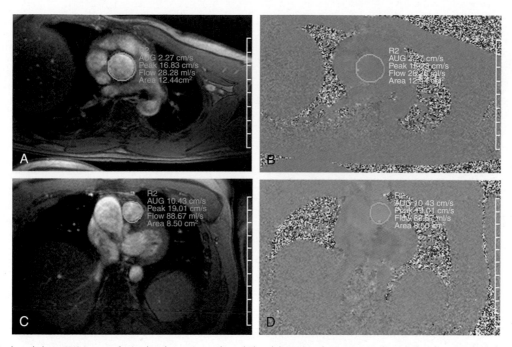

FIGURE 7–6 Magnitude and phase CMR images obtained at the aortic root (**A** and **B**) and the main pulmonary artery (**C** and **D**). Left ventricular (LV) and right ventricular (RV) stroke volumes are calculated as the product of area by velocity. In patients with aortic regurgitation regurgitant volume may be determined as the difference between LV and RV forward stroke volumes. (See text for details.)

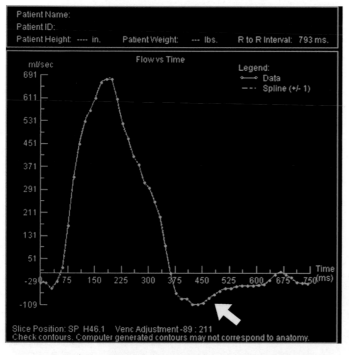

FIGURE 7–7 Phase-contrast velocity–encoded flow obtained at the ascending aorta in a patient with moderate aortic regurgitation. *Arrow* indicates the regurgitant flow in diastole.

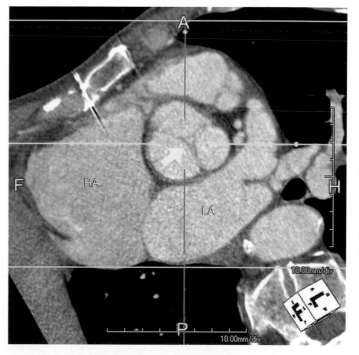

FIGURE 7–8 CCT cross-sectional view of the aortic valve obtained in a patient with aortic regurgitation. The *arrow* indicates the area of incomplete leaflet coaptation.

of lack of coaptation may be visualized in diastolic phase reconstructions centrally or at the commissures, often providing accurate visualization of the anatomical regurgitant orifice (Figure 7-8). The severity of aortic regurgitation cannot be accurately established by CT, because this modality cannot visualize flow. However, in cases of severe regurgitation, CT may demonstrate left ventricular dilatation and/or a significant difference between the left and right ventricular stroke volumes.

In aortic regurgitation due to enlargement of the aortic root, the regurgitant orifice is typically located centrally (Figure 7-9). Other etiologies that can be depicted include interposition of an intimal flap in dissection, valve distortion or perforation in endocarditis, or leaflet prolapse, often observed in dissection and Marfan syndrome. CMR may evaluate the thickness and compliance of the aortic root. In many patients, the presence of edema may suggest the diagnosis of an inflammatory process such as giant cell arteritis. It is increasingly

7

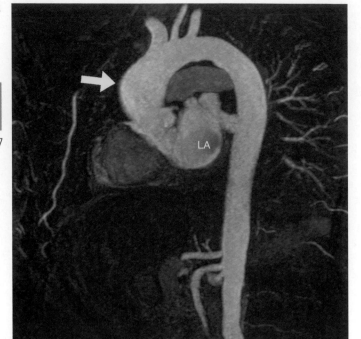

FIGURE 7–9 Contrast-enhanced magnetic resonance angiogram demonstrating a dilated aortic root (*arrow*) in a patient with aortic regurgitation. LA, left atrium.

being recognized that many patients with aortic regurgitation have an aortopathy. Thus, it has been suggested that treatment should involve aortic root replacement in many instances even in the absence of severe aortic root dilatation.

The thoracic aorta and main branches may be imaged by CMR using either ECG-gated static spin-echo (black-blood), gradient-echo (cine white-blood), and/or contrast-enhanced magnetic resonance angiography. Each technique has several potential advantages and disadvantages. Spin-echo and gradient-echo images are acquired in multiple two-dimensional planes, whereas contrast-enhanced magnetic resonance angiography is done in a three-dimensional reconstruction, which allows reorientation and measurements in any direction and plane. Magnetic resonance angiography

may, however, result in overestimation of the aortic root size because of cardiac motion artifacts. This technique provides the measurement of the lumen, whereas the others provide the external diameter.

CT is accepted as the most accurate method for obtaining measurements of the aorta, owing to its high isotropic spatial resolution. With the use of ECG gating, motion artifacts are virtually eliminated. One important disadvantage, however, is the required radiation exposure, a consideration for younger patients undergoing serial follow-up.

Measurements of the thoracic aorta are typically performed at multiple levels, including the annulus, sinus of Valsalva, sinotubular junction, mid-ascending (pulmonary artery bifurcation) arch, and mid-thoracic levels. Measurements are typically done from outside to outside edge, at end-diastole, and in oblique planes perpendicular to the long axial orientation of each segment. Off-line digital measurements performed in computer workstations with three-dimensional reconstruction capability have helped to eliminate the overestimation that often occurs when measurements were performed from plain films in straight axial orientation.

Mitral Regurgitation

Mitral regurgitant volume may be determined by CMR as the difference between (1) forward stroke volume across the mitral and aortic annulus, (2) LV and RV stroke volume, and (3) LV stroke volume and forward aortic stroke volume. The estimation of forward volume flow through the mitral annulus has shown accuracy of 90% but may be unreliable in patients with eccentric jets or atrial fibrillation. Accordingly, the quantitative assessment of mitral regurgitant volume is most commonly calculated as the difference between the LV stroke volume, as determined by planimetry, and the forward flow in the ascending aorta. The accuracy for this technique has been reported as 91% and the interobserver reproducibility as 90%.

CMR is particularly useful for the evaluation of patients with ischemic mitral regurgitation. CMR studies have shown a strong relationship between LV end-systolic volume, interpapillary muscle distance, anterior mitral annulus to medial and lateral papillary muscle distance, and functional ischemic mitral regurgitation[71,72] Mitral systolic tenting area and scarring of the anterolateral region (Figure 7-10) have been shown to be independent predictors of mitral regurgitation severity.[73]

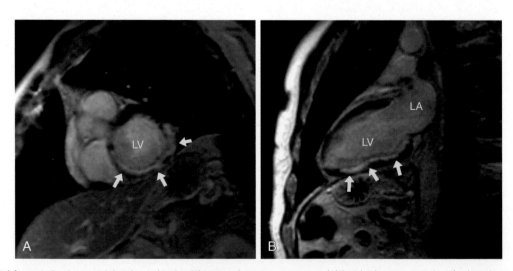

FIGURE 7–10 CMR left ventricular short-axis (**A**) and two-chamber (**B**) images showing near-transmural delayed enhancement in the inferolateral segments (*arrows*) in a patient with mitral regurgitation and previous myocardial infarction. LA, left atrium; LV, left ventricle.

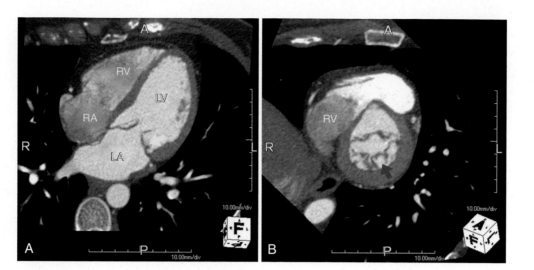

FIGURE 7–11 CCT four-chamber (**A**) and short-axis (**B**) images demonstrating thickened leaflets (*arrows*) in a patient with mitral valve prolapse.

In patients with mitral valve prolapse, CCT can demonstrate the presence of leaflet thickening or the degree and location of prolapse (Figure 7-11). In patients with mitral regurgitation due to annular enlargement, dimensions of the annulus can be accurately quantified, and a central area of insufficient leaflet coaptation may be observed. Although quantifying mitral regurgitation severity may be difficult, a recent study suggested that planimetry of the regurgitant orifice by CCT correlates well with echocardiographic grading of mitral regurgitation severity.[74] An alternative approach validated for EBCT includes quantification of cardiac output with the flow mode by the indicator dilution method, and LV volumetric calculations in the cine mode. The regurgitant fraction is obtained from the difference between these two measurements.[75]

Pulmonary and Tricuspid Valve Regurgitation

Management decisions in patients with right-side regurgitant lesions are usually more difficult than in patients with mitral and/or aortic regurgitation. Although previously these were always considered benign, we now know that many patients experience severe RV dysfunction and irreversible heart failure. Evaluation of RV function is notoriously difficult. RV volumes and ejection fraction are less reproducible than LV measurements. Geometrical assumptions are usually erroneous because the geometry of the right ventricle is distorted with chronic pressure and/or volume overload. The quantification of tricuspid and pulmonic valve regurgitation by echocardiography has not been as thoroughly validated. CMR provides accurate determination of RV volumes and ejection fraction because volume determinations do not require any specific geometric assumptions. The accuracy rates for velocity mapping of pulmonary regurgitant volume and regurgitant fraction by CMR have been reported to be 78% and 76%, respectively (Figure 7-12).[76]

As discussed previously, CCT is unreliable for evaluation of valvular regurgitation. Nevertheless, dilatation and contrast opacification of the inferior vena cava and hepatic veins may be seen in patients with severe tricuspid regurgitation.[77]

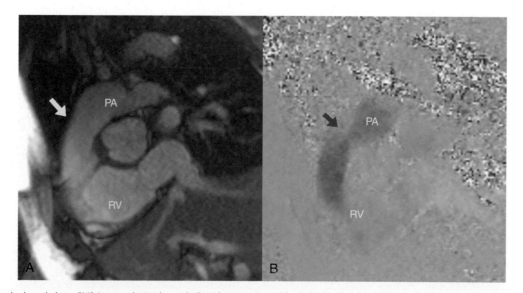

FIGURE 7–12 Magnitude and phase CMR images obtained at early diastole in a patient with corrected tetralogy of Fallot and severe pulmonary regurgitation. *Arrows* indicate the location of the pulmonary valve regurgitant orifice. PA, pulmonary artery; RV, right ventricle.

At a magnetic field strength of 1.5 Tesla, all valvular prostheses, except some ball-and-cage models can be safely imaged.[78] Most prosthetic valves are visible on bright-blood MRI as areas of signal loss (Figure 7-13). The extent of the artifact depends on the type of prosthesis, magnetic field strength, and type of sequence used. The assessment of mechanical valve prosthesis dysfunction may be limited, and intra- or periprosthetic regurgitation may be easily hidden by the signal loss around the prosthesis. CMR has shown good agreement with TEE in separating pathologic from physiologic and paravalvular from transvalvular prosthetic valve regurgitation.[79] Measurement of prosthetic valve gradients and evaluation of flow profiles with phase-contrast velocity–encoded CMR also have been reported.[80]

Many of the aforementioned features of native valvular heart disease apply also to the evaluation of cardiac bioprostheses (Figure 7-14). CCT is particularly useful for the evaluation of some types of mechanical valves. In prosthesis with two discs, these should open symmetrically. In those with a single disc, the angle of opening can also be measured. Finally, heterografts and homografts can be evaluated completely, including the distal anastomosis and the patency of the coronary arteries if these were reimplanted (Figure 7-15).

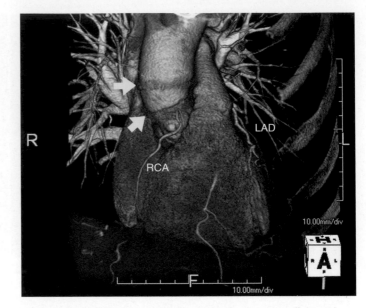

FIGURE 7–15 CCT volume-rendered image showing the suture cuffs (arrows) of an interposed aortic graft in a patient with repaired aortic valve and aortic root aneurysm.

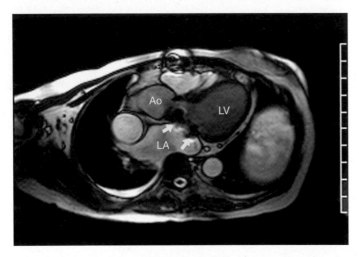

FIGURE 7–13 Cine CMR end-diastolic image obtained from a patient with aortic bioprosthesis and mitral homograft. *Arrows* indicate the artifacts caused by the metallic rings. Ao, aorta; LA, left atrium; LV, left ventricle.

INFECTIVE ENDOCARDITIS

The diagnosis of infective endocarditis usually relies on the visualization of vegetations and TTE and TEE are usually superior to CCT because of higher temporal resolution. Vegetations are often mobile and thus require imaging at high temporal resolution. However, CCT can be particularly useful in the demonstration of perivalvular abscesses as fluid-filled collections.[81] Aortic valve vegetations and complications of endocarditis may be recognized on MRI in some patients.[82,83]

EVALUATION OF THE CORONARY ARTERIES

The most common primary indication for CCT is the assessment of the coronary arteries. The accuracy of CT coronary angiography has been reported in recent studies, with slightly lower diagnostic yield in patients with aortic stenosis because of the frequent coexistence of both aortic and coronary

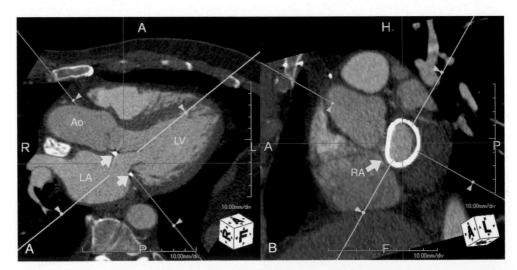

FIGURE 7–14 CCT long-axis (**A**) and short-axis view (**B**) from a patient with a prosthetic mitral annuloplasty ring (*arrow*). Ao, aorta; LA, left atrium; LV, left ventricle; RA, right atrium.

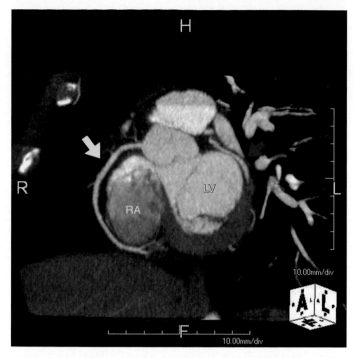

FIGURE 7-16 CCT sagittal image demonstrating a normal right coronary artery (*yellow arrow*) in a patient with mitral valve prolapse before repair surgery. A segment of the left circumflex artery is also seen (*red arrow*). RA, right atrium.

calcification.[84,85] These studies have demonstrated high negative predictive value but lower positive predictive value for the detection of significant coronary stenosis. Thus, patients who have been referred for surgical repair of valvular lesions and demonstrate absence of significant coronary stenosis by CCT may safely avoid the need for invasive coronary angiography. On the other hand, patients who seem to have greater than a mild degree of luminal stenosis or extensive calcifications need to have a confirmatory catheterization. For this reason, it is prudent to consider CT for this application only in selected patients with low or intermediate pretest probability (Figure 7-16). In patients with aortic valve endocarditis with highly mobile vegetations, CCT offers an alternative to invasive coronary angiography.

SUMMARY

CMR and CCT imaging are useful and complementary methods for the evaluation of valvular disease. However, the limitations of these techniques need to be considered in selection of patients who may derive a benefit. In CMR, choosing the correct value for the velocity-encoding gradient is important because the range must be appropriate to encompass the expected peak velocities. If these are set too low, the peak gradient may be underestimated. Conversely, when the value is set too high, sensitivity for slow flow is reduced. Selecting the correct plane of interrogation is important, because the maximal velocity will be detected at a specific spatial location and in a plane perpendicular to the direction of flow. High spatial and temporal resolutions are important to localize the peak velocity. Improved spatial resolution can be achieved by decreasing the field of view or increasing the acquisition matrix. Temporal resolution is much lower than in Doppler echocardiography; thus, peak velocities may occasionally be underestimated. CMR, however, has the advantage of not being limited to specific acoustic windows for interrogation, which is the main limitation of Doppler echocardiography. CMR and CT are superior to echocardiography for the assessment of ventricular function and aortic dimensions.

1. Barkhausen J, Ruehm SG, Goyen M, et al: MR evaluation of ventricular function: true fast imaging with steady-state free precession versus fast low-angle shot cine MR imaging: feasibility study. Radiology 2001;219:264-269.
2. Bellenger NG, Burgess MI, Ray SG, et al: Comparison of left ventricular ejection fraction and volumes in heart failure by echocardiography, radionuclide ventriculography and cardiovascular magnetic resonance. Are they interchangeable? Eur Heart J 2000;21:1387-1396.
3. Grothues F, Smith GC, Moon JC, et al: Comparison of interstudy reproducibility of cardiovascular magnetic resonance with two-dimensional echocardiography in normal subjects and in patients with heart failure or left ventricular hypertrophy. Am J Cardiol 2002;90:29-34.
4. Møgelvang J, Stockholm KH, Saunamäki K, et al: Assessment of left ventricular volumes by magnetic resonance in comparison with radionuclide angiography, contrast angiography and echocardiography. Eur Heart J 1992;13:1677-1683.
5. Markiewicz W, Sechtem U, Kirby R, et al: Measurement of ventricular volumes in the dog by nuclear magnetic resonance imaging. J Am Coll Cardiol 1987;10:170-177.
6. Katz J, Milliken MC, Stray-Gundersen J, et al: Estimation of human myocardial mass with MR imaging. Radiology 1988;169:495-498.
7. Ostrzega E, Maddahi J, Honma H, et al: Quantification of left ventricular myocardial mass in humans by nuclear magnetic resonance imaging. Am Heart J 1989;117:444-452.
8. Keller AM, Peshock RM, Malloy CR, et al: In vivo measurement of myocardial mass using nuclear magnetic resonance imaging. J Am Coll Cardiol 1986;8:113-117.
9. Shapiro EP, Rogers WJ, Beyar R, et al: Determination of left ventricular mass by magnetic resonance imaging in hearts deformed by acute infarction. Circulation 1989;79:706-711.
10. Semelka RC, Tomei E, Wagner S, et al: Normal left ventricular dimensions and function: interstudy reproducibility of measurements with cine MR imaging. Ann Thorac Surg 1990;174:763-768.
11. Young AA, Orr R, Smaill BH, Dell'Italia LJ: Three-dimensional changes in left and right ventricular geometry in chronic mitral regurgitation. Am J Physiol 1996;271:H2689-H2700.
12. Doherty NE III, Seelos KC, Suzuki J, et al: Application of cine nuclear magnetic resonance imaging for sequential evaluation of response to angiotensin-converting enzyme inhibitor therapy in dilated cardiomyopathy. J Am Coll Cardiol 1992;19:1294-1302.
13. Bellenger NG, Davies LC, Francis JM, et al: Reduction in sample size for studies of remodeling in heart failure by the use of cardiovascular magnetic resonance. J Cardiovasc Magn Reson 2000;2:271-278.
14. Bellenger NG, Rajappan K, Rahman SL, et al: Effects of carvedilol on left ventricular remodeling in chronic stable heart failure: a cardiovascular magnetic resonance study. Heart 2004;90:760-764.
15. Auffermann W, Wagner S, Holt WW, et al: Noninvasive determination of left ventricular output and wall stress in volume overload and in myocardial disease by cine magnetic resonance imaging. Am Heart J 1991;121:1750-1758.
16. Rumberger JA, Reiring AJ, Rees MR, et al: Quantitation of left ventricular mass and volume in normal patients using cine computed tomography. J Am Coll Cardiol 1986;7:173.
17. Orakzai SH, Orakzai RH, Nasir K, Budoff MJ: Assessment of cardiac function using multidetector row computed tomography. J Comput Assist Tomogr 2006;30:555-563.
18. Rihal CS, Nishimura RA, Rumberger JA, Tajik AJ: Quantitative echocardiography: a comparison with ultrafast computed tomography in patients with chronic aortic regurgitation. J Heart Valve Dis 1994;3:417-424.
19. Karwatowski SP, Brecker SJ, Yang GZ, et al: A comparison of left ventricular myocardial velocity in diastole measured by magnetic resonance and left ventricular filling measured by Doppler echocardiography. Eur Heart J 1996;17:795-802.
20. Kim WY, Walker PG, Pedersen EM, et al: Left ventricular blood flow patterns in normal subjects: a quantitative analysis by three-dimensional magnetic resonance velocity mapping. J Am Coll Cardiol 1995; 26:224-238.
21. Hartiala JJ, Mostbeck GH, Foster E, et al: Velocity-encoded cine MRI in the evaluation of left ventricular diastolic function: measurement of mitral valve and pulmonary vein flow velocities and flow volume across the mitral valve. Am Heart J 1993;125:1054-1066.
22. Hartiala JJ, Foster E, Fujita N, et al: Evaluation of left atrial contribution to left ventricular filling in aortic stenosis by velocity-encoded cine MRI. Am Heart J 1994;127:593-600.
23. Grothues F, Moon JC, Bellenger NG, et al: Interstudy reproducibility of right ventricular volumes, function, and mass with cardiovascular magnetic resonance. Am Heart J 2004;147:218-223.
24. Pattynama PM, Lamb HJ, Van der Velde EA, et al: Reproducibility of MRI-derived measurements of right ventricular volumes and myocardial mass. Magn Reson Imaging 1995;13:53-63.
25. Markiewicz W, Sechtem U, Higgins CB: Evaluation of the right ventricle by magnetic resonance imaging. Am Heart J 1987;113:8-15.
26. Møgelvang J, Stubgaard M, Thomsen C, Henriksen O: Evaluation of right ventricular volumes measured by magnetic resonance imaging. Eur Heart J 1988;9:529-533.
27. Doherty NE, Fujita N, Caputo GR, Higgins CB: Measurement of right ventricular mass in normal and dilated cardiomyopathic ventricles using cine magnetic resonance imaging. Am J Cardiol 1992;69:1223-1228.
28. Mackey ES, Sandler MP, Campbell RM, et al: Right ventricular myocardial mass quantification with magnetic resonance imaging. Am J Cardiol 1990;65:529-532.
29. Helbing WA, de Roos A: Clinical applications of cardiac magnetic resonance imaging after repair of tetralogy of Fallot. Pediatr Cardiol 2000;21:70-79.
30. Helbing WA, de Roos A: Optimal imaging in assessment of right ventricular function in tetralogy of Fallot with pulmonary regurgitation. Am J Cardiol 1998;82:1561-1562.
31. Evans AJ, Blinder RA, Herfkens RJ, et al: Effects of turbulence on signal intensity in gradient echo images. Invest Radiol 1988; 23:512-518.
32. Globits S, Higgins CB: Assessment of valvular heart disease by magnetic resonance imaging. Am Heart J 1995;129:369-381.
33. Søndergaard L, Stahlberg F, Thomsen C, et al: Accuracy and precision of MR velocity mapping in measurement of stenotic cross-sectional area, flow rate, and pressure gradient. J Magn Reson Imaging 1993;3:433-437.

7

34. Danielsen R, Nordrehaug JE, Vik-Mo H: Factors affecting Doppler echocardiographic valve area assessment in aortic stenosis. Am J Cardiol 1989;63:1107-1111.

35. John AS, Dill T, Brandt RR, et al: Magnetic resonance to assess the aortic valve area in aortic stenosis: how does it compare to current diagnostic standards? J Am Coll Cardiol 2003;42:519-526.

36. Koos R, Mahnken AH, Kuhl HP, et al: Quantification of aortic valve calcification using multislice spiral computed tomography: comparison with atomic absorption spectroscopy. Invest Radiol 2006;41:485-489.

37. Messika-Zeitoun D, Aubry M-C, Detaint D, et al: Evaluation and clinical implications of aortic valve calcification measured by electron-beam computed tomography. Circulation 2004;110:356-362.

38. Budoff MJ, Takasu J, Katz R, et al: Reproducibility of CT measurements of aortic valve calcification, mitral annulus calcification, and aortic wall calcification in the multi-ethnic study of atherosclerosis. Acad Radiol 2006;13:166-172.

39. Alkadhi H, Wildermuth S, Plass A, et al: Aortic stenosis: comparative evaluation of 16-detector row CT and echocardiography. Radiology 2006;240:47-55.

40. Feuchtner GM, Dichtl W, Friedrich GJ, et al: Multislice computed tomography for detection of patients with aortic valve stenosis and quantification of severity. J Am Coll Cardiol 2006;47:1410-1417.

41. Casolo GC, Zampa V, Rega L, et al: Evaluation of mitral stenosis by cine magnetic resonance imaging. Am Heart J 1992;123:1252-1260.

42. Kilner PJ, Manzara CC, Mohiaddin RH, et al: Magnetic resonance jet velocity mapping in mitral and aortic valve stenosis. Circulation 1993;87:1239-1248.

43. Heidenreich PA, Steffens J, Fujita N, et al: Evaluation of mitral stenosis with velocity-encoded cine-magnetic resonance imaging. Am J Cardiol 1995;75:365-369.

44. Lin SJ, Brown PA, Watkins MP, et al: Quantification of stenotic mitral valve area with magnetic resonance imaging and comparison with Doppler ultrasound. J Am Coll Cardiol 2004;44:133-137.

45. White ML, Grover MM, Weiss RM, et al: Prediction of change in mitral valve area after mitral balloon commissurotomy using cine computed tomography. Invest Radiol 1994;29:827-833.

46. Messika-Zeitoun D, Serfaty JM, Laissy JP, et al: Assessment of the mitral valve area in patients with mitral stenosis by multislice computed tomography. J Am Coll Cardiol 2006;48:411-413.

47. Mirowitz SA, Gutierrez FR: MR and CT diagnosis of carcinoid heart disease. Chest 1993;103:630-631.

48. Schievano S, Coats L, Migliavacca F, et al: Variations in right ventricular outflow tract morphology following repair of congenital heart disease: implications for percutaneous pulmonary valve implantation. J Cardiovasc Magn Reson 2007;9:687-695.

49. Sondergaard L, Lindvig K, Hildebrandt P, et al: Quantification of aortic regurgitation by magnetic resonance velocity mapping. Am Heart J 1993;125:1081-1090.

50. Ambrosi P, Faugere G, Desfossez L, et al: Assessment of aortic regurgitation severity by magnetic resonance imaging of the thoracic aorta. Eur Heart J 1995;16:406-409.

51. Honda N, Machida K, Hashimoto M, et al: Aortic regurgitation: quantitation with MR imaging velocity mapping. Radiology 1993;186:189-194.

52. Kizilbash AM, Hundley WG, Willett DL, et al: Comparison of quantitative Doppler with magnetic resonance imaging for assessment of the severity of mitral regurgitation. Am J Cardiol 1998;81:792-795.

53. Hundley WG, Hong FL, Willard JE, et al: Magnetic resonance imaging assessment of the severity of mitral regurgitation: comparison with invasive techniques. Circulation 1995;92:1151-1158.

54. Wagner S, Auffermann W, Buser P, et al: Diagnostic accuracy and estimation of the severity of valvular regurgitation from the signal void on cine magnetic resonance images. Am Heart J 1989;118:760-767.

55. Aurigemma G, Reichek N, Schiebler M, Axel L: Evaluation of aortic regurgitation by cardiac cine magnetic resonance imaging: planar analysis and comparison to Doppler echocardiography. Cardiology 1991;78:340-347.

56. Yoshida K, Yoshikawa J, Hozumi T, et al: Assessment of aortic regurgitation by the acceleration flow signal void proximal to the leaking orifice in cinemagnetic resonance imaging. Circulation 1991;83:1951-1955.

57. Cranney GB, Benjelloun H, Perry GJ, et al: Rapid assessment of aortic regurgitation and left ventricular function using cine nuclear magnetic resonance imaging and the proximal convergence zone. Am J Cardiol 1993;71:1074-1081.

58. Sechtem U, Pflugfelder PW, Gould RG, et al: Measurement of right and left ventricular volumes in healthy individuals with cine MR imaging. Radiology 1987;163:697-702.

59. Lorenz CH, Walker ES, Morgan VL, et al: Normal human right and left ventricular mass, systolic function, and gender differences by cine magnetic resonance imaging. J Cardiovasc Magn Reson 1999;1:7-21.

60. Sechtem U, Pflugfelder PW, Cassidy MM, et al: Mitral or aortic regurgitation: quantification of regurgitant volumes with cine MR imaging. Ann Thorac Surg 1988;167:425-430.

61. Underwood SR, Klipstein RH, Firmin DN, et al: Magnetic resonance assessment of aortic and mitral regurgitation. Br Heart J 1986;56:455-462.

62. Sechtem U, Pflugfelder PW, Cassidy MM, et al: Mitral or aortic regurgitation: quantification of regurgitant volumes with cine MR imaging. Radiology 1988;167:425-430.

63. Fujita N, Chazouilleres AF, Hartiala JJ, et al: Quantification of mitral regurgitation by velocity-encoded cine nuclear magnetic resonance imaging [see comments]. J Am Coll Cardiol 1994;23:951-958.

64. Reiter SJ, Rumberger JA, Stanford W, Marcus ML: Quantitative determination of aortic regurgitant volumes in dogs by ultrafast computed tomography. Circulation 1987;76:728-735.

65. Kaminaga T, Naito H, Takamiya M, Nishimura T: Quantitative evaluation of mitral regurgitation with ultrafast CT. J Comput Assist Tomogr 1994;18:239-242.

66. Ambrosi P, Faugere G, Desfossez L, et al: Assessment of aortic regurgitation severity by magnetic resonance imaging of the thoracic aorta. Eur Heart J 1995;16:406-409.

67. Bogren HG, Klipstein RH, Firmin DN, et al: Quantitation of antegrade and retrograde blood flow in the human aorta by magnetic resonance velocity mapping. Am Heart J 1989;117:1214-1222.

68. Chatzimavroudis GP, Oshinski JN, Franch RH, et al: Quantification of the aortic regurgitant volume with magnetic resonance phase velocity mapping: a clinical investigation of the importance of imaging slice location. J Heart Valve Dis 1998;7:94-101.

69. Dulce MC, Mostbeck GH, O'Sullivan M, et al: Severity of aortic regurgitation: interstudy reproducibility of measurements with velocity-encoded cine MR imaging. Radiology 1992;185:235-240.

70. Globits S, Blake L, Bourne M, et al: Assessment of hemodynamic effects of angiotensin-converting enzyme inhibitor therapy in chronic aortic regurgitation by using velocity-encoded cine magnetic resonance imaging. Am Heart J 1996;131:289-293.

71. Yu HY, Su MY, Liao TY, et al: Functional mitral regurgitation in chronic ischemic coronary artery disease: analysis of geometric alterations of mitral apparatus with magnetic resonance imaging. J Thorac Cardiovasc Surg 2004;128:543-551.

72. Kaji S, Nasu M, Yamamuro A, et al: Annular geometry in patients with chronic ischemic mitral regurgitation: three-dimensional magnetic resonance imaging study. Circulation 2005;112:409-414.

73. Srichai MB, Grimm RA, Stillman AE, et al: Ischemic mitral regurgitation: impact of the left ventricle and mitral valve in patients with left ventricular systolic dysfunction. Ann Thorac Surg 2005;80:170-178.

74. Alkadhi H, Wildermuth S, Bettex DA, et al: Mitral regurgitation: quantification with 16-detector row CT—initial experience. Radiology 2005;238:454-463.

75. Lembcke A, Borges AC, Dushe S, et al: Assessment of mitral valve regurgitation at electron-beam CT: comparison with Doppler echocardiography. Radiology 2005;236:47-55.

76. Rebergen SA, Chin JGJ, Ottenkamp J, et al: Pulmonary regurgitation in the late postoperative follow-up of tetralogy of Fallot: volumetric quantitation by nuclear magnetic resonance velocity mapping. Circulation 1993;88:2257-2266.

77. Collins MA, Pidgeon JW, Fitzgerald R: Computed tomography manifestations of tricuspid regurgitation. Br J Radiol 1995;68:1058-1060.

78. Shellock FG, Crues JV: MR procedures: biologic effects, safety, and patient care. Radiology 2004;232:635-652

79. Deutsch HJ, Bachmann R, Sechtem U, et al: Regurgitant flow in cardiac valve prostheses: diagnostic value of gradient echo nuclear magnetic resonance imaging in reference to transesophageal two-dimensional color Doppler echocardiography. J Am Coll Cardiol 1992;19:1500-1507.

80. Di Cesare E, Enrici RM, Paparoni S, et al: Low-field magnetic resonance imaging in the evaluation of mechanical and biological heart valve function. Eur J Radiol 1995;20:224-228.

81. Gilkeson RC, Markowitz AH, Balgude A, Sachs PB: MDCT evaluation of aortic valvular disease. AJR Am J Roentgenol 2006;186:350-360.

82. Caduff JH, Hernandez RJ, Ludomirsky A: MR visualization of aortic valve vegetations. J Comput Assist Tomogr 1996;20:613-615.

83. Winkler ML, Higgins CB: MRI of perivalvular infectious pseudoaneurysms. AJR Am J Roentgenol 1986;147:253-256.

84. Meijboom WB, Mollet NR, Van Mieghem CA, et al: Pre-operative computed tomography coronary angiography to detect significant coronary artery disease in patients referred for cardiac valve surgery. J Am Coll Cardiol 2006;48:1658-1665.

85. Gilard M, Cornily J-C, Pennec P-Y, et al: Accuracy of multislice computed tomography in the preoperative assessment of coronary disease in patients with aortic valve stenosis. J Am Coll Cardiol 2006;47:2020-2024.

Basic Principles of Medical Therapy in the Patient with Valvular Heart Disease

Catherine M. Otto

KEY POINTS

- Many adverse outcomes in adults with valvular heart disease are due to sequelae of the disease process including atrial fibrillation, embolic events, left ventricular dysfunction, pulmonary hypertension, and endocarditis.
- Medical therapy in adults with valvular heart disease focuses on prevention and treatment of complications because there are no specific therapies to prevent progression of the valve disease itself.
- Endocarditis prophylaxis guidelines no longer recommend antibiotics for native valve disease, although treatment in adults with prosthetic valves is still recommended.
- Periodic evaluation of disease severity and the left ventricular response to chronic volume and/or pressure overload allows optimal timing of surgical and percutaneous interventions.
- General health maintenance is important, including evaluation and treatment of coronary disease risk factors, regular exercise, standard immunizations, and optimal dental care.
- Management of concurrent cardiovascular disease—hypertension, coronary disease, arrhythmias, and heart failure—follows standard approaches with modification, as needed, based on the potential confounding effects of valve hemodynamics.
- In patients with valvular disease undergoing noncardiac surgery, management focuses on an accurate assessment of disease severity and symptom status, with appropriate hemodynamic monitoring and optimization of loading conditions in the perioperative period.
- Evaluation of coronary anatomy usually is needed before valve surgery because of the high prevalence of coronary disease and improved surgical outcomes with concurrent coronary revascularization.

In patients with valvular heart disease, the basic principles of management are to (1) obtain an accurate diagnosis of the specific valvular lesion and quantitative disease severity using Doppler echocardiography, (2) prevent complications of the disease process, such as endocarditis, atrial fibrillation, and embolic events, (3) periodically reevaluate ventricular size and function to identify early ventricular dysfunction and optimize the timing of surgical intervention, (4) provide optimal management of associated conditions, and (5) provide patient education regarding the disease process, expected outcomes, and potential medical or surgical therapies.

DIAGNOSIS OF VALVE DISEASE

Valvular heart disease may first be diagnosed in the setting of an acute medical event, such as heart failure, pulmonary edema, atrial fibrillation, or infective endocarditis. More often, the diagnosis of valvular heart disease is initially suspected before the onset of overt symptoms based on the physical examination finding of a cardiac murmur; during screening in families with a history of a genetic disorder; or based on abnormal findings on an electrocardiogram, chest radiograph, or echocardiogram requested for unrelated reasons. Worldwide, valvular heart disease is first diagnosed in many patients when a cardiac murmur is heard during an episode of acute rheumatic fever.

In patients with a cardiac murmur, the first step is clinical assessment based on the history and physical examination.[1-3] If clinical evaluation indicates a high likelihood of significant valvular disease, the next step is echocardiography to confirm the diagnosis and evaluate valve anatomy and function.[4,5] A condensed version of indications for echocardiography in patients with suspected or known valve disease is shown in Table 8-1.[6]

In a patient with cardiac or respiratory symptoms and a cardiac murmur on auscultation, it is prudent to obtain an echocardiogram to evaluate for possible valvular disease. When symptoms are present, it is difficult to reliably exclude significant valvular disease on physical examination as findings may be subtle.[7] For example, some patients with severe aortic stenosis have only a grade 2 or 3 murmur on examination,

TABLE 8–1 | **Indications for Echocardiography in Adults with Suspected or Known Valvular Heart Disease**

Suspected valvular disease
Cardiac murmur in a patient with cardiorespiratory symptoms
Murmur suggestive of structural heart disease, even if asymptomatic
  Diastolic murmur
  Continuous murmur
  Holosystolic or late systolic murmur
  Murmur associated with an ejection click or radiation to neck or back
  Grade 3 or louder mid-peaking systolic murmur

Native valve disease
Stenosis
  Initial diagnosis and assessment of hemodynamic severity
  Assessment of left and right ventricular size, function, and hemodynamics
  Reevaluation for changing signs or symptoms
  Assessment of changes in valve or ventricular function during pregnancy
  Periodic reevaluation
  Assessment of pulmonary pressures with exercise in patients with mitral stenosis when there is a discrepancy between symptoms and resting
    hemodynamics
  TEE before percutaneous valvotomy in mitral stenosis patients
Regurgitation
  Initial diagnosis and assessment of hemodynamic severity
  Initial evaluation of left and right ventricular size, function, and hemodynamics
  Assessment of aortic regurgitation when aortic root enlargement is present
  Reevaluation with a change in symptoms
  Periodic reevaluation, even in asymptomatic patients
  Reassessment of valve and ventricular function during pregnancy
Mitral valve prolapse
  Assessment of leaflet morphology, hemodynamic severity, and ventricular compensation
Infective endocarditis*
  Detection of valvular vegetations with or without positive blood cultures
  Characterization of hemodynamic severity with known endocarditis
  Detection of complications, such as abscesses, fistulas, or shunts
  Reevaluation in high-risk patients (virulent organism, clinical deterioration, persistent or recurrent fever, new murmur, persistent bacteremia)

Interventions for valvular disease
Selection of alternate therapies for mitral valve disease (balloon valvuloplasty, surgical valve repair versus replacement)*
Monitoring interventional techniques in the catheterization laboratory (ICE, TEE, or TTE)
Intraoperative TEE for valve repair surgery
Intraoperative TEE for stentless bioprosthetic, homograft, or autograft valve replacement surgery
Intraoperative TEE for valve surgery of infective endocarditis

Prosthetic valves
Baseline postoperative study (hospital discharge or 2-4 wk)
Annual evaluation of bioprosthetic valves after 5 yr of implantation
Changing clinical signs and symptoms or suspected prosthetic valve dysfunction*
Prosthetic valve endocarditis
  Detection of endocarditis and characterization of valve and ventricular function
  Detection of endocarditis complications and reevaluation in complex endocarditis*
  Persistent fever without bacteremia or a new murmur*
  Bacteremia without known source*

*TEE usually required.
ICE, intracardiac echocardiography; TEE, transesophageal echocardiography; TTE, transthoracic echocardiography.
Summarized from Bonow RO, Carabello BA, Chatterjee K, et al: ACC/AHA 2006 guidelines for the management of patients with valvular heart disease: a report of the American
  College of Cardiology/American Heart Association Task Force on Practice Guidelines. J Am Coll Cardiol 2006 August 1;48(3):e1-e148.

and the carotid upstroke may appear normal because of coexisting atherosclerosis.[8-10] Diagnosis may be even more difficult in other situations. For example, only 50% of patients with acute mitral regurgitation have an audible murmur.[11]

In *asymptomatic* patients with a murmur on physical examination, those with a benign flow murmur should be distinguished from those with a pathologic murmur.[12] Although there are no absolutely reliable criteria for making this distinction, a reasonable estimate of the pretest likelihood of disease can be derived from the history and physical examination findings. Flow murmurs, defined as audible systolic murmurs in the absence of structural heart disease, are most common in younger patients and those with high output states. Thus, a flow murmur is a normal finding in pregnancy, being recognized in more than 80% of pregnant women.[4,5] Flow murmurs also are likely in patients who are anemic or febrile. Typically, a flow murmur is systolic, low intensity (grade 1 to 2), loudest at the base with little radiation, ends before the second heart sound, and is crescendo-decrescendo or "ejection" shaped with an early systolic peak. These murmurs are related to rapid ejection into the aorta or pulmonary artery in patients with normal valve function, high flow rates, and good transmission of sound to the chest wall.[2,3,13,14] The yield of echocardiography is very low in asymptomatic patients with a typical flow murmur on examination, no cardiac history, and no cardiac symptoms on careful questioning.

In contrast, echocardiographic examination usually is appropriate in asymptomatic patients with a diastolic or continuous murmur, a systolic murmur of grade 3 or higher, an ejection click or mid-systolic click, a holosystolic (rather than ejection) murmur, or an atypical pattern of radiation, even if the patient is asymptomatic. To some extent, the loudness of the murmur correlates with disease severity but is not reliable for decision making in an individual patient.[15,16] Echocardiography allows differentiation of valve disease from a flow murmur, identification of the specific valve involved, definition of the etiology of valve disease, and quantitation of the hemodynamic severity of the lesion along with left ventricular size and function. On the basis of these data, the expected prognosis, need for preventative measures, and timing of subsequent examinations (if any) can be determined.

In older adults, distinguishing a benign from a pathologic murmur is more difficult than in younger patients because many older patients have some degree of aortic valve sclerosis or mild mitral regurgitation that can be appreciated on auscultation and many have mild symptoms that may or may not be related to heart disease.[9,17-20] In this setting, a baseline echocardiogram may be prudent. The finding of aortic sclerosis is associated with an increased risk of adverse cardiovascular events, and some patients will have progressive valve obstruction. A soft mitral regurgitant murmur is most likely associated with mild to moderate regurgitation due to mitral annular calcification, but establishing the diagnosis with a baseline echocardiogram and excluding other causes of mitral regurgitation, such as ischemic disease or mitral valve prolapse, is appropriate.

Although echocardiography is the primary diagnostic modality used for evaluation of valve disease, cardiac magnetic resonance imaging and cardiac computed tomographic imaging are useful in some patients as discussed in Chapter 7. Diagnostic cardiac catheterization continues to be useful in selected patients, particularly when echocardiographic data are nondiagnostic or discrepant with other clinical data, as discussed in Chapter 6.

PREVENTATIVE MEASURES

Diagnosis and Prevention of Rheumatic Fever

Rheumatic fever is a multiorgan inflammatory disease that occurs 10 days to 3 weeks after group A streptococcal pharyngitis. The clinical diagnosis is based on the conjunction of an antecedent streptococcal throat infection and classic manifestations of the disease including carditis, polyarthritis, chorea, erythema marginatum, and subcutaneous nodules.[21-23] Clinical guidelines for the diagnosis of rheumatic fever allow increased specificity as many of the manifestations of rheumatic fever are seen in other conditions as well (Table 8-2). Some studies show that strict adherence to these guidelines may result in underdiagnoses, and additional echocardiographic criteria have been suggested.[22,24] Although these guidelines are helpful in the initial diagnosis of rheumatic fever, exceptions do occur so that consideration of the diagnosis is of central importance in the recognition of this disease.

The carditis associated with rheumatic fever is a pancarditis; there may be involvement of the pericardium, myocardium, and valvular tissue. Rheumatic disease preferentially affects the mitral valve with mitral regurgitation being characteristic of the acute episode whereas mitral stenosis is characteristic of the long-term effect of the disease process.[25] It has been suggested that echocardiography can improve the early diagnosis of rheumatic fever by detection of valvular regurgitation.[26] However, because a slight degree of mitral regurgitation is common in normal individuals, overdiagnosis should be avoided.

Primary prevention of rheumatic fever is based on treatment of streptococcal pharyngitis with appropriate antibiotics

TABLE 8–2	Updated Jones Criteria for the Diagnosis of Initial Attacks of Rheumatic Fever

Major criteria
Carditis (may involve endocardium, myocardium, and pericardium)
Polyarthritis (most frequent manifestation, usually migratory)
Chorea (documentation of recent group A streptococcal infection may be difficult)
Erythema marginatum (distinctive, evanescent rash on trunk and proximal extremities)
Subcutaneous nodules (firm, painless nodule on extensor surfaces of elbows, knees, and wrists)

Minor criteria
Clinical findings (arthralgia, fever)
Laboratory findings (elevated erythrocyte sedimentation rate or C-reactive protein)
Electrocardiography (prolonged PR interval)

Evidence of antecedent group A streptococcal infection
Positive throat culture or rapid streptococci antigen test
Elevated or rising streptococcal antibody titer

High probability of rheumatic fever
2 major criteria or
1 major plus 2 minor criteria
PLUS evidence of preceding group A streptococcal infection

Modified from Dajani et al: JAMA 1995;268:2069 as updated in Ferrieri P: Circulation 2002;106:2521.

for a sufficient length of time.[21,27] Patients with a history of rheumatic fever have a high risk for recurrent disease, leading to repeated episodes of valvulitis and increased damage to the valvular apparatus. Because recurrent streptococcal infections may be asymptomatic, secondary prevention is based on the use of continuous antibiotic therapy (Table 8-3). The risk of recurrent disease is highest in those exposed to streptococcal infections (contact with children or crowded situations) and in economically disadvantaged groups. A longer duration of secondary prevention is recommended in patients with evidence of carditis or persistent valvular disease than in those with no evidence of valvular damage.

TABLE 8–3	Recommendations for Prevention of Rheumatic Fever

Primary prevention (treatment of group A streptococcal tonsillopharyngitis)
Benzathine penicillin G 900,000 U plus 300,000 U procaine penicillin IM OR
Penicillin V 250 mg (children) or
500 mg (adolescents and adults)
orally 2-3 times daily for 10 days

For pts allergic to penicillin:
Erythromycin estolate 20-40 mg/kg/day (maximum 1 g/d) or
erythromycin ethylsuccinate 40 mg/kg/d (maximum 1 g/d)
in 2-4 divided oral doses daily for 10 days

Secondary prevention (of recurrent rheumatic fever)
Benzathine penicillin G 1.2 million U IM every 4 wk (every 3 wk in high-risk situations)
OR
Penicillin V 250 mg twice daily PO
OR
Sulfadiazine 500 mg/day (patients <27 kg) or 1000 mg daily (patients >27 kg)
For patients allergic to penicillin and sulfadiazine: Erythromycin 250 mg twice daily PO

Duration of secondary prophylaxis
Rheumatic fever with severe valve disease and/or after valve surgery: Lifelong
Rheumatic fever with mild regurgitation: At least 10 yr or until age 25 yr
Rheumatic fever without carditis: 5 yr or until age 18 yr, whichever is longer

IM, intramuscularly; PO, orally.
Modified from from Dajani et al: JAMA 1995;268:2069, and World Health Organization Technical Report 2001;923.

Prevention of Infective Endocarditis

Infective endocarditis occurs when bacteremia results in bacterial adherence and proliferation at sites of platelet and fibrin deposition on disrupted endothelial surfaces. Patients with native and prosthetic heart valve disease have an increased risk for infective endocarditis because of endothelial disruption on the valve leaflets due to high velocity and turbulent blood flow patterns (see Chapter 22). About 50% of patients with endocarditis have underlying native valve disease, and endocarditis may precipitate the diagnosis of valve disease in a previously asymptomatic patient.

Prevention of bacterial endocarditis is based on short-term antibiotic therapy at times of anticipated bacteremia in patients with the highest risk of endocarditis. The American Heart Association has published revised guidelines for groups of patients with the highest risk (Table 8-4), procedures likely to cause significant bacteremia (Table 8-5), and appropriate antibiotic regimens for dental procedures (Table 8-6).[28] Prophylaxis for other procedures should include antibiotics active against the organisms most likely to be present as detailed in these guidelines. Antibiotics also are recommended at the time of surgical implantation of prosthetic cardiac valves or other intracardiac material.

Current guidelines no longer recommend endocarditis prophylaxis for patients with native valvular heart disease based on a careful review of the published literature and expert opinion.[28,29] The key elements underlying the current recommendations are (1) the recognition that bacteremia due to normal daily activities, such as tooth brushing, flossing, and chewing, is much more frequent than bacteremia related to dental procedures, (2) the lack of controlled studies showing that short-term use of antibiotics at the time of anticipated bacteremia prevents endocarditis and estimates of total benefit are exceedingly small, (3) the risk of an adverse reaction to the antibiotic is higher than any potential benefit, and (4) the most important factor in reducing daily bacteremia is maintaining optimal oral health and hygiene, including regular dental care.[30-32]

Prevention of Embolic Events

Prevention of embolic events in patients with valvular heart disease, particularly those with mitral stenosis or atrial fibrillation, is a key component of optimal medical therapy

TABLE 8–4	Cardiac Conditions for Which Endocarditis Prophylaxis for Dental Procedures Is Reasonable
Prosthetic cardiac valve or prosthetic material used for cardiac valve repair*	
Previous infective endocarditis	

Congenital Heart Disease (CHD)
  Unrepaired cyanotic CHD including palliative shunts and conduits
  Completely repaired CHD with prosthetic material or device, whether placed by surgery or catheter intervention, during the first 6 months after the procedure‡
  Repaired CHD with residual defects at the site or adjacent to the site of a prosthetic patch or prosthetic device (which inhibit endothelialization)	

Cardiac transplant recipients who develop cardiac valvulopathy	

*Prophylaxis is not needed for patients with coronary artery stents only.

†Except for the conditions listed, antibiotic prophylaxis is no longer recommended for any other form of CHD.

‡Prophylaxis is reasonable because endothelization of prosthetic material occurs within 6 months after the procedure.

From Wilson W, Taubert KA, Gewitz M, et al: Prevention of infective endocarditis: guidelines from the American Heart Association. Circulation 2007;116:1736-1754, with permission.

TABLE 8–5	Dental or Surgical Procedures for Which Endocarditis Prophylaxis is Recommended

Prophylaxis recommended for patients meeting criteria in Table 8-4

All dental procedures that involve manipulation of gingival tissue or the periapical region of teeth or perforation of the oral mucosa (Class IIa, LOE C)

Invasive procedures of the respiratory tract that involve incision or biopsy, including tonsillectomy and adenoidectomy (Class IIa, LOE C)

Infections of the GI or GU tract, including an antibiotic active against enterococci (Class IIb, LOE B)

Elective cystoscopy or other urinary tract manipulation only in patients with an enterococcal urinary tract infection or colonization, using an agent active against enterococci (Class IIb, LOE B)

Procedures on infected skin or musculoskeletal tissue including agents active against staphylococci and β-hemolytic streptococci (Class IIb, LOE C)

Prophylaxis recommended for ALL patients

Surgical placement of prosthetic heart valves or prosthetic intravascular or intracardiac material, (Class I, LOE B) using a first-generation cephalosporin (Class I, LOE A) or vancomycin at centers with high prevalence of methicillin-resistant *Staphylococcus epidermidis* (Class IIb, LOE C). Prophylaxis should begin immediately before surgery and be continued for <48 hr (Class IIa, LOE B).

Prophylaxis solely to prevent endocarditis NOT needed

Minor dental procedures
  Routine anesthetic injections through noninfected tissue
  Dental radiographs
  Placement, removal, or adjustment of prosthodontic or orthodontic appliances
  Placement of orthodontic brackets
  Shedding of deciduous teeth
  Bleeding from trauma to the lips and/or oral mucosa
Respiratory procedures
  Bronchoscopy without incision of the respiratory tract mucosa
GU or GI procedures
  All GI and GU procedures, including diagnostic esophagogastroduodenoscopy or colonoscopy
  Vaginal delivery and hysterectomy
Skin and musculoskeletal procedures
  Tattooing
  Body piercing

LOE, level of evidence; GI, gastrointestinal; GU, genitourinary.

American College of Cardiology/American Heart Association classification of recommendations (I, IIa, IIb) and level of evidence (A, B, C) are used (see Appendix A).

Summarized from Wilson W, Taubert KA, Gewitz, M et al: Prevention of infective endocarditis: guidelines from the American Heart Association. Circulation 2007; 116:1736-1754.

(Table 8-7).[6,33-38] The consequences of a systemic embolic event can be devastating and may occur even in previously asymptomatic patients. Systemic embolism usually is due to left atrial thrombus formation in patients with low blood flow in a dilated left atrial chamber, with or without concurrent atrial fibrillation (Figure 8-1).[39-44] Embolic events due to calcific debris from the aortic or mitral valves are much less common.[45,46]

Anticoagulation Clinics

Therapy for prevention of embolic events in patients with valvular heart disease may include antiplatelet agents or chronic warfarin anticoagulation. Warfarin therapy is monitored using the international normalized ratio (INR) as it provides a consistent measure of the degree of anticoagulation. Management by hospital-based anticoagulation clinics results in low complication rates and appears to be cost-effective. Long-term management is equally effective with periodic direct patient contact and with telephone encounters.[47-50] The typical anticoagulation clinic is staffed by pharmacists, with special expertise in anticoagulation management, using written policies and procedures developed in collaboration with the responsible physicians.

TABLE 8–6	American Heart Association Recommendations for Endocarditis Prophylaxis for Dental Procedures		
		Regimen: Single Dose 30-60 min before Procedure	
Situation	**Agent**	**Adults**	**Children**
Oral	Amoxicillin	2.0 g	50 mg/kg
Unable to take oral medications	Ampicillin OR	2.0 g IM or IV	50mg/kg IM or IV
	Cefazolin or ceftriaxone	1g IM or IV	50mg/kg IM or IV
Allergic to penicillins or ampicillin—oral	Cephalexin*† OR	2g	50mg/kg
	Clindamycin OR	600mg	20mg/kg
	Azithromycin or clarithromycin	Adults 500 mg; children 15 mg/kg orally 1 hr before procedure	15mg/kg
Allergic to penicillins or ampicillin and unable to take oral medications	Cefazolin or ceftriaxone† OR	1g IM or IV	50mg/kg IM or IV
	Clindamycin	600mg IM or IV	20mg/kg IM or IV

*Or other first- or second-generation oral cephalosporin in equivalent adult or pediatric dosage.

†Cephalosporins should not be used in an individual with anaphylaxis, angioedema, or urticaria with penicillin or ampicillin.

IM intramuscularly; IV, intravenously.

From Wilson W, Taubert KA, Gewitz M et al: Prevention of infective endocarditis: guidelines from the American Heart Association. Circulation 2007;116:1736-1754, with permission.

TABLE 8–7	Recommendations for Anticoagulation Therapy in Patients with Native Valvular Heart Disease
Valve Lesion	**Recommendation**
Mitral valve disease with AF	Warfarin, INR 2.0-3.0
Rheumatic mitral valve stenosis	
Paroxysmal, persistent or permanent AF	Warfarin, INR 2.0-3.0
Previous embolic event or LA thrombus (even with NSR)	Warfarin, INR 2.0-3.0
Recurrent systemic emboli despite adequate anticoagulation	Add aspirin 80-100 mg qd OR dipyridamole 400 mg qd OR ticlopidine 250 mg bid
Mitral valve prolapse	
TIAs	Long-term (75-325 mg qd) aspirin
AF at age <65 yr with no other risk factors	Long-term (75-325 mg qd) aspirin
AF plus at least 1 other risk factor (age >65 yr, hypertension, MR murmur, or history of CHF)	Warfarin, INR 2.0-3.0
CVA with AF, MR, or LA thrombus	Warfarin, INR 2.0-3.0
Infective endocarditis	
Native valve or tissue prosthesis	Anticoagulation therapy contraindicated
Mechanical valve	Continue or restart anticoagulation (heparin or warfarin) as soon as neurologic condition allows
Nonbacterial thrombotic endocarditis*	
With systemic emboli	Heparin anticoagulation
Debilitating disease with aseptic vegetations on echocardiography	Heparin anticoagulation

*This recommendation is not guideline based but is based on review of references cited.

AF, atrial fibrillation; CHF, congestive heart failure; CVA, cardiovascular accident; INR, international normalized ratio; LA, left atrial; MR, mitral regurgitation; NSR, normal sinus rhythm; TIA, transient ischemic attack.

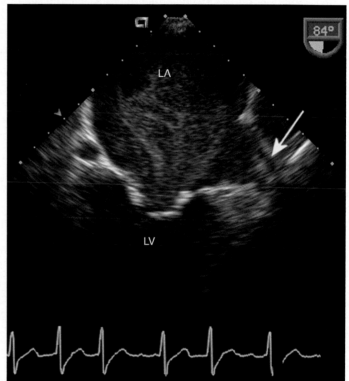

FIGURE 8–1 Example of spontaneous left atrial contrast on transesophageal imaging, using a two-chamber view, in a patient with rheumatic mitral stenosis. The arrow indicates the left atrial appendage with a possible thrombus. LA, left atrium; LV, left ventricle. *(From Otto CM: Textbook of Clinical Echocardiography, 3rd ed. Philadelphia, Saunders, 2004, with permission.)*

Another option is self-management of anticoagulation by the patient with a small home monitoring device that uses a fingerstick blood sample. In randomized trials, conventional therapy versus home management showed similar rates of anticoagulation control, with an INR in the therapeutic range about two thirds of the time in both groups, but the rate of major complications was lower in the home management group.[51,52] A meta-analysis of 14 randomized studies of home monitoring of warfarin therapy demonstrated lower rates of thromboembolic events, all-cause mortality, and major hemorrhage.[53] All of these authors emphasize that home monitoring is only appropriate in selected patients and requires careful education and supervision.[54]

At the initiation of therapy, a target INR and acceptable range are defined by the referring physician for each patient on the basis of published guidelines and clinical factors unique to that patient. The pharmacist interviews each patient with specific attention to current medications, diet, lifestyle, and any other factors that may have an impact on long-term anticoagulation therapy. In addition, patient education about anticoagulation, possible dietary and drug interactions, recognition of complications of therapy, and the need for careful monitoring of the INR is provided verbally and using a variety of media (such as pamphlets, recorded presentations, and computer-based material).

Typically, the INR is measured weekly (or more frequently) at the initiation of therapy with an interval of 4 weeks for patients maintained on a stable therapeutic regimen. At each visit, the timing of the next INR measurement is determined on the basis of the current INR and any trends over the past several visits. In addition, further patient education and counseling are provided as needed. The pharmacist monitors concurrent medical therapy for any potential drug interaction, and the patient or physician can contact the pharmacist before starting new prescription or nonprescription medications either to avoid possible interactions by choosing an alternate agent or to alert the pharmacist of the need for more frequent INR determinations if an effect is likely (Figures 8-2 and 8-3).

Minor bleeding complications may be managed by the anticoagulation clinic in consultation with the physician, depending on the specific protocol at each institution. If major bleeding episodes or thromboembolic events occur, the patient is triaged promptly for acute medical care. The anticoagulation clinic also manages changes in therapy necessitated by surgical or invasive procedures, using protocols developed in conjunction with the referring physician.

Anticoagulation in Patients with Native Valve Disease

Valvular heart disease patients with paroxysmal, persistent, or permanent atrial fibrillation should be treated with warfarin to maintain an INR of 2.0 to 3.0.[55] In mitral stenosis, warfarin anticoagulation is also recommended in patients with a previous embolic event or a left atrial thrombus, even if in sinus rhythm (Figure 8-4).[6,56-59] Some data support the use of warfarin anticoagulation in patients with mitral stenosis who have sinus rhythm with a left atrial dimension greater than 55 mm and in those with prominent spontaneous contrast on echocardiography, because of the high risk of atrial thrombus formation even in the absence of

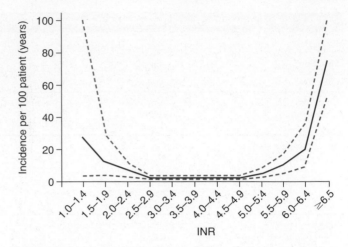

FIGURE 8–3 International normalized ratio (INR)-specific incidence of all adverse events (all episodes of thromboembolism, all major bleeding episodes, and unclassified stroke). The dotted lines indicate the 95% confidence interval. *(From Cannegieter SC, Rosendaal FR, Wintzen AR, et al: Optimal oral anticoagulant therapy in patients with mechanical heart valves. N Engl J Med 1995;333:11-17, with permission.)*

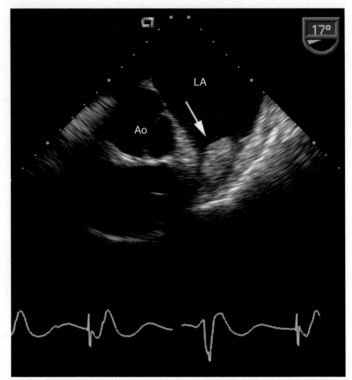

FIGURE 8–4 Example of a left atrial thrombus *(arrow)* on transesophageal imaging in a short axis view at the level of the aortic valve. Ao, aorta, LA, left atrium. *(From Otto CM, Schwaegler RG: Echocardiography Review Guide. Philadelphia, Saunders, 2008, with permission.)*

atrial fibrillation,[60-62] but this clinical decision is influenced by the severity of stenosis and the presence of comorbid conditions. Anticoagulation is not indicated for patients with aortic valve disease or asymptomatic mitral valve prolapse because of the low risk of embolic events with these lesions. Although elderly patients with mitral annular calcification appear to have a higher risk for embolic events, there is no evidence that anticoagulation is beneficial in the absence of concurrent atrial fibrillation.[63-66] If patients with mitral valve prolapse have unexplained transient ischemic attacks, treatment with aspirin is recommended. Long-term warfarin anticoagulation is indicated in patients with mitral

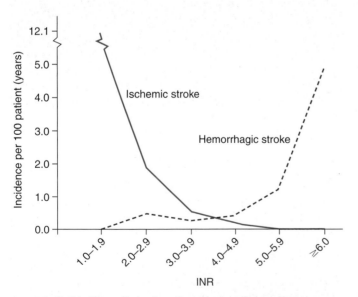

FIGURE 8–2 Incidence of ischemic and hemorrhagic stroke according to international normalized ratio (INR) category. *(From Cannegieter SC, Rosendaal FR, Wintzen AR, et al: Optimal oral anticoagulant therapy in patients with mechanical heart valves. N Engl J Med 1995;333:11-17, with permission.)*

valve prolapse, with or without a documented systemic embolic event, who are in atrial fibrillation if the patient has at least one other risk factor (age older than 65 years, mitral regurgitation, or left atrial thrombus).

In younger patients (<65 years) with mitral value prolapse and atrial fibrillation, aspirin therapy is recommended unless there is a history of stroke, hypertension, mitral regurgitation, or left atrial thrombus, situations in which warfarin is appropriate. However, some clinicians would also consider warfarin therapy in patients with mitral valve prolapse with a stroke and excessive leaflet thickening (>5 mm) or redundancy (even without atrial fibrillation or other risk factors) and in those with persistent transient ischemic attacks despite aspirin.[6]

In patients with infective endocarditis, anticoagulation should be avoided in general, given an increased risk of hemorrhagic transformation of embolic stroke in these patients and the lack of evidence of benefit.[67,68] The major exception to the avoidance of anticoagulation in endocarditis is the presence of a mechanical valve. In this situation, most studies suggest that chronic anticoagulation should be continued, unless the patient develops a stroke.[69-71] The choice of intravenous heparin, so that anticoagulation can be promptly stopped in the event of a stroke, versus warfarin therapy is controversial and depends on the specific clinical circumstances of each patient. If warfarin is used, close monitoring is needed as many antibiotics affect its metabolism.

General Health Maintenance

Adults with mild to moderate asymptomatic valvular heart disease should be encouraged to maintain a normal body weight and to remain physically fit with regular dynamic physical activity. There are no restrictions on participation in competitive sports for asymptomatic patients with valvular heart disease who are in sinus rhythm, have normal left ventricular size and systolic function, and have normal pulmonary pressures at rest and with exercise. Even those with severe asymptomatic valve disease should also be encouraged to participate in regular low-level aerobic activity although participation in competitive sports and strenuous activity should be avoided as summarized in Table 8-8.[72] Recommendations regarding competitive sports are more problematic in patients

with moderate disease and should be individualized on the basis of the presence of left ventricular dilation or dysfunction and the patient's hemodynamic response to exercise. Patients receiving chronic anticoagulation for atrial fibrillation should avoid sports with the potential for bodily contact or falls.

Both pneumococcal and annual influenza vaccination are recommended for all adults older than age 65 and are especially important in patients with valvular disease as the increased hemodynamic demands of an acute infection may lead to cardiac decompensation.[73] In younger patients with valve disease, routine immunization is indicated only if coexisting conditions associated with immunocompromise are present.

Patients with valvular disease should have an assessment of risk factors for coronary artery disease and aggressive risk factor modification as appropriate. Because aortic valve sclerosis is associated with an increased risk of myocardial infarction and cardiac death, the finding of aortic sclerosis on echocardiography should prompt a careful evaluation and initiation of treatment for known cardiac risk factors. In addition, many patients with valvular disease will eventually need surgical intervention, and both surgical mortality and morbidity rates are markedly increased when coronary disease complicates valvular heart disease. The negative impact of coexisting coronary disease is particularly striking for mitral regurgitation, with coronary disease conferring a fourfold increase in surgical mortality[74] and a 5-year survival one half that of patients without coronary disease.[75] In aortic stenosis, concurrent coronary disease is associated with an approximate doubling of surgical mortality.[74,76-79]

MONITORING DISEASE PROGRESSION

Periodic noninvasive monitoring is essential for optimal timing of interventions in patients with valvular heart disease. Disease progression may be evident as changes in valve anatomy or motion; an increase in the severity of valve stenosis or regurgitation; left ventricular dilation, hypertrophy, or dysfunction in response to pressure and/or volume overload; or secondary effects of the valvular lesion, such as pulmonary hypertension or atrial fibrillation. The frequency of periodic evaluations, if tailored to each patient, depends on the severity of the lesion at the initial evaluation, the known natural history of the disease, indications for surgical intervention, and other clinical factors. Clearly, there is no simple set of rules that defines the optimal or most cost-effective frequency of evaluation. However, on the basis of our current understanding of the natural history of valve disease, a framework for periodic evaluation can be devised (Table 8-9). First, an initial complete diagnostic echocardiographic study is performed to define disease severity, left ventricular size and systolic function, pulmonary pressures, and any associated abnormalities. Next, a basic frequency of repeat examination is suggested for each valve lesion depending on the severity of valve disease and, for valve regurgitation, on the left ventricular response to chronic volume overload.

However, the specific timing of repeat studies may need to be modified, depending on interim changes in symptoms or physical examination findings, new onset of atrial fibrillation, evidence for progressive left ventricular dilation or early contractile dysfunction, or evidence of increasing pulmonary pressures. For example, an apparent increase in ventricular dimensions in a patient with chronic regurgitation prompts a repeat evaluation at a shorter time interval to distinguish a pathologic change from normal physiologic or measurement variation. Similarly, a change in symptom status in a patient with myxomatous mitral valve disease warrants reevaluation as a sudden change in regurgitant severity due to chordal rupture may have occurred. In addition, more frequent

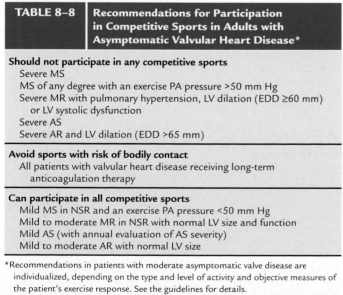

TABLE 8–8	Recommendations for Participation in Competitive Sports in Adults with Asymptomatic Valvular Heart Disease*

Should not participate in any competitive sports
Severe MS
MS of any degree with an exercise PA pressure >50 mm Hg
Severe MR with pulmonary hypertension, LV dilation (EDD ≥60 mm) or LV systolic dysfunction
Severe AS
Severe AR and LV dilation (EDD >65 mm)

Avoid sports with risk of bodily contact
All patients with valvular heart disease receiving long-term anticoagulation therapy

Can participate in all competitive sports
Mild MS in NSR and an exercise PA pressure <50 mm Hg
Mild to moderate MR in NSR with normal LV size and function
Mild AS (with annual evaluation of AS severity)
Mild to moderate AR with normal LV size

*Recommendations in patients with moderate asymptomatic valve disease are individualized, depending on the type and level of activity and objective measures of the patient's exercise response. See the guidelines for details.
AR, aortic regurgitation; LV, left ventricular; EDD, end-diastolic dimension; MR, mitral regurgitation; MS, mitral stenosis; NSR, normal sinus rhythm; PA, pulmonary artery.
Summarized from Bonow RO, Cheitlin MD, Crawford MH, Douglas PS: Task Force 3: valvular heart disease. J Am Coll Cardiol 2005;45:1334-1340.

TABLE 8–9 | **Framework for Periodic Echocardiography in Patients with Valvular Heart Disease**

Step 1. Initial diagnostic study
A comprehensive baseline echocardiographic and Doppler examination. Transesophageal imaging should be considered if transthoracic images are nondiagnostic.

Step 2. Basic frequency of examination
The basic frequency of echocardiographic examination provides a starting point for each patient, which will be modified as appropriate in steps 3 and 4 below.

Valve Lesion	Severity	Basic Frequency
Aortic stenosis	Mild (V_{max} <3.0 m/s)	3-5 yr
	Moderate (V_{max} 3-4 m/s)	1-2 yr
	Severe (V_{max} >4.0 m/s)	Annually
Aortic regurgitation	Mild	2-3 yr
	Moderate, normal LV size	1-2 yr
	Severe, normal LV size	Annually
	Severe, LV dilation	6-12 mo
Mitral stenosis	Mild (MVA >2.0 cm²)	2-3 yr
	Moderate (MVA 1-2 cm²)	Annually
	Severe (MVA <1.0 cm²)	6-12 mo
Mitral regurgitation	Mild	2-3 yr
	Moderate	1-2 yr
	Severe, normal LV size	Annually
	Severe, change in LV size or function	6 mo

Step 3. Modifiers of examination frequency
Increase frequency
   Interim change in symptoms or physical examination findings
   New onset atrial fibrillation
   Evidence for progressive LV dilation and/or early contractile dysfunction
   Evidence for increasing pulmonary pressures
Decrease frequency
   Stable findings over 2-3 examination intervals

Step 4. Special Situations
Preoperative for noncardiac surgery
Pregnancy
Monitoring interventional procedures
Assessment of complications and hemodynamic results after an intervention
Intraoperative transesophageal monitoring

LV, left ventricular; MVA, mitral valve area.

examinations are warranted when quantitative parameters are approaching the values defined as optimal for timing of surgical intervention.

In other clinical situations, reevaluation may be indicated to assess hemodynamics under changing physiologic conditions (such as during pregnancy), to guide a surgical or interventional procedure, or to assess results and complications after an intervention. In patients with comorbid diseases, such as those undergoing noncardiac surgery, a repeat echocardiographic examination may be needed to assist in medical and/or surgical management.

MEDICAL THERAPY

Primary Treatment of Valve Disease

Ideally, the treatment of valvular heart disease should be directed towards the underlying disease process affecting valve anatomy and function. Worldwide, primary prevention of rheumatic heart disease would have a dramatic impact on the incidence of valvular heart disease. In patients with rheumatic heart disease, prevention of recurrent episodes of rheumatic fever is critical for preventing further valve damage and progressive disease. However, there currently are no specific therapies available to prevent or reverse the primary disease processes in other types of valve disease.

The recent recognition that calcific valve disease is an active disease process with similarities to atherosclerosis has led to the hypothesis that disease progression might be prevented by lipid-lowering therapy. Although retrospective data were promising, prospective randomized trials did not show benefit of lipid lowering therapy for prevention of hemodynamic progression of calcific aortic stenosis and did not decrease the rate of valve replacement surgery[80-83] (see Chapters 3 and 9).

There are no specific medical therapies to prevent development or progression of valve regurgitation. However, it often is possible to avoid the irreversible consequences of chronic regurgitation, specifically prevention of left ventricular dilation and systolic dysfunction, left atrial enlargement, atrial fibrillation, and pulmonary hypertension. Currently, this goal is achieved primarily through sequential noninvasive monitoring that allows surgical intervention before irreversible changes have occurred.

Prevention of Left Ventricular Contractile Dysfunction

As discussed in Chapter 4, the basic response of the left ventricle to the chronic volume overload imposed by aortic or mitral regurgitation is an increase in chamber size. Initially, left ventricular systolic function is normal; however, with long-standing disease, contractile dysfunction may supervene and may not improve after intervention to correct the regurgitant lesion. Although most patients develop symptoms that prompt consideration of valve surgery, in a subset of patients, left ventricular dysfunction occurs before symptom onset.[84] Thus, a major focus of the medical management of patients with chronic valvular regurgitation is periodic noninvasive evaluation to monitor left ventricular size and systolic function. The rationale for sequential monitoring is that surgical intervention can be performed just before (or soon after) the onset of contractile dysfunction.

A more elusive goal in the medical therapy of patients with chronic regurgitation is to prevent or delay progressive left ventricular dilation and contractile dysfunction, thus delaying the need for surgical intervention. Afterload reduction therapy improves acute hemodynamics, but clinical studies have yielded variable results on the potential benefit of afterload reduction to prevent progressive left ventricular dilation in response to chronic aortic or mitral regurgitations (see Chapters 4, 10, and 15). There currently are no class I indications for afterload reduction therapy in nonhypertensive adults with chronic asymptomatic aortic or mitral regurgitation.[6,85] However, adults with chronic regurgitation and an elevated blood pressure, which is common in this patient group, should receive appropriate antihypertensive therapy.

In patients with valvular aortic stenosis, the development of left ventricular contractile dysfunction is uncommon, and the timing of surgical intervention is based on the symptom onset rather than on changes in left ventricular geometry or function.[86] There are no known medical therapies to prevent or modify the development of left ventricular hypertrophy in adults with aortic stenosis, and it is not clear that preventing this adaptive response would improve outcome (see Chapter 4). There also has been considerable interest in the changes in diastolic ventricular dysfunction that occur in patients in aortic stenosis.[87-89] It has been hypothesized that surgical intervention before the development of irreversible changes in the myocardium might improve long-term clinical outcome.[90,91] Again, however, there is no medical therapy known to prevent diastolic dysfunction in patients with pressure overload hypertrophy.

Prevention of Left Atrial Enlargement and Atrial Fibrillation

Progressive left atrial enlargement and atrial fibrillation typically complicate the clinical course of mitral valve disease. Both mitral regurgitation and mitral stenosis are associated with left atrial dilation because of the pressure and/or volume overload of the left atrium.[92-94] Atrial fibrillation occurs frequently, particularly in older patients, and in those with severe and long-standing disease.[95-98] Atrial enlargement and fibrillation occasionally complicate aortic valve disease, typically late in the disease course, and may worsen hemodynamics substantially owing to loss of the atrial contribution to ventricular filling.[99]

Medically, there is no specific therapy to prevent these complications of the disease process, although it has been proposed that earlier surgical or percutaneous intervention might prevent atrial enlargement and eventual atrial fibrillation. Surgical intervention for mitral regurgitation soon after the onset of atrial fibrillation (within 3 months) is more likely to restore sinus rhythm than surgical intervention in patients with atrial fibrillation of longer duration but still is not uniformly successful.[100] In patients with mitral stenosis, atrial fibrillation usually recurs or persists after intervention.[97,101,102]

Prevention of Pulmonary Hypertension

The chronic elevation in left atrial pressure associated with mitral valve disease results in a passive increase in pulmonary pressures that resolves when left atrial pressure decreases after surgical or percutaneous intervention. However, reactive changes in the pulmonary vasculature may become superimposed on this passive rise in pressure with secondary histologic changes leading to irreversible pulmonary hypertension (see Chapter 14). Intervention before the onset of irreversible changes is desirable to avoid long-term complications of right heart failure. In some patients, an excessive rise in pulmonary pressures with exercise may be the first clue that intervention is needed to prevent further irreversible changes in the pulmonary vasculature.[103,104]

Symptoms Due to Valve Disease

Although the goal in management of patients with valvular disease is mechanical intervention prior to or at symptom onset, some patients have persistent symptoms after intervention, have symptoms only in response to a superimposed hemodynamic stress (such as pregnancy), or are not candidates for surgical or percutaneous intervention. In these situations, medical therapy is based primarily on adjustment of loading conditions and control of heart rate and rhythm.

Patients with pulmonary congestion are treated with diuretics to decrease left atrial and pulmonary venous pressures whether elevated left atrial pressures are due to left ventricular dysfunction, mitral regurgitation, or mitral stenosis. However, when mitral stenosis is present, care is needed to ensure that left atrial pressures allow adequate left ventricular diastolic filling across the narrowed valve. In patients with aortic stenosis, diuretics should be used cautiously as pulmonary congestion often is due to diastolic dysfunction rather than to volume overload. The further decrease in ventricular diastolic volume induced by diuretics may worsen symptoms as mid-cavity ventricular obstruction develops in the small, hypertrophied, hyperdynamic left ventricle.

Afterload reduction is most beneficial for treatment of heart failure symptoms in patients with acute aortic or mitral regurgitation. With acute regurgitation, a continuous intravenous infusion of nitroprusside may be used. In patients with acute mitral regurgitation, intraaortic balloon counterpulsation provides effective afterload reduction while maintaining coronary diastolic perfusion pressures. However an intraaortic balloon is contraindicated with aortic regurgitation because the increase in aortic diastolic pressure results in more severe valve regurgitation. In symptomatic patients with chronic regurgitation, standard therapy for heart failure is reasonable, including afterload reduction, only if surgery is not an option or if heart failure occurs in the setting of a reversible hemodynamic stress. In patients with mitral stenosis, afterload reduction is not helpful as the ventricle typically is small with normal systolic function.

In the past, there was concern that afterload reduction in adults with severe aortic stenosis might result in a precipitous fall in blood pressure due to peripheral vasodilation because only a fixed stroke volume can be pumped though the rigid orifice.[105,106] However, more recent studies suggest that cautious use of afterload reduction is well tolerated and may be beneficial.[107,108] Other studies suggest that valve area is not fixed, but instead there is a greater degree of leaflet motion when cardiac output is increased.[109,110] In particular, when there is coexisting left ventricular dysfunction, the decrease in systemic vascular resistance may lead to improved left ventricular contractility and an increase in left ventricular output due to increased opening of the valve leaflets.[111]

MANAGEMENT OF CONCURRENT CARDIOVASCULAR CONDITIONS

Hypertension

Concurrent hypertension is common in adults, with a prevalence close to 50% in those older than 65 years. Thus, many patients with valve disease also have hypertension, which should be treated per the JNC-7 or other established guidelines.[112] Treatment of hypertension is well tolerated with mitral valve disease so that modification in therapy is rarely needed because of the valve lesions.

Treatment of hypertension in patients with aortic valve disease is especially important to reduce total ventricular afterload, which includes both the load imposed by the valve lesions and the systemic vascular resistance. With aortic regurgitation, two factors are important in treatment of hypertension. First, severe aortic regurgitation is characterized by a wide pulse pressure; overtreatment of the high systolic pressure, which is due to a large total stroke volume, may result in excessively low diastolic pressures. In theory, lowering blood pressure could compromise diastolic coronary blood flow. Second, therapy that lowers heart rate may result in higher systolic blood pressure attributable to an even larger stroke volume with a longer diastolic filling period. Thus, if a β-blocker is used, additional therapy with an afterload reducing agent may be need.

With aortic stenosis, treatment of hypertension should follow standard approaches except that therapy should be initiated at low doses and slowly titrated to the therapeutic dose to avoid hypotension. Diuretics should be avoided, particularly in elderly women with aortic stenosis who typically have a small hypertrophic ventricle, because any decrease in preload will reduce forward cardiac output. Despite concerns in the past that systemic vasodilation might result in hypotension because of a lack of a compensatory increase in stroke volume across the narrowed valve as systemic resistance decreases, in fact, angiotensin-converting enzyme inhibitor therapy is well tolerated in adults with moderate aortic stenosis.[113] Afterload reduction therapy has been proposed as having potential, but unproven, benefits for preservation of ventricular systolic and diastolic function in aortic stenosis.[114] The presence of hypertension may affect the accuracy of measures of aortic stenosis severity so that blood pressure should be controlled before assessment of valve disease severity.[115-118]

Coronary Artery Disease

Coronary artery disease also is common in adults with valvular heart disease, as expected on the basis of age, sex, and clinical risk factors in this patient group.[119] In patients undergoing valve surgery, coronary angiography is needed in most patients because concurrent coronary artery bypass grafting is recommended when significant disease is present. Similarly, the timing of valve intervention may be affected by the presence and severity of coronary disease, particularly when a patient with asymptomatic aortic stenosis is referred for valve surgery (Table 8-10).

TABLE 8–10	Indications for Coronary Angiography in Adults with Valvular Heart Disease
Before surgical or percutaneous valve procedures in patients with 　Chest pain 　Objective evidence of ischemia 　Decreased left ventricular systolic function 　History of coronary disease 　Coronary risk factors (including age)*	
Men ≥35 yr	
Postmenopausal women	
Women ≥35 yr with coronary risk factors	
Mild to moderate valve disease in patients with 　Progressive angina 　Objective evidence of ischemia 　Decreased left ventricular systolic function 　Congestive heart failure	

*Patients undergoing percutaneous balloon valvotomy do not need coronary angiography solely on the basis of coronary disease risk factors.
Summarized from Class I indications in 2006 American College of Cardiology/American Heart Association Guidelines.[6]

In adults with asymptomatic valve disease, prevention of coronary disease based on risk factor evaluation and modification is essential. When symptoms, in particular angina, occur, it may be difficult to distinguish whether symptoms are due to coronary or valve disease.[120] The resting electrocardiogram often shows left ventricular hypertrophy and ST changes due to valve disease. Both exercise and pharmacologic stress testing are less accurate for detection of coronary stenoses when valve disease is present because exercise duration may be limited by valve, not coronary, disease and coronary flow patterns are affected by valve hemodynamics.[121-124] Thus, direct imaging of coronary anatomy, usually by coronary angiography but alternatively with high resolution computed tomographic imaging, may be needed. If the cause of symptoms remains unclear after consideration of the severity of valve and coronary disease, it may be appropriate to consider a percutaneous coronary intervention. If symptoms resolve, continued treatment of coronary disease is reasonable; persistent symptoms suggest that the cause is the valve disease. Standard approaches to percutaneous and medical therapy of coronary disease are appropriate in adults with valvular heart disease.

Aortic Root Disease

Aortic valve dysfunction may be due to or associated with abnormalities of the aortic root. In adults with a bicuspid valve, aortic root dilation is common, and there is an increased risk of aortic dissection. In adults with a primary abnormality of the aortic root, such as Marfan syndrome, aortic regurgitation may be the result of aortic dilation with relatively normal valve anatomy. Tomographic imaging with a wide field of view, either cardiac computed tomography or cardiac magnetic resonance, typically is needed in addition to echocardiography for evaluation and monitoring of disease severity. In both of these situations, the aortic root involvement may be the primary driver of the frequency of imaging and the timing of surgical intervention. In addition, β-blockers are reasonable therapy in adults with a bicuspid aortic valve and aortic dilation (diameter 40 to 50 mm) when surgery is not yet indicated.[6]

Arrhythmias

In patients with valvular heart disease and atrial fibrillation, restoration and maintenance of sinus rhythm is of high priority both to prevent atrial thrombus formation (as discussed above) and to preserve the atrial contribution to left ventricular diastolic filling. Approaches to restoring and maintaining sinus rhythm are no different from those in patients without valve disease other than the increased awareness of embolic risk and the need for appropriate anticoagulation (see Table 8-7).[125] There is increasing interest in the use of atrial fibrillation ablation procedures at the time of surgical intervention.[126-128] Atrial fibrillation ablation is unlikely to be successful when significant valve disease is present unless the hemodynamic abnormality also is corrected. Often the onset of atrial fibrillation is the first sign of hemodynamic decompensation with chronic slowly progressive valve diseases.

When sinus rhythm cannot be maintained, the ventricular rate is controlled using standard approaches. Rate control is especially important in patients with mitral stenosis as a shortened diastolic filling time may result in a symptomatic decrease in forward cardiac output.[129,130]

Even when sinus rhythm is present, heart rate control may be needed in patients with valvular heart disease. For example, the increased heart rate (and shortened diastolic filling time) associated with pregnancy in a patient with mitral stenosis leads to inadequate ventricular filling and a reduced cardiac output. Slowing the heart rate with a β-blocker improves diastolic filling and restores a normal cardiac output.[131,132] Another example is the elderly patient with aortic stenosis. These elderly patients may develop bradycardia due to calcification of the conduction system with heart block or sick sinus syndrome, which further reduces the total cardiac output across the stenotic valve, leading to cardiac symptoms. Symptoms due to bradycardia resolve after placement of a pacer, possibly allowing deferral of aortic valve surgery.

There is an increased risk of sudden death in patients with valvular heart disease and significant left ventricular dilation or dysfunction due to chronic aortic regurgitation,[133] which is prevented by aortic valve replacement. Mitral valve prolapse also is associated with an increased risk of sudden death but antiarrhythmic therapy or placement of an automated implanted defibrillator is based on standard indications for these procedures, not on the presence of valve disease alone.[134]

Heart Failure

Heart failure due to valve stenosis or regurgitation is an indication for surgical or percutaneous intervention with either aortic or mitral valve disease. When severe valve disease is present, it is likely that heart failure is due to the valve lesion. For example, severe aortic regurgitation results in left ventricular dilation and systolic dysfunction. With prompt valve replacement, ventricular size and function return to normal.

However, when only mild to moderate valve disease is present and there is evidence of heart failure, evaluation for other causes is appropriate. The combination of moderate to severe aortic stenosis and moderate to severe left ventricular dysfunction is a particular clinical challenge as it can be difficult to distinguish whether aortic stenosis resulted in ventricular dysfunction or whether the poor ventricular function contributes to reduce aortic valve opening (see Chapter 9).

When heart failure is not due to valve dysfunction, standard approaches to medical therapy and continued sequential monitoring of valve disease are reasonable. Therapy may need to be started at low doses and titrated upward slowly when aortic stenosis is present to avoid hypotension due to an abrupt change in systemic vascular resistance. Evaluation of volume status should include consideration of the effects of valve dysfunction on ventricular filling, as well as standard parameters. For example, when mitral stenosis is present, the left ventricle may still be underfilled when central venous and pulmonary venous pressures are elevated.

Heart failure also may be the cause of valve dysfunction. For example, primary ventricular dilation and dysfunction result in secondary (or functional) mitral regurgitation due to distortion of the normal mitral annular-ventricular geometry, even when the mitral valve is structurally normal. In these patients, treatment of ventricular dysfunction may result in a decrease in regurgitant severity (see Chapter 16).

NONCARDIAC SURGERY IN PATIENTS WITH VALVE DISEASE

Most adults with valvular heart disease can safely undergo noncardiac surgery, particularly when only mild or moderate disease is present.[135] The key principles in management of patients with valvular heart disease undergoing noncardiac surgery are as follows:
- Accurate assessment of the severity of valve disease
- Evaluation of symptom status
- Hemodynamic monitoring in the perioperative period
- Optimization of loading conditions

Most adverse outcomes with noncardiac surgery in adults with valve disease are due to failure to recognize the presence of valve disease preoperatively.[136] When valve disease is suspected on the basis of history or physical examination findings, echocardiography is appropriate to identify and define the severity of any valve lesions.

In asymptomatic patients, valve regurgitation is generally well tolerated during noncardiac surgery, even if severe. However, patients with moderate to severe left-sided valve obstruction are at higher risk because an elevated preload results in pulmonary edema, and low preload results in hypotension due to a low cardiac output. Peripheral vasodilation also is poorly tolerated because of the inability to increase stroke volume when systemic vascular resistance falls. In asymptomatic patients with stenotic lesions, invasive hemodynamic monitoring often is helpful beginning in the preoperative setting, to allow optimization of loading conditions, and continuing for 48 to 72 hours postoperatively during the period of major changes in volume status. Intraoperative echocardiography and participation of an experienced cardiac anesthesiologist also are recommended. When left-sided valve obstruction is very severe, relief of stenosis before noncardiac surgery may be considered, depending on the urgency of the noncardiac surgery and on whether a percutaneous approach to relief of valve obstruction is possible.[137]

Symptoms due to valve disease are an indication for a corrective valve procedure. Thus, elective noncardiac surgery should be deferred until after treatment of the valve lesions whenever possible. With urgent surgery, symptomatic valve regurgitation is managed using standard heart failure regimens based on hemodynamic parameters. Symptomatic severe left-sided valve obstruction can sometimes be managed with the combination of invasive hemodynamic monitoring, intraoperative echocardiography, and an experienced cardiac anesthesiologist. However, with mitral stenosis, percutaneous valvotomy should be considered if valve anatomy is suitable and there is no left atrial thrombus. With severe symptomatic aortic stenosis, balloon valvotomy or percutaneous valve implantation may be considered with severe stenosis and an urgent noncardiac surgical procedure. Management of valvular heart disease during pregnancy is discussed in Chapter 25.

PATIENT EDUCATION

Patient education is the key to compliance with periodic noninvasive monitoring, prevention of complications, and the early recognition of symptoms in patients with valvular heart disease. Each patient should understand the expected long-term prognosis, potential complications, typical symptoms, rationale for sequential monitoring, and indications for surgical intervention. Appropriate education avoids needless concern and prompts early reporting of symptoms, allowing optimal timing of surgical intervention. Increasingly, patients are actively involved in decisions about timing of surgery and choice of intervention.

Patients also should be knowledgeable about the risk of infective endocarditis and the importance of maintaining optimal oral hygiene, including regular dental care. Education about the clinical presentation of endocarditis and the importance of obtaining blood cultures before antibiotics are started allows the patient to make sure that primary care physicians consider the possibility of endocarditis with a febrile illness. Patients with a prosthetic valve should be aware of situations in which endocarditis prophylaxis is needed, and the specific antibiotic regimen to be taken.

Patients receiving long term anticoagulation therapy need both education and a reliable and available source for consultation regarding warfarin dose, interactions with other medications, and prompt evaluation of any complications.

All patients with valvular heart disease should be evaluated for risk factors for coronary artery disease and should receive education and appropriate therapy for coronary risk factor reduction.

Because the risk of pregnancy in patients with valvular heart disease ranges from normal to very high, this risk should be estimated and discussed with the patient (see Chapter 25). In patients with very high-risk valve lesions, surgical correction before a planned pregnancy may be considered. In women receiving long-term anticoagulation, the issue of warfarin versus heparin anticoagulation during pregnancy is addressed prior to planned pregnancy, whenever possible. In addition, contraception options should be reviewed in all women with valvular disease.

In patients with inherited forms of valve disease, such as Marfan syndrome, the physician should make every effort to ensure that other family members are screened for the disease. With the increased understanding of the genetic basis of myxomatous mitral valve disease and bicuspid aortic valves, screening of family members also may be appropriate for patients with these conditions, particularly if there is a family history of sudden death or aortic dissection.

REFERENCES

1. Giuliani ER, Brandenburg RO, Fuster V: Evaluation of cardiac murmurs. Cardiovasc Clin 1980;10:1-18.
2. Perloff JK: Physical Examination of the Heart and Circulation. Philadelphia, Saunders, 1982.
3. Abrams J: Synopsis of Cardiac Physical Diagnosis. Philadelphia:, Lea & Febiger; 1989.
4. Mishra M, Chambers JB, Jackson G: Murmurs in pregnancy: an audit of echocardiography. BMJ 1992;304:1413-1444.
5. Northcote RJ, Knight PV, Ballantyne D: Systolic murmurs in pregnancy: value of echocardiographic assessment. Clin Cardiol 1985;8:327-328.
6. Bonow RO, Carabello BA, Chatterjee K, et al: ACC/AHA 2006 guidelines for the management of patients with valvular heart disease: a report of the American College of Cardiology/American Heart Association Task Force on Practice Guidelines. J Am Coll Cardiol 2006;48:e1-e148.
7. Jaffe WM, Roche AHG, Coverdale HA, et al: Clinical evaluation versus Doppler echocardiography in the quantitative assessment of valvular heart disease. Circulation 1988;78:267-275.
8. Lombard JT, Selzer A: Valvular aortic stenosis: a clinical and hemodynamic profile of patients. Ann Intern Med 1987;106:292-298.
9. Aronow WS, Kronzon I: Correlation of prevalence and severity of valvular aortic stenosis determined by continuous-wave Doppler echocardiography with physical signs of aortic stenosis in patients aged 62 to 100 years with aortic systolic ejection murmurs. Am J Cardiol 1987;60:399-401.
10. Forssell G, Jonasson R, Orinius E: Identifying severe aortic valvular stenosis by bedside examination. Acta Med Scand 1985;218:397-400.
11. Sutton GC, Craige E: Clinical signs of severe acute mitral regurgitation. Am J Cardiol 1967;20:141-144.
12. Etchells E, Bell C, Robb K: Does this patient have an abnormal systolic murmur? JAMA 1997;277:564-571.
13. Murgo JP: Systolic ejection murmurs in the era of modern cardiology: what do we really know? J Am Coll Cardiol 1998;32:1596-1602.
14. Spooner PH, Perry MP, Brandenburg RO, Pennock GD: Increased intraventricular velocities: an unrecognized cause of systolic murmur in adults. J Am Coll Cardiol 1998;32:1589-1595.
15. Desjardins VA, Enriquez Sarano M, Tajik AJ, et al: Intensity of murmurs correlates with severity of valvular regurgitation. Am J Med 1996;100:149-156.
16. Munt B, Legget ME, Kraft CD, et al: Physical examination in valvular aortic stenosis: correlation with stenosis severity and prediction of clinical outcome. Am Heart J 1999;137:298-306.
17. Etchells E, Glenns V, Shadowitz S, et al: A bedside clinical prediction rule for detecting moderate or severe aortic stenosis. J Gen Intern Med 1998;13:699-704.
18. Sainsbury R, White T, Wray R: Echocardiography in elderly patients with systolic murmurs. Age Ageing 1981;10:225-230.
19. Vigna C, Impagliatelli M, Russo A, et al: Systolic ejection murmurs in the elderly: aortic valve and carotid arteries echo-Doppler findings. Angiology 1991;42:455-461.
20. Wong M, Tei C, Shah PM: Degenerative calcific valvular disease and systolic murmurs in the elderly. J Am Geriatr Soc 1983;31:156-163.
21. Dajani A, Taubert K, Ferrieri P, et al: Treatment of acute streptococcal pharyngitis and prevention of rheumatic fever: a statement for health professionals. Committee on Rheumatic Fever, Endocarditis, and Kawasaki Disease of the Council on Cardiovascular Disease in the Young, the American Heart Association. Pediatrics 1995;96:1758-1764.
22. Ferrieri P: Proceedings of the Jones Criteria workshop. Circulation 2002;106: 2521-2523.
23. Meira ZM, Goulart EM, Colosimo EA, Mota CC: Long term follow up of rheumatic fever and predictors of severe rheumatic valvar disease in Brazilian children and adolescents. Heart 2005;91:1019-1022.
24. Carapetis JR, Currie BJ: Rheumatic fever in a high incidence population: the importance of monoarthritis and low grade fever. Arch Dis Child 2001;85:223-227.
25. Marcus RH, Sareli P, Pocock WA, Barlow JB: The spectrum of severe rheumatic mitral valve disease in a developing country: correlations among clinical presentation, surgical pathologic findings, and hemodynamic sequelae. Ann Intern Med 1994;120:177-183.
26. Abernethy M, Bass N, Sharpe N, et al: Doppler echocardiography and the early diagnosis of carditis in acute rheumatic fever. Aust N Z J Med 1994;24:530-535.
27. World Health Organization: Rheumatic fever and rheumatic heart disease: report of a WHO expert consultation. WHO Technical Report Series 2001:923.
28. Wilson W, Taubert KA, Gewitz M, et al: Prevention of Infective Endocarditis. Guidelines From the American Heart Association. A guideline from the American Heart Association Rheumatic Fever, Endocarditis, and Kawasaki Disease Committee, Council on Cardiovascular Disease in the Young, and the Council on Clinical Cardiology, Council on Cardiovascular Surgery and Anesthesia, and the Quality of Care and Outcomes Research Interdisciplinary Working Group. Circulation 2007;116:1736-1754.
29. Gould FK, Elliott TS, Foweraker J, et al: Guidelines for the prevention of endocarditis: report of the Working Party of the British Society for Antimicrobial Chemotherapy. J Antimicrob Chemother 2006;57:1035-1042.
30. Duval X, Alla F, Hoen B, et al: Estimated risk of endocarditis in adults with predisposing cardiac conditions undergoing dental procedures with or without antibiotic prophylaxis. Clin Infect Dis 2006;42:e102-e107.
31. Seto TB: The case for infectious endocarditis prophylaxis: time to move forward. Arch Intern Med 2007;167:327-330.
32. Morris AM: Coming clean with antibiotic prophylaxis for infective endocarditis. Arch Intern Med 2007;167:330-332.
33. Levine HJ, Gaasch WH: Vasoactive drugs in chronic regurgitant lesions of the mitral and aortic valves. J Am Coll Cardiol 1996;28:1083-1091.
34. Stein PD, Alpert JS, Copeland J, et al: Antithrombotic therapy in patients with mechanical and biological prosthetic heart valves [published erratum appears in Chest 1996;109:592]. Chest 1995;108(4 Suppl):371S-379S.
35. Vongpatanasin W, Hillis LD, Lange RA: Prosthetic heart valves. N Engl J Med 1996;335:407-416.
36. Cannegieter SC, Rosendaal FR, Wintzen AR, et al: Optimal oral anticoagulant therapy in patients with mechanical heart valves. N Engl J Med 1995;333:11-17.
37. Altman R, Rouvier J, Gurfinkel E, et al: Comparison of high-dose with low-dose aspirin in patients with mechanical heart valve replacement treated with oral anticoagulant. Circulation 1996;94:2113-2116.
38. Acar J, Iung B, Boissel JP, et al: AREVA: multicenter randomized comparison of low-dose versus standard-dose anticoagulation in patients with mechanical prosthetic heart valves. Circulation 1996;94:2107-2112.
39. Aberg H: Atrial fibrillation. I. A study of atrial thrombosis and systemic embolism in a necropsy material. Acta Med Scand 1969;185:373-379.
40. Hwang JJ, Li YH, Lin JM, et al: Left atrial appendage function determined by transesophageal echocardiography in patients with rheumatic mitral valve disease. Cardiology 1994;85:121-128.
41. Coulshed N, Epstein EJ, McKendrick CS, et al: Systemic embolism in mitral valve disease. Br Heart J 1970;32:26-34.
42. Hinton RC, Kistler JP, Fallon JT, et al: Influence of etiology of atrial fibrillation on incidence of systemic embolism. Am J Cardiol 1977;40:509-513.
43. Wolf PA, Dawber TR, Thomas HE Jr, Kannel WB: Epidemiologic assessment of chronic atrial fibrillation and risk of stroke: the Framingham study. Neurology 1978;28: 973-977.
44. Chiang CW, Lo SK, Kuo CT, et al: Noninvasive predictors of systemic embolism in mitral stenosis: an echocardiographic and clinical study of 500 patients. Chest 1994;106:396-399.
45. Brockmeier LB, Adolph RJ, Gustin BW, et al: Calcium emboli to the retinal artery in calcific aortic stenosis. Am Heart J 1981;101:32-37.
46. Pleet AB, Massey EW, Vengrow ME: TIA, stroke, and the bicuspid aortic valve. Neurology 1981;31:1540-1542.
47. Wilson SJ, Wells PS, Kovacs MJ, et al: Comparing the quality of oral anticoagulant management by anticoagulation clinics and by family physicians: a randomized controlled trial. CMAJ 2003;169:293-298.
48. Anderson RJ: Cost analysis of a managed care decentralized outpatient pharmacy anticoagulation service. J Manag Care Pharm 2004;10:159-165.
49. Fitzmaurice DA, Hobbs FD, Murray ET, et al: Oral anticoagulation management in primary care with the use of computerized decision support and near-patient testing: a randomized, controlled trial. Arch Intern Med 2000;160:2343-2348.
50. Wittkowsky AK, Nutescu EA, Blackburn J, et al: Outcomes of oral anticoagulant therapy managed by telephone vs in-office visits in an anticoagulation clinic setting. Chest 2006;130:1385-1389.
51. Beyth RJ, Quinn L, Landefeld CS: A multicomponent intervention to prevent major bleeding complications in older patients receiving warfarin: a randomized, controlled trial. Ann Intern Med 2000;133:687-695.
52. Menendez-Jandula B, Souto JC, Oliver A, et al: Comparing self managment of oral anticoagulant therapy with clinic management: a randomize trial. Ann Intern Med 2005;142:1-10.
53. Heneghan C, Onso-Coello P, Garcia-Alamino JM, et al: Self-monitoring of oral anticoagulation: a systematic review and meta-analysis. Lancet 2006;367:404-411.
54. Ansell JE: Is self-management of oral anticoagulation a feasible and safe option?. Nat Clin Pract Cardiovasc Med 2005;2:240-241.
55. Hylek EM, Skates SJ, Sheehan MA, Singer DE: An analysis of the lowest effective intensity of prophylactic anticoagulation for patients with nonrheumatic atrial fibrillation. N Engl J Med 1996;335:540-546.
56. Fleming HA: Anticoagulants in rheumatic heart-disease. Lancet 1971;2:486.
57. Petersen P, Boysen G, Godtfredsen J, et al: Placebo-controlled, randomised trial of warfarin and aspirin for prevention of thromboembolic complications in chronic atrial fibrillation: the Copenhagen AFASAK study. Lancet 1989;1:175-179.
58. Preliminary report of the Stroke Prevention in Atrial Fibrillation Study. N Engl J Med 1990;322:863-868.
59. Warfarin versus aspirin for prevention of thromboembolism in atrial fibrillation: Stroke Prevention in Atrial Fibrillation II Study. Lancet 1994;343:687-691.
60. Fatkin D, Kelly RP, Feneley MP: Relations between left atrial appendage blood flow velocity, spontaneous echocardiographic contrast and thromboembolic risk in vivo. J Am Coll Cardiol 1994;23:961-969.

61. Black IW, Hopkins AP, Lee LC, Walsh WF: Left atrial spontaneous echo contrast: a clinical and echocardiographic analysis. J Am Coll Cardiol 1991;18:398-404.
62. Bernhardt P, Schmidt H, Hammerstingl C, et al: Patients with atrial fibrillation and dense spontaneous echo contrast at high risk a prospective and serial follow-up over 12 months with transesophageal echocardiography and cerebral magnetic resonance imaging. J Am Coll Cardiol 2005;45:1807-1812.
63. de Bono DP, Warlow CP: Mitral-annulus calcification and cerebral or retinal ischaemia. Lancet 1979;2:383-385.
64. Fulkerson PK, Beaver BM, Auseon JC, Graber HL: Calcification of the mitral annulus: etiology, clinical associations, complications and therapy. Am J Med 1979;66:967-977.
65. Benjamin EJ, Plehn JF, D'Agostino RB, et al: Mitral annular calcification and the risk of storke in an elderly cohort. N Engl J Med 1992;327:374-379.
66. Hart RG, Easton JD: Mitral valve prolapse and cerebral infarction. Stroke 1982;13: 429-430.
67. Salem DN, Stein PD, Al Ahmad A, et al: Antithrombotic therapy in valvular heart disease—native and prosthetic: the Seventh ACCP Conference on Antithrombotic and Thrombolytic Therapy. Chest 2004;126(3 Suppl):457S-482S.
68. Tornos P, Almirante B, Mirabet S, et al: Infective endocarditis due to *Staphylococcus aureus*: deleterious effect of anticoagulant therapy. Arch Intern Med 1999;159: 473-475.
69. Wilson WR, Geraci JE, Danielson GK, et al: Anticoagulant therapy and central nervous system complications in patients with prosthetic valve endocarditis. Circulation 1978;57:1004-1007.
70. Leport C, Vilde JL, Bricaire F, et al: Fifty cases of late prosthetic valve endocarditis: improvement in prognosis over a 15 year period. Br Heart J 1987;58:66-71.
71. Delahaye JP, Poncet P, Malquarti V, et al: Cerebrovascular accidents in infective endocarditis: role of anticoagulation. Eur Heart J 1990;11:1074-1078.
72. Bonow RO, Cheitlin MD, Crawford MH, Douglas PS: Task Force 3: valvular heart disease. J Am Coll Cardiol 2005;45:1334-1340.
73. Recommended Adult Immunization Schedule—United States, October 2006–September 2007. MMWR Recomm Rep 2006;55:Q1-Q4.
74. Fremes SE, Goldman BS, Ivanov J, et al: Valvular surgery in the elderly. Circulation 1989;80(Suppl I):I77-I90.
75. Hendren WG, Nemec JJ, Lytle BW, et al: Mitral valve repair for ischemic mitral insufficiency. Ann Thorac Surg 1991;52:1246-1251.
76. Craver JM, Weintraub WS, Jones EL, et al: Predictors of mortality, complications, and length of stay in aortic valve replacement for aortic stenosis. Circulation 1988;78:I85-I90.
77. Freeman WK, Schaff HV, O'Brien PC, et al: Cardiac surgery in the octogenarian: perioperative outcome and clinical follow-up. J Am Coll Cardiol 1991;18:29-35.
78. Culliford AT, Galloway AC, Colvin SB, et al: Aortic valve replacement for aortic stenosis in persons aged 80 years and over. Am J Cardiol 1991;67:1256-1260.
79. Elayda MA, Hall RJ, Reul RM, et al: Aortic valve replacement in patients 80 years and older: operative risks and long-term results. Circulation 1993;88:II1-II16.
80. Moura LM, Ramos SF, Zamorano JL, et al: Rosuvastatin affecting aortic valve endothelium to slow the progression of aortic stenosis. J Am Coll Cardiol 2007;49:554-561.
81. Cowell SJ, Newby DE, Prescott RJ, et al: A randomized trial of intensive lipid-lowering therapy in calcific aortic stenosis. N Engl J Med 2005;352:2389-2397.
82. Rossebø AB, Pedersen TR, Boman K, Brudi P, Chambers JB, Egstrup K, Gerdts E, Gohlke-Bärwolf C, Holme I, Kesäniemi YA, Malbecq W, Nienaber CA, Ray S, Skjaerpe T, Wachtell K, Willenheimer R; SEAS Investigators. Intensive lipid lowering with simvastatin and ezetimibe in aortic stenosis. N Engl J Med. 2008;359:1343-56.
83. Chan KL, Teo K, Tam J, Dumesnil JG: Rationale, design, and baseline characteristics of a randomized trial to assess the effect of cholesterol lowering on the progression of aortic stenosis: the Aortic Stenosis Progression Observation: Measuring Effects of Rosuvastatin (ASTRONOMER) trial. Am Heart J 2007;153:925-931.
84. Otto CM: Timing of intervention in chronic valve regurgitation: the role of echocardiography. In: Otto CM (ed): The Practice of Clinical Echocardiography, 3rd ed. Philadelphia, Saunders-Elsevier, 2007:430-458.
85. Vahanian A, Baumgartner H, Bax J, et al: Guidelines on the management of valvular heart disease: The Task Force on the Management of Valvular Heart Disease of the European Society of Cardiology. Eur Heart J 2007;28:230-268.
86. Otto CM, Burwash IG, Legget ME, et al: A prospective study of asymptomatic valvular aortic stenosis: clinical, echocardiographic, and exercise predictors of outcome. Circulation 1997;95:2262-2270.
87. Douglas PS, Otto CM, Mickel MC, et al: Gender differences in left ventricular geometry and function in patients undergoing balloon dilation of the aortic valve for isolated aortic stenosis. Br Heart J 1995;73:548-554.
88. Villari B, Campbell SE, Hess OM, et al: Influence of collagen network on left ventricular systolic and diastolic function in aortic valve disease. J Am Coll Cardiol 1993;22:1477-1484.
89. Villari B, Campbell SE, Schneider J, et al: Sex-dependent differences in left ventricular function and structure in chronic pressure overload. Eur Heart J 1995;16:1410-1419.
90. Lund O, Nielsen TT, Pilegaard HK, et al: The influence of coronary artery disease and bypass grafting on early and late survival after valve replacement for aortic stenosis. J Thorac Cardiovasc Surg 1990;100:327-337.
91. Carabello BA: Timing of valve replacement in aortic stenosis: moving closer to perfection [editorial; comment]. Circulation 1997;95:2241-2243.
92. Pape LA, Price JM, Alpert JS, et al: Relation of left atrial size to pulmonary capillary wedge pressure in severe mitral regurgitation. Cardiology 1991;78:297-303.
93. Burwash IG, Blackmore GL, Koilpillai CJ: Usefulness of left atrial and left ventricular chamber sizes as predictors of the severity of mitral regurgitation. Am J Cardiol 1992;70:774-779.
94. Sanfilippo AJ, Abascal VM, Sheehan M, et al: Atrial enlargement as a consequence of atrial fibrillation: a prospective echocardiographic study. Circulation 1990;82: 792-797.
95. Deverall PB, Olley PM, Smith DR, et al: Incidence of systemic embolism before and after mitral valvotomy. Thorax 1968;23:530-536.
96. Arora R, Kalra GS, Murty GS, et al: Percutaneous transatrial mitral commissurotomy: immediate and intermediate results. J Am Coll Cardiol 1994;23:1327-1332.
97. Multicenter experience with balloon mitral commissurotomy. NHLBI Balloon Valvuloplasty Registry Report on immediate and 30-day follow-up results. The National Heart, Lung, and Blood Institute Balloon Valvuloplasty Registry Participants. Circulation 1992;85:448-461.
98. Tuzcu EM, Block PC, Griffin BP, et al: Immediate and long-term outcome of percutaneous mitral valvotomy in patients 65 years and older. Circulation 1992;85:963-971.
99. Braunwald E, Frahm CJ: Studies on Starling's law of the heart. IV. Observations on the hemodynamic functions of the left atrium in man. Circulation 1961;24:633.
100. Chua YL, Schaff HV, Orszulak TA, Morris JJ: Outcome of mitral valve repair in patients with preoperative atrial fibrillation: should the maze procedure be combined with mitral valvuloplasty?. J Thorac Cardiovasc Surg 1994;107:408-415.
101. Pan M, Medina A, Su'arez de Lezo J, et al: Factors determining late success after mitral balloon valvulotomy. Am J Cardiol 1993;71:1181-1185.
102. Vahanian A, Michel PL, Cormier B, et al: Immediate and mid-term results of percutaneous mitral commissurotomy. Eur Heart J 1991;12(Suppl B):84-89.
103. Tunick PA, Freedberg RS, Gargiulo A, Kronzon I: Exercise Doppler echocardiography as an aid to clinical decision making in mitral valve disease. J Am Soc Echocardiogr 1992;5:225-230.
104. Leavitt JI, Coats MH, Falk RH: Effects of exercise on transmitral gradient and pulmonary artery pressure in patients with mitral stenosis or a prosthetic mitral valve: a Doppler echocardiographic study. J Am Coll Cardiol 1991;17:1520-1526.
105. Richards AM, Nicholls MG, Ikram H, et al: Syncope in aortic valvular stenosis. Lancet 1984;2:1113-1116.
106. Johnson AM: Aortic stenosis, sudden death, and the left ventricular baroceptors. Br Heart J 1971;33:1-5.
107. Khot UN, Novaro GM, Popovic ZB, et al: Nitroprusside in critically ill patients with left ventricular dysfunction and aortic stenosis. N Engl J Med 2003;348:1756-1763.
108. Chockalingam A, Venkatesan S, Subramaniam T, et al: Safety and efficacy of angiotensin-converting enzyme inhibitors in symptomatic severe aortic stenosis: Symptomatic Cardiac Obstruction—Pilot Study of Enalapril in Aortic Stenosis (SCOPE-AS). Am Heart J 2004;147:E19.
109. Bermejo J, Antoranz JC, Burwash IG, et al: In-vivo analysis of the instantaneous transvalvular pressure difference-flow relationship in aortic valve stenosis: implications of unsteady fluid-dynamics for the clinical assessment of disease severity. J Heart Valve Dis 2002;11:557-566.
110. Burwash IG, Thomas DD, Sadahiro M, et al: Dependence of Gorlin formula and continuity equation valve areas on transvalvular volume flow rate in valvular aortic stenosis. Circulation 1994;89:827-835.
111. Zile MR, Gaasch WH: Heart failure in aortic stenosis—improving diagnosis and treatment. N Engl J Med 2003;348:1735-1736.
112. Chobanian AV, Bakris GL, Black HR, et al: The Seventh Report of the Joint National Committee on Prevention, Detection, Evaluation, and Treatment of High Blood Pressure: the JNC 7 report. JAMA 2003;289:2560-2572.
113. O'Brien KD, Zhao XQ, Shavelle DM, et al: Hemodynamic effects of the angiotensin-converting enzyme inhibitor, ramipril, in patients with mild to moderate aortic stenosis and preserved left ventricular function. J Investig Med 2004;52:185-191.
114. Routledge HC, Townend JN: ACE inhibition in aortic stenosis: dangerous medicine or golden opportunity?. J Hum Hypertens 2001;15:659-667.
115. Kadem L, Dumesnil JG, Rieu R, et al: Impact of systemic hypertension on the assessment of aortic stenosis. Heart 2005;91:354-361.
116. Otto CM: Valvular aortic stenosis: disease severity and timing of intervention. J Am Coll Cardiol 2006;47:2141-2151.
117. Bermejo J: The effects of hypertension on aortic valve stenosis. Heart 2005;91: 280-282.
118. Little SH, Chan KL, Burwash IG: Impact of blood pressure on the Doppler echocardiographic assessment of severity of aortic stenosis. Heart 2007;93:848-855.
119. Grundy SM, Pasternak R, Greenland P, et al: Assessment of cardiovascular risk by use of multiple-risk-factor assessment equations: a statement for healthcare professionals from the American Heart Association and the American College of Cardiology. Circulation 1999;100:1481-1492.
120. Julius BK, Spillmann M, Vassalli G, et al: Angina pectoris in patients with aortic stenosis and normal coronary arteries: mechanisms and pathophysiological concepts. Circulation 1997;95:892-898.
121. Kupari M, Virtanen KS, Turto H, et al: Exclusion of coronary artery disease by exercise thallium-201 tomography in patients with aortic stenosis. Am J Cardiol 1992;70:635-640.
122. Baroni M, Maffei S, Terrazzi M, et al: Mechanisms of regional ischaemic changes during dipyridamole echocardiography in patients with severe aortic valve stenosis and normal coronary arteries. Heart 1996;75:492-497.
123. Rask P, Karp KL, Eriksson MP, Moore T: Dipyridamole thallium-201 single photon emission tomography in aortic stenosis: gender differences. Eur J Nucl Med 1995;22:1155-1162.
124. Samuels B, Kiat H, Friedman JD, Berman DS: Adenosine pharmacologic stress myocardial perfusion tomographic imaging in patients with significant aortic stenosis: diagnostic efficacy and comparison of clinical, hemodynamic and electrocardiographic variable with 100 age-matched control subjects. J Am Coll Cardiol 1995;25:99-106.
125. Fuster V, Ryden LE, Asinger RW, et al: ACC/AHA/ESC Guidelines for the Management of Patients With Atrial Fibrillation: Executive Summary: a report of the American College of Cardiology/American Heart Association Task Force on Practice Guidelines and the European Society of Cardiology Committee for Practice Guidelines and Policy Conferences (Committee to Develop Guidelines for the Management of Patients With Atrial Fibrillation) developed in collaboration with the North American Society of Pacing and Electrophysiology. Circulation 2001;104:2118-2150.
126. Gillinov AM, Bakaeen F, McCarthy PM, et al: Surgery for paroxysmal atrial fibrillation in the setting of mitral valve disease: a role for pulmonary vein isolation?. Ann Thorac Surg 2006;81:19-26.

126

127. Gaita F, Riccardi R, Caponi D, et al: Linear cryoablation of the left atrium versus pulmonary vein cryoisolation in patients with permanent atrial fibrillation and valvular heart disease: correlation of electroanatomic mapping and long-term clinical results. Circulation 2005;111:136-142.

128. Doty JR, Doty DB, Jones KW, et al: Comparison of standard maze III and radiofrequency Maze operations for treatment of atrial fibrillation. J Thorac Cardiovasc Surg 2007;133:1037-1044.

129. Patel JJ, Dyer RB, Mitha AS: -Adrenergic blockade does not improve effort tolerance in patients with mitral stenosis in sinus rhythm. Eur Heart J 1995;16:1264-1268.

130. Ashcom TL, Johns JP, Bailey SR, Rubal BJ: Effects of chronic β-blockade on rest and exercise hemodynamics in mitral stenosis. Cathet Cardiovasc Diagn 1995;35:110-115.

131. Stoll BC, Ashcom TL, Johns JP, et al: Effects of atenolol on rest and exercise hemodynamics in patients with mitral stenosis. Am J Cardiol 1995;75:482-484.

132. al Kasab SM, Sabag T, al Zaibag M, et al: β-Adrenergic receptor blockade in the management of pregnant women with mitral stenosis. Am J Obstet Gynecol 1990;163:137-140.

133. Bonow RO, Rosing DR, McIntosh CL, et al: The natural history of asymptomatic patients with aortic regurgitation and normal left ventricular function. Circulation 1983;68:509-517.

134. Grigioni F, Enriquez-Sarano M, Ling LH, et al: Sudden death in mitral regurgitation due to flail leaflet. J Am Coll Cardiol 1999;34:2078-2085.

135. Fleisher LA, Beckman JA, Brown KA, et al: ACC/AHA 2006 guideline update on perioperative cardiovascular evaluation for noncardiac surgery: focused update on perioperative β-blocker therapy: a report of the American College of Cardiology/American Heart Association Task Force on Practice Guidelines (Writing Committee to Update the 2002 Guidelines on Perioperative Cardiovascular Evaluation for Noncardiac Surgery): developed in collaboration with the American Society of Echocardiography, American Society of Nuclear Cardiology, Heart Rhythm Society, Society of Cardiovascular Anesthesiologists, Society for Cardiovascular Angiography and Interventions, and Society for Vascular Medicine and Biology. Circulation 2006;113:2662-2674.

136. Rohde LE, Polanczyk CA, Goldman L, et al: Usefulness of transthoracic echocardiography as a tool for risk stratification of patients undergoing major noncardiac surgery. Am J Cardiol 2001;87:505-509.

137. Torsher LC, Shub C, Rettke SR, Brown DL: Risk of patients with severe aortic stenosis undergoing noncardiac surgery. Am J Cardiol 1998;81:448-452.

CHAPTER 9

Aortic Stenosis

Raphael Rosenhek and Helmut Baumgartner

KEY POINTS

- Aortic stenosis is the most frequent valvular heart disease in North America and Europe.
- Aortic stenosis is associated with high morbidity and mortality.
- Echocardiography is the key diagnostic tool for diagnosis, quantification of stenosis severity, and assessment of secondary changes.
- Aortic stenosis is a progressive disease, and the possibility of rapid hemodynamic progression needs to be considered.
- Symptomatic patients (dyspnea, angina, dizziness/syncope with exertion) require urgent surgery.
- A watchful waiting approach is generally safe in asymptomatic patients but should include regular echocardiographic and clinical examinations.
- Risk stratification is useful in asymptomatic patients. It should include measurement of calcification and hemodynamic progression and exercise testing in physically active patients. It permits identification of patients who may benefit from early elective surgery.
- So far, there is no established medical therapy for aortic stenosis.

PATHOPHYSIOLOGY

The primary determinant of disease severity in patients with valvular aortic stenosis is the degree of obstruction to left ventricular outflow. In addition, valve obstruction leads to secondary effects on the left ventricle, peripheral vasculature, and coronary artery blood flow that affect both the clinical presentation of disease and subsequent outcome.

Valvular Hemodynamics

Pressure Gradients

Obstruction at the aortic valve level results in an increased antegrade velocity across the narrowed valve corresponding to the systolic pressure gradient between the left ventricle and aorta (Figure 9-1). For any given transvalvular volume flow rate, both antegrade velocity and transaortic pressure gradient increase with increasing degrees of valvular narrowing. However, for any given valve area, the magnitude of increase in jet velocity and pressure gradient varies with the volume flow rate across the valve. Thus, patients with severe stenosis and a low stroke volume (e.g., with left ventricular systolic dysfunction) have only a moderate increase in antegrade velocity and systolic pressure gradient, whereas those with moderate stenosis and a high transaortic flow rate (e.g., with coexisting aortic regurgitation) have a high jet velocity and systolic pressure gradient.

The rate of rise and fall of the antegrade velocity and the timing of the pressure gradient across the valve also are related to disease severity. With mild stenosis, the maximum velocity and maximum pressure difference across the valve occur in early systole, before the peak volume flow rate across the valve, at a time point corresponding to the maximum rate of flow acceleration.[1,2] As stenosis becomes more severe, the maximum velocity and pressure difference occur later in systole, eventually coinciding with the maximum volume flow rate across the valve. In aortic stenosis, left ventricular pressure exceeds aortic pressure throughout most of systole, but the pressure gradient is reversed in late systole. In an animal model of aortic stenosis, the normalized time to pressure crossover was $93 \pm 13\%$ for a stenotic valve compared with $69 \pm 36\%$ for a normal aortic valve (Figure 9-2).[3] In addition to stenosis severity, the shape of the velocity curve and timing of the pressure gradient may be affected by other factors that alter left ventricular or aortic pressure, such as coexisting aortic regurgitation or an increased systemic vascular resistance.

The antegrade (or jet) velocity across the aortic valve usually is described in terms of the maximum instantaneous velocity, typically occurring in early systole to midsystole. The maximum instantaneous velocity corresponds to the maximum instantaneous pressure gradient across the valve as stated in the Bernoulli equation. Although theoretically more complicated, the relationship can be simplified for most clinical applications so that the pressure gradient is equal to the velocity squared multiplied by 4 (i.e., "simplified Bernoulli equation").[3-6] At cardiac catheterization, the difference between peak left ventricular and peak aortic

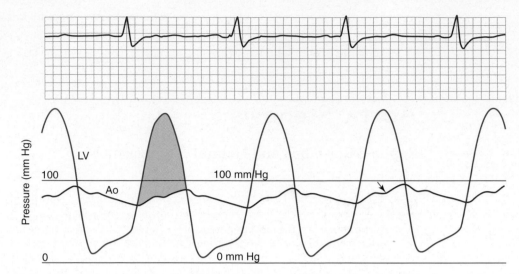

FIGURE 9–1 Left ventricular and aortic pressure tracings in a 47-year-old man with a congenitally bicuspid valve and new onset of congestive heart failure symptoms. The peak-to-peak pressure gradient is 100 mmHg with a mean transaortic pressure gradient of 62 mmHg. Aortic valve area, calculated by the continuity equation, is 0.5 cm². Note the marked delay and decrease in the aortic pressure waveform upstroke.

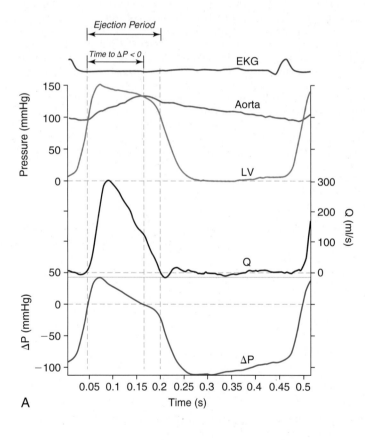

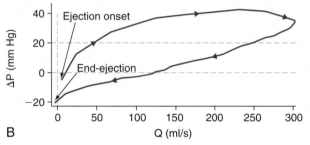

FIGURE 9–2 (**A**) Simultaneous instantaneous tracings of the electrocardiogram (EKG), aortic and left ventricular (LV) pressure, transvalvular volume flow rate (Q) and transvalvular pressures gradient (ΔP) are plotted against time in an animal model of aortic valve stenosis. The LV ejection period occurs between the onset of aortic flow (simultaneous to LV-aortic pressure crossover) until transaortic Q returns to zero. During late ejection, ΔP is negative. The time of ΔP reversal is shown and, normalized to the duration of the ejection period, is 73% for this beat. (**B**) Phase diagram of ΔP-Q for the same beat to demonstrate the nonlinearity and time dependence of the ΔP-Q relationship. (*From Bermejo J, Antoranz JC, Burwash IG, et al: In-vivo analysis of the instantaneous transvalvular pressure difference-flow relationship in aortic valve stenosis: implications of unsteady fluid-dynamics for the clinical assessment of disease severity. J Heart Valve Dis 2002;11:557-566, with permission.*)

pressures (the peak-to-peak gradient) often is reported. Because the peak left ventricular and aortic pressures usually are not simultaneous, the difference between these two pressures is not a physiologic measurement and does not correspond to the maximum or any other instantaneous Doppler velocity.

Mean transaortic pressure gradients can be derived from Doppler data or invasive pressure recordings by averaging the instantaneous pressure gradients over the systolic ejection period. In adults with valvular aortic stenosis, maximum and mean pressure gradients are linearly related, with a close correlation.[7,8] However, the relationship between maximum and mean gradient depends on the shape of the velocity curve, which varies with stenosis severity and flow rate. Thus, digitizing the pressure or velocity curve with calculation of the mean gradient is most precise. This can easily be done by computer-assisted quantitation packages integrated into current echocardiography instruments. Measurement of mean transaortic gradient correlates well by invasive and noninvasive assessment and is useful for clinical decision making.

The phenomenon of pressure recovery distal to the stenotic valve contributes to some of the confusion surrounding comparisons of invasive and noninvasive transaortic gradients because Doppler velocities reflect the pressure drop in the orifice itself, whereas catheter pressure data may include pressure recovery distal to the orifice, depending on the exact location of the catheter relative to the stenotic orifice.[9-11] The geometry of the flow obstruction in aortic stenosis with its abrupt widening from the stenotic orifice to a comparatively large ascending aorta causes extensive turbulence with dissipation of kinetic energy into heat. This turbulence precludes the occurrence of pressure recovery of a clinically relevant magnitude in the majority of patients. Only in the case of a small aorta with a favorable orifice to cross-sectional aortic area ratio, which reduces the degree of turbulence, will pressure recovery reach a magnitude that causes clinically relevant differences between the Doppler gradient (pressure drop from ventricle to vena contracta) and net pressure gradient (drop from ventricular to distal, recovered pressure).[9,11] In the clinical setting, this situation becomes likely when the aortic root diameter is smaller than 3 cm.[11,12] With significant pressure recovery, the Doppler gradient overestimates the pathophysiologic consequence of a stenosis. In this case less proximal pressure and, respectively, workload are required to maintain an adequate peripheral pressure compared with a clinical setting with the same Doppler gradient but no pressure recovery.

In vitro data indicate that the recovered pressure drop is directly related to the energy loss that determines ventricular pump work, and it has been suggested that energy loss may be a better measure of stenosis severity than the gradient across the orifice.[13,14] The calculation of energy loss includes both the transvalvular pressure gradient and the ratio of effective orifice area to aortic root dimension.[14]

Valve Area

Aortic valve area is defined as the extent of aortic valve opening in systole and provides a clinically useful measure of stenosis severity that is less dependent on volume flow rate than pressure gradients. Valve area can be calculated from Doppler data using the continuity equation based on the principle that the volume flow rates are equal just proximal to and in the stenotic orifice.[15-18] Aortic valve area is calculated from determination of the stroke volume just proximal to the valve, based on measurement of left ventricular outflow tract diameter and velocity, divided by the velocity-time integral of maximum aortic jet velocity (Figure 9-3). Valve area also can be calculated at cardiac catheterization, using the Gorlin equation, based on measurement of transaortic volume flow rate and mean systolic pressure gradient across the valve.[19-23]

There has been considerable controversy regarding the relative accuracy of Doppler continuity and catheterization Gorlin formula valve areas calculations. In addition to technical differences between invasive and Doppler measures of valve area and the potential sources of error in each approach, these approaches differ in that Doppler valve areas represent the physiologic orifice area, also called effective orifice area (the narrowest cross-sectional area of flow, i.e., the vena contracta), whereas Gorlin formula valve areas represent the anatomic or geometric orifice area (see Chapter 6).[24,25] Depending on stenosis morphology, which determines the magnitude of flow contraction, the effective orifice area is only 70% to 90% of the geometric area.[26] Nevertheless, both valve area measurements reflect the same basic underlying physiologic parameter, and both provide useful data for clinical decision making when performed correctly. However, it has to be taken into account that valve area must decrease markedly to less than 2 cm^2 before it causes hemodynamic consequences with occurrence of a pressure drop (gradient). When the valve area decreases toward 1 cm^2 and below, very small changes in orifice area cause marked changes in gradient and hemodynamic burden. In considering

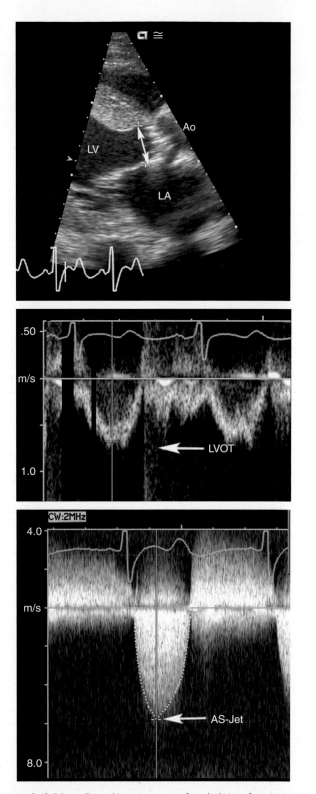

FIGURE 9-3 Echocardiographic measurements for calculation of continuity equation valve area. *Top,* parasternal long axis view for measurement of left ventricular outflow tract diameter (*arrow*). *Middle,* left ventricular outflow velocity recorded from an apical view with the pulsed Doppler sample volume positioned just proximal to the stenotic aortic valve. *Bottom,* continuous wave Doppler recording of the aortic stenosis jet from an apical approach showing a maximum velocity of 5.2 m/s. Continuity equation aortic valve area is 0.9 cm^2. Ao, aorta; AS, aortic stenosis; LA, left atrium; LV, left ventricle; LVOT, left ventricle outflow tract.

the required precision, neither Doppler echocardiography nor catheterization is accurate enough to produce a calculated valve area number that can be relied on by itself for clinical decisions. Thus, final judgment of stenosis severity should always be based on velocity and gradient, as well as valve area, with additional consideration of the given flow state.

Although less flow-dependent than pressure gradients, aortic valve area also varies with transaortic volume flow rate, especially in patients with calcific stenosis.[27-30] The unfused commissures allow variation in the degree of valve opening, depending on the interaction between the stiffness of the cusps and the force directed against the valve in systole.[23,31-36] The variable opening of stiff aortic valve leaflets is not surprising given the common echocardiographic observation in patients with dilated cardiomyopathy that changes in flow rate are associated with changes in the extent of aortic cusp opening, even in the absence of leaflet thickening. With aortic valve stenosis the increase in left ventricular outflow velocity with exercise may result in an increase in the extent of valve opening if the leaflets still have some degree of flexibility. Initial concerns that the observed increase was related to the mathematical assumptions of the calculations or to changes in the fluid dynamics across the valve have been resolved by direct observation of valve opening[37] so that most investigators now concur that leaflet opening varies with flow rate. With disease progression, the gradual increase in the degree of leaflet thickening and calcification eventually reaches a point at which valve area is fixed over the physiologic range of force that can be generated by the left ventricle.

The time course of valve opening or the rate of change in valve area during a single cardiac cycle reflects valve stiffness, inertia, and elasticity.[38] Stenotic aortic valves open and close more slowly than normal valves,[39] and the rate of change in valve area during systole is a predictor of clinical outcome.[40]

Flow dependence of the valve area becomes particularly important in the presence of low cardiac output; most frequently due to left ventricular dysfunction. Reduced opening forces may then cause a mildly or moderately stenotic valve to open to a valve area less than 1cm². The term *pseudosevere stenosis* has been proposed for this condition.[41,42] The transvalvular gradient is typically low (mean gradient <30 to 40 mmHg) in this situation (low-flow, low-gradient aortic stenosis). Although many patients with reduced left ventricular function in a late stage of severe aortic stenosis (afterload mismatch, see below) maintain a surprisingly high gradient (>40 mmHg mean gradient),[43] some of them may also present with low gradients just because of severe flow reduction. Low-dose dobutamine can be used during echocardiography to stimulate myocardial contraction and increase flow rate. With increasing flow one would assume that valve area increases with little change in gradient in the presence of pseudosevere stenosis, whereas primarily velocity and gradient should increase with less change in valve area when there is fixed severe stenosis.[42] The test, of course, requires that there is indeed contractile reserve.

In addition to flow-related changes in geometric orifice area, it has been suggested that effective orifice area may increase with flow even without changes in anatomic area.[44] At normal flow rates, the kinetic energy of the fluid crossing the obstruction is sufficient to break down the vortex structures generated downstream from the stenosis and thus enables the formation of a large and well-established flow jet. However, at low flow rates, the reduction in kinetic energy may predispose to the formation of vortices, which tend then to squeeze the flow jet and thus the vena contracta, resulting in a smaller effective orifice.[44] The phenomenon is certainly less important in the presence of very small orifices but may become clinically relevant in moderately severe low-flow aortic stenosis. These findings once more emphasize that clinical judgment should not only rely on the absolute value of calculated valve area but also take into account all available hemodynamic and morphologic information.[45]

Other Indices of Stenosis Severity

Some investigators have explored the concept of valve resistance as a measure of aortic stenosis severity.[36,46,47] Because valve resistance is calculated as the simple ratio of pressure gradient to flow across the valve, the underlying assumption of this approach is that there is a linear relationship between pressure gradient and transvalvular flow rate. This assumption is inconsistent with the Bernoulli equation, which assumes a quadratic relationship between pressure gradient and flow rate. Although some disagreement persists as to the exact relationship between pressure and flow across a stenotic valve; in fact, careful fluid dynamic studies support the concept of a quadratic relationship.[48] Although experimental studies suggest that valve resistance provides better discrimination of the degree of valve stiffness for valves 100 to 200 times stiffer than normal, in the clinical setting, disease progression and symptoms occur in the range of valve stiffness from 20 to 100 times normal, a range in which valve area provides better quantitation of disease severity.[49] Valve resistance has also been proposed for the evaluation of low-flow, low-gradient aortic stenosis, arguing that it was less flow dependent.[46] However, this concept is not supported by fluid dynamics theory, experimental studies, or clinical observation.[34,48,50] These studies convincingly demonstrated that valve resistance has no advantages compared with valve area with regard to flow dependence. In fact, valve resistance may obscure actual changes in valve area because resistance changes only slightly despite significant changes in valve area with increasing flow rate, making resistance even less useful for the evaluation of aortic stenosis. As a matter of fact, an increase in flow must necessarily result in an increase in resistance unless it is compensated for by a concomitant increase in effective valve area.[11,50] In addition, the calculation of valve "resistance" has no clear advantages over jet velocities, pressure gradients, and valve areas in predicting clinical outcome.[51,52]

Compared with mitral stenosis, the fluid dynamics of aortic stenosis are more complex in that the pressure gradient and volume flow rate across the valve depend on the force of left ventricular contraction as well as on the characteristics of the valve itself. Thus, another approach to describing aortic stenosis severity is to estimate the total work performed by the ventricle in opening the aortic valve. In concept, total left ventricular stroke work is calculated as the integral of flow times pressure. Effective stroke work (aortic pressure times flow) then is subtracted to yield the stroke work "lost" across the valve.[53,54] Although left ventricular stroke work loss does correlate with other measures of stenosis severity, it also varies with flow rate (even when normalized for stroke volume), is an unfamiliar concept for most physicians, and offers no obvious clinical advantages. In addition, the calculation of stroke work loss mainly accounts for the potential energy components of total work, whereas kinetic energy losses, which are more difficult to estimate, may be even more important in valvular aortic stenosis.[34]

Because aortic valve hemodynamics depend on aortic valve anatomy, left ventricular mechanics, and the characteristics of the vascular system downstream from the valve, a complete description of aortic stenosis severity would include all three of these components. Obviously, this type of descriptor is conceptually complex and may be difficult to derive in the clinical setting. A step toward an integrated descriptor of aortic stenosis severity is the concept of ventricular-vascular coupling with the inclusion of components to describe the effect of the abnormal valve in the system.[55] Preliminary studies in this area are of interest but are not yet clinically applicable.

Left Ventricular Pressure Overload

The basic response of the left ventricle to the chronic and gradually progressive pressure overload of valvular aortic stenosis is concentric hypertrophy. However, not all patients develop hypertrophy, even with severe stenosis, and there are significant gender differences in the degree and pattern of hypertrophy.[56-59] In pathophysiologic terms, the increase in wall thickness occurs as a mechanism to maintain normal wall stress as left ventricular pressure rises (see Chapter 4). Typically, contractility is normal, and ejection fraction is preserved until late in the disease course. However, even when contractility is normal, left ventricular systolic performance may appear to be impaired in patients with severe outflow obstruction for at least three reasons. First, ejection fraction may decline because of the excessive increase in afterload, often termed *afterload mismatch*. Second, ventricular preload may be shifted to the left on the Starling curve because of a small, hypertrophied, noncompliant ventricle. Third, the temporal sequence of myocardial contraction often is asynchronous in pressure overload hypertrophy with an "uncoordinated" ventricular contraction. The resultant fall in the peak rate of circumferential shortening correlates with an increase in systolic wall stress.[60] This pattern of discordant contraction and the apparent decrease in ventricular function resolves after relief of aortic stenosis.

When left ventricular mass measurements are normalized for body size and gender, hypertrophy is seen in 54% of men and 81% of women with aortic stenosis.[57] The pattern of hypertrophy in women with aortic stenosis is characterized by a small ventricular chamber with increased wall thickness, normal or hypercontractile systolic function, and early diastolic dysfunction.[56-59,61] In men with aortic stenosis, the more common pattern is a normal or only mildly increased wall thickness and impaired systolic function.

Diastolic dysfunction occurs early in the disease course of aortic stenosis[62] in association with an increase in the total collagen volume of the myocardium and an increase in the orthogonal collagen fiber network.[63] As for ventricular hypertrophy, significant gender differences in diastolic function are seen. Specifically, men have a higher constant of myocardial stiffness in association with a greater degree of endocardial fibrosis and an abnormal myocardial collagen pattern.[61] Age also affects the severity of diastolic dysfunction with more severe left ventricular hypertrophy and diastolic dysfunction seen in elderly patients (older than 65 years).[64]

The Peripheral and Pulmonary Vasculature

In patients with aortic stenosis, the need to correct for peripheral amplification, if femoral artery rather than central aortic pressures are used for invasive calculation of valve area, has long been recognized.[65] However, there are few data on the influence of systemic factors on valve or ventricular function in these patients. Whereas left ventricular afterload is predominantly affected by the severity of obstruction at the valvular level, both factors internal to the left ventricle and characteristics of the systemic vascular circuit also contribute to total afterload.[55] To date, few studies have evaluated the impact of systemic vascular resistance (or impedance), wave reflections, or aortic elastance on the hemodynamics of valvular aortic stenosis.

Mild pulmonary hypertension is common in patients with isolated aortic stenosis when patients are followed prospectively.[52] In a series of 388 symptomatic patients with isolated aortic stenosis, mild pulmonary hypertension was present in 35%, moderate in 50%, and severe (systolic pressure > 50 mm Hg) in 15%.[66] In addition, a higher prevalence of moderate to severe pulmonary hypertension (as high as 71% of patients) has been noted in some surgical series.[67] The degree of pulmonary hypertension correlates with left ventricular end-diastolic pressure, but not with the severity of aortic stenosis or left ventricular ejection fraction.[66] The presence of pulmonary hypertension is a risk factor for cardiac surgery,[68] but pulmonary pressures usually return to normal after valve replacement for aortic stenosis, even when severely elevated.[67,69]

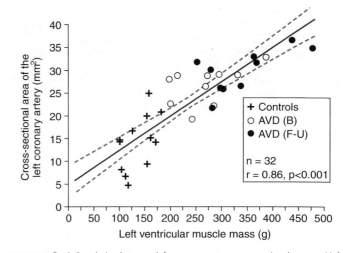

FIGURE 9–4 Correlation between left coronary artery cross-sectional area and left ventricular mass in 12 control subjects and 10 patients with aortic valve disease (AVD) at baseline (B) and follow-up (F-U). *(From Villari B, Hess OM, Moccetti D, et al: Effect of progression of left ventricular hypertrophy on coronary artery dimensions in aortic valve disease. J Am Coll Cardiol 1992;20: 1073-1079, with permission.)*

Coronary Blood Flow

Abnormalities in coronary blood flow, even in the absence of significant coronary atherosclerosis, contribute to the clinical presentation and long-term outcome of patients with valvular aortic stenosis. Although coronary artery size and thus blood flow are increased in patients with aortic stenosis, the increase in coronary artery size often is inadequate for the increase in muscle mass and, in addition, coronary flow reserve is limited (Figure 9-4).[70-73] Coronary flow reserve is most impaired in the subendocardium with the severity of impairment related to aortic stenosis severity.[74] After aortic valve replacement, coronary flow reserve improves in conjunction with regression of left ventricular hypertrophy.[75] Left ventricular hypertrophy also is associated with decreased capillary density and increased diffusion distances.[76] Other factors that may affect coronary blood flow in patients with aortic stenosis include decreased diastolic perfusion time, impaired early diastolic relaxation, and increased diastolic wall stresses, all leading to a reduction in subendocardial blood flow.[77]

Transthoracic echocardiographic evaluation of phasic coronary blood flow in adults with aortic stenosis shows reversal of early systolic flow and delayed forward flow in diastole with resolution of both these abnormalities after aortic valve replacement.[78] These findings were further elucidated in both transthoracic and transesophageal echocardiographic studies, which showed that systolic coronary flow decreases in inverse relationship to the increase in left ventricular wall stress, whereas diastolic flow increases in direct relationship to the transaortic pressure gradient, with these changes being particularly marked in symptomatic patients.[79,80] Coronary flow, measured by an intracoronary Doppler flow catheter, also shows retrograde systolic flow at rest, which correlates with the peak transaortic pressure gradient.[81] With stress induced by pacing and/or dobutamine, retrograde systolic flow increases, total systolic flow decreases, and forward diastolic flow increases, compared with values in normal control subjects in whom both systolic and diastolic flow increased proportionately.[81] These data suggest that an inadequate increase in total coronary blood flow in response to stress may contribute to the clinical presentation of aortic stenosis, specifically the symptom of angina in patients with normal coronary arteries.

A further imbalance in myocardial oxygen demand and supply occurs late in the disease course as left ventricular wall stress (and oxygen demands) increases out of proportion to the increase in coronary blood flow.[82] Angina, in the absence of

132 coexisting coronary artery disease, is associated with increased left ventricular wall stress due to inadequate hypertrophy in conjunction with increased ventricular systolic pressures.[76] This increase in wall stress leads to an increase in myocardial oxygen consumption. The combination of increased myocardial oxygen demand and limited coronary blood flow leads to myocardial ischemia and symptoms of coronary insufficiency.

Exercise Physiology

Even asymptomatic patients with aortic stenosis have a slight decrease in exercise tolerance compared with normative age standards. The hemodynamic response to exercise is characterized by a normal increase in heart rate to age-predicted maximums, but only a 50% increase in cardiac output. The increase in cardiac output is mediated by an increase in heart rate as stroke volume is unchanged or decreases slightly with upright exercise.[28,29,34,35,53,83] Although total stroke volume does not increase, there is an increase in the maximum instantaneous and mean systolic flow rates across the aortic valve because the systolic ejection period shortens owing to the increase in heart rate (Figure 9-5). Transaortic velocity, maximum gradient, and mean gradient increase as the flow rate increases, although the degree of increase often is less than predicted by the resting valve area.[28,29,35,36,84]

Measures of left ventricular diastolic function also are abnormal with exercise in adults with aortic stenosis. Based on micromanometer pressure recordings, resting diastolic pressures are elevated, diastolic pressures increase further with exercise, and both the rate of diastolic pressure decay and the isovolumic contraction interval fail to decrease with exercise, compared with values in normal control subjects.[85]

With exercise, valve area increases, on average by 0.2 cm², accounting for the smaller increase in jet velocity and gradient than expected for resting valve area (Figure 9-6).[28,29,35] The increase in valve area with exercise allows ejection of a relatively normal stroke volume across the valve and an appropriate increase in cardiac output. As the disease becomes more severe and the leaflets become more rigid and stiff, the degree of valve opening is progressively limited, resulting in a decrease in transaortic stroke volume and a failure of cardiac output to increase adequately with exercise.[29,34]

The increase in valve stiffness at adequate cardiac output results in a higher increase in gradient with exercise, which has been shown to be a predictor in outcome.[86]

CLINICAL PRESENTATION

Clinical History

Valvular aortic stenosis is a gradually progressive disease, and patients remain asymptomatic for many years.[87-91] Aortic stenosis typically is first diagnosed based on the finding of a systolic murmur on auscultation. Because the increase in hemodynamic severity occurs slowly, many patients fail to recognize early symptoms, emphasizing the importance of patient education in medical management, including a discussion of the classic symptoms of aortic stenosis (e.g., heart failure, angina, and syncope). In addition, the clinician must carefully question the patient to elicit symptoms, specifically asking the patient to compare current activity levels with activities at a set time point in the past. In particular, older patients often unconsciously tend to avoid activities that may cause symptoms and then still describe themselves as asymptomatic.

The most common initial symptom of valvular aortic stenosis is decreased exercise tolerance due to exertional dyspnea or fatigue.[52,92] The mechanism of this symptom most often is an elevated left ventricular end-diastolic pressure due to a noncompliant, hypertrophied ventricle.[93] Exercise intolerance also may be due to left ventricular systolic dysfunction or coexisting coronary artery disease in some patients. Over time, exertional dyspnea may progress to frank heart failure with resting symptoms seen with long-standing severe valvular obstruction. Some patients present with the sudden onset of heart failure or pulmonary edema, often related to an acute infectious process, anemia, or other hemodynamic stress or to new onset atrial fibrillation.

Exertional angina also is a common initial symptom in adults with valvular aortic stenosis due to an increase in oxygen demand by the hypertrophied myocardium, even in the absence of coexisting epicardial coronary artery disease.[52,92] Again, angina may be precipitated by other hemodynamic stresses, such as pregnancy, anemia, or a febrile disease.

The third classic symptom of aortic stenosis is exertional lightheadedness or syncope. Several potential mechanisms of syncope in aortic stenosis have been proposed including ventricular arrhythmias and left ventricular systolic dysfunction, but the most likely mechanism is an acute drop in blood pressure due to an inappropriate left ventricular baroreceptor response.[94-96] The elevated ventricular pressure activates baroreceptors, which mediate peripheral vasodilation.

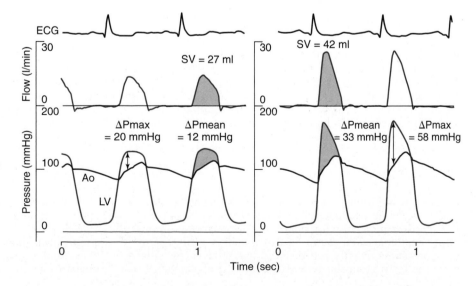

FIGURE 9–5 Hemodynamic recordings at two different volume flow rates in an animal model of valvular aortic stenosis. The electrocardiogram (ECG) recording is displayed on top, instantaneous volume flow rate in the middle, and left ventricular (LV) and aortic (Ao) pressures at the bottom. ΔPmax indicates maximum instantaneous pressure gradient; ΔPmean, mean pressure gradient; SV, stroke volume. *(From Burwash IG, Thomas DD, Sadahiro M, et al: Dependence of Gorlin formula and continuity equation valve areas on transvalvular volume flow rate in valvular aortic stenosis. Circulation 1994;89:827-835, with permission.)*

9

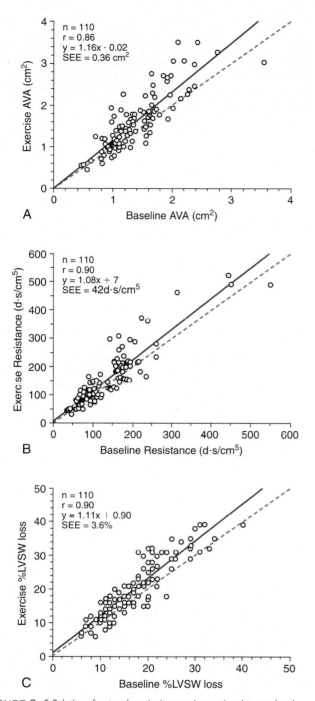

FIGURE 9–6 Relation of rest and continuity equation aortic valve area (*top*), aortic valve resistance (*middle*), and percent left ventricular stroke work loss (*bottom*) in 110 exercise studies in adults with asymptomatic valvular aortic stenosis. The slopes of the regression lines (*solid line*) are greater than the slope of the line of identity (*dashed line*), demonstrating an increase in all three indices with exercise. AVA, aortic valve area; LVSW, left ventricular stroke work. (*From Burwash IG, Pearlman AS, Kraft CD, et al: Flow dependence of measures of aortic stenosis severity during exercise. J Am Coll Cardiol 1994;24:1342-1350, with permission.*)

In the setting of a restricted aortic orifice, cardiac output fails to rise so that blood pressure falls, and the patient loses consciousness.

Physical Examination

The key features in the physical examination of patients with suspected aortic stenosis are palpation of the carotid pulse contour and amplitude; auscultation of the location, loudness, timing, and radiation of the systolic murmur; assessment of

the splitting of the second heart sound, and examination for signs of heart failure.[97,98]

The timing and amplitude of the carotid pulse contour reflect central aortic pressure. As aortic stenosis becomes more severe, the peak aortic pressure occurs later in systole (pulsus tardus) and the pulse amplitude is decreased (pulsus parvus). Both the timing and amplitude of the carotid pulse correlate with aortic stenosis severity.[99,100] However, the pulse contour is affected by factors other than stenosis severity, particularly in adult patients.[101] The pulse amplitude may be diminished with a reduced cardiac output and only mild to moderate stenosis due to the low volume flow rate into the aorta, although the timing of the impulse typically is normal in this situation. Conversely, the pulse amplitude and timing may appear to be normal with coexisting atherosclerosis as the stiff vessels lead to a rapid and excessive rise in aortic pressure even when severe stenosis is present. Thus, a slow-rising, low-amplitude carotid pulse has a relatively high specificity for the diagnosis of severe valvular obstruction. However, sensitivity is poor and severe stenosis cannot be excluded in adults with an apparently normal carotid upstroke.

The systolic murmur of aortic stenosis most often is loudest at the base, over the right second intercostal space. In general, the loudness of the murmur correlates with jet velocity or pressure gradient.[100,102,103] The presence of systolic thrill in the aortic region (i.e., a grade IV murmur) is highly specific for severe valvular obstruction. Conversely, severe stenosis is unlikely with a grade 1 murmur. Unfortunately, there is considerable overlap in disease severity with intermediate murmur grades (II-III) so that further evaluation is needed, depending on the clinical setting.[92,100] Besides the systolic pressure gradient across the valve, the loudness of the murmur is modulated by the volume flow rate across the valve, transmission of the murmur to the chest wall, and direction of the turbulent jet. Thus, even with severe stenosis the murmur may be soft if cardiac output is low or if obesity or lung disease diminishes its transmission to the chest wall.

The murmur of aortic stenosis radiates to the carotid arteries in the majority of patients as the turbulent jet is directed superiorly into the ascending aorta, allowing transmission of sound through the aorta to the carotid arteries. In a minority of patients, the murmur radiates to the apex, a pattern referred to as the Gallavardin phenomenon.[104]

The murmur of aortic stenosis has a crescendo-decrescendo pattern of amplitude corresponding to the shape of the pressure difference between the left ventricle and aortic during the ejection period. As stenosis becomes more severe, the maximum instantaneous gradient occurs later in systole so that a late-peaking murmur is recognized on auscultation. Conditions that are associated with a high transaortic volume flow rate such as aortic regurgitation may lead to early peaking of the murmur. Thus, whereas a late peaking murmur is quite specific for the presence of severe stenosis, sensitivity is low.

The second heart sound in severe aortic stenosis typically is single as the aortic component is inaudible because of the impaired motion of the thickened valve leaflets. Earlier in the disease course, the second heart sound may show reversed splitting with respiration due to a prolonged left ventricular ejection time.

An S4 gallop may be recognized in many patients with aortic stenosis, reflecting an increased atrial contribution to ventricular filling.[105] Other physical examination findings in patients with aortic stenosis depend on whether hemodynamic decompensation has occurred, leading to typical signs of heart failure.

Chest Radiography and Electrocardiography

The chest radiograph may be entirely normal in patients with valvular aortic stenosis, although dilation of the ascending aorta may be seen in some patients, even early in the disease

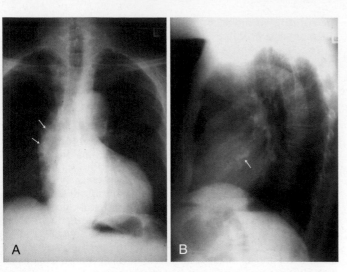

9

FIGURE 9–7 A, Chest radiograph in an adult with valvular aortic stenosis showing a normal cardiac silhouette with mild dilation of the ascending aorta (double arrow). **B,** In the lateral view, calcification of the aortic valve is seen (arrow).

course. Such aortic dilation has previously been called "post-stenotic." However, it is not related to hemodynamic severity and seems to be caused by intrinsic abnormalities of the aortic wall rather than by the stenosis itself, particularly in patients with bicuspid valves.[106] The cardiac silhouette typically is normal because left ventricular hypertrophy due to increased wall thickness with a normal chamber dimension is not evident on a standard chest film (Figure 9-7). Calcification of the aortic valve rarely is evident on chest radiography but may be seen using fluoroscopy in a high percentage of patients with severe valvular obstruction.[107] Mitral annular calcification, which often accompanies degenerative aortic valve disease, also may be seen. With long-standing disease, left ventricular dilation and signs of heart failure are present. Radiographic findings of pulmonary hypertension also may be evident late in the disease course.

The classic electrocardiographic finding in aortic stenosis is left ventricular hypertrophy. However, many adults and children with severe aortic stenosis do not have electrocardiographic criteria for left ventricular hypertrophy.[108,109] Other nonspecific electrocardiographic changes in adults with aortic stenosis include left atrial enlargement, left axis deviation, and left bundle branch block. Although early studies suggested that T-wave changes correlated with the degree of aortic stenosis, this finding has not been reliable in clinical practice.[110,111]

Electrocardiographic changes with exercise, specifically ST depression, are common in adults with aortic stenosis. Significant (>1 mm) flat or downsloping ST depression is observed in about two thirds of patients, even with only mild to moderate valve obstruction. Even when the resting electrocardiograph is normal, half of the patients still have ST depression with exercise. The presence or severity of ST changes with exercise in adults with aortic stenosis does not correlate with the presence or absence of epicardial coronary artery disease.[52]

Echocardiography

The standard echocardiographic evaluation of a patient with known or suspected aortic stenosis includes assessment of stenosis severity, the degree of coexisting aortic regurgitation, left ventricular size and function, estimation of pulmonary pressures, and identification of any other cardiac abnormalities.[52] With an experienced examiner, diagnostic data are obtained on transthoracic examination in nearly all (>99%) patients even when ultrasound tissue penetration is poor. Transesophageal imaging rarely is needed and can be misleading because of the inability to align the Doppler beam parallel to the aortic jet. Transesophageal imaging does allow two-dimensional planimetry of the valve area[31,112-114] which can be useful in the operating room. Care is needed with the use of this approach, given the nonplanarity and irregular stellate shape of the orifice and the reverberations and shadowing due to valve calcification.[115] Because of these limitations transesophageal imaging with planimetry of the valve area is currently not recommended as the first-line diagnostic method for the assessment of aortic stenosis severity. It has to be kept in mind that flow markedly contracts, in particular in the case of abrupt narrowing, which is generally the case in calcific aortic stenosis, so that planimetered valve area will be significantly larger than the functional (effective) orifice area.[26] Depending on individual stenosis morphology, effective orifice area will only be 70% to 90% of the anatomic orifice.

The most clinically useful measures of stenosis severity are maximum aortic jet velocity, mean pressure gradient (highly flow dependent), and continuity equation valve area (less flow dependent). For more details see Valvular Hemodynamics above. As discussed in Chapter 5, accurate Doppler data acquisition in patients with aortic stenosis requires trained and experienced sonographers and physicians with meticulous attention to the technical details of imaging and Doppler flow recording. A suboptimal examination may lead to underestimation of stenosis severity resulting from failure to obtain a parallel intercept angle between the continuous wave Doppler beam and the high-velocity aortic jet or less frequently due to erroneous recording of the outflow tract velocity. Conversely, stenosis severity may be overestimated owing to erroneous recording of the mitral regurgitation velocity, failure to account for increased subvalvular velocity (i.e., >1 m/s) in the Bernoulli equation or selection of nonrepresentative velocity recordings in the presence of arrhythmias (post-extrasystolic beat, after short/long RR interval in atrial fibrillation). Doppler gradients also may be misleading in the presence of an aorta smaller than 30 mm in diameter due to pressure recovery.[11,12] Doppler gradients measure the conversion of pressure to kinetic energy induced by the stenosis. When significant pressure recovery is present, the overall energy loss (i.e., net pressure decrease measured after pressure recovery), which determines the left ventricular pressure required to maintain a given systemic pressure and therefore the actual hemodynamic burden, is significantly overestimated by the Doppler measurement.

Calculation of valve area by the continuity equation also has limitations. The outflow tract velocity used in the equation may not be representative for the entire cross-section or may not be measured at the same site where cross-sectional area is calculated. The latter is usually derived from the outflow tract diameter, assuming a circular shape. However, the outflow tract is usually oval in shape, which causes some underestimation of the area and consequently of flow and valve area.[116] In addition, anatomic valve area and effective orifice area, are somewhat flow dependent (see Valvular Hemodynamics above). Despite these potential limitations, the validity and accuracy of Doppler measures of aortic stenosis severity for clinical purposes are well established both in comparison to catheterization data[5,6,117-121] and in terms of clinical outcome.[8,52] Nevertheless, it has to be emphasized that the above-mentioned limitations must be kept in mind in clinical practice and that careful consideration of all three measurements in conjunction with other findings such as valve morphology and left ventricular function should be the basis for the final judgment of stenosis severity that will guide clinical management.

Several other echocardiographic measures of stenosis severity have been proposed but have not gained widespread clinical acceptance, and none have been shown to have incremental diagnostic value in predicting patient outcome, compared with measurement of jet velocity, pressure gradient, and aortic valve area.

Coexisting aortic regurgitation is present in 70% to 80% of adults with predominant aortic stenosis.[7,52]

Left ventricular chamber dimensions and volumes, wall thickness, left ventricular mass, and ejection fraction and diastolic dysfunction are calculated using standard techniques as described in Chapter 5. Left ventricular meridional and circumferential wall stress can be calculated from echocardiographic data in conjunction with a cuff blood pressure measurement as described in Chapter 5. However, while useful in clinical research studies, wall stress calculations are rarely performed routinely as these measurements are tedious to obtain and their clinical utility has not yet been convincingly demonstrated.

Other important information derived from the echocardiographic examination include left atrial size, pulmonary artery systolic pressure, right ventricular size and systolic function, and mitral valve anatomy and function. Mitral annular calcification is seen in about 50% of adults with aortic stenosis,[52] and about 90% of patients have mild coexisting mitral regurgitation, with a smaller number having moderate mitral regurgitation. In patients with rheumatic disease, evaluation of the severity of mitral stenosis and/or regurgitation also is needed for clinical decision making.

Stress Testing

Traditionally, valvular aortic stenosis has been considered to be a contraindication to stress testing. However, recent studies suggest that stress testing can be performed with a low likelihood of complications in selected patients if they are monitored closely during the stress test. In several series of patients with minimal or absent symptoms, no serious complications have been reported.[34,52,122] However, even in this patient group, exertional hypotension occurs in about 10%; the majority have significant ST segment depression with exercise, and ventricular ectopy is common.[34,52,123,124] Because these series have focused on asymptomatic patients, it is important to assess symptom status before stress testing, with deferment of the test in patients with definite symptoms. The study should be promptly stopped for any decline in blood pressure, symptom onset, or the occurrence of significant arrhythmias.

Probably the most common indication for stress testing in patients with valvular aortic stenosis is an objective measure of exercise capacity in the asymptomatic patient to define the parameters of a safe exercise program for that individual. Although patients with aortic stenosis should not participate in competitive sports or extremely vigorous activities, moderate levels of recreational activity are usually well tolerated in asymptomatic individuals.[125,126]

Exercise testing also may be used to clarify symptom status in patients with equivocal symptoms, denial of apparent symptoms, or a decrease in exercise tolerance that is perceived by other family members. Exercise testing has also been shown to allow risk stratification and predict outcome in asymptomatic patients with severe aortic stenosis. A normal exercise test indicates a very low likelihood of symptom development or other complications within the following 6 to 12 months.[127-129] On the other hand, clear symptoms on exercise indicate a high likelihood of symptom development or other complications within 12 months in physically active patients, particularly those younger than 70 years.[129] Shortness of breath during exercise in patients with little physical activity in daily life, particularly elderly patients, may, however, be a nonspecific finding. Abnormal blood pressure response and/or ST segment depression previously thought to predict outcome[128,130] were more recently found to have a low positive predictive value.[129]

As in other types of cardiac disease, there has been considerable interest in the use of stress testing for detection of coexisting coronary artery disease in patients with valvular aortic stenosis. Exercise electrocardiography is not helpful as most patients have significant ST depression with exertion even in the absence of criteria for left ventricular hypertrophy on the electrocardiogram and in the absence of significant coronary artery disease.[52] Radionuclide stress imaging studies have shown more promise with a fair sensitivity and specificity for detection of coronary artery disease. Although there are few data on the utility of stress echocardiography for detection of coronary artery disease in adults with aortic stenosis, experience indicates that it is insensitive, possibly owing to diffuse subendocardial ischemia obscuring regional dysfunction. However, regional wall motion abnormalities appear to be specific for severe coronary obstruction in the rare patient with a positive result.

Several investigators have suggested that the changes in hemodynamics during a stress study might provide a better index of stenosis severity than a single resting value. Specifically, impending symptom onset can be identified by a fixed valve area that fails to increase with an increase in transaortic volume flow rate. Although clinical studies comparing groups of patients support this hypothesis and provide insight into the pathophysiology of the disease process, exercise stress testing to evaluate changes in valve area is not helpful in clinical decision making in individual patients for several reasons.[34,131] First, recording aortic stenosis jet and outflow tract velocities immediately after exercise is technically demanding and subject to considerable acquisition and measurement error, especially when performed by less experienced laboratories. Second, the magnitude of the hemodynamic changes seen with exercise or pharmacologic stress is similar to the expected measurement variability, even in the most experienced laboratories, limiting evaluation of individual patients, although group comparisons may be statistically valid. Third, the results do not affect clinical decision making, because the timing of surgical intervention is based on symptom status and resting measures of stenosis severity in most patients with valvular aortic stenosis.

Although the increase in mean pressure gradient with exercise has been reported to predict outcome and provide information beyond a regular exercise test,[86] more data are required to validate this finding before recommending its use in clinical practice.

Evaluation of the change in valve area with changes in flow rate in response to intravenous infusion of dobutamine may be helpful in the subgroup of patients with aortic stenosis and coexisting significant left ventricular systolic dysfunction who present with a low gradient but small valve area.[42,131-137] Although more data are required to confirm that the distinction between truly severe and pseudosevere aortic stenosis is a useful guide to clinical management, contractile reserve (defined as stroke volume increase of 20% or greater) has been shown to be a potent predictor of outcome.[134] However, contractile reserve was surprisingly not found to be an independent predictor of postoperative left ventricular function.[138] Although more likely to die perioperatively, patients who survived aortic valve replacement who had no contractile reserve before surgery were found to have an increase in ejection fraction similar to that of those with contractile reserve.[138]

In the majority of patients with valvular aortic stenosis, diagnostic data, including quantitation of stenosis severity, can be obtained noninvasively by Doppler echocardiography. Invasive measurement of the transaortic gradient and calculation of valve area using the Gorlin formula is needed only in patients for whom echocardiographic data are nondiagnostic or are not congruent with other clinical data. As with any diagnostic modality, careful attention to technical details at cardiac catheterization is needed for accurate quantitation of aortic stenosis severity, as discussed in Chapter 6. In particular, simultaneous pressure recordings with proper location of the catheter tips in the left ventricle and ascending aorta are crucial. Invasive cardiac output calculation also has its limitations. For example, associated aortic regurgitation may result in a significant difference between transvalvular flow and effective stroke volume, which has to be considered when valve area is calculated. Finally, the Gorlin equation with various simplified assumptions may result in inaccurate valve area estimates.[139]

Coronary angiography often is indicated to ascertain whether anginal symptoms are due to coexisting coronary disease in patients with mild or moderate aortic stenosis. With severe aortic stenosis coronary angiography usually is needed before aortic valve surgery, unless the pretest likelihood of disease is extremely low, as, for example, in a young women with congenital aortic stenosis. The role of multislice computed tomography for the preoperative evaluation of coronary arteries requires further investigation. However, proper visualization of all major coronary branches with good-quality normal multislice computed tomography may make a preoperative invasive angiography redundant.

DISEASE COURSE

Clinical Outcome

Asymptomatic Patients

In adults with valvular aortic stenosis, obstruction to left ventricular outflow develops gradually over many years.[88,90,91] In many patients aortic stenosis is coincidentally diagnosed when echocardiography is performed for other reasons or after the finding of a systolic murmur on examination, while they are still asymptomatic. Asymptomatic patients are found across the whole spectrum of aortic stenosis severity including a significant number of patients with severe aortic stenosis. In some patients a substantial decrease in valve area and an increase in transaortic velocity occurs before symptom onset. The occurrence of symptoms clearly presents a turning point in the natural history of the disease (Table 9-1).

Patients with congenital aortic stenosis may become symptomatic in early childhood or adolescence; in particular, patients with unicuspid valves tend to present with early symptoms. Later, at a young adult age (typically between 20 and 30 years), these patients may also present with symptoms due to restenosis after a surgical valvotomy in childhood.[140,141] In patients with a congenital bicuspid stenotic aortic valve, surgery is typically performed at 50 to 70 years of age.[142-144] In the adult patient with degenerative calcific valve disease, symptom onset may already occur at 50 years of age but usually occurs in elderly patients aged 70 to 90 years.[144] Rheumatic aortic stenosis becomes symptomatic over a wider age range, with patients most often presenting between 20 and 50 years of age.

In the absence of overt symptoms, clinical outcome is excellent (Figure 9-8). However, some investigators suggest that irreversible changes of the ventricular myocardium occur even before symptom onset.[145]

When following asymptomatic patients with aortic stenosis conservatively, the risk of sudden death is one of the major concerns. In three studies in which significant numbers of patients with nonsevere stenosis were included, no sudden death was reported. Otto et al[52] followed 123 patients with an average peak velocity of 3.6 ± 0.6 m/s for 30 months. The two other series with 51[146] and 37 patients[147] had follow-up periods of 1.5 and 2.0 years, respectively. Only two studies reported the outcome of larger cohorts of patients with severe stenosis exclusively as defined by a peak aortic jet velocity of 4.0 m/s or greater. Pellikka et al[148] observed two sudden deaths among 113 patients during a mean follow-up of 20 months. Both patients, however, had developed symptoms at least 3 months before death. In a recently published study, which is the largest to date, 11 sudden deaths were observed among 622 patients who had been followed for a mean of 5.4 years.[149] However, as the authors stated, medical follow-up was limited in about half of the patients. It thus remained unclear in this study whether these patients had eventually developed symptoms in the months before the event. Rosenhek et al[150] reported one sudden death that was not preceded by any symptoms among 104 patients followed for 27 months on average. Thus, sudden death may indeed occur even in the absence of preceding symptoms in patients with aortic stenosis, but this appears to be a very uncommon event with a rate of probably less than 1% per year during the asymptomatic phase of the disease. Finally, one has to consider that sudden death has even been reported after successful valve replacement with an incidence of about 0.3%; thus, this risk cannot be entirely eliminated by surgical treatment.[151,152]

Overall a watchful waiting strategy, which consists of regularly following patients as long as they are asymptomatic and referring them for surgery once they become symptomatic results in good survival that is not statistically different from that of an age- and gender-matched control population (Figure 9-9).[150]

Risk Stratification in Asymptomatic Patients

In initially asymptomatic patients, the rate of symptom onset ranges from less than 1% to 15% per year. Predictors of symptom onset include older age, male gender, aortic stenosis severity, and functional status. One of the most important predictors of outcome in patients with aortic stenosis is the degree of stenosis severity. The necessity for subsequent aortic valve surgery is directly related to peak aortic jet velocity over the whole spectrum of disease with event rates being lowest in patients with mild stenosis, followed by moderate and severe stenosis.[52,150,153] The rate of symptom onset is about 8% per year in those with a jet velocity less than 3.0 m/s, 17% per year in those with a jet velocity of 3 to 4 m/s, and 40% per year in those with a jet velocity more than 4.0 m/s (Figure 9-10).

Significant calcification, age, and the presence of coronary artery disease are associated with higher event rates in patients with mild to moderate aortic stenosis (Figure 9-11).[153] In addition, the rate of increase in aortic jet velocity over time is a strong predictor of clinical outcome.[52,150,153-155] In severe asymptomatic aortic stenosis, the rate of symptom onset is higher in patients older than 50 years and in those with significant valve calcification, suggesting that calcific disease progresses more rapidly than rheumatic aortic valve stenosis.[150,156] Among 126 patients with asymptomatic severe aortic stenosis, it was shown that the presence of a moderately to severely calcified aortic valve was associated with a significantly increased event rate, and 80% of these patients developed symptoms warranting aortic valve replacement or died within 4 years (Figure 9-12).[150] The combination of a calcified aortic valve with rapid hemodynamic progression, defined as an increase in peak aortic jet velocity of more than 0.3 m/s within 1 year identified a patient group at particularly high risk with an event rate of 79% within 2 years (Figure 9-13).[150] The echocardiographic determination of aortic valve calcification has the advantage of being fast and easily

TABLE 9–1 | **Natural History of Valvular Aortic Stenosis**

Series	Entry Criteria	n	Age (yr)	AS Severity	Mean Follow-up	Actuarial Survival
Symptomatic patients						
Frank, 1973[88]	ΔP_{peak} ≥50 mmHg or AVI <0.7 cm²/m²	15	32–59	AVI 0.4 ± 0.1 cm²/m²	>2 yr	50% at 5 yr 10% at 9 yr
Chizner, 1980[87]	Cardiac cath, no AVR	42	22–77	AVA 0.7 ± 0.3 (0.2–1.1) cm²	5.4 yr	36% at 5 yr 20% at 9 yr
O'Keefe, 1987[163]	Severe aortic stenosis, no AVR, age ≥60 yr	50	Mean 77 (60–89)	V_{max} 4.5 m/s, AVA 0.6 (0.3–8) cm²	1.7 yr	37% at 2 yr 5% at 3 yr
Turina, 1987[159]	Cardiac cath, no AVR	125	43 (16–73)	Mean ΔP 60 mmHg	6.6 yr	12% at 5 yr
Horstkotte, 1988[140]	Refused surgery	35		Severe AS (AVA <0.8 cm²)		18% at 5 yr
Kelly, 1988[146]	V_{max} ≥3.6 m/s	39	72 ± 11	ΔP 68±19 mmHg	15±10 months	60% at 2 yr
Asymptomatic patients						
Turina, 1987[159]		65		Mean ΔP 57 mmHg AVA 0.76 cm²		76% at 5 yr
Horstkotte, 1988[140]	Cath for other reasons	142		Mild AS (AVA >1.5 cm²)		92% at 10 yr
	Cath for other reasons	236		Moderate AS (AVA 0.8–1.5 cm²)		80% at 10 yr
Kelly, 1988[146]	V_{max} ≥3.6 m/s	51	63 ± 19	ΔP 68 ± 19	15 ± 10 mo	90% at 2 yr
Pellikka, 1990[148]	Doppler V_{max} ≥4 m/s	143	72 (40–94)	V_{max} 4.4 (4–6.4) m/s	20 mo	74% at 2 yr 62% remained symptom free
Kennedy, 1991[162]	Moderate AS at cath, no AVR	66	67 ± 10	AVA 0.92 ± 0.13 cm²	35 mo	59% at 4 yr
Otto, 1997[52]	Abnormal valve with V_{max} >2.6 m/s	123	63 ± 16	V_{max} <3 m/s V_{max} 3–4 m/s V_{max} >4 m/s	2.5 ± 1.4 yr	84 ± 16% at 2 yr 66 ± 13% 21 ± 18%
Rosenhek, 2000[150]	V_{max} ≥4.0 m/s	128	60 ±18	Mean V_{max} 5.0 ± 0.6 m/s	1.8 ± 1.5 yr	67 ± 5% at 1 yr 33 ± 5% at 4 yr
Rosenhek, 2004[153]	V_{max} 2.5–3.9 m/s	176	58 ± 19	V_{max} 3.1 ± 0.4 m/s	4.0 ± 1.6 yr	95% at 1 yr 75% at 2 yr 60% at 5 yr
Pellikka, 2005[149]	V_{max} ≥4.0 m/s	622	72 ± 11	V_{max} 4.4 ± 0.4 m/s	5.4 ± 4.0 yr	82% at 1 yr 67% at 2 yr 33% at 5 yr

AS, aortic stenosis; AVA, aortic valve area; AVI, aortic valve index; AVR, aortic valve replacement; cath, catheterization; ΔP, pressure gradient; V_{max}, maximum aortic jet velocity.

FIGURE 9–8 Event-free survival (left panel) and overall survival (right panel) in hemodynamically severe aortic stenosis and combined lesions or with aortic regurgitation red circles in severely symptomatic (solid lines) and asymptomatic or mildly symptomatic patients (dashed lines). *(From Turina J, Hess O, Sepulcri F, Krayenbuehl HP: Spontaneous course of aortic valve disease. Eur Heart J 1987;8:471-483, with permission.)*

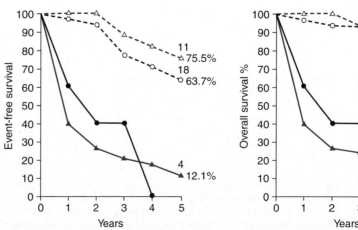

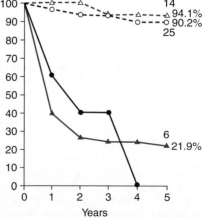

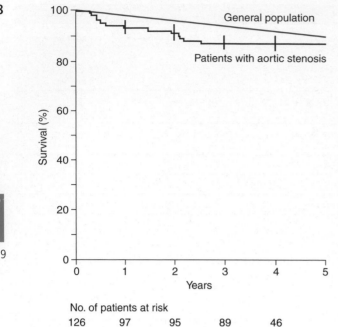

No. of patients at risk

| 126 | 97 | 95 | 89 | 46 |

FIGURE 9–9 Kaplan-Meier analysis of overall survival among 126 patients with asymptomatic but severe aortic stenosis compared with age- and sex-matched persons in the general population. This analysis included perioperative and postoperative deaths among patients who required valve replacement during follow-up. The vertical bars indicate standard errors. *(From Rosenhek R, Binder T, Porenta G, et al: Predictors of outcome in severe, asymptomatic aortic stenosis. N Engl J Med 2000;343:611-617, with permission.)*

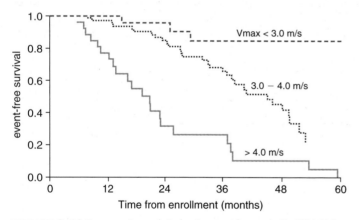

FIGURE 9–10 Cox regression analysis showing event-free survival in 123 initially asymptomatic adults with valvular aortic stenosis, defined by aortic jet velocity at entry (P < 0.001 by log-rank test). *(From Otto CM, Burwash IG, Legget ME, et al: Prospective study of asymptomatic valvular aortic stenosis: Clinical, echocardiographic, and exercise predictors of outcome. Circulation 1997;95:2262-2270, with permission.)*

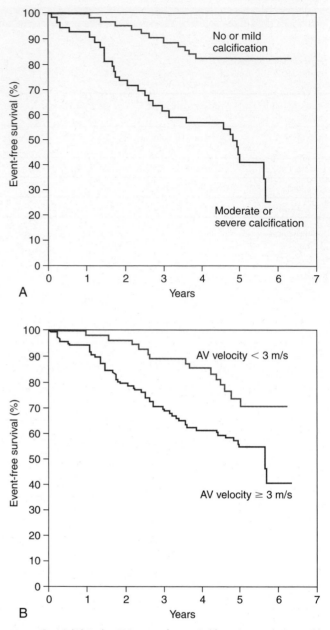

FIGURE 9–11 (**A**) Kaplan-Meier event-free survival for patients with no or mild calcification compared with patients having moderate or severe aortic valve (AV) calcification (P = 0.0001). (**B**) Kaplan-Meier event-free survival for patients with an aortic jet velocity less than 3 m/s compared with patients having a jet velocity of 3 m/s at study entry (P = 0.008). *(From Rosenhek R, Klaar U, Schemper M, et al: Mild and moderate aortic stenosis: Natural history and risk stratification by echocardiography. Eur Heart J 2004;25:199-205, with permission.)*

obtainable at the moment of the echocardiographic examination. Although being a semiquantitative method, the differentiation between no or mild versus moderate to severe calcification can be easily performed. The finding that aortic valve calcification is associated with a poor outcome was also confirmed by a study that assessed the degree of aortic valve calcification by electron beam tomography.[157]

Lancellotti et al[86] assessed the value of exercise Doppler echocardiographic measurements in 69 patients with severe asymptomatic aortic stenosis.[86] In this study, an exercise-induced increase in the mean transaortic gradient of 18 mmHg or greater (Figure 9-14), abnormal results on an exercise test, and an aortic valve area of less than 0.75 cm² were significant

predictors of subsequent events in multivariate analysis, and all had an incremental value when occurring together. Still these findings need confirmation in larger studies.

Interestingly, there is a wide range of hemodynamic severity at symptom onset in adults with valvular aortic stenosis.[52,140,158,159] In the Balloon Valvuloplasty Registry, aortic jet velocities ranged from 2.3 to 6.6 (mean 4.4 ± 0.8) m/s, mean transaortic pressure gradients from 13 to 120 (mean 48 ± 18) mmHg, and aortic valve areas from 0.1 to 1.4 (mean 0.6 ± 0.2) cm², even though all these patients were symptomatic.[7] In this study, there may have been bias toward overestimation of disease severity at symptom onset because some patients may have been symptomatic for several months or years before study entry. However, a prospective study of initially asymptomatic adults with valvular aortic stenosis also showed a wide range of hemodynamic severity at symptom

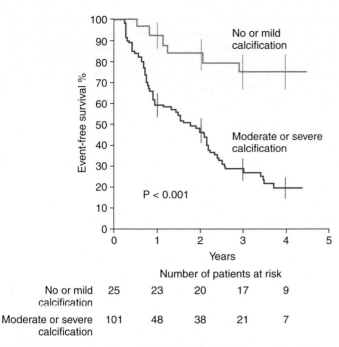

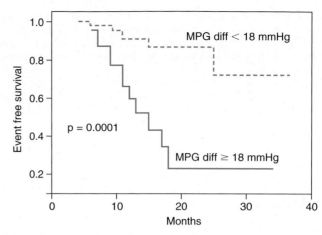

FIGURE 9–12 Kaplan-Meier analysis of event-free survival among 25 patients with no or mild aortic valve calcification compared with 101 patients with moderate or severe calcification. All patients had an aortic jet velocity of at least 4 m/s at study entry. The vertical bars indicate standard errors. *(From Rosenhek R, Binder T, Porenta G, et al: Predictors of outcome in severe, asymptomatic aortic stenosis. N Engl J Med 2000;343:611-617, with permission.)*

FIGURE 9–14 Event-free survival curves according to exercise-induced changes in mean transaortic pressure gradient (MPG) in 69 consecutive patients with severe aortic stenosis. *(From Lancellotti P, Lebois F, Simon M, et al: Prognostic importance of quantitative exercise Doppler echocardiography in asymptomatic valvular aortic stenosis. Circulation 2005;112:1377-1382, with permission.)*

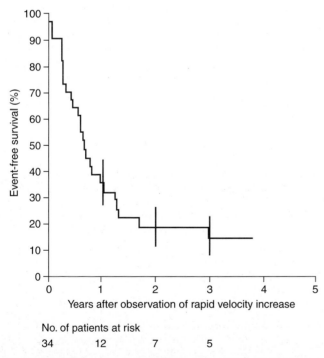

FIGURE 9–13 Kaplan-Meier analysis of event-free survival among 34 patients with moderate or severe calcification of the aortic valve and a rapid increase in aortic-jet velocity (at least 0.3 m/s within 1 year). In this analysis, follow-up started with the visit at which the rapid increase was identified. The vertical bars indicate standard errors. *(From Rosenhek R, Binder T, Porenta G, et al: Predictors of outcome in severe, asymptomatic aortic stenosis. N Engl J Med 2000;343:611-617, with permission.)*

onset with an average jet velocity of 4.6 ± 0.8 m/s, a mean transaortic gradient of 49 ± 18 mmHg, and a valve area of 0.93 ± 0.31 cm². [52] The range of hemodynamic severity at symptom onset is similar if indexed to body surface area, indicating that these differences between patients are not simply due to differences in body size. Other clinical series also show a

substantial overlap in hemodynamic severity in symptomatic versus asymptomatic patients.[140,159]

These clinical observations support the hypothesis that symptom onset is due to the interaction of valve stiffness, left ventricular ejection force, and the metabolic requirements in each individual. Symptoms typically occur initially with conditions that increase total tissue oxygen demands, such as exertion, pregnancy, febrile illness, or anemia, owing to the inability of the heart to increase cardiac output across the narrowed valve. Thus, the specific degree of valve narrowing associated with clinical symptoms shows considerable individual variability. In addition, concurrent conditions such as aortic regurgitation or coronary artery disease also modify the specific degree of hemodynamic perturbation associated with symptoms. Because operative mortality for aortic valve replacement surgery has decreased considerably over the last years, the threshold defining severe aortic stenosis has also been lowered. In the recently updated guidelines from the American College of Cardiology (ACC)/American Heart Association (AHA) and the European Society of Cardiology (ESC), a valve area less than 1.0 cm² is used to define severe stenosis.[160,161] The threshold used for the mean gradient is discrepant, with 40 mmHg proposed by the ACC/AHA and 50 mmHg by the ESC guidelines. In this intermediate range, the presence of symptoms should be considered a manifestation of severe symptomatic aortic stenosis.

Symptomatic Patients

Once definite symptoms of aortic stenosis are present, outcome is very poor without surgical intervention. Autopsy studies performed before aortic valve replacement were available, and more recent series of adults who refused surgical intervention indicate survival rates with severe symptomatic aortic stenosis of only 15% to 50% at 5 years.[87,140,146,159,162-164] Using data from earlier autopsy series it was projected that the average time from symptom onset to death is 2 years for patients with exertional syncope, 3 years for patients with heart failure symptoms, and 5 years for those with angina.[88-90,165,166] Although the retrospective nature of these studies does not support such a clear differentiation of clinical outcome according to underlying symptoms, it is indisputable that outcome is very poor in the presence of any symptom. More intense symptoms are associated with worse outcome. This finding emphasizes the importance of patient education, the need for periodic clinical evaluation, and the importance of intervention for any symptom due to aortic stenosis.

In adults with symptomatic aortic stenosis, predictors of survival are transaortic velocity or gradient, functional status, left ventricular systolic function, comorbid disease, and gender.[164] When symptoms due to severe aortic stenosis are present, prognosis is better in the presence of a high gradient (or jet velocity), because a low gradient and transaortic velocity in the setting of severe valve narrowing is the reflection of a reduced cardiac output.

Symptomatic patients refusing aortic valve replacement have a shortened survival and a suboptimal quality of life. Not surprisingly, brain natriuretic peptide (BNP) levels predict survival in this group of patients.[167] Often these patients have symptoms with minimal exertion or at rest, and many have recurrent hospital admissions for decompensated heart failure. Medical therapy may alleviate episodes of acute decompensation, for example, the use of diuretics for acute pulmonary edema, but does not prevent recurrent episodes of decompensation or prolong life.

Aortic Sclerosis and Mild to Moderate Aortic Stenosis

In a recent community-based study it was shown that the presence of aortic valve sclerosis, defined as focal valve thickening without outflow obstruction, is associated with significantly increased cardiovascular and all-cause mortality.[168] Mild to moderate aortic stenosis also is associated with increased cardiovascular mortality.[52,153] Thus, aortic sclerosis and mild to moderate aortic stenosis have to be viewed as predictors of a poor overall prognosis.

The prognosis of patients with non-severe aortic stenosis is influenced by hemodynamic progression of the disease. A recent analysis of the Cardiovascular Health Study showed that a progression of aortic sclerosis to aortic stenosis occurs in about 9% of patients within 5 years.[169] The interval between observing aortic valve "sclerosis" on echocardiography and clinical evidence of severe stenosis may be as short as 5 years.[170] In addition, the progression to severe, hemodynamically significant stenosis is common and may be more rapid than previously assumed.[153]

Hemodynamic Progression

An understanding of the progressive nature of aortic stenosis and the rate of increase in disease severity is fundamental for appropriate patient management and individualization of follow-up intervals in patients who have mild or moderate aortic

stenosis. Researchers have aimed to define hemodynamic progression of aortic stenosis during the phase before symptom onset, to predict prognosis, to identify predictors of rapid disease progression, and to increase our understanding of the relationship between hemodynamic severity and symptom onset.

Early data on the hemodynamic progression of valvular aortic stenosis was derived from studies of patients who had undergone two or more cardiac catheterizations.[171-176] The fact that only patients who did not die or undergo valve replacement after the first catheterization and yet required a second catheterization for clinical indications are included in these series clearly resulted in a selection bias. Yet, these studies demonstrated variable rates of disease progression.

The availability of an accurate, noninvasive method to evaluate hemodynamic severity has allowed larger and more detailed studies on the rate of hemodynamic progression[40,147,150,153,155,177-181] (Table 9-2). Recent intervention studies, designed to assess the effects of statin therapy in halting or delaying the progression of aortic stenosis, provide additional information on hemodynamic progression[182-186] (Table 9-3). Overall, these studies show an average rate of increase in mean pressure gradient of about 8 mmHg per year and a decrease in valve area between 0.15 cm² per year. In these studies, the average rate of increase in aortic jet maximum velocity ranged from 0.2 to 0.4 m/s/year. However, marked individual variability in the rate of hemodynamic progression was observed. Factors predicting rapid hemodynamic progression are the presence of a calcified aortic valve, coronary artery disease, and age (Figure 9-15).[153] Although Doppler echocardiographic studies have the advantage of larger patient numbers and potentially less selection bias (a repeat echocardiographic study is likely to be requested more often than a repeat cardiac catheterization), many of these studies are retrospective with the data extracted from on-going clinical databases. Thus, patients with rapid progression, those developing symptoms, or those requiring surgical intervention may be over-represented. Conversely, repeat studies may not have been performed in clinically stable patients. Some of these biases may have been avoided in the results of more recent prospective studies.[52,150,184,187]

As the disease progresses, increasing obstruction to left ventricular outflow most often is reflected by a decrease in valve area and an increase in jet velocity and pressure

TABLE 9–2	Hemodynamic Progression of Valvular Aortic Stenosis (Selected Catheter and Echocardiographic Studies)						
Author, Year	Clinical Status at Entry	Type of Study	n	Mean Follow-up (yr)	Increase in Mean Δ P (mmHg/yr)	Increase in V_{max} (m/s/yr)	Decrease in AVA (cm²/yr)
Catheter studies							
Bogart, 1979[171]	2 cardiac caths	Retrospective	11	4.9	11.6 (1.2 to 24)		0.2 (0.02–0.6)
Cheitlin, 1979[172]	2 cardiac caths	Retrospective	29	4	8.4 (−12 to 45)		
Wagner, 1982[176]	2 cardiac caths	Retrospective	50	3.5	"Rapid" (n = 21)		0.32 ± 0.20
					"Slow" (n = 29)		0.02 ± 0.13
Jonasson, 1983[174]	Calcific AS	Retrospective	26	9			0.1
Nestico, 1983[176]	2 cardiac caths	Retrospective	29	5.9	0.8 (−8 to 10.4)		0.05 (0 to 0.5)
Davies, 1991[173]	2 cardiac caths	Retrospective	47		6.5 (−10 to 38)		
Echocardiographic studies							
Otto, 1989[178]	Asymptomatic	Prospective	42	1.7	8 (−7 to 23)	0.36 ± 0.31	0.1 (0 to 0.5)
Roger, 1990[181]	AS on echo	Retrospective	112	2.1		0.23 ± 0.37	
Faggiano, 1992[170]	AS on echo	Prospective	45	1.5		0.4 ± 0.3	0.1 ± 0.13 (−0.7 to 0.1)
Peter, 1993[180]	AS on echo	Retrospective	49	2.7	7.2		
Brener, 1995[177]	AS on echo	Retrospective	394	6.3			0.14
Otto, 1997[52]	Asymptomatic	Prospective	123	2.5	7 ± 7	0.32 ± 0.34	0.12 ± 0.19
Bahler, 1999[155]	AS on echo	Retrospective	91	1.8	2.8	0.2	0.04
Palta, 2000[179]	AS on echo	Retrospective	170	1.9			0.10 ± 0.27
Rosenhek, 2000[150]	AS on echo with V_{max} >4.0 m/s	Prospective	128	1.8	Slow	0.14 ± 0.18	
					Rapid	0.45 ± 0.38	
Rosenhek, 2004[153]	AS on echo with V_{max} 2.5–3.9 m/s	Retrospective	176	3.8		0.24 ± 0.30	

AS, aortic stenosis; cath, catheterization; echo, echocardiogram.

TABLE 9-3 Hemodynamic Progression of Valvular Aortic Stenosis (Selected Echocardiographic Intervention Studies)

Author, Year	Clinical Status at Entry	Type of Study	n	Mean Follow-up (years)	Intervention	Increase in V_{max} (m/s/yr)	Decrease in AVA (cm²/yr)	p-values
Novaro, 2001[185]	AS on echo with AVA 1.0–1.8 cm²	Retrospective	174	1.7	Statin therapy No statin		0.06 ± 0.16 0.11 ± 0.18	0.03
Bellamy, 2002[183]	AS on echo with AVA <2.0 cm²	Retrospective	156	3.7	Statin therapy No statin		0.04 ± 0.15 0.09 ± 0.17	0.04
Rosenhek, 2004[186]	AS on echo with V_{max} >2.5 m/s	Retrospective	211	2.0	Statin therapy No statin	0.1 ± 0.41 0.39 ± 0.42		0.0001
Cowell (SALTIRE), 2005[184]	AS on echo with V_{max} >2.5 m/s	Prospective	134	2.1	Statin therapy Placebo	0.2 ± 0.21 0.2 ± 0.21	0.08 ± 0.11 0.08 ± 0.11	0.95
Moura, 2007[187]	AS on echo with AVA 1.0–1.5 cm²	Prospective	121	1.4	Statin therapy No statin	0.4 ± 0.38 0.24 ± 0.30	0.05 ± 0.12 0.1 ± 0.09	0.007
Rossebø (SEAS) 2008[256]	As on echo with V_{max} 2.5–4.0 m/s	Prospective	1873	4.35	Stain + Ezetimibe therapy Placebo	0.15 ± 0.01 m/s/yr* (simvastatin+ezetimibe) and 0.16 ± 0.01 m/s/yr* (placebo)	0.03 ± 0.01 cm²/yr* (simvastatin+ezetimibe) and 0.03 ± 0.01 cm²/yr* (placebo)	0.83

AS, aortic stenosis; AVA, aortic valve area; echo, echocardiogram.

*Data are expressed as mean ± SE

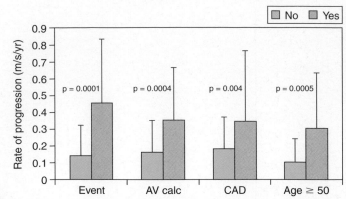

FIGURE 9–15 Rates of hemodynamic progression expressed as increase in peak aortic jet velocity among patients with mild to moderate aortic stenosis. AV calc, calcified aortic valve; CAD, coronary artery disease. *(From Rosenhek R, Klaar U, Schemper M, et al: Mild and moderate aortic stenosis: Natural history and risk stratification by echocardiography. Eur Heart J 2004;25:199-205, with permission.)*

9

gradient. However, if there is a concurrent decrease in transaortic volume flow rate, a decrease in valve area alone may be seen with no change in jet velocity or transaortic gradient. This situation may occur due to comorbid disease, such as increasing mitral regurgitation or myocardial infarction, but may also be due to a decrease of left ventricular function late in the disease course. On the other hand, an increase in jet velocity and pressure gradient with no change in valve area may be observed if transaortic stroke volume is increased due to hyperdynamic states (e.g., anemia, fever, pregnancy) or increasing aortic regurgitation.

In general, the rate of hemodynamic progression is fairly linear. However, in some patients there is evidence for more abrupt progression preceding the appearance of symptoms. This might be the point at which leaflet stiffness exceeds the capacity of ventricular ejection force to adequately open the valve.

Associated Clinical Factors

The presence of calcific aortic stenosis is associated with clinical factors similar to those associated with atherosclerosis. Several studies have also suggested that aortic stenosis and atherosclerosis have a number of risk factors such as hypercholesterolemia, elevated lipoprotein(a), smoking, hypertension, and diabetes in common.[103,188-192] In addition, the rate of hemodynamic progression of aortic stenosis is related to a history of smoking[193] and serum calcium levels.[179] The difficulty in establishing a relationship between disease progression and other clinical factors may relate to the relatively small sample size of the data available. Nevertheless, these clinical factors might be triggers in the disease pathogenesis, which is now recognized to be an active, calcific process (see Chapter 3).

Coexisting Coronary Artery Disease

About 50% of adults undergoing valve replacement for aortic stenosis have significant coronary artery disease. The concurrence of valvular aortic stenosis and coronary artery disease both complicates diagnosis and management in individual patients and complicates interpretation of outcome studies.

Clinical evaluation is hampered by the fact that angina may be due to isolated aortic stenosis or to coexisting coronary artery disease. Only between 20% and 60% of patients with aortic stenosis and symptoms of angina have coronary disease, whereas 0% to 54% (mean 16%) of those without angina also have significant coronary artery disease.[194] In the patient with previously asymptomatic aortic stenosis, it

is difficult to ascertain whether the onset of angina is due to the severe valvular stenosis or whether angina is due to coexisting coronary artery disease. Alcalai et al[195] described a series of 38 consecutive symptomatic patients with significant aortic stenosis and coronary artery disease who underwent percutaneous coronary intervention (surgery was not performed because of patient preference, high surgical risk, or physician recommendation). After the intervention 35 of these patients reported relief of their symptoms.

On a general basis, even though the origin of the symptoms might not always be unequivocally attributable to the stenosis, aortic valve replacement should not be deferred in symptomatic patients with severe stenosis because of the unfavorable natural history of severe symptomatic aortic stenosis. When stenosis severity is intermediate, decision making is more difficult, especially given that symptoms can occur with a relatively wide range of stenosis severity. Often, coronary angiography is needed to clarify the contribution of coronary disease to symptoms in these patients. The decision should incorporate coronary morphology, severity of aortic stenosis and progression rates that can be expected.

In clinical studies of the natural history of aortic stenosis, it rarely is possible to separate outcomes due to coexisting coronary disease from those due to valvular obstruction given the high rate of concordance for these diseases. Note that of the 4 cardiac deaths in a prospective study of 123 adults with asymptomatic aortic stenosis, 2 were due to coexisting coronary artery disease, whereas the other 2 patients had severe aortic stenosis but refused aortic valve replacement.[52]

Coronary angiography is routinely performed before planned surgical intervention. The operative mortality for patients with aortic stenosis and coexisting coronary artery disease ranges from 1.1% to 4.8% if coronary artery bypass grafting is performed at the time of valve replacement but may be as high as 4% to 13.2% when no revascularization is performed in the setting of significant coronary disease, most likely related to inadequate myocardial perfusion immediately after cardiopulmonary bypass and in the early postoperative period.[145,196] Noninvasive tests generally are of limited use in the preoperative assessment. Older patients with calcific aortic stenosis, who often have a significant risk profile and a high rate of associated coronary artery disease, in particular, should systematically undergo preoperative coronary angiography. Ruling out the presence of coronary artery disease by computed tomography angiography might be an option in younger patients at low risk for the presence of coronary artery disease.

SURGICAL INTERVENTION AND POSTOPERATIVE OUTCOME

Timing of Surgical Intervention

Symptom Onset

Surgical intervention for aortic stenosis is indicated at symptom onset in adults, given the dramatic improvement in survival with surgical versus medical therapy and the high likelihood of symptom relief after valve replacement. Surgery can be deferred in asymptomatic adults because survival and clinical outcome are excellent without surgical intervention. The only clinical difficulty with this approach is defining at what point the patient can be considered symptomatic.

Symptom onset in adults is so gradual that many patients fail to recognize early symptoms and first present for medical attention with a syncopal episode, frank congestive heart failure, or unstable angina. Surgical intervention clearly is needed in these patients. In contrast, patients followed prospectively who are educated about the possible symptoms tend to present with a history of gradually decreasing exercise tolerance and increasing exertional dyspnea that is elicited only by focused and detailed questions. Physical examination typically shows severe aortic stenosis but fails to reveal evidence of hemodynamic decompensation. Thus, it often is unclear whether these patients are truly symptomatic or whether these nonspecific symptoms are due to age, intercurrent illness, or comorbid conditions.

In general, if severe aortic stenosis is present by echocardiography or catheterization, even mild symptoms should be considered to be due to aortic stenosis, and the patient should be referred promptly for surgical intervention. Support for this approach includes natural history studies showing the high rate of symptom onset and death with Doppler evidence of severe stenosis so that even if surgery is deferred initially, the patient is likely to develop more severe symptoms requiring surgical intervention within a relatively short time period.[52,197,198] Additional support for surgical intervention for mild symptoms is the increasing evidence that systolic dysfunction may be irreversible in some patients with aortic stenosis and that nearly all patients have significant diastolic dysfunction that persists for several years after valve replacement. Some investigators suggest that even earlier intervention is needed (e.g., in the asymptomatic patient) to prevent the secondary left ventricular changes of this disease process.[145]

Another clinical difficulty in the timing of surgical intervention in aortic stenosis is determining whether symptoms are caused by aortic stenosis when the degree of obstruction is not severe. In the patient with symptoms, such as angina, but only mild valve obstruction, it is clear that aortic stenosis is not the cause of the symptoms. However, when symptoms are present and stenosis appears "moderate," the relationship between the valve obstruction and symptoms is less clear, especially given the observation that there is substantial overlap in hemodynamic severity between symptomatic and asymptomatic patients. There is no simple method to establish a cause-effect relationship between valve obstruction and symptoms in these patients. A careful history and search for alternate causes of symptoms may resolve the issue. If not, exercise testing for objective evaluation of exercise tolerance, hemodynamic response, and symptoms may be helpful.

Surgery in Asymptomatic Patients

Although there is consensus now that surgery is indicated in symptomatic aortic stenosis even if symptoms are mild,[160,161] the management of asymptomatic aortic stenosis remains a matter of controversy.[199] The only exception is the very rare asymptomatic patient with impaired left ventricular systolic function that cannot be explained by other causes. Despite the data showing overall good outcome for all other truly asymptomatic patients and the low risk of sudden death during the asymptomatic phase of disease, many physicians are reluctant to follow these patients for several reasons: There is the above-mentioned difficulty to clearly distinguish between asymptomatic and mildly symptomatic status and the fact that patients frequently do not present immediately when symptoms develop. Furthermore, operative risk significantly increases with symptoms and their severity. A large surgical registry reported operative mortality of less than 2% for patients in New York Heart Association class I or II compared with 3.7% and 7% for patients in functional classes III and IV, respectively.[200] In addition, there remains concern that severe myocardial hypertrophy and fibrosis may develop during the asymptomatic phase and preclude a later optimal surgical outcome although solid data to support this hypothesis are still lacking. Nevertheless, because it seems unlikely from current data that the potential benefit of valve replacement in asymptomatic patients can outweigh the risk of surgery and the long-term risk of prosthesis-related complications in all patients, surgery for severe aortic stenosis can certainly not be recommended in general before symptom onset. However, risk stratification should be considered to select patients who are likely to benefit from elective surgery. Because these indications are less well established, they are currently listed as IIa and IIb indications with slight differences between American and European practice guidelines.[160,161] Patients with a high likelihood of rapid progression can be identified by moderate to severe calcification of the valve, older age, the presence of coronary artery disease, and an observed rapid increase in transvalvular velocity.[150,153] Of those patients with notably calcified valves who have in addition an increase in transaortic velocity of 0.3 m/s or greater from one visit to the following visit within 1 year, 80% have been reported to either develop symptoms or die within 2 years.[150] Those patients may be considered for surgery despite being asymptomatic. Stress testing as a predictor of outcome has been discussed above. Patients with normal exercise capacity can be considered low risk and safely followed. Symptom development during an exercise test indicates surgery, particularly in physically active patients (class I in Europe and IIb in North America). However, it has to be kept in mind that breathlessness on exercise may be difficult to interpret in patients with only low physical activity, particularly elderly patients, making decisions more difficult. Asymptomatic patients with a fall in blood pressure to less than baseline during exercise testing may also be considered for surgery. Arrhythmias on exercise and severe left ventricular hypertrophy are more controversial.[160,161] Although plasma concentrations of cardiac neurohormones have been shown to predict outcome in aortic stenosis, these data have been considered too preliminary by both expert committees to include such measurements in current recommendations. In a series of asymptomatic patients with severe aortic stenosis, those with BNP concentrations greater than 130 pg/ml or N-terminal BNP concentrations greater than 80 pmol/l were unlikely to develop symptoms within the following 9 months (symptom-free survival close to 90%), whereas those with higher concentrations frequently required surgery within this time period (symptom-free survival <50%).[201] Furthermore, high plasma levels of neurohormones have been reported to be associated with high operative mortality and worse postoperative outcome with regard to left ventricular function and symptomatic status.[201] Finally, neurohormones may help to better distinguish between asymptomatic and early symptomatic states or to relate shortness of breath to aortic stenosis in patients with an additional pulmonary cause of this symptom. Regulation of BNP expression and production is certainly complex, and BNP levels cannot be expected to reflect directly one myocardial or hemodynamic feature. Nevertheless, in aortic stenosis, besides a possible role of increased left ventricular mass or systolic load, diastolic stretch load is likely to be the key mechanical stimulus triggering on-and-off BNP expression and production.[202,203] In this instance, BNP appears to predict the actual hemodynamic state of an individual patient and to reflect noninvasively the transition from a compensated to decompensated state.[202] Recommendations for surgery in the current American[160] and European[161] guidelines are summarized in Table 9-4 and in Figures 9-16 and 9-17.

Surgical Intervention in Elderly Patients

Operative mortality is relatively high in older adults, variously identified as those older than 70, 75, or 80 years, with rates of 5% to 15%. In addition, there is a higher rate of complications in elderly patients, including preoperative myocardial infarction in 3% to 8% and cerebrovascular events in up to 11% of patients.[204-214] Although some investigators suggest that elderly patients are more likely to have a prolonged hospitalization, require more extensive rehabilitation, and require interim or long-term skilled nursing care, a case-control study of younger and older adults found no difference in use of hospital resources between these age groups.[214]

Indication Class	Evidence Level	ACC/AHA Guidelines[160]	ESC Guidelines[161]
TABLE 9-4		**Indications for Aortic Valve Replacement in Aortic Stenosis as Recommended by Current Practice Guidelines**	
I	B	Symptomatic pt. with severe AS	Symptomatic pt. with severe AS
	C	Pt. with severe AS and EF <0.50	Pt. with severe AS and EF <0.50
	C	Pt. with severe AS undergoing CABG or surgery on the aorta or other heart valves	Pt. with severe AS undergoing CABG or surgery on the aorta or other heart valves
	C		Asympt. pt. developing symptoms during exercise test
IIa	C	Pt. with moderate AS undergoing CABG or surgery on the aorta or other heart valves	Pt. with moderate AS undergoing CABG or surgery on the aorta or other heart valves
	C		Asympt. pt. with severe AS and fall of blood pressure below baseline during exercise test
	C		Asympt. pt. with severe AS and moderate to severe valve calcification and peak velocity progression ≥0.3m/s per year
	C		AS with low gradient (<40 mmHg) with LV dysfunction and contractile reserve
IIb	C	Asympt. pt. with severe AS and abnormal response to exercise (e.g., development of symptoms or asympt. hypotension)	Asympt. pt. with severe AS and complex ventricular arrhythmias during exercise test
	C	Asympt. pt. with severe AS and high likelihood of rapid progression (age, calcification, and CAD) or if surgery might be delayed at the time of symptom onset)	Asympt. pt. with severe AS and excessive LV hypertrophy (≥15 mm) unless this is due to hypertension
	C	Pt. with mild AS undergoing CABG when there is evidence, such as moderate to severe calcification, that progression may be rapid	AS with low gradient (<40 mmHg) and LV dysfunction without contractile reserve
	C	Asympt. pt. with extremely severe AS (valve area <0.6 cm², mean gradient >60 mmHg, jet velocity >5 m/s) when expected operative mortality ≤1%	

ACC, American College of Cardiology; AHA, American Heart Association; AS, aortic stenosis; asympt., asymptomatic; CABG, coronary artery bypass graft surgery; CAD, coronary artery disease; EF, ejection fraction; ESC, European Society of Cardiology; LV, left ventricle, pt., patient.

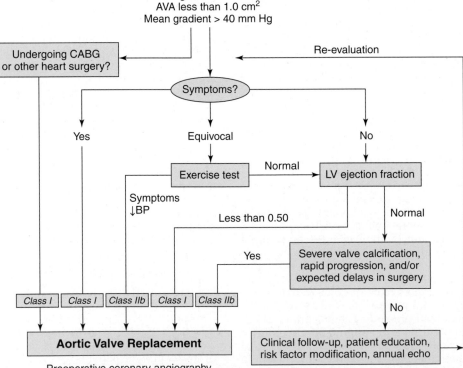

FIGURE 9–16 Algorithm representing the management strategy for patients with severe aortic stenosis from the American College of Cardiology/American Heart Association Guidelines. Preoperative coronary angiography should be performed routinely as determined by age, symptoms, and coronary risk factors. Cardiac catheterization and angiography may also be helpful when there is discordance between clinical findings and echocardiography. AVA, aortic valve area; BP, blood pressure; CABG, coronary artery bypass graft surgery; echo, echocardiography; LV, left ventricular; Vmax, maximal velocity across aortic valve by Doppler echocardiography.

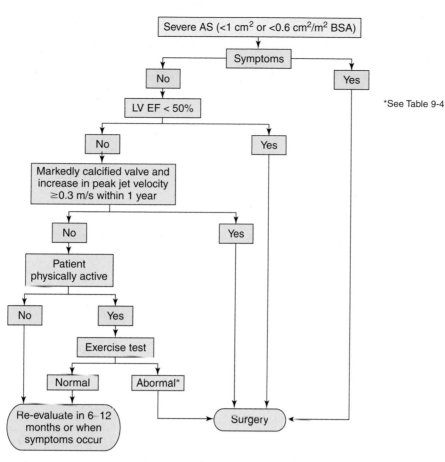

FIGURE 9–17 Algorithm representing the management strategy for patients with severe aortic stenosis from the European Society of Cardiology Guidelines. AS, aortic stenosis; BSA, body surface area; EF, ejection fraction; LV, left ventricle. *(From Vahanian A, Baumgartner H, Bax J, et al: Guidelines on the management of valvular heart disease: The Task Force on the Management of Valvular Heart Disease of the European Society of Cardiology. Eur Heart J 2007;28:230-268, with permission.)*

Although surgical mortality is higher in elderly patients, life expectancy is still significantly prolonged after valve replacement. When surgical intervention in elderly patients is considered, it is helpful to consult age-adjusted life tables so that expected survival after surgery (similar to that of age-matched adults without aortic stenosis) can be compared with the expected survival without surgical intervention. In an analysis looking at relative survival, defined as the observed compared with the expected survival for age, outcome in elderly adults was excellent after aortic valve replacement with a 10-year relative survival of 100%.[211] Because symptomatic aortic stenosis has such a high mortality rate without surgery, valve replacement remains the procedure of choice even in octogenarians. As an example, using a decision analysis model, Wong et al[215] showed that an 87-year-old woman with severe symptomatic aortic stenosis, coronary artery disease, and depressed left ventricular systolic function would have a life expectancy of 5.1 years with valve replacement and bypass grafting versus 1.6 years with medical therapy.

Surgical intervention also improves quality of life because elderly patients who refuse surgical intervention typically have recurrent hospital admissions for heart failure and have a very limited exercise tolerance and functional status between hospitalizations. The use of quality adjusted life years in the decision model described above highlights this point showing a quality adjusted life year value of 5.0 years with surgery versus 1.1 years with medical therapy.[215]

Despite convincing data on the benefits of aortic valve surgery in elderly patients, the rate of referral of elderly patients for aortic valve surgery is low with studies estimating that about 33% of appropriate candidates are referred for surgical intervention.[216] Inappropriate reasons often are used to justify deferring valve surgery, such as older age, poor left ventricular function, and response to medical therapy, indicating that improved education of primary care physicians about the benefits of intervention in this age group is needed.[216] Another reason for not referring elderly patients for surgery is the frequent presence of comorbidities. The operative risks can be estimated with readily available and well-validated online risk calculators from the Society of Thoracic Surgeons (http://www.sts.org) and the European Sytem for Cardiac Operative Risk Evaluation (http://www.euroscore.org). For patients with predicted high surgical mortality, less invasive alternative techniques of valve implantation have been developed (see Chapter 13).

Aortic Valve Replacement at the Time of Coronary Artery Bypass Surgery

Given that many patients with aortic stenosis also have significant coronary artery disease, it is not surprising that in some patients surgical intervention is required for coronary disease before the development of severe valvular obstruction. Subsequent progression of stenosis severity then leads to the need for aortic valve surgery at a later date in many of these patients. Unfortunately, the operative mortality for aortic valve replacement in patients with previous cardiac surgery is very high, ranging from 14% to 30%, although long-term outcome is more promising, with an approximate 5-year survival rate of 75%.[217,218]

One study with a long interval (9 years) between the two surgical procedures reported that there was no evidence of aortic stenosis at the time of the initial procedure.[217] However, in a study with a shorter time interval (6 years) between surgical procedures, it was noted that evidence of mild to moderate aortic stenosis was present at the first procedure in many patients.[219] These observations have generated controversy about the role of aortic valve replacement for mild to moderate aortic stenosis in patients undergoing coronary bypass procedures. The rationale for not replacing the aortic valve is based on the hypothesis that disease progression is slow and does not occur in all patients so that valve surgery may never be needed or can be deferred to a much later date. The rationale for "prophylactic" replacement of the aortic valve is that disease progression is inevitable so that a second surgical intervention will be needed at a predictable time point, depending on baseline stenosis severity. Recent studies on the natural history of mild to moderate aortic stenosis support the latter of these two rationales and suggest that prophylactic valve replacement be considered when the aortic valve is anatomically abnormal and the antegrade velocity is increased. The rate of hemodynamic progression in specific subgroups appears to be quite predictable, even though there is some variability in the individual rate of progression.[52,147]

In asymptomatic patients with an anatomically abnormal aortic valve and an aortic jet velocity more than 4.0 m/s, almost 80% need aortic valve replacement within 2 years, suggesting that valve surgery at the time of coronary artery surgery is appropriate to prevent early reoperation. In asymptomatic patients with a jet velocity between 3 and 4 m/s, the rate of valve replacement still is high with about 40% requiring valve surgery by 2 years and nearly 80% needing surgery within 5 years. In this group, the decision about prophylactic valve replacement should be individualized, depending on the jet velocity within this range, the degree of valve calcification on two-dimensional echocardiography and on fluoroscopy, and other clinical factors, such as age, comorbid disease, and patient preference. When aortic sclerosis is present but the jet velocity is less than 3.0 m/s, it is appropriate to defer valvular intervention as the rate of symptom development is considerably slower, being only 16% at 2 years.

This approach will be refined as additional data on the natural history of mild to moderate aortic stenosis become available and also will be modified as improved surgical procedures for aortic stenosis are developed. Because the major reasons to postpone valve replacement in a patient already undergoing cardiac surgery include the increased operative risk, the complications and inconvenience of long-term anticoagulation, suboptimal prosthetic valve hemodynamics, and the risk of prosthetic valve dysfunction or infection, improvements in any of these factors might tip the balance toward earlier intervention. Conversely, the use of minimally invasive surgical approaches might argue against performing valve surgery until it is absolutely necessary, because the coronary and valve procedures are performed from different approaches. In any case, a history of aortic valve disease or a pathologic murmur on auscultation mandates a careful evaluation of valve anatomy and function in the patient undergoing coronary artery surgery. When Doppler echocardiography shows moderate or severe disease, concurrent aortic valve surgery should be considered.

Aortic Stenosis with Left Ventricular Systolic Dysfunction

Left ventricular systolic dysfunction is a risk factor for operative mortality with valve replacement for aortic stenosis with threefold higher mortality in elderly patients with an ejection fraction less than 20% compared with those with an ejection fraction more than 60% (15% versus 6%).[209] However, clinical outcome is even worse without surgical intervention with a 12-month survival of only 20% to 50% in adults with aortic stenosis and severely reduced left ventricular function.[164] When left ventricular systolic dysfunction is due to increased afterload with normal myocardial contractility, systolic function is expected to improve after relief of outflow obstruction. Even with superimposed myocardial dysfunction, ventricular ejection performance should improve due to the afterload-reducing effect of valve replacement.[220] In a series

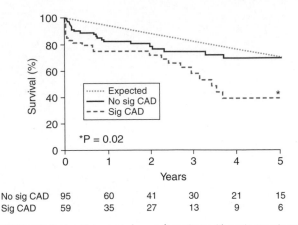

FIGURE 9–18 Kaplan-Meier survival curves for patients with aortic stenosis and reduced left ventricular function with and without significant coronary artery disease (two-vessel disease or greater or left main coronary disease) in comparison with expected survival. Number of patients alive at each point is shown on the x-axis. CAD, coronary artery disease. *(From Connolly HM, Oh JK, Orszulak TA, et al: Aortic valve replacement for aortic stenosis with severe left ventricular dysfunction: prognostic indicators. Circulation 1997;95:2395-2400, with permission.)*

of 154 patients with severe aortic stenosis and an ejection fraction of 35% or less, operative mortality was only 9%. Even though more than 50% of these patients had concurrent coronary artery bypass grafting, most had an improved ejection fraction and decreased symptoms after surgical intervention (Figure 9-18).[43]

In patients with severe aortic stenosis, a low gradient, and left ventricular dysfunction, dobutamine stress echocardiography has been suggested as an approach to distinguish those with contractile reserve from those unlikely to benefit from surgical intervention.[133] Although this approach may be useful in some patients, caution is warranted as there are not sufficient outcome studies addressing whether this approach should be used to deny surgical intervention in any of these patients. Patients with a small aortic valve area and a low transvalvular mean gradient (<30 mmHg) have poor outcomes with surgical therapy, with operative mortality of 21% and a 3-year survival of only 62% compared with 68% in patients with aortic stenosis, left ventricular dysfunction, and a mean gradient of 30 mmHg or greater.[221] However, those who survive surgery have improved functional status, and ejection fraction improves by about 10 ejection fraction units. In another nonrandomized comparison of medical versus surgical therapy for low-gradient aortic stenosis, survival was 78% at 4 years in the surgical group compared with 15% in the medical group (Figure 9-19).[222] More recently, a multicenter registry of patients with low-flow, low-gradient aortic stenosis reported that patients without contractile reserve had a markedly worse outcome compared with those with contractile reserve. However, survival was better with valve replacement even in the absence of contractile reserve (Figure 9-20).[134] More importantly, survivors showed similar improvement in left ventricular function regardless of the presence of contractile reserve.[138] Thus, although surgical risk is high, given the dismal outcome with medical therapy, surgical intervention may be considered in patients with low-flow, low-gradient severe aortic stenosis even without contractile reserve, particularly when other alternatives such as heart transplantation are not an option.

Operative Mortality and Long-Term Survival

Currently, the operative mortality of aortic valve replacement for aortic stenosis is low, and long-term outcomes after aortic valve surgery are excellent. Nevertheless, increased operative mortality can be expected in elderly patients and in the presence of comorbidity.[200] This topic is discussed in further detail in Chapter 12.

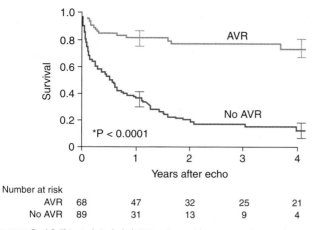

Number at risk

AVR	68	47	32	25	21
No AVR	89	31	13	9	4

FIGURE 9–19 This study included 157 patients with severe aortic stenosis (valve area ≤0.75 cm²), a left ventricular ejection fraction of 35% or less and a mean gradient of 30 mm Hg or less. Aortic valve replacement (AVR) was performed in 68 and 89 were treated medically. Survival by Kaplan-Meier analysis among all patients in the AVR and no AVR groups ($P < 0.0001$). The number of patients at risk during follow-up is shown on the x-axis. Echo, echocardiography. *(From Pereira JJ, Lauer MS, Bashir M, et al: Survival after aortic valve replacement for severe aortic stenosis with low transvalvular gradients and severe left ventricular dysfunction. J Am Coll Cardiol 2002;39:1356-1363, with permission.)*

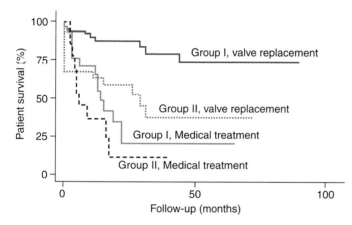

FIGURE 9–20 Kaplan-Meier survival estimates of 136 consecutive patients with low-flow, low-gradient aortic stenosis. Group I (n = 92) represents patients with contractile reserve determined by low-dose dobutamine echocardiography. Group II represents the group of patients with absent contractile reserve (n = 44). Survival estimates are represented according to contractile reserve and treatment strategy (aortic valve replacement versus medical therapy). *(From Monin JL, Quere JP, Monchi M, et al: Low-gradient aortic stenosis: operative risk stratification and predictors for long-term outcome: a multicenter study using dobutamine stress hemodynamics. Circulation 2003;108:319–324, with permission.)*

LEFT VENTRICULAR CHANGES

Postoperative Intracavitary Obstruction

In a subset of patients with aortic stenosis, dynamic midventricular outflow obstruction occurs in the early postoperative period. Intracavitary obstruction is most likely in the presence of a small hypertrophied left ventricle with preserved systolic function. After valve replacement, the acute decrease in left ventricular afterload results in hyperdynamic ventricular function with midcavity obstruction. These patients do not have asymmetric septal hypertrophy and systolic anterior motion of the mitral valve is only rarely seen. The late-peaking systolic velocity curve may have maximum velocities ranging from 1.8 to 6.8 m/s, corresponding to maximum gradients of 13 to 185 mmHg.[223-225] The mean gradients

corresponding to these maximum velocities are lower than those seen with valvular obstruction, given the late-peaking shape of the velocity curve with low velocities in early systole and midsystole.

Dynamic outflow obstruction is more likely in the early postoperative period, being recognized in as many as 50% of patients immediately after surgery and in about 14% of patients when echocardiography is performed within 10 days of surgery, averaging about 25% of patients overall.[223-225] In patients without evidence for obstruction at rest, an intracavitary gradient can be induced in an additional 13% using a nitroprusside and/or dobutamine infusion to decrease afterload and increase contractility.[224]

It is important to recognize dynamic intracavitary obstruction as these patients often have significant hypotension and dyspnea due to an impaired outflow from the small, hyperdynamic left ventricle. Prevention and treatment depend on maintaining an adequate preload and increasing (rather than further decreasing) afterload. Patients with postoperative obstruction have a prolonged hospital course.[224] Some studies showed no differences in 1-year survival rates,[224] whereas other studies suggested that excessive ventricular hypertrophy, specifically in women, is associated with increased postoperative mortality.[226]

Left Ventricular Systolic Function

Left ventricular ejection performance improves after aortic valve replacement because of the favorable effects of valve surgery on afterload. A small increase in ejection fraction is seen even in patients with a normal preoperative ejection fraction and a dramatic increase in ejection fraction may be seen in patients with impaired systolic function at baseline.[227,228]

When preoperative ventricular function is normal, about 90% of patients have preserved systolic function postoperatively.[229] Ventricular ejection performance predictably improves after relief of aortic stenosis if the cause of impaired ventricular function was increased afterload due to valvular obstruction. Intraoperative transesophageal echocardiographic studies suggest that end-systolic wall stress decreases within 30 minutes of aortic valve replacement.[230] Even when preoperative left ventricular function is severely impaired with an ejection fraction less than 35%, an improvement of left ventricular function can be expected in the majority of patients.[221] However, the degree of improvement is minimal if irreversible changes in the myocardium are present, for example, in patients with previous myocardial infarction or a cardiomyopathy.

Nevertheless, despite pathophysiologic arguments that ventricular function should improve after surgery for aortic stenosis, it is preferable to operate before the onset of ventricular dysfunction.[145] Although most patients with aortic stenosis followed prospectively have definite symptoms before there is any evidence of ventricular dysfunction, an occasional patient will have the onset of left ventricular systolic dysfunction as the cause of symptom onset

Regression of Left Ventricular Hypertrophy

Left ventricular hypertrophy gradually resolves after surgery for aortic stenosis (Figure 9-21).[61,231] However, in most patients, some degree of left ventricular hypertrophy persists indefinitely after aortic valve replacement and might be a marker of irreversible myocardial damage.[232] The pathophysiology of persistent hypertrophy probably is multifactorial with both permanent structural changes in the myocardium and the persistent, although less severe, outflow obstruction imposed by the prosthetic valve.

Persistent Diastolic Dysfunction Postoperatively

The muscular component of left ventricular hypertrophy resolves more rapidly than the fibrous component so that early and up to 2 years after valve replacement the proportion

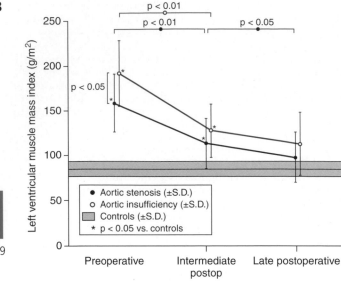

FIGURE 9–21 Left ventricular muscle mass index in patients with aortic stenosis preoperatively (red line) and in those with aortic insufficiency (blue line) preoperatively at the intermediate postoperative study (1.6 ± 0.5 years), and late postoperatively (8.1 ± 2 years) after aortic valve replacement. Whereas the greatest fall in muscle mass index occurred by 1 to 2 years after aortic valve surgery, significant further reductions continued to occur. *(From Monrad ES, Hess OM, Murakami T, et al: Time course of regression of left ventricular hypertrophy after aortic valve replacement. Circulation 1988;77:1345-1355, with permission.)*

of fibrous tissue in the myocardium increases compared with the amount of myocardium. This relative increase in fibrous tissue is associated with an increase in myocardial stiffness early after valve replacement and a decrease in early diastolic relaxation rate, concurrent with a reduction in the degree of left ventricular hypertrophy.[61,233]

The interstitial fibrosis component of ventricular hypertrophy regresses slowly so that balance between muscular and nonmuscular tissue does not normalize for several years after surgery. The prolonged persistence of diastolic dysfunction after surgery for aortic stenosis has significant clinical implications in terms of exercise capacity and functional status.[234] As surgical approaches to aortic stenosis improve in the future, the question as to whether surgery should be performed earlier in the disease course to prevent diastolic dysfunction will need to be addressed.

Exercise Capacity and Functional Status

After aortic valve replacement, in the absence of coexisting left ventricular dysfunction or uncorrected coronary artery disease, nearly all patients have resolution of symptoms of angina, syncope, dizziness, or overt heart failure. Most patients also report an improvement in functional class with all 6-month survivors being in New York Heart Association class I or II in a series of patients older than 80 years.[214] Improvement in symptomatic status can also generally be expected to occur in the majority of patients having a depressed preoperative left ventricular function.[221,222]

In a prospective study of 34 patients undergoing valve replacement for aortic stenosis, although left ventricular systolic function improved and left ventricular mass decreased, there was no objective improvement in treadmill exercise performance at 8 and 20 months after surgery, which might be attributable to persistent diastolic dysfunction.[228] Preoperative peak systolic strain rate has recently been suggested to predict reverse remodeling with a cutoff value of more than 2 seconds^{-1} predicting favorable symptomatic recovery after aortic valve replacement.[235]

MEDICAL THERAPY

In asymptomatic patients with valvular aortic stenosis, medical therapy is focused on prevention of complications, patient education, and prompt recognition of symptom onset. Once symptoms supervene, surgical intervention is needed to improve outcome and relieve symptoms. Pharmacologic therapy alone is appropriate only in those symptomatic patients who are not candidates for surgery because of comorbid conditions or those who refuse surgical intervention.

Noninvasive Follow-up

Echocardiographic evaluation is indicated at the time of diagnosis to ensure that valvular stenosis is present, to quantitate disease severity, and to evaluate any coexisting lesions. Many patients with an aortic outflow murmur have either no obstruction or only minimal sclerotic changes of the valve leaflets with only a minor increase in antegrade velocity. Because some of these patients may progress to aortic stenosis, routine repeat examinations at extended intervals are recommendable.

Once the initial diagnosis of aortic stenosis has been confirmed, the frequency of noninvasive follow-up is tailored to disease severity and other clinical factors for each individual patient. Because the timing of surgical intervention is based on symptom onset, it is essential to follow the patient's functional status. Patient education with the aim of recognizing and promptly reporting the typical symptoms of aortic stenosis is fundamental in patients with severe but also in mild to moderate aortic stenosis because rapid progression and symptomatic deterioration is not infrequent. Further risk stratification should be performed by assessing the degree of aortic valve calcification and hemodynamic progression.

Repeat echocardiographic examination is indicated for any change in clinical status and before any major noncardiac surgical procedures or events (such as pregnancy). In the absence of new symptoms, routine evaluation every 6 to 12 months is appropriate for patients with moderate or severe stenosis (aortic jet velocity >3.0 m/s). With mild aortic stenosis (jet velocity 2.0–3.0 m/s), evaluation every 2 to 3 years is reasonable in the absence of any change in clinical status or physical examination findings. The objective of the follow-up visit is best summarized in an editorial by Catherine Otto entitled "Aortic Stenosis—Listen to the Patient, Look at the Valve."[236]

Management of Arterial Hypertension

Approximately 40% of patients with aortic stenosis have concomitant hypertension.[52,153] Because patients with aortic stenosis are a population at high risk for cardiovascular events,[153,168] hypertension is a risk factor that needs to be addressed. In addition, the presence of arterial hypertension results in increased left ventricular wall stress.

Hypertension needs to be treated cautiously in patients with aortic stenosis, and negative inotropic drugs such as β-blockers should be avoided. There is also a concern that vasodilators may lead to a reduction of the coronary perfusion pressure. Classically, the use of angiotensin-converting enzyme (ACE) inhibitors in aortic stenosis was considered to be contraindicated.[237]

Although not designed to assess the safety of ACE inhibitor use in patients with aortic stenosis, the findings of a retrospective study indicate that a significant number of patients with aortic stenosis seen in daily clinical practice receive treatment with ACE inhibitors because of concomitant arterial hypertension (102 of 211 patients).[186] The observation that a significant number of patients with documented aortic stenosis receive ACE inhibitors is also shared by O'Brien et al.[238] Among 235 patients with aortic stenosis screened by echocardiography, 71 were already on treatment with an ACE inhibitor. In an additional 13 patients, who had mild-to-moderate aortic stenosis with preserved ventricular function, initiation of ACE inhibitor therapy was safe and well tolerated.[238]

In the Symptomatic Cardiac Obstruction-Pilot Study of Enalapril in Aortic Stenosis (SCOPE-AS) trial, symptomatic patients with severe aortic stenosis and normal left ventricular function who were not candidates for surgery, were randomly assigned to treatment with enalapril or placebo.[239] ACE inhibitors were well tolerated in these patients; however, patients, having reduced left ventricular functions, were prone to develop hypotension.

Finally, Jimenez-Candil et al[240] designed an elegant drug withdrawal study. Twenty patients with moderate to severe aortic stenosis already receiving an ACE inhibitor were included.[240] Both the withdrawal and the careful reintroduction of the drug were well tolerated. While taking the ACE inhibitor, patients had a lower blood pressure, higher transvalvular gradients but kept an unchanged exercise capacity and symptomatic status.

These data suggest that ACE inhibitor therapy may be cautiously used in patients with aortic stenosis. When following a patient with aortic stenosis who is taking antihypertensive medication, one has to consider that with increasing severity of stenosis, a reduction in the dosage of the antihypertensive drug might be necessary, because hypertension may become less accentuated and hypotension may even develop as a result of further narrowing of the aortic valve.

Prevention of Endocarditis

The recently updated guidelines for prevention of infective endocarditis no longer recommend antibiotic prophylaxis in patients with valvular aortic stenosis unless a patient has experienced a previous episode of infective endocarditis.[241] However, antibiotic prophylaxis is still recommended in patients with prosthetic heart valves. The considerations underlying this change are discussed in Chapter 8.

Management during Periods of Hemodynamic Stress

Asymptomatic patients with severe valvular aortic stenosis undergoing noncardiac surgery are at risk of decompensation, with development of symptoms and potential hemodynamic instability. These concerns also apply to patients with aortic stenosis with an intercurrent illness, particularly if it is accompanied by fever or anemia, and to the increased hemodynamic demands of pregnancy in a women with aortic stenosis. Several factors contribute to clinical decompensation in these situations, including changes in blood volume, fluid balance shifts, increased metabolic demands, decreased myocardial oxygen delivery, pain, and increased sympathetic system activity. During pregnancy hemodynamic changes include increases in cardiac output, heart rate, and blood volume and a decrease in systemic vascular resistance.[242] Additional physiologic changes occur during labor (further increases in cardiac output, in heart rate, and in blood pressure as well as an increase in systemic vascular resistance) and after the delivery of the placenta (increase in afterload and preload).[242] Whenever possible, aortic stenosis severity should be evaluated before pregnancy or a surgical procedure.

If aortic stenosis is very severe, suggesting impending symptom onset, surgical relief before pregnancy or noncardiac surgery should be considered. Pregnancy in patients with severe aortic stenosis is associated with significant maternal morbidity and a high necessity of cardiac surgery after pregnancy.[243-245] Two earlier studies described an acceptable operative risk for noncardiac surgery performed in patients with

severe aortic stenosis in whom valve replacement was refused or who were judged to be at too high risk.[246,247] On the other hand, severe aortic stenosis has been reported to significantly increase the risks for perioperative mortality and nonfatal myocardial infarction.[248] In this study, the risk of perioperative mortality was associated with a high risk score for coronary artery disease, suggesting that a screening for coronary artery disease is helpful for the assessment of the operative risk. In any case meticulous planning and monitoring in the perioperative period is required.

Patients with asymptomatic mild or moderate aortic stenosis can successfully undergo noncardiac surgery or pregnancy; however, they need close care.[151,244,245,249] Echocardiographic evaluation of stenosis severity and left ventricular function is essential. Procedures need to be planned (e.g., induction of labor rather than spontaneous labor) to allow invasive hemodynamic monitoring and to allow prevention or alleviation of pain (e.g., using an epidural anesthetic for vaginal delivery). Invasive hemodynamic monitoring is required to optimize loading conditions both during the procedure and in the postoperative period. It is especially important to continue monitoring postoperatively until fluid shifts have stabilized.

With use of this approach, adults with aortic stenosis have undergone noncardiac surgery with an acceptable mortality and morbidity[249] and women with aortic stenosis can undergo a successful pregnancy with delivery of a normal infant with low maternal mortality and morbidity.[151,244,245] The development of a second superimposed hemodynamic stress, such as a febrile illness, during pregnancy in a woman with aortic stenosis may tip the balance toward hemodynamic instability. In our experience these patients have been managed with monitoring in the intensive care unit, but surgical intervention during pregnancy may be needed in extreme cases.[141,250]

Prevention of Disease Progression

The similarities between aortic stenosis and atherosclerosis in terms of associated clinical factors, histopathological changes, and clinical outcomes indicate that calcific aortic stenosis is an active disease process that may be amenable to medical therapy (see Chapter 3). Specifically, it has been hypothesized that therapies for associated factors such as hyperlipidemia, inflammation, or calcification might slow or prevent disease progression. Experimental studies appear to support this concept. Rajamannan et al[251] demonstrated in a rabbit model that hypercholesterolemia-induced changes of the aortic valve were reversed when atorvastatin was administered. An association of ACE with low-density lipoprotein was shown in sclerotic and stenotic but not in normal human aortic valves.[252] Furthermore, in a retrospective study, O'Brien et al[253] found an association between the use of ACE inhibitors and a lower rate of aortic valve calcium accumulation as determined by electron beam computed tomographic scans.[253] However, another retrospective study showed no effect of ACE inhibitors on echocardiographically determined hemodynamic progression.[186]

Although four retrospective studies reported significantly slower rates of hemodynamic progression in patients receiving treatment with statins[182,183,185,186] these studies did not provide conclusive evidence as to whether the effect of statin therapy is dependent on cholesterol lowering. Whereas Novaro et al[185] reported an association between aortic stenosis progression and cholesterol levels, Bellamy et al[183] did not observe such an association in their analysis. Similarly, the rate of hemodynamic progression was unrelated to cholesterol levels, among both the statin-treated and the untreated patients in our study.[186] These findings initiated the hypothesis that the effects of statins at the valvular level may be caused by their pleiotropic or anti-inflammatory properties rather than by their cholesterol-lowering effect. The retrospective analysis by Rosenhek et al[186] is also unique for inclusion of patients with severe aortic stenosis and demonstrated that statins may slow hemodynamic progression in both mild to moderate as well as severe aortic stenosis and that the beneficial effects of statin therapy therefore may not be restricted to the early disease stages. Because a rapid increase in peak aortic jet velocity among patients with severe aortic stenosis and moderately to severely calcified valves results in a poor outcome,[150] slowing disease progression in these patients may still beneficially alter their outcome with respect to the development of symptoms and the necessity for surgery.

However, the Scottish Aortic Stenosis and Lipid Lowering Trial, Impact on Regression (SALTIRE) trial, which was the first prospective study to randomly assign patients with aortic stenosis to receive placebo or 80 mg of atorvastatin yielded a negative result after a mean follow-up of 26 months.[184] With 155 patients the study size was similar to that of the retrospective trials and also the follow-up duration was similar. The major difference with this study, however, was that patients who actually had hyperlipidemia were excluded as it was judged to be unethical to deprive these patients of statin therapy.[254]

The recent Rosuvastatin Affecting Aortic Valve Endothelium (RAAVE) trial is a prospective study for which a different approach has been chosen. Hypercholesterolemic patients were treated with rosuvastatin according to current hyperlipidemia management guidelines.[187] A significantly slower rate of progression was observed for patients receiving statin therapy. Furthermore, a correlation between change in low-density lipoprotein cholesterol levels during therapy and hemodynamic progression of aortic stenosis was found.

The largest prospective study that has been published to date is the SEAS trial in which 1873 patients were randomized to receive either 40mg of simvastatin plus 10 mg of ezetimibe or placebo.[256] After a mean follow-up duration of 52 months, no significant difference in hemodynamic progression was observed between the treatment and the placebo arms of the study. As in the SALTIRE trial, patients with hyperlipidemia, were not included, so as not to withhold a lipid-lowering therapy from them. The currently available data therefore support aggressive control of hyperlipidemia (using statins as a first-line therapy) in all patients with aortic sclerosis and stenosis. However, no data are available to support lipid-lowering therapies in patients with aortic stenosis who have normal cholesterol levels.

There are two other aspects with regard to statin therapy in patients with aortic stenosis. Because patients with aortic stenosis and even patients with aortic sclerosis are known to have increased cardiovascular morbidity and mortality,[168] statin therapy might ultimately be beneficial. Shah et al.[255] demonstrated that patients with known coronary artery disease with a sclerotic aortic valve not receiving statin therapy had a 2.4-fold increased risk for the occurrence of a myocardial infarction compared with patients with a normal aortic valve. They also showed that this risk might be attenuated by statins. In the SEAS trial[256], there were fewer ischemic cardiovascular events in the treatment arm than in the placebo group (15.7% versus 20.1%, p=0.02) with a significantly lower incidence of the necessity for coronary artery bypass grafting in the treated patients (7.3% versus 10.8%, p=0.02). Furthermore, because symptoms might be triggered by progressive coronary artery disease in some patients with aortic stenosis, symptom onset might be delayed by statin therapy.

The results from larger randomized trials are needed to provide an answer to these questions. In addition, the stage of disease at which an initiation of therapy is most beneficial needs yet to be defined, should therapy prove to be effective. The expectation is that early initiation of therapy might be advantageous.

REFERENCES

1. Clark C: Relation between pressure difference across the aortic valve and left ventricular outflow. Cardiovasc Res 1978;12:276-287.
2. Pasipoularides A: Clinical assessment of ventricular ejection dynamics with and without outflow obstruction. J Am Coll Cardiol 1990;15:859-882.
3. Bermejo J, Antoranz JC, Burwash IG, et al: In-vivo analysis of the instantaneous transvalvular pressure difference-flow relationship in aortic valve stenosis: implications of unsteady fluid-dynamics for the clinical assessment of disease severity. J Heart Valve Dis 2002;11:557-566.
4. Otto CM, Pearlman AS, Gardner CL, et al: Experimental validation of Doppler echocardiographic measurement of volume flow through the stenotic aortic valve. Circulation 1988;78:435-441.
5. Hatle L, Angelsen BA, Tromsdal A: Non-invasive assessment of aortic stenosis by Doppler ultrasound. Br Heart J 1980;43:284-292.
6. Currie PJ, Seward JB, Reeder GS, et al: Continuous-wave Doppler echocardiographic assessment of severity of calcific aortic stenosis a simultaneous Doppler-catheter correlative study in 100 adult patients. Circulation 1985;71:1162-1169.
7. Otto CM, Nishimura RA, Davis KB, et al: Doppler echocardiographic findings in adults with severe symptomatic valvular aortic stenosis: Balloon Valvuloplasty Registry Echocardiographers. Am J Cardiol 1991;68:1477-1484.
8. Otto CM, Pearlman AS: Doppler echocardiography in adults with symptomatic aortic stenosis: diagnostic utility and cost-effectiveness. Arch Intern Med 1988;148: 2553-2560.
9. Laskey WK, Kussmaul WG: Pressure recovery in aortic valve stenosis. Circulation 1994;89:116-121.
10. Levine RA, Jimoh A, Cape EG, et al: Pressure recovery distal to a stenosis: potential cause of gradient "overestimation" by Doppler echocardiography. J Am Coll Cardiol 1989;13:706-715.
11. Niederberger J, Schima H, Maurer G, Baumgartner H: Importance of pressure recovery for the assessment of aortic stenosis by Doppler ultrasound: role of aortic size, aortic valve area, and direction of the stenotic jet in vitro. Circulation 1996;94:1934-1940.
12. Baumgartner H, Stefenelli T, Niederberger J, et al: "Overestimation" of catheter gradients by Doppler ultrasound in patients with aortic stenosis: a predictable manifestation of pressure recovery. J Am Coll Cardiol 1999;33:1655-1661.
13. Heinrich RS, Fontaine AA, Grimes RY, et al: Experimental analysis of fluid mechanical energy losses in aortic valve stenosis: importance of pressure recovery. Ann Biomed Eng 1996;24:685-694.
14. Garcia D, Pibarot P, Dumesnil JG, et al: Assessment of aortic valve stenosis severity: a new index based on the energy loss concept. Circulation 2000;101:765-771.
15. Otto CM, Pearlman AS, Comess KA, et al: Determination of the stenotic aortic valve area in adults using Doppler echocardiography. J Am Coll Cardiol 1986;7:509-517.
16. Zoghbi WA, Farmer KL, Soto JG, et al: Accurate noninvasive quantification of stenotic aortic valve area by Doppler echocardiography. Circulation 1986;73:452-459.
17. Teirstein P, Yeager M, Yock PG, Popp RL: Doppler echocardiographic measurement of aortic valve area in aortic stenosis: a noninvasive application of the Gorlin formula. J Am Coll Cardiol 1986;8:1059-1065.
18. Ohlsson J, Wranne B: Noninvasive assessment of valve area in patients with aortic stenosis. J Am Coll Cardiol 1986;7:501-508.
19. Gorlin R, Gorlin SG: Hydraulic formula for calculation of the area of the stenotic mitral valve, other cardiac valves, and central circulatory shunts. I. Am Heart J 1951;41:1-29.
20. Cannon SR, Richards KL, Crawford MH, et al: Inadequacy of the Gorlin formula for predicting prosthetic valve area. Am J Cardiol 1988;62:113-116.
21. Cannon SR, Richards KL, Crawford M: Hydraulic estimation of stenotic orifice area: a correction of the Gorlin formula. Circulation 1985;71:1170-1178.
22. Richards KL, Cannon SR, Miller JF, Crawford MH: Calculation of aortic valve area by Doppler echocardiography: a direct application of the continuity equation. Circulation 1986;73:964-969.
23. Segal J, Lerner DJ, Miller DC, et al: When should Doppler-determined valve area be better than the Gorlin formula? Variation in hydraulic constants in low flow states. J Am Coll Cardiol 1987;9:1294-305.
24. Dumesnil JG, Yoganathan AP: Theoretical and practical differences between the Gorlin formula and the continuity equation for calculating aortic and mitral valve areas. Am J Cardiol 1991;67:1268-1272.
25. Gorlin R, Gorlin WB: Further reconciliation between pathoanatomy and pathophysiology of stenotic cardiac valves. J Am Coll Cardiol 1990;15:1181-1182.
26. Gilon D, Cape EG, Handschumacher MD, et al: Effect of three-dimensional valve shape on the hemodynamics of aortic stenosis: three-dimensional echocardiographic stereolithography and patient studies. J Am Coll Cardiol 2002;40:1479-1486.
27. Montarello JK, Perakis AC, Rosenthal E, et al: Normal and stenotic human aortic valve opening: in vitro assessment of orifice area changes with flow. Eur Heart J 1990;11: 484-491.
28. Bache RJ, Wang Y, Jorgensen CR: Hemodynamic effects of exercise in isolated valvular aortic stenosis. Circulation 1971;44:1003-1013.
29. Otto CM, Pearlman AS, Kraft CD, et al: Physiologic changes with maximal exercise in asymptomatic valvular aortic stenosis assessed by Doppler echocardiography. J Am Coll Cardiol 1992;20:1160-1167.
30. Shively BK, Charlton GA, Crawford MH, Chaney RK: Flow dependence of valve area in aortic stenosis: relation to valve morphology. J Am Coll Cardiol 1998;31:654-660.
31. Tardif JC, Rodrigues AG, Hardy JF, et al: Simultaneous determination of aortic valve area by the Gorlin formula and by transesophageal echocardiography under different transvalvular flow conditions: evidence that anatomic aortic valve area does not change with variations in flow in aortic stenosis. J Am Coll Cardiol 1997;29:1296-302.
32. Badano L, Cassottano P, Bertoli D, et al: Changes in effective aortic valve area during ejection in adults with aortic stenosis. Am J Cardiol 1996;78:1023-1028.
33. Bermejo J, Garcia-Fernandez MA, Torrecilla EG, et al: Effects of dobutamine on Doppler echocardiographic indexes of aortic stenosis. J Am Coll Cardiol 1996;28:1206-1213.

34. Burwash IG, Pearlman AS, Kraft CD, et al: Flow dependence of measures of aortic stenosis severity during exercise. J Am Coll Cardiol 1994;24:1342-1350.
35. Burwash IG, Thomas DD, Sadahiro M, et al: Dependence of Gorlin formula and continuity equation valve areas on transvalvular volume flow rate in valvular aortic stenosis. Circulation 1994;89:827-835.
36. Casale PN, Palacios IF, Abascal VM, et al: Effects of dobutamine on Gorlin and continuity equation valve areas and valve resistance in valvular aortic stenosis. Am J Cardiol 1992;70:1175-1179.
37. Chambers JB, Sprigings DC, Cochrane T, et al: Continuity equation and Gorlin formula compared with directly observed orifice area in native and prosthetic aortic valves. Br Heart J 1992;67:193-199.
38. Bermejo J, Antoranz JC, Garcia-Fernandez MA, et al: Flow dynamics of stenotic aortic valves assessed by signal processing of Doppler spectrograms. Am J Cardiol 2000;85:611-617.
39. Arsenault M, Masani N, Magni G, et al: Variation of anatomic valve area during ejection in patients with valvular aortic stenosis evaluated by two-dimensional echocardiographic planimetry: comparison with traditional Doppler data. J Am Coll Cardiol 1998;32:1931-1937.
40. Lester SJ, McElhinney DB, Miller JP, et al: Rate of change in aortic valve area during a cardiac cycle can predict the rate of hemodynamic progression of aortic stenosis. Circulation 2000;101:1947-1952.
41. Carabello BA, Green LH, Grossman W, et al: Hemodynamic determinants of prognosis of aortic valve replacement in critical aortic stenosis and advanced congestive heart failure. Circulation 1980;62:42-48.
42. deFilippi CR, Willett DL, Brickner ME, et al: Usefulness of dobutamine echocardiography in distinguishing severe from nonsevere valvular aortic stenosis in patients with depressed left ventricular function and low transvalvular gradients. Am J Cardiol 1995;75:191-194.
43. Connolly HM, Oh JK, Orszulak TA, et al: Aortic valve replacement for aortic stenosis with severe left ventricular dysfunction: prognostic indicators. Circulation 1997;95:2395-2400.
44. Kadem L, Rieu R, Dumesnil JG, et al: Flow-dependent changes in Doppler-derived aortic valve effective orifice area are real and not due to artifact. J Am Coll Cardiol 2006;47:131-137.
45. Baumgartner H: Hemodynamic assessment of aortic stenosis: are there still lessons to learn. J Am Coll Cardiol 2006;47:138-140.
46. Cannon JD Jr, Zile MR, Crawford FA Jr, Carabello BA: Aortic valve resistance as an adjunct to the Gorlin formula in assessing the severity of aortic stenosis in symptomatic patients. J Am Coll Cardiol 1992;20:1517-1523.
47. Ford LE, Feldman T, Chiu YC, Carroll JD: Hemodynamic resistance as a measure of functional impairment in aortic valvular stenosis. Circ Res 1990;66:1-7.
48. Voelker W, Reul H, Nienhaus G, et al: Comparison of valvular resistance, stroke work loss, and Gorlin valve area for quantification of aortic stenosis: an in vitro study in a pulsatile aortic flow model. Circulation 1995;91:1196-204.
49. Frank A, Chung C: The aortic valve hemodynamics under degenerative leaflet calcification: a computer modeling approach. Bioeng Conf 2001;50:655-675.
50. Blais C, Pibarot P, Dumesnil JG, et al: Comparison of valve resistance with effective orifice area regarding flow dependence. Am J Cardiol 2001;88:45-52.
51. Burwash IG, Hay KM, Chan KL: Hemodynamic stability of valve area, valve resistance, and stroke work loss in aortic stenosis: a comparative analysis. J Am Soc Echocardiogr 2002;15:814-822.
52. Otto CM, Burwash IG, Legget ME, et al: Prospective study of asymptomatic valvular aortic stenosis: clinical, echocardiographic, and exercise predictors of outcome. Circulation 1997;95:2262-2270.
53. Sprigings DC, Chambers JB, Cochrane T, et al: Ventricular stroke work loss: validation of a method of quantifying the severity of aortic stenosis and derivation of an orifice formula. J Am Coll Cardiol 1990;16:1608-1614.
54. Tobin JR Jr, Rahimtoola SH, Blundell PE, Swan HJ: Percentage of left ventricular stroke work loss: a simple hemodynamic concept for estimation of severity in valvular aortic stenosis. Circulation 1967;35:868-879.
55. Laskey WK, Kussmaul WG, Noordergraaf A: Valvular and systemic arterial hemodynamics in aortic valve stenosis: a model-based approach. Circulation 1995;92:1473-1478.
56. Carroll JD, Carroll EP, Feldman T, et al: Sex-associated differences in left ventricular function in aortic stenosis of the elderly. Circulation 1992;86:1099-107.
57. Douglas PS, Otto CM, Mickel MC, et al: Gender differences in left ventricle geometry and function in patients undergoing balloon dilatation of the aortic valve for isolated aortic stenosis. NHLBI Balloon Valvuloplasty Registry. Br Heart J 1995;73:548-554.
58. Aurigemma GP, Silver KH, McLaughlin M, et al: Impact of chamber geometry and gender on left ventricular systolic function in patients >60 years of age with aortic stenosis. Am J Cardiol 1994;74:794-798.
59. Legget ME, Kuusisto J, Healy NL, et al: Gender differences in left ventricular function at rest and with exercise in asymptomatic aortic stenosis. Am Heart J 1996;131:94-100.
60. Jin XY, Pepper JR, Gibson DG: Effects of incoordination on left ventricular force-velocity relation in aortic stenosis. Heart 1996;76:495-501.
61. Villari B, Campbell SE, Schneider J, et al: Sex-dependent differences in left ventricular function and structure in chronic pressure overload. Eur Heart J 1995;16:1410-1419.
62. Douglas PS, Berko B, Lesh M, Reichek N: Alterations in diastolic function in response to progressive left ventricular hypertrophy. J Am Coll Cardiol 1989;13:461-467.
63. Villari B, Campbell SE, Hess OM, et al: Influence of collagen network on left ventricular systolic and diastolic function in aortic valve disease. J Am Coll Cardiol 1993;22:1477-1484.
64. Villari B, Vassalli G, Schneider J, et al: Age dependency of left ventricular diastolic function in pressure overload hypertrophy. J Am Coll Cardiol 1997;29:181-186.
65. Folland ED, Parisi AF, Carbone C: Is peripheral arterial pressure a satisfactory substitute for ascending aortic pressure when measuring aortic valve gradients? J Am Coll Cardiol 1984;4:1207-1212.
66. Faggiano P, Antonini-Canterin F, Ribichini F, et al: Pulmonary artery hypertension in adult patients with symptomatic valvular aortic stenosis. Am J Cardiol 2000;85:204-208.
67. Tracy GP, Proctor MS, Hizny CS: Reversibility of pulmonary artery hypertension in aortic stenosis after aortic valve replacement. Ann Thorac Surg 1990;50:89-93.
68. Aragam JR, Folland ED, Lapsley D, et al: Cause and impact of pulmonary hypertension in isolated aortic stenosis on operative mortality for aortic valve replacement in men. Am J Cardiol 1992;69:1365-1367.
69. Snopek G, Pogorzelska H, Zielinski T, et al: Valve replacement for aortic stenosis with severe congestive heart failure and pulmonary hypertension. J Heart Valve Dis 1996;5:268-272.
70. Kaufmann P, Vassalli G, Lupi-Wagner S, et al: Coronary artery dimensions in primary and secondary left ventricular hypertrophy. J Am Coll Cardiol 1996;28:745-750.
71. Marcus ML, Doty DB, Hiratzka LF, et al: Decreased coronary reserve a mechanism for angina pectoris in patients with aortic stenosis: and normal coronary arteries. N Engl J Med 1982;307:1362-1366.
72. Nadell R, DePace NL, Ren JF, et al: Myocardial oxygen supply/demand ratio in aortic stenosis: hemodynamic and echocardiographic evaluation of patients with and without angina pectoris. J Am Coll Cardiol 1983;2:258-262.
73. Villari B, Hess OM, Kaufmann P, et al: Effect of aortic valve stenosis (pressure overload) and regurgitation (volume overload) on left ventricular systolic and diastolic function. Am J Cardiol 1992;69:927-934.
74. Rajappan K, Rimoldi OE, Dutka DP, et al: Mechanisms of coronary microcirculatory dysfunction in patients with aortic stenosis and angiographically normal coronary arteries. Circulation 2002;105:470-476.
75. Hildick-Smith DJ, Shapiro LM: Coronary flow reserve improves after aortic valve replacement for aortic stenosis: an adenosine transthoracic echocardiography study. J Am Coll Cardiol 2000;36:1889-1896.
76. Julius BK, Spillmann M, Vassalli G, et al: Angina pectoris in patients with aortic stenosis and normal coronary arteries: mechanisms and pathophysiological concepts. Circulation 1997;95:892-898.
77. Gould KL: Why angina pectoris in aortic stenosis. Circulation 1997;95:790-792.
78. Kenny A, Wisbey CR, Shapiro LM: Profiles of coronary blood flow velocity in patients with aortic stenosis and the effect of valve replacement: a transthoracic echocardiographic study. Br Heart J 1994;71:57-62.
79. Omran H, Fehske W, Rabahieh R, et al: Relation between symptoms and profiles of coronary artery blood flow velocities in patients with aortic valve stenosis: a study using transoesophageal Doppler echocardiography. Heart 1996;75:377-383.
80. Isaaz K, Bruntz JF, Paris D, et al: Abnormal coronary flow velocity pattern in patients with left ventricular hypertrophy, angina pectoris, and normal coronary arteries: a transesophageal Doppler echocardiographic study. Am Heart J 1994;128:500-510.
81. Petropoulakis PN, Kyriakidis MK, Tentolouris CA, et al: Changes in phasic coronary blood flow velocity profile in relation to changes in hemodynamic parameters during stress in patients with aortic valve stenosis. Circulation 1995;92:1437-1447.
82. Smucker ML, Tedesco CL, Manning SB, et al: Demonstration of an imbalance between coronary perfusion and excessive load as a mechanism of ischemia during stress in patients with aortic stenosis. Circulation 1988;78:573-582.
83. Anderson FL, Tsagaris TJ, Tikoff G, et al: Hemodynamic effects of exercise in patients with aortic stenosis. Am J Med 1969;46:872-885.
84. Ettinger PO, Frank MJ, Levinson GE: Hemodynamics at rest and during exercise in combined aortic stenosis and insufficiency. Circulation 1972;45:267-276.
85. Movsowitz C, Kussmaul WG, Laskey WK: Left ventricular diastolic response to exercise in valvular aortic stenosis. Am J Cardiol 1996;77:275-280.
86. Lancellotti P, Lebois F, Simon M, et al: Prognostic importance of quantitative exercise Doppler echocardiography in asymptomatic valvular aortic stenosis. Circulation 2005;112:I377-I382.
87. Chizner MA, Pearle DL, deLeon AC Jr: The natural history of aortic stenosis in adults. Am Heart J 1980;99:419-424.
88. Frank S, Johnson A, Ross J Jr: Natural history of valvular aortic stenosis. Br Heart J 1973;35:41-46.
89. Rapaport E: Natural history of aortic and mitral valve disease. Am J Cardiol 1975;35:221-227.
90. Ross J Jr, Braunwald E: Aortic stenosis. Circulation 1968;38:61-67.
91. Selzer A: Changing aspects of the natural history of valvular aortic stenosis. N Engl J Med 1987;317:91-98.
92. Lombard JT, Selzer A: Valvular aortic stenosis: a clinical and hemodynamic profile of patients. Ann Intern Med 1987;106:292-298.
93. Faggiano P, Sabatini T, Rusconi C, et al: Abnormalities of left ventricular filling in valvular aortic stenosis: usefulness of combined evaluation of pulmonary veins and mitral flow by means of transthoracic Doppler echocardiography. Int J Cardiol 1995;49:77-85.
94. Johnson AM: Aortic stenosis, sudden death, and the left ventricular baroceptors. Br Heart J 1971;33:1-5.
95. Richards AM, Nicholls MG, Ikram H, et al: Syncope in aortic valvular stenosis. Lancet 1984;2:1113-1116.
96. Schwartz LS, Goldfischer J, Sprague GJ, Schwartz SP: Syncope and sudden death in aortic stenosis. Am J Cardiol 1969;23:647-658.
97. Eddleman EE Jr, Frommeyer WB Jr, Lyle DP, et al: Critical analysis of clinical factors in estimating severity of aortic valve disease. Am J Cardiol 1973;31:687-695.
98. Jaffe WM, Roche AH, Coverdale HA, et al: Clinical evaluation versus Doppler echocardiography in the quantitative assessment of valvular heart disease. Circulation 1988;78:267-275.
99. Bonner AJ Jr, Sacks HN, Tavel ME: Assessing the severity of aortic stenosis by phonocardiography and external carotid pulse recordings. Circulation 1973;48:247-252.
100. Munt B, Legget ME, Kraft CD, et al: Physical examination in valvular aortic stenosis: correlation with stenosis severity and prediction of clinical outcome. Am Heart J 1999;137:298-306.
101. Judge TP, Kennedy JW: Estimation of aortic regurgitation by diastolic pulse wave analysis. Circulation 1970;41:659-665.

102. Aronow WS, Kronzon I: Prevalence and severity of valvular aortic stenosis determined by Doppler echocardiography and its association with echocardiographic and electrocardiographic left ventricular hypertrophy and physical signs of aortic stenosis in elderly patients. Am J Cardiol 1991;67:776-777.
103. Aronow WS, Schwartz KS, Koenigsberg M: Correlation of serum lipids, calcium and phosphorus, diabetes mellitus, aortic valve stenosis and history of systemic hypertension with presence or absence of mitral anular calcium in persons older than 62 years in a long-term health care facility. Am J Cardiol 1987;59:381-382.
104. Perloff J: Physical examination of the heart and circulation. WB Saunders, Philadephia 1982.
105. Caulfield WH, de Leon AC Jr, Porloff JK, Steelman RD: The clinical significance of the fourth heart sound in aortic stenosis. Am J Cardiol 1971;28:179-182.
106. Bonderman D, Gharehbaghi-Schnell E, Wollenek G, et al: Mechanisms underlying aortic dilatation in congenital aortic valve malformation. Circulation 1999;99:2138-2143.
107. Szamosi A, Wassberg B: Radiologic detection of aortic stenosis. Acta Radiol Diagn (Stockh) 1983;24:201-207.
108. Braunwald E, Goldblatt A, Aygen MM, et al: Congenital aortic stenosis. I. Clinical and hemodynamic findings in 100 patients. II. Surgical treatment and the results of operation. Circulation 1963;27:426-462.
109. Hugenholtz PG, Lees MM, Nadas AS: The scalar electrocardiogram, vectorcardiogram, and exercise electrocardiogram in the assessment of congenital aortic stenosis. Circulation 1962;26:79-91.
110. Abdin ZH: The electrocardiogram in aortic stenosis. Br Heart J 1958;20:31-40.
111. Fowler RS: Ventricular repolarization in congenital aortic stenosis. Am Heart J 1965;70:603-611.
112. Kim KS, Maxted W, Nanda NC, et al: Comparison of multiplane and biplane transesophageal echocardiography in the assessment of aortic stenosis. Am J Cardiol 1997;79:436-441.
113. Cormier B, Iung B, Porte JM, et al: Value of multiplane transesophageal echocardiography in determining aortic valve area in aortic stenosis. Am J Cardiol 1996;77: 882-885.
114. Tribouilloy C, Shen WF, Peltier M, et al: Quantitation of aortic valve area in aortic stenosis with multiplane transesophageal echocardiography: comparison with monoplane transesophageal approach. Am Heart J 1994;128:526-532.
115. Bernard Y, Meneveau N, Vuillemenot A, et al: Planimetry of aortic valve area using multiplane transoesophageal echocardiography is not a reliable method for assessing severity of aortic stenosis. Heart 1997;78:68-73.
116. Baumgartner H, Khan S, DeRobertis M, et al: Discrepancies between Doppler and catheter gradients in aortic prosthetic valves in vitro: a manifestation of localized gradients and pressure recovery. Circulation 1990;82:1467-1475.
117. Callahan MJ, Tajik AJ, Su-Fan Q, Bove AA: Validation of instantaneous pressure gradients measured by continuous-wave Doppler in experimentally induced aortic stenosis. Am J Cardiol 1985;56:989-993.
118. Simpson IA, Houston AB, Sheldon CD, et al: Clinical value of Doppler echocardiography in the assessment of adults with aortic stenosis. Br Heart J 1985;53:636-639.
119. Burwash IG, Forbes AD, Sadahiro M, et al: Echocardiographic volume flow and stenosis severity measures with changing flow rate in aortic stenosis. Am J Physiol 1993;265:H1734-H1743.
120. Smith MD, Dawson PL, Elion JL, et al: Correlation of continuous wave Doppler velocities with cardiac catheterization gradients: an experimental model of aortic stenosis. J Am Coll Cardiol 1985;6:1306-1314.
121. Smith MD, Kwan OL, DeMaria AN: Value and limitations of continuous-wave Doppler echocardiography in estimating severity of valvular stenosis. JAMA 1986;255: 3145-3151.
122. Clyne CA, Arrighi JA, Maron BJ, et al: Systemic and left ventricular responses to exercise stress in asymptomatic patients with valvular aortic stenosis. Am J Cardiol 1991;68:1469-1476.
123. Atterhog JH, Jonsson B, Samuelsson R: Exercise testing: a prospective study of complication rates. Am Heart J 1979;98:572-579.
124. Atwood JE, Kawanishi S, Myers J, Froelicher VF: Exercise testing in patients with aortic stenosis. Chest 1988;93:1083-1087.
125. Bonow RO, Cheitlin MD, Crawford MH, Douglas PS: Task Force 3: valvular heart disease. J Am Coll Cardiol 2005;45:1334-1340.
126. Maron BJ, Thompson PD, Puffer JC, et al: Cardiovascular preparticipation screening of competitive athletes. A statement for health professionals from the Sudden Death Committee (clinical cardiology) and Congenital Cardiac Defects Committee (cardiovascular disease in the young), American Heart Association. Circulation 1996;94:850-856.
127. Alborino D, Hoffmann JL, Fournet PC, Bloch A: Value of exercise testing to evaluate the indication for surgery in asymptomatic patients with valvular aortic stenosis. J Heart Valve Dis 2002;11:204-209.
128. Amato MC, Moffa PJ, Werner KE, Ramires JA: Treatment decision in asymptomatic aortic valve stenosis: role of exercise testing. Heart 2001;86:381-386.
129. Das P, Rimington H, Chambers J: Exercise testing to stratify risk in aortic stenosis. Eur Heart J 2005;26:1309-1313.
130. Iung B, Gohlke-Barwolf C, Tornos P, et al: Recommendations on the management of the asymptomatic patient with valvular heart disease. Eur Heart J 2002;23:1252-1266.
131. Otto CM: Clinical practice: evaluation and management of chronic mitral regurgitation. N Engl J Med 2001;345:740-746.
132. Lin SS, Roger VL, Pascoe R, et al: Dobutamine stress Doppler hemodynamics in patients with aortic stenosis: feasibility, safety, and surgical correlations. Am Heart J 1998;136:1010-1016.
133. Monin JL, Monchi M, Gest V, et al: Aortic stenosis with severe left ventricular dysfunction and low transvalvular pressure gradients: risk stratification by low-dose dobutamine echocardiography. J Am Coll Cardiol 2001;37:2101-2107.
134. Monin JL, Quere JP, Monchi M, et al: Low-gradient aortic stenosis: operative risk stratification and predictors for long-term outcome: a multicenter study using dobutamine stress hemodynamics. Circulation 2003;108:319-324.
135. Nishimura RA, Grantham JA, Connolly HM, et al: Low-output, low-gradient aortic stenosis in patients with depressed left ventricular systolic function: the clinical utility of the dobutamine challenge in the catheterization laboratory. Circulation 2002;106:809-813.
136. Schwammenthal E, Vered Z, Moshkowitz Y, et al: Dobutamine echocardiography in patients with aortic stenosis and left ventricular dysfunction: predicting outcome as a function of management strategy. Chest 2001;119:1766-1777.
137. Takeda S, Rimington H, Chambers J: The relation between transaortic pressure difference and flow during dobutamine stress echocardiography in patients with aortic stenosis. Heart 1999;82:11-14.
138. Quere JP, Monin JL, Levy F, et al: Influence of preoperative left ventricular contractile reserve on postoperative ejection fraction in low-gradient aortic stenosis. Circulation 2006;113:1738-1744.
139. Baumgartner H, Khan SS, DeRobertis M, et al: Doppler assessment of prosthetic valve orifice area: an in vitro study. Circulation 1992;85:2275-2283.
140. Horstkotte D, Loogen F: The natural history of aortic valve stenosis. Eur Heart J 1988;9(Suppl E):57-64.
141. Lao TT, Adelman AG, Sermer M, Colman JM: Balloon valvuloplasty for congenital aortic stenosis in pregnancy. Br J Obstet Gynaecol 1993;100:1141-1142.
142. Beppu S, Suzuki S, Matsuda H, et al: Rapidity of progression of aortic stenosis in patients with congenital bicuspid aortic valves. Am J Cardiol 1993;71:322-327.
143. Pachulski RT, Chan KL: Progression of aortic valve dysfunction in 51 adult patients with congenital bicuspid aortic valve: assessment and follow up by Doppler echocardiography. Br Heart J 1993;69:237-240.
144. Roberts WC, Ko JM: Frequency by decades of unicuspid, bicuspid, and tricuspid aortic valves in adults having isolated aortic valve replacement for aortic stenosis, with or without associated aortic regurgitation. Circulation 2005;111:920-925.
145. Lund O, Nielsen TT, Pilegaard HK, et al: The influence of coronary artery disease and bypass grafting on early and late survival after valve replacement for aortic stenosis. J Thorac Cardiovasc Surg 1990;100:327-337.
146. Kelly TA, Rothbart RM, Cooper CM, et al: Comparison of outcome of asymptomatic to symptomatic patients older than 20 years of age with valvular aortic stenosis. Am J Cardiol 1988;61:123-130.
147. Faggiano P, Ghizzoni G, Sorgato A, et al: Rate of progression of valvular aortic stenosis in adults. Am J Cardiol 1992;70:229-233.
148. Pellikka PA, Nishimura RA, Bailey KR, Tajik AJ: The natural history of adults with asymptomatic, hemodynamically significant aortic stenosis. J Am Coll Cardiol 1990;15:1012-1017.
149. Pellikka PA, Sarano ME, Nishimura RA, et al: Outcome of 622 adults with asymptomatic, hemodynamically significant aortic stenosis during prolonged follow-up. Circulation 2005;111:3290-3295.
150. Rosenhek R, Binder T, Porenta G, et al: Predictors of outcome in severe, asymptomatic aortic stenosis. N Engl J Med 2000;343:611-617.
151. Easterling TR, Chadwick HS, Otto CM, Benedetti TJ: Aortic stenosis in pregnancy. Obstet Gynecol 1988;72:113-118.
152. Keane JF, Driscoll DJ, Gersony WM, et al: Second natural history study of congenital heart defects: results of treatment of patients with aortic valvar stenosis. Circulation 1993;87:I16-27.
153. Rosenhek R, Klaar U, Schemper M, et al: Mild and moderate aortic stenosis; natural history and risk stratification by echocardiography. Eur Heart J 2004;25:199-205.
154. Antonini-Canterin F, Faggiano P, Zanuttini D, Ribichini F: Is aortic valve resistance more clinically meaningful than valve area in aortic stenosis? Heart 1999;82:9-10.
155. Bahler RC, Desser DR, Finkelhor RS, et al: Factors leading to progression of valvular aortic stenosis. Am J Cardiol 1999;84:1044-1048.
156. Vaturi M, Porter A, Adler Y, et al: The natural history of aortic valve disease after mitral valve surgery. J Am Coll Cardiol 1999;33:2003-2008.
157. Messika-Zeitoun D, Aubry MC, Detaint D, et al: Evaluation and clinical implications of aortic valve calcification measured by electron-beam computed tomography. Circulation 2004;110:356-362.
158. Archer SL, Mike DK, Hetland MB, et al: Usefulness of mean aortic valve gradient and left ventricular diastolic filling pattern for distinguishing symptomatic from asymptomatic patients. Am J Cardiol 1994;73:275-281.
159. Turina J, Hess O, Sepulcri F, Krayenbuehl HP: Spontaneous course of aortic valve disease. Eur Heart J 1987;8:471-483.
160. Bonow RO, Carabello BA, Chatterjee K, et al: ACC/AHA 2006 guidelines for the management of patients with valvular heart disease: a report of the American College of Cardiology/American Heart Association Task Force on Practice Guidelines (writing Committee to Revise the 1998 guidelines for the management of patients with valvular heart disease) developed in collaboration with the Society of Cardiovascular Anesthesiologists endorsed by the Society for Cardiovascular Angiography and Interventions and the Society of Thoracic Surgeons. J Am Coll Cardiol 2006;48: e1-e148.
161. Vahanian A, Baumgartner H, Bax J, et al: Guidelines on the management of valvular heart disease: the Task Force on the Management of Valvular Heart Disease of the European Society of Cardiology. Eur Heart J 2007;28:230-268.
162. Kennedy KD, Nishimura RA, Holmes DR Jr, Bailey KR. Natural history of moderate aortic stenosis. J Am Coll Cardiol 1991;17:313-319.
163. O'Keefe JH Jr, Vlietstra RE, Bailey KR, Holmes DR Jr: Natural history of candidates for balloon aortic valvuloplasty. Mayo Clin Proc 1987;62:986-991.
164. Otto CM, Mickel MC, Kennedy JW, et al: Three-year outcome after balloon aortic valvuloplasty: insights into prognosis of valvular aortic stenosis. Circulation 1994; 89:642-650.
165. Bergeron J, Abelmann WH, Vazquez-Milan H, Ellis LB: Aortic stenosis; clinical manifestations and course of the disease; review of one hundred proved cases. AMA Arch Intern Med 1954;94:911-924.
166. Mitchell AM, Sackett CH, Hunzicker WJ, Levine SA: The clinical features of aortic stenosis. Am Heart J 1954;48:684-720.

167. Nessmith MG, Fukuta H, Brucks S, Little WC: Usefulness of an elevated B-type natriuretic peptide in predicting survival in patients with aortic stenosis treated without surgery. Am J Cardiol 2005;96:1445-1448.
168. Otto CM, Lind BK, Kitzman DW, et al: Association of aortic-valve sclerosis with cardiovascular mortality and morbidity in the elderly. N Engl J Med 1999;341:142-147.
169. Novaro GM, Katz R, Aviles RJ, et al: Clinical factors, but not C-reactive protein, predict progression of calcific aortic-valve disease: the Cardiovascular Health Study. J Am Coll Cardiol 2007;50:1992-1998.
170. Faggiano P, Antonini-Canterin F, Erlicher A, et al: Progression of aortic valve sclerosis to aortic stenosis. Am J Cardiol 2003;91:99-101.
171. Bogart DB, Murphy BL, Wong BY, et al: Progression of aortic stenosis. Chest 1979;76:391-396.
172. Cheitlin MD, Gertz EW, Brundage BH, et al: Rate of progression of severity of valvular aortic stenosis in the adult. Am Heart J 1979;98:689-700.
173. Davies SW, Gershlick AH, Balcon R: Progression of valvar aortic stenosis: a long-term retrospective study. Eur Heart J 1991;12:10-14.
174. Jonasson R, Jonsson B, Nordlander R, et al: Rate of progression of severity of valvular aortic stenosis. Acta Med Scand 1983;213:51-54.
175. Nestico PF, DePace NL, Kimbiris D, et al: Progression of isolated aortic stenosis: analysis of 29 patients having more than 1 cardiac catheterization. Am J Cardiol 1983;52:1054-1058.
176. Wagner S, Selzer A: Patterns of progression of aortic stenosis: a longitudinal hemodynamic study. Circulation 1982;65:709-712.
177. Brener SJ, Duffy CI, Thomas JD, Stewart WJ: Progression of aortic stenosis in 394 patients: relation to changes in myocardial and mitral valve dysfunction. J Am Coll Cardiol 1995;25:305-310.
178. Otto CM, Pearlman AS, Gardner CL: Hemodynamic progression of aortic stenosis in adults assessed by Doppler echocardiography. J Am Coll Cardiol 1989;13:545-550.
179. Palta S, Pai AM, Gill KS, Pai RG: New insights into the progression of aortic stenosis: implications for secondary prevention. Circulation 2000;101:2497-502.
180. Peter M, Hoffmann A, Parker C, et al: Progression of aortic stenosis Role of age and concomitant coronary artery disease. Chest 1993;103:1715-1719.
181. Roger VL, Tajik AJ, Bailey KR, et al: Progression of aortic stenosis in adults: new appraisal using Doppler echocardiography. Am Heart J 1990;119:331-338.
182. Aronow WS, Ahn C, Kronzon I, Goldman ME: Association of coronary risk factors and use of statins with progression of mild valvular aortic stenosis in older persons. Am J Cardiol 2001;88:693-695.
183. Bellamy MF, Pellikka PA, Klarich KW, et al: Association of cholesterol levels, hydroxymethylglutaryl coenzyme-A reductase inhibitor treatment, and progression of aortic stenosis in the community. J Am Coll Cardiol 2002;40:1723-1730.
184. Cowell SJ, Newby DE, Prescott RJ, et al: A randomized trial of intensive lipid lowering therapy in calcific aortic stenosis. N Engl J Med 2005;352:2389-2397.
185. Novaro GM, Tiong IY, Pearce GL, et al: Effect of hydroxymethylglutaryl coenzyme a reductase inhibitors on the progression of calcific aortic stenosis. Circulation 2001;104:2205-2209.
186. Rosenhek R, Rader F, Loho N, et al: Statins but not angiotensin-converting enzyme inhibitors delay progression of aortic stenosis. Circulation 2004;110:1291-1295.
187. Moura LM, Ramos SF, Zamorano JL, et al: Rosuvastatin affecting aortic valve endothelium to slow the progression of aortic stenosis. J Am Coll Cardiol 2007;49:554-561.
188. Isner JM, Sours HE, Paris AL, et al: Sudden, unexpected death in avid dieters using the liquid-protein-modified-fast diet: observations in 17 patients and the role of the prolonged QT interval. Circulation 1979;60:1401-1412.
189. Deutscher S, Rockette HE, Krishnaswami V: Diabetes and hypercholesterolemia among patients with calcific aortic stenosis. J Chronic Dis 1984;37:407-415.
190. Mohler ER, Sheridan MJ, Nichols R, et al: Development and progression of aortic valve stenosis: atherosclerosis risk factors—a causal relationship? A clinical morphologic study. Clin Cardiol 1991;14:995-999.
191. Sprecher DL, Schaefer EJ, Kent KM, et al: Cardiovascular features of homozygous familial hypercholesterolemia: analysis of 16 patients. Am J Cardiol 1984;54:20-30.
192. Wilmshurst PT, Stevenson RN, Griffiths H, Lord JRr: A case-control investigation of the relation between hyperlipidaemia and calcific aortic valve stenosis. Heart 1997;78:475-479.
193. Ngo MV, Gottdiener JS, Fletcher RD, et al: Smoking and obesity are associated with the progression of aortic stenosis. Am J Geriatr Cardiol 2001;10:86-90.
194. Georgeson S, Meyer KB, Pauker SG: Decision analysis in clinical cardiology: when is coronary angiography required in aortic stenosis? J Am Coll Cardiol 1990;15:751-762.
195. Alcalai R, Viola N, Mosseri M, et al: The value of percutaneous coronary intervention in aortic valve stenosis with coronary artery disease. Am J Med 2007;120:185 e7-e13.
196. Iung B, Drissi MF, Michel PL, et al: Prognosis of valve replacement for aortic stenosis with or without coexisting coronary heart disease: a comparative study. J Heart Valve Dis 1993;2:430-439.
197. Carabello BA: Timing of valve replacement in aortic stenosis: moving closer to perfection. Circulation 1997;95:2241-2243.
198. Faggiano P, Aurigemma GP, Rusconi C, Gaasch WH: Progression of valvular aortic stenosis in adults: literature review and clinical implications. Am Heart J 1996;132:408-417.
199. Rosenhek R, Maurer G, Baumgartner H: Should early elective surgery be performed in patients with severe but asymptomatic aortic stenosis? Eur Heart J 2002;23:1417-1421.
200. STS U.S. cardiac surgery database: 1997 aortic valve replacement patients: preoperative risk variables. Chicago: Society of Thoracic Surgeons, 2000. Available at http://www.ctsnet.org/doc/3031.
201 Bergler-Klein J, Klaar U, Heger M, et al: Natriuretic peptides predict symptom-free survival and postoperative outcome in severe aortic stenosis. Circulation 2004;109:2302-2308.
202. Iwanaga Y, Nishi I, Furuichi S, et al: B-type natriuretic peptide strongly reflects diastolic wall stress in patients with chronic heart failure: comparison between systolic and diastolic heart failure. J Am Coll Cardiol 2006;47:742-748.
203. Vanderheyden M, Goethals M, Verstreken S, et al: Wall stress modulates brain natriuretic peptide production in pressure overload cardiomyopathy. J Am Coll Cardiol 2004;44:2349-2354.
204. Azariades M, Fessler CL, Ahmad A, Starr A: Aortic valve replacement in patients over 80 years of age a comparative standard for balloon valvuloplasty. Eur J Cardiothorac Surg 1991;5:373-377.
205. Craver JM, Weintraub WS, Jones EL, et al: Predictors of mortality, complications, and length of stay in aortic valve replacement for aortic stenosis. Circulation 1988;78:I85-I90.
206. Culliford AT, Galloway AC, Colvin SB, et al: Aortic valve replacement for aortic stenosis in persons aged 80 years and over. Am J Cardiol 1991;67:1256-1260.
207. Elayda MA, Hall RJ, Reul RM, et al: Aortic valve replacement in patients 80 years and older. Operative risks and long-term results. Circulation 1993;88:II11-II16.
208. Freeman WK, Schaff HV, O'Brien PC, et al: Cardiac surgery in the octogenarian: perioperative outcome and clinical follow-up. J Am Coll Cardiol 1991;18:29-35.
209. Fremes SE, Goldman BS, Ivanov J, et al: Valvular surgery in the elderly. Circulation 1989;80:I77-I90.
210. Kirklin JK, Naftel DC, Blackstone EH, et al: Risk factors for mortality after primary combined valvular and coronary artery surgery. Circulation 1989;79:I185-I190.
211. Kvidal P, Bergstrom R, Horte LG, Stahle E: Observed and relative survival after aortic valve replacement. J Am Coll Cardiol 2000;35:747-756.
212. Levinson JR, Akins CW, Buckley MJ, et al: Octogenarians with aortic stenosis: outcome after aortic valve replacement. Circulation 1989;80:I49-I56.
213. Logeais Y, Langanay T, Roussin R, et al: Surgery for aortic stenosis in elderly patients: a study of surgical risk and predictive factors. Circulation 1994;90:2891-2898.
214. Olsson M, Granstrom L, Lindblom D, et al: Aortic valve replacement in octogenarians with aortic stenosis: a case-control study. J Am Coll Cardiol 1992;20:1512-1516.
215. Wong JB, Salem DN, Pauker SG: You're never too old. N Engl J Med 1993;328:971-975.
216. Iung B, Cachier A, Baron G, et al: Decision-making in elderly patients with severe aortic stenosis: why are so many denied surgery? Eur Heart J 2005;26:2714-2720.
217. Fighali SF, Avendano A, Elayda MA, et al: Early and late mortality of patients undergoing aortic valve replacement after previous coronary artery bypass graft surgery. Circulation 1995;92:II163-II168.
218. Sethi GK, Miller DC, Souchek J, et al: Clinical, hemodynamic, and angiographic predictors of operative mortality in patients undergoing single valve replacement. Veterans Administration Cooperative Study on Valvular Heart Disease. J Thorac Cardiovasc Surg 1987;93:884-897.
219. Collins JJ Jr, Aranki SF: Management of mild aortic stenosis during coronary artery bypass graft surgery. J Card Surg 1994;9:145-147.
220. Thibault GE: Too old for what? N Engl J Med 1993;328:946-950.
221. Connolly HM, Oh JK, Schaff HV, et al: Severe aortic stenosis with low transvalvular gradient and severe left ventricular dysfunction: result of aortic valve replacement in 52 patients. Circulation 2000;101:1940-1946.
222. Pereira JJ, Lauer MS, Bashir M, et al: Survival after aortic valve replacement for severe aortic stenosis with low transvalvular gradients and severe left ventricular dysfunction. J Am Coll Cardiol 2002;39:1356-1363.
223. Aurigemma G, Battista S, Orsinelli D, et al: Abnormal left ventricular intracavitary flow acceleration in patients undergoing aortic valve replacement for aortic stenosis: a marker for high postoperative morbidity and mortality. Circulation 1992;86:926-936.
224. Bartunek J, Sys SU, Rodrigues AC, et al: Abnormal systolic intraventricular flow velocities after valve replacement for aortic stenosis: mechanisms, predictive factors, and prognostic significance. Circulation 1996;93:712-719.
225. Wiseth R, Samstad S, Rossvoll O, et al: Cross-sectional left ventricular outflow tract velocities before and after aortic valve replacement: a comparative study with two-dimensional Doppler ultrasound. J Am Soc Echocardiogr 1993;6:279-285.
226. Orsinelli DA, Aurigemma GP, Battista S, et al: Left ventricular hypertrophy and mortality after aortic valve replacement for aortic stenosis: a high risk subgroup identified by preoperative relative wall thickness. J Am Coll Cardiol 1993;22:1679-1683.
227. Harpole DH, Jones RH: Serial assessment of ventricular performance after valve replacement for aortic stenosis. J Thorac Cardiovasc Surg 1990;99:645-650.
228. Munt BI, Legget ME, Healy NL, et al: Effects of aortic valve replacement on exercise duration and functional status in adults with valvular aortic stenosis. Can J Cardiol 1997;13:346-350.
229. Hwang MH, Hammermeister KE, Oprian C, et al: Preoperative identification of patients likely to have left ventricular dysfunction after aortic valve replacement: participants in the Veterans Administration Cooperative Study on Valvular Heart Disease. Circulation 1989;80:I65-I76.
230. Jin XY, Pepper JR, Brecker SJ, et al: Early changes in left ventricular function after aortic valve replacement for isolated aortic stenosis. Am J Cardiol 1994;74:1142-1146.
231. Monrad ES, Hess OM, Murakami T, et al: Time course of regression of left ventricular hypertrophy after aortic valve replacement. Circulation 1988;77:1345-1355.
232. Lund O, Erlandsen M: Changes in left ventricular function and mass during serial investigations after valve replacement for aortic stenosis. J Heart Valve Dis 2000;9:583-593.
233. Gilchrist IC, Waxman HL, Kurnik PB: Improvement in early diastolic filling dynamics after aortic valve replacement. Am J Cardiol 1990;66:1124-1129.
234. Villari B, Vassalli G, Betocchi S, et al: Normalization of left ventricular nonuniformity late after valve replacement for aortic stenosis. Am J Cardiol 1996;78:66-71.
235. Bauer F, Mghaiet F, Dervaux N, et al: Preoperative tissue Doppler imaging differentiates beneficial from detrimental left ventricular hypertrophy in patients with surgical aortic stenosis: a postoperative morbidity study. Heart 2008;94:1440-1445.
236. Otto CM: Aortic stenosis—listen to the patient, look at the valve. N Engl J Med 2000;343:652-654.
237. Carabello BA, Stewart WJ, Crawford FA: Aortic valve disease. In Topol E (ed): Textbook of Cardiovascular Medicine. Baltimore, Lippincott Williams & Wilkins, 1998:533-555.
238. O'Brien KD, Zhao XQ, Shavelle DM, et al: Hemodynamic effects of the angiotensin-converting enzyme inhibitor, ramipril, in patients with mild to moderate aortic stenosis and preserved left ventricular function. J Investig Med 2004;52:185-191.
239. Chockalingam A, Venkatesan S, Subramaniam T, et al: Safety and efficacy of angiotensin-converting enzyme inhibitors in symptomatic severe aortic stenosis: Symptomatic Cardiac Obstruction-Pilot Study of Enalapril in Aortic Stenosis (SCOPE-AS). Am Heart J 2004;147:E19.

154

240. Jimenez-Candil J, Bermejo J, Yotti R, et al: Effects of angiotensin converting enzyme inhibitors in hypertensive patients with aortic valve stenosis: a drug withdrawal study. Heart 2005;91:1311-1318.

241. Wilson W, Taubert KA, Gewitz M, et al: Prevention of infective endocarditis: guidelines from the American Heart Association: a guideline from the American Heart Association Rheumatic Fever, Endocarditis, and Kawasaki Disease Committee, Council on Cardiovascular Disease in the Young, and the Council on Clinical Cardiology, Council on Cardiovascular Surgery and Anesthesia, and the Quality of Care and Outcomes Research Interdisciplinary Working Group. Circulation 2007;116:1736-1754.

242. Stout KK, Otto CM: Pregnancy in women with valvular heart disease. Heart 2007;93:552-558.

243. Elkayam U, Bitar F: Valvular heart disease and pregnancy. Part I: native valves. J Am Coll Cardiol 2005;46:223-230.

244. Hameed A, Karaalp IS, Tummala PP, et al: The effect of valvular heart disease on maternal and fetal outcome of pregnancy. J Am Coll Cardiol 2001;37:893-899.

245. Silversides CK, Colman JM, Sermer M, et al: Early and intermediate-term outcomes of pregnancy with congenital aortic stenosis. Am J Cardiol 2003;91:1386-1389.

246. Raymer K, Yang H: Patients with aortic stenosis: cardiac complications in non-cardiac surgery. Can J Anaesth 1998;45:855-859.

247. Torsher LC, Shub C, Rettke SR, Brown DL: Risk of patients with severe aortic stenosis undergoing noncardiac surgery. Am J Cardiol 1998;81:448-452.

248. Kertai MD, Bountioukos M, Boersma E, et al: Aortic stenosis: an underestimated risk factor for perioperative complications in patients undergoing noncardiac surgery. Am J Med 2004;116:8-13.

249. O'Keefe JH Jr, Shub C, Rettke SR: Risk of noncardiac surgical procedures in patients with aortic stenosis. Mayo Clin Proc 1989;64:400-405.

250. Ben-Ami M, Battino S, Rosenfeld T, et al: Aortic valve replacement during pregnancy: a case report and review of the literature. Acta Obstet Gynecol Scand 1990;69:651-653.

251. Rajamannan NM, Subramaniam M, Springett M, et al: Atorvastatin inhibits hypercholesterolemia-induced cellular proliferation and bone matrix production in the rabbit aortic valve. Circulation 2002;105:2660-2665.

252. O'Brien KD, Shavelle DM, Caulfield MT, et al: Association of angiotensin-converting enzyme with low-density lipoprotein in aortic valvular lesions and in human plasma. Circulation 2002;106:2224-2230.

253. O'Brien KD, Probstfield JL, Caulfield MT, et al: Angiotensin-converting enzyme inhibitors and change in aortic valve calcium. Arch Intern Med 2005;165:858-862.

254. Rosenhek R: Statins for aortic stenosis. N Engl J Med 2005;352:2441-2443.

255. Shah SJ, Ristow B, Ali S, et al Acute myocardial infarction in patients with versus without aortic valve sclerosis and effect of statin therapy (from the Heart and Soul Study). Am J Cardiol 2007;99:1128-1133.

256. Rossebo AB, Pedersen TR, Boman K, et al: Intensive lipid lowering with simvastatin and ezetimibe in aortic stenosis. N Engl J Med 2008;359:1343-1356.

Aortic Regurgitation

Pilar Tornos and Robert O. Bonow

KEY POINTS

- The majority of causes of aortic regurgitation produce chronic volume overload with slow indolent left ventricular dilatation and a prolonged asymptomatic phase.
- Patients with acute aortic regurgitation often present with hypotension and tachycardia, and many of the characteristic physical findings of chronic volume overload are modified or absent.
- In chronic aortic regurgitation, excessive preload and excessive afterload may overcome the ability of the left ventricle to compensate via hypertrophy and recruitment of preload reserve, leading to left ventricular systolic dysfunction. This may occur in the absence of symptoms.
- Left ventricular systolic function (ejection fraction) and end-systolic dimension (or volume) are the most important determinants of survival and functional recovery after aortic valve replacement.
- Indications for aortic valve replacement include development of (a) symptoms, (b) left ventricular systolic dysfunction, (c) excessive left ventricular dilatation, and/or (d) severe dilatation of the aortic root or ascending aorta.
- In patients with AR due to enlargement of the aorta or aortic root, the natural history of the disease and thus the timing and choice of surgical intervention are often based on the degree and rate of aortic or aortic root dilatation rather than on the left ventricular response to aortic regurgitation.

ETIOLOGY

Pure aortic regurgitation (AR) has multiple causes, many of which arise from primary abnormalities of the aortic valve leaflets. The most frequent causes include congenital abnormalities of the aortic valve (most notably bicuspid valves (Figure 10-1), but also unicuspid, tricuspid, and quadricuspid valves), rheumatic disease, infective endocarditis, calcific degeneration, and myxomatous degeneration. Other common causes of AR represent diseases of the aorta without direct involvement of the aortic valve, as in systemic hypertension, idiopathic annuloaortic ectasia, aortic dissection, and Marfan syndrome.[1,2]

Less common causes of AR include traumatic injuries to the aortic valve, aortitis occurring in ankylosing spondylitis, syphilitic infection, rheumatoid arthritis, osteogenesis imperfecta, giant cell aortitis, Takayasu disease, Ehlers Danlos syndrome, and Reiter syndrome. AR can also occur in patients with discrete subaortic stenosis and a ventricular septal defect with prolapse of an aortic cusp, ruptured aneurysms of the sinuses of Valsalva, and fenestrated aortic cusps.[3] AR has also been described as complicating balloon aortic valvuloplasty,[4,5] and anorectic drugs have been reported to cause AR.[6] However, in many patients with AR the precise etiology is unclear. In a recent pathologic study of a surgical series of excised aortic valves, up to 34% cases of pure AR were considered of unclear etiology.[2] In the recent Euro Heart Survey for Valvular Diseases, AR represented 13.3% of patients with single native left-sided disease: of these, 15.2% were considered of congenital origin, and the same percentage was observed for rheumatic origin.[7]

The majority of these lesions produce chronic AR, with slow, insidious left ventricular (LV) dilatation and a prolonged asymptomatic phase. Other lesions, in particular, infective endocarditis, aortic dissection, and trauma, more often produce acute severe AR with sudden elevation of LV filling pressures, pulmonary edema, and reduction in cardiac output.

ACUTE AORTIC REGURGITATION

Pathophysiology

In acute severe AR the sudden large regurgitant volume is imposed on a left ventricle of normal size that has not had time to adjust to the volume overload. Thus, the acute increase in diastolic flow into the nondilated left ventricle leads to a marked elevation in end-diastolic pressure due to a rightward shift along the normal LV diastolic pressure-volume curve. In severe cases, the increased ventricular pressures during the diastolic filling period in conjunction with the decrease in the aortic diastolic pressure leads to a rapid equalization of aortic and LV pressures at end-diastole (Figure 10-2).[8-10]

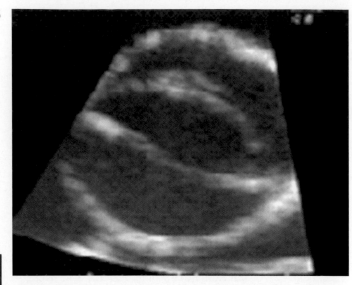

FIGURE 10–1 Transthoracic parasternal short-axis view showing a bicuspid aortic valve.

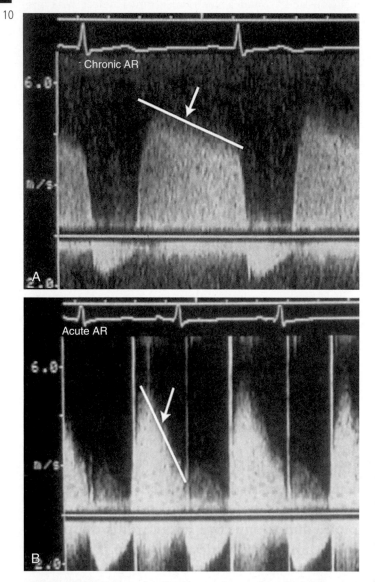

FIGURE 10–2 Continuous wave Doppler curves from a patient with chronic compensated aortic regurgitation (AR) due to a bicuspid aortic valve **(A)** and in a patient with acute aortic regurgitation due to endocarditis **(B)**. Note the steeper deceleration slope (*arrow*) in the acute case corresponding to the equalization of left ventricular and aortic pressures. In addition, regurgitation is more severe in the acute case, as evidenced by the increased density of the signal relative to the antegrade velocity signal.

With acute regurgitation, forward cardiac output is decreased because the total stroke volume of the nondilated ventricle now includes both regurgitant and forward stroke volume. Compensatory tachycardia may partially correct this decline in forward stroke volume, but it is often insufficient to maintain cardiac output, and hence patients may present in cardiogenic shock. Pulmonary edema results from the markedly elevated LV end-diastolic pressure and concomitant elevation of pulmonary venous pressure. In addition, coronary flow reserve is acutely diminished, which may lead to subendocardial ischemia. As the LV end-diastolic pressure approaches the diastolic aortic and coronary artery pressures, myocardial perfusion pressure in the subendocardium is diminished, at a time when myocardial oxygen demand is increased owing to the effects of increased afterload and tachycardia.[10]

Diagnosis

Many of the characteristic physical findings of chronic volume overload are modified or absent when valvular regurgitation is acute. Therefore, the severity of AR can be underestimated. Because of the acute hemodynamic deterioration, patients with acute AR are often tachycardic and tachypneic and have pulmonary edema. However, LV size may be normal on physical examination, and cardiomegaly may be absent on chest radiography. In addition, pulse pressure may not be increased because systolic pressure is reduced in relation to the decrease in forward stroke volume and diastolic pressure equilibrates with the elevated LV diastolic pressure. In the absence of a widened pulse pressure, the characteristic peripheral signs of AR are absent. Although a diastolic murmur is usually present, it can be soft and short because the rapidly rising LV diastolic pressure reduces the aortic-ventricular pressure gradient. The murmur is thus often poorly heard.[11]

Echocardiography is indispensable in confirming the presence and severity of the AR, assessing its cause, and determining whether there is a rapid equilibration of aortic and LV diastolic pressure. Evidence for rapid pressure equilibration includes a short AR diastolic half-time (<300 ms), a short mitral deceleration time (<150 ms) or premature closure of the mitral valve (Figure 10-3).

Transesophageal echocardiography is indicated when aortic dissection, acute endocarditis, or trauma is suspected (Figure 10-4). Computed tomography or cardiac magnetic resonance can be used in some settings if either of these will lead to a more rapid diagnosis than can be achieved by transesophageal echocardiography.[12-14]

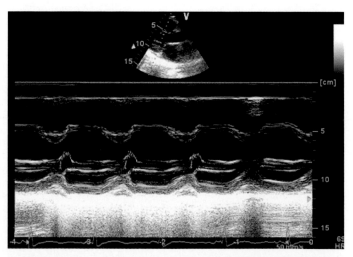

FIGURE 10-3 Transthoracic parasternal long-axis view showing early closure of the mitral valve by M-mode echocardiography in a patient with acute aortic regurgitation due to infective endocarditis.

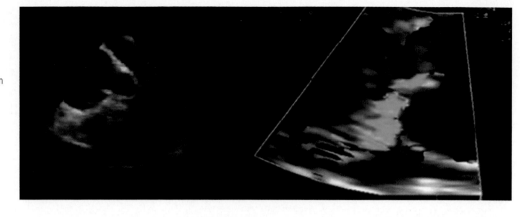

FIGURE 10–4 Transesophageal echocardiogram showing the intimal flap prolapsing into the left ventricular outflow tract in a case of aortic dissection (*left*). Eccentric aortic regurgitation in the same patient (*right*).

Management

Death due to pulmonary edema, ventricular arrhythmias, electromechanical dissociation, or circulatory collapse is common in acute, severe AR. Thus, patients require emergency or urgent surgery for correction of the underlying disease process and relief of the acute volume overload. Intra-aortic balloon counterpulsation is contraindicated. In patients with acute AR due to an ascending aortic dissection, prompt surgical intervention is needed, including a composite replacement of the aorta along with an aortic valve or a valve-sparing reimplantation technique.[15-17] In severe acute AR due to infective endocarditis, patients need immediate initiation of antibiotics and aggressive medical treatment. If the hemodynamic situation does not immediately improve, emergency aortic valve replacement (AVR) may be life-saving. If the clinical situation stabilizes, surgery can be postponed for a few days under strict medical supervision to allow a few days of antibiotic treatment before surgical correction.[18-20]

CHRONIC AORTIC REGURGITATION

Pathophysiology

The left ventricle responds to the volume load of chronic AR with a series of compensatory mechanisms, including an increase in end-diastolic volume, an increase in chamber compliance that accommodates the increased volume without an increase in filling pressures, and a combination of eccentric and concentric hypertrophy. The central hemodynamic feature of chronic AR is combined volume and pressure overload of the left ventricle.[21-23] Because total LV stroke volume equals forward plus regurgitant stroke volume, normal cardiac output is maintained by an increase in total stroke volume corresponding to the severity of regurgitation. This increase in total stroke volume is achieved by progressive ventricular dilatation, with increased end-diastolic and end-systolic volumes. The greater diastolic volume permits the ventricle to eject a large total stroke volume, thus keeping forward stroke volume in the normal range. This is accomplished though rearrangement of myocardial fibers with the addition of new sarcomeres and development of eccentric LV hypertrophy.[24] As a result, preload at the sarcomere level remains normal or near normal, and the ventricle retains its preload reserve. The enhanced total stroke volume is achieved though normal performance of each contractile unit along the enlarged circumference.[25] Thus, LV ejection performance is normal, and ejection phase indexes such as ejection fraction (EF) and fractional shortening remain in the normal range. However, the enlarged chamber size with the associated increase in systolic wall stress also results in a stimulus for further hypertrophy.[26] Despite an increase in end-systolic dimension and pressure early in the course of the disease, end-systolic wall stress is maintained in the normal range by a compensatory increase in wall thickness. Thus, patients with compensated chronic AR have substantial increases in LV mass as well as LV volumes, and EF and end-systolic elastance tend to be normal. As the disease progresses, recruitment of preload reserve and compensatory hypertrophy permit the left ventricle to maintain normal ejection performance despite the elevated afterload.[22,27,28] The majority of patients remain asymptomatic during this compensated phase, which may last for decades. During this compensated phase, ejection phase indexes of LV systolic function at rest are normal. It is recognized, however, that other indices of LV function may not be normal. It is further recognized that the transition to LV dysfunction represents a continuum and that there is no single hemodynamic measurement that represents the absolute boundary between normal LV systolic function and LV systolic dysfunction.

In a large subset of patients, the balance between afterload excess, preload reserve, and hypertrophy cannot be maintained indefinitely. Preload reserve may be exhausted and/or the hypertrophic response may be inadequate[29] so that further increases in afterload result in a reduction in EF, first into the low normal range and then below normal. Impaired contractility may also contribute to this process. Patients often develop dyspnea at this point in the natural history. In addition, diminished coronary blood flow reserve in the hypertrophied myocardium may result in exertional angina.[30] However, this transition may be more insidious, and it is possible for patients to remain asymptomatic even when severe LV dysfunction has developed.

LV systolic dysfunction (defined as an EF below normal at rest) is initially a reversible phenomenon related predominantly to afterload excess, and full recovery of LV size and function is possible with AVR.[31-42] With time, during which the left ventricle develops progressive chamber enlargement and a more spherical geometry, depressed myocardial contractility predominates over excessive loading as the cause of progressive dysfunction. Contractile dysfunction can progress to the extent that the full benefit of surgical correction of the regurgitant lesion in terms of recovery of LV function and improved survival can no longer be achieved. A number of studies have identified LV systolic function and end-systolic size as the most important determinants of survival and postoperative recovery of LV function in patients undergoing AVR for chronic AR.[43-64] Studies of predictors of surgical outcome are listed in Table 10-1. Among patients undergoing AVR for chronic AR with preoperative LV systolic dysfunction, several factors are associated with worse functional and survival results after the operation (Table 10-2).

Clinical Presentation

Clinical History

AR is diagnosed in many patients before symptom onset based on the finding on physical examination of a diastolic murmur, the discovery of an enlarged cardiac silhouette on

TABLE 10–1 | **Preoperative Predictors of Surgical Outcome in Aortic Regurgitation**

Author, Year	Study Design	No. of Patients	Outcome Assessed	Findings
Cunha et al., 1980	Retrospective	86	Survival	High-risk group identified by preoperative echocardiographic LV FS <0.30. Mortality also significantly associated with preoperative ESD. Among patients with FS <0.30, mortality higher in NYHA FC III-IV than in FC I-II.
Forman et al., 1980	Retrospective	90	Survival	High-risk group identified by preoperative angiographic LV EF <0.50.
Henry at al., 1980	Prospective	50	Survival	High-risk group identified by preoperative echocardiographic LV FS <0.25 and/or ESD >55 mm.
Greves et al., 1981	Retrospective	45	Survival	High-risk group identified by preoperative angiographic LV EF <0.45 and/or CI <2.5 L/min. Among patients with EF <0.45, mortality higher in NYHA FC III-IV than in FC I-II.
Kumpuris et al., 1982	Prospective	43	Survival, heart failure, LV function	Persistent LV dilatation after AVR predicted by preoperative echocardiographic LV ESD, radius/thickness ratio and end-systolic wall stress. All deaths occurred in patients with persistent LV dilatation.
Fioretti et al., 1983	Retrospective	47	LV function	Persistent LV dysfunction predicted by preoperative EDD ≥75 mm and/or ESD ≥55 mm.
Gaasch et al., 1983	Prospective	32	Symptoms, LV function	Persistent LV dilatation after AVR predicted by echocardiographic LV ESD ≥2.6 cm/m² and radius/thickness ratio ≥3.8. Trend toward worse survival in patients with persistent LV dilatation.
Stone et al., 1984	Prospective	113	LV function	Normal LV function after AVR predicted by preoperative LV FS ≥0.26, ESD <55 mm, and EDD <80 mm. No preoperative variable predicted postoperative LV function.
Bonow et al., 1985, 1988	Prospective	80	Survival, LV function	Postoperative survival and LV function predicted by preoperative LV EF, FS, and ESD. High-risk group identified by subnormal EF at rest. Among patients with subnormal EF, poor exercise tolerance and prolonged duration of LV dysfunction identified the highest-risk group.
Daniel et al., 1985	Retrospective	84	Survival, symptoms, LV function	Outcome after AVR predicted by preoperative LV FS and ESD. Survival at 2.5 years was 90.5% with FS >0.25 and ESD ≤55 mm but only 70% with ESD ≥55 mm and FS ≤25%.
Cormier et al., 1986	Prospective	73	Survival	High-risk group identified by preoperative LV EF <0.40 and ESD ≥55 mm.
Sheiban et al., 1986	Retrospective	84	Survival	High-risk group identified by preoperative LV EF <0.50 and ESD >55 mm.
Carabello et al., 1987	Retrospective	14	LV function	Postoperative LV EF predicted by preoperative ESD, FS, EDD, and radius/thickness ratio.
Taniguchi et al., 1987	Retrospective	62	Survival	High-risk group identified by preoperative ESV >200 mL/m² and/or EF <0.40.
Michel et al., 1995	Retrospective	286	LV function	Postoperative LV dysfunction predicted by preoperative LV EF, FS, ESD, and EDD.
Klodas et al., 1996, 1997	Retrospective	289	Survival	High-risk group identified by symptom severity and preoperative EF <0.50.
Turina et al., 1998	Retrospective	192	Survival	High-risk group identified by symptom severity, low EF, and elevated end-diastolic volume.
Tornos et al., 2006	Prospective	170	Survival	High risk identified by symptom severity, low EF, and elevated EDD and ESD.

AVR, aortic valve replacement; CI, cardiac index; EDD, end-diastolic dimension; EF, ejection fraction; ESD, end-systolic dimension; ESV, end-systolic volume; FC, functional class; FS, fractional shortening; LV, left ventricular; NYHA, New York Heart Association.

From Bonow RO, Carabello BA, Chatterjee K, et al: ACC/AHA 2006 guidelines for the management of patients with valvular heart disease: A report of the American College of Cardiology/American Heart Association Task Force on Practice Guidelines. J Am Coll Cardiol 2006;48:e1-e148, with permission.

TABLE 10–2	Factors Predictive of Reduced Postoperative Survival and Recovery of Left Ventricular Function in Patients with Aortic Regurgitation and Preoperative Left Ventricular Systolic Dysfunction

Severity of preoperative symptoms or reduced exercise tolerance
Severity of depression of LV ejection fraction
Duration of preoperative LV systolic dysfunction

LV, left ventricular.

From Bonow RO, Carabello BA, Chatterjee K, et al: ACC/AHA 2006 guidelines for the management of patients with valvular heart disease: a report of the American College of Cardiology/American Heart Association Task Force on Practice Guidelines. J Am Coll Cardiol 2006;48:e1-e148, with permission.

chest radiography, or evidence of LV hypertrophy on electrocardiography. The most common initial symptom in patients with chronic severe AR is exertional dyspnea, most likely due to an elevated LV end-diastolic pressure with exercise.[65] Because chronic AR has a slowly progressive course, the gradual decrease in exercise capacity may not be recognized as abnormal by the patient, and therefore very careful questioning is often needed to elicit evidence of a subtle decrease in functional status. In patients in whom symptoms are doubtful or equivocal, exercise testing may be valuable in assessing functional capacity. Patients with severe LV dysfunction can present with symptoms of overt heart failure including dyspnea at rest, orthopnea, and pulmonary edema. The acute onset of heart failure symptoms can occur in patients with chronic disease owing to an acute increase in the severity of regurgitation, for example, in patients with infective endocarditis or aortic dissection. In some patients, an uncomfortable awareness of the heartbeat or palpitations, related to the increased pulse pressure, is the earliest complaint that leads to the diagnosis of AR.

Angina may occur, even in the absence of atherosclerotic coronary artery disease, because of decreased myocardial perfusion pressure, increased myocardial oxygen demand, and decreased ratio of coronary artery size to myocardial mass. Syncope or sudden death, although rare, can occur in AR. Sudden death has been reported in association with extreme degrees of LV dilatation.[66]

Physical Examination

In patients with mild or moderate AR, the only finding on physical examination may be the diastolic murmur, but in many patients there is also a systolic outflow murmur related to the increased stroke volume, and often the systolic murmur is more apparent than the diastolic murmur. Physical examination is able to elicit most cases of severe AR by the combination of the cardiac murmurs, the widened pulse pressure on blood pressure measurement, and peripheral findings related to this widened pulse pressure. Classically, in severe AR systolic arterial pressure is elevated and diastolic pressure is abnormally low, but the blood pressure may remain normal in many patients with severe AR.[67] The apical impulse is diffuse and hyperdynamic and is displaced laterally and inferiorly because of the LV dilatation. The carotid pulse is bounding with a more rapid rate of pressure rise in early systole as well as an increase in the amplitude of the systolic pressure curve. A bisferiens carotid pulse may be present.[68] In patients with very severe AR, the head may bob forward with each heartbeat (DuMusset sign). The classic peripheral signs of AR are only present in patients with severe and chronic regurgitation and reflect the increased pulse pressure. These include the water-hammer or collapsing pulse (Corrigan pulse),[69] systolic pulsation of the fingernail bed on gentle pressure (Quincke pulse),[70] and a systolic and diastolic bruit over the femoral arteries on gentle compression by the stethoscope (Duroziez sign), a manifestation of the reversal of flow in the descending aorta.

A short midsystolic murmur related to the increased ejection rate and stroke volume may be audible at the base of the heart and transmitted to the carotid vessels. The aortic regurgitant murmur is one of high frequency that begins immediately after S2, continues to S1, and has a decrescendo intensity. The murmur is best heard along the left sternal border in the third or fourth intercostal space with valve leaflet abnormalities, whereas with aortic root disease a selective radiation along the right sternal border is common.[71] However, the diastolic murmur is often not recognized on physical examination. Compared with Doppler echocardiography or aortic angiography, the sensitivity of auscultation for detection of AR is 37% to 73% with a specificity of 85% to 92%.[72-74] The loudness of the murmur correlates with disease severity to some extent.[75] Another classic finding in patients with severe chronic AR is the Austin-Flint murmur, a low pitched mid-diastolic rumble that mimics the murmur of mitral stenosis.[76] Comparisons of Doppler echocardiographic findings with physical examination suggest that this diastolic murmur is related to the severity of AR with a jet directed toward the anterior mitral leaflet or LV free wall, causing vibrations recognized on auscultation as a low-pitched diastolic rumble.[77-79]

The physical findings in acute AR differ from those of chronic regurgitation in parallel with the different hemodynamics of acute versus chronic disease (Table 10-3).

Electrocardiography and Chest Radiography

The electrocardiogram (ECG) findings in patients with AR include voltage criteria for LV hypertrophy and associated repolarization abnormalities. A strain pattern on the resting ECG correlates strongly with abnormal LV dimensions, mass, and wall stress.[80-82] However, some patients with severe AR and pathologic LV hypertrophy do not meet ECG criteria for LV hypertrophy.[83] When the ECG is normal at rest, flat and or downsloping ST depression may develop with exercise, even

TABLE 10–3	Chronic Compensated, Decompensated, and Acute Aortic Regurgitation		
Characteristics	Chronic Compensated	Chronic Decompensated	Acute
Etiology	Valvular or aortic root abnormalities		Dissection, endocarditis, trauma
Physiology			
LV volume	Increased (ESD <55 mm)	Increased (ESD >55 mm)	Normal
Ejection fraction	Normal (>55%)	Normal or decreased	Normal or decreased
LV EDP	Normal	Normal	Increased
Physical examination			
Diastolic murmur	High-pitched, decrescendo, holodiastolic	High-pitched, decrescendo, holodiastolic	Low-pitched, harsh, early diastolic
Pulse pressure	Wide	Wide	Normal
LV impulse	Enlarged	Enlarged	Normal
Peripheral signs of AR	Present	Present	Absent
Clinical presentation	Asymptomatic	Gradual onset of symptoms, typically exertional	Sudden onset, pulmonary edema and hypotension

AR, aortic regurgitation; EDP, end-diastolic pressure; ESD, end-systolic dimension; LV, left ventricular.

in the absence of coronary artery disease, and is associated with an increased LV systolic dimension.[84] Ventricular ectopic beats and nonsustained ventricular arrhythmias are also relatively common in AR, with a significant correlation with LV hypertrophy and function.[85]

The chest radiograph shows an enlarged silhouette due to LV dilatation. Aortic root enlargement is also frequently present due to primary diseases of the aorta or dilatation secondary to the increased flow. Both evidence of LV hypertrophy on the ECG and cardiac size on the chest radiograph have been shown to be predictors of outcome after AVR.[86-90] However, neither the ECG nor the chest radiogram offers sufficiently precise data to be useful in clinical decision making or sequential follow-up of patients with AR.

Echocardiography

After the history and physical examination, echocardiography is the most important examination in patients with AR. Echocardiography is used to diagnose and estimate the severity of regurgitation using color Doppler (width of regurgitant jet) (Figure 10-5) and continuous wave Doppler (rate of decline of aortic regurgitant flow and holodiastolic flow reversal in the descending aorta) (Figure 10-6).[91-93] These indices are influenced by loading conditions and the compliance of the ascending aorta and the left ventricle. Quantitative Doppler echocardiography, using the continuity equation or analysis of proximal isovelocity surface area is less sensitive to loading conditions[94,95] and provides measures of regurgitant volume, regurgitant fraction, and effective regurgitant orifice. These measures have become the preferred method for assessing severity of AR.[91] The criteria for defining severe AR are shown in Table 10-4. Echocardiography is also performed to determine the mechanisms of regurgitation, describe the valve anatomy, and determine the feasibility of valve repair. An important role of echocardiography is to provide precise and reproducible measures of LV dimensions, volumes, and systolic performance, and therefore it is the cornerstone for clinical decision-making and serial follow-up of patients with chronic AR (Figure 10-7). Indexing for body surface area is especially recommended in women and men of small body size.[61,96] Serial echocardiographic evaluation of LV size and function should take into account the potential of confounding factors of interval changes in instrumentation, variability in recording and measuring the data, variability in loading conditions and physiologic variability. When a change is detected it is prudent to repeat the examination to confirm the magnitude and direction of the change. Good-quality echocardiograms and data confirmation are essential before recommending surgery in asymptomatic patients. Echocardiography should also be used to image the aorta at four different levels: annulus, sinuses of Valsalva, sinotubular junction, and ascending aorta (Figure 10-8). Transesophageal echocardiography may be performed

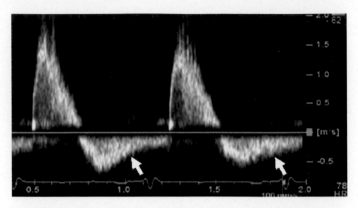

FIGURE 10–6 Pulsed Doppler in the abdominal aorta showing pandiastolic regurgitant flow (*arrows*).

TABLE 10–4	Criteria for the Definition of Severe Aortic Regurgitation
Specific signs	Central jet, width ≥65% of left ventricular outflow tract Vena contracta >0.6 cm
Supportive signs	Pressure half-time <200 ms Holodiastolic aortic flow reversal in descending aorta Moderate or greater left ventricular enlargement

Quantitative parameters
  Regurgitant volume
  Regurgitant fraction
  Effective regurgitant orifice area
	
	≥60 mL/beat
	≥50%
	≥0.30 cm²

From Zoghbi WA, Enriquez-Sarano M, Foster E, et al: Recommendations for evaluation of the severity of native valvular regurgitation with two-dimensional and Doppler echocardiography. J Am Soc Echocardiogr 2003;16:777-802, with permission.

to better define the anatomy of the valve and ascending aorta, especially when an aortic pathologic lesion is suspected or valve-sparing intervention is considered.[97]

Other Imaging Modalities

Cardiac Magnetic Resonance. In patients with indeterminant echocardiographic findings, cardiac magnetic resonance (CMR) is a reliable tool for assessment of the severity of AR.[98,99] Magnetic resonance phase-contrast sequences perpendicular to the aortic valve allow accurate antegrade and retrograde blood flow measurements in the ascending aorta[100] so that the severity of AR by calculation of regurgitant volume, peak velocity, and regurgitant fraction can be assessed.[101,102] In addition, cine CMR sequences, such as steady-state free precession techniques, permit visualization of the aortic valve in a chosen plane with excellent image

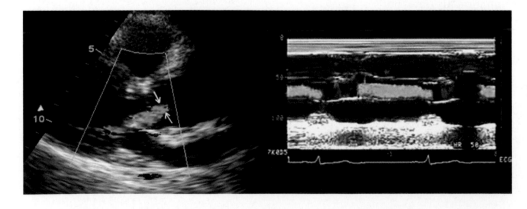

FIGURE 10–5 Parasternal long-axis view showing the vena contracta of the regurgitant flow by Doppler in a patient with severe aortic regurgitation (*left*). Color M-mode in the same patient showing the width of the regurgitant jet (*right*).

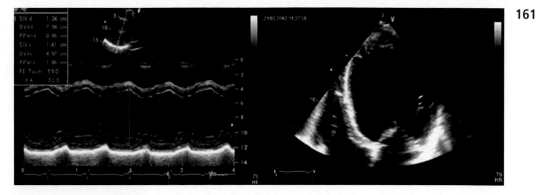

FIGURE 10-7 Transthoracic parasternal long-axis view showing enlargement of left ventricular end-diastolic and end-systolic dimensions in a patient with severe chronic aortic regurgitation (*left*). Apical four-chamber view of the same patient showing a spherical enlargement of the left ventricle (*right*).

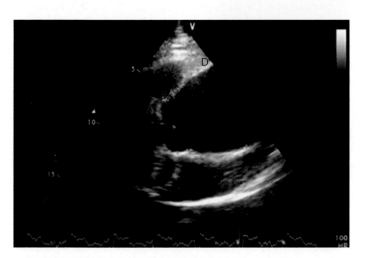

FIGURE 10-8 Parasternal long-axis view showing enlargement of the aortic root and ascending aorta at the level of the annulus **(A)**, sinuses of Valsalva **(B)**, sinotubular junction **(C)**, and ascending aorta **(D)**.

quality. Cine CMR also aids in determination of the morphology of the valve, and valve area can be measured by planimetry methods (Figure 10-9).[101-106] Moreover, by using serial short axis slices of the left ventricle it is possible to calculate LV volumes, mass, and EF very accurately. Several studies have shown that CMR is an excellent technique to monitor LV volumes and EF with a high degree of interobserver reproducibility ($r = 0.96-0.99$).[107] Finally, using contrast agents (gadolinium-diethylenetriaminepentaacetic acid) and different magnetic resonance angiography sequences or three-dimensional whole-chest steady-state free precession sequences (without contrast), aortic root and ascending aortic anatomy and diameters can also be determined. Therefore, CMR is a useful technique to obtain a global evaluation of patients with AR, to determine the evolution of the regurgitation and its impact on LV volume and function, to assess aortic root and ascending aortic anatomy, and to decide the optimum time for surgery.[108]

Cardiac Computed Tomography. Recently the utility of 64-slice multidetector computed tomography (CT) has been investigated in patients with AR. Aortic root and

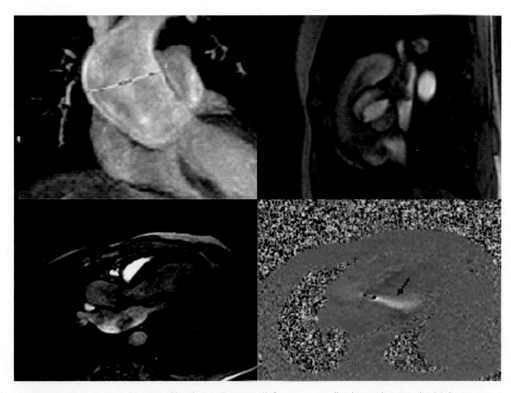

FIGURE 10-9 Cardiac magnetic resonance images showing a dilated ascending aorta (*left upper panel*), a bicuspid aortic valve (*right upper panel*), and the regurgitant jet with a phase-contrast sequence (*bottom panels*) in a patient with aortic regurgitation.

LV parameters by CT correlate well with corresponding measurements by transthoracic echocardiography.[109] Direct planimetry of the aortic valve anatomic regurgitant orifice accurately detects and quantifies AR.[110] CT coronary angiography is also useful for the detection of coronary artery disease in patients with AR.[111]

Radionuclide Angiography. Radionuclide ventriculograms can provide accurate measurements of LV EF and semiquantitative assessment of LV volumes and thus can be used as an alternative technique to echocardiography in patients with suboptimal echocardiograms or in patients showing discrepancies between clinical and echocardiographic data.[112]

Exercise Testing

Exercise stress testing is useful for assessing functional capacity and symptomatic responses in patients with equivocal symptoms. It is also useful in patients with AR before participation in athletic activities. Several investigators have suggested that exercise testing, with or without concurrent imaging, may help to identify patients with early systolic LV dysfunction. On exercise electrocardiography the finding of at least 1.0 mm of ST segment depression is associated with a lower resting and exercise EF, a higher wall stress, and a greater end-systolic dimension compared to those with no ST segment changes with exercise.[113,114] Reduced maximal oxygen consumption and aerobic threshold are also predictive of moderate to severe LV dysfunction, suggesting that cardiopulmonary stress testing may be useful in some patients.[115,116]

Echocardiography can be used to measure the incremental change in LV dimensions and EF with exercise in patients with AR. Measurements of the change in EF with exercise echocardiography reflect contractile reserve, and may be more predictive of clinical outcome than resting EF.[117,118] Similarly an increase in radionuclide EF with exercise of at least 5 EF units correlates with preserved LV systolic function, whereas any decrease or increase of less than 5 units indicates elevated end-systolic wall stress, increased end-systolic dimension, and impaired systolic function[112] At the present time the role of exercise testing must be individualized. It may be helpful when there is a discrepancy between the clinical presentation and the resting echocardiographic findings. However, clinical decisions should not be based solely on changes in EF with exercise nor on data from stress echocardiography, because these indices have not been adequately validated.

Natural History

There is no information regarding the natural history of mild AR. There is also little information in the literature regarding the progression from mild to moderate and severe regurgitation. It has been postulated that decreased aortic distensibility with age contributes to progressive AR due to the increase in LV afterload.[119] Doppler measures of jet width and regurgitant orifice area suggest that there is progressive enlargement of the regurgitant orifice over time.[120] One echocardiographic study showed that the severity of regurgitation increased in 30% of patients with at least two echocardiographic studies with associated increases in severity of LV dilatation, and the greatest increases in LV volumes and mass were observed in those with severe AR.[121]

Patients with Normal Left Ventricular Systolic Function

The data regarding the natural history of asymptomatic patients with severe AR and normal LV systolic function were analyzed in the formulation of the American College of Cardiology (ACC)/American Heart Association (AHA) guidelines on valvular heart disease,[122] which included a review of nine published series that involved a total of 593 such patients (Table 10-5).[66,123-130] These studies consistently showed that patients can remain asymptomatic with preserved LV function for a considerable period of time. The rate of progression to symptoms and/or LV dysfunction averaged 4.3% per year. Sudden death occurred in 7 of the 593 patients, for an average mortality rate of less than 0.2% per year. The available data also show that the rate of development of LV dysfunction, defined as EF at rest below normal, occurs at a rate of 1.2% per year.

Despite the low likelihood of patients developing asymptomatic LV dysfunction, it should be emphasized that this occurred in more than one fourth of patients in these series before the onset of warning symptoms. Thus, in the serial evaluation of patients, assessing symptomatic status alone is insufficient, and quantitative assessment of LV size and function is indispensable. The natural history studies have also defined variables that predict development of symptoms or LV dysfunction. These variables are age, LV end-diastolic dimension or volume, LV end-systolic dimension or volume, and LV EF during exercise.[66,125,126,129] In two multivariate analysis[66,130] only age and end-systolic dimensions on the initial study were independent predictors of outcome, as were the rate of increase in end-systolic dimension and decrease in resting EF during longitudinal studies. During a mean follow-up period of 8 years, patients with initial end-systolic dimensions greater than 50 mm had a likelihood of death, symptoms, and/or LV dysfunction of 19% per year. In those with end-systolic dimensions of 40 to 50 mm, the likelihood was 6% per year and when the dimensions were less than 40 mm it was zero. In a third study, the change in EF with exercise was the strongest determinant of outcome on multivariate analysis.[129]

A tenth study of asymptomatic patients with normal LV systolic function, published after the 2006 ACC/AHA guidelines, reported a higher clinical event rate and also a higher mortality rate.[131] This study, in which quantitative measurement of severity of AR was obtained with Doppler echocardiography, reported that patients with severe AR (using the definitions shown in Table 10-4) had a much higher mortality risk and a higher likelihood of AVR than patients with less severe AR. The measures of AR severity were stronger predictors of outcome than LV EF or any of the measures of LV dilatation. Importantly, the annual mortality rate in this 10th study of patients with initially normal EF was 2.2%,[131] which is 10-fold higher than the average 0.2% per year mortality rate of the other previous 9 studies.[122] This higher mortality rate may be explained by the greater age of the patients in this latter study (60 years), which is more than 20 years older than the average age of patients in the other studies (39 years). This finding suggests that severe AR in older patients, who have stiffer arteries and stiffer left ventricles, may be more poorly tolerated than AR in younger patients.

Patients with Left Ventricular Systolic Dysfunction

Data in asymptomatic patients with depressed LV function are limited, but it has been estimated that the average rate of symptom onset in such patients is greater than 25% per year.[132-134] Symptoms caused by AR are a strong predictor of clinical outcome.[135] The data developed in the presurgical era indicate that patients with dyspnea, angina, or overt heart failure have a poor outcome with medical therapy, with annual mortality rates of greater than 10% in those with angina and 20% in those with heart failure.[90,136,137]

Medical Management

Role of Vasodilator Therapy

Vasodilator therapy has been designed to reduce regurgitant volume, and hence reduce LV volumes and wall stress. These effects could theoretically be beneficial in AR by preserving LV function and reducing LV mass. Vasodilators are useful in patients with severe AR and symptoms and/or LV dysfunction who are considered poor candidates

Author, Year	No. of Patients	Mean Follow-up (yr)	Progression to Symptoms, Death, or LV Dysfunction Rate/Year (%)	Progression to Asymptomatic LV Dysfunction		Mortality (No of Patients)	Comments
				n	Rate/Year (%)		
Bonow et al., 1983, 1991	104	8.0	3.8	4	0.5	2	Outcome predicted by LV ESD, EDD, change in EF with exercise, and rate of change in ESD and EF at rest with time.
Scognamiglio et al., 1986*	30	4.7	2.1	3	2.1	0	Three patients developing asymptomatic LV dysfunction had lower initial PAP/ESV ratios and trend toward higher LV ESD and EDD and lower FS.
Siemienczuk et al., 1989	50	3.7	4.0	1	0.5	0	Patients included those receiving placebo and medical dropouts in a randomized drug trial; included some patients with NYHA FC II symptoms; outcome predicted by LV ESV, EDV, change in EF with exercise, and end-systolic wall stress.
Scognamiglio et al., 1994*	74	6.0	5.7	15	3.4	0	All patients received digoxin as part of a randomized trial.
Tornos et al., 1995	101	4.6	3.0	6	1.3	0	Outcome predicted by pulse pressure, LV ESD, EDD, and EF at rest.
Ishii et al., 1996	27	14.2	3.6	—	—	0	Development of symptoms predicted by systolic BP, LV ESD, EDD, mass index, and wall thickness. LV function not reported in all patients.
Borer et al., 1998	104	7.3	6.2	7	0.9	4	20% of patients in NYHA FC II; outcome predicted by initial FC II symptoms, change in LV EF with exercise, LV ESD, and LV FS.
Tarasoutchi et al., 2003	72	10	4.7	1	0.1	0	Development of symptoms predicted by LV ESD and EDD. LV function not reported in all patients.
Evangelista et al., 2005	31	7	3.6	—	—	1	Placebo control group in 7-year vasodilator clinical trial.
Average	593	6.6	4.3	37	1.2	(0.18%/yr)	

*Two studies by same authors involved separate patient groups.

BP, blood pressure; EDD, end-diastolic dimension; EDV, end-diastolic volume; EF, ejection fraction; ESD, end-systolic dimension; ESV, end-systolic volume; FC, functional class; FS, fractional shortening; LV, left ventricular; NYHA, New York Heart Association; PAP, pulmonary artery pressure.

From Bonow RO, Carabello BA, Chatterjee K, et al: ACC/AHA 2006 guidelines for the management of patients with valvular heart disease: a report of the American College of Cardiology/American Heart Association Task Force on Practice Guidelines. J Am Coll Cardiol 2006;48:e1-e148, with permission.

for surgery because of severe comorbidities. Vasodilators are also useful for improving the hemodynamic profile in patients with severe heart failure symptoms before AVR. The most controversial role of vasodilators is their use to alter the natural history of asymptomatic patients with preserved LV systolic function and prolong the compensated phase of the disease. If vasodilator therapy successfully delays decompensation of the left ventricle, it would postpone the need for surgery. Several studies with small numbers of patients and short-term follow-up periods showed different beneficial effects of vasodilators on hemodynamic and echocardiographic parameters of LV function.[138-146] Regarding long-term effects, only one study reported that long-acting nifedipine therapy produced a reduction in LV dimensions and an increase in EF,[126] and two studies demonstrated improvement in hemodynamic parameters with enalapril and quinapril, particularly when accompanied by a drop in blood pressure.[139,145] A more recent randomized clinical trial using nifedipine, enalapril, or no treatment in asymptomatic patients with severe AR and normal LV function failed to demonstrate any significant benefit of such therapy; vasodilators did not delay the need for AVR

after an extended follow-up period and did not result in a reduction in regurgitant volume or beneficial effect on LV size or function (Figure 10-10).[67] Thus, there is no consensus regarding the role of vasodilator therapy. If such therapy is used in asymptomatic patients with severe AR, the goal should be to reduce systolic blood pressure, and drug dosage should be increased until a measurable decrease in blood pressure is achieved.

Prevention of Endocarditis

Patients with AR should be instructed in the importance of good oral hygiene and regular dental cleaning and examinations. Patients should also be instructed on early reporting of unexplained fever lasting for more than 1 week and on the importance of refraining from self-medication with antibiotics in the case of fever. According to the 2007 AHA guidelines on endocarditis prevention, antibiotic prophylaxis before dental work or other invasive procedures is no longer recommended in patients with AR or other forms of native valve disease. Antibiotic prophylaxis is only recommended in patients with AR who have a previous history of endocarditis.[147]

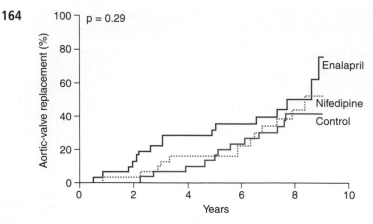

FIGURE 10–10 Progression to aortic valve replacement in initially asymptomatic patients with aortic regurgitation randomly assigned to treatment with enalapril, nifedipine, or placebo. *(From Evangelista A, Tornos P, Sambola A, et al: Long-term vasodilator therapy in patients with severe aortic regurgitation. N Engl J Med 2005;353:1342-1349, with permission.)*

Serial Evaluations

The aim of serial evaluation of asymptomatic patients with chronic AR is to detect the onset of clinical symptoms and to assess objective changes in LV function and size that can occur in the absence of symptoms to determine the optimal time for surgery. Patients with mild to moderate AR can be seen on a yearly basis with echocardiograms performed every 2 years. Patients with severe AR in whom the chronic nature of the regurgitation is uncertain when they are first seen should be reevaluated within 2 to 3 months to be certain that their condition is stable and that a subacute process with rapid progression is not underway. Once the chronicity and stability of the regurgitation have been established, the frequency of the clinical re-evaluation and repeat of examinations will depend on the severity of the regurgitation, the degree of LV dilation, and the level of systolic function at rest. In patients with severe AR, those with normal EF at rest (>50%) and moderate degrees of LV dilatation (end-diastolic dimension of 60 to 65 mm) may be seen every 6 months. During every visit a careful clinical history should be obtained. An exercise test is useful if symptoms are equivocal. Echocardiographic measurements should also be obtained yearly. In patient with more severe dilation, with end-diastolic dimensions approaching 70 mm, it is wise to recommend clinical evaluations and repeat echocardiography measurements every 6 months or even more frequently if a progressive dilatation or decline in EF is detected. Echocardiography should also be performed when there is a real or suspected change in the clinical situation in patients with severe AR. Some authors recommend the use of stress echocardiography and brain natriuretic peptide measurements to document earlier stages of LV dysfunction,[148-151] although the clinical relevance of such findings needs further validation. CMR or radionuclide angiography can be used in the serial assessment as an alternative to echocardiography, particularly in patients with technically suboptimal echocardiograms.

In patients with aortic root dilatation, serial echocardiograms should include accurate measurements of the aorta. Indexing for body surface area is recommended, especially in patients of small body size and in women.[152,153] CMR or CT is also a good alternative for following the severity of aortic dilatation.

Indications for Surgery

The surgical management in AR usually requires AVR. In highly selected patients and in surgical centers of excellence, there is increasing experience in aortic valve repair.[154-156] In younger patients, some groups use the pulmonic autograft procedure (the Ross procedure).[157,158] The indications for surgery on the aortic valve are the same irrespective of the surgical technique used.

The goals of the operation are to improve outcome, to diminish symptoms, to prevent the development of postoperative heart failure and cardiac death, and to avoid aortic complications in patients who present with aortic aneurysms. Several investigators[39-41,43,46,48-50,52-60,62,63] have identified preoperative predictors of patient outcome and LV function AVR for chronic AR. The most consistent of these measures have been the functional class, EF, and end-systolic dimension (see Table 10–1). On the basis of robust observational evidence, the recommended indications for surgical intervention for severe AR are similar in both the ACC/AHA and the European Society of Cardiology guidelines (Figures 10-11 and 10-12).[122,159]

Symptom onset is an indication for surgery, irrespective of LV function. When the LV systolic function is normal and the patient experiences symptoms, every effort should be made to clearly relate the symptoms to the AR. Especially when the symptoms are mild, such as New York Heart Association functional class II dyspnea, clinical judgment is necessary, and in this setting the role of exercise testing is valuable. However, in patients with LV dilatation and progressive enlargement in chamber size or decline in EF on serial studies, the beginning of even mild symptoms is a clear indication for AVR.

In symptomatic patients with decreased LV systolic function (subnormal EF), surgery is definitely indicated. Several studies have shown that the long-term outcome is excellent if patients with depressed LV systolic function undergo AVR when asymptomatic or only mildly symptomatic or with mild degrees of LV dysfunction.[41,50,63] Therefore, every effort should be made to refer patients for surgery at this stage. Postoperative survival and the likelihood of recovery of systolic function will be worse in patients with preoperative New York Heart Association functional class III-IV symptoms[160] or with extremely enlarged ventricles (>55 mm at end-systole) and/or very poor EF (<30%).[63,161] However, even in those very ill patients, AVR and subsequent medical treatment is a better alternative than long-term medical therapy alone or cardiac transplantation. Recent data, demonstrating a significant decrease in operative and long-term postoperative mortality in patients with AR and severe preoperative LV dysfunction, reinforces this opinion.[64]

Surgery should also be considered in asymptomatic patients with severe AR and impaired LV function at rest, defined as resting EF less than 50% and/or extreme degrees of LV dilatation (end-diastolic diameter ≥70 to 75 mm and end-systolic diameter ≥50 to 55 mm).[162-167] In these patients, the likelihood that symptoms will develop in the short-term is high, whereas perioperative mortality is very low, and the postoperative long-term results are excellent. Good-quality echocardiograms and data confirmation with repeated measurements are necessary before surgery is recommended for asymptomatic patients.

In patients with AR undergoing other cardiac operations, such as coronary bypass surgery or mitral valve surgery, the decision to replace the aortic valve should be individualized according to the severity of AR, age, and overall clinical situation. If the AR is severe, AVR is almost always indicated,[122] whereas AVR can be postponed in most patients when the AR is mild.

Concomitant Aortic Root Disease

In patients with AR due to enlargement of the aorta or aortic root, the natural history of the disease and thus the timing and choice of surgical intervention are often based on the

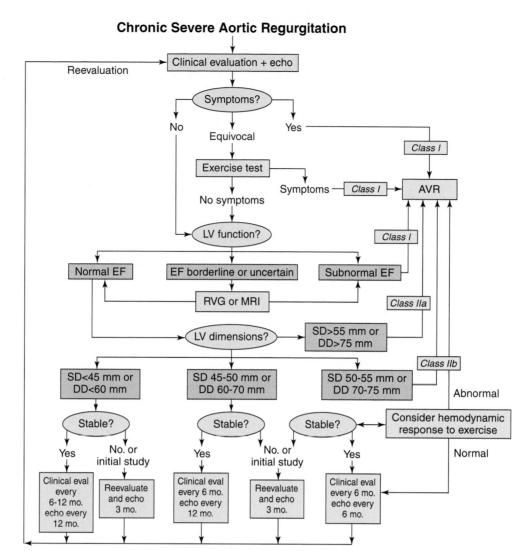

FIGURE 10–11 Management strategy for patients with chronic severe aortic regurgitation. Preoperative coronary angiography should be performed routinely as determined by age, symptoms, and coronary risk factors. Cardiac catheterization and angiography may also be helpful when there is discordance between clinical findings and echocardiography. "Stable" refers to stable echocardiographic measurements. In some centers, serial follow-up may be performed with radionuclide ventriculography or cardiac magnetic resonance rather than echocardiography to assess left ventricular volume and systolic function. DD, end-diastolic dimension; ESD, end-systolic dimension; LV, left ventricular; MRI, magnetic resonance imaging; RVG, radionuclide ventriculography. *(From Bonow RO, Carabello BA, Chatterjee K, et al: ACC/AHA 2006 guidelines for the management of patients with valvular heart disease: a report of the American College of Cardiology/American Heart Association Task Force on Practice Guidelines. J Am Coll Cardiol 2006;48:e1–e148, with permission.)*

degree and rate of aortic or aortic root dilation rather than on the LV response to AR. These patients include patients with Marfan syndrome, patients with bicuspid aortic valves, and patients with annuloaortic ectasia.

When AR is mild, management decisions should focus on the underlying aortic and aortic root disease. In other patients in whom the AR is more severe, both conditions should be considered in decision making.

In patients with Marfan syndrome, β-blockers slow the progression of aortic dilatation.[168] However, in patients with severe AR β-blockers should be used cautiously because the lengthening of diastole increases the regurgitant volume. Enalapril has also been used to delay aortic dilatation in patients with Marfan syndrome.[169] Recent animal models of Marfan syndrome have shown a beneficial effect of the angiotensin receptor blocker losartan in normalizing the aortic root growth and aortic wall architecture,[170] and a clinical trial comparing the effects of atenolol and losartan is currently underway.[171] Whether the same beneficial effect of β-blockers or other drugs occurs in patients with bicuspid aortic valves and aortic dilatation is unknown.

The rationale for an aggressive surgical approach in patients with aortic dilatation and only mild AR is better defined in patients with Marfan syndrome than in patients with bicuspid valves or annuloaortic ectasia.[152] Aortic root dilatation greater than 55 mm should be considered a surgical indication irrespective of the degree and etiology of AR. In patients with Marfan syndrome or bicuspid valves, lower degrees of root dilatation (>45 and >50 mm, respectively) have been proposed as indicators for surgery, especially when there is a rapid increase in aortic diameter between serial measurements (5 mm per year) or a family history of aortic dissection.[122,159,172-175] For patients who have reached the recommended indications for surgery based on severity of AR, a lower threshold can be used for combining surgery on the ascending aorta.[122] In patients with borderline indications the decision to replace the ascending aorta also relies on perioperative surgical findings regarding the thickness of the aortic valve and the status of the rest of the aorta. Both the ACC/AHA and the European guidelines also consider that lower thresholds of aortic diameters can be used for indicating surgery if valve repair can be performed by experienced surgeons.[122,159]

10

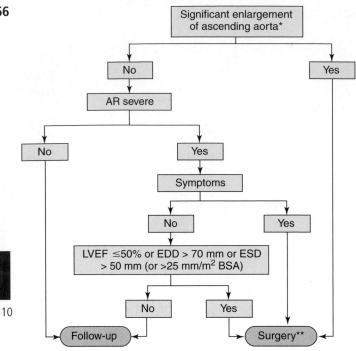

FIGURE 10–12 Management of aortic regurgitation. AR, aortic regurgitation; BSA, body surface area; EDD, end-diastolic dimension; EF, ejection fraction; ESD, end-systolic dimension; LV, left ventricular. *(From Vahanian A, Baumgartner H, Bax J, et al: Guidelines on the management of valvular heart disease: the Task Force on the Management of Valvular Heart Disease of the European Society of Cardiology. Eur Heart J 2007;28:230–268, with permission.)*

REFERENCES

1. Olson LJ, Subramanian R, Edwards WD: Surgical pathology of pure aortic insufficiency: a study of 255 cases. Mayo Clin Proc 1984;59:835-841.
2. Roberts WC, KO JM, Moore TR, Jones WH: Causes of pure aortic regurgitation in patients having isolated aortic valve replacement in a single US tertiary hospital (1993-2005). Circulation 2006;114:422-429.
3. Baszyk H, Witkiewicz AJ, Edwards WD: Acute aortic regurgitation due to spontaneous rupture of a fenestrated cusp: report in a 65 year old man and review of seven additional cases. Cardiovasc Pathol 1999;8:213-216.
4. Sadaniantz A, Malhotra R, Korr KS: Transient acute severe aortic regurgitation complicating balloon aortic valvuloplasty. Cath Cardiovasc Diagn 1989;17:186-189.
5. Alexopoulos D, Sherman W: Unusual presentation of acute aortic regurgitation following percutaneous balloon valvuloplasty. Am Heart J 1988;1161622-1623.
6. Connolly HM, Crary JL, McGoon MD, et al: Valvular heart disease associated with fenfluramine-phentermine. N Engl J Med 1997;337;581-588.
7. Iung B, Baron G, Butchart EG: A prospective survey of patients with valvular heart disease in Europe: The Euro Heart Survey on Valvular Heart Disease. Eur Heart J 2003;24:1231-1243.
8. Dervan J, Goldberg S: Acute aortic regurgitation: pathophysiology and management. Cardiovasc Clin 1986;16:281-288.
9. Morganroth J, Perloff JK, Zeldis SM, Dunkman WB: Acute severe aortic regurgitation: pathophysiology, clinical recognition and management. Ann Intern Med 1977;87:223-232.
10. Ardehali A, Segal J, Cheitlin MD: Coronary blood flow reserve in acute aortic regurgitation. J Am Coll Cardiol 1995;25:1387-1392.
11. Mann T, McLaurin L, Grossman W, Craige E: Assessing the hemodynamic severity of acute aortic regurgitation due to infective endocarditis. N Engl J Med 1975;293:108-113.
12. Cigarroa JE, Isselbacher EM, DeSanctis RW, Eagle KA: Diagnostic imaging in the evaluation of suspected aortic dissection: old standards and new directions. N Engl J Med 1993;328:35-43.
13. Nienaber CA, von Kokolitsch Y, Nicholas V, et al: The diagnosis of thoracic aortic dissection by non invasive imaging procedures. N Engl J Med 1993;328:1-9.
14. Mith MD, Cassidy JM, Souther S, et al: Transesophageal echocardiography in the diagnosis of traumatic rupture of the aorta. N Engl J Med 1995;332;356-362.
15. David TE, Feindel CM: An aortic valve-sparing operation for patients with aortic incompetence and aneurysm of the ascending aorta. J Thorac Cardiovasc Surg 1992;103:617-622.
16. Graeter TP, Langer F, Nikoloudakis N, et al: Valve-preserving operations in acute aortic dissection type A. Ann Thorac Surg 2000;70:1460-1465.
17. Kallenbach K, Oelze T, Salcher R, et al: Evolving strategies for treatment of acute aortic dissection type A. Circulation 2004;110(Suppl II):II-243-II-249.
18. Habib G, Avierinos JF, Thuny F: Aortic valve endocarditis: is there an optimal surgical timing? Curr Opin Cardiol 2007;22:77-83.
19. Cabell CH, Abrutyn E, Fowler VG, et al: Use of surgery in patients with native valve endocarditis: results from the international collaboration on endocarditis merged database. Am Heart J 2005;150:1092-1098.
20. Aksoy O, Sexton DJ, Wang A, et al: Early surgery in patients with infective endocarditis: a propensity score analysis. Clin Infect Dis 2007;44:364-372.
21. Carabello BA: Aortic regurgitation. a lesion with similarities to both aortic stenosis and mitral regurgitation. Circulation 1990;82:1051-1053.
22. Ross J Jr: Afterload mismatch in aortic and mitral valve disease: implications for surgical therapy J Am Coll Cardiol 1985;5:811-826.
23. Borow KM: Surgical outcome in chronic aortic regurgitation: a physiologic framework for assessing preoperative predictors. J Am Coll Cardiol 1987;10:1165-1170.
24. Grossman W, Jones D, McLaurin LP: Wall stress and patterns of hypertrophy in the human left ventricle. J Clin Invest 1975;56:56-64.
25. Ross J Jr, McCullagh WH: Nature of enhanced performance of the dilated left ventricle in the dog during chronic volume overloading. Circ Res 1972;30:549-556.
26. Wisenbaugh T, Spann JF, Carabello BA: Differences in myocardial performance and load between patients with similar amounts of chronic aortic versus chronic mitral regurgitation. J Am Coll Cardiol 1984;3:916-923.
27. Ricci DR: Afterload mismatch and preload reserve in chronic aortic regurgitation. Circulation 1982;66:862-834.
28. Rigolin VH, Bonow RO: Hemodynamic characteristics and progression to heart failure in regurgitant lesions. Heart Fail Clin 2007;2:453-460.
29. Gaasch WH: Left ventricular radius to wall thickness ratio. Am J Cardiol 1979;43:1189-1194.
30. Nitenberg A, Foult JM, Blanchet F, Rahali M: Coronary flow and resistance reserve in patients with chronic aortic regurgitation, angina pectoris and normal coronary arteries. J Am Coll Cardiol 1988;11:478-486.
31. Gaasch WH, Andrias CW, Levine HJ: Chronic aortic regurgitation: the effect of aortic valve replacement on left ventricular volume, mass and function. Circulation 1978;58:825-836.
32. Schwarz F, Flameng W, Langebartels F, et al: Impaired left ventricular function in chronic aortic valve disease: survival and function after replacement by Bjork Shiley prosthesis. Circulation 1979;60:48-58.
33. Borer JS, Rosing DR, Kent KM, et al: Left ventricular function at rest and during exercise after aortic valve replacement in patients with aortic regurgitation. Am J Cardiol 1979;44:1297-1305.
34. Clark DG, McAnulty JH, Rahimtoola SH: Valve replacement in aortic insufficiency with left ventricular dysfunction. Circulation 1980;61:411-421.
35. Toussaint C, Cribier A, Cazor JL, et al: Hemodynamic and angiographic evaluation of aortic regurgitation 8 and 27 months after aortic valve replacement. Circulation 1981;64:456-463.
36. Carroll JD, Gaasch WH, Zile MR, Levine HJ: Serial changes in left ventricular function after correction of chronic aortic regurgitation: dependence on early changes in preload and subsequent regression of hypertrophy. Am J Cardiol 1983;51:476-482.
37. Bonow RO, Rosing DR, Maron BJ, et al: Reversal of left ventricular dysfunction after aortic valve replacement for chronic aortic regurgitation: influence of duration of preoperative left ventricular dysfunction. Circulation 1984;70:570-579.
38. Fioretti P, Roclandt J, Sclavo M, et al: Postoperative regression of left ventricular dimensions in aortic insufficiency: a long term echocardiographic study. J Am Coll Cardiol 1985;5:856-861.
39. Carabello BA, Usher BW, Hendrix GH, et al: Predictors of outcome for aortic valve replacement in patients with aortic regurgitation and left ventricular dysfunction: a change in the measuring stick. J Am Coll Cardiol 1987;10:991-997.
40. Taniguchi K, Nakano S, Hirose H, et al: Preoperative left ventricular function: minimal requirement for successful late results of valve replacement for aortic regurgitation. J Am Coll Cardiol 1987;10:510-518.
41. Bonow RO, Dodd JT, Maron BJ, et al: Long term serial changes in left ventricular function and reversal of ventricular dilatation after valve replacement for chronic aortic regurgitation. Circulation 1988;78:1108-1120.
42. Borer JS, Herrold EM, Hochreiter C, et al: Natural history of left ventricular performance at rest and during exercise after aortic valve replacement for aortic regurgitation. Circulation 1991;84(Suppl III):III-133-III-139.
43. Cohn PF, Gorlin R, Cohn LH, Collins JJ Jr: Left ventricular ejection fraction as a prognostic guide in surgical treatment of coronary and valvular disease. Am J Cardiol 1974;34:136-141.
44. Copeland JG, Grepp RB, Stinson EB, Shumway NE: Long term follow-up after isolated aortic valve replacement. J Thorac Cardiovasc Surg 1977;74:875-889.
45. Herreman F, Amcur A, de Vernejoul F, et al: Pre and postoperative hemodynamic and cineangiographic assessment of left ventricular function in patients with aortic regurgitation. Am Heart J 1979;98:63-72.
46. Cuhna CL, Giuliani ER, Fuster V, et al: Preoperative M mode echocardiography as predictor of surgical results in chronic aortic insufficiency. J Thorac Cardiovasc Surg 1980;79:256-265.
47. Forman R, Firth BG, Barnard MS: Prognostic significance of preoperative left ventricular ejection fraction and valve lesion in patients with aortic valve replacement. Am J Cardiol 1980;45:1120-1125.
48. Greves J, Rahimtoola SH, McAnulty JH, et al: Preoperative criteria predictive of late survival following valve replacement for severe aortic regurgitation. Am Heart J 1981;101:300-308.
49. Gaasch WH, Carroll JD, Levine H, Cristicello MG: Chronic aortic regurgitation: prognostic value of left ventricular end-systolic dimension and end-diastolic radius/thickness ratio. J Am Coll Cardiol 1983;1:775-782.
50. Bonow RO, Picone AL, McIntosh CL, et al: Survival and functional results after valve replacement for aortic regurgitation from 1976 to 1983: impact of preoperative left ventricular function. Circulation 1985;72:1244-1256.
51. Carabello BA, Williams H, Gaasch AK, et al: Hemodynamic predictors of outcome in patients undergoing valve replacement. Circulation 1986;72:1244-1256.

52. Michel PL, Iung B, Abou JS, et al: The effect of left ventricular systolic function on long term survival in mitral and aortic regurgitation. J Heart Valve Dis 1995;4(Suppl 2): S160-S168.
53. Henry WL, Bonow RO, Borer JS, et al: Observations on the optimum time for operative intervention for aortic regurgitation. I. Evaluation of the results of aortic valve replacement in symptomatic patients. Circulation 1980;61:471-483.
54. Kumpuris AG, Quinones MA, Waggoner AD, et al: Importance of preoperative hypertrophy, wall stress and end-systolic dimension as echocardiographic predictors of normalization of left ventricular dilatation after valve replacement in symptomatic patients. Am J Cardiol 1982;49:1091-1100.
55. Fioretti P, Roelandt J, Bos RJ, et al: Echocardiography in chronic aortic insufficiency: is valve replacement too late when left ventricular end systolic dimension reaches 55 mm? Circulation 1983;67:216-221.
56. Stone PH, Clark RD, Goldschlager N, et al: Determinants of prognosis of patients with aortic regurgitation who undergo aortic valve replacement. J Am Coll Cardiol 1984;3:1118-1126.
57. Daniel WG, Hood WP Jr, Siart A, et al: Chronic aortic regurgitation: reassessment of the prognostic value of preoperative left ventricular end systolic dimension and fractional shortening. Circulation 1985;7:669-680.
58. Cormier B, Vahanian A, Luxereaux P, et al: Should asymptomatic or mildly symptomatic aortic regurgitation be operated on? Z Kardiol 1986;75(Suppl 2):141-145.
59. Sheiban I, Trevi GP, Carassotto D, et al: Aortic valve replacement in patients with aortic incompetence: preoperative parameters influencing long term results. Z Kardiol 1986;75(Suppl 2):146-154.
60. Klodas E, Enriquez-Sarano M, Tajik AJ, et al: Aortic regurgitation complicated by extreme left ventricular dilation: long-term outcome after surgical correction. J Am Coll Cardiol 1996;27:670-677.
61. Klodas E, Enriquez-Sarano M, Tajik AJ, et al: Optimizing timing of surgical correction in patients with severe aortic regurgitation: role of symptoms. J Am Coll Cardiol 1997;30:746-752.
62. Turina J, Milinic J, Seifert B, Turina M: Valve replacement in chronic aortic regurgitation: true predictors of survival after extended follow-up. Circulation 1998;98 (Suppl II):II-100-II-106.
63. Tornos P, Sambola A, Permanyer-Miralda G, et al: Long term outcome of surgically treated aortic regurgitation: influence of guidelines adherence toward early surgery. J Am Coll Cardiol 2006;47:1012-1017.
64. Bhudia SK McCarthy PM, Kumpati GS, et al: Improved outcomes after aortic valve surgery for chronic aortic regurgitation with severe left ventricular dysfunction. J Am Coll Cardiol 2007;49:1465-1471.
65. Kawanishi DT, McKay CR, Chandraratna PA, et al: Cardiovascular response to dynamic exercise in patients with chronic symptomatic mild to moderate and severe aortic regurgitation. Circulation 1986;73:62-72.
66. Bonow RO, Lakatos E, Maron BJ, Epstein SE: Serial long-term assessment of the natural history of asymptomatic patients with chronic aortic regurgitation and normal left ventricular systolic function. Circulation 1991;84:1625-1635.
67. Evangelista A, Tornos P, Sambola A, et al: Long-term vasodilator therapy in patients with severe aortic regurgitation. N Engl J Med 2005;353:1342-1349.
68. Perloff JK: Physical Examination of the Heart and Circulation. Philadelphia, WB Saunders, 1982.
69. Corrigan DJ: On permanent patency of the mouth of the aorta, or inadequacy of the aortic valve. Edinburgh Med Surg 1832;37:225
70. Quincke H: Observations on capillary and venous pulse. Berl Klin Wochenschr 1868;5:357 [translated in Willius FA, Keys TE (eds): Classics of Cardiology. New York, Dover, 1961].
71. Harvey WP, Corrado MA, Perloff JK: Right sided murmurs of aortic insufficiency (diastolic murmurs better heard to the right of the sternum than to the left). Am J Med Sci 1963;245:533
72. Grayburn PA, Smith MD, Handshoe R, et al: Detection of aortic insufficiency by standard echocardiography, pulsed Doppler echocardiography and auscultation: a comparison of accuracies. Ann Intern Med 186;104:599-605.
73. Kinney EL: Causes of false-negative auscultation of regurgitant lesions: a Doppler echocardiographic study of 294 patients. J Gen Intern Med 1988;3:429-434.
74. Aronow WS, Krozon I: Correlation of prevalence and severity of aortic regurgitation detected by pulsed Doppler echocardiography with the murmur of aortic regurgitation in elderly patients in a long term health facility. Am J Cardiol 1989;63:128-129.
75. Desjardin VA, Enriquez Sarano M, Tajik AJ, et al: Intensity of murmurs correlates with severity of valvular regurgitation. Am J Med 1996;100:149-156.
76. Flint A: On cardiac murmurs. Am J Med Sci 1862;44:29-55.
77. Emi S, Fukuda N, Oki T, et al: Genesis of the Austin Flint murmur: relation to mitral flow and aortic regurgitant flow dynamics. J Am Coll Cardiol 1993;21:1399-1405.
78. Rahko PS: Doppler and echocardiography characteristics of patients having an Austin Flint murmur. Circulation 1991;83:1940-1950.
79. Landzberg JS, Pflugfelder PW, Cassidy MM, et al: Etiology of the Austin Flint murmur. J Am Coll Cardiol 1992;20:408-413.
80. Roman MJ, Kligfield P, Devereux RB, et al: Geometric and functional correlates of electrocardiographic repolarization and voltage abnormalities in aortic regurgitation. J Am Coll Cardiol 197;9:500-508.
81. Chen J, Okin PM, Roman MJ, et al: Combined rest and exercise electrocardiographic repolarization findings in relation to structural and functional abnormalities in symptomatic aortic regurgitation. Am Heart J 1996;132:343-347.
82. Kligfield P, Ameisen O, Okin PM, et al: Relationship of the electrocardiographic response to exercise to geometric and functional findings in aortic regurgitation. Am Heart J 1987;113:1097-1102.
83. Reichek N, Deverex RB: Left ventricular hypertrophy: relationship of anatomic, echocardiographic and electrocardiographic findings. Circulation 1981;63:1391-1398.
84. Bishop N, Boyle R, Watson DA, et al: Aortic valve disease and the ST/heart rate relationship: a longitudinal study before and after aortic valve replacement. J Electrocardiol 1988;21:31-37.
85. Martinez Useros C, Tornos P, Montoyo J, et al: Ventricular arrhythmias in aortic valve disease: a further marker of impaired ventricular function. Int J Cardiol 1992;34: 49-56.
86. Samuels DA, Curfman GD, Friedlich AL, et al: Valve replacement for aortic regurgitation: long term follow up with factors that influence the results. Circulation 1979;60:647-654.
87. Acar J, Luxereau P, Ducimetiere P, et al: Prognosis of surgically treated chronic aortic valve disease: predictive indicators of early postoperative risk and long term survival based on 439 cases. J Thorac Cardiovasc Surg 1981;82:114-126.
88. Isom OW, Dembrow JM, Glassman E, et al: Factors influencing long-term survival after isolated aortic valve replacement. Circulation 1974;50:154-162.
89. Hirshfield JW, Epstein SE, Roberts AJ, et al: Indices predicting long-term survival after valve replacement in patients with aortic regurgitation and patients with aortic stenosis. Circulation 1974;50:1190-1199.
90. Spagnuolo M, Kloth H, Taranta A, et al: Natural history of rheumatic aortic regurgitation: criteria predictive of death, congestive heart failure and angina in young patients. Circulation 1971:44:368-380.
91. Zoghbi WA, Enriquez-Sarano M, Foster E, et al: Recommendations for evaluation of the severity of native valvular regurgitation with two-dimensional and Doppler echocardiography. J Am Soc Echocardiogr 2003;16:777-802.
92. Evangelista A, Garcia del Castillo H, Calvo F, et al: Strategy for optimal aortic regurgitation quantification by Doppler echocardiography: agreement among different methods. Am Heart J 2000;139:773-781.
93. Teague SM, Heinsimer JA, Anderson JL, et al: Quantification of aortic regurgitation utilizing continuous wave Doppler ultrasound. J Am Coll Cardiol 1986;8:592-599.
94. Labovitz AJ, Ferrara RP, Kern MJ, et al: Quantitative evaluation of aortic insufficiency by continuous wave Doppler echocardiography. J Am Coll Cardiol 1986;8:1341-1347.
95. Xic GY, Berk MR, Smith MD, DeMaria AN: A simplified method for determining regurgitant fraction by Doppler echocardiography in patients with aortic regurgitation. J Am Coll Cardiol 1994;24:1041-1045.
96. Sambola A, Tornos P, Ferreira I, Evangelista A: Prognostic value of preoperative indexed end-systolic left ventricular diameter in the outcome after surgery in patients with chronic aortic regurgitation. Am Heart J 2008;155:1114-1120.
97. deWaroux JB, Pouleur AC, Goffinet C, et al: Functional anatomy of aortic regurgitation: accuracy, prediction of surgical repairability and outcome implications of transesophageal echocardiography. Ciculation 2007;116(suppl I):I-264-I-269.
98. Debl K, Djavidani B, Buchner S, et al: Assessment of the anatomic regurgitant orifice in aortic regurgitation: a clinical magnetic resonance imaging study. Heart 2007;94:e8.
99. Gentchos GE, Tischler MD, Christian TF: Imaging and quantifying valvular heart disease using magnetic resonance techniques. Curr Treat Options Cardiovasc Med 2006;8:453-460.
100. Chatzimavroudis GP, Oshinski JN, Franch RH, et al: Evaluation of the precision of magnetic resonance phase velocitymapping for blood flow measurements. J Cardiovasc Magn Reson 2001;3:11-19.
101. Kozerke S, Schwitter J, Pedersen EM, Boesiger P: Aortic and mitral regurgitation quantification using moving slice velocity mapping. J Magn Reson Imaging 2001;14:106-112.
102. Chatzimavroudis GP, Oshinski JN, Franch RH, et al: Quantification of the aortic regurgitant volume with magnetic resonance phase velocity mapping: a clinical investigation of the importance of imaging slice location. J Heart Valve Dis 1998;7:94-101.
103. Friedrich MG, Schulz-Menger J, Poetsch T, et al: Quantification of valvular aortic stenosis by magnetic resonance imaging. Am Heart J 2002;144:329-334.
104. John AS, Dill T, Brandt RR, et al: Magnetic resonance to assess the aortic valve area in aortic stenosis: how does it compare to current diagnostic standards. J Am Coll Cardiol 2003;42:519-526.
105. Kupfahl C, Honold M, Meinhardt G, et al: Evaluation of aortic stenosis by cardiovascular magnetic resonance imaging: comparison with established routine clinical techniques. Heart 2004;90:893-901.
106. Debl K, Djavidani B, Seitz J, et al: Planimetry of aortic valve area in aortic stenosis by magnetic resonance imaging. Invest Radiol 2005;40:631-636.
107. Doherty NE 3rd, Seelos KC, Sazuki J, et al: Application of cine MR imaging for sequential evaluation of response to angiotensin converting enzyme inhibitor therapy in dilated cardiomyopathy. J Am Coll Cardiol 1992;19:1294-1302.
108. Masci PG, Dymarkowski S, Bogaert J: Valvular heart disease: what does cardiovascular MRI add. Eur Radiol 2008;18:197-208.
109. Alkadhi H, Desbioller L, Husmann L, et al: Aortic regurgitation: assessment with 64 section CT. Radiology 2007;245:111-121.
110. Jassal DS, Shapiro MD, Neilan TG, et al: 64-slice multidetector computed tomography (MDTC) for detection of aortic regurgitation and quantification of severity. Invest Radiol 2007;42:507-512.
111. Scheffeld H, Leschkas S, Plass A, et al: Accuracy of 64-slice computed tomography for the preoperative detection of coronary artery disease in patients with chronic aortic regurgitation. Am J Cardiol 2007;100:701-706.
112. Iskandrian AS, Heo J: Radionuclide angiographic evaluation of left ventricular performance at rest and exercise response in aortic regurgitation. Am J Cardiol 1985;55:428-431.
113. Misra M, Thakur R, Bhandari K, Puri VK: Value of treadmill exercise test in asymptomatic and minimally symptomatic patients with chronic severe aortic regurgitation. Int J Cardiol 1987;15:309-316.
114. Scriven AJ, Lipkin DP, Fox KM, Poole Wilson PA: Maximal oxygen uptake in severe aortic regurgitation: a different view of left ventricular function. Am Heart J 1990;120:902-909.
115. Weber KT, Janicki JS, McElroy PA: Cardiopulmonary exercise testing in the evaluation of mitral and aortic valve incompetence. Herz 1986;11:88-96.
116. Yousuf A, Khan N, Askhar M, et al: Echocardiography studies during stress testing using cold pressor test combined with hand grip exercise in asymptomatic paients with severe aortic regurgitation. Can J Cardiol 1986;2:200-205.
117. Wahi S, Haluska B, Pasquet A, et al: Exercise echocardiography predicts development of left ventricular dysfunction in medically and surgically treated patients with asymptomatic aortic regurgitation. Heart 2000;84:606-614.

118. Wu WC: Evaluation of aortic valve disorders using stress echocardiography. Echocardiography 2004;21:459-466.

119. Wilson RA, McDonald RW, Bristow JD, et al: Correlates of aortic distensibility in chronic aortic regurgitation and relation to progression to surgery. J Am Coll Cardiol 1992;19:259-265.

120. Rimold SC, Orav EJ, Come PC, et al: Progressive enlargement of the regurgitant orifice in patients with chronic aortic regurgitation. J Am Soc Echocardiogr 1998;11:259-265.

121. Padial LR, Oliver A, Vivaldi M, et al: Doppler echocardiographic assessment of progression of aortic regurgitation. Am J Cardiol 1997;80:306-314.

122. Bonow RO, Carabello BA, Chatterjee K, et al: ACC/AHA 2006 guidelines for the management of patients with valvular heart disease: a report of the American College of Cardiology/American Heart Association Task Force on Practice Guidelines. J Am Coll Cardiol 2006;48:e1-e148.

123. Bonow RO, Rosing DR, McIntosh CL, et al: The natural history of asymptomatic patients with aortic regurgitation and normal left ventricular function. Circulation 1983;68:509-515.

124. Scognamiglio R, Fasoli G, Dalla Volta S: Progression of myocardial dysfunction in asymptomatic patients with severe aortic insufficiency. Clin Cardiol 1986;9:151-156.

125. Siemienczuk D, Greenberg B, Morris C, et al: Chronic aortic insufficiency: factors associated with progression to aortic valve replacement. Ann Intern Med 1989;110:587-592.

126. Scognamiglio R, Rahimtoola SH, Fasoli G, et al: Nifedipine in asymptomatic patients with severe aortic regurgitation and normal left ventricular function. N Engl J Med 1994;331:689-694.

127. Tornos MP, Olona M, Permanyer-Miralda G, et al: Clinical outcome of severe asymptomatic chronic aortic regurgitation: a long term prospective follow up study. Am Heart J 1995;130:333-339.

128. Ishii K, Hirota Y, Suwa M, et al: Natural history and left ventricular response in chronic aortic regurgitation. Am J Cardiol 1996;78:357-361.

129. Borer JS, Hochreiter C, Herrold E, et al: Prediction of indications for valve replacement among asymptomatic or minimally symptomatic patients with chronic aortic regurgitation and normal left ventricular performance. Circulation 1998;97:525-534.

130. Tarasoutchi F, Grinberg M, Spina GS, et al: Ten year clinical laboratory follow up after application of a symptom-based therapeutic strategy to patients with severe aortic regurgitation of predominant rheumatic etiology. J Am Coll Cardiol 2003;41:1316-1324.

131. Detaint D, Messika-Zeitoun D, Maalouf J, et al: Quantitative echocardiographic determinants of clinical outcome in asymptomatic patients with aortic regurgitation: a prospective study. J Am Coll Cardiol Imaging 2008;1:1-11.

132. Henry WL, Bonow RO, Rosing DR, Epstein SE: Observations on the optimum time for operative intervention for aortic regurgitation. II. Serial echocardiographic evaluation of asymptomatic patients. Circulation 1980;61:484-492.

133. McDonald IG, Jelinck VM: Serial M mode echocardiography in severe aortic regurgitation. Circulation 1980;62:1291-1296.

134. Bonow RO: Radionuclide angiography in the management of asymptomatic aortic regurgitation. Circulation 1991;84(suppl I):I-296-I-302.

135. Dujardin KS, Enriquez-Sarano M, Schaff HV, et al: Mortality and morbidity of aortic regurgitation in clinical practice: a long-term follow up study. Circulation 1999;99:1851-1857.

136. Hegglin R, Scheu H, Rothlin M: Aortic insufficiency. Circulation 1968;38:77-92.

137. Rapaport E: Natural history of aortic and mitral valve disease. Am J Cardiol 1975;35:221-227.

138. Greenberg BH, Massie B, Bristow JD, et al: Long term vasodilator therapy of chronic aortic insufficiency: a randomized double-blinded, placebo controlled clinical trial. Circulation 1988;78:92-103.

139. Schon HR, Dorn R, Barthel P, Schomig A: Effects of 12 month quinapril therapy in asymptomatic patients with chronic aortic regurgitation. J Heart Valve Dis 1994;3:500-509.

140. Sondegaard L, Aldershvile J, Hildebrant P, et al: Vasodilatation with felodipine in chronic asymptomatic aortic regurgitation. Am Heart J 2000;139:667-674.

141. Greenberg BH, DeMots H, Murphy E, Rahimtoola SH: Mechanism for improved cardiac performance with arteriolar dilators in aortic insufficiency. Circulation 1981;63:263-268.

142. Greenberg BH, DeMots H, Murphy E, Rahimtoola SH: Beneficial effects of hydralazine on rest and exercise hemodynamics in patients with chronic severe aortic insufficiency. Circulation 1980;62:49-55.

143. Fioretti P, Benussi B, Scardi S, et al: Afterload reduction with nifedipine in aortic insufficiency. Am J Cardiol 1982;49:1728-1732.

144. Scognamiglio R, Fasoli G, Ponchia A, Dalla Volta S: Long term nifedipine unloading therapy in asymptomatic patients with chronic severe aortic regurgitation. J Am Coll Cardiol 1990;1:424-429.

145. Lin M, Chiang H, Lin S, et al: Vasodilator therapy in chronic asymptomatic aortic regurgitation: enalapril versus hydralazine therapy. J Am Coll Cardiol 1994;24:1046-1053.

146. Alehan D, Özkulu B: Beneficial effects of 1 year captopril therapy in children with chronic aortic regurgitation who have no symptoms. Am Heart J 1998;135:598-603.

147. Wilson W, Taubert KA, Gewitz M, et al: Prevention of infective endocarditis: a guideline from the American Heart Association Rheumatic Fever, Endocarditis, and Kawasaki Disease Committee, Council on Cardiovascular Disease in the Young, and the Council on Clinical Cardiology, Council on Cardiovascular Surgery and Anesthesia, and the Quality of Care and Outcomes Research Interdisciplinary Working Group. Circulation 2007;116:1736-1754.

148. Gabriel RS, Kerr AJ, Sharma V, et al: B-type natriuretic peptide and left ventricular dysfunction on exercise echocardiography in patients with chronic aortic regurgitation. Heart 2008;94:897-902.

149. Weber M, Arnold R, Rau M, et al: Relation of N terminal pro-B-type natriuretic peptide to progression of aortic valve disease. Eur Heart J 2005;26:1023-1030.

150. Eimer MJ, Ekery DL, Rigolin VH, et al: Elevated B type natriuretic peptide in asymptomatic men with chronic aortic regurgitation and preserved left ventricular function. Am J Cardiol 2004;94:676-678.

151. Weber M, Hausen M, Arnold R, et al: Diagnostic and prognostic value of N terminal pro-B-type natriuretic peptide (NT-proBNP) in patients with aortic regurgitation. Int J Cardiol 2008;127:321-327.

152. Judge DP, Dietz HC: Marfan's syndrome. Lancet 2005;366:1965-1976.

153. Davies RR, Goldstein LJ, Coady MA, et al: Yearly rupture or dissection rates for thoracic aneurysms: simple prediction based on size. Ann Thorac Surg 2002;73:1-27.

154. El Khoury G, Vanoverschelde JL, Glineur D, et al: Repair of bicuspid aortic valves in patients with aortic regurgitation. Circulation 2006;114(suppl I):I-610-I-616.

155. Gleason TG: Current perspective on aortic valve repair and valve-sparing aortic root replacement. Semin Thorac Cardiovasc Surg 2006;18:154-164.

156. Izumoto H, Kawazoe K, Oka T, et al: Aortic valve repair for aortic regurgitation: intermediate-term results in patients with tricuspid morphology. J Heart Valve Dis 2006;15:163-173.

157. Hanke T, Stierle U, Boehm JO, et al: Autograft regurgitation and aortic root dimensions after the Ross procedure: the German Ross Registry experience. Circulation 2007;116(suppl I):I-251-I-258.

158. Chiappini B, Absil B, Rubay J, et al: The Ross procedure: clinical and echocardiographic follow up in 219 consecutive patients. Ann Thorac Surg 2007;83:1285-1289.

159 Vahanian A, Baumgartner H, Bax J, et al: Guidelines on the management of valvular heart disease: the Task Force on the Management of Valvular Heart Disease of the European Society of Cardiology. Eur Heart J 2007;28:230-268.

160. Dujardin KS, Enriquez-Sarano M, Schaff HV, et al: Mortality and morbidity of aortic regurgitation in clinical practice: a long term follow up study. Circulation 1999;99:1851-1857.

161. Bonow RO, Nikas D, Elefteriades JA: Valve replacement for regurgitant lesions of the aortic or mitral valve in advanced left ventricular dysfunction. Cardiol Clin 1995;13:73-83.

162. Nishimura RA, McGoon MD, Schaff HV, Giuliani ER: Chronic aortic regurgitation: indications for operation 1988. Mayo Clin Proc 1988;63:270-280.

163. Carabello BA: The changing unnatural history of valvular regurgitation. Ann Thorac Surg 1992;53:191-199.

164. Gaasch WH, Sundaram M, Meyer TE: Managing asymptomatic patients with chronic aortic regurgitation. Chest 1997;111:1702-1709.

165. Bonow RO: Chronic aortic regurgitation: role of medical therapy and optimal timing for surgery. Cardiol Clin 1998;16:449-461.

166. Borer JS, Bonow RO: Contemporary approach to aortic and mitral regurgitation. Circulation 2003;108:2432-2438.

167. Enriquez-Sarano M, Tajik AJ: Clinical practice: aortic regurgitation. N Engl J Med 2004;351:1539-1546.

168. Shores J, Berger KR, Murphy EA, Pyeritz RE: Progression of aortic dilatation and the benefit of long term β-adrenergic blockade in Marfan's syndrome. N Engl J Med 1994;330:1335-1341.

169. Yetman AT, Bornemeier RA, McCrindle BW: Usefulness of enalapril versus propranolol or atenolol for prevention of aortic dilatation in patients with Marfan syndrome. Am J Cardiol 2005;95:1125-1127.

170. Habashi JP, Judge DP, Holm TM, et al: Losartan, an AT1 antagonist, prevents aortic aneurysm in a mouse model of Marfan syndrome. Science 2006;312:117-121.

171. Lacro R, Dietz HC, Wruck LM, et al: Rationale and design of a randomized clinical trial of beta-blocker therapy (atenolol) versus angiotensin II receptor blocker therapy (losartan) in individuals with Marfan syndrome. Am Heart J 2007;154:624-631.

172. Silverman DI, Gray J, Roman MJ: Family history of severe cardiovascular disease in Marfan syndrome associated with increased aortic diameter and decreased survival. J Am Coll Cardiol 1995;26:1062-1067.

173. Davies RR, Gallo A, Coady MA, et al: Novel measurements of relative aortic size predicts rupture of thoracic aortic aneurysm. Ann Thorac Surg 2006;81:169-177.

174. Davies RR, Goldstein LJ, Coady MA, et al: Yearly rupture or dissection rates for thoracic aortic aneurysms: simple prediction based on size. Ann Thorac Surg 2002;73:17-27.

175. Bonow RO: Bicuspid aortic valves and dilated aortas: a critical review of the critical review of the ACC/AHA guidelines recommendations. Am J Cardiol 2008;102:111-114.

10

CHAPTER 11

The Bicuspid Aortic Valve

Alan C. Braverman, Michael A. Beardslee

KEY POINTS

- The bicuspid valve is one of the most common congenital heart defects, affecting approximately 1% of the population.
- Familial occurrence of a bicuspid aortic valve is noted in 9% of first-degree relatives. When familial, the bicuspid aortic valve is inherited in an autosomal dominant pattern with incomplete penetrance.
- Most patients with bicuspid aortic valves will require surgical therapy for the valve and/or the aorta during their lifetime.
- Approximately 50% of severe aortic stenosis in adults is related to a bicuspid aortic valve.
- A bicuspid aortic valve may coexist with a number of other congenital cardiovascular defects and occurs in 50% of patients with coarctation of the aorta. Individuals with a bicuspid valve and coarctation of the aorta have an increased risk of aortic complications.
- When the transthoracic echocardiogram is not diagnostic, a transesophageal echocardiogram or magnetic resonance imaging may be useful for diagnosis of a bicuspid aortic valve.
- Ascending aortic dilatation occurs commonly in bicuspid aortic valve disease, even in the absence of aortic stenosis or regurgitation.
- The aortopathy of bicuspid aortic valve disease is associated with cystic medial degeneration and an increased risk of aortic dissection bicuspid aortic valve patients.
- After bicuspid aortic valve replacement, the patient is still at risk for aortic root complications including aneurysm formation and dissection. Surveillance of the aortic root late after bicuspid aortic valve replacement is imperative.

The bicuspid aortic valve (BAV) affects approximately 1% of the population and is one of the most common congenital heart disorders. Occurrence of a BAV may be sporadic or may be inherited as an autosomal dominant condition with incomplete penetrance. Significant valvular lesions including aortic stenosis and regurgitation and an increased risk of endocarditis may complicate the BAV from youth to old age. BAV disease is associated with an intrinsic defect in the aortic wall, which includes metalloproteinase activation and smooth muscle cell apoptosis. The aortopathy of BAV disease is associated with an increased risk for ascending aortic dilatation, aneurysm formation, and aortic dissection. The majority of people with a BAV will develop a complication from the valve and/or the aortic root during their lifetime, requiring continued surveillance and eventual surgical intervention. Advances in molecular genetics, imaging, and surgery have greatly improved the understanding and management of the BAV and associated aortopathy.

HISTORY

It has been long recognized that the BAV is an important cause of valvular heart disease. Leonardo da Vinci sketched the bicuspid variant of the aortic valve more than 400 years ago (Figure 11-1).[1] In 1844, Paget recognized the clinical sequelae of the BAV, and in 1858 Peacock observed that these valves develop obstructive lesions and incompetence.[2] Osler's landmark report of 18 cases of BAV in 1886 emphasized the frequent complication of infective endocarditis with this lesion.[3] In the 1950s, it was observed that aortic stenosis occurred in the setting of BAV as the result of an intrinsic property of the valve rather than from rheumatic disease.[4-6] Autopsy studies established the BAV as the most common congenital anomaly of the heart.[1,3] The association of congenital BAV with diseases of the aorta was first recorded by Abbott in 1927.[7] The relationship between abnormal aortic valve structure and aortic root disease was emphasized by Larson and Edwards, who noted in 1984[8] that BAV was associated with a ninefold greater risk of aortic dissection.

Developments in cardiac imaging in the 20th century and, in particular, echocardiography, have clarified the prevalence of BAV in the general population. Progress in molecular biology and genetics has begun to elucidate the basic mechanisms of BAV and the associated aortopathy.

169

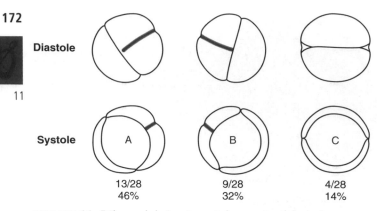

FIGURE 11–5 The morphologic pattern noted on parasternal short-axis echocardiography of 28 patients with bicuspid aortic valves. *(From Brandenburg RO, Tajik AJ, Edwards WD, et al: Accuracy of 2 dimensional echocardiographic diagnosis of congenitally bicuspid aortic valve: Echocardiographic-anatomic correlation in 115 patients. Am J Cardiol 1983;51:1469-1473, reproduced with permission.)*

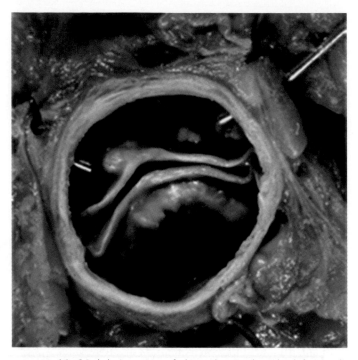

FIGURE 11–6 Pathologic specimen of a bicuspid aortic valve with calcification of the leaflets. Probes are present in the coronary arteries. *(Photograph courtesy of Dr. Jeffrey Saffitz.)*

leaflet fusion was the most common morphologic variant (similar to pattern A in Figure 11-4).[31] Pattern B, or the fusion of the right coronary and noncoronary leaflet was more likely to be associated with aortic stenosis or regurgitation in this pediatric series. Pattern C (fusion of the left coronary and noncoronary cusps) was the least common morphologic variant. In a surgical pathological study of 542 BAVs, 86% were noted to have pattern A, 12% pattern B, and 3% pattern C.[21] Although the patterns demonstrated schematically in Figure 11-2 are the most common ones seen, there is significant variability in the morphology of the BAV.[29]

The valve orientation of a BAV may be predictive of clinical outcomes. Fusion of the right and noncoronary valve leaflets has been associated with more rapid progression of aortic stenosis and regurgitation than fusion of the right and left coronary leaflets.[32] In addition, leaflet orientation in BAV may also be predictive of aortic elastic properties.[33]

Calcium deposition and the development of fibrosis of the BAV increases with age and is largely confined to the raphe and base of the cusp (Figure 11-6).[2,34] The calcification process that occurs in the BAV is comparable in its cellular and molecular mechanism to that of a tricuspid aortic valve (TAV); however, the processes occur in an accelerated manner.[35] BAVs demonstrate folding or wrinkling of the valve tissue and increased doming of the leaflets during the cardiac cycle.[36] Currents of turbulence were also noted to be present in BAVs, even when the leaflets were not stenotic. As a result of multiple mechanisms, the majority of patients with BAVs will require valve surgery during the course of their lifetime.[37] In a recent series, more than half of patients referred for surgery for isolated aortic valve stenosis were noted to have a BAV.[38]

PREVALENCE

The prevalence of BAVs is approximately 1% of the population with at least a 2:1 male/female ratio. Before noninvasive imaging was available, autopsy studies provided the earliest data regarding the prevalence of BAVs in the general population and are summarized in Table 11-1.[2,39-42]

In a retrospective analysis of 85 confirmed necropsy cases of BAV, 13 cases were not associated with any significant stenosis, regurgitation, or underlying structural heart disease, giving a likely prevalence of 0.9% for the asymptomatic adult population of the United States.[2] However, if the number of diseased BAVs found were included in the estimate, the true prevalence was estimated to approach 2% of the population.[2] In the largest reported necropsy series involving 21,417 consecutive cases, 293 cases were noted to have a BAV for a prevalence rate of 1.37%.[42]

The development of echocardiography has significantly increased understanding of the prevalence of the BAV in the general population. In an echocardiography screening of 817 asymptomatic children, a BAV was found in 4 (0.5%) with 3 of these being in boys.[39] In an echocardiography study of 1075 neonates, the prevalence of the BAV was 4.6 per 1000 live births (7.1 per 1000 males and 1.9 per 1000 females).[43] Of 20,946 military recruits in Italy, the prevalence of the BAV was 0.8%. This is probably an underestimation, as only those

TABLE 11–1	Prevalence of Bicuspid Aortic Valve in Reported Necropsy Studies		
Author	**Year**	**Study Population (n)**	**Bicuspid Aortic Valve Prevalence (%)**
Osler	1886	800	1.2
Lewis and Grant	1923	215	1.39
Wauchope	1928	9,966	0.5
Grant et al	1928	1,350	0.89
Gross	1937	5,000	0.56
Roberts	1970	1,440	0.9
Larson and Edwards	1984	21,417	1.37
Datta et al	1988	8,800	0.59
Pauperio et al	1999	2,000	0.65

Adapted from Basso C, Boschello M, Perrone C et al: An echocardiographic survey of primary school children for bicuspid aortic valve. Am J Cardiol 2004;93:661-663, with permission.

with an abnormal history, physical examination, or electro-cardiogram underwent echocardiograms.[44]

Certain groups have a much higher prevalence of BAVs than the general population. Greater than 50% of patients with coarctation of the aorta (CoA) are noted to have BAVs.[45] In addition, females with Turner syndrome are noted to have a high prevalence of BAVs.[46-48]

GENETICS

Case reports describing the familial clustering of the BAV and reports of BAVs in monozygotic twins underscored the genetic predisposition for a BAV.[49-53] In a study of 41 families in which one family member had a surgically proven BAV, 15% of the families were noted to have more than 1 BAV in another family member.[54] In families in whom more than one member had aortic valve disease, 24% of relatives had evidence of aortic valve disease probably due to a BAV.[55] In large family studies, the prevalence of BAVs in first-degree relatives of an individual with a BAV has been reported to be approximately 9%.[56,57] By using variance component methodology, the heritability (h^2) of the BAV was calculated to be 89%.[57] The inheritance pattern is consistent with an autosomal dominant pattern with reduced penetrance.[56,57] Diverse genes with dissimilar inheritance patterns in families are considered responsible.[57]

The specific gene loci or products responsible for the development of BAVs, whether structural proteins or those with vital roles in cardiac development, have yet to be discovered. Animal models with a BAV have provided insight into potential pathogenetic mechanisms, including abnormalities in endothelial nitric oxide synthase, NKX2.5, and *NOTCH* signaling.[9] Human studies have demonstrated the genetic influences on left-sided outflow lesions including hypoplastic left heart and BAVs.[9,58] Detailed phenotyping has identified an increased prevalence of BAVs in probands and family members of patients with hypoplastic left hearts, providing support for the idea that a hypoplastic left heart is allelic to the BAV.[58] *NOTCH1* mutations have been found in a small number of families with BAVs and BAVs with ascending aortic aneurysms.[9]

THE BICUSPID AORTIC VALVE AND ASSOCIATED CARDIOVASCULAR LESIONS

In most instances, the BAV is an isolated cardiovascular finding. However, the BAV may coexist with a number of other congenital cardiovascular defects (Table 11-2). The presence of a BAV may account for significant morbidity associated with these syndromes and should prompt a rigorous search for related cardiovascular defects. Conversely, the presence of any of the following lesions should also prompt a further search for the presence of a BAV.

Coarctation of the Aorta

CoA can be either "simple" (isolated defect) or "complex" (associated with other intracardiac or extracardiac defects). A BAV occurs in 25% to 75% of complex CoA (Figure 11-7). The BAV accompanying CoA has been described as "equally bicuspid" with two symmetric sinuses of Valsalva.[59] Morphologic analysis of the BAV has demonstrated increased frequency of fusion of the left and right coronary cusps in the presence of CoA.[60] Identification of a BAV in patients with coarctation is vital as its presence confers a substantially increased risk for aortic dissection.[34,61] In addition, valvular complications from the BAV such as aortic stenosis or regurgitation as well as ascending aortic aneurysm are more prevalent in subjects with both CoA and a BAV.[62]

TABLE 11–2	Bicuspid Aortic Valve and Associated Cardiovascular Conditions	
Condition	**Incidence of BAV (%)**	**Comments**
Coarctation of the aorta	50	BAV confers increased risk of aortic complications
Turner syndrome	30	Most frequent cardiac abnormality; right-left cusp fusion most common
Supravalvular aortic stenosis	30	Usually part of William syndrome
Subvalvular aortic stenosis	23	May result in significant aortic regurgitation
Patent ductus arteriosus	Unknown	Usually diagnosed in childhood/infancy
Sinus of Valsalva aneurysm	15-20	Frequently asymptomatic; most commonly involves right coronary sinus
Ventricular septal defect	30	May result in significant aortic regurgitation
Shone's complex	60-85	Series of left-sided obstructive lesion
Ascending aortic dilatation	Common	BAV is one of the most common associates of a dilated ascending aorta

BAV, bicuspid aortic valve.

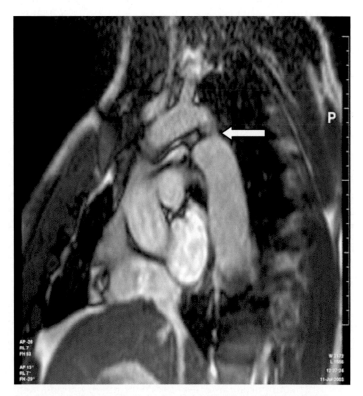

FIGURE 11–7 Representative cardiovascular magnetic resonance imaging of a patient with coarctation of the aorta. Note the typical postductal stenosis (*arrow*). (*From Braverman AC, Guven H, Beardslee MA, et al: The bicuspid aortic valve. Curr Prob Cardiol 2005;30:470-522.*)

Although patients with CoA are often diagnosed and treated at an early age, those individuals with a BAV require long-term follow-up of not only the coarctation repair but also of the BAV and ascending aorta.[62,63] In one large series of patients who were operated on for CoA, 41% of reoperations were primarily for valvular indications.[63] It is therefore imperative that these patients receive meticulous follow-up with routine radiographic and echocardiographic assessment.[64]

Turner Syndrome

11 Turner syndrome is characterized by complete or partial absence of one X chromosome. Turner syndrome is due to the 45 XO karyotype about 50% of the time, whereas the remainder of the time it is due to 45 XO/XX mosaicism or other X chromosomal abnormalities. Cardiovascular defects are commonly identified in patients with Turner syndrome with the earliest description by Morgagni.[65] Cardiovascular defects occur in up to 75% of patients with Turner syndrome.[46] The BAV is noted in up to 30% of those with Turner syndrome and is the most common cardiovascular malformation.[45,48,66] Other vascular defects include partial anomalous pulmonary venous return, CoA and pseudo-CoA, and persistent left superior vena cava.[67]

In patients with Turner syndrome, a preponderance of BAVs are due to fusion of right and left coronary cusps (anteroposterior orientation). The presence of a BAV is associated with larger aortic dimensions at the annulus, sinuses, sinotubular junction, and ascending aorta.[48] Patients with Turner syndrome may have a shortened life expectancy with cardiovascular causes being the most common cause of death.[68] In addition, patients with Turner syndrome have short stature, making ascending aortic dimensions significantly dilated relative to body surface area. Previously established guidelines regarding indications for elective aortic surgery in the setting of ascending aortic dilatation are not applicable to patients with Turner syndrome, and surgery is recommended at smaller aortic dimensions.[69] Intensive screening for the BAV and other cardiovascular abnormalities as well as serial echocardiographic and radiographic follow-up is important in Turner syndrome.

Associated Congenital Heart Malformations

Patent Ductus Arteriosus

Patent ductus arteriosus is usually an isolated lesion but has been associated with the BAV especially in the pediatric population.[70,71] The prevalence of this association is less in the adult population, probably because of the identification and treatment of the patent ductus arteriosus at a young age. Adults with treated patent ductus arteriosus warrant further evaluation to assess for the presence of the BAV.

Supravalvular Aortic Stenosis/William Syndrome

Supravalvular aortic stenosis can be seen in isolation, although approximately 60% of patients with supravalvular aortic stenosis have William-Beuren syndrome characterized by elfin facies, short stature, stellate iris, peripheral pulmonic stenosis, arterial hypertension, hypercalcemia, CoA, and renal artery stenosis.[59] These findings suggest that supravalvular aortic stenosis is not merely an isolated aortic defect but is more likely part of a diffuse arteriopathy. A significant number of individuals (35% to 50%) have abnormal aortic valves and up to 30% have a bicuspid valve.[72] The presence of a BAV is important as rates of reoperation in patients with supravalvular aortic stenosis are much higher in the presence of a BAV than with a TAV (56% versus 19%).[73]

Ventricular Septal Defect

Ventricular septal defect (VSD) is the most common congenital defect occurring in children and may occur in isolation or in association with more complex congenital lesions. BAV is associated with VSD in the adult patients in up to 30% of patients.[74,75] Perimembranous VSDs may result in aortic regurgitation because of partial aortic leaflet prolapse into the defect.

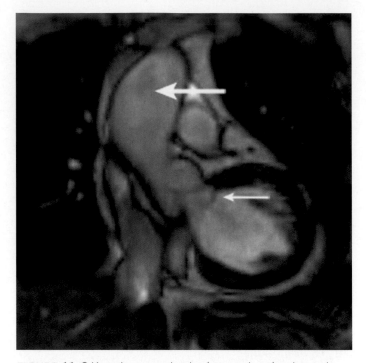

FIGURE 11–8 Magnetic resonance imaging demonstrating subaortic stenosis (*small lower arrow*) and a moderately dilated ascending aorta (*larger upper arrow*). A bicuspid aortic valve is also present (not shown).

In addition, surgical repair of the VSD may cause structural change in the aortic valve, resulting in valvular insufficiency.

Subvalvular Aortic Stenosis

Subvalvular aortic stenosis may be due to either a discrete fibrous membrane (90% of patients) or a long muscular tunnel-like stenosis of the left ventricular outflow tract. A BAV is present in up to 23% of patients with subvalvular aortic stenosis (Figure 11-8). The subvalvular stenosis frequently results in aortic regurgitation owing to the deleterious effects of the high-velocity systolic outflow tract jet on the undersurface of the aortic valve. Once significant aortic regurgitation occurs, relief of the outflow tract obstruction does little to affect the progression of the valvular insufficiency. Interestingly, BAVs in the presence of subvalvular aortic stenosis are not more prone to aortic regurgitation than TAVs.[76]

Sinus of Valsalva Aneurysm

Sinus of Valsalva aneurysm is a rare defect that may be diagnosed incidentally but may also rupture suddenly, causing chest pain, heart failure, sudden death, or compression or destruction of neighboring cardiac structures. A BAV is seen in 15% to 20% of patients with sinus of Valsalva aneurysms (Figure 11-9).

Shone's Complex

Shone's complex is a congenital anomaly consisting of a series of left heart obstructive lesions including supravalvular mitral ring, parachute mitral valve, subaortic stenosis, and CoA (Figure 11-10). A BAV is noted in 60% to 84% of patients.[77,78] Although the degree of mitral valve dysfunction and pulmonary hypertension frequently seem to dictate clinical survival postoperatively, aortic valvular disease is a common indication for reoperation.

Coronary Artery Anomalies

Congenital coronary anomalies have been described in association with BAVs. Left coronary artery dominance is present in 24% to 57% of patients. In addition, BAVs are associated with a shorter left main coronary artery compared with TAVs.[26,27,79-81]

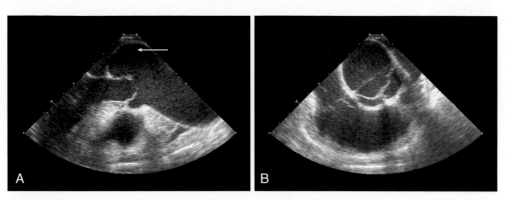

FIGURE 11–9 Transesophageal echocardiogram of a bicuspid aortic valve (BAV) and sinus of Valsalva aneurysm. **A,** Transesophageal echocardiogram long-axis view demonstrating aneurysm of the noncoronary cusp. **B,** Short-axis image demonstrating BAV and dilated aortic sinus.

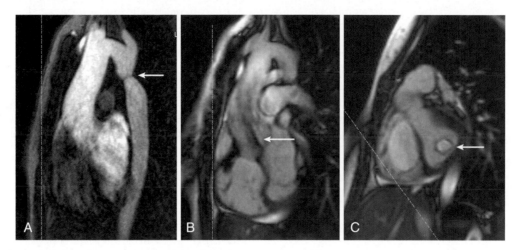

FIGURE 11–10 Cardiovascular magnetic resonance imaging of Shone's complex. **A,** Coarctation of the aorta. **B,** Bicuspid aortic valve with moderate stenosis and mildly dilated ascending aorta. **C,** Typical appearance of a mildly stenotic parachute mitral valve.

Other isolated congenital coronary artery anomalies have been reported in the presence of a BAV.[82-84] Thus, consideration should be given to definition of the coronary anatomy with either catheter-based or computed CT coronary angiography before elective valve surgery to prevent coronary injury and provide for adequate myocardial protection intraoperatively.

CLINICAL PRESENTATION

Physical Examination

A majority of younger patients with an isolated BAV are asymptomatic, with the BAV often diagnosed incidentally when a systolic ejection sound or murmur is noted or by echocardiography. In adults, the auscultatory findings depend on the degree of stenosis or regurgitation present. A functionally normal BAV will have an ejection sound followed by an early peaking systolic flow murmur. The ejection sound is a reflection of the sudden cephalad movement of the dome-shaped bicuspid valve in systole and generally correlates with valve leaflet mobility.[59]

In the setting of progressive aortic stenosis, the ejection murmur becomes harsher and later peaking. This is accompanied by a displaced and sustained left ventricular impulse and decreased arterial pulses. The ejection sound diminishes as the valve cusps become more immobile. In the setting of an incompetent BAV, the examination varies with the severity of the lesion. An ejection sound is typically present with mild to moderate aortic regurgitation and absent when severe regurgitation is present.[59,85-87] With significant aortic regurgitation,

a typical early diastolic decrescendo murmur is best heard at the left lower sternal border. When the murmur of aortic regurgitation is heard loudest at the right midsternal border, concern should arise for the presence of a dilated ascending aorta complicating the BAV.

Give the frequent association of the BAV with other cardiovascular lesions, routine physical examination should include auscultation for the presence of VSD and CoA. Bilateral upper extremity and lower extremity blood pressures as well as palpation for radial-femoral pulse delay should be included in the examination.

Chest Radiography

The plain chest radiograph may provide significant clues as to the presence of a BAV and any significant hemodynamic sequelae related to valvular complications or associated vascular lesions. Often, however, results may be entirely unremarkable. With an isolated stenotic BAV, the lung fields are usually clear. Aortic valve calcification may be detected on the plain film and is best seen on the lateral projection.[88] A complete or partial ring with or without a calcified central raphe characterizes the distinctive pattern of calcification of the BAV. In general, left ventricular size remains normal unless advanced heart failure is present.[87,88] In the setting of a chronically regurgitant BAV, an enlarged cardiac silhouette may be noted. A dilated aortic root may be present, even in the absence of significant valvular lesions. When CoA is associated with the BAV, rib notching and convexity of the proximal descending aorta are often present.[87]

In light of the clinical significance of a BAV, echocardiographic identification and characterization are imperative. There are a number of distinct echocardiographic features of the BAV that assist in making this diagnosis (Table 11-3).[30] Care must be taken to assess the valve in both systole and diastole. In patients with a prominent raphe, the valve may appear trileaflet in diastole; however, the distinct elliptical or "football"-shaped orifice will be visualized in systole, indicating that the raphe is not a functional commissure (Figure 11-11).

The leaflets of a BAV are often thickened and calcified out of proportion to one's age. Prominent systolic doming of the leaflets and eccentric valve closure are often noted on the parasternal long-axis views.[89,90] It is noteworthy, however, that up to 25% of BAVs may not demonstrate eccentric closure, and, conversely, tricuspid aortic valves may infrequently have eccentric closure. The presence of leaflet redundancy when viewed in the parasternal and apical long-axis views should suggest the presence of a BAV.

Valvular calcification is a function of age, increasing significantly after age 40. It is important to note that significant calcification may limit the degree of systolic doming and in addition give the appearance of a stenotic trileaflet valve on short-axis views.

When poor acoustic windows or technical limitations prohibit adequate leaflet visualization, the opening pattern of the valve may aid in the diagnosis. The BAV tends to open from the center and separate at the commissures in a curvilinear fashion similar to a rope going slack from the center,[91] whereas tricuspid aortic valve leaflets maintain a straighter shape in diastole, pivoting from their point of annular insertion.

In the diagnosis of a BAV, the transthoracic echocardiogram has a sensitivity of 78%, a specificity of 96%, and a predictive accuracy of 93%[30]; however, both false-negative and false-positive results do occur. A prominent raphe may often give the appearance of a third coaptation line, suggesting a trileaflet valve. Conversely, the aortic valve may appear bicuspid when one of the cusps is diminutive.[91] Ascending aortic enlargement should trigger a careful evaluation for a BAV (Figure 11-12).[92]

Valvular Complications

Once a BAV is detected, the echocardiogram should include a formal assessment for valvular complications. Aortic stenosis tends to occur at a younger age, particularly when the aortic cusps are asymmetric or there is fusion of the right-left cusps (anteroposterior position).[34] Because of the eccentric nature of the systolic jet in BAV stenosis, interrogation of the jet via the right parasternal window may yield the highest gradients. Patients with BAVs often have larger left ventricular outflow tracts. Thus, use of the continuity equation may yield larger calculated valve areas, potentially underestimating the hemodynamic severity. The use of serial gradients and velocity-time integral ratios may more accurately reflect the hemodynamic burden in these patients.[93] Patients with BAVs may have symptomatic valvular disease with aortic valve areas of greater than $1.0\,cm^2$. Many of these patients have combined valvular lesions with aortic stenosis and regurgitation, and these may also be responsible for symptom onset with a relatively larger valve area.

Aortic regurgitation may be the main clinical manifestation of a BAV in the adolescent or young adult. Aortic regurgitation in the BAV may be a result of leaflet fibrosis with retraction of the commissural margins of the leaflets, cusp prolapse, aneurysmal root enlargement, aortic dissection, or valvular destruction from endocarditis. In addition, the presence of a ventricular septal defect, subaortic

TABLE 11–3	Echocardiographic Features of Bicuspid Aortic Valve

Systolic doming
Eccentric valve closure
Leaflet redundancy
Presence of raphe (often calcified)
Elliptical ("football") shaped systolic orifice
Distinct opening pattern: opens from the center and separates at the commissures in a curvilinear fashion
Dilated ascending aorta

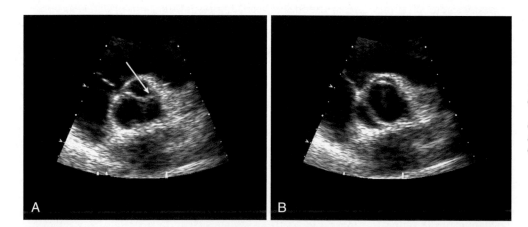

FIGURE 11–11 Transthoracic echocardiogram of bicuspid aortic valve. **A,** Short-axis view of the bicuspid aortic valve in diastole demonstrating asymmetrical sinuses and a raphe, **B,** Bicuspid aortic valve in systole with elliptical opening pattern.

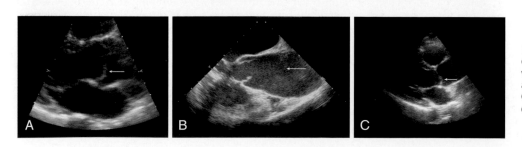

FIGURE 11–12 Transthoracic echocardiographic features of a bicuspid aortic valve. **A,** Prominent systolic doming of the aortic valve leaflets, **B,** Dilated ascending aorta. **C,** Eccentric closure of the aortic valve (*arrow* denotes coaptation point).

membrane, or sinus of Valsalva aneurysm may result in aortic regurgitation. Endocarditis accounts for up to 50% of cases of severe BAV regurgitation and may be the presenting symptom in patients with previously undiagnosed BAVs.

Associated Lesions

When a BAV is present, the echocardiographic examination should include a routine evaluation for the presence of coexisting vascular lesions (see Table 11-2). Care should be taken to assess for the presence of VSD, CoA, and aortic root pathologic conditions (sinus of Valsalva aneurysm, supravalvular aortic stenosis, aortic root aneurysm, aortic dissection, and left ventricular outflow tract abnormalities). The standard examination should include an interrogation of the distal aortic arch via suprasternal notch views to assess for the presence of CoA.

Transesophageal Echocardiography

In up to 25% of patients, the morphology of the aortic valve cannot be accurately determined by transthoracic echocardiography. Transesophageal echocardiography (TEE) is useful in such patients for diagnosis of a BAV. Multiplane TEE is highly accurate for detecting BAVs with a reported sensitivity of 87% and a specificity of 91% (Figure 11-13).[94] The sensitivity of TEE approaches 100% when little valvular calcification is present. In the presence of moderate to severe valvular calcification, however, the sensitivity of TEE is lower.[95]

TEE also provides vital information in patients with BAVs who have coexisting cardiovascular malformations including aortic root abnormalities (ascending aortic aneurysm and dissection, sinus of Valsalva aneurysm, and supravalvular stenosis), outflow tract defects (subvalvular stenosis and membranous VSD), and valvular complications (aortic stenosis, regurgitation, and endocarditis).

Magnetic Resonance Imaging and Computed Tomography

Cardiovascular magnetic resonance imaging (MRI) represents a vital noninvasive complementary diagnostic modality to standard echocardiography in the diagnosis and management of BAV. MRI probably has both high diagnostic sensitivity and specificity compared with standard echocardiography although few data exist in this regard (Figure 11-14). MRI correlates well with both echocardiographic and invasive catheter-based techniques for evaluation of stenotic and regurgitant valvular lesions.[96,97]

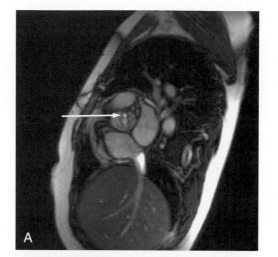

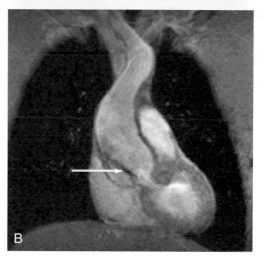

FIGURE 11–14 Cardiovascular magnetic resonance imaging in the bicuspid aortic valve. **A,** Short-axis view of the bicuspid aortic valve (BAV) (*arrow*). **B,** Long-axis image of a stenotic BAV and concomitant dilated ascending aorta. Note the turbulent flow from the stenotic valve striking the anterior aortic wall (*arrow*). *(From Braverman AC, Guven H, Beardslee MA, et al: The bicuspid aortic valve. Curr Prob Cardiol 2005;30:470-522, reproduced by permission.)*

MRI is also an important diagnostic modality in the assessment of associated vascular sequelae and congenital lesions, many of which are suboptimally visualized and defined by standard echocardiography. Routine MRI or computed tomography follow-up is warranted in the presence of aortic root aneurysm and CoA. Multidetector computed tomography has been shown to accurately identify BAVs and assess aortic valve area via planimetry compared with MRI, TEE, and transthoracic echocardiography (Figure 11-15).[98]

DISEASE COURSE AND OUTCOMES

Given its prevalence, the BAV accounts for more adverse outcomes than all other congenital heart defects combined. Much of the natural history, however, has been derived from autopsy data or surgical series. More recent studies, using improved surgical and noninvasive diagnostic techniques, contain relatively few patients with congenital aortic valve disease. Thus, the natural history of the BAV is less well defined, but it can be altered by valvular complications, vascular complications, and complications due to associated cardiovascular lesions. Early reports and autopsy data have described the incidence of fatal valvular and aortic complications.[2,37,99] In the present era, these numbers are probably lower.

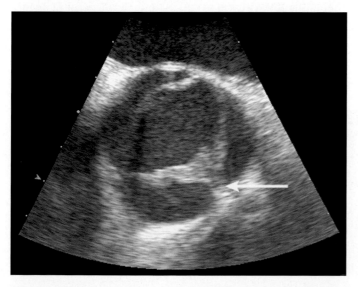

FIGURE 11–13 Transesophageal echocardiogram of a bicuspid aortic valve with a raphe (*arrow*).

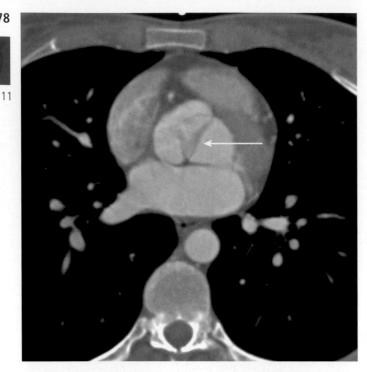

FIGURE 11–15 Cardiac computed tomography short-axis image of the bicuspid aortic valve (*arrow*). *(From Braverman AC, Guven H, Beardslee MA, et al: The bicuspid aortic valve. Curr Prob Cardiol 2005;30:470-522, reproduced by permission.)*

Aortic Stenosis

The reported incidence of aortic stenosis complicating BAV in autopsy series has ranged from 15% to 75%.[2,37,99] Surgical pathologic series indicate that the incidence of aortic stenosis with BAV is between 5% and 50%.[34,38,100,101] At present, approximately 50% of cases of severe aortic stenosis in adults are related to BAVs.[38] Progression of BAV stenosis is age related with fibrosis beginning in the second decade and calcification progressing significantly after the fourth decade. The morphology of the BAV as well as traditional risk factors for atherosclerotic disease and gender seem to play a role in the progression of aortic stenosis in the BAV.

The valve orientation may be predictive of a subsequent valvular pathologic lesion. In children and adolescents, fusion of the right and noncoronary cusps (right-left morphology) correlated highly with both aortic stenosis and regurgitation, whereas fusion of the right and left cusps (anteroposterior morphology) correlated strongly with the presence of CoA.[32] Interestingly, in adult studies, the presence of the anterior-posterior morphology (fusion of right and left cusps) predisposes one to more rapid progression of aortic stenosis.[34,102] This discrepancy may be due in part to selection bias with fewer children with fusion of right-noncusps reaching adulthood without prior surgical correction.

Traditional risk factors for atherosclerosis may play a role in the progression of aortic stenosis. Valvular calcification, once thought to be a function solely of aging, histologically shares the same features as atherosclerotic lesions, namely lipid deposits, neoangiogenesis, and inflammatory cells.[103] Cigarette smoking and hypercholesterolemia are risk factors for progression to severe aortic stenosis.[103-105] These risk factors may represent targets for therapy to slow the progression of valvular stenosis. Preliminary evidence suggests that therapy with 3-hydroxy-3-methylglutaryl-coenzyme A reductase inhibitors may slow the progression of valvular stenosis, and studies are currently underway to help clarify this issue.[106,107]

BAV stenosis progresses more rapidly than TAV stenosis. Patients with BAVs generally undergo surgery for aortic stenosis 5 to 10 years earlier than those with TAV stenosis. Anteroposterior cusp orientation and eccentric cusps may predict more rapid progression of stenosis.[108] Early observational studies showed that one third of initially asymptomatic patients with a BAV experience significant valvular deterioration during 2 to 11 years of follow-up.[1,109]

Aortic Regurgitation

In adults, aortic regurgitation may coexist with stenosis but is often only mild to moderate in degree. Isolated aortic regurgitation may be more common in the child or adolescent. Even more pronounced than with BAV aortic stenosis, an increased frequency of isolated aortic regurgitation is seen in men.[21] With the BAV, aortic regurgitation may be due to cusp prolapse, fibrotic retraction of the leaflets, endocarditis, or annular dilatation in the setting of aortic dilatation or dissection.[110] The BAV is the most common cause of aortic regurgitation requiring valve replacement. Aortic valve replacement due to BAV regurgitation occurs much earlier in life (typically at 20 at 50 years of age) compared with valve replacement due to BAV stenosis. In large surgical series of patients undergoing aortic valve replacement for aortic regurgitation, 15% to 20% of BAVs require valve replacements because of aortic regurgitation.[21]

Infective Endocarditis

Infective endocarditis is a potentially catastrophic complication of the BAV (Figure 11-16). Although the exact incidence and prevalence are unknown, selected case series reported a 10% to 30% incidence of endocarditis in patients with BAVs.[34] More than one third of pathologic specimens of aortic valves with endocarditis were BAVs.[41] The true incidence

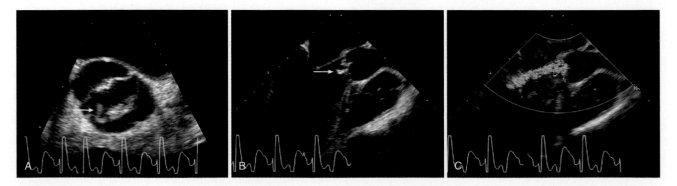

FIGURE 11–16 Transesophageal echo images of infective endocarditis complicating the bicuspid aortic valve (BAV). **A,** Short-axis view of BAV with vegetations (*arrow*). **B,** Long-axis view of BAV with vegetations (*arrow*). **C,** Color flow long-axis images showing severe, eccentric aortic regurgitation due to endocarditis and BAV.

is likely to be less, and more recent estimates place the population risk for endocarditis closer to 3%.[37] Endocarditis accounts for up to 60% of the cases of severe aortic regurgitation in patients with BAVs, most commonly because of cusp perforation.[34] Acute endocarditis may be the initial diagnosis of BAV in previously asymptomatic patients. BAV endocarditis has a very high complication rate, requiring surgical correction more often than TAV endocarditis.[111]

The overall risk of infective endocarditis in BAVs is difficult to quantify. The lifetime risk for development of endocarditis in patients with congenital aortic stenosis has been estimated to be 271 in 100,000 patient years. For reference, the lifetime risk for the general population with no known cardiac defect is 5 per 100,000 patient years. The population with the highest risk population (patients after replacement of infected prosthetic valves) has an estimated risk of 2160 per 100,000 patient years.[112,113] The recently published American Heart Association/American College of Cardiology guidelines for the prevention of endocarditis no longer endorse preprocedural antibiotic prophylaxis in the setting of an isolated BAV, instead recommending a focus on improved dental care and oral health in those predisposed to the development of infective endocarditis.[114]

PREGNANCY AND THE BICUSPID AORTIC VALVE

In general, severe left heart obstruction (symptomatic or not) is poorly tolerated in pregnancy. Likewise, severely regurgitant left-sided valve lesions with class III or IV symptoms are associated with significant peripartal risk.[115]

In the presence of severe congenital aortic stenosis, clinical deterioration and cardiovascular complications occur in 10% to 30% of pregnancies accompanied by a high rate of therapeutic abortions with a relatively low complication rate among women with only mild to moderate aortic stenosis.[116,117] Despite the low to moderate complication rate during pregnancy, up to 40% of mothers with severe aortic stenosis required surgical intervention during short-term follow-up.[117] Sudden clinical deterioration during pregnancy, including worsening heart failure, angina, and arrhythmias, require prompt intervention and are associated with an increase in both maternal and fetal risk. Thus, in women at high risk (severe valvular stenosis or class III/IV symptoms), pregnancy should be proscribed until surgical correction is achieved.[118] Interventions during pregnancy in the form of percutaneous balloon valvuloplasty and valve replacement have been reported. Cardiac surgery requiring cardiopulmonary bypass during pregnancy carries a significant risk of fetal distress, fetal wastage, and subsequent growth retardation.[119-121]

Women with mild to moderate aortic stenosis or class I/II symptoms with aortic regurgitation generally tolerate pregnancy well. Parents should be counseled regarding the risk of congenital cardiac defects in their offspring (6% to 7%).[122]

Pregnancy may predispose women to an increased risk for aortic pathologic conditions due to hormone-induced histologic changes in the aortic wall coupled with the hemodynamic stress of pregnancy. The presence of a BAV and its concomitant risk for aortic pathologic conditions may place some women at risk for aortic complications during pregnancy. In one series of 50 women with aortic dissection during pregnancy, 5 women had BAVs.[123] For those woman at increased risk (aortic dimension >4 cm or an increase in aortic root size during pregnancy), close monitoring is required, especially during and up to 3 months after pregnancy. Use of β-blockers may be beneficial but can result in low birth weight and therefore close monitoring of fetal development is required. Cesarean section may be warranted in those women with significantly dilated aortas. Unfortunately, outcome data are lacking in this area. The presence of CoA may further increase peripartal risk for dissection. In recent series, maternal outcomes were satisfactory with only one dissection reported in a patient with Turner syndrome.[124,125] Nevertheless, prepregnancy counseling in addition to thorough evaluation of the CoA (repaired or not) is warranted.

ABNORMALITIES OF THE AORTIC WALL ASSOCIATED WITH THE BICUSPID AORTIC VALVE

The BAV is associated with various disorders of the thoracic aorta, including CoA and aortic dissection.[126,127] Aortic root dilatation has been recognized to be a frequent complication of the BAV, even in the absence of aortic stenosis or regurgitation. The aortic wall abnormality complicating the BAV may occur independently of any hemodynamically significant valvular disease. However, the relative role of intrinsic aortic wall defects and hemodynamic stress on aortic dilatation in BAVs has been debated. In a computer simulation model, the BAV is intrinsically stenotic with turbulent flow present even in the absence of a transvalvular gradient.[128]

The term "poststenotic dilatation" has often been used for an enlarged aortic root associated with aortic valve disease (especially AS). However, recent experience suggests an alternative explanation.[92] An enlarged aortic root is seen infrequently in patient with trileaflet aortic valve disease. In contrast, the BAV is much more commonly associated with a dilated proximal aorta and must be considered one of the most common etiologies of aortic root enlargement.[92] In a survey of aortic root size in severe aortic stenosis, patients with severe BAV stenosis had significantly larger aortic root diameters than those with TAV stenosis.[129] Thus, the notion of post stenotic dilatation should be dispelled.

Coarctation of the Aorta

The BAV is associated with CoA in approximately 50% of patients (see Figure 11-7).[34,45,61] CoA is associated with an increased risk of aortic dissection. Whereas arterial hypertension often complicates CoA, it is not the only explanation for the increased risk of aortic dissection in these patients. Inherent abnormalities of the aortic wall are also important in the pathogenesis of dissection. In the presurgical era, aortic dissection was the cause of death in 19% to 27% of patients with CoA.[34,61] Importantly, when a BAV was present with CoA, aortic dissection occurred in approximately 50% of patients.[34,61,62] In a series of 235 patients with CoA, 57% had a congenital BAV.[61,62] The presence of a BAV was the strongest clinical predictor of subsequent aortic wall complications (ascending aortic aneurysm, descending aortic aneurysm, aortic dissection, and aortic rupture) in patients with CoA (Figure 11-17).[62] Furthermore, the aortic wall abnormalities were not confined to the ascending aorta, suggesting that the aortopathy involves the thoracic aorta more diffusely.[62]

Aortic Dissection

The BAV is a risk factor for aortic dissection independent of hypertension or CoA (Figure 11-18). In autopsy series of aortic dissection, the BAV is present in 7% to 9% of patients.[8,34] In clinical series of aortic dissection, the BAV is also present in 7% of patients.[34] A BAV is described in up to 15% of patients with an ascending aortic dissection.[10] In the patient with an aortic dissection (particularly an ascending aortic dissection), one must diligently search for the presence of a BAV. This is particularly true for the young patient and the normotensive patient with dissection. In individuals younger than 40 years who sustained an aortic dissection,

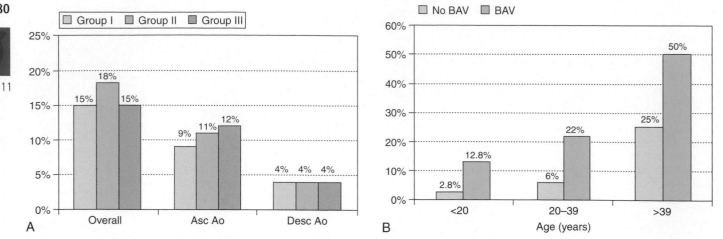

FIGURE 11–17 A, Prevalence of aortic complications and ascending (Asc Ao) or descending (Desc Ao) aortic aneurysm in adults with coarctation of the aorta, according to management: surgery (group I), transcatheter intervention (group II), or not previously repaired (group III). B, Prevalence of aortic wall complications in patients with coarctation of the aorta when these patients were classified according to age and coexistence of bicuspid aortic valve. (From Oliver JM, Gallego P, Gonzalez A, et al: Risk factors for aortic complications in adults with coarctation of the aorta. J Am Coll Cardiol 2004;44:1641-1647, reproduced by permission.)

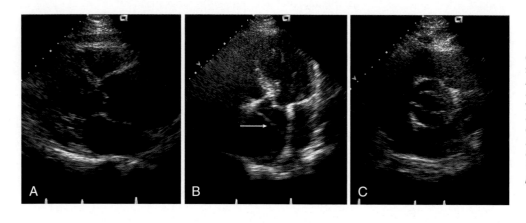

FIGURE 11–18 Transthoracic echocardiogram of a bicuspid aortic valve with severe aortic root dilatation and aortic dissection. A, Parasternal long-axis view with severe aortic root dilatation. B, Apical five-chamber view demonstrating the intimal flap (arrow) and a dilated aortic root. C, Short-axis view demonstrating the bicuspid aortic valve. (From Braverman AC, Guven H, Beardslee MA, et al: The bicuspid aortic valve. Curr Prob Cardiol 2005;30:470-522, reproduced by permission.)

28% had a BAV.[130] In the International Registry of Aortic Dissection, 68 of 951 patients with acute dissection were younger than 40 years.[131] Notably, a BAV was present in 9% of these young patients with dissection, but only in 1% of the patients older than 40 years.[131] Aortic dissection occurs at a younger age in patients with a BAV. When dissection complicates the BAV, the average age of the patient is 54 years compared with 62 years for the patient with a trileaflet aortic valve and aortic dissection.[132] Aortic dissection occurs 5 to 10 times more commonly in patients with a BAV than in those with a TAV.[8] When aortic dissection occurs in the presence of a BAV, the valve is usually functionally normal.[34] Aortic dissection may also occur with BAV stenosis or regurgitation and may occur late after aortic valve replacement.[133] In addition to aortic dissection, the BAV has also been associated with spontaneous cervicocephalic arterial dissection, extending the association of arterial medial abnormalities to the cervical arteries.[134]

Aortic Medial Disease and Aortic Root Dilatation

The aortic wall abnormalities that complicate the BAV have led many to theorize the presence of a common underlying developmental defect involving the aortic valve and aortic wall in patients with a BAV, which includes cystic medial necrosis.[48,61,127] To investigate whether aortic wall structural abnormalities underlie the aortopathy of BAV disease, the presence of a pathologic or clinical correlate of aortic wall fragility must be demonstrated[135] Noninvasive imaging studies

and histopathologic examinations using tissue samples have been performed to address these issues.

Echocardiograms in patients with functionally normal BAVs have demonstrated significantly greater aortic root diameters compared with those in control subjects (Figure 11-19).[135,136] The degree of aortic enlargement is greater in those with aortic regurgitation than in those with stenotic or functionally normal BAVs.[136-139] Distinct types of aortic enlargement may be present in the patient with a BAV. Differing from the aortic enlargement pattern in Marfan syndrome (which typically involves the sinuses of Valsalva), the enlargement with a BAV may arise in the sinuses, the proximal ascending aorta, or the mid-ascending aorta.[138,139] In some patients, the aortic arch is also enlarged. In patients with a BAV, aortic root dilatation is more prevalent in older age groups, and the aortic dimension is usually largest in the ascending aorta above the sinuses.[139] Leaflet orientation in the BAV may play a role in the various aortic root shapes/phenotypes in the patient with a BAV.[140] Other echocardiographic surveys have not demonstrated a relationship between cusp orientation and aortic dilatation.[139]

Even young children with BAVs have aortic root dilatation compared with control children.[139-142] The dilatation is most pronounced in the tubular portion of the ascending aorta and is larger than normal at all measured levels and independent of any functional abnormality of the BAV.[141]

In one large echocardiographic survey, when a dilated aortic root was discovered on echocardiogram, 20% of these patients were found to have a BAV.[143] Variables related to the presence of a BAV included age older than 65 years, aortic stenosis, and normotension.[143]

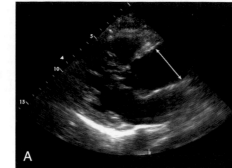
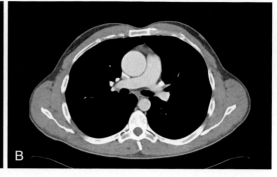

FIGURE 11–19 Aortic root aneurysm complicating a functionally normal bicuspid aortic valve. **A,** Transthoracic echocardiogram of a 4.9-cm ascending aorta. **B,** Corresponding computed tomographic image of the aortic root aneurysm.

Thus, careful assessment of the entire thoracic aorta is important in evaluating each patient with a BAV. In many patients, this involves imaging with computed tomography or MRI to better visualize the ascending aorta. These data support the view that a BAV and aortic root dilatation may reflect a common developmental defect.[48] In addition, these studies dispel the notion of poststenotic dilatation as the etiology of aortic root enlargement in the setting of a BAV.

Noninvasive evaluation of aortic wall elastic properties using MRI has demonstrated reduced aortic elasticity and aortic root distensibility in patients with nonstenotic BAVs.[144] The elastic tissue properties of the BAV aorta may be related to cusp orientation. Compared with those with right-left leaflet orientation, patients with anterior-posterior leaflets had larger aortic diameters and a higher aortic stiffness index and lower distensibility.[33]

There are few data regarding progression of aortic dilatation in the setting of a BAV. In a study of children with BAV, more than one third developed significant aortic enlargement during follow-up. Elevated aortic valve gradients or right-noncoronary commissural fusion was associated with accelerated growth.[145] In one study of children with BAVs, the mean rate of ascending aortic growth was 1.2 mm/year.[146] In a retrospective study of adult patients with BAVs evaluated by echocardiogram, the mean rate of aortic diameter progression was 0.5 mm/year at the sinuses of Valsalva and 0.9 mm/year at the ascending aorta.[147] The prevalence of aortic root dilatation increased during the study. Others have reported the growth of the ascending aorta in adults with BAVs to be from 0.2 mm/year[148] to 0.86 mm/year.[149] BAV aortic root aneurysms grow faster than aneurysms associated with a trileaflet aortic valve. The rate of growth is greater for those with associated aortic stenosis.[150] Of 304 BAV operations at a single institution, 90 (30%) patients had ascending aortic aneurysms of at least 5 cm.[23]

Cystic Medial Necrosis

The histologic abnormality underlying aortic root complications in BAV is cystic medial necrosis, which has been demonstrated in the aortic wall of patients with BAV, even without significant aneurysm formation (Figure 11-20).[151,152]

The pulmonary autograft has been noted to dilate in some patients with BAV who have a dilated aortic root before performance of the Ross procedure.[151] Because the pulmonary trunk shares a common embryologic origin with the aorta (the conotruncus), it was theorized to be affected in a similar manner. Cystic medial necrosis in both the aorta and pulmonary trunk has been demonstrated to be much more severe in patients with BAVs compared with patients with trileaflet aortic valves. Although others have not reported late autograft dilatation after the Ross procedure for BAV disease,[153] concerns have been raised about the appropriateness of the Ross procedure for patients with BAV disease and ascending aortic enlargement.[151]

Cystic medial necrosis has been demonstrated in multiple types of congenital heart disease. In the majority of patients with BAVs requiring surgery, moderate or severe grades of aortic cystic medial necrosis is present.[154] In patients with CoA and BAV, histologic examination demonstrates identical medial abnormalities both proximal and distal to the CoA, implying that the abnormalities were not hemodynamically mediated.[154]

Apoptosis is a mechanism that may underlie aortic medial layer smooth muscle cell loss, leading to aneurysm formation in patients with BAVs.[152-155] Massive focal apoptosis has been observed in the medial layers of patients with BAV, whether or not aortic dilatation was present.[155] Compared with TAV aneurysms, BAV aneurysms exhibit a distinct pattern of medial destruction, elastic fragmentation, and increased apoptosis.[156]

Differences in matrix metalloproteinases (MMPs) and endogenous inhibitors are observed in ascending aortic aneurysms of patients with BAVs compared with aneurysms associated with TAVS.[157-161] Elevated MMP-2 expression has been demonstrated in the BAV aorta, whereas MMP-9 activity was normal.[157,160] It has been theorized that the abnormal elastic properties, dilatation, and fragmentation of elastic components within the aortic wall of patients with BAVs may be associated with the increased expression of matrix-degrading proteins.[159]

FIGURE 11–20 Elastic tissue stain of aortic media from a normal aorta from a patient with a trileaflet aortic valve patient demonstrating normal elastic fiber orientation (labeled Normal aorta) and elastic stain from a patient with a bicuspid aortic valve and aortic root aneurysm demonstrating cystic medial degeneration (labeled Aortic aneurysm). *(From Braverman AC, Guven H, Beardslee MA, et al: The bicuspid aortic valve. Curr Prob Cardiol 2005;30:470-522, reproduced by permission.)*

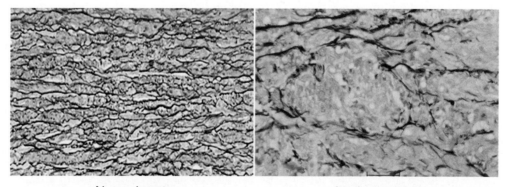

Normal aorta   Aortic aneurysm

Fibrillin-1 content is reduced in BAV aortas (and pulmonary arteries) compared with that seen in TAV aortas.[157] In the mouse model of Marfan syndrome (fibrillin-1-deficient mouse), increased MMP activity is associated with matrix fragmentation and reduced structural integrity of the aorta.[162] It is not known whether abnormal fibrillin content in BAV aortas is a primary or secondary effect.[162] Matrix proteins have been examined in patients with aortic root aneurysms who have a BAV and compared with those in patients with aneurysms associated with Marfan syndrome.[157] Reduced extracellular deposition and altered quantities of matrix proteins are associated with a similar degree of increased apoptosis in vascular smooth muscle cells from those with BAV aneurysms and those with Marfan syndrome.[158] These studies suggest that a differential extracellular matrix proteolytic cascade exists within the aorta of patients with BAVs and ascending aortic aneurysms as opposed to TAVs and aneurysms. However, these data do not provide insight into the potential cause and effect relationship between MMP expression and aortic root dilatation.[157,160]

Aortic Complications after Valve Replacement

Late aortic complications have been reported after BAV replacement.[133,163,164] Compared with patients with TAVs, patients with BAVs had an increased number of aortic complications years after aortic valve replacement including aortic dissection, late aneurysm formation, and sudden death.[134] In addition, late echocardiography surveillance demonstrated significantly larger ascending aortas in the patients with BAVs.[133]

The ascending aorta continues to dilate after valve replacement in patients with BAVs, but does not dilate after valve replacement in patient with TAVs.[133,163] The patients with BAVs with and without valve replacement showed a similar progression of dilatation.[163] Borger et al[164] reported 10-year follow-up in 201 patients who underwent aortic valve replacement for a BAV without ascending aorta replacement. Ascending aortic size was less than 4.0 cm in 57%, 4.0 to 4.4 cm in 32%, and 4.5 to 4.9 cm in 11% of patients. All aortas greater than 5.0 cm were replaced at the primary operation, which included 17% of all patients with BAVs. During follow-up, 18 patients (9%) required late ascending aortic replacement with a mean ± SD aortic diameter of 58 ± 9 mm. Freedom from ascending aortic complications, including late aneurysm repair, dissection, or sudden death was 78% ± 6%, 81% ± 6%, and 43% ± 15% in the three increasing size groups, respectively (Figure 11-21).[164]

These studies highlight the importance of continuous surveillance of the ascending aorta in patients with BAVs after valve surgery. Patients with BAVs remain at risk for aortic root dilatation, aneurysm formation, and aortic dissection after aortic valve replacement.[127] This fact has implications for the management of the aortic root, regarding timing of prophylactic root replacement, in patients with BAVs undergoing valve surgery.[134,165,166] Current American Heart Association/American College of Cardiology Guidelines for the management of the aortic root in BAV disease are listed in Table 11-4.[118]

FAMILIAL BICUSPID AORTIC VALVE AND ASCENDING AORTIC ANEURYSMS

The BAV may be hereditary or familial, with studies demonstrating the occurrence of a BAV in approximately 9% of first-degree relatives of affected individuals.[56,57] Aneurysms associated with the BAV may also be familial.[165,166] A comprehensive evaluation of multiple pedigrees segregating BAVs with ascending aortic aneurysms revealed a high incidence of individuals with ascending aneurysms alone, suggesting that BAVs and ascending aortic aneurysm are both primary manifestations of a single gene defect with variable expression. Linkage to chromosome 15q has been identified in families segregating BAVs and ascending aortic aneurysms.[165] Potential loci at 18q, 5q, and 13q have also been suggested for BAVs and aortic aneurysms.[167]

In a prospective evaluation of 13 families with BAVs and ascending aortic aneurysms, 6 of 13 had at least two family members with both a BAV and a thoracic aortic aneurysm, often in successive generations.[166] Either partial penetrance (BAV alone) or complete nonpenetrance was observed in obligate carriers. Notably, all 13 families had at least 1 family member with a thoracic aortic aneurysm in the absence of a BAV. Of the 96 comprehensively evaluated relatives of affected probands, 45 (47%) had an aortic aneurysm with or without a BAV. Aortic dilatation was maximal above the sinotubular junction in 11 of 13 families. Aortic dissection was observed in 7 of 13 families and occurred in individuals with or without BAVs. These data are consistent with BAV as an autosomal dominant disorder with variable expressivity and incomplete penetrance.[166] Altered transforming growth factor-β signaling has been hypothesized in BAV aneurysm disease.[166] These authors suggest that all family members, including those without a BAV, undergo follow-up using imaging protocols that specifically assess aortic segments beyond the sinotubular junction.[166]

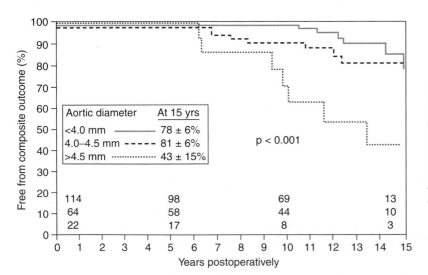

FIGURE 11–21 Kaplan-Meier curves for freedom from ascending aortic complications according to the three groups of patients with bicuspid aortic valves undergoing valve replacement surgery. Patients with an ascending aortic diameter of 4.5 cm or greater had a significantly increased risk of future aortic complications (aneurysm, dissection, or sudden death) (*P* <.001). *(From Borger MA, Preston M, Ivanov J, et al: Should the ascending aorta be replaced more frequently in patients with bicuspid aortic valve disease? J Thorac Cardiovasc Surg 2004;128:677-683, reproduced by permission.)*

TABLE 11-4	ACC/AHA Guidelines for Managing Bicuspid Aortic Valve with Dilated Ascending Aorta

Class I

1. Patients with known bicuspid aortic valves should undergo an initial transthoracic echocardiogram to assess the diameters of the aortic root and ascending aorta. (Level of Evidence: B)

2. Cardiac magnetic resonance imaging or cardiac computed tomography is indicated in patients with bicuspid aortic valves when morphology of the aortic root or ascending aorta cannot be assessed accurately by echocardiography. (Level of Evidence: C)

3. Patients with bicuspid aortic valves and dilatation of the aortic root or ascending aorta (diameter >4.0 cm*) should undergo serial evaluation of aortic root/ascending aorta size and morphology by echocardiography, cardiac magnetic resonance, or computed tomography on a yearly basis. (Level of Evidence: C)

4. Surgery to repair the aortic root or replace the ascending aorta is indicated in patients with bicuspid aortic valves if the diameter of the aortic root or ascending aorta is greater than 5.0 cm* or if the rate of increase in diameter is 0.5 cm/year or more. (Level of Evidence: C)

5. In patients with bicuspid valves undergoing aortic valve replacement because of severe aortic stenosis or aortic regurgitation (see Sections III-A-6 and III-B-2-g), repair of the aortic root or replacement of the ascending aorta is indicated if the diameter of the aortic root or ascending aorta is greater than 4.5 cm.* (Level of Evidence: C)

Class IIa

1. It is reasonable to give β-adrenergic blocking agents to patients with bicuspid valves and dilated aortic roots (diameter greater than 4.0 cm*) who are not candidates for surgical correction and who do not have moderate to severe AR. (Level of Evidence: C)

2. Cardiac magnetic resonance imaging or cardiac computed tomography is reasonable in patients with bicuspid aortic valves when aortic root dilatation is detected by echocardiography to further quantify severity of dilatation and involvement of the ascending aorta. (Level of Evidence: B)

*Consider lower threshold values for patients of small stature of either gender.
From Bonow RO, Carabello B, Chatterjee K, et al: ACC/AHA 2006 Guidelines for the Management of Patients with Valvular Heart Disease: a report of the American College of Cardiology/American Heart Association Task Force on Practice Guidelines (Writing Committee to Revise the 1998 Guidelines for the Management of Patients with Valvular Heart Disease). J Am Coll Cardiol 2006:48:e1-e148.

NOTCH1 mutations have been found in a small number of families with BAVs and BAVs with ascending aortic aneurysms.[9,168,169] In the families with *NOTCH1* mutations, the BAV is stenotic and calcified. However, most families with BAVs and aortic aneurysms do not have associated calcific aortic stenosis, raising the possibility of alternative genetic explanations for the majority with BAVs and associated aortic aneurysms.[170]

SURGICAL TREATMENT OF THE BICUSPID AORTIC VALVE AND ASCENDING AORTA

The indications for replacement of a BAV with stenosis or regurgitation are well established.[118] However, patients undergoing aortic valve replacement for BAVs are often young, making the decision to implant a mechanical versus a bioprosthetic valve more complex.[127,171] Valve repair in the BAV is occasionally performed in carefully selected patients, but durability of the repair remains a concern.[172-175] The decision of when to perform prophylactic aortic root replacement is also complex.[133,163,164,169,171] It is recommended that patients with BAV with ascending aortic aneurysms exceeding 4.5 cm undergo simultaneous aortic replacement at the time of aortic valve replacement.[118,127,164] In patients with BAVs and normal valve function, aortic aneurysm resection is recommended when the diameter of the aorta exceeds 5 cm or is associated

with rapid growth.[118] Gender and body surface area may also be important factors in the timing of ascending aortic surgery.[176]

For patients who require simultaneous valve and ascending aortic replacement for BAV, surgical options include (1) valve replacement and separate supracoronary graft replacement of the ascending aorta leaving the sinuses intact, (2) aortic valve and root replacement with a composite valve-graft conduit and coronary reimplantation, (3) valve-sparing root replacement and (4) reduction aortoplasty.[110,127] Reduction aortoplasty is controversial in the management of BAV and aortic dilatation because of concerns about risk for recurrent dilation and is not recommended.[110] Patients with supracoronary grafts are at risk for late sinus enlargement although long-term results are often satisfactory.[177] The Ross procedure (pulmonary autograft) is an alternative to prosthetic valve replacement in BAV disease.[153] However, reports of late autograft dilatation raise important concerns about the appropriateness of this procedure for adult patients, especially those with significant annular or aortic dilatation.[110,127,151,178-180]

RECOMMENDATIONS FOR MANAGEMENT OF THE PATIENT WITH A BICUSPID AORTIC VALVE

Complex relationships between the BAV and intrinsic valvular lesions exist as well as associated aortopathy, which may lead to significant morbidity and mortality (Figure 11-22). There are several important steps in the long-term management of the patient with a BAV. First, the patient must be correctly identified as having this lesion by echocardiogram. Once the lesion is recognized, the patient must be educated about the potential for valve lesion progression, the risk of infective endocarditis, and the possibility of aortic aneurysm formation and risk of aortic dissection (when appropriate). Good dental hygiene is critical for the patient with a BAV.

Because the BAV may be familial, the clinician should strongly consider screening all first-degree relatives of the patient to evaluate for BAV. This step is especially important when an ascending aortic aneurysm or dissection complicates the BAV. The person with a BAV should undergo serial clinical and echocardiography follow-up over his or her lifespan detect complications from the BAV and aortic root and appropriately time surgical intervention. Computed tomography or MRI is indicated in patients with BAVs when the morphologic characteristics of the aortic root or ascending aorta cannot be assessed accurately by echocardiography and to evaluate further the dilated aorta visualized by echocardiography.[118]

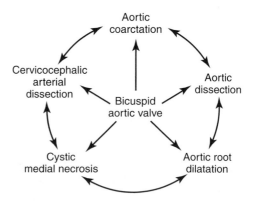

FIGURE 11-22 Schematic diagram of interrelationships of the bicuspid aortic valve and aortic and arterial wall abnormalities. *(From Schievink WI, Mikri B: Familial aorto-cervicocephalic arterial dissections and congenitally bicuspid aortic valve. Stroke 1995:26:1935-1940, reproduced by permission.)*

Because the aortic valve lesion may respond favorably to risk factor modification, the patient with a BAV should follow a sensible diet, avoid cigarette smoking, and receive treatment for hypertension and hyperlipidemia. Studies are ongoing to evaluate the relationship between aortic valve function and long-term cholesterol management. It is not yet known whether cholesterol lowering with medications over many years will have a favorable impact on the bicuspid aortic valve.

The BAV is associated with abnormal aortic elastic properties and a risk of aneurysm formation. Patients should be counseled about this possibility and in many instances given guidelines to avoid strenuous isometric activities such as weightlifting and other competitive athletics.[181] It is recommended that β-blocker therapy be instituted when the aortic root exceeds 4.0 cm in the patient with a BAV who does not have moderate to severe aortic regurgitation.[118] This therapy may have a benefit by lessening the hemodynamic stress on the aortic root. The recommendation is based on the data for the effect of β-blocker therapy on aortic growth in Marfan syndrome, but one must recognize that there are no long-term data on the use of prophylactic β-adrenergic blockade in the treatment of BAV root enlargement.[118,126] When patients with BAV disease are followed, the clinician must image the aortic root over time. When the aorta is 4.0 to 4.5 cm, imaging should be done yearly with echocardiography and, if necessary, computed tomography or MRI to document stability. If the aorta is 4.5 to 5.0 cm, imaging should be done every 6 to 12 months to document stability, depending on the individual patient. Timely surgical treatment of valve lesions and aortic root aneurysms is critical to the longevity of the patient with a BAV. For appropriate surgical candidates, surgical resection of the dilated root is recommended when the aortic dimension reaches or exceeds ≈5 cm.[118] Because the aortic root dimension depends on body surface area and size, use of a nomogram is necessary to evaluate the size of the aorta in different age groups.[182] The risk of aortic root complications may not be the same for all individuals. Those with Turner syndrome and certain familial aortic aneurysm syndromes have an increased risk, and surgery should be performed at smaller aortic root dimensions. Individuals of different body size and gender may have different risks. Although not validated in a large population, a nomogram may be helpful in certain individuals to estimate risk of dissection and timing of prophylactic aortic root resection.[183] Finally, even after surgical replacement of the BAV, the patient is at risk for future aortic root dilation, aneurysm formation, and dissection and must undergo imaging surveillance over time.

REFERENCES

1. Mills P, Leech G, Davies M, et al: The natural history of a non-stenotic bicuspid aortic valve. Br Heart J 1978;40:951-957.
2. Roberts W: The congenitally bicuspid aortic valve: a study of 85 autopsy cases. Am J Cardiol 1970;26:72-83.
3. Wauchope G: The clinical importance of variations in the number of cusps forming the aortic and pulmonary valves. Q J Med 1928;21:383-399.
4. Campbell M, Dauntze R: Congenital aortic valvular stenosis. Br Heart J 1953;15;175-194.
5. Smith D, Matthews M: Aortic valvular stenosis with coarctation of the aorta: with special reference to the development of aortic stenosis upon congenital bicuspid valves. Br Heart J 1955;17:198-206.
6. Bacon A, Matthews M: Congenital bicuspid aortic valves and the aetiology of isolated aortic valvular stenosis. Q J Med 1959;28:545-560.
7. Acierno LJ: The History of Cardiology. Pearl River, NY, Parthenon Publishing Group; 1994:96.
8. Larson EW, Edwards WD: Risk factors for aortic dissection: a necropsy study of 161 cases. Am J Cardiol 1984;53:849-855.
9. Garg V: Molecular genetics of aortic valve disease. Curr Opin Cardiol 2006;21:180-184.
10. Sans-Coma V, Fernandez B, Duran AC, et al: Fusion of valve cushions as a key factor in the formation of congenital bicuspid aortic valves in Syrian hamsters. Anat Rec 1996;244:490-498.
11. Fernández B, Fernandez MC, Durán AC, et al: Anatomy and formation of congenital bicuspid and quadricuspid pulmonary valves in Syrian hamsters. Anat Rec 1998;250:70-79.
12. Mancuso D, Basso C, Cardaioli P, Thiene G: Clefted bicuspid aortic valve. Cardiovasc Path 2002;11:217-220.
13. Duran AC, Frescura V, Sans-Coma V, et al: Bicuspid aortic valves in hearts with other congenital heart disease. J Heart Valve Dis 1995;4:581-590.
14. Kappetein AP, Gittenberger-de Groot AC, Zwinderman AH, et al: The neural crest as a possible pathogenetic factor in coarctation of the aorta and bicuspid aortic valve. J Thorac Cardiovasc Surg 1991;102:830-836.
15. Sumida H, Akimoto N, Nakamura H: Distribution of the neural crest cells in the heart of birds: A three dimensional analysis. Anat Embryol 1989;180:29-35.
16. Takamura K, Okishima T, Ohdo S, Hayakawa K: Association of cephalic neural crest cells with cardiovascular development, particularly that of the semilunar valves. Anat Embryol 1990;182:263-270.
17. Eisenberg LM, Markwald RR: Molecular regulation of atrioventricular valvuloseptal morphogenesis. Circ Res 1995;77:1-6.
18. Fedak PW, Verma S, Tirone DE, et al: Clinical and pathophysiological implications of a bicuspid aortic valve. Circulation 2002;106:900-904.
19. Lee TC, Zhao YD, Courtman DW, Stewart DJ: Abnormal aortic valve development in mice lacking endothelial nitric oxide synthase. Circulation 2000;101:2345-2348.
20. Aicher D, Urbich C, Zeiher A, et al: Endothelial nitric oxide synthase in bicuspid aortic valve disease. Ann Thorac Surg 2007;83:1290-1294.
21. Sabet HY, Edwards WD, Tazelaar HD, Daly RC: Congenitally bicuspid aortic valves: a surgical pathology study of 542 cases and a literature review of 2,715 additional cases. Mayo Clin Proc 1999;74:14-26.
22. Pomerance A: Pathogenesis of aortic stenosis and its relation to age. Br Heart J 1972;34:569-574.
23. Sievers HH, Schmidtke C: A classification system for the bicuspid aortic valve from 304 surgical specimens. J Thorac Cardiovasc Surg 2007;133:1226-1233.
24. Yener N, Oktar GL, Erer D, et al: Bicuspid aortic valve. Ann Thorac Cardiovasc Surg 2002;8;264-267.
25. Clarke DR, Bishop DA: Congenital malformation of the aortic valve and left ventricular outflow tract. In Baue AE (ed): Glenn's Thoracic and Cardiovascular Surgery, 6th ed. Norwalk, CT, Appleton & Lange, 996:1221-1242.
26. Murphy ES, Rosch J, Rahimtoola S: The frequency and significance of coronary arterial dominance in isolated aortic stenosis. Am J Cardiol 1977;39:505-509.
27. Hutchins GM, Nazarian IH, Bulkley BH: Association of left dominant coronary arterial system with congenital bicuspid aortic valve. Am J Cardiol 1978;42:57-59.
28. Olson LJ, Subramanian R, Edwards WD: Surgical pathology of pure aortic insufficiency: a study of 225 cases. Mayo Clin Proc 1984;59:835-841.
29. Angelini A, Ho SY, Anderson RH, et al: The morphology of the normal aortic valve as compared with the aortic valve having two leaflets. J Thorac Cardiovasc Surg 1989;98:362-367.
30. Brandenburg RO, Tajik AJ, Edwards WD, et al: Accuracy of 2 dimensional echocardiographic diagnosis of congenitally bicuspid aortic valve: echocardiographic-anatomic correlation in 115 patients. Am J Cardiol 1983;51:1469-1473.
31. Fernandes SM, Sanders SP, Khairy P, et al: Morphology of bicuspid aortic valve in children and adolescents. J Am Coll Cardiol 2004;44:1648-1651.
32. Fernandes SM, Khairy P, Sanders SP, Colan SD: Bicuspid aortic valve morphology and interventions in the young. J Am Coll Cardiol 2007;49:2211-2214.
33. Schaefer BM, Lewin MB, Stout KK, et al: Usefulness of bicuspid aortic valve phenotype to predict elastic properties of the ascending aorta. Am J Cardiol 2007;99:686-690.
34. Ward C: Clinical significance of the bicuspid aortic valve. Heart 2000;83:81-85.
35. Wallby L, Janerot-Sjoberg B, Steffensen T, Broqvist M: T lymphocyte infiltration in non-rheumatic aortic stenosis: a comparative descriptive study between tricuspid and bicuspid aortic valves. Heart 2002;88:348-351.
36. Robiscsek F, Thubrikar MJ, Cook JW, Fowler B: The congenitally bicuspid aortic valve: How does it function? Why does it fail? Ann Thor Surg 2004;77:177-185.
37. Lewin MB, Otto CM: The Bicuspid aortic valve: adverse outcomes from infancy to old age. Circulation 2005;111:832-834.
38. Roberts WC, Ko JM: Frequency of unicuspid, bicuspid and tricuspid aortic valves by decade in adults having aortic valve replacement for isolated aortic stenosis. Circulation 2005;111:920-925.
39. Basso C, Boschello M, Perrone C, et al: An echocardiographic survey of primary school children for bicuspid aortic valve. Am J Cardiol 2004;93:661-663.
40. Grant W: On the condition of fusion of two segments of the semilunar valves. Montreal Gen Hosp Rep 1880;1:233.
41. Lewis T, Grant RT: Observations relating to subacute infective endocarditis. Heart 1923;10:21-29.
42. Larson EW, Edwards WD: Risk factors for aortic dissection: a necropsy study of 161 cases. Am J Cardiol 1984;53:849-855.
43. Tutar E, Ekicki F, Atalay S, Nacar N: The prevalence of bicuspid aortic valve in newborns by echocardiographic screening. Am Heart J 2005;150:513-515.
44. Nistri S, Basso C, et al: Frequency of bicuspid aortic valve in young male conscripts by echocardiogram. Am J Cardiol 2005;96:718-721.
45. Roos-Hesselink JW, Scholzel BE, Heijdra RJ, et al: Aortic valve and aortic arch pathology after coarctation repair. Heart 2003;89:1074-1077.
46. Ostberg JE, Brookes JAS, McCarthy C, et al: A comparison of echocardiography and magnetic resonance imaging in cardiovascular screening of adults with turner syndrome. J Clin Endocrinol Metab 2004;89:5966-5971.
47. Sybert VP: Cardiovascular malformations and complications in Turner syndrome. Pediatrics 1998;101:E11.
48. Sachdev V, Matura LA, Sidenko S, et al: Aortic valve disease in Turner syndrome. J Am Coll Cardiol 2008;51:1904-1909.
49. McKusick V: Association of congenital bicuspid aortic valve and Erdheim's cystic medial necrosis. Lancet 1972;1:1026-1027.
50. Gale AN, McKusick VA, Hutchins GH, Gott VL: Familial congenital bicuspid aortic valve. Chest 1977;72:668-670.

51. Godden DJ, Sandhu PS, Kerr F: Stenosed bicuspid aortic valves in twins. Eur Heart J 1987;8:316-318.

52. McDonald K, Maurer BJ: Familial aortic valve disease: evidence for a genetic influence? Eur Heart J 1989;19:676-677.

53. Brown C, Sane DC, Kitzman DW: Bicuspid aortic valves in monozygotic twins. Echocardiography 2003;20:183-184.

54. Emmanuel R, Withers R, O'Brien K, et al: Congenitally bicuspid aortic valves, clinicogenetic study of 41 families. Br Heart J 1978;40:1402-1407.

55. Glick BN, Roberts WC: Congenitally bicuspid aortic valve in multiple family members. Am J Cardiol 1994;73:400-404.

56. Huntington K, Hunter A, Chan K: A prospective study to assess the frequency of familial clustering of congenital bicuspid aortic valve. J Am Coll Cardiol 1997;30:1809-1812.

57. Cripe L, Andelfinger G, Martin LJ, et al: Bicuspid aortic valve is heritable. J Am Coll Cardiol 2004;44:138-143.

58. Hinton RB, Martin LJ, Tabangin ME, et al: Hypoplastic left heart syndrome is heritable. J Am Coll Cardiol 2007;50:1590-1595.

59. Perloff JK: The Clinical Recognition of Congenital Heart Disease, 4th ed. Philadelphia, WB Saunders, 1994.

60. Fernandes SM, Sanders SP, Khairy P, et al: Morphology of bicuspid aortic valve in children and adolescents. J Am Coll Cardiol 2004;44:1648-1651.

61. Abbott ME: Coarctation of the aorta of adult type; statistical study and historical retrospect of 200 recorded cases with autopsy; of stenosis or obliteration of descending arch in subjects above age of two years. Am Heart J 3:574, 1928.

62. Oliver JM, Gallego P, Gonzalez A, et al: Risk factors for aortic complications in adults with coarctation of the aorta. J Am Coll Cardiol 2004;44:1641-1647.

63. Cohen M, Fuster V, Steele PM, et al: Coarctation of the aorta: long-term follow-up and prediction of outcome after surgical correction. Circulation 1989;80:840-845.

64. Attenhofer Jost CH, Schaff HV, Connolly HM, et al: Spectrum of reoperations after repair of aortic coarctation: importance of an individualized approach because of coexistent cardiovascular disease. Mayo Clin Proc 2002;77:646-653.

65. Morgagni JB: De sedibus et causis morborum. 1760, Epist 18, article 6.

66. Miller MJ, Geffner ME, Lippe BM, et al: Echocardiography reveals a high incidence of bicuspid aortic valve in Turner syndrome. J Pediatr 1983;102:47-50.

67. Ho VB, Bakalov VK, Cooley M, et al: Major vascular anomalies in Turner syndrome: prevalence and magnetic resonance angiographic features. Circulation 2004;110:1694-1700.

68. Price WH, Clayton JF, Collyer S, et al: Mortality ratios, life expectancy, and causes of death in patients with Turner's syndrome. J Epidemiol Commun Health 1986;40:97-102.

69. Matura LA, Ho VB, Rosing D, Bondy CA: Aortic dilation and dissection in Turner Syndrome. Circulation 2007;116:1-7.

70. Glower DD, Bashore TM, Spritzer CE: Congenital aortic stenosis and patent ductus arteriosus in the adult. Ann Thorac Surg 1992;54:368-370.

71. Deshpande J, Kinare SG: The bicuspid aortic valve—an autopsy study. Indian J Pathol Microbiol 1991;34:112-118.

72. Sugayama SM, Moises RL, Wagenfur J, et al: Williams-Beuren syndrome: cardiovascular abnormalities in 20 patients diagnosed with fluorescent in situ hybridization. Arq Bras Cardiol 2003;81:462-473.

73. Delius RE, Samyn MM, Behrendt DM, et al: Should a bicuspid aortic valve be replaced in the presence of subvalvar or supravalvar aortic stenosis? Ann Thorac Surg 1998;66:1337-1342.

74. Oppenheimer-Dekker A, Gittenberger-de Groot AC, Bartelings MM: Abnormal architecture of the ventricles in hearts with an overriding aortic valve and a perimembranous ventricular septal defect. Int J Cardiol 1985;9:341-355.

75. Neumayer U, Stone S, Somerville J: Small ventricular septal defects in the adult. Eur Heart J 1998;9:1573-1582.

76. Aboulhosn J, Child JS: Left ventricular outflow obstruction: subaortic stenosis, bicuspid aortic valve, supravalvar aortic stenosis, and coarctation of the aorta. Circulation 2006;114;2412-2422.

77. Bolling SF, Iannettoni MD, Dick M: Shone's anomaly: operative results and late outcome. Ann Thorac Surg 1990;49:887-893.

78. Brauner RA, Laks H, Drinkwater DC, et al: Multiple left heart obstructions (Shone's anomaly) with mitral valve involvement: Long-term surgical outcome. Ann Thorac Surg 1997;64:721-729.

79. Scholz DG, Lynch JA, Willerscheidt AB, et al: Coronary arterial dominance associated with congenital bicuspid aortic valve. Arch Pathol Lab Med 1980;104:417-418.

80. Higgins CB, Wexler L: Reversal of dominance of the coronary arterial system in isolated aortic stenosis and bicuspid aortic valve. Circulation 1975;52:292-296.

81. Lerer PK, Edwards WD: Coronary arterial anatomy in bicuspid aortic valve: necropsy study of 100 hearts. Br Heart J 1981;45:142-147.

82. Tejada JG, Albarran A, Hernandez F, et al: Anomalous coronary artery origin associated with bicuspid aortic valve in a patient with rheumatic mitral stenosis: a case report. Angiology 2001;52:649-652.

83. Takahashi M, Ikeda U, Shimada K, et al: Rare association of congenital bicuspid aortic valve, annuloaortic ectasia, and anomalous origin of the left circumflex coronary artery. Cardiology 1994;84:61-64.

84. Doty DB: Anomalous origin of the left circumflex coronary artery associated with bicuspid aortic valve. J Thorac Cardiovasc Surg 2001;122:842-843.

85. Gatzoulis MA, Webb GD, Daubeney PE: Diagnosis and Management of Adult Congenital Heart Disease. Philadelphia, Churchill Livingstone, 2003:258.

86. Perloff JK, Braunwald E: Physical examination of the heart. In Braunwald E (ed): Heart Disease: A Textbook of Cardiovascular Medicine, 5th ed. Philadelphia, WB Saunders, 1997:15-53.

87. Brickner ME, Hillis LD, Lange RA: Congenital heart disease in adults. N Engl J Med 2000;342:334-342.

88. Steiner RM, Reddy GP, Flicker S: Congenital cardiovascular disease in the adult patient: imaging update. J Thorac Imaging 2002;17:1-17.

89. Fowles RE, Martin RP, Abrams JM, et al: Two dimensional echocardiographic features of bicuspid aortic valve. Chest 1979;75:434-440.

90. Nanda NC, Gramiak R: Echocardiographic recognition of the congenital bicuspid aortic valve. Circulation 1974;49:870-875.

91. Weyman AE, Griffin BP: Left ventricular outflow tract: the aortic valve, aorta and subvalvular outflow tract. In Weyman AE (ed): Principles and Practice of Echocardiography, 2nd ed. Philadelphia, Lea and Febiger, 1994:505-508.

92. Boyer J, Gutierez F, Braverman AC: Approach to the dilated aortic root. Curr Opin Cardiol 2004;19:563-569.

93. Ahmed S, Honos GN, Walling AD, et al: Clinical outcome and echocardiographic predictors of aortic valve replacement in patients with bicuspid aortic valve. J Am Soc Echocardiogr 2007;20:998-1003.

94. Espinal M, Fuisz AR, Nanda NC, et al: Sensitivity and specificity of transesophageal echocardiography for determination of aortic valve morphology. Am Heart J 2000;139:1071-1076.

95. Makkar A, Siddiqui TS, Stoddard MF, et al: Impact of valvular calcification on the diagnostic accuracy of transesophageal echocardiography for the detection of congenital aortic valve malformation. Echocardiography 2007;24:745-749.

96. John AS, Dill T, Brandt RR, et al: Magnetic resonance to assess the aortic valve area in aortic stenosis: how does it compare to current diagnostic standards? J Am Coll Cardiol 2003;43:519-526.

97. Caruthers SD, Shiow JL, Brown P, et al: Practical value of cardiac magnetic resonance imaging for clinical quantification of aortic valve stenosis—comparison with echocardiography. Circulation 2003;108:2236-2243.

98. Pouler AC, le Polain de Waroux JB, et al: Aortic valve area assessment: multidetector CT compared with cine MR imaging and transthoracic and transesophageal echocardiography. Radiology 2007;244:745-754.

99. Fenoglio JJ, McAllister HA, DeCastro CM, et al: Congenital bicuspid aortic valve after age 20. Am J Cardiol 1997;39:164-169.

100. Subramanian R, Olson LJ, Edwards WD: Surgical pathology of pure aortic stenosis: a study of 374 cases. Mayo Clin Proc 1984;59:683-690.

101. Turri M, Thiene G, Bortolotti U, et al: Surgical pathology of aortic valve disease: a study based on 602 specimens. Eur J Cardiothorac Surg 1990;4:556-560.

102. Novaro GM, Tiong IY, Pearce GL, et al: Features and predictors of ascending aortic dilatation in association with a congenital bicuspid aortic valve. Am J Cardiol 2003;92:1:99-101.

103. Mohler ER: Are atherosclerotic processes involved in aortic-valve calcification? Lancet 2000;356:524-525.

104. Stewart BF, Siscovik D, Lind BK: Clinical factors associated with calcific aortic valve disease. J Am Coll Cardiol 1997:29:630-634.

105. Chan KL, Ghani M, Woodend K, Burwash IG: Case-controlled study to assess risk factors for aortic stenosis in congenitally bicuspid aortic valve. Am J Cardiol. 2001;88:690-693.

106. Novaro GM, Tiong IY, Pearce GL, et al: Effect of hydroxymethylglutaryl coenzyme A reductase inhibitors on the progression of calcific aortic stenosis. Circulation 2001;104:2205-2209.

107. Wu B, Elmariah S, Kaplan FS, et al: Paradoxical effects of statins on aortic valve myofibroblasts and osteoblasts. Arterioscler Thromb Vasc Biol 2005;25:592-597.

108. Beppu S, Suzuki S, Matsuda H, et al: Rapidity of progression of aortic stenosis in patients with congenital bicuspid aortic valve. Am J Cardiol 1993;71:322-327.

109. Pachulski RT, Chan KL: Progression of aortic valve dysfunction in 51 adult patients with congenital bicuspid aortic valve. Br Heart J 1993;69:237-240.

110. Fedak PWM, David TE, et al: Bicuspid aortic valve disease: recent insights in pathophysiology and treatment. Expert Rev Cardiovasc Ther 2005;3:295-308.

111. Lamas GC, Eykyn SJ: Bicuspid aortic valve—a silent danger: analysis of 50 cases of infective endocarditis. Clin Inf Dis 2000;30:336-341.

112. Gersony WM, Hayes CJ, Driscoll DJ, et al: Bacterial endocarditis in patients with aortic stenosis, pulmonary stenosis, or ventricular septal defect. Circulation 1993;87(Suppl):I-121-I-126.

113. Steckelberg JM, Wilson WR: Risk factors for infective endocarditis. Infect Dis Clin North Am 1993;7:9-19.

114. Wilson W, Taubert KA, Gewitz M, et al: Prevention of infective endocarditis: guidelines from the American Heart Association: a guideline from the American Heart Association Rheumatic Fever, Endocarditis, and Kawasaki Disease Committee, Council on Cardiovascular Disease in the Young, and the Council on Clinical Cardiology, Council on Cardiovascular Surgery and Anesthesia, and the Quality of Care and Outcomes Research Interdisciplinary Working Group. Circulation 2007;116:1736-1754.

115. Siu SC, Sermer M, Colman JM, et al: Prospective multicenter study of pregnancy outcomes in women with heart disease. Circulation 2001;104:515-552.

116. Lao TT, Sermer M, Magee L, et al: Congential aortic stenosis. Am J Obstet Gynecol 1993;169:540-545.

117. Silversides C, Colman JM, Sermer M, et al: Early and intermediate—term outcomes of pregnancy with congenital aortic stenosis. Am J Cardiol 2003;91:1386-1389.

118. Bonow RO, Carabello B, Chatterjee K, et al: ACC/AHA 2006 Guidelines for the Management of Patients with Valvular Heart Disease: a report of the American College of Cardiology/American Heart Association Task Force on Practice Guidelines (Writing Committee to Revise the 1998 Guidelines for the Management of Patients with Valvular Heart Disease). J Am Coll Cardiol 2006:48:e1-e148.

119. Banning AP, Pearson JF, Hall RJ: Role of balloon dilatation of the aortic valve in pregnant patients with severe aortic stenosis. Br Heart J 1993;70:544-545.

120. Sullivan HJ: Valvular heart surgery during pregnancy. Surg Clin North Am 1995;75:59-75.

121. Goldstein I, Jakobi P, Gutterman E, et al: Umbilical artery flow velocity during maternal cardiopulmonary bypass. Ann Thorac Surg 1995;60:1116-1118.

122. Brickner ME. Valvar aortic stenosis. In Gatzoulis MA, Webb GD, Daubeney PE (ed.): Diagnosis and Management of Adult Congenital Heart Disease. Philadelphia, Churchill Livingstone, 2003.

123. Immer FF, Bansi AG Alexsandra S, et al: Aortic dissection in pregnancy: analysis of risk factors and outcome. Ann Thorac Surg 2003;76:309-314.

124. Beauchesne LM, Connolly HM, Ammash NM, Warnes CA: Coarctation of the aorta: outcome of pregnancy. J Am Coll Cardiol 2001;38:1728-1733.

125. Vriend JW, Drenthen W, Pieper PG, et al: Outcome of pregnancy in patients after repair of aortic coarctation. Eur Heart J 2005;26:2173-2178.

126. Braverman AC: Bicuspid aortic valve and associated aortic wall abnormalities. Curr Opin Cardiol 1996;11:501-503.

127. Braverman AC, Guven H, Beardslee MA, et al: The bicuspid aortic valve. Curr Prob Cardiol 2005;30:470-522.

128. Robicsek F, Thubrikar MJ, Cook JW, Fowler B: The congenitally bicuspid aortic valve: how does it function? Why does it fail? Ann Thorac Surg 2004;77:177-185.

129. Morgan-Hughes GJ, Roobottom CA, Owens PE, Marshall AJ: Dilatation of the aorta in pure, severe bicuspid aortic valve stenosis. Am Heart J 2004;147:736-740.

130. Gore I: Dissecting aneurysm of the aorta in persons under forty years of age. Arch Pathol 1953;55:1-13.

131. Januzzi JL, Isselbacher EM, Fattori R, et al: Characterizing the young patient with aortic dissection: results from the international registry of aortic dissection (IRAD). J Am Coll Cardiol 2004;43:665-669.

132. Roberts CS, Roberts WC: Dissection of the aorta associated with congenital malformation of the aortic valve. J Am Coll Cardiol 1991;17:712-716.

133. Russo CF, Mazzetti S, Garatti A, et al: Aortic complications after bicuspid aortic valve replacement: long-term results. Ann Thorac Surg 2002;74:S1773-6.

134. Schievink WI, Mikri B: Familial aorto-cervicocephalic arterial dissections and congenitally bicuspid aortic valve. Stroke 1995;26:1935-1940.

135. Pachulski RT, Winberg AL, Chan KL: Aortic aneurysm in patients with functionally normal or minimally stenotic bicuspid aortic valve. Am J Cardiol 1991;67:781-782.

136. Hahn RT, Roman MJ, Mogtader AH, Devereux RB: Association of aortic dilation with regurgitant, stenotic and functionally normal bicuspid aortic valves. J Am Coll Cardiol 1992;19:283-288.

137. Cecconi M, Nistri S, Quarti A, Manfrin M, et al: Aortic dilatation in patients with bicuspid aortic valve. J Cardiovasc Med 2006;7:11-20.

138. Nkomo VT, Enrique-Sarano M, Ammash NM, et al: Bicuspid aortic valve associated with aortic dilatation: a community-based study. Arterioscler Thromb Vasc Biol 2003;23:351-356.

139. Cecconi M, Manfrin M, Moraca A, et al: Aortic dimensions in patients with bicuspid aortic valve without significant valve dysfunction. Am J Cardiol 2005;95:292-294.

140. Schaefer BM, Lewin MB, Stout KK, et al: The bicuspid aortic valve: an integrated phenotypic classification of leaflet morphology and aortic root shape. Heart 2008;94:1634-1638.

141. Gurvitz M, Chang RK, Drant S, Allada V: Frequency of aortic root dilation in children with a bicuspid aortic valve. Am J Cardiol 2004;94:1337-1340.

142. Basso C, Boschello M, Perrone C, et al: An echocardiographic survey of primary school children for bicuspid aortic valve. Am J Cardiol 2004;93:661-663.

143. Alegret JM, Duran I, Palazon O, et al: Prevalence of and predictors of bicuspid aortic valves in patients with dilated aortic roots. Am J Cardiol 2003;91:619-622.

144. Grotenhuis HB, Ottenkamp J, Westenberg JJM, et al: Reduced aortic elasticity and dilatation are associated with aortic regurgitation and left ventricular hypertrophy in nonstenotic bicuspid aortic valves. J Am Coll Cardiol 2007;49:1660-1665.

145. Holmes KW, Lehmann CU, Dalal D, et al: Progressive dilation of the ascending aorta in children with isolated bicuspid aortic valve. Am J Cardiol 2007;99:978-983.

146. Beroukhim BS, Kruzick TL, Taylor AL, et al: Progression of aortic dilation in children with a functionally normal bicuspid aortic valve. Am J Cardiol 2006;98:828-830.

147. Ferencik M, Pape LA: Changes in size of the ascending aorta and aortic valve function with time in patients with congenitally bicuspid aortic valves. Am J Cardiol 2003;92:43-46.

148. Novaro GM, Griffin BP: Congenital bicuspid aortic valve and rate of ascending aortic dilatation. Am J Cardiol 2003;92:525-526.

149. La Canna G, Ficarra E, Tsagalau E, et al: Progression rate of ascending aortic dilation in patients with normally functioning bicuspid and tricuspid aortic valves. Am J Cardiol 2006;98:249-253.

150. Davies RR, Kaple RK, Mandapati D, et al: Natural history of ascending aortic aneurysms in the setting of an unreplaced bicuspid aortic valve. Ann Thorac Surg 2007;83:1338-1344.

151. de Sa M, Moshkovitz Y, Butany J, David TE: Histologic abnormalities of the ascending aorta and pulmonary trunk in patients with bicuspid aortic valve disease: clinical relevance to the Ross procedure. J Thorac Cardiovasc Surg 1999;118:588-594.

152. Fedak PWM, Verma S, David TE, et al: Clinical and pathophysiological implications of a bicuspid aortic valve. Circulation 2002;106:900-904.

153. Luciani GB, Mazzucco A: Aortic root disease after the Ross procedure. Curr Opin Cardiol 2006;21:555-560.

154. Niwa K, Perloff JK, Bhuta SM, et al: Structural abnormalities of great arterial walls in congenital heart disease. Circulation 2001;103:393-400.

155. Bonderman D, Gharehbaghi-Schell E, Wollenek G, et al: Mechanisms underlying aortic dilatation in congenital aortic valve malformation. Circulation 1999;99:2138-2143.

156. Schmid FX, Bielenberg K, Schneider A, et al: Ascending aortic aneurysm associated with bicuspid and tricuspid aortic valve: involvement and clinical relevance of smooth muscle cell apoptosis and expression of cell death-initiating proteins. Eur J Cardiothorac Surg 2003;23:537-543.

157. Fedak PWM, de Sa MPL, Verma S, et al: Vascular matrix remodeling in patients with bicuspid aortic valve malformations: implications for aortic dilatation. J Thorac Cardiovasc Surg 2003;126:797-806.

158. Nataatmadja M, West M, West J, et al: Abnormal extracellular matrix protein transport associated with increased apoptosis of vascular smooth muscle cells in Marfan syndrome and bicuspid aortic valve thoracic aortic aneurysm. Circulation 2003;108(Suppl II):II-329-II-34.

159. Boyum J, Fellinger EK, Schmoker JD, et al: Matrix metalloproteinase activity in thoracic aortic aneurysms associated with bicuspid and tricuspid aortic valves. J Thorac Cardiovasc Surg 2004;127:686-691.

160. LeMaire SA, Wang X, Wilks JA, et al: Matrix metalloproteinases in ascending aortic aneurysms: bicuspid versus trileaflet aortic valves. J Surg Res 2005;123:40-48.

161. Ikonomidis JS, Jones JA, Barbour JR, et al: Expression of matrix metalloproteinases and endogenous inhibitors within ascending aortic aneurysms of patients with bicuspid or tricuspid aortic valves. J Thorac Cardiovasc Surg 2007;133:1028-1036.

162. Pereira L, Lee SY, Gayraud B, et al: Pathogenetic sequence for aneurysm revealed in mice underexpressing fibrillin-1. Proc Natl Acad Sci USA 1999;96:3819-3823.

163. Yasuda H, Nakatani S, Stugaard M, et al: Failure to prevent progressive dilation of ascending aorta by aortic valve replacement in patients with bicuspid aortic valve: comparison with tricuspid aortic valve. Circulation 2003;108: (suppl II):II-291-II-294.

164. Borger MA, Preston M, Ivanov J, et al: Should the ascending aorta be replaced more frequently in patients with bicuspid aortic valve disease? J Thorac Cardiovasc Surg 2004;128:677-683.

165. Goh DL, Han LF, Judge DP, et al: Linkage of familial bicuspid aortic valve with aortic aneurysm to chromosome 15q (abstract). Am Soc Hum Genet 2002;71(Suppl):211.

166. Loscalzo ML, Goh D, Loeys B, et al: Familial thoracic aortic dilation and bicommissural aortic valve: a prospective analysis of the natural history and inheritance. Am J Med Genet A 2007;143A:1960-1967.

167. Martin L, Ramachandran V, Cripe L, et al: Evidence in favor of linkage to human chromosomal regions 18q, 5q, and 13q for bicuspid aortic valve and associated cardiovascular malformations. Hum Genet 2007;121:275-284.

168. Mohamed SA, Aherrahrou Z, Liptau H, et al: Novel missense mutations (p.T596M and p.P1797H) in *NOTCH1* in patients with bicuspid aortic valve Biochem Biophys Res Commun 2006;345:1460-1465.

169. McKeller SH, Tester DJ, Yagubyan M, et al: Novel *NOTCH1* mutations in patients with bicuspid aortic valve disease and thoracic aortic aneurysms. J Thorac Cardiovasc Surg 2007;134:290-296.

170. Kent KC, Loscalzo ML, Goh DLM, et al: Genotype-phenotype correlation in patients with bicuspid aortic valve and aneurysm (abstract 1759W). Am Soc Hum Genet Oct 23-27, 2007. San Diego, CA 2007.

171. Gaudiani VA, Grunkemeier GL, Castro LJ, et al: The risks and benefits of re-operative aortic valve replacement. Heart Surg Forum 2004;7:E170-173.

172. Minakata K, Schaff HV, Zehr KJ, et al: Is repair of aortic valve regurgitation a safe alternative to valve replacement? J Thorac Cardiovasc Surg 2004;127:645-653.

173. Svensson LG, Longoria J, Kimmel WA, Nadolny E: Management of aortic valve disease during aortic surgery. Ann Thorac Surg 2000;69:778-784.

174. Davierwala PM, David TE, Armstrong S, Ivanov J: Aortic valve repair versus replacement in bicuspid aortic valve disease. J Heart Valve Dis 2003;12:679-686.

175. Coady MA, Rizzo JA, Hammond GL, et al: What is the appropriate size criterion for resection of thoracic aortic aneurysms? J Thorac Cardiovasc Surg 1997;113:476-491.

176. Svensson LG, Lim KH, Lytle BW, Cosgrove DM: Relationship of aortic cross-sectional area to height ratio and the risk of aortic dissection in patients with bicuspid aortic valves. J Thorac Cardiovasc Surg 2003;126:892-893.

177. Sundt TM, Mora BN, Moon MR, et al: Options for repair of a bicuspid aortic valve and ascending aortic aneurysm. Ann Thorac Surg 2000;69:1333-1337.

178. Kouchoukos NT, Masetti P, Nickerson NJ, et al: The Ross procedure: long-term clinical and echocardiographic follow-up. Ann Thorac Surg 2004;78:773-781.

179. Sundt TM, Moon MR, Xu H: Reoperation for dilatation of the pulmonary autograft after the Ross procedure. J Thorac Cardiovasc Surg 2001;122:1249-1252.

180. David TE, Omran A, Ivanov J, et al: Dilation of the pulmonary autograft after the Ross procedure. J Thorac Cardiovasc Surg 2000;119:210-220.

181. Maron BJ, Ackerman MJ, Nishimura RA, et al: Task Force 4: HCM and other cardiomyopathies, mitral valve prolapse, myocarditis, and Marfan syndrome. J Am Coll Cardiol 2005;45:1340-1345.

182. Roman MJ, Devereux R, Kramer-Fox R, O'Ranghlin J: Two-dimensional aortic root dimensions in normal children and adults. Am J Cardiol 1989;64:507-512.

183. Svennson LG, Lim KH, Lytle BW, et al: Relationship of aortic cross-sectional area to height ratio and the risk of aortic dissection in patients with bicuspid aortic valves. J Thorac Cardiovasc Surg 2003;126:892-893.

Surgical Approach to Aortic Valve Disease

Paul Stelzer and David H. Adams

KEY POINTS

- The choice of operative treatment for diseases of the aortic valve and aortic root must be individualized with special consideration given to patient age, lifestyle, and concomitant diseases.
- The guiding principle in aortic valve and root surgery is to restore the functional unit of the root, extending from the left ventricular outflow tract to the sinotubular ridge.
- Aortic valve repair is essentially a treatment only for aortic regurgitation, and bicuspid valves are better candidates for repair than tricuspid valves.
- The Ross procedure remains an operation for specialized centers because of its technical challenges and small number of patients young enough to justify its use. Candidates for this option should be referred to such centers.
- Complex aortic root surgery can be done more safely and with more predictable results by surgeons in centers that have a solid depth of experience with these more technically demanding procedures.

The guiding principle in aortic valve and root surgery is to restore the functional unit of the root. This means restoration of the entire structure from the left ventricular (LV) outflow tract (LVOT) to the sinotubular ridge with the complex, beautiful interaction of the sinuses and leaflets, and the dynamic changes in annular and sinotubular dimensions that mark the cycle of systole and diastole (Figure 12-1). Although some compromises are often necessary, failure to consider the entire unit may result in short- and long-term consequences. A thorough understanding of the surgical principles and options is relevant as we move beyond the consideration of early results and focus on very long-term outcomes after valvular heart surgery. Because none of the surgical alternatives for a specific patient are truly curative or associated with guaranteed durability or freedom from adverse events, a clear understanding of the many options available to treat aortic valve disease is mandatory in the modern era.

FUNDAMENTAL PRINCIPLES

It has become increasingly clear that surgery has an impact on aortic valve and root physiology that may affect long-term results. This may include factors that limit leaflet durability or impair coronary flow reserve[1] with implications for exercise capacity and longevity. The newer concepts of leaflet stress and energy loss may be as important as gradients and valve areas.[2] In addition, leaving abnormal stresses on living or biologic leaflets may limit the durability of the procedure, be it repair or replacement.[3] The more laminar the flow, the less trauma there is to the living elements of the root. The decision to replace a diseased aortic valve must always take into consideration the flow characteristics of the proposed replacement device.[4]

Surgery has always involved the concept of changing anatomic abnormalities with adverse physiologic consequences in such a way as to minimize or reverse those consequences. Unfortunately, many operations necessarily substitute a different anatomic abnormality for the problem instead of restoring normal anatomy. An appreciation for the complex anatomy of the normal aortic root and the favorable physiologic impact of the normal interaction of all of its elements has led to considerable interest in preservation, reconstruction, and imitation of these elements in modern surgery of the aortic root. These concepts have been particularly important in younger patients with aortic valve and root disease. Advances in imaging have demonstrated the very limited zone of semilunar leaflet coaptation and have allowed accurate measurements of the root at multiple levels to assess suitability for various repair and replacement options (see Figure 12-1). Marked calcification of the aortic tissues in some patients can present unique challenges forcing choices that are much less ideal but must be considered when "theoretically better" alternatives are impractical. A valve conduit from the LV apex to the descending or supraceliac aorta is an example of such a solution to a bad aortic root situation.

The setting in which maximal restoration or imitation of the normal anatomy is needed most is in the very young patient

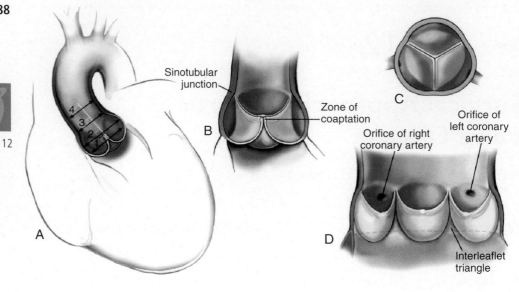

FIGURE 12-1 Normal anatomy of the aortic root. **A**, Important measurements include annulus (1), sinus diameter (2), sinotubular junction (3), and ascending aortic diameter (4). **B**, Coaptation area is limited to 1 to 2 mm in the normal aortic valve. **C**, The diastolic anatomic equivalent of the short-axis echo view "Mercedes" sign. **D**, The coronal insertion line of the aortic leaflets leaves triangular areas under each commissure that can be plicated down to increase coaptation in some incompetent valves.

with a long life expectancy. Probably only the Ross operation can approach true restoration of normal anatomy because of its use of completely living elements in all parts of the new aortic root. Root remodeling or reimplantation procedures can preserve the cusps and their relationships to one another but impose alternative sinus geometry with implications for coronary flow and closing forces on the leaflets. The modifications that create "pseudo-sinuses" or use a graft with a sinus segment incorporated into its design may be of benefit in this regard but may introduce other technical issues in the process.[5] Primary leaflet repair techniques can also be used in very specific circumstances but also introduce less predictable effects on leaflet stress and durability.

The field of aortic valve surgery has expanded substantially from the early days of choosing between simple mechanical or bioprosthetic aortic valve replacement (AVR). Today many options are available for a specific patient and must be considered, with full consideration of root pathology as well as optimal valve performance. For example, it has been increasingly apparent that simply replacing the aortic valve leaflets with a mechanical or bioprosthetic valve in a very dilated root or leaving a 5.0-cm ascending aorta behind is a formula for future disaster. The physics of excessive wall tension must be addressed, usually by replacing these abnormal tissues. Conversely, a good valve that has been rendered incompetent by ascending aortic or root dilatation or even by acute aortic dissection can often be restored to normal function by appropriate valve-sparing root reconstruction and aortic grafting. These are not simple procedures but in experienced hands offer the possibility of preserving and restoring normal function to the native, living aortic leaflets

with the potential for long-term freedom from both anticoagulation and reoperation. In this chapter, we will review the spectrum of surgical options for patients with pathologic aortic valve and root conditions, with an emphasis on nonthrombogenic alternatives including valve repair, valve sparing, and biologic replacement options.

AORTIC VALVE LEAFLET REPAIR TECHNIQUES

Surgical aortic valvotomy for critical aortic stenosis (AS) is a pediatric cardiac surgical procedure relegated to history by the advent of balloon aortic valvuloplasty. Balloon dilatation works well in the very young but has been associated with rapid recurrence, occasional disastrous aortic regurgitation (AR), and frequent femoral arterial complications in elderly patients, in whom its use is still justified in special temporizing situations. Attempts to perform open surgical decalcification of the stenotic aortic valve have been abandoned because of early development of severe AR after the calcium is removed.

Aortic valve repair, then, is essentially a treatment only for AR. In patients without major root disease, this goal can sometimes be accomplished with a simple commissuroplasty (Figure 12-2). The annulus is narrowed selectively below the commissures to increase coaptation. The knots are placed on the outside of the aorta to prevent trauma to the leaflets. This technique is most applicable to the posterior (left-noncoronary) commissure where the triangle is completely fibrous.

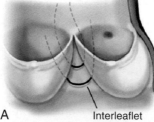
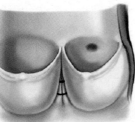
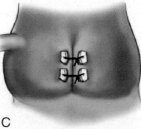

FIGURE 12-2 Aortic commissuroplasty. The wide interleaflet triangle is narrowed with sutures that plicate this area to increase coaptation.

The right-left commissure is completely muscular and is less accessible because of the close adherence of the aorta to the pulmonary artery in this area. The anterior (right-noncoronary) commissure is limited by the conduction system, which can be compromised if sutures are placed too low in the membranous septum located here.

More sophisticated techniques include extending leaflets, shortening the free edges to prevent prolapse,[6] or even converting a bicuspid valve into a three-leaflet arrangement (Figures 12-3 through 12-6). Bicuspid valves have actually been better candidates for repair than tricuspid valves. In rare cases of healed endocarditis, a leaflet perforation can be repaired with a patch of autologous pericardium (Figure 12-7). These methods have been particularly useful in children in whom AVR should be delayed as long as possible to allow adult size constraints to apply. Experience with these repair techniques is limited, and long-term follow-up is not available. They are certainly worth consideration, however,

in the very young patient to avoid anticoagulation and preserve later replacement options. Part of the strategy in these patients should always be to close the pericardium or place a pericardial substitute to minimize the risk of subsequent surgery.

AORTIC VALVE REPLACEMENT

In the absence of root disease, the usual treatment for critical and/or symptomatic AS is surgical AVR. With the patient on cardiopulmonary bypass, the aorta is clamped, and myocardial protection is assured. Aortotomy exposes the diseased valve, which is excised. The annulus is debrided carefully and measured with appropriate sizing devices. The most common replacement choices are mechanical and animal tissue devices (Figure 12-8). More sophisticated alternatives have their place, and each option will be discussed in detail.

Mechanical Valves

Mechanical AVR or replacement of the entire aortic root with a mechanical valved conduit has been an alternative since the 1960s. There has been considerable evolution in the devices from the early ball-in-cage devices to the present single or bileaflet tilting disk valves. A handful of the first Starr-Edwards valves are still serving their recipients 40 years later, but the vast majority of patients with these ball-in-cage devices did not survive for 20 years. Kaplan-Meier survival was only 23% at 20 years and 8% at 30 years.[7] Efforts to make these devices less thrombogenic have been intense, but they all require life-long anticoagulation. The Medtronic-Hall valve serves as an example of the modern single disk valve, and long-term follow-up in Oslo demonstrates a 24.9% survival at 25 years with particularly good results in those younger than 18 years at implant who had 95% 15-year and 88% 20-year survival.[8] The St. Jude bileaflet device has been used for the largest number of implants worldwide with the longest track record. Despite major differences in design and flow patterns,[9] the single and bileaflet valves have performed in very similar ways, and a recent editorial regards them as essentially equivalent.[10] A 10-year randomized trial of two different bileaflet devices (St. Jude and Carbo-Medics) showed no significant differences in outcomes between the two.[11] The intrinsic durability of these devices still makes them the least likely to require reoperation of any valve alternative, be it AVR or repair. However, the only class I indication for a mechanical aortic valve in

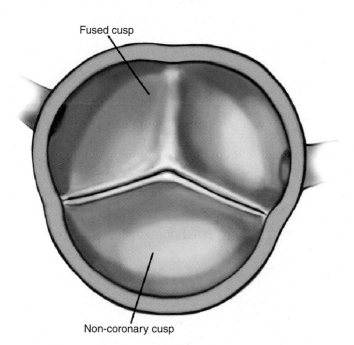

FIGURE 12–3 Bicuspid valve. The most common configuration is really a fusion of two leaflets (most often right and left coronary leaflets) with a rudimentary commissure or raphe where the normal commissure would be.

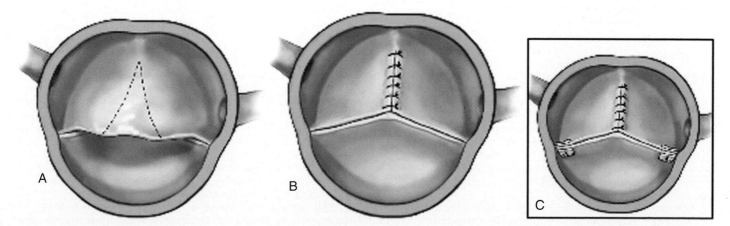

FIGURE 12–4 Resection of leaflet prolapse. The redundant central portion of the larger (fused) leaflet is resected and closed primarily to restore normal coaptation level. If both leaflets prolapse, the commissures can be shortened with pledgeted sutures as well.

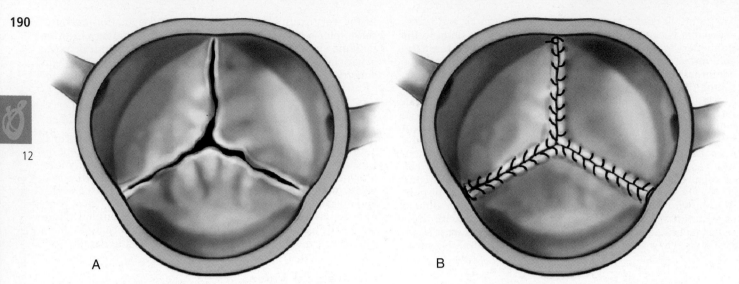

FIGURE 12–5 Leaflet shortening. Continuous over-and-over suture from commissure to commissure is one method for shortening leaflets; 6-0 Gore-Tex is suggested for this maneuver with the knots placed outside the aorta.

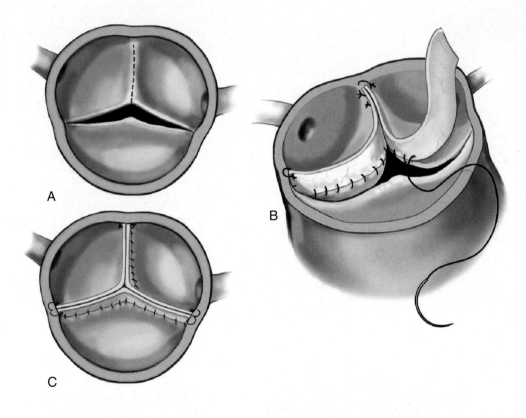

FIGURE 12–6 Tricuspidization. The rudimentary commissure is opened to make three leaflets out of two. The edges of all three are then extended with autologous pericardium attached to the aortic wall at each end to increase the coaptation surface.

current guidelines is the presence of a mechanical mitral or tricuspid valve (level of evidence C).[12] An extension of this principle is that a mechanical valve is a logical choice if the patient is already committed to life-long warfarin for chronic deep venous thrombosis, pulmonary emboli, or atrial fibrillation. The other situation most likely to justify this type of valve is Marfan syndrome in a young patient with an unsalvageable aortic valve, especially if root replacement is required. The long-term results in this high-risk population are quite good.[13]

The mechanical valves currently available are quite hemodynamically efficient, but they are also intrinsically rigid. This rigidity puts stress on the extremes of the coronal shape of the native annulus, which may increase the likelihood of

sutures pulling through to cause a paravalvular leak. The low-lying left main ostium is also more at risk of obstruction from a mechanical valve, which can ride up over the posterior annulus into a position that compromises this orifice (see Figure 12-1). Care must be taken when the mechanical valve is implanted to prevent this from happening. The surgical techniques for accomplishing this task are well defined and easily reproducible. Orientation of the mechanism is adjustable in most devices after implantation to optimize the opening angle for the leaflets (Figure 12-9).

The biggest issue with a mechanical valve is still the double-edged sword of thromboembolic phenomena and anticoagulant-related hemorrhage. Despite the fact that the mechanical valve has been the mainstay of treatment in

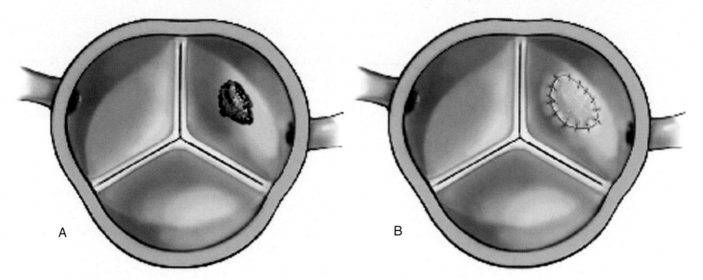

FIGURE 12–7 Repair of healed endocarditis. A simple leaflet perforation can be repaired with an autologous pericardial patch.

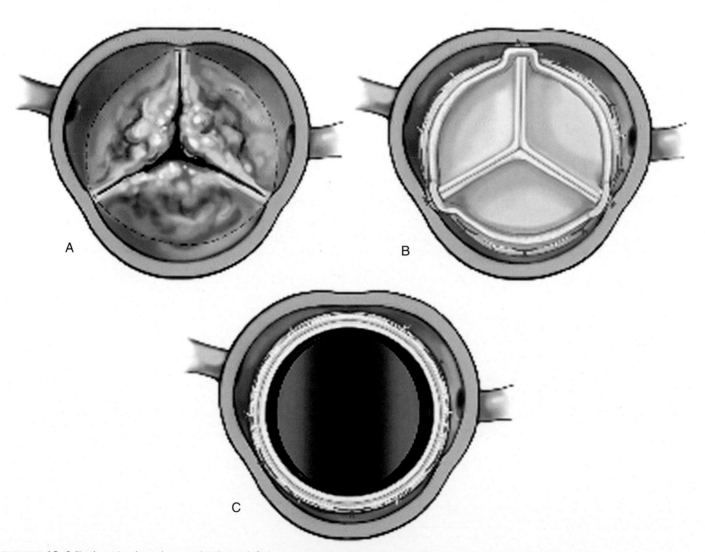

FIGURE 12–8 Simple aortic valve replacement (AVR). **A**, Calcified native aortic valve. **B**, Stented tissue valve replacement. **C**, Mechanical AVR in place.

12

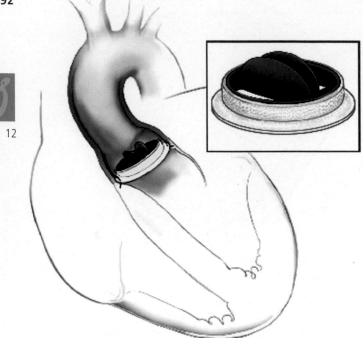

FIGURE 12–9 Mechanical valve. The Pyrolite carbon disks are seen enclosed in a circular housing covered by a cloth sewing ring which allows attachment to the aortic annulus.

the past, it has always been recognized as another disease (Figure 12-10).[14] This has been the primary reason that AVR has been delayed in most young patients until absolutely necessary. The dual issues of thromboembolic phenomena and anticoagulant-related hemorrhage have a never-ending linearized incidence of 1% to 2%/patient-year for each. The long-term risks of these complications have been well documented by Grunkemeier et al.[15] That risk is highest in the first few months after surgery, but it never goes away. That total of 2% to 4%/patient-year is the reason that by 15 years a patient with a mechanical valve has a 40% chance of death or a serious complication, and by 20 years the actuarial freedom from either valve-related mortality or morbidity is only 32%. The myth that mechanical valves never require another operation is dispelled by the data demonstrating a 20-year actuarial risk of 10% that reoperation will be precipitated by endocarditis, paravalvular leak, pannus ingrowth, valve thrombosis, or insoluble problems with thromboembolic or anticoagulant-related hemorrhage issues.[16] All of these possibilities must be considered when the mechanical valve option is discussed with patients, especially if their lifestyles may put them at increased risk of bleeding or if a serious reliability issue could make international normalized ratio monitoring and medication compliance difficult.

Stented Tissue Valves

Stented porcine and bovine pericardial tissue valves have increasingly become the aortic valves of choice because of their ease of implantation and low rates of thromboembolism without anticoagulation. These valves are constructed by attaching the animal tissue to a support frame (stent) that has a cloth sewing ring into which surgical sutures can easily be placed and securely tied (Figure 12-11). Several generations of tissue treatment have evolved since the first porcine valves of the 1960s. Results with second-generation valves have been quite good[17] and third-generation tissue technology has improved the durability of these valves to allow forecasting of durability in the 15- to 20-year range. Unfortunately, durability is still inversely related to age (Figure 12-12).[18]

The increased safety of both primary and reoperative AVR has made the bioprosthesis an increasingly attractive alternative and explains the major shift from mechanical valves to tissue valves in the last decade. Even in the setting of chronic atrial fibrillation, it has been shown that stented tissue valves have lower complication and better survival rates than mechanical valves.[19] These valves are easily implanted by most cardiac surgeons using standard techniques that have proven reliable for many years. The softer, usually scalloped, sewing ring of these valves makes implantation at or in the native annulus easier than with a rigid mechanical valve. The hemodynamic characteristics of these valves are quite good in larger sizes but progressively less so at sizes less than 23 mm. The latest iteration of the pericardial valve incorporates a thinner sewing ring that may enhance hemodynamics in small sizes and allow a slightly larger size valve to be implanted.[20]

Stentless Tissue Valves

Stentless porcine and pericardial valves have been available for more than 15 years but have been slow to reach widespread use. The more difficult implant techniques for these

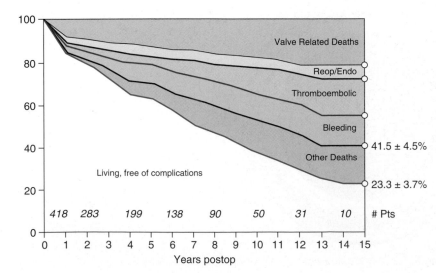

FIGURE 12–10 Event-free survival with mechanical valve. *(Adapted from Zellner JL, Kratz JM, Crumbley AJ 3rd, et al: Long-term experience with the St. Jude Medical valve prosthesis. Ann Thorac Surg 1999;68:1210-1218, used with permission.)*

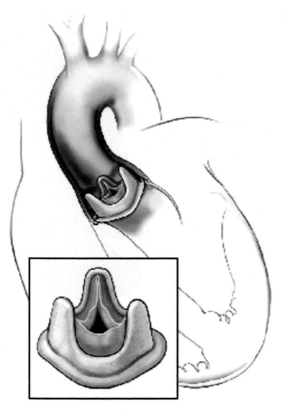

FIGURE 12–11 Stented bioprosthetic aortic valve. The heterologous tissue leaflets are attached to the supporting frame with incorporated sewing ring.

prospective trial of stentless versus conventional stented tissue valves demonstrated a survival advantage and decrease in thromboembolic phenomena with stentless valves.[22] Other authors have not seen similar benefits in their clinical experience.[23,24] The first stentless valve[25] was designed for a fully scalloped subcoronary implant. This implant required a proximal suture line (roughly circular) based at the nadir of the aortic annulus, well below the high points of the commissures. A second (distal) suture line was then required to attach the top edge of the device to the native aortic wall coursing below the coronary ostia and up above the commissural posts. The fact that newer stentless devices have been provided as a complete bioprosthetic root allows their use as a full root replacement as well as a modified subcoronary implant preserving the noncoronary sinus (Figure 12-13).

A hybrid technique called root inclusion is also possible. For surgeons not experienced in aortic root surgery, the option of replacing the aortic root is seldom chosen in elective circumstances. However, for those with solid root experience, root replacement with a stentless device not only gives better hemodynamics but also invariably allows a larger sized valve to be implanted.[26] As with any root replacement operation, this operation requires mobilization and reimplantation of the coronary ostia, which requires judgment and skill (Figure 12-14). The potential for bleeding from inaccessible suture lines must also be recognized and addressed by careful technique and gentle tissue handling. The additional time required for root replacement must be considered as well, but this is not excessive in the presence of good myocardial protection. The one situation that is a relative contraindication to a stentless valve is the presence of severe aortic wall calcification around the coronary ostia. These areas must allow sutures to penetrate for

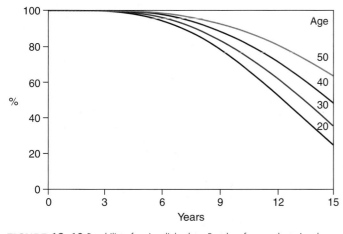

FIGURE 12–12 Durability of pericardial valves. Freedom from explantation due to structural deterioration as a function of age. *(Adapted from Svensson LG, Blackstone EH, Cosgrove DM 3rd: Surgical options in young adults with aortic valve disease. Curr Probl Cardiol 2003;28:417-480, used with permission.)*

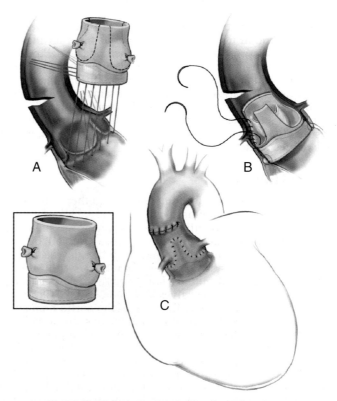

FIGURE 12–13 Modified subcoronary stentless valve implantation. **A**, Proximal, interrupted suture line in a circular plane at or below annulus. **B**, Distal, continuous polypropylene suture line attaching residual aortic wall to native aortic wall running below the coronary ostia and preserving the porcine noncoronary sinus. **C**, Aortotomy closed showing relationship of distal suture line to coronary ostia.

valves have discouraged many surgeons from using them. This difficulty is particularly true for surgeons in low-volume centers where it is difficult for them to garner adequate experience to be comfortable with these devices. The primary advantage of the stentless devices is the fuller use of the outflow tract diameter by eliminating the sewing ring that takes up space, thus resulting in faster and more complete resolution of LV hypertrophy and greater LV mass regression than are seen with the standard stented valves.[21] A randomized

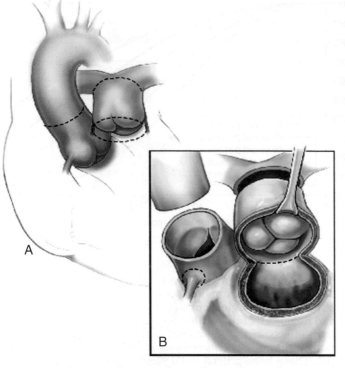

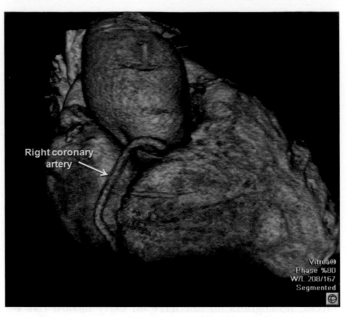

FIGURE 12–20 Dilated autograft root. Computed tomography angiogram reconstruction of pulmonary autograft root showing distal radial and longitudinal expansion of the pulmonary root but no dilatation at the supported proximal end.

FIGURE 12–18 Ross procedure. Incision lines are illustrated for aortic (transverse and distal) and pulmonary roots. The distal pulmonary incision is made first to allow inspection of the valve and to allow accurate placement of the proximal incision below the annulus.

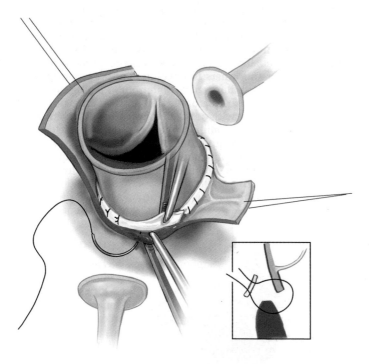

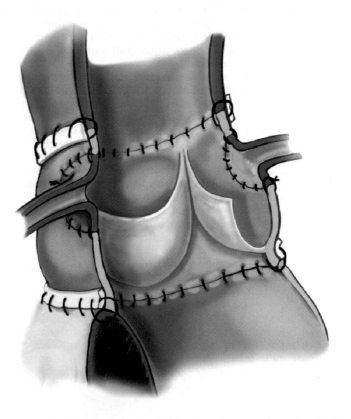

FIGURE 12–19 Annular support of the autograft. A measured length felt strip is incorporated into the proximal autograft suture line (interrupted or continuous) to prevent late dilatation at this level. Inset shows the sutures placed directly under the hinge point of the pulmonary leaflet.

FIGURE 12–21 Supported autograft. Felt strips are incorporated at both proximal and distal suture lines with the distal support right at the sinotubular junction.

aortic root tissue can provide an additional layer of thickness especially in the noncoronary sinus to prevent primary sinus dilatation while maintaining the flexibility and shape of the normal sinus aorta (Figure 12-22). Another alternative is to enclose the entire autograft in a piece of vascular tube graft, but this must not be too tight (Figure 12-23). This method is appropriate in patients with a true root aneurysm or marked thinning of the sinuses of Valsalva. With use of either of these support methods, compromise of neoaortic root height, which can result in leaflet prolapse and incompetence, must be avoided. Some have proposed returning to the intra-aortic cylinder technique to preserve the external support of the

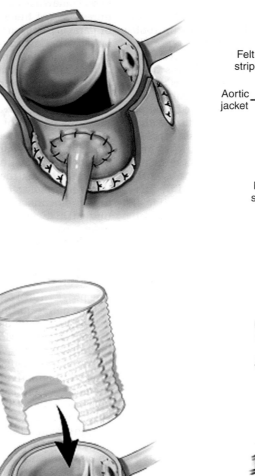

FIGURE 12–22 Autograft with native jacket. The native aortic wall from the noncoronary sinus and the "pillar" between coronary buttons is preserved and used to enclose the autograft by attaching them in the distal suture line along with the felt strip.

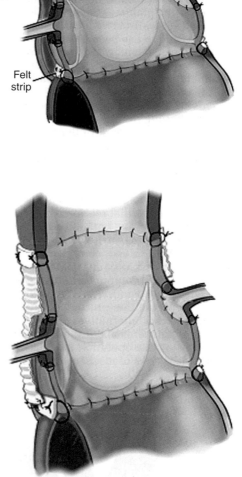

Felt strip

Aortic jacket

Felt strip

FIGURE 12–23 Autograft with Dacron jacket. The entire autograft is enclosed in a generous-diameter vascular graft attached to the felt strip proximally and included with the felt strip in the distal anastomosis.

native aortic root.[42] Unfortunately, the native aortic root is often too small or too big to use without tailoring, and if it is normal, external support is probably not necessary. A comparison of the full root and the subcoronary techniques from two centers in Germany that actively perform the Ross procedure showed no difference in midterm follow-up results.[43] The distal aorta can also be a problem if a dilated segment is left behind. A much lower threshold for resection and graft repair minimizes this risk. Aortorrhaphy may also be appropriate for aortas between 3.5 and 5.0 cm in diameter with the aim of a final diameter of 3.5 cm or less.[44] Aortas at highest risk are those greater than 5.0 cm in diameter especially if the patient has had previous coarctation repair. This combination of defects is a clinical marker for aortopathy and should be noted.[45]

In summary, the Ross procedure in experienced hands offers a survival advantage over use of alternative valves[46] and completely restores normal hemodynamics for the young person desiring extreme physical activity such as competitive athletics.[47,48] It can be offered to those with life expectancy greater than 20 to 25 years who want to avoid anticoagulation and have the benefit of optimal hemodynamics.[49]

Risk at further surgery is minimized by closing the pericardium (or using a substitute) at the primary procedure. The living autograft tissue is soft and pliable, making it easy to work inside this structure or even replace it completely if necessary. The pulmonary homograft on the right side of the heart can calcify over time and shrink, but this is rarely significant if the original graft is oversized. Sievers et al[50] have tried to reduce this shrinkage by removing all of the muscle from the inflow end replacing it with Gore-Tex. It remains to be seen whether this strategy will be successful in the long-term. The advent of percutaneous pulmonary valve replacement offers hope for extending the life of the homograft without further surgery.[51] Use of this device has none of the coronary, neurologic, or femoral arterial access issues of a percutaneous aortic valve, but similar durability concerns will remain until better tissue technology is available. Tissue engineering of potential substitutes for the right ventricular outflow tract offers the hope of other alternatives that will increase the appeal of the Ross procedure in the future. Clearly, the Ross procedure will always remain an operation for specialized centers because of its technically challenging nature and the small number of patients young enough to justify its use. Candidates for this option should be referred to such centers.

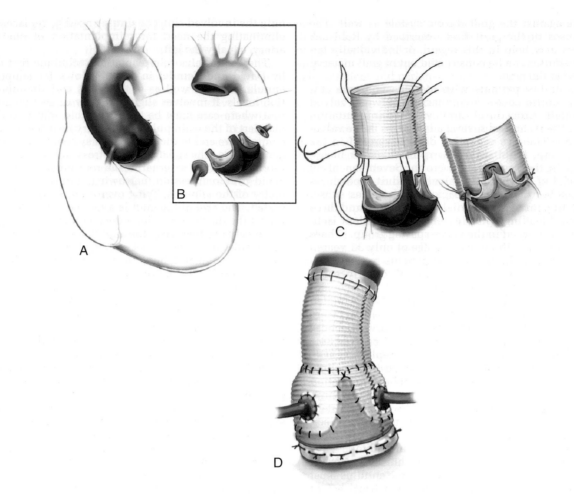

FIGURE 12–27 David procedure. Aneurysmal root (**A**) is resected (**B**) including sinuses of Valsalva with coronary "buttons" mobilized away. **C**, Subannular sutures (six to eight) are placed. Commissural posts are drawn up inside the valve and the annular sutures are passed through the proximal end of the graft. **D**, Annular sutures are tied gently. Then the valve is reimplanted with continuous 5-0 polypropylene suture inside the graft. Aortic continuity is reestablished with another graft of a size appropriate to the desired sinotubular junction and proximal arch.

to be worth sparing. If extensive leaflet resection, extension, shortening, or tailoring is required, the short- and long-term success of the operation is less predictable. Obviously, there is no substitute for experience and judgment during surgery to make the decision about saving or replacing a valve in any given patient. Reference centers with appropriately committed and capable personnel are most likely to succeed in this regard.

Aicher et al[59] reported a 10-year experience with 274 remodeling operations including 193 with three-leaflet valves and 81 with bicuspid valves. Hospital mortality was 3.6% overall. At 10 years, freedom from grade II or greater AR was 91% in bicuspid and 87% in the patients with three-leaflet valves. Of nine valves that required reoperation, three were successfully rescued with repair. One insight from this experience was that cusp prolapse should be addressed aggressively during the original procedure to avoid problems with AR. In other centers, the results have been best when the valve is normal and does not require any repair at all.

Root Enlargement/Prevention of Mismatch

Any device used to replace the aortic valve that must be implanted within the limited confines of the LVOT is intrinsically obstructive to some extent. The sewing ring that houses the valve allows surgeons to attach it to the annulus but takes up a finite amount of space. This necessarily reduces the effective diameter of the outflow tract available for blood flow and the "hourglass" effect creates turbulence that is not present

in the normal aortic root. For most patients, this decrement in effective valve opening area is not a problem because the cardiac output demands placed upon this orifice are limited by age and lifestyle. It becomes an issue in very active young people or in individuals of any age when the LVOT is only 19 mm. The concept of effective orifice area index was introduced to allow comparison and analysis of the potential for this prosthesis-patient mismatch (PPM) among various body sizes. The effective orifice area of the proposed valve is divided by the body surface area of the patient. Normal is an effective orifice area index greater than $0.85\,cm^2/m^2$, moderate PPM is between 0.65 and $0.84\,cm^2/m^2$, and severe PPM is less than $0.65\,cm^2/m^2$. With this definition, it is troubling to note that the majority of stented tissue valves and many mechanical valves implanted in the United States each year (typically 21- to 23-mm valves) are moderately mismatched. (It could also be noted that AVR is NOT a treatment for obesity.)

Although it may be argued that elderly patients do not require the hemodynamics of a marathon runner, there are some data to suggest that the very worst ventricles may need the advantage of a large effective orifice area the most. Mortality for AVR in patients with severe LV dysfunction rises from 3% when there is no PPM to 6% with moderate PPM and 26% with severe PPM.[60] Even the generally more efficient bileaflet mechanical valves can be problematic in the smaller sizes. Severe mismatch proved to be an independent predictor of death and congestive heart failure in a recent Mayo Clinic study with the St. Jude valve.[61] In contrast to these reports, the long-term mortality in those who survive AVR to leave the hospital was found to be unaffected by prosthesis size in a review of the large Cleveland Clinic database.[62] A more recent study seeking to clarify this question showed mixed results, with PPM adversely affecting only certain groups such as patients younger than age 60 or patients with mechanical valves whose body surface area was greater than 2.1.[63]

Typically, in the operating room transesophageal echocardiography (TEE) is readily available to measure the annular dimension available for valve implantation. On preoperative TTE, the LVOT diameter in the parasternal long-axis view is a good approximation to the size valve that can be implanted (Figure 12-28). When this value is greater than 21 mm, a valve size of at least 21 mm can be used, but when the valve size is 19 mm or less, consideration must be given to alternatives that enlarge or at least do not decrease this opening. The full root replacement option is one choice and is discussed elsewhere in this chapter. The other choice is to enlarge the root to allow implantation of a larger stented device.

Root enlargement procedures described by Nicks et al,[64] Manouguian et al,[65] and Konno et al[66] are all ways of dividing one element of the LVOT and expanding it with a patch. In the Konno procedure the ventricular septum is divided right under the right-left commissure, and this procedure is typically used only in pediatric patients in whom the right ventricular outflow tract is also being addressed. The other two procedures make room in the area of the fibrous continuity between the aortic and mitral valves at or near the commissure between the left and noncoronary leaflets. Cutting across the annulus at this level can be extended all the way down into the anterior mitral leaflet itself if necessary. A patch of pericardial tissue or prosthetic material is sewn into the defect to expand the circumference of the aortic annulus. The left atrial roof is often opened in the process, and this is also patched closed. The wall of the aorta must also be patched (Figure 12-29).

By the time all this patching is done, the time factor and risk of bleeding from the extra suture lines are about the same as those for a root replacement so it is understandable that an experienced root surgeon would prefer to do the root replacement. The one situation in which the root enlargement is worth considering is when calcification around the coronary ostia might preclude safe coronary reimplantation. Root enlargement is also useful in patients with combined aortic and mitral disease in whom both inflow and outflow tracts are very limited in size. In this situation a cut across the annulus of both valves and out onto the left atrial roof opens up both widely. A larger mitral valve replacement device can be placed through this approach, leaving about one third of its circumference to sew to the center of a boomerang-shaped patch, one blade of which closes the atrial roof. The aortic

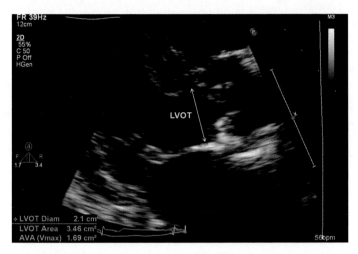

FIGURE 12–28 Left ventricular outflow tract (LVOT) dimension. The parasternal long-axis view is shown, demonstrating the measurement of LVOT from the hinge point of the anterior mitral leaflet to the basal septum parallel to the annulus of the aortic valve.

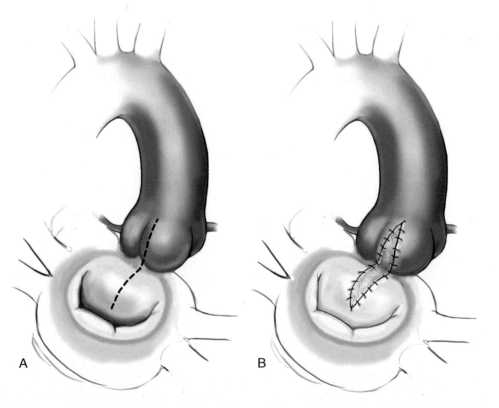

FIGURE 12–29 Root enlargement. Incision in the noncoronary sinus (A) is carried down into the anterior mitral leaflet. A patch of pericardium (B) is used to expand the leaflet, annulus, and aortic wall to allow implantation of a larger aortic valve.

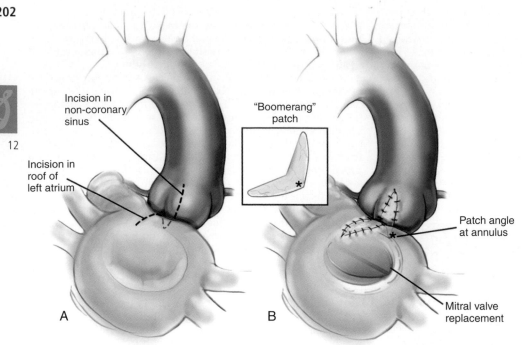

device is then placed with about one third of its sutures also placed in the patch, which then is used to expand the lateral aortic wall (Figure 12-30).

SPECIAL CHALLENGES IN AORTIC ROOT SURGERY

Aortic Dissection

Aortic dissection remains one of the few true emergencies in the world of cardiac surgery. The risk of death in the first 24 to 72 hours exceeds 50% for dissection involving the intrapericardial aorta. It is important to distinguish this type of dissection from the far less life-threatening descending aortic dissection (type B) for which the risk of surgery exceeds that of medical therapy unless there is evidence of rupture or continued critical expansion of the false lumen. The ascending aortic dissection can be lethal because of any one or a combination of three crucial elements: pericardial tamponade, acute coronary compromise, and acute AR.

Because the adventitia is very thin, when elastic tissue degeneration of the media allows blood to get between the intima and adventitia, it can easily leak through the wall into the pericardial space even without frank rupture of the aorta. This leakage fills the pericardium to the point of tamponade at which diastolic filling is impaired and cardiac output is dramatically compromised. Hypotension, shock, and death will follow unless the dissection is promptly recognized and treated. Pericardiocentesis should be avoided except in rare circumstances when shock is present on presentation and fails to respond to volume therapy. Complete rupture of the aortic wall is almost always immediately fatal if this occurs in the ascending aorta, but a slow leak can allow time to rescue the patient. Echocardiographic evidence of significant pericardial fluid with or without tamponade criteria in the presence of acute type A dissection is an indication for an emergency operation without any further tests such as computed tomography (CT), cardiac magnetic resonance, or cardiac catheterization.

Coronary blood flow can be compressed by pressure in the false channel if the dissection extends around the coronary ostium. This compression is more likely to affect the right coronary artery with right ventricular implications than the left. When the left coronary artery is affected, the course is often rapidly fatal, hence, the desirability of prompt treatment of the dissection before this can occur.

The commissures of the aortic valve are suspended by the intima of the aortic root and as the dissection separates the intima from the adventitia in this area, the commissures are displaced centrally and downward causing prolapse of the leaflets and acute AR. This is poorly tolerated by the unprepared left ventricle, and pulmonary edema can develop rapidly. Usually, the commissure between the right and left leaflets is spared. The posterior (left-non) commissure is affected more often than the anterior (right-non) commissure.

In general, this acute AR can be corrected by resuspending the commissures in the process of repairing the dissection, and AVR is not required. Valve-sparing root replacement is possible in this situation but takes longer and still involves reassembling the intima and adventitia at the commissural levels.

Failure of the initial attempt to save the valve may precipitate the need for complete root replacement, which can also be done. This is more challenging because the potential for dissection involving the coronary ostia (usually the right) makes reimplantation of the ostia more perilous.

Standard repair of ascending aortic dissection involves graft replacement of the ascending aorta with an open anastomosis into the proximal arch. This is done with the patient on cardiopulmonary bypass with profound hypothermia and circulatory arrest for the arch anastomosis. Earlier repairs using an aortic cross-clamp were complicated by additional intimal injury from the clamp so the current standard is to use an open technique to avoid this problem. This technique also allows the surgeon to view the arch anatomy to repair or exclude any additional tears that might affect flow to the critical arch branches. It should be noted that the object of surgery for acute type A dissection is not necessarily to eliminate the dissection because there are usually multiple reentry points along the course of the distal aorta. The object of the operation is to eliminate the development of the three lethal complications just discussed. A persistent false lumen is present in approximately 70% of patients with type A dissections after ascending aortic repair. The operation essentially converts the type A to a type B dissection, which is then treated medically. The operation moves the concern out of the pericardial space.

Peripheral arterial cannulation before opening of the pericardium is generally the safest approach in these patients. Most surgeons use a femoral artery approach. Axillary cannulation can also be used but has not been shown to have any advantage over the simpler, faster femoral cannulation in this particular disease.[67] The dissected ascending aorta is certainly treacherous for direct aortic cannulation, but with TEE guidance, this has been shown to be possible.[68] In the presence of significant pericardial effusion, it is wise to heparinize and to have the peripheral artery cannulated before the pericardium is opened. These measures allow blood to be drained quickly if relief of the tamponade results in a sudden rise in blood pressure, which can convert a small leak into a free rupture of the aorta. For this reason, slow release of the pericardium with careful attention to blood pressure is indicated. Once the pericardium is opened safely, the atrium can be cannulated for venous return so femoral venous cannulation is rarely required. Cardiopulmonary bypass is begun and cooling is undertaken to prepare for circulatory arrest. The presence of AR makes LV venting imperative in this situation. When fibrillation occurs, the vent may be inadequate, and systemic perfusion may be compromised by the shunt so the dissected aorta can be clamped at a point proximal to where it will later be resected and repaired. Malperfusion of the head vessels can sometimes occur at this point or earlier and can be detected by a acute drop in brain saturations or right radial pressure. This must be addressed immediately to avoid anoxic brain injury. Fenestrating the intima distal to the clamp is the easiest solution. Direct cannulation with perfusion of the head vessels is the alternative. Axillary cannulation might avoid this problem, but the incidence of neurologic injury has not been lowered by routine use of this approach.

Once the aorta is clamped, work on the proximal aortic root can begin while systemic cooling continues. When the target temperature is reached, the distal ascending aorta is resected, and the layers of the arch are reassembled and attached to an appropriate size vascular graft as an open anastomosis under deep hypothermic circulatory arrest. A thin layer of biologic glue between the dissected layers has been helpful but must be placed carefully to avoid systemic and cerebral consequences. The use of felt reinforcement should be encouraged with generous, gentle bites of continuous polypropylene suture tightened carefully in these delicate tissues. Once the distal anastomosis is completed, air is evacuated and antegrade systemic perfusion via the axillary artery or through the graft itself is resumed. Grafts with a perfusion sidearm are commercially available to simplify this. (Cerebral protection during the time of arrest can be aided by selective antegrade perfusion via an axillary cannula with clamping of the innominate artery or retrogradely via the superior vena cava.) Warming is begun while the proximal end of the graft is attached to the aortic root (Figure 12-31). Alternatively, a separate piece of graft can be placed to the root during cooling and then the two grafts can be attached to one another at the end.

In experienced hands the patient with an acute type A dissection who gets to the operating room alive has a 90% chance of going home alive without major morbidity. There are risks of stroke, renal failure, and bleeding, which are higher than those with other kinds of aortic root surgery, but the lethal consequences of not operating clearly justify prompt surgery.

Aortic Valve Replacement after Previous Coronary Artery Bypass Grafting

Patients with aortic valve disease have frequently undergone coronary bypass grafting (CABG) without AVR, and many of these have progression of AS which requires treatment several years after the bypass surgery. This situation has led to a lower threshold for AVR in the older population, particularly when moderate AS is present, at the time of bypass surgery. The durability of current bioprosthetic valves in this population makes this a reasonable strategy. For those who require AVR after bypass surgery, sternal reentry and access to the aortic root may be hazardous. Careful preoperative assessment with graft and native vessel angiography is essential. The use of multidetector (64-slice) CT angiography has allowed very helpful three-dimensional reconstructions of the retrosternal topography to plan these operations safely as well. CT is not a complete substitute for coronary angiography so both may be required.

The group at New York-Presbyterian Weill Cornell Medical Center led by Girardi published an excellent review of aortic operations on patients with previous cardiac surgery of

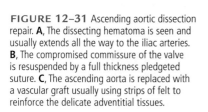

FIGURE 12–31 Ascending aortic dissection repair. **A,** The dissecting hematoma is seen and usually extends all the way to the iliac arteries. **B,** The compromised commissure of the valve is resuspended by a full thickness pledgeted suture. **C,** The ascending aorta is replaced with a vascular graft usually using strips of felt to reinforce the delicate adventitial tissues.

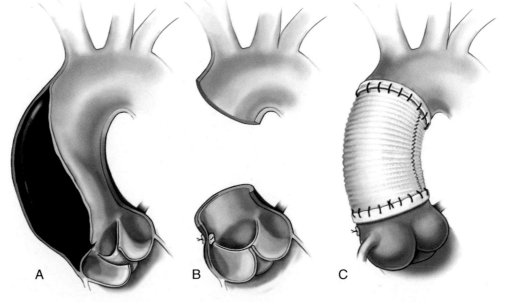

various kinds[69] and relied heavily on the CT scan for evidence of aortic adherence to the posterior sternal table. When this is found, axillary or femoral cannulation with cardiopulmonary bypass and cooling before sternal reentry can allow for brief deep hypothermic circulatory arrest to get in and get control of what might otherwise be a life-threatening hemorrhage with cerebral hypoperfusion and devastating neurologic consequences. They recognized that significant LV distention can occur during the asystole that accompanies hypothermia even without much AR. The left ventricle can be decompressed with apical venting via a small left anterior thoracotomy incision.

One of the key aspects of reoperation with patent bypass grafts is the myocardial protection strategy. Many of these patients will have a patent left internal mammary artery (LIMA) to the left anterior descending coronary artery, which must be protected during the procedure. Previously, the entire heart would be dissected out and the LIMA isolated and clamped with a vascular Bulldog clamp to allow cardioplegia solution to cool the entire heart. More recently, it has been documented that the entire left side of the heart can be left stuck in adhesions and the LIMA allowed to run the entire time without ever finding it or clamping it.[70] This tactic makes injury to the vessel extremely unlikely unless it was allowed to drift over the midline or become adherent to the chest wall after takedown. Moderate systemic hypothermia combined with frequent retrograde cardioplegia is a reasonable approach. The distribution of the LIMA is not the problem as the left anterior descending coronary artery territory is protected by continuous antegrade blood flow. The issue is how to keep the LIMA from washing cardioplegia solution out of the rest of the heart; hence the need for more frequent or continuous retrograde perfusion.

The approach of femero-femoral bypass and cooling before sternotomy is probably not the best approach because of the risk of retrograde embolization from the femoral artery in aortas of elderly patients. Most patients can have the sternum opened without bypass, or axillary artery cannulation can be used to avoid the femoral approach with its problems.

The increasing need for these operations because of the aging population makes this a wise strategy to consider.

Aortic Root Aneurysm after Previous Heart Surgery

If the entire aortic root and ascending aorta must be replaced after previous CABG, this can be accomplished with a modification of the running LIMA approach. Systemic cooling is taken to 18 °C and a hemiarch graft is placed with the patient under deep hypothermic circulatory arrest. Rewarming is begun slowly while the root replacement is done (usually with biologic methods) in the standard fashion. If there is a usable island of native aorta with multiple proximal vein grafts attached, this can be taken off the specimen and reimplanted in the wall of the aortic graft. Alternatively, old vein grafts can be reimplanted separately. An interposition graft of new vein is sometimes required (Figure 12-32). Obviously, if new disease of grafts or native vessels requires additional bypass grafting, the strategy must be altered, but a hybrid approach with interventional methods is worth considering if only one or two branches need revascularization.

One way to avoid these reoperations is to be more aggressive about resecting dilated aortas in patients with bicuspid valves. Certainly no aorta greater than 4.5 cm should be left behind when a bicuspid valve is replaced or repaired, but this number should probably be dropped to 4.0 cm and perhaps as low as 3.5 cm. This aggressive approach, when used by Griepp and colleagues put patients with root replacement for bicuspid valve disease on a virtually normal life expectancy curve with an extremely rare need for distal aortic surgery.[71]

The Porcelain Aorta

In some patients atherosclerosis of the ascending aorta is so extensive that the entire wall is heavily calcified and clamping is impossible (Figure 12-33). Some of these aortas have a soft spot where cannulation may be possible, but others do

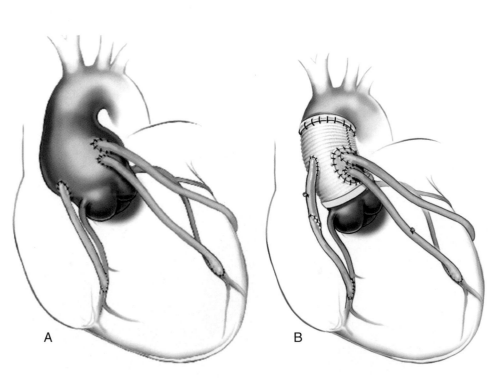

FIGURE 12–32 Aneurysm after bypass grafting. **A**, Patent grafts arise from a new ascending aneurysm. **B**, The right coronary graft is extended with a new segment of saphenous vein. The left-sided grafts are reimplanted as a single island of native aorta.

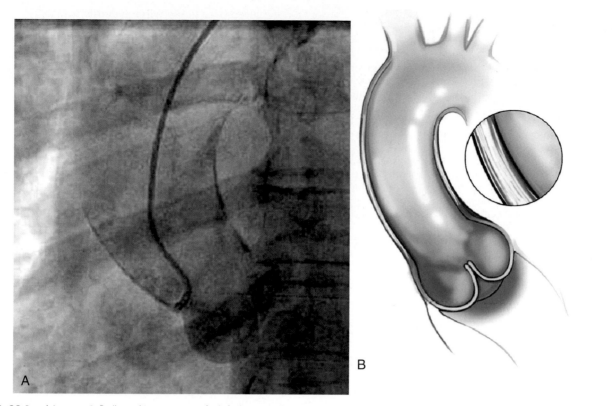

FIGURE 12-33 Porcelain aorta. **A**, Radiographic appearance of calcified aortic wall at catheterization. A dense strip of calcification is seen in both the greater and lesser curvature in this left anterior oblique aortogram. **B**, Artist's conception of the calcified wall seen in cutaway view with close-up inset.

not and axillary cannulation may be required. Whereas coronary work can be done without a pump or on a fibrillating heart and other valve work can be done without clamping the aorta, the aortic valve normally cannot be replaced without opening the aorta. The operative strategy has been to use systemic cooling to deep hypothermia and then use circulatory arrest. In rare instances, the aorta can be opened safely at the root, the valve quickly replaced, and the aortotomy closed all under one period of circulatory arrest. In general, the time required to do this is excessive or the root itself is too calcified to allow a safe aortotomy, so graft replacement of the ascending aorta is typically required. The graft is then clamped, and circulation is resumed while the valve or root is replaced. In the past, surgery on these patients was aborted, and the chest was closed without completion of the procedure. The deep hypothermic circulatory arrest alternative makes surgery possible, but the risk of stroke and other morbid events is still high. The presence of severe AR is an even bigger problem, because it is impossible to cool the patient adequately to protect the central nervous system. In this situation, direct antegrade cannulation and perfusion of the head vessels may be required. In the absence of AR, construction of a valved conduit from the apex of the left ventricle to the descending or supraceliac abdominal aorta is another alternative that can be entertained. Unfortunately, severe ascending aortic disease is often a marker for even worse descending aortic atherosclerosis, which makes this option less appealing. Clearly, these patients may be better served by percutaneous or transapical approaches to AVR in the future as this technology develops.

The severely atherosclerotic aorta with mobile soft plaque is even more dangerous than the calcified aorta because there is no radiographic warning, and significant disease can be hidden from TEE by the trachea (Figure 12-34). Epiaortic ultrasound can be very helpful in detecting this problem and avoiding dislodgement of debris by cannulation. Clearly, axillary artery cannulation is preferable in this situation and a

"no-touch" technique should be used with cooling and circulatory arrest with graft replacement of this diseased aorta before anything else.

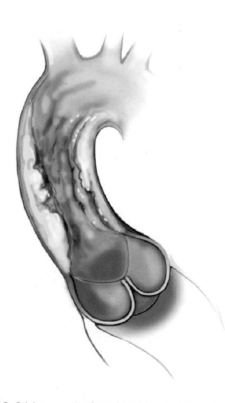

FIGURE 12-34 Severe aortic atherosclerosis. Massive intimal disease is shown that makes cannulation and clamping impossible. Complete replacement is necessary.

Minimally Invasive Approaches

A variety of less invasive approaches to aortic valve and root disease have been tried in the last decade. Some of these, like the vertical parasternal approach, have been abandoned because of chest wall healing problems. The upper partial sternotomy has been the most popular. Proponents of the technique claim less bleeding, less pain, faster recovery time, and shorter hospital and intensive care unit stays.[72] The primary advantage of less invasive cardiac operations, however, has always been cosmetic. Using the upper half of a standard sternotomy incision is not much of an advantage in this regard. Maintaining some degree of chest wall integrity may be an advantage in a patient with severe chronic obstructive pulmonary disease, but the partial sternotomy can be as difficult to close and as painful as a full sternotomy. The exposure to the aortic root is quite good and allows standard aortic cannulation, but venous cannulation is often done from the groin (percutaneously). Myocardial protection may be limited by the inability to cannulate the coronary sinus for retrograde cardioplegia and the rewarming effect of leaving the heart enclosed in a warmer chest than can be achieved with a full sternotomy using topical ice and an insulation pad behind the heart using direct distal septal temperature monitoring to be sure it is cold. Despite these limitations, in experienced hands the less invasive aortic valve operation has been extremely safe and effective even in reoperation situations.[73]

Percutaneous/Transapical Approaches

The heart-lung machine is needed for most operations on the aortic valve and root, so this degree of "invasion" has been unavoidable. The newest approaches to simple AVR, however, involve the use of a stent-supported tissue valve that is placed over guide wires percutaneously via the groin[74] or via the LV apex.[75] The latter is done in the operating room with TEE, fluoroscopy, and a small left anterior thoracotomy to pass the delivery system through the ventricle straight up to the root (Figure 12-35). This may well be the procedure of choice in very high-risk patients such as those in whom trials are currently being conducted.[76]

Improvements in delivery systems and techniques are anticipated as well as in the devices/materials for the actual valve replacement. Current tissues are prepared in ways similar to those used for the first generation of porcine and bovine valves from the 1970s, and durability cannot be expected to be as good as that for the third-generation tissue valves currently placed by open methods. Issues regarding potential migration of these devices or impingement on coronary ostia over time remain to be delineated. The anticipated high risk of embolic consequences from the heavily calcified valves treated in this fashion has fortunately (and surprisingly) not materialized. The risk is equivalent to that of balloon aortic valvuloplasty which is part of this replacement technique. The high recurrence of stenosis that made valvuloplasty so ineffective is prevented by the support of the stent intrinsic to the replacement device. Theoretically, this technique could be repeated or used as an alternative in reoperation after a stented tissue aortic valve,[77] but questions arise regarding the safety and efficacy of this approach. The issue of coronary obstruction by the anatomic proximity of the ostia toward which the stent material displaces heavily calcified leaflets has been less than anticipated, and the incidence of embolic stroke, as in simple balloon aortic valvuloplasty, has been surprisingly low.

If it is necessary to remove one of these devices with open surgery (for endocarditis, for example), there is no experience upon which to base risk assessment. For all of these reasons, use of these devices will probably be restricted to older patients with limited life expectancy, who are deemed to have excessive risk for open surgical treatment.

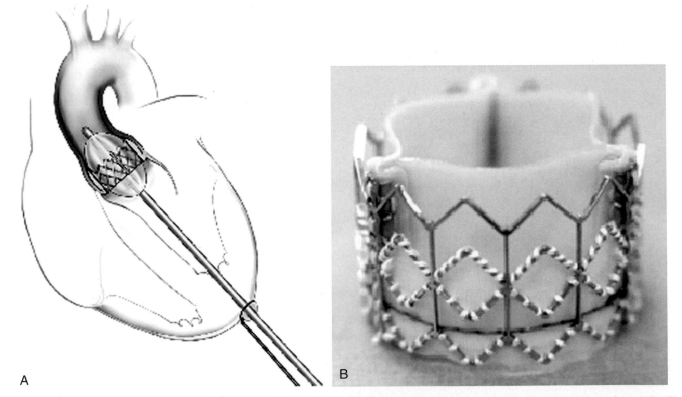

A

B

FIGURE 12–35 Transapical aortic valve replacement. **A,** The concept of replacing the aortic valve via apical puncture is shown. **B,** A stent-mounted tissue valve is deployed in this procedure.

RISK OF SURGERY

Morbidity and mortality are inescapable realities with any disease and any treatment course, but they tend to be more acute and easily measurable in cardiac surgery because of the relatively immediate time course of these events. With steady improvement in anesthesia, perfusion, and intensive care as well as refinement of operative techniques, it has become increasingly apparent that the risk of these adverse events is most often due to patient-specific factors as opposed to the specific kind of operation performed. The surgeon's choices are limited by the anatomy, urgency, and concomitant diseases, both cardiac and noncardiac, in any given patient. Morbidity from AVR mimics that with other forms of cardiac surgery. Stroke, infection, and bleeding rates are all less than 2% of patients in the modern era.

Today the expected mortality for a simple AVR should be between 2% and 4%. A review of valve surgery reported to the Society of Thoracic Surgeons national database from 1994 through 2003 showed a mortality rate of 23.8% for those requiring emergency operations and nearly 45% for those described as "salvage procedures."[78] Advanced age, reoperation, endocarditis, coronary artery disease, and female gender were all factors adversely increasing the odds ratio for death, as were specific comorbid conditions such as renal failure or the presence of multiple comorbidities. The overall mortality for patients undergoing AVR (50% of whom had concomitant CABG) averaged 5.7%. For those who had aortic root replacement (10,274) or valve-sparing root reconstruction (821), the mortality rate was 11.1% with only 21% requiring CABG but 64% requiring "other" additional procedures. The treatment of aortic aneurysm with composite root and ascending aortic replacement had a 10.5% mortality risk. These differences led the authors of this review to point out a subgroup of just more than 5000 patients who had no specific aortic root pathologic lesion documented but still were treated with root replacement including 2152 stentless porcine or aortic homograft roots and 545 mechanical valved conduits. Interestingly this review specifically identified the Ross root replacements as having the lowest mortality risk (2.8%) reported for any valve procedure in the entire report, suggesting that surgical experience and patient selection are very important determinants of outcomes.

One point that has become increasingly clear is that complex aortic root surgery can be done more safely by surgeons in centers that have a solid depth of experience with these more technically demanding procedures. With the exception of acute aortic dissection, most patients who are candidates for root reconstruction or replacement can and should be identified and referred to centers with this kind of experience.

CONCLUSION

In summary, diseases of the aortic valve and root can be treated with a high degree of safety and effectiveness by a wide variety of surgical methods. It is no longer the simple choice of biologic or mechanical AVR as often represented in the Guidelines.[12] The choice of operative treatment must be individualized with special consideration given to patient age (life expectancy), lifestyle, and concomitant diseases. The presence of additional valvular and coronary disease must always be considered along with the myocardial functional capacity to tolerate any planned surgical procedure. Most operations are not emergencies. Thus, there is time for thorough discussion of the options with patients and planning for appropriate care. That may include consideration for referral to specialized centers of excellence where greater experience can offer safer and more durable outcomes in complex root surgery when the need for this is anticipated by preoperative imaging or clinical circumstances. More and more, younger patients in particular will be well informed and involved in making the important choices regarding their care. A very high standard of success is their expectation and is an achievable goal. As none of the aortic valve operations "cure" the younger patient, it is becoming increasingly apparent that reference referral for operations such as valve-sparing procedures or the Ross procedure should be offered to patients with an anticipated long life expectancy.

REFERENCES

1. Bakhtiary F, Schiemann M, Dzemali O, et al: Impact of patient-prosthesis mismatch and aortic valve design on coronary flow reserve after aortic valve replacement. J Am Coll Cardiol 2007;49:790-796.
2. Garcia D, Pibarot P, Dumesnil JG, et al: Assessment of aortic valve stenosis severity: a new index based on the energy loss concept. Circulation 2000;101:765-771.
3. Robicsek F, Thubrikar MJ: Role of sinus wall compliance in aortic leaflet function. Am J Cardiol 1999;84:944-946.
4. Otto CM: Valvular aortic stenosis: disease severity and timing of intervention. J Am Coll Cardiol 2006;47:2141-2151.
5. Thubrikar MJ, Robisek F, Gong GG, Fowler BL: A new aortic root prosthesis with compliant sinuses for valve-sparing operations. Ann Thorac Surg 2001;71(5 Suppl): S318-S322.
6. El Khoury G, Vanoverschelde JL, Glineur D, et al: Repair of aortic valve prolapse: experience with 44 patients. Eur J Cardiothorac Surg 2004;26:628-633.
7. Gao G, Wu Y, Grunkemeier GL, et al: Forty-year survival with the Starr-Edwards aortic valve prosthesis. J Heart Valve Dis 2004;13:91-96.
8. Svennevig JL, Abdelnoor M, Nitter-Hauge S: Twenty-five-year experience with the Medtronic-Hall valve prosthesis in the aortic position: a follow-up cohort study of 816 consecutive patients. Circulation 2007;116:1795-1800.
9. Mottl-Link S, Wolf I, Hastenteufel M, et al: Non-invasive assessment of differences between bileaflet and tilting-disc aortic valve prostheses by 3D-Doppler profiles. Interact Cardiovasc Thorac Surg 2005;4:383-387.
10. Vlahakes GJ: Mechanical heart valves: the test of time. Circulation 2007;116: 1759-1760.
11. Bryan AJ, Rogers CA, Bayliss K, et al: Prospective randomized comparison of CarboMedics and St. Jude Medical bileaflet mechanical heart valve prostheses: ten-year follow-up. J Thorac Cardiovasc Surg 2007;133:614-622.
12. Bonow RO, Carabello BA, Chatterjee K, et al: ACC/AHA 2006 guidelines for the management of patients with valvular heart disease: a report of the American College of Cardiology/American Heart Association Task Force on Practice Guidelines (writing Committee to Revise the 1998 guidelines for the management of patients with valvular heart disease) developed in collaboration with the Society of Cardiovascular Anesthesiologists endorsed by the Society for Cardiovascular Angiography and Interventions and the Society of Thoracic Surgeons. J Am Coll Cardiol 2006;48:e1-148.
13. Gott VL, Cameron DE, Alejo DE, et al: Aortic root replacement in 271 Marfan patients: a 24-year experience. Ann Thorac Surg 2002;73:438-443.
14. Zellner JL, Kratz JM, Crumbley AJ 3rd, et al: Long-term experience with the St. Jude Medical valve prosthesis. Ann Thorac Surg 1999;68:1210-1218.
15. Grunkemeier GL, Li HH, Naftel DC, et al: Long-term performance of heart valve prostheses. Curr Probl Cardiol 2000;25:73-154.
16. Ikonomidis JS, Kratz JM, Crumbley AJ 3rd, et al: Twenty-year experience with the St. Jude Medical mechanical valve prosthesis. J Thorac Cardiovasc Surg 2003;126: 2022-2031.
17. Borger MA, Ivanov J, Armstrong S, et al: Twenty-year results of the Hancock II bioprosthesis. J Heart Valve Dis 2006;15:49-55; discussion 55-46.
18. Svensson LG, Blackstone EH, Cosgrove DM 3rd: Surgical options in young adults with aortic valve disease. Curr Probl Cardiol 2003;28:417-480.
19. Jamieson WR, Miyagishima RT, Henderson C, Germann E: Bioprostheses with atrial fibrillation and mechanical prostheses in aortic valve replacement. Thorac Cardiovasc Surg 2005;53:150-153.
20. Borger MA, Nette AF, Maganti M, Feindel CM: Carpentier-Edwards Perimount Magna valve versus Medtronic Hancock II: a matched hemodynamic comparison. Ann Thorac Surg 2007;83:2054-2058.
21. Borger MA, Carson SM, Ivanov J, et al: Stentless aortic valves are hemodynamically superior to stented valves during mid-term follow-up: a large retrospective study. Ann Thorac Surg 2005;80:2180-2185.
22. Lehmann S, Walther T, Kempfert J, et al: Stentless versus conventional xenograft aortic valve replacement: midterm results of a prospectively randomized trial. Ann Thorac Surg 2007;84:467-472.
23. Cohen G, Christakis GT, Joyner CD, et al: Are stentless valves hemodynamically superior to stented valves? A prospective randomized trial. Ann Thorac Surg 2002;73: 767-778.
24. Doss M, Martens S, Wood JP, et al: Performance of stentless versus stented aortic valve bioprostheses in the elderly patient: a prospective randomized trial. Eur J Cardiothorac Surg 2003;23:299-304.
25. David TE, Pollick C, Bos J: Aortic valve replacement with stentless porcine aortic bioprosthesis. J Thorac Cardiovasc Surg 1990;99:113-118.
26. Kon ND, Cordell AR, Adair SM, et al: Aortic root replacement with the freestyle stentless porcine aortic root bioprosthesis. Ann Thorac Surg 1999;67:1609-1616.
27. David TE, Ivanov J, Eriksson MJ, et al: Dilation of the sinotubular junction causes aortic insufficiency after aortic valve replacement with the Toronto SPV bioprosthesis. J Thorac Cardiovasc Surg 2001;122:929-934.

28. Palka P, Harrocks S, Lange A, et al: Primary aortic valve replacement with cryopreserved aortic allograft: an echocardiographic follow-up study of 570 patients. Circulation 2002;105:61-66.

29. O'Brien MF, Harrocks S, Stafford EG, et al: The homograft aortic valve: a 29-year, 99.3% follow up of 1,022 valve replacements. J Heart Valve Dis 2001;10:334-344.

30. Takkenberg JJ, van Herwerden LA, Eijkemans MJ, et al: Evolution of allograft aortic valve replacement over 13 years: results of 275 procedures. Eur J Cardiothorac Surg 2002;21:683-691.

31. Smedira NG, Blackstone EH, Roselli EE, et al: Are allografts the biologic valve of choice for aortic valve replacement in nonelderly patients? Comparison of explantation for structural valve deterioration of allograft and pericardial prostheses. J Thorac Cardiovasc Surg 2006;131:558-564.

32. Yankah AC, Pasic M, Klose H, et al: Homograft reconstruction of the aortic root for endocarditis with periannular abscess: a 17-year study. Eur J Cardiothorac Surg 2005;28:69-75.

33. Avierinos JF, Thuny F, Chalvignac V, et al: Surgical treatment of active aortic endocarditis: homografts are not the cornerstone of outcome. Ann Thorac Surg 2007;84:1935-1942.

34. McGiffin DC, Galbraith AJ, McLachlan GJ, et al: Aortic valve infection: risk factors for death and recurrent endocarditis after aortic valve replacement. J Thorac Cardiovasc Surg 1992;104:511-520.

35. Ross DN: Replacement of aortic and mitral valves with a pulmonary autograft. Lancet 1967;2:956-958.

36. Stelzer P, Jones DJ, Elkins RC: Aortic root replacement with pulmonary autograft. Circulation 1989;80(5 Pt 2):III209-III213.

37. Kouchoukos NT, Masetti P, Nickerson NJ, et al: The Ross procedure: long-term clinical and echocardiographic follow-up. Ann Thorac Surg 2004;78:773-781.

38. Brown JW, Ruzmetov M, Rodefeld MD, et al: Incidence of and risk factors for pulmonary autograft dilation after Ross aortic valve replacement. Ann Thorac Surg 2007;83:1781-1789.

39. Elkins RC, Lane MM, McCue C. Pulmonary autograft reoperation: incidence and management. Ann Thorac Surg 1996;62:450-455.

40. Klieverik LM, Takkenberg JJ, Bekkers JA, et al: The Ross operation: a Trojan horse? Eur Heart J 2007;28:1993-2000.

41. Stelzer P: Reoperation for dilatation of the pulmonary autograft after the Ross procedure. J Thorac Cardiovasc Surg 2002;124:417-418.

42. Sievers H, Dahmen G, Graf B, et al: Midterm results of the Ross procedure preserving the patient's aortic root. Circulation 2003;108(Suppl 1):II55-II60.

43. Bohm JO, Botha CA, Hemmer W, et al: Hemodynamic performance following the Ross operation: comparison of two different techniques. J Heart Valve Dis 2004;13:174-181.

44. Bauer M, Pasic M, Schaffarzyk R, et al: Reduction aortoplasty for dilatation of the ascending aorta in patients with bicuspid aortic valve. Ann Thorac Surg 2002;73:720-723.

45. Roos-Hesselink JW, Schölzel BE, Heijdra RJ, et al: Aortic valve and aortic arch pathology after coarctation repair Heart 2003;89:1074-1077.

46. Yacoub MH, Klieverik LM, Melina G, et al: An evaluation of the Ross operation in adults. J Heart Valve Dis 2006;15:531-539.

47. Oury JH, Doty DB, Oswalt JD, et al: Cardiopulmonary response to maximal exercise in young athletes following the Ross procedure. Ann Thorac Surg 1998;66(6 Suppl):S153-S154.

48. Pibarot P, Dumesnil JG, Briand M, et al: Hemodynamic performance during maximum exercise in adult patients with the Ross operation and comparison with normal controls and patients with aortic bioprostheses. Am J Cardiol 2000;86:982-988.

49. Al-Halees Z, Pieters F, Qadoura F, et al: The Ross procedure is the procedure of choice for congenital aortic valve disease. J Thorac Cardiovasc Surg 2002;123:437-442.

50. Schmidtke C, Dahmen G, Graf B, Sievers HH: Pulmonary homograft muscle reduction to reduce the risk of homograft stenosis in the Ross procedure. J Thorac Cardiovasc Surg 2007;133:190-195.

51. Khambadkone S, Bonhoeffer P: Nonsurgical pulmonary valve replacement: why, when, and how? Catheter Cardiovasc Interv 2004;62:401-408.

52. Bentall H, De Bono A: A technique for complete replacement of the ascending aorta. Thorax 1968;23:338-339.

53. Etz CD, Homann TM, Rane N, et al: Aortic root reconstruction with a bioprosthetic valved conduit: a consecutive series of 275 procedures. J Thorac Cardiovasc Surg 2007;133:1455-1463.

54. Kvitting JP, Ebbers T, Wigstrom L, et al: Flow patterns in the aortic root and the aorta studied with time-resolved, 3-dimensional, phase-contrast magnetic resonance imaging: implications for aortic valve-sparing surgery. J Thorac Cardiovasc Surg 2004;127:1602-1607.

55. Karck M, Kallenbach K, Hagl C, et al: Aortic root surgery in Marfan syndrome: comparison of aortic valve-sparing reimplantation versus composite grafting. J Thorac Cardiovasc Surg 2004;127:391-398.

56. David TE, Feindel CM. An aortic valve-sparing operation for patients with aortic incompetence and aneurysm of the ascending aorta. J Thorac Cardiovasc Surg 1992;103:617-622.

57. David TE, Feidel CM, Webb GD, et al: Aortic valve preservation in patients with aortic root aneurysm: results of the reimplantation technique. Ann Thorac Surg 2007;63:S732-S735.

58. Demers P, Miller DC: Simple modification of "T. David-V" valve-sparing aortic root replacement to create graft pseudosinuses. Ann Thorac Surg 2004;78:1479-1481.

59. Aicher D, Langer F, Lausberg H, et al: Aortic root remodeling: ten-year experience with 274 patients. J Thorac Cardiovasc Surg 2007;134:909-915.

60. Blais C, Dumesnil JG, Baillot R, et al: Impact of valve prosthesis-patient mismatch on short-term mortality after aortic valve replacement. Circulation 2003;108:983-988.

61. Mohty D, Malouf JF, Girard SE, et al: Impact of prosthesis-patient mismatch on long-term survival in patients with small St. Jude Medical mechanical prostheses in the aortic position. Circulation 2006;113:420-426.

62. Blackstone EH, Cosgrove DM, Jamieson WR, et al: Prosthesis size and long-term survival after aortic valve replacement. J Thorac Cardiovasc Surg 2003;126:783-796.

63. Moon MR, Pasque MK, Munfakh NA, et al: Prosthesis-patient mismatch after aortic valve replacement: impact of age and body size on late survival. Ann Thorac Surg 2006;81:481-488.

64. Nicks R, Cartmill T, Bernstein L: Hypoplasia of the aortic root: the problem of aortic valve replacement. Thorax 1970;25:339-346.

65. Manouguian S, Seybold-Epting W: Patch enlargement of the aortic valve ring by extending the aortic incision into the anterior mitral leaflet: new operative technique. J Thorac Cardiovasc Surg 1979;78:402-412.

66. Konno S, Imai Y, Iida Y, et al. A new method for prosthetic valve replacement in congenital aortic stenosis associated with hypoplasia of the aortic valve ring. J Thorac Cardiovasc Surg 1975;70:909-917.

67. Fusco DS, Shaw RK, Tranquilli M, et al: Femoral cannulation is safe for type A dissection repair. Ann Thorac Surg 2004;78:1285-1289.

68. Reece TB, Tribble CG, Smith RL, Singh RR, Stiles BM, Peeler BB, et al. Central cannulation is safe in acute aortic dissection repair. J Thorac Cardiovasc Surg 2007;133:428-434.

69. Girardi LN, Krieger KH, Mack CA, et al: Reoperations on the ascending aorta and aortic root in patients with previous cardiac surgery. Ann Thorac Surg 2006;82:1407-1412.

70. Byrne JG, Karavas AN, Filsoufi F, et al: Aortic valve surgery after previous coronary artery bypass grafting with functioning internal mammary artery grafts. Ann Thorac Surg 2002;73:779-784.

71. Etz CD, Homann TM, Silovitz D, et al: Long-term survival after the Bentall procedure in 206 patients with bicuspid aortic valve. Ann Thorac Surg 2007;84:1186-1193.

72. Bonacchi M, Priffi E, Giunti G, et al: Does ministernotomy improve postoperative outcome in aortic valve operation? A prospective randomized study. Ann Thorac Surg 2002;73:460-465.

73. Mihaljevic T, Cohn LH, Unic D, et al: One thousand minimally invasive valve operations: early and late results. Ann Surg 2004;240:529-534.

74. Cribier A, Eltchaninoff H, Tron C, et al: Treatment of calcific aortic stenosis with the percutaneous heart valve: mid-term follow-up from the initial feasibility studies: the French experience. J Am Coll Cardiol 2006;47:1214-1223.

75. Webb JG, Lichtenstein S. Transcatheter percutaneous and transapical aortic valve replacement. Semin Thorac Cardiovasc Surg 2007;19:304-310.

76. Walther T, Simon P, Dewey T, et al: Transapical minimally invasive aortic valve implantation: multicenter experience. Circulation 2007;116(11 Suppl):I240-I245.

77. Walther T, Falk V, Dewey T, et al: Valve-in-a-valve concept for transcatheter minimally invasive repeat xenograft implantation. J Am Coll Cardiol 2007;50:56-60.

78. Rankin JS, Hammill BG, Ferguson TB Jr, et al: Determinants of operative mortality in valvular heart surgery. J Thorac Cardiovasc Surg 2006;131:547-557.

CHAPTER 13

Percutaneous Aortic Valve Implantation

Brad Munt

KEY POINTS

- The field of percutaneous aortic valve implantation is rapidly evolving.
- Definitive therapy of valvular aortic stenosis requires relief of obstruction to left ventricular ejection.
- Currently, open surgical aortic valve replacement (or repair in rare instances) is the most commonly used modality and offers excellent long-term results.
- Approximately one third of patients with symptomatic aortic stenosis are denied traditional surgery.
- Interest in a percutaneous approach to aortic valve implantation started with animal work of Andersen et al. Cribier et al. are credited with the first implantation in humans.
- Two types of aortic valves for percutaneous implantation have been used in a significant number of patients: balloon-expandable and self-expanding.
- Percutaneous aortic valve implantation was successful in more than 90% of patients in recent series.
- Medium term outcomes after percutaneous aortic valve implantation show good hemodynamic and clinical results.
- Alternatives to percutaneous aortic valve implantation include surgical aortic valve replacement, aortic balloon valvuloplasty, aortic balloon valvuloplasty followed by external beam radiation, and apical to aortic conduit.
- The Placement of AoRTic traNscathetER Valve (PARTNER) trial using the Edwards Sapien transcatheter valve systems is ongoing and should provide information on the safety and effectiveness of the device and delivery systems in patients with severe symptomatic aortic stenosis at high surgical risk for aortic valve replacement and in patients who are not candidates for surgery.

Definitive therapy of valvular aortic stenosis requires relief of obstruction to left ventricular ejection. Currently, open surgical aortic valve replacement (or repair in rare instances) is the most commonly used modality and offers excellent long-term results.[1] However, given the aging of the population, the frequency of patients presenting for reoperation, and medical advances that have allowed patients with comorbidities to survive and present with valvular aortic stenosis, a significant number of patients are deemed to have excessive risk for traditional surgery. Percutaneous techniques, therefore, were developed initially to offer relief of obstruction to left ventricular ejection in patients who were not candidates for surgery. Initial results with aortic balloon valvuloplasty were disappointing, with neither long-term hemodynamic nor clinical improvement noted.[2] The need for alternative treatment options including percutaneous aortic valve implantation is demonstrated by the Euro Heart Survey on Valvular Heart Disease, in which up to one third of patients with symptomatic aortic stenosis were denied traditional surgery.[3]

Interest in a percutaneous approach to aortic valve implantation started with the animal work of Andersen et al,[4] followed by work of a number of groups. Cribier et al.[5] are credited with the first implantation in humans. These pioneers led the development of percutaneous techniques for aortic valve implantation and have opened a new era in the therapy of patients with valvular aortic stenosis.

PATIENT SELECTION FOR PERCUTANEOUS AORTIC VALVE IMPLANTATION

No randomized trials of surgical versus percutaneous implantation of an aortic prosthesis have been reported, although at least one such study is underway (the Placement of AoRTic traNscathetER valve [PARTNER] trial, see ongoing trials section below). Therefore, to date, candidates for percutaneous aortic valve implantation have primarily included patients with a contraindication to or high risk for surgical aortic valve replacement.[6-9] This profile was demonstrated in one series[7] of patients who underwent percutaneous aortic valve implantation with a balloon-expandable valve via a transfemoral approach; the mean age was 82 ± 7 years (range, 62 to 94 years) with a logistic EuroSCORE (used to predict operative mortality) of 28%. Comorbidities included coronary artery disease in 72%, moderate to severe mitral regurgitation in 48%, severe lung disease in 32%, prior thoracotomy in 34%, porcelain aorta in 16%, severe

TABLE 13–1 | **Indications and Contraindications for Percutaneous Aortic Valve Implantation**

Indications

Severe symptomatic valvular aortic stenosis (generally an aortic valve area <0.7 cm²/m² body surface area) with one or more of the following

High risk for conventional aortic valve surgery (generally a logistic EuroScore >20% or Society of Thoracic Surgeons score >10)

Porcelain aorta

Previous (usually multiple) thoracotomies or radiation therapy with anatomy that would make repeat thoracotomy not an option

Severe pulmonary disease (forced expiratory volume <1 L/sec)

Cirrhosis of the liver

Contraindications

Patients in whom a conventional surgical aortic valve procedure can be done at acceptable risk (except patients enrolled in a trial of percutaneous versus conventional aortic valve implantation)

An aortic annulus too small or too large for the prosthesis

An ascending aorta (specifically at the sinotubular junction) too large for the prosthesis (applies to the CoreValve prosthesis)

Severe iliofemoral disease (vessel size too small to accommodate the sheath, these patients can be considered for implantation with a transapical transcatheter technique, an antegrade technique, or subclavian approach)

Patients in whom relief of their aortic stenosis will not improve their quality or prolong their life

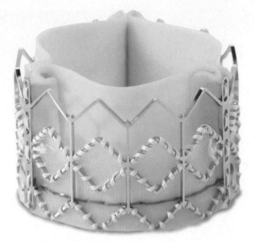

FIGURE 13–1 Edwards Sapien balloon expandable transcatheter heart valve shown with the leaflets in the open (systolic) position. The valve consists of a tubular slotted stainless steel stent with attached bovine pericardial leaflets and a fabric cuff. The ventricular end of the valve is marked with the green suture. *(Courtesy of Edwards Lifesciences, Irvine, CA.)*

pulmonary hypertension in 18%, prior cerebral ischemic events in 12%, and severe debility in 22%. In another series[9] in which a balloon-expandable valve with a transapical tran-scatheter technique was implanted, patients had a mean age of 81 ± 6 years with 75% women. The logistic EuroSCORE was 27 ± 14%. Comorbidities included coronary artery disease in 37%, prior cardiac surgery in 17%, prior cerebral ischemic events in 15%, and prior recent myocardial infarction in 12%. These demographics should be kept in mind when the results of the procedure are evaluated.

Contraindications to percutaneous aortic valve implantation partially depend on the technique of implantation used. Current indications and contraindications are presented in Table 13-1.

It must be emphasized that percutaneous aortic valve implantation is a rapidly advancing field and that limited experience exists in patient selection to date; selection criteria will undoubtedly evolve as experience accrues.

PERCUTANEOUS AORTIC VALVE DESIGNS

Two types of aortic valves for percutaneous implantation have been used in a significant number of patients: balloon-expandable and self-expanding.

Balloon-Expandable Percutaneous Aortic Valves

Balloon-expandable prostheses with published human implantation data include the first-generation Cribier-Edwards valve and the slightly modified second generation Sapien valve (both from Edwards Lifesciences, Irvine, CA) (Figure 13-1). The Sapien valve is available in 23- and 26-mm sizes (referring to the valve diameter). The 23-mm valve is 14.5 mm in length when fully expanded and the 26-mm is 16 mm in length. The valve consists of a tubular slotted stain-less steel stent with attached bovine pericardial leaflets and a fabric cuff (initially the leaflets were equine pericardium). In vitro testing has repeatedly shown the durability of the valve to be greater than 200 million cycles corresponding to more than 5 years of life.[10]

On September 5, 2007, Edwards Lifesciences announced that it had received CE Mark approval for European commercial sales of its Edwards Sapien transcatheter aortic heart valve technology with the RetroFlex transfemoral delivery system. On March 5, 2008, Edwards announced that the first three human implants of a next-generation Edwards transcatheter aortic heart valve was performed at St. Paul's Hospital in Vancouver, BC, Canada. This next-generation balloon-expandable pericardial tissue valve features a cobalt chromium alloy frame that reduces the profile by 4 to 5 F over the Sapien delivery system.

Implantation

Percutaneous Transvenous and Transarterial Techniques. The largest clinical experience is with the Edwards Lifesciences series of balloon-expandable aortic valves. This valve is available in a 23- and 26-mm size (referring to the fully expanded stent diameter: the 23-mm valve is 14.5 cm in length and the 26-mm valve is 16 mm in length) (see Figure 13-1). The initial implantation technique involved an antegrade approach to the native aortic valve with trans-venous access to the right atrium and a transseptal puncture for access to the left atrium followed by passage of the valve across the mitral valve and positioning in the aortic annulus.[5,11] Our group and others found this technique technically challenging, and we therefore developed a transfemoral retrograde technique that we now use routinely in the majority of our implants.[6]

Before valve implantation, patients undergo transthoracic echocardiography, iliofemoral contrast angiography, and coronary angiography. Computed tomography of the iliofemoral system is performed if a decision on the adequacy of arterial access cannot be made from angiography alone. If, in the opinion of the interventional cardiologist, the iliofemoral system is too small, diseased, or tortuous to safely reach the aortic valve, the patient will be considered for a transapical transcatheter approach (see below). An iliofemoral diameter of 8 mm or larger is considered adequate for using the transfemoral approach with the 22-F sheath and 9 mm for the 24-F sheath; patients with short segments of noncalcified focal stenosis less than these diameters are not excluded. Significant obstructive coronary artery disease is treated percutaneously as per American College of Cardiology/American Heart Association guidelines in a separate procedure usually during the coronary angiogram or in a separate setting before the aortic valve implantation.

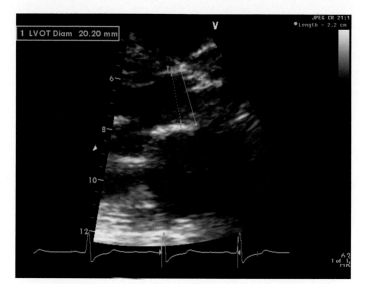

FIGURE 13–2 Measurement of the aortic annulus diameter at the cusp insertion on transthoracic echocardiography. The annulus measures 22 mm and the left ventricular outflow tract (LVOT) measures 20 mm. The measurement of this annulus by transesophageal echocardiography is presented in Figure 13-3.

The aortic annulus diameter at the level of the aortic cusp insertion is measured on a transthoracic echocardiogram if possible (Figure 13-2); patients are currently excluded if the diameter is less than 18 mm or greater than 26 mm. If an accurate diameter cannot be measured on the transthoracic echocardiogram (in our experience this included 5% to 10% of patients), a transesophageal echocardiogram is performed and the annulus diameter is measured (Figure 13-3). There is a tendency for the diameters we measure on a transesophageal echocardiogram to be larger than those we measure on a transthoracic echocardiogram (Figure 13-4).

Valve implantation is performed in the cardiac catheterization laboratory or hybrid operating room, usually with general anesthesia and fluoroscopy and transesophageal echocardiography. Patients are premedicated with aspirin, clopidogrel, and vancomycin. Unfractionated heparin is given to maintain an activated clotting time greater than 250 seconds. Anesthesia is maintained using conventional techniques with short-acting vasopressors to maintain adequate perfusion pressure during the procedure: the importance of skilled anesthesia management in

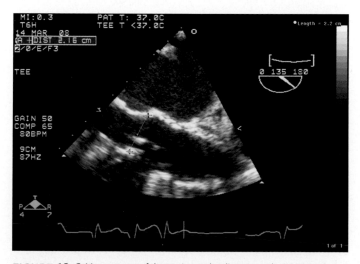

FIGURE 13–3 Measurement of the aortic annulus diameter at the cusp insertion on transesophageal echocardiography. The annulus measures 22 mm. The measurement of this annulus by transthoracic echocardiography is presented in Figure 13-2.

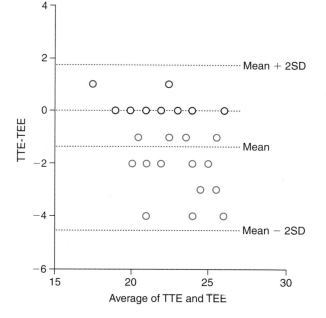

The mean difference (TTE-TEE) is −1.36 mm (2 SD −4.48 to +1.75 mm)

FIGURE 13–4 Bland-Altman plot illustrating the difference between the aortic annulus diameter by transthoracic (TTE) and transesophageal echocardiography (TEE). The red circles indicate larger dimensions by transthoracic imaging, the black circles indicate agreement, and the green circles indicate larger dimensions by transesophageal echocardiography. *(From Moss RR, Ivans E, Pasupati S, et al: Role of echocardiography in percutaneous aortic valve implantation. J Am Coll Cardiol Imaging 2008;1:15-24, with permission.)*

these procedures cannot be overestimated. Sheaths are placed percutaneously in both femoral arteries and one femoral vein. If a percutaneous closure of the femoral artery is planned a preclosure strategy is used with a commercial suture-based closure device to place but not tie the sutures (i.e., Prostar XL suture-mediated closure; Abbott Vascular, Redwood City, CA). An aortic root angiogram is performed to outline the aortic root anatomy and facilitate valve positioning.

The aortic annulus size at the aortic cusp insertion is measured on a transesophageal echocardiogram; we usually measure in the midesophageal long-axis view at approximately 130° of probe rotation (see Figure 13-3). We generally implant a 23-mm valve in annuli that measure 18 to 22 mm in diameter and a 26-mm valve in annuli that measure 23 to 26 mm. An intraprocedural diameter greater than 26 mm was measured in only one patient; in this patient the annulus measured 28 mm on a intraprocedural transesophageal echocardiogram after measuring 26 mm on a transthoracic echocardiogram, and a 26-mm valve was implanted without serious complication (mild paravalvular aortic regurgitation was seen). Rapid right ventricular pacing is tested as pacing is used to reduce ejection forces and reduce cardiac motion during valve deployment. A balloon aortic valvuloplasty is then performed by standard techniques with a balloon slightly smaller than the planned prosthesis size.

Next a femoral access site is dilated to allow placement of either a 22-F (for a 23-mm valve) or 24-F (for a 26-mm valve) sheath. The valve is then mechanically crimped onto the delivery catheter. With a steerable guiding catheter (Figure 13-5), the balloon-mounted valve is passed retrograde into the aorta and positioned across the aortic valve. Correct positioning coaxial to the aortic root so that the fabric valve cuff is at the correct level is imperative (the ventricular aspect of the prosthetic valve is placed 3 to 4 mm ventricular to the insertion point of the native aortic cusps into the aorta before balloon inflation; we aim for the final position

13

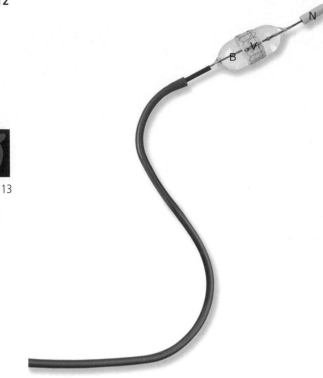

FIGURE 13–5 Edwards Retroflex II delivery catheter for percutaneous, transcatheter aortic valve implantation with an Edwards Sapien valve mounted on an inflated balloon. Note the yellow nose cone designed to allow easier crossing of the stenotic native aortic valve. The green suture line marks the ventricular end of the valve. C, delivery catheter; B, inflated balloon; V, valve; N, nose cone. *(Courtesy of Edwards Lifesciences, Irvine, CA.)*

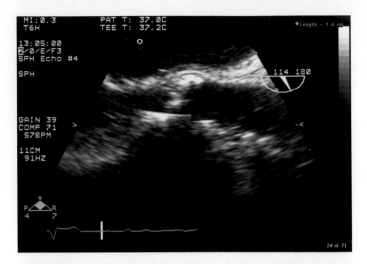

FIGURE 13–6 Transesophageal echocardiogram of a 26-mm Edwards Sapien valve positioned "too ventricularly" for proper deployment. The 16-mm length of the stent is measured on the image. The ventricular end of the stent is approximately 8 mm from the native valve cusp insertion into the aorta; the correct position is 3 to 4 mm.

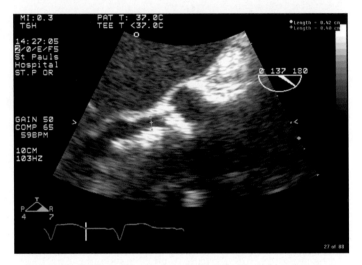

FIGURE 13–7 Transesophageal echocardiogram of a 23-mm Edwards Sapien valve positioned 4 mm from the native aortic valve cusp insertion into the aorta. The aortic end of the valve stent is not well seen. The green line marks the ventricular end of the valve stent; the blue line measures the 4-mm distance from the calcified native aortic valve cusp to the ventricular end of the stent. This is correct valve positioning before balloon inflation.

of the ventricular aspect of the prosthetic valve to be 2 mm ventricular to the insertion point of the native aortic cusps into the aorta). Positioning is accomplished with a combination of fluoroscopic, aortic root angiographic, and transesophageal echocardiographic imaging. Because the valve tends to move "aortically" during balloon inflation, we try to position the ventricular end of the valve 3 to 4 mm ventricular to the native aortic cusp insertion point in the aorta before final deployment (Figures 13-6 and 13-7). Some indication of the degree of prosthetic valve movement expected during balloon inflation can be obtained during the aortic balloon valvuloplasty that is also done with rapid right ventricular pacing.

Once a suitable valve position is confirmed using a consensus of fluoroscopic, angiographic, and echocardiographic imaging, the valve is deployed by inflating the balloon. If there is more than mild paravalvular aortic regurgitation after initial deployment, a repeat balloon dilation of the valve can be performed. After the procedure, the femoral access site is closed either surgically or with a commercial percutaneous closure device (i.e., Prostar XL suture-mediated closure).

Transapical Transcatheter Balloon-Expandable Valve Implantation. Although not truly percutaneous, a left ventricular transapical transcatheter approach to implantation of a balloon-expandable aortic valve has been developed to offer therapy to patients who do not have adequate transfemoral access.[9,10] Once again, patients are premedicated with aspirin, clopidogrel, and vancomycin. The procedure is performed in an operating room under fluoroscopic and transesophageal echocardiography guidance. We size the valves the same as for transfemoral implantation. We generally implant a 23-mm valve in annuli that measure 18 to 22 mm in diameter and a 26-mm valve in annuli that measure 23 to 26 mm.

Preprocedure imaging is identical to that performed for the retrograde femoral approach, and the same valves (Edwards Sapien) are used. After induction of general anesthesia with a double lumen intubation, the apex of the patient's left ventricle is identified using palpation and fluoroscopy. A 5- to 8-cm anterolateral thoracotomy incision is made to enter the pleural space overlying the apex. The pericardium overlying the left ventricular apex is opened, and the thin portion of the left ventricular apex is identified by simultaneous palpation and transesophageal echocardiography imaging. Paired orthogonal U-shaped sutures with pledgets are placed into the myocardium and passed through tensioning tourniquets. A 7-F sheath is placed through the apex into the left ventricle using a standard needle puncture and over-the-wire technique. Care is taken to avoid air entry into the left ventricle. Unfractionated heparin is given to achieve an activated clotting time greater than 250 seconds.

A stiff wire is introduced through the sheath into the left ventricle and advanced through the aortic valve and into the descending aorta. A pigtail catheter is placed via a femoral artery to perform aortic root angiography as required. The 7-F sheath is exchanged for a 14-F sheath, and an aortic balloon valvuloplasty is performed using rapid pacing. The 14-F sheath is replaced with a 24-F sheath. The prosthesis that has been mechanically crimped onto the balloon-tipped steerable catheter (Figure 13-8) is introduced through this larger sheath, positioned coaxial to the aortic root so that the fabric valve cuff is at the correct level. The ventricular aspect of the prosthetic valve should be 3 to 4 mm ventricular to the insertion point of the native aortic cusps into the aorta before balloon inflation; we aim for the final position of the ventricular aspect of the prosthetic valve to be 2 mm ventricular to the insertion point of the native aortic cusps into the aorta. Positioning is

accomplished with a combination of fluoroscopic, aortic root angiographic, and transesophageal echocardiographic imaging. Because the valve tends to move aortically during balloon inflation, we try to place the ventricular end of the valve 3 to 4 mm ventricular to the aortic cusp insertion point in the aorta before final deployment. The valve is then deployed by inflating the balloon with rapid pacing. If more than mild paravalvular aortic regurgitation is present, another balloon dilation of the valve can be performed. At this point, the sheath is removed, and homeostasis is secured with the previously placed pledgeted sutures. The pericardium is approximated, drainage tubes are placed, and the chest incision is closed.

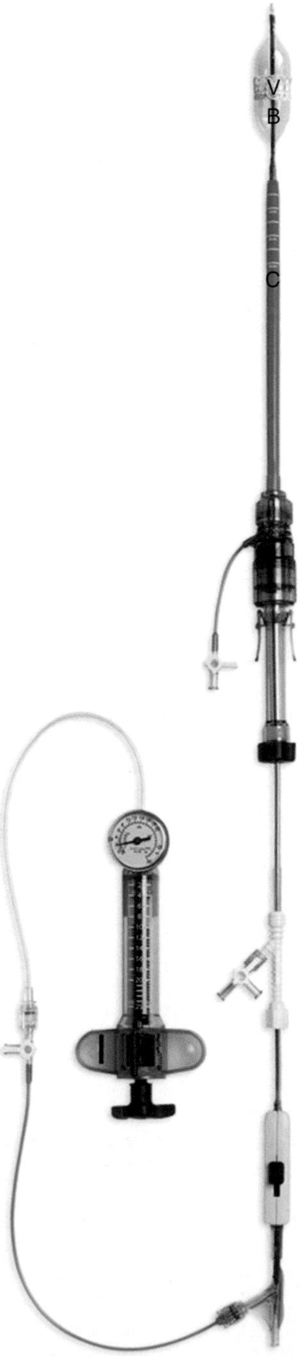

Procedural Success and Complications

After an initial learning curve of approximately 25 procedures with the transfemoral approach and fewer with the transapical approach (when the transapical approach is performed by a team involving cardiac surgeons and cardiologists with interventional and echocardiographic expertise), excellent rates of procedural success with low intraprocedural mortality can be achieved. The standard complications of interventional cardiovascular procedures, valve implantation, and anesthesia as well as some rate of unsuccessful implantation should be expected with percutaneous aortic valve procedures. Vascular access complications occur more often than with other interventional procedures, and are more severe with transfemoral procedures because of the large size of the sheaths. Transapical, transcatheter techniques will also have the complications associated with a limited thoracotomy.

The unsuccessful implantation in 7 of the initial 50 transfemoral procedures[7] done at St. Paul's Hospital was reported to be due to an inability to pass the iliac artery in 1 patient, inability to cross the aortic valve in 3 patients, a defective prototype delivery catheter in 1 patient, and malpositioning in 2 patients. Other complications are presented in Table 13-2 No patient needed emergency cardiac surgery or developed endocarditis. Complications in the first 100 patients receiving implants at St. Paul's Hospital,[12] a series that includes the 50 transfemoral procedures presented in Table 13-3, included malposition of the aortic prosthesis in 3% of patients and a periprocedural cardiovascular accidents (CVA) in 4%.

Procedural success overall in 43 of 50 patients receiving implants at a single center (86% overall: 76% in the first 25 patients and 96% in the second 25 patients) with the transfemoral approach has been reported.[7]

The results for the first 100 patients receiving implants at St. Paul's Hospital in Vancouver with the Sapien series of

FIGURE 13–8 Edwards Acsendra delivery system for transapical, transcatheter aortic valve implantation with an Edwards Sapien valve mounted on an inflated balloon. C, delivery catheter; B, inflated balloon; V, valve; I, balloon inflation mechanism. (*Courtesy of Edwards Lifesciences, Irvine, CA.*)

TABLE 13–2	Outcome and Complications of Transfemoral Aortic Valve Implantation in 50 Patients
Characteristic	***n* (%)**
Procedural success	43 (86)
Stroke	2 (4)
Myocardial infarction	1 (2)
Ventricular fibrillation	2 (4)
Heart block, new and sustained	2 (4)
Tamponade*	1 (2)
Transfusion >3 units	9 (18)
Emergency cardiac surgery	0 (0)
Endocarditis	0 (0)
Death, intraprocedural	1 (2)
Death, 30 days	6 (12)
Death, stroke, or myocardial infarction at 30 days	8 (16)

*Complication of postprocedural implantation of a permanent pacemaker.

From Webb JG, Pasupati S, Humphries K, et al: Percutaneous transarterial aortic valve replacement in selected high-risk patients with aortic stenosis. Circulation 2007; 116:755-763, with permission.

TABLE 13–3	Postoperative Outcome and Follow-up of 59 Consecutive Patients Undergoing Attempted Implantation of an Edwards Sapien Transcatheter Heart Valve Prosthesis by a Transapical Minimally Invasive Approach
Intubation time, median (hr)	6
Same day extubation, n (%)	37 (62.7)
Intensive card unit stay, median (hr)	20
Postoperative complications	
None	11
Stroke	2
Pleural effusion	18
Supraventricular arrhythmia	18
Transient hemofiltration	8
Tracheostomy	8
Cardiopulmonary resuscitation (successful)	4 (3)
Pericardial effusion	3
Rethoracotomy (chest wall/diffuse bleeding)	8 (7)
30-day mortality, n (%)	8 (13.6)
In-hospital mortality, n (%)	8 (13.6)
Follow-up mortality, n (%)	5 (9.8)
Overall mortality, n (%)	13 (22%)
Follow-up interval, days	110 ± 77

From Wather T, Simon P, Dewey T, et al: Transapical minimally invasive aortic valve implantation: Multicenter experience. Circulation 2007;116:1240-1245, with permission.

TABLE 13–4	Echocardiographic Results at Follow-up of Consecutive Patients Undergoing Attempted Implantation of an Edwards Sapien Transcatheter Heart Valve Prosthesis by a Transapical Minimally Invasive Approach
n	40
V_{max} (m/sec)	2.0 ± 0.6 (1.81-2.19)
ΔP_{max} (mmHg)	18 ± 11 (14.9-21.1)
ΔP_{mean} (mmHg)	9 ± 6 (7.3-10.7)
Grade of aortic incompetence	
None	14
Trace	11
Mild (1 degree)	12
Moderate (1-2 degrees)	2
Severe (2 degrees or higher)	1
Paravalvular incompetence	17/26

Numbers in parentheses are 95% confidence interval

ΔP_{mean}, mean transvalvular pressure gradient; ΔP_{max}, maximum transvalvular pressure gradient; V_{max}, maximum transvalvular blood flow velocity.

From Wather T, Simon P, Dewey T, et al: Transapical minimally invasive aortic valve implantation: Multicenter experience. Circulation 2007; 116:1240-1245, used with permission.

valves has been reported in abstract form.[12] Implantation in 74 patients was attempted with the transfemoral approach, and 26 patients had a transapical approach. The mean age was 83 years (range, 58 to 97 years) with 56% males. Data are presented based on the sequence of procedures performed: the first 1 to 25, the next 26 to 50, and the most recent 51 to 74 transfemoral and 1 to 26 transapical procedures. Procedural success was 91% overall (76%, 96%, 96%, and 96%, respectively). Malposition occurred in 3 patients (8%, 0%, 0%, and 4%). A periprocedural CVA occurred in 4% with 1 patient in each group. Intraprocedural mortality was 2% (4%, 0%, 0%, and 4%). The logistic EuroSCORE was 33% (26%, 30%, 36%, and 38%); the actual operative (30-day) mortality was 15% (16%, 8%, 12%, and 24%).

Postoperative complications and outcome of a surgical series[9] of 59 attempted transapical transcatheter valve implantations with a 90% initial success rate are presented in Table 13-3.

Immediate Hemodynamic Results

Gradients and aortic valve areas appear better than expected compared to biologic valves surgically implanted in similar sized annuli; however, this result occurs at a cost of higher rates of aortic regurgitation than with conventional biologic aortic valve replacements.[7-9,12,13] Based on 100 patients receiving implants at St. Paul's Hospital,[12] hemodynamics improved from baseline values of 0.6 ± 0.2 cm² aortic valve area and 46 ± 16 mm Hg mean transaortic systolic gradient to values at hospital discharge (median discharge on day 5 after the procedure; interquartile range, 4 to 12 days) of 1.7 ± 0.4 cm² for aortic valve area and 10 ± 5 mmHg for the mean transaortic systolic gradient. Median aortic regurgitation grade was mild (interquartile range, trace to mild) at baseline and at discharge; no patient had severe aortic regurgitation. In a transapical transcatheter series,[9] hemodynamics (by transthoracic echocardiography) at discharge showed a mean gradient of 9 ± 6 mm Hg; the preoperative gradients were not stated in the article but preoperative aortic valve area was 0.2 to 0.9 cm². Aortic

regurgitation was reported as none in 14 patients, trace in 11 patients, mild in 12 patients, moderate in 2 patients, and severe in 1 patient (Table 13-4).

Long-Term Outcome

Because most percutaneous aortic valves have been implanted in patients deemed to have excessive risk for conventional surgery, comparing long-term outcomes between conventional surgery and percutaneous implantation is difficult. We have experienced good valve durability and preserved hemodynamics in the patients we have followed. The PARTNER trial should provide valuable data comparing a conventional to a percutaneous approach (see ongoing trials section below).

In the series of 50 transfemoral procedures at St. Paul's Hospital[7] at 359 days of follow-up (interquartile range, 60 to 371 days), 35 of 43 (81%) patients undergoing successful transcatheter aortic valve replacement remained alive. Figure 13-9 illustrates the Kaplan-Meier survival after percutaneous valve implantation. Structural valve deterioration was not observed during follow-up. Of the 37 patients who reached a 1-month follow-up with an implanted prosthesis, 70% were in New York Heart Association class III and 16% were in class IV before the procedure; 1 month after the procedure 11% of patients were in class III, and no patient was in class IV ($P < 0.01$) (Figure 13-10E). Improvements were also seen in left ventricular systolic function with an ejection fraction less than 40% in 21% of patients before the procedure but only 12% of patients at discharge ($P < 0.01$). Mitral regurgitation was also reduced with moderate or severe mitral regurgitation in 53% of patients before the procedure compared to 33% at discharge ($P < 0.01$) (see Figure 13-10).

In the 7 of 50 patients, in whom the initial transfemoral percutaneous aortic valve implantation procedure was not successful[7] (6 of these 7 patients did have a balloon aortic valvuloplasty performed as part of the attempted valve implantation), subsequent aortic valve procedures were performed in 3 patients. In each patient, the reason was ongoing symptomatic aortic stenosis after the unsuccessful transcatheter procedure. Repeat valve procedures consisted of 1 transapical transcatheter aortic valve implantation, 1 conventional surgical aortic valve replacement, and 1 reattempted transfemoral transcatheter implantation. All 3 procedures were successful with all 3 patients remaining alive at the 30-day postprocedure follow-up.

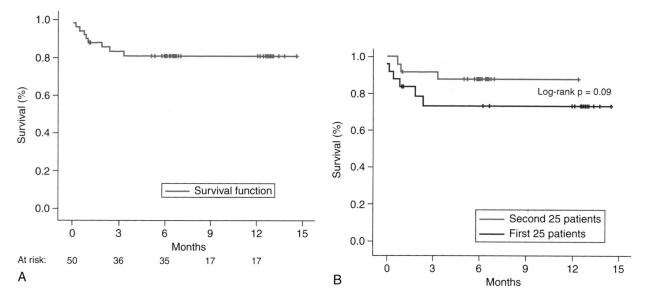

FIGURE 13–9 Kaplan-Meier survival. **A,** First consecutive 50 transarterial aortic valve implantation patients done at St. Paul's Hospital in Vancouver, BC, Canada. Logistic EuroSCORE mortality estimate was 28%. **B,** First 25 patients versus second 25 patients for 50 transarterial aortic valve implantations done at St. Paul's Hospital. Logistic EuroSCORE estimates were 26% and 30%, respectively. In this series the Cribier Edwards valve (Edwards Lifesciences, Irvine, CA) was implanted. *(From Webb JG, Pasupati S, Humphries K, et al: Percutaneous transarterial aortic valve replacement in selected high-risk patients with aortic stenosis. Circulation 2007;116:755-763, with permission.)*

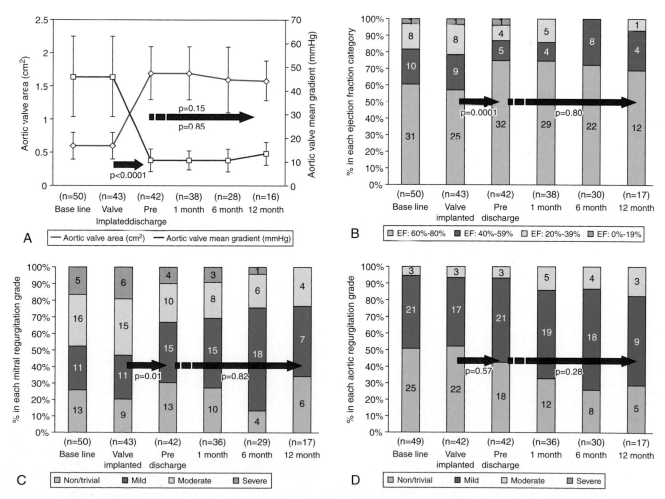

FIGURE 13–10 Follow-up of functional class and echocardiographic parameters of the first consecutive 50 transarterial aortic valve implantations done at St. Paul's Hospital in Vancouver, BC, Canada. **A,** Time trends in aortic valve area and aortic valve mean gradient (error bars indicate ± 1 SD). **B,** Time trend in left ventricular ejection fraction (EF). **C,** Time trend in mitral regurgitation. **D,** Time trend in aortic regurgitation.

Continued

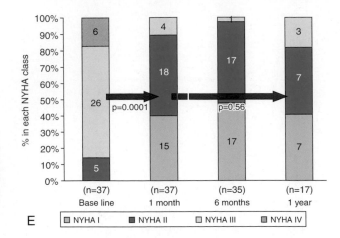

E

FIGURE 13–10 Cont'd—E, New York Heart Association (NYHA) functional class in patients who reached the 1-month follow-up. In this series the Cribier Edwards valve (Edwards Lifesciences, Irvine, CA) was implanted. *(From Webb JG, Pasupati S, Humphries K, et al: Percutaneous transarterial aortic valve replacement in selected high-risk patients with aortic stenosis. Circulation 2007;116:755-763, with permission.)*

Postoperative complications and outcome of a surgical series of 59 attempted transapical transcatheter aortic valve implantations are presented in Table 13-3.

Self-Expanding Valves

Self-expanding valves with published human implantation data include the CoreValve series of prosthesis (CoreValve Inc., Irvine, CA) (Figure 13-11). The 26-mm inflow size (small valve) is intended for patients with an aortic annulus measuring between 20 and 23 mm and the 29-mm inflow size (large valve) is intended for patients with an aortic annulus

measuring between 24 and 27 mm. The CoreValve technology features a multilevel frame with pericardial leaflets. The term "frame" is used rather than stent because by engineering definition, a stent exhibits the same radial force at every point of its peripheral circumference; the CoreValve frame exhibits three entirely different radial and hoop strength levels at different parts of its peripheral circumference.

Other self-expanding valves are also in development but have no published data on human implantation as yet. An example is the JenaValve.[14] This valve incorporates a tissue valve in a frame with positioning hoops. This design is claimed to allow accurate positioning of the valve through the use of the positioning hoops, shortening of the valve frame to facilitate passage through the aortic arch, and the ability to reposition the valve after the frame is initially deployed.

Implantation

The largest experience is with the CoreValve series of self-expanding aortic valves.[15] Initial protocols had patients undergo transthoracic and transesophageal echocardiography, carotid and arteriovenous duplex ultrasonography, computed tomography angiography, coronary angiography, and left ventriculography. Cardiac magnetic resonance imaging was performed in selected patients. Patients were premedicated with aspirin and clopidogrel, and unfractionated heparin was given to achieve an activated clotting time of 300 to 350 seconds. Later protocols have patients undergo transthoracic echocardiography and cardiac catheterization only before the procedure. Activated clotting time targets have been modified to greater than 250 seconds.

With the first- and second-generation devices (25- and 21-F, respectively) the procedure was performed with general anesthesia and with hemodynamic support (extracorporeal percutaneous femorofemoral bypass or tandem heart or extracorporeal membrane oxygenation) and with transesophageal echocardiography. Extracorporeal circulatory support, when used with first- and second-generation devices, was activated just before valve placement and stopped after removal of the delivery catheter and confirmation of adequate valve function. Vascular access was obtained to the common iliac artery, common femoral artery, or subclavian artery with surgical cutdown and repair.

The current valve (third-generation) is delivered through an 18-F system (Figure 13-12); the majority of the procedures are

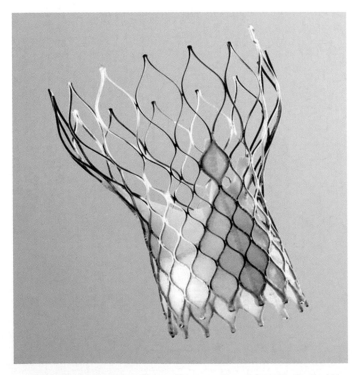

FIGURE 13–11 CoreValve self-expanding transcatheter heart valve. The CoreValve technology features a multilevel frame with pericardial leaflets *(Courtesy of CoreValve Inc., Irvine, CA.)*

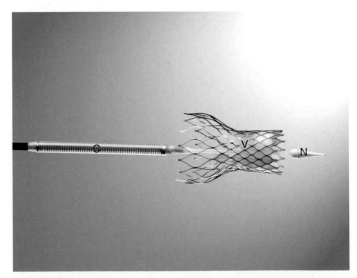

FIGURE 13–12 CoreValve self-expanding transcatheter heart valve and third-generation delivery system. The valve is shown in the deployed position after being extruded from the delivery catheter. The system features a nosecone for easier crossing of the native aortic valve. C, delivery catheter; V, valve; N, nosecone. *(Courtesy of CoreValve Inc., Irvine, CA.)*

performed with local anesthesia with preclosure of the femoral artery (a commercial suture-based closure device is used to place but not tie the sutures preprocedure, i.e., Prostat XL suture-mediated closure). Fluoroscopy guidance only is used without any mechanical hemodynamic support or rapid pacing.

Preimplantation balloon valvuloplasty is performed with a 20- to 25-mm balloon under rapid pacing. A stiff guide wire is then placed in the left ventricle, and the valve is deployed. The CoreValve prosthesis can also be implanted via a transapical, transcatheter technique.[16]

The JenaValve has only been implanted in animals.[14] Implantation involves a retrograde approach to the aortic valve; the positioning hoops are released in the ascending aorta by a retraction of an encasement that permits the protrusion of the valve only as far as the cusps of the original aortic valve. Once the hoops are positioned behind the commissures of the native valve, the prosthetic valve is released by retraction of a retaining jacket. The native valve is compressed against the aortic wall and "sandwiched" between the positioning hoops and the new valve. At this stage, the position can be checked and only after further retraction of the retaining jacket and an additional check of the fit is the JenaValve implant finally released.

Procedural Success and Complications

Similar to results with balloon-expandable aortic valves, excellent rates of procedural success with low intraprocedural mortality can be achieved with self-expanding valves after an initial learning curve. Within the framework of the safety and efficacy studies, 76 of 86 patients (88%) received implants successfully with a combination of retrograde percutaneous access either with or without standard surgical cutdown of the common iliac artery, the common femoral artery, or the subclavian artery. Mean age was 82 ± 6 years. The Logistic EuroSCORE was 22%. A periprocedural CVA occurred in 10% of patients, and procedural mortality (defined as within 48 hours of the procedure) was 6%. Further data are presented in Table 13-5.

Since publication of this series, CoreValve reported that CE Mark approval for the 18-F percutaneous aortic valve replacement ReValving System for both small and large valves was received in mid-2007. The CoreValve system CE Mark-approved indication is "aortic stenosis in high risk patients" within the criteria parameters of the safety and efficacy trials (i.e., 80 years of age or older or Logistic EuroScore >20 or 65 years of age and at least one of a specific list of comorbidities). As of February 14, 2008, a CoreValve registry indicated a mean age of 81 years and a 98% procedural success rate. Because of device size reduction, current ReValving procedures are performed under local anesthesia, without the use of surgical cutdown/repair (with preclosing) and without hemodynamic support or artificially accelerating the heart rate during the valve delivery. Total procedure time (defined as patient arrives to patient leaves laboratory) is typically between 1 and 1½ hours. A valve-in-valve procedure using the CoreValve prosthesis has been reported in a patient with severe aortic regurgitation through a degenerated tissue aortic prosthesis.[17] As of March 12, 2008, CoreValve indicated that more than 700 patients had received implants with its percutaneous aortic valve replacement system and that clinical evaluation was continuing at 38 centers in 12 countries in Europe.

Immediate Hemodynamic Results

The hemodynamics of balloon-expandable aortic valves are better than comparably sized surgically implanted tissue valves, however, this result occurs at a cost of higher rates of aortic regurgitation than with conventional biological aortic valve implantation. Pre- and postimplantation mean systolic gradients across the aortic prosthesis in a series of 86 patients[15] are presented in Figure 13-13. Aortic regurgitation remained unchanged or was reduced in 51 (66%) patients after the procedure. A worsening of the preinterventional aortic regurgitation grade after the procedure to grade 2 was noted in 15 (20%) patients and from 0 to grade 1 in 11 (14%) patients. All aortic regurgitation was due to paravalvular leakages as determined by echocardiography. Severe postprocedural aortic regurgitation (grade 3 or 4) was not present in any patient. After 30 days, the overall grade of aortic regurgitation remained unchanged.

TABLE 13-5	Procedural Major Adverse Cardiac and Cerebral Events (MACCE) in Patients Implanted with the CoreValve Series of Prosthesis		
	Overall (*n* = 86)	21-F (*n* = 50)	18-F (*n* = 36)
Death, *n* (%)	5 (6)	2 (4)	3 (8)
Stroke, *n* (%)	9 (10)	5 (10)	4 (11)
Major, *n* (%)	3 (4)	2 (4)	1 (3)
Minor, *n* (%)	6 (7)	3 (6)	3 (8)
Myocardial infarction, *n* (%)	0	0	0
Cardiac tamponade			
Procedure related	6 (7)	1 (2)	5 (14)
After conversion to surgery	2 (2)	2 (4)	0
Aortic dissection, *n* (%)	0	0	0
Coronary flow impairment, *n* (%)	0	0	0
Conversion to surgery or valvuloplasty, *n* (%)	8 (9)	6 (12)	2 (6)
Procedural MACCE, *n* (%)	22 (26)	11 (22)	11 (28)
Procedural MACCE, excluding conversions*, *n* (%)	14 (18)	5 (11)	9 (26)
Combined death, stroke, and myocardial infarction, *n* (%)	14 (17)	7 (14)	7 (19)
Procedural success, *n* (%)	64 (74)	39 (78)	25 (69)

Based on 78 patients with device success.

From Grube E, Schuler G, Buellesfeld L, et al: Percutaneous aortic valve replacement for severe aortic stenosis in high-risk patients using the second- and current third-generation self-expanding CoreValve prosthesis: device success and 30-day clinical outcome. J Am Coll Cardiol 2007; 50:69-76, with permission.

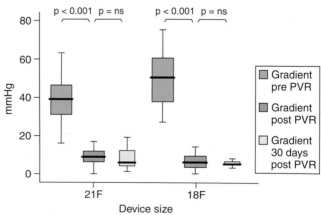

FIGURE 13-13 Mean gradient before versus after implantation of the CoreValve prosthesis (CoreValve Inc., Irvine, CA) versus 30-day follow-up (for patients with procedural success). PVR, percutaneous valve replacement. *(From Grube E, Schuler G, Buellesfeld L, et al: Percutaneous aortic valve replacement for severe aortic stenosis in high-risk patients using the second- and current third-generation self-expanding CoreValve prosthesis: device success and 30-day clinical outcome. J Am Coll Cardiol 2007;50:69-76, with permission.)*

The overall mortality rate at 30 days was 12% in the intent-to-treat population with a combined rate of death, stroke, and myocardial infarction of 22%.[15] With the analysis restricted to patients with device and procedural success, the 30 day mortality was 5%, with a 9% combined rate of death, stroke and myocardial infarction. A decline from a mean New York Heart Association functional class of 2.85 ± 0.73 before to 1.85 ± 0.60 after valve implantation ($P < 0.001$) was reported.

ALTERNATIVES TO PERCUTANEOUS AORTIC VALVE IMPLANTATION

Surgical Aortic Valve Replacement

Surgical aortic valve replacement should be considered in all patients regardless of age. One-, 2-, and 5-year survival rates among selected patients older than 80 years undergoing aortic valve replacement of 87%, 78%, and 68%, respectively, have been reported.[18] In general, I would advocate consideration for surgical aortic valve replacement (or entry into a randomized trial of surgical replacement versus percutaneous aortic valve implantation) in all patients who have a predicted rate of surgical mortality or serious irreversible morbidity of less than 40%.

Aortic Balloon Valvuloplasty

Suggested indications for aortic balloon valvuloplasty include hemodynamically significant aortic stenosis and any of the following: bridge to surgical aortic valve replacement in hemodynamically unstable patients; increased perioperative risk (Society of Thoracic Surgeons score >15), anticipated survival less than 3 years, age in the late 80s or 90s and patient preference for an aortic valvuloplasty over surgical replacement; severe comorbidities such as porcelain aorta, severe lung disease, and others for which the surgeon prefers not to operate; and severe neuromuscular or arthritic conditions that would limit the patient's ability to undergo postoperative rehabilitation.[19] In general, we now implant a percutaneous aortic valve in the majority of these patients.

We reserve aortic balloon valvuloplasty for the rare hemodynamically unstable patient as a bridge to a decision to provide more definitive therapy of their aortic stenosis, for patients with a predicted survival from noncardiac causes measured in weeks to a few months, or for patients who have a contraindication to percutaneous aortic valve implantation in whom we feel relief of the aortic obstruction will improve their quality of life (e.g., a patient with severe aortic stenosis and a metastatic gastrointestinal malignancy who requires a palliative abdominal operative procedure for symptom relief that can only be safely performed if the aortic stenosis gradient is reduced).

Aortic Balloon Valvuloplasty Followed by External Beam Radiation

Balloon aortic valvuloplasty for calcific aortic stenosis has been largely abandoned because of high restenosis rates.[20] Radiation therapy is useful for preventing restenosis after vascular interventions.[21,22] A 20-patient study evaluating external beam radiation to prevent restenosis after aortic balloon valvuloplasty in elderly patients (age 89 ± 4 years) with calcific aortic stenosis has been reported (RADAR pilot trial).[23] Total radiation doses of 12 to 18 Gy were delivered in fractions over a 3- to 5-day period after balloon aortic valvuloplasty. The 1-year follow-up is reported. There were no complications related to external beam radiation. Twelve patients survived to 1 year (60%). One patient underwent aortic valve replacement; no patient had repeated aortic balloon valvuloplasty.

Four of the survivors had restenosis (defined as loss of >50% of the initial increase in aortic valve area).

Apical to Aortic Conduit

Several small series reporting the use of a valved conduit between the left ventricular apex and the aorta for treatment of patients in whom a standard surgical aortic valve replacement was contraindicated have been reported.

In one series, from 2002 through 2005, 13 patients (mean age, 75 ± 8.7 years; 8 men) with severe calcific aortic stenosis had insertions of an apical aortic valved conduit because of a porcelain aorta ($n = 4$), previous coronary bypass grafting ($n = 6$), or both ($n = 3$).[24] An off-pump technique was used in 9 patients; a mini-extracorporeal circulation system was used in 4 patients. Mean intensive care unit stay was 2 ± 2.7 days, and mean hospital stay was 12 ± 8 days. The 30-day mortality was 15%. Mortality later than 30 days postoperatively was 23% (follow-up from 6 to 33 months). The remaining 8 patients are reported to be in New York Heart Association class I or II at follow-up. Echocardiography shows a low gradient over the valved conduit in survivors.

Another series reported results from procedures performed between 1995 and 2003.[25] Thirteen patients (mean age 71 years) underwent an apical aortic conduit for severe symptomatic aortic stenosis (mean valve area 0.65 ± 0.02 cm²). Indications for apical aortic conduit were heavily calcified ascending aorta and aortic root, patent retrosternal mammary grafts, calcified ascending aorta and aortic root plus patent retrosternal mammary graft, retrosternal colonic interposition, and multiple previous sternotomies. The procedures were performed under cardiopulmonary bypass through a left thoracotomy ($n = 10$), median sternotomy ($n = 2$), or bilateral thoracotomy ($n = 1$). Hearts were kept beating ($n = 5$) or fibrillated ($n = 7$). Circulatory arrest was used in one patient. Three patients (23%) died in the hospital; the mean hospital stay was 26 days. At a mean follow-up of 2.1 years, four (31%) late deaths have been reported.

ONGOING TRIALS

The PARTNER trial is sponsored by Edwards Lifesciences, Duke University, and the Harvard Clinical Research Institute. The study will use Edwards Sapien transcatheter valve systems (Edwards Lifesciences). The purpose of the study is to determine the safety and effectiveness of the device and delivery systems in patients with severe symptomatic aortic stenosis in two study populations: (A) patients with high surgical risk for aortic valve replacement and (B) non-surgical patients. In study population A, patients will be randomly assigned to implantation of an Edwards Sapien transcatheter valve versus surgical aortic valve replacement. In study population B, patients will be randomly assigned to implantation of an Edwards Sapien transcatheter valve versus medical management and/or balloon aortic valvuloplasty. Investigators plan to enroll 600 patients by December 2008. The primary outcome will be freedom from death. Further trial details are listed in Table 13-6.

Acknowledgment and Disclosure

The author acknowledges Stephanie, Duncan, Meredith, Benjamin, and Oliver for their love and support; the physicians, nurses, and other staff involved in the percutaneous aortic valve program at St. Paul's Hospital for making the program possible; the sonographers at St. Paul's Hospital for keeping me interested and honest in the pursuit of echocardiographic knowledge and techniques; and Adam Dashe at Edwards Lifesciences LLC (Irvine, CA) and Rob Michiels at CoreValve Inc. (Irvine, CA) for providing images.
Dr. Munt has received consulting fees and travel support from Edwards Lifesciences.

TABLE 13–6 | Details of the Placement of AoRTic traNscathetER Valve (PARTNER) Trial

Primary Outcome Measures:

Freedom from death (Cohort A: Edwards Sapien valve vs. other surgical valve) [Time frame: 1 year]
Freedom from death (Cohort B: Edwards Sapien valve vs. medical therapy) [Time frame: duration of study]

Secondary Outcome Measures:

Functional improvement from baseline per New York Heart Association functional classification (Cohort A and Cohort B) [Time frame: 30 days, 6 months, 1 year]
Freedom from major adverse cardiac events defined as death, myocardial infarction, stroke, or aortic valve reintervention (Cohort A and Cohort B) [Time frame: 30 days, 6 months, 1 year]
Evidence of prosthetic valve dysfunction (hemolysis, infection, thrombosis, severe paravalvular leak, or migration) (Cohort A) [Time frame: 30 days, 6 months, 1 year]
Length of index hospital stay (Cohort A) [Time frame: number of days hospitalized]
Total hospital days from the index procedure to 1 year postprocedure. (Cohort A) [Time frame: 1 year]
Improved quality of life from baseline to 30 days, 6 months, and 1 year (Cohort A and Cohort B) [Time Frame: 30 days, 6 months, 1 year]
Improved valve function demonstrated by a responder analysis showing the percentage of patients in each treatment group who have a greater than 50% improvement in aortic valve area at 30 days, 6 months, and 12 months. (Cohort A and Cohort B) [Time Frame: 30 days, 6 months, 1 year]
Total hospital days from the index procedure or randomization in to control arm for medical management patients to 1 year postprocedure or randomization (Cohort B) [Time Frame: 1 year]

Inclusion Criteria Cohort A

1. Patients must have comorbidities such that the surgeon and cardiologist principle investigators concur that the predicted risk of operative mortality is 15% and a minimum Society of Thoracic Surgeons score of 10.
2. Patient has senile degenerative aortic valve stenosis with echocardiographically derived mean gradient >40 mmHg and/or jet velocity >4.0 m/sec or an initial aortic valve area of <0.8 cm^2.
3. Patient is symptomatic from his/her aortic valve stenosis, as demonstrated by New York Heart Association functional class II or greater.
4. The subject or the subject's legal representative has been informed of the nature of the study, agrees to its provisions and has provided written informed consent as approved by the institutional review board of the respective clinical site.
5. The subject and the treating physician agree that the subject will return for all required postprocedure follow-up visits.

Cohort B: All candidates for Cohort B of this study must meet 2, 3, 4, 5 of the above criteria and

6. The subject, after formal consultations by a cardiologist and two cardiovascular surgeons, agrees that medical factors preclude operation, based on a conclusion that the probability of death or serious, irreversible morbidity exceeds the probability of meaningful improvement. Specifically, the probability of death or serious, irreversible morbidity should exceed 50%.

Exclusion Criteria

Evidence of an acute myocardial infarction ≤1month before the intended treatment
Aortic valve is a congenital unicuspid or bicuspid valve or is noncalcified
Mixed aortic valve disease (aortic stenosis and aortic regurgitation with predominant aortic regurgitation >3+)
Any therapeutic invasive cardiac procedure, other than balloon aortic valvuloplasty, performed within 30 days of the index procedure (or 6 months if the procedure was a drug eluting coronary stent implantation)
Preexisting prosthetic heart valve in any position, prosthetic ring, or severe (>3+) mitral insufficiency
Blood dyscrasias as defined: leukopenia, acute anemia, thrombocytopenia, history of bleeding diathesis, or coagulopathy
Untreated clinically significant coronary artery disease requiring revascularization
Hemodynamic instability requiring inotropic support or mechanical heart assistance
Need for emergency surgery for any reason
Hypertrophic cardiomyopathy with or without obstruction
Severe ventricular dysfunction with left ventricular ejection fraction <20%.
Echocardiographic evidence of intracardiac mass, thrombus, or vegetation
Active peptic ulcer or upper gastrointestinal bleeding within the prior 3 months
A known hypersensitivity or contraindication to aspirin, heparin, ticlopidine, or clopidogrel or sensitivity to contrast media, which cannot be adequately premedicated
Native aortic annulus size <16 mm or >24 mm per the baseline echo as estimated by the left ventricular outflow tract
Patient has been offered surgery but has refused surgery
Recent (within 6 months) cardiovascular accident or a transient ischemic attack
Renal insufficiency and/or end-stage renal disease requiring chronic dialysis
Life expectancy <12 months due to noncardiac comorbid conditions
Significant aortic disease, including abdominal aortic or thoracic aneurysm defined as maximal luminal diameter ≥5 cm; marked tortuosity (hyperacute bend), aortic arch atheroma, or narrowing (especially with calcification and surface irregularities) of the abdominal or thoracic aorta, severe "unfolding" and tortuosity of the thoracic aorta
Ileofemoral vessel characteristics that would preclude safe placement of 22-F or 24-F introducer sheath such as severe obstructive calcification, severe tortuosity, or vessels size <7 mm in diameter
Currently participating in an investigational drug or another device study.

220 REFERENCES

1. Bonow R, Carabello B, Kanu C, et al: ACC/AHA 2006 guidelines for the management of patients with valvular heart disease: a report of the American College of Cardiology/American Heart Association Task Force on Practice Guidelines (writing committee to revise the 1998 Guidelines for the Management of Patients with Valvular Heart Disease): developed in collaboration with the Society of Cardiovascular Anesthesiologists: endorsed by the Society for Cardiovascular Angiography and Interventions and the Society of Thoracic Surgeons. Circulation 2006;114:e84-e231.

2. Otto CM, Mickel MC, Kennedy JW, et al: Three-year outcome after balloon aortic valvuloplasty. Insights into prognosis of valvular aortic stenosis. Circulation 1994;89: 642-650.

3. Iung B, Cachier A, Baron G: Decision-making in elderly patients with severe aortic stenosis: why are so many denied surgery?. Eur Heart J 2005;26:704-708.

4. Andersen H, Knudsen L, Hasenkam J: Transluminal implantation of artificial heart valves: description of a new expandable aortic valve and initial results with implantation by catheter technique in closed chest pigs. Eur Heart J 1992;13:704-708.

5. Cribier A, Eltchaninoff H, Bash A, et al: Percutaneous transcatheter implantation of an aortic valve prosthesis for calcific aortic stenosis: first human case description. Circulation 2002;106:3006-3008.

6. Webb J, Chandavimol M, Thompson C, et al: Percutaneous aortic valve implantation retrograde from the femoral artery. Circulation 2006;113:842-850.

7. Webb J, Pasupati S, Humphries K, et al: Percutaneous transarterial aortic valve replacement in selected high-risk patients with aortic stenosis. Circulation 2007;116:755-763.

8. Grube E, Laborde J, Gerckens U, et al: Percutaneous implantation of the CoreValve self-expanding valve prosthesis in high-risk patients with aortic valve disease the Siegburg first-in-man study. Circulation 2006;114:1616-1624.

9. Walther T, Simon P, Dewey T, et al: Transapical minimally invasive aortic valve implantation: multicenter experience. Circulation 2007;116:I240-I245.

10. Lichtenstein S, Cheung A, Ye J, et al: Transapical transcatheter aortic valve implantation in humans: initial clinical experience. Circulation 2006;114:591-596.

11. Cribier A, Eltchaninoff H, Tron C, et al: Early experience with percutaneous transcatheter implantation of heart valve prosthesis for the treatment of end-stage inoperable patients with calcific aortic stenosis. J Am Coll Cardiol 2004;43:698-703.

12. Pasupati S, Humphries K, AlAli A, et al: Balloon expandable aortic valve implantation: the first 100 Canadian patients. Circulation 2007;116:II-357.

13. Rosenhek R, Binder T, Maurer G, Baumgartner H: Normal values for Doppler echocardiographic assessment of heart valve prostheses. J Am Soc Echocardiogr 2003;16: 1116-1127.

14. Figulla H, Ferrari M: Percutaneously implantable aortic valve: the JenaValve concept evolution. Herz 2006;31:685-687.

15. Grube E, Schuler G, Buellesfeld L, et al: Percutaneous aortic valve replacement for severe aortic stenosis in high-risk patients using the second- and current third-generation self-expanding CoreValve prosthesis: device success and 30-day clinical outcome. J Am Coll Cardiol 2007;50:69-76.

16. Lange R, Schreiber C, Gotz W, et al: First successful transapical aortic valve implantation with the CoreValve ReValving system: a case report. Heart Surg Forum 2007;10: E478-E479.

17. Wenaweser P, Buellesfeld L, Gerckens U, Grube E: Percutaneous aortic valve replacement for severe aortic regurgitation in degenerated bioprosthesis: the first valve in valve procedure using the CoreValve ReValving system. Catheter Cardiovasc Interv 2007;70:760-764.

18. Varadarajan P, Kapoor N, Bansal R, Pai R: Survival in elderly patients with severe aortic stenosis is dramatically improved by aortic valve replacement: results from a cohort of 277 patients aged greater than or equal to 80 years. Eur J Cardiothorac Surg 2006;30:722-727.

19. Hara H, Pedersen W, Ladich E, et al: Percutaneous balloon aortic valvuloplasty revisited: time for a renaissance? Circulation 2007;115:e334-e338.

20. Hashimoto H, Tamura T, Ikari Y, et al: Comparison of aortic valve replacement and percutaneous aortic balloon valvuloplasty for elderly patients with aortic stenosis. Jpn Circ J 1996;60:142-148.

21. Verin V, Popowski Y, de Bruyne B, et al: Endoluminal beta-radiation therapy for the prevention of coronary restenosis after balloon angioplasty. The Dose-Finding Study Group. N Engl J Med 2001;344:243-249.

22. Hagenaars T, A Po I, van Sambeek M, et al: Gamma radiation induces positive vascular remodeling after balloon angioplasty: a prospective, randomized intravascular ultrasound scan study. J Vasc Surg 2002;36:318-324.

23. Pedersen W, Van Tassel R, Pierce T, et al: Radiation following percutaneous balloon aortic valvuloplasty to prevent restenosis (RADAR pilot trial). Catheter Cardiovasc Interv 2006;68:183-192.

24. Lockowandt U: Apicoaortic valved conduit: potential for progress? J Thorac Cardiovasc Surg 2006;132:796-801.

25. Crestanello J, Zehr K, Daly R, et al: Is there a role for the left ventricle apical-aortic conduit for acquired aortic stenosis? J Heart Valve Dis 2004;13:57-63.

13

CHAPTER **14**

Rheumatic Mitral Valve Disease

Bernard Iung and Alec Vahanian

KEY POINTS

- Despite the decrease in the incidence of rheumatic heart diseases, mitral stenosis remains prevalent in industrialized countries. It occurs frequently and is underdiagnosed in developing countries.
- Clinical assessment is paramount in detecting mitral stenosis in asymptomatic patients and to evaluate symptoms.
- Planimetry using 2-dimensional echocardiography is the reference measurement for valve area.
- Intervention is needed in symptomatic patients who have mitral stenosis with a valve area less than 1.5 cm².
- Balloon mitral commissurotomy can be considered in selected asymptomatic patients who have mitral stenosis with a valve area less than 1.5 cm², particularly those who have a high risk for thromboembolism.
- The choice between balloon mitral commissurotomy and surgery should be individualized and based not only on valve anatomy but also on other clinical and echocardiographic characteristics.
- Balloon mitral commissurotomy and surgery are complementary techniques, which should be used at different times of the evolution of mitral stenosis.

Despite the decrease in the incidence of rheumatic heart disease, mitral stenosis (MS) remains prevalent, even in industrialized countries. The main purpose in evaluation of patients with MS is to determine the optimal timing of intervention as well as the most appropriate treatment approach. The treatment of MS has been reoriented from a surgical to a percutaneous approach with the development of balloon mitral commissurotomy (BMC). Large series reporting long-term follow-up after BMC have contributed to improving the level of evidence of decision making for interventions in MS, as attested to by contemporary guidelines.

PATHOPHYSIOLOGY

Mechanisms of Valve Obstruction

Unlike other heart valve diseases, MS occurs in most cases as a consequence of rheumatic fever.[1] The main mechanism of stenosis is commissural fusion. Posterior leaflet thickening and restriction are almost constant but have limited hemodynamic consequences. Thickening and rigidity of the anterior leaflet and/or the subvalvular apparatus can also contribute to stenosis (Figure 14-1).[2] Commissural fusion results in a fixed mitral orifice when stenosis is severe, whereas valve area may vary with flow rate once commissures have been opened after BMC.[3]

Degenerative mitral annular calcification occurs frequently in elderly individuals but has few or no hemodynamic consequences in most patients. Significant stenosis seldom occurs and is related to restriction of both leaflets because of extensive calcification, without commissural fusion.

Other etiologies of mitral stenosis are rare. Congenital MS is mainly the consequence of abnormalities of the subvalvular apparatus. Inflammatory diseases (e.g., systemic lupus erythematosus), infiltrative diseases, carcinoid heart disease, and drug-induced valve diseases are characterized by a predominance of leaflet thickening and restriction, whereas commissures are seldom fused.

The predominance of a rheumatic etiology explains why the prevalence of MS has decreased in industrialized countries.[4] However, it still accounts for approximately 10% of native valve diseases and affects young immigrants or older patients in Europe and North America.[1] Conversely, the prevalence of rheumatic heart disease remains high in developing countries, with an estimated prevalence between 1 and 5 per 1000 in children according to clinical data and 10 times higher when systematic echocardiographic screening is used.[5,6]

Hemodynamic Consequences of Mitral Stenosis

Mitral Gradient

The first consequence of MS is an increase in the diastolic mitral pressure gradient, which depends on mitral valve area but also on other factors such as transvalvular flow and heart rate.[7] For a given valve area, mean mitral gradient increases when cardiac output increases or when tachycardia reduces the length of the diastolic filling period. Atrial contraction contributes to the increase of transmitral flow in

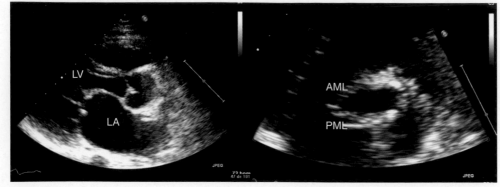

FIGURE 14–1 Mitral stenosis. Transthoracic echocardiography, parasternal long-axis (*left*) and short-axis (*right*) views. Both leaflets are moderately thickened with a pliable anterior leaflet on the long-axis view and fusion of both commissures on the short-axis view. LA, left atrium; LV, left ventricle; Ao, aorta; AML, anterior mitral leaflet; PML, posterior mitral leaflet.

end-diastole and, therefore, of mitral gradient. Severe MS may thus be associated with a low gradient in patients with low cardiac output, particularly those who are in chronic atrial fibrillation.

Left Atrium

The trans-mitral pressure gradient causes an increase in left atrial pressure. Chronic left atrial pressure overload leads to enlargement of the left atrium, according to the severity and chronicity of MS, although it is subject to significant interpatient variability. Atrial enlargement favors the occurrence of atrial fibrillation.

The other consequence of MS is blood stasis in the left atrium and, upstream, a decrease in systolic pulmonary vein flow.[8] The severity of blood stasis can be assessed using Doppler echocardiography by the intensity of left atrial spontaneous contrast and low flow velocities in the left atrial appendage in patients in sinus rhythm. Blood stasis and left atrial appendage flow velocities are considerably impaired when atrial fibrillation occurs, thereby increasing the risk of thrombosis. The left atrial appendage is the most frequent location of left atrial thrombus (Figure 14-2).[9]

Thrombus formation is also associated with local abnormalities of hemostasis, particularly increases in fibrinopeptide A and the thrombin-antithrombin III complex.[10]

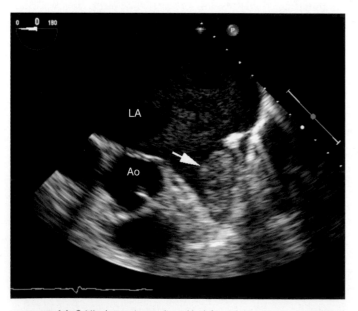

FIGURE 14–2 Mitral stenosis complicated by left atrial thrombus. Transesophageal echocardiography. Thrombus is located in the left appendage (*arrow*). The left atrium is enlarged with swirling spontaneous echo contrast. LA, left atrium; Ao, aorta.

Pulmonary Circulation

A constant mechanism of pulmonary hypertension in MS is the passive rise in pulmonary artery pressure after the increase in left atrial pressure. In addition, pulmonary hypertension can be worsened in certain patients by an increase in pulmonary vascular resistance, which results in gradient greater than 10 mmHg between diastolic pulmonary pressure and left atrial pressure. Increased pulmonary vascular resistance involves vasoconstriction and structural changes of the pulmonary arterial wall.

Vasoconstriction seems to involve endothelium-dependent vascular tone regulation as shown by the decrease in pulmonary vascular resistance after inhaled nitric oxide and the probable synthesis of endothelin I in the pulmonary circulation.[11,12]

The sequence of histologic changes in pulmonary hypertension due to MS is characterized initially by medial thickening in muscular arteries and arterioles, followed by intimal thickening.[13] These changes are likely to be reversible with a decrease in pulmonary pressures. More severe pulmonary hypertension is associated with fibrinoid necrosis and arteritis, loss of smooth muscle cell nuclei, fibrin deposition in the arterial wall, and the presence of inflammatory cells. The pathologic hallmark of end-stage, irreversible pulmonary hypertension is the plexiform lesion. The plexiform lesion consists of aneurysmal dilation of the arterial wall with a plexus of glomus-like thin-walled channels branching to join with adjacent capillaries. Nonspecific parenchymal changes due to irreversible pulmonary hypertension include pulmonary hemosiderosis and cholesterol granuloma formation.

In a multivariate analysis comprising 744 patients with severe MS, factors associated with pulmonary vascular bed gradient were mitral gradient, left ventricular end-diastolic pressure, mitral valve area, and a history of chronic pulmonary disease.[14] These numerous factors explain the wide range in pulmonary pressures for any given degree of MS.

Right Heart

Chronic pulmonary hypertension leads to right ventricular hypertrophy, right ventricular dilation, and right heart failure. This process may be exacerbated by significant tricuspid regurgitation due either to rheumatic involvement of the tricuspid valve or to annular dilation secondary to right ventricular enlargement. Although pulmonary hypertension presumably is the cause of right heart dysfunction, there is a poor correlation between pulmonary pressures and right ventricular failure in patients with MS.[15]

Left Ventricle

Left ventricular size is generally normal or moderately reduced in MS. The main consequence of MS on the left ventricle is impaired diastolic filling. Compared with normal subjects, patients with MS have a prolongation of early diastolic filling and an increased contribution of left atrial contraction. Loss of atrial contraction explains the severe hemodynamic impairment that occurs with the onset of atrial fibrillation. Left ventricular filling may also be impaired by right ventricular pressure or volume overload causing abnormal septal motion.

Although left ventricular contractility typically is normal in isolated MS, forward stroke volume may be reduced owing to low filling volumes across the stenotic mitral valve. In addition, the left ventricular ejection fraction is impaired in 5% to 10% of patients in the absence of another cause, specifically other valve or coronary artery disease.[16] This impairment does not seem to be explained by abnormal loading conditions because left ventricular dysfunction generally persists after the relief of MS.

Exercise Physiology

Hemodynamic changes during exercise provide additional insights on the multiple factors interacting with the severity of the stenosis to determine its repercussions. The increase in transmitral gradient at exercise is the consequence of the shortening of the diastolic filling period, and it determines an upstream increase in pulmonary artery pressure. However, changes in mitral gradient and pulmonary artery pressure are highly variable for a given degree of stenosis.[17,18] This heterogencity may be explained by differences in the change in stroke volume during exercise[19] and by differences in atrioventricular compliance.[20]

An increase in stroke volume during exercise, as in normal patients, is associated with an increase in mitral valve area during exercise, which is observed in patients who have a moderate impairment of valve anatomy. Conversely, in patients with a severe impairment of valve anatomy, stroke volume does not increase or even decreases during exercise. Net atrioventricular compliance is the strongest determinant of left atrial and pulmonary artery pressures at rest, more than valve area, gradient, or pulmonary vascular resistance.[21] A low net compliance is mainly the consequence of a low compliance of the left atrium, and it is also associated, even more than at rest, with a higher pulmonary artery pressure at exercise and more severe symptoms.[20]

CLINICAL PRESENTATION

History

Dyspnea is the most frequent symptom of MS, and its presence has prognostic value. However, onset of dyspnea may be difficult to assess, given the slowly progressive course of the disease. Patients frequently adapt their level of activity to their functional capacity and do not complain of dyspnea despite objective effort limitation. This situation underlines the need for a careful discussion with the patient and relatives, taking into account her (or his) lifestyle and comparing the evolution of activity levels over time.[22-24] Paroxysmal dyspnea should always be looked for because it could be triggered not only by intermittent atrial fibrillation but also by emotional stress, sexual intercourse, or fever even in patients with few or no symptoms with exercise. Paroxysmal cough or hemoptysis occurs seldom but should be searched for, particularly in young patients during effort.

Patients sometimes complain more of fatigue rather than of dyspnea, especially older patients and/or those who have advanced heart disease with chronic atrial fibrillation. Asthenia and abdominal pain are suggestive of right heart failure. It is now unusual to observe hoarseness due to compression of the left recurrent laryngeal nerve by the enlarged left atrium.

Complications, such as atrial fibrillation or embolic events, may reveal MS in previously asymptomatic patients. Pregnancy is a common cause of decompensation of previously well tolerated MS, because the increase in cardiac output and tachycardia causes a sharp increase in mitral gradient and pulmonary artery pressure during the second trimester.

The search for comorbidity as a cause of symptom onset is important in older patients, who account for a growing part of patients with MS in industrialized countries.[25,26]

Physical Examination

Auscultation reveals a loud first heart sound and an opening snap in early diastole, just after the second heart sound, followed by a holodiastolic decrescendo rumbling murmur which increases in intensity at end-diastole in patients in sinus rhythm (Figure 14-3). The murmur is often difficult to identify because it is localized and of low acoustic frequency. Thus, careful auscultation is needed, using the bell of the stethoscope at different points around the apical impulse with the patient in the left lateral decubitus position.

The loudness of the murmur depends on the intensity of the transmitral gradient. A loud murmur with a thrill suggests severe stenosis. Conversely, a low-intensity murmur does not exclude severe stenosis in patients with low cardiac output. The duration of the interval between the second aortic sound and the opening snap is shortened in severe stenosis, because increased left atrial pressure causes earlier opening of the mitral valve.[7] The intensity of the first sound and the opening snap may be diminished in patients with extensive calcification limiting leaflet motion.

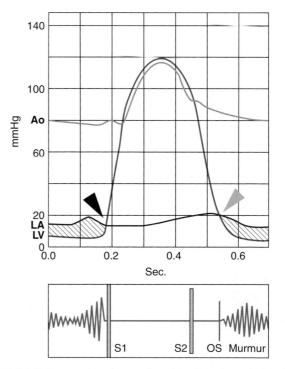

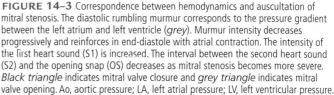

FIGURE 14–3 Correspondence between hemodynamics and auscultation of mitral stenosis. The diastolic rumbling murmur corresponds to the pressure gradient between the left atrium and left ventricle (*grey*). Murmur intensity decreases progressively and reinforces in end-diastole with atrial contraction. The intensity of the first heart sound (S1) is increased. The interval between the second heart sound (S2) and the opening snap (OS) decreases as mitral stenosis becomes more severe. *Black triangle* indicates mitral valve closure and *grey triangle* indicates mitral valve opening. Ao, aortic pressure; LA, left atrial pressure; LV, left ventricular pressure.

Auscultation should also be used to search for a holosystolic murmur at the apex suggesting concurrent mitral regurgitation (MR). The holosystolic murmur of tricuspid regurgitation is usually located at the xiphoid but may be heard near the apex when the right ventricle is enlarged. It is differentiated from a murmur of MR by its respiratory variation. It is important to pay attention to even a low-intensity, midsystolic murmur, which attests to associated aortic stenosis, the severity of which tends to be underestimated when combined with MS.

A diastolic murmur at the left sternal border is more likely to be the consequence of aortic rather than pulmonic regurgitation. The second pulmonary sound is louder in patients with pulmonary hypertension.

Auscultation is also the first means of detecting arrhythmias, which should be confirmed by an electrocardiogram.

Clinical signs of left-sided heart failure, in particular pulmonary rales, are present in patients with severe symptoms. Signs of right heart failure are observed in patients with severe and, often, long-standing disease, including hepatomegaly, which may be pulsatile in patients with severe tricuspid regurgitation; peripheral edema; and jugular venous distension, which is the most specific sign. "Mitral facies" is characterized by patchy flushing of the cheeks and has become rare because it is only encountered in patients with long-standing, untreated MS.

Chest Radiography and Electrocardiography

The first abnormality of the cardiac silhouette on a chest radiograph is left atrial enlargement characterized by a left atrial double density and prominence of the left atrial appendage (Figure 14-4). Pulmonary hypertension causes dilation of the pulmonary artery trunk and branches. Heart size is normal at this stage. Severe chronic MS leads to right ventricular and right atrial enlargement and cardiomegaly. Pulmonary vascular redistribution and, later, interstitial edema are early

radiographic signs of elevated left atrial pressure, which are often seen even in patients with moderate symptoms and without clinical signs of heart failure. Alveolar edema is a sign of acute hemodynamic decompensation. A lateral chest radiograph is useful for diagnosing right ventricular enlargement, mild pleural effusion, and mitral valve calcification, which is detected by fluoroscopy with a higher sensitivity.

Left atrial enlargement is the only electrocardiographic abnormality at an early stage. Right atrial and right ventricular enlargement with right axis deviation and right bundle branch block are observed in more advanced diseases associated with severe and/or long-standing pulmonary hypertension. Electrocardiography plays a major role in the detection of atrial arrhythmias, i.e., frequent atrial premature beats and transient or persistent atrial fibrillation or, less frequently, atrial flutter or atrial tachycardia.

ECHOCARDIOGRAPHY

Echocardiography is the cornerstone in the evaluation of suspected or known MS to confirm the diagnosis, evaluate the severity and consequences of valve lesions, and assess valve anatomy and associated diseases.[27] Echocardiographic techniques are detailed in Chapter 5.

The diagnostic features of rheumatic mitral valve disease are leaflet thickening and decreased mobility, commissural fusion, and involvement of the subvalvular apparatus.

Assessment of Severity

The parasternal short-axis view enables planimetry to be performed, which is the reference standard for mitral valve area.[28,29] It is the only direct measurement of valve area and thereby is independent of loading conditions and associated heart diseases (Figure 14-5). However, technical expertise is needed to scan the mitral valve apparatus to position the measurement plane at the leaflet tip. Positioning the

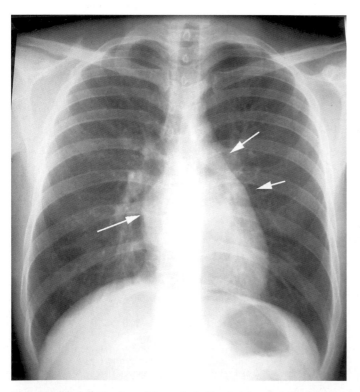

FIGURE 14–4 Chest radiograph in a patient with mitral stenosis. Left atrium is enlarged (*right-side arrow* and *inferior left-side arrows*). There is a moderate enlargement of pulmonary trunk (*superior left-side arrow*) and branches. Heart size is normal, and lung fields are clear.

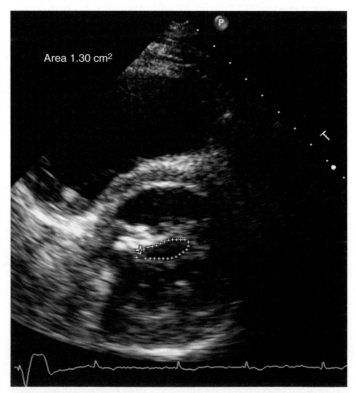

Area 1.30 cm²

FIGURE 14–5 Planimetry of mitral stenosis (transthoracic echocardiography, parasternal short-axis view). Valve area is 1.3 cm². Both commissures are fused and the anterior leaflet is thickened beside the internal commissure.

measurement plane can be facilitated with the use of three-dimensional echocardiography, which improves reproducibility in this setting, particularly when for less experienced echocardiographers.[30-32] Planimetry is also useful during BMC to monitor the procedure and immediately after BMC when it is the most reliable technique. However, planimetry may be difficult and may not even be feasible in patients with an irregular and heavily calcified orifice or in patients with poor echogenicity.

Besides planimetry, the parasternal short-axis view assesses commissural fusion. This is of particular importance to differentiate rheumatic MS from other types of MS, in particular degenerative MS, in which commissures are not fused, and to determine the feasibility of balloon or surgical commissurotomy. The assessment of commissural opening is also an additional indication of the efficacy of BMC during and after the procedure as well as during late follow-up. The assessment of the commissural opening is more accurate using three-dimensional than two-dimensional echocardiography (Figure 14-6).[32]

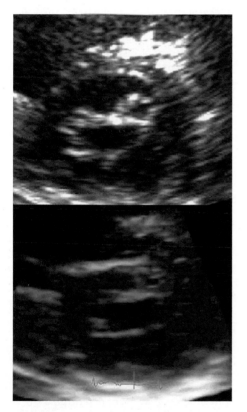

FIGURE 14–6 Assessment of commissural opening after balloon mitral commissurotomy in the same patient using two-dimensional (*top panel*) and real-time three-dimensional (*bottom panel*) echocardiography (parasternal short-axis view). (*Courtesy of Dr. Messika-Zeitoun*).

The pressure half-time method is generally easier to perform and is therefore widely used. However, it may be misleading in cases of aortic regurgitation or abnormal compliance of cardiac chambers and immediately after BMC.[33-36] The most significant discrepancies with planimetry are observed in patients older than 60 years and in those in atrial fibrillation.[36]

The continuity equation is not valid in cases of associated significant mitral or aortic regurgitation. Its accuracy and reproducibility are limited, given the number of measurements involved.[37]

Use of the proximal isovelocity surface area is technically demanding and requires multiple measurements. Its accuracy can be improved using M-mode echocardiography.[38]

Mean mitral gradient, as assessed by pulsed or continuous wave Doppler, is not a reliable measurement to assess the severity of MS, because it is highly dependent on flow conditions. However, its value should be consistent with valve area, and it has prognostic value after BMC.

The consistency of results for planimetry, the pressure half-time method, and gradient should always be checked, keeping in mind the limitations of the different measurements (Figure 14-7).[22,23,39] The continuity equation and proximal isovelocity surface area are not used routinely but may be useful when other methods lead to uncertain or discordant findings.

Mitral valve area is considered significantly narrowed when valve area is less than 1.5 cm^2.[22,23] This corresponds to the value above which hemodynamics are not affected at rest. The interpretation of valve area should take into account body size, even if no definite value indexed on body surface area is advised in guidelines (Table 14-1).

Mitral valve resistance has been proposed as an alternative measurement of the severity of valve obstruction.[40] Although it is a good predictor of pulmonary artery pressure, it has not superseded valve area as the marker of MS severity.

Assessment of Valve Morphology

The analysis of the morphology of valve leaflets and subvalvular apparatus using bidimensional echocardiography is a key feature for diagnosis of MS and has also important implications for the potential of progression and, in particular, the choice of the most appropriate intervention when needed.[41]

Echocardiographic evaluation assesses leaflet thickening (significant if ≥5 mm), leaflet mobility in the long-axis parasternal view, and calcification, which is best confirmed by fluoroscopic examination. The parasternal short-axis view is paramount, not only for planimetry but also to evaluate the homogeneity of the impairment of the mitral orifice, focusing on commissural areas. Long-axis parasternal and apical views enable impairment of the subvalvular apparatus (thickening and/or shortening of chordae) to be assessed, although it tends to be underestimated compared with anatomic findings.

Valvular and subvalvular lesions are usually combined in scores. The Wilkins score grades each of the following components of mitral apparatus from 1 to 4: leaflet mobility,

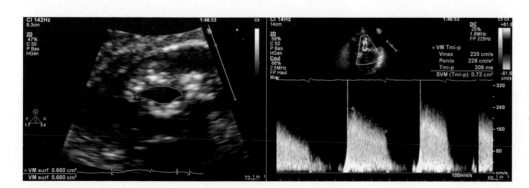

FIGURE 14–7 Consistency between different methods used to assess the severity of mitral stenosis in a patient in atrial fibrillation. Valve area is estimated to be 0.66 cm^2 using two-dimensional planimetry (*left*) and 0.72 cm^2 using Doppler pressure half-time (*right*).

TABLE 14–1	Classification of the Severity of Mitral Stenosis[22]		
	Mild	**Moderate**	**Severe**
Mean gradient (mmHg)*	<5	5-10	>10
Pulmonary artery pressure (mmHg)	<30	30-50	>50
Valve area (cm²)	>1.5	1.0-1.5	<1.0

*Valve gradients are flow dependent and when used as estimates of severity of valve stenosis should be assessed with knowledge of cardiac output of forward flow across the valve.

TABLE 14–3	Assessment of Mitral Valve Anatomy According to the Cormier Score[43]
Echocardiographic Group	**Mitral Valve Anatomy**
Group 1	Pliable noncalcified anterior mitral leaflet and mild subvalvular disease (i.e., thin chordae ≥10 mm long)
Group 2	Pliable noncalcified anterior mitral leaflet and severe subvalvular disease (i.e., thickened chordae <10 mm long)
Group 3	Calcification of mitral valve of any extent, as assessed by fluoroscopy, whatever the state of subvalvular apparatus

thickness, calcification, and impairment of subvalvular apparatus (Table 14-2).[42] The final scores range from 4 to 16. An alternative approach is to assess the whole mitral valve anatomy according to the best surgical alternative, leading to classification in three groups (Table 14-3).[43]

These two scores share limitations related to the lack of a detailed location of calcification and leaflet thickening, particularly in relation to commissural areas, which are likely to influence the results of BMC.[44-46] In addition, they tend to underestimate the weight of subvalvular apparatus impairment.[47] Other scoring systems include a more detailed approach, with the aim of achieving better prediction of the results of BMC.[48-51] However, besides concerns related to their reproducibility, they still lack validation in large prospective series, and, thus, are not widely used in current practice. Therefore, no comparative evaluation of different scoring systems enables a particular one to be recommended.[52] In addition, it is unlikely that a single scoring system could combine reproducibility and accurate prediction of the results of mitral commissurotomy. The echocardiographer is advised to use a method with which he or she is familiar and which includes the assessment of valve morphology, among other clinical and echocardiographic findings.

Consequences of Mitral Stenosis

For quantitation of left atrial enlargement, time-motion measurement is the most widely used method, but it lacks accuracy. Estimation of left atrial area or volume using bidimensional echocardiography is preferred.

Systolic pulmonary artery pressure is estimated from the velocity of Doppler tricuspid flow. Diastolic and mean pulmonary artery pressures can be derived from pulmonary flow.

Mitral Regurgitation

For quantitation of associated MR different semiquantitative and quantitative measurements should be combined with a check for consistency. An accurate evaluation using quantitative methods is of particular importance for moderate regurgitation because it may have important implications for the choice of the type of intervention.[22,23,53]

Associated Lesions

Rheumatic aortic valve disease is frequently associated with MS. Decreased stroke volume due to MS may lead to underestimation of aortic stenosis because of a low gradient. Valve area should be quantitated using the continuity equation and/or planimetry of the aortic valve.

Functional tricuspid regurgitation is caused by enlargement of the right heart chambers due to pulmonary hypertension without rheumatic lesions of the valve. The quantitation of tricuspid regurgitation is less well established than that for left-sided heart valve diseases, and it is highly dependent on loading conditions. The diameter of the tricuspid annulus seems to be a better marker of the persistence of severe tricuspid regurgitation after the treatment of MS.[23,54] However, further standardization of its measurement is needed. Rheumatic tricuspid disease is less frequent. It is characterized by thickening and decreased mobility of tricuspid leaflets and may combine stenosis and regurgitation.

Thromboembolic Risk

Transesophageal echocardiography (TEE) has a much higher sensitivity than transthoracic echocardiography for detecting left atrial thrombus particularly in the left atrial appendage. TEE is therefore mandatory before BMC. TEE is also useful for assessing left atrial spontaneous contrast, which is a strong predictor of thromboembolic risk in patients with MS.[55]

Stress Testing

Semisupine bicycle ergometry enables hemodynamic changes to be sequentially assessed for increasing workload and particularly for mean mitral gradient and estimated systolic pulmonary artery pressure (Figure 14-8). It is useful in patients whose symptoms are equivocal or discordant with the severity of MS. However, thresholds of mitral gradient and pulmonary

TABLE 14–2	Assessment of Mitral Valve Anatomy According to the Wilkins Score[42]			
Grade	**Mobility**	**Thickening**	**Calcification**	**Subvalvular Thickening**
1	Highly mobile valve with only leaflet tips restricted	Leaflets near normal in thickness (4-5 mm)	A single area of increased echo brightness	Minimal thickening just below the mitral leaflets
2	Leaflet mid and base portions have normal mobility	Mid leaflets normal, considerable thickening of margins (5-8 mm)	Scattered areas of brightness confined to leaflet margins	Thickening of chordal structures extending to one of the chordal length
3	Valve continues to move forward in diastole, mainly from the base	Thickening extending through the entire leaflet (5-8 mm)	Brightness extending into the mid portions of the leaflets	Thickening extended to distal third of the chords
4	No or minimal forward movement of the leaflets in diastole	Considerable thickening of all leaflet tissue (>8-10 mm)	Extensive brightness throughout much of the leaflet tissue	Extensive thickening and shortening of all chordal structures extending down to the papillary muscles

The total score is the sum of the four items and ranges between 4 and 16.

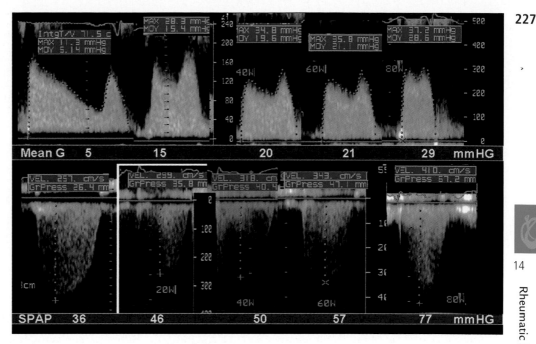

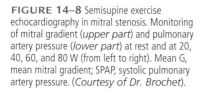

FIGURE 14–8 Semisupine exercise echocardiography in mitral stenosis. Monitoring of mitral gradient (*upper part*) and pulmonary artery pressure (*lower part*) at rest and at 20, 40, 60, and 80 W (from left to right). Mean G, mean mitral gradient; SPAP, systolic pulmonary artery pressure. (*Courtesy of Dr. Brochet*).

artery pressure, as stated in guidelines to consider intervention in asymptomatic patients, rely on low levels of evidence and are frequently achieved in practice.[22,23]

Dobutamine stress echocardiography, although less physiologic than exercise echocardiography, increases mean gradient and systolic pulmonary artery pressure.[56] It has been shown to have a prognostic value in one study.[57]

Other Noninvasive Investigations

Preliminary reports suggest that magnetic resonance imaging and multislice computed tomography are reliable alternate techniques to perform planimetry of the mitral valve.[58,59] Although the availability of such techniques is limited, they may be helpful when echocardiographic imaging is of poor quality.

Cardiac Catheterization

There is now little interest in the use of right and left heart cardiac catheterization to calculate mitral valve area using the Gorlin formula. The validity of the Gorlin formula is questionable when cardiac output is decreased and immediately after BMC.[60,61] Thus, invasive evaluation of the severity of MS is only justified in patients for whom echocardiography results are inconclusive.[22,23]

Cardiac catheterization remains, however, the only technique to calculate pulmonary vascular resistance, which may be useful to assess the risk of surgery in patients with severe pulmonary hypertension. In current practice, the main indication for invasive investigations is the assessment of associated coronary disease using coronary angiography. Monitoring of the results of BMC is now done mainly with intra-procedure echocardiography particularly when the Inoue stepwise technique is used.

NATURAL HISTORY

Onset and Progression of Valvular Lesions

MS develops over many years after acute rheumatic fever. It is difficult to evaluate the course of the disease because rheumatic fever is not always diagnosed, is often subject to recurrences, and is subject to highly variable evolution according to the country considered. A majority of patients with initial rheumatic carditis will develop chronic rheumatic valve disease. A prospective study using echocardiography identified three risk factors for progression toward chronic rheumatic valve disease: the severity of carditis, recurrences of acute rheumatic fever, and mother's low educational level.[62] The course of the disease is particularly rapid in countries where rheumatic fever is endemic, leading to severe MS in young adults, adolescents, and even children.[63] Conversely, MS frequently occurs in adults older than 50 years in Western countries. This pattern is illustrated by series of BMCs, in which mean age is around 30 years in Asia or North Africa and between 40 and 60 years in Europe or the United States.

The progression of MS has been evaluated in series including serial hemodynamic or echocardiographic evaluations.[64-66] These studies are subject to bias because all of them were retrospective and included a limited number of patients. They reported an average decrease of 0.01 cm²/year; however, this result reflects a mix between patients in whom valve area remained stable, accounting for between one third and two thirds, and patients experiencing progression with an annual decrease in valve area ranging between 0.1 and 0.3 cm². Impairment of valve anatomy (Wilkins score ≥8) and a peak mitral gradient of 10 mmHg or greater were identified as predictors of a more rapid progression of MS.[65]

Clinical Outcome without Intervention

As in other valve diseases, studies on natural history are frequently old, retrospective, and subject to inclusion bias. Despite these limitations, which may explain differences in estimations, there is agreement on the poor prognosis of MS when patients become symptomatic, with 10-year survival rates ranging from 34% to 61% and 20-year rates between 14% and 21%.[67,68] A more recent series reported 44% survival at 5 years in patients refusing intervention.[69] Survival is highly influenced by the evolutive stage of the disease, particularly symptoms and atrial fibrillation. Asymptomatic patients have a 20-year survival of greater than 80%; however, approximately half of them become symptomatic after 10 years.[67] Clinical deterioration is sudden in approximately half of the patients. The leading cause of death is heart failure in about 60% of patients, followed by thromboembolic complications in about 20%.[68]

Complications

Atrial fibrillation is a frequent complication of MS, and it is largely related to left atrial enlargement. However, its frequency is only partly related to the severity of stenosis.[70] As in the general population, the frequency of atrial fibrillation is also strongly dependent on patient age.[25]

The use of systematic Holter electrocardiographic monitoring has shown that half of patients with MS in sinus rhythm had atrial arrhythmias; although 95% were asymptomatic, 14% of them had embolic complications. The three factors predictive of atrial arrhythmias were age, left atrial diameter, and valve calcification.[71]

Atrial fibrillation considerably worsens the consequences of MS. The lack of atrial contraction and the shortening of the diastolic filling period further impair hemodynamics and may cause acute decompensation such as pulmonary edema.[72] The other consequence is the increase in blood stasis in the left atrium, which increases the thromboembolic risk. The Framingham study estimated a 17-fold increase in the risk of stroke in patients with atrial fibrillation and MS compared with a 5-fold increased risk for atrial fibrillation in the absence of mitral valve disease. Finally, atrial fibrillation is associated with an increased mortality in MS.[73]

Annual linearized risk of thromboembolism in atrial fibrillation without anticoagulant therapy has been estimated to be 3.6% for moderate MS and 5.7% for severe MS. The corresponding figures for patients in sinus rhythm were 0.25% for moderate MS and 0.85% for severe MS.[69] In patients with atrial fibrillation, most embolic complications originate from left atrial thrombosis, which is located in the left atrial appendage.[69] Embolic events are cerebral in location in 60% to 70% of patients, leave sequelae in 30% to 45% of patients, and are prone to recurrence.[74] Left atrial spontaneous contrast as assessed by TEE plays a particular important role in risk stratification for thromboembolic risk in MS.[75]

MEDICAL THERAPY

The goals of medical therapy are to prevent rheumatic fever, to improve symptoms, and to decrease the thromboembolic risk. These should be considered in conjunction with a close follow-up to enable timely intervention when needed.

Prevention of Rheumatic Fever

Primary prevention is based on adequate antibiotic treatment of streptococcal pharyngitis. Secondary prevention is based on the use of continuous antibiotic therapy.[76] Although painful, intramuscular injection of benzathine penicillin every 3 weeks has the advantage of better compliance than daily oral treatment, particularly in young patients and in developing countries. Antibiotic prophylaxis of rheumatic fever is advised for up to 25 years in patients with rheumatic carditis. Once rheumatic valve disease has occurred, no medical treatment has been shown to be able to slow the progression of MS.

The prevention of infective endocarditis has been recently reoriented toward reduced indications for antibiotic prophylaxis, which is no longer advised in native heart valve diseases. On the other hand, the importance of general hygiene measures is stressed, particularly regarding dental and cutaneous hygiene.[77]

Treatment of Symptoms

The occurrence of dyspnea in a patient with MS should first lead the clinician to consider intervention. Medical treatment of symptomatic MS includes diuretics to relieve congestion and β-blockers to lengthen the diastolic filling period.

β-Blockers are particularly useful in pregnant women, enabling a dramatic decrease in mean gradient and pulmonary artery pressure in most women.[78] However, β-blockers do not seem to improve exercise tolerance in MS.[79,80]

In patients with MS and atrial fibrillation, restoration of sinus rhythm is superior to rate control to improve indices of functional capacity and quality of life.[81] When atrial fibrillation cannot be converted in sinus rhythm, rate control is obtained using digitalis and/or β-blockers.

Prevention of Thromboembolism

Unlike in patients with nonvalvular atrial fibrillation, there are no randomized trials on the efficacy of anticoagulant therapy in MS with or without atrial arrhythmias. Permanent or paroxysmal atrial fibrillation is a class I indication for oral anticoagulation, regardless of stenosis severity, in the American College of Cardiology/American Heart Association (ACC/AHA) as well as the European Society of Cardiology (ESC) guidelines.[22,23] In a retrospective study, oral anticoagulation decreased the annual risk of thromboembolism in patients with MS and atrial fibrillation from 5.7% to 1.0% for severe MS and from 3.6% to 0.9% for moderate MS.[69]

In patients with MS in sinus rhythm, the annual risk of thromboembolism decreased from 0.85% to 0.10% for severe MS and from 0.25% to 0.10% for moderate MS.[69] Given the risk of bleeding inherent to oral anticoagulation, the analysis of risk and benefits does not support systematic anticoagulant therapy in patients with MS in sinus rhythm. Anticoagulant therapy is advised in selected patients with MS in sinus rhythm who have a high risk for thromboembolic events according to the following criteria. Prior embolism and left atrial thrombus are class I recommendations for oral anticoagulation in the ACC/AHA and ESC guidelines. Dense spontaneous contrast and enlargement of the left atrium are class IIa recommendations in the ESC guidelines and IIb in ACC/AHA guidelines. Target international normalized ratio is 2.5, i.e., a range between 2.0 and 3.0. Aspirin or other antiplatelet drugs alone are not valid alternatives to decrease thromboembolic risk in patients with MS.[22,23]

A randomized trial showed a benefit with use of a combination of an antiplatelet drug with low-dose oral anticoagulation compared with conventional anticoagulation, but this result requires further confirmation.[82]

Pharmacological or electrical cardioversion should be attempted in patients with nonsevere MS who have persistent atrial fibrillation. In most patients with severe MS, cardioversion should be postponed until after the intervention on the mitral valve, because it is unlikely to allow sustained restoration of sinus rhythm in the absence of intervention.

Modalities of Follow-up

Follow-up timing should be adapted to the severity of MS, symptoms, and potential complications. Clinical follow-up should include a search for symptoms and clinical signs of examination suggesting complications, particularly transient ischemic attacks, which may not be spontaneously reported by the patient. Auscultation may reveal an increase in the severity of MS or arrhythmia.

In asymptomatic patients with significant MS in whom intervention is not planned, systematic clinical and echocardiographic follow-up is performed yearly. In patients with moderate MS, follow-up intervals can be longer, in particular for echocardiography, which may be performed at 2- to 3-year intervals.

The patient should be educated to identify interim changes in symptoms, which should lead to a prompt visit. Women should be informed of the risks inherent to pregnancy. Appropriate contraception should be used, and BMC may be indicated if a patient with MS and a valve area less than 1.5 cm², even without symptoms, desires pregnancy.

Follow-up should adapted to circumstances that increase the risk of complications, such as pregnancy and infections. Repeated echocardiographic examinations at 1- to 2-month intervals are useful during the second and third trimesters of pregnancy to monitor mean gradient and pulmonary artery pressure. Follow-up after successful BMC is the same as that for asymptomatic patients. The follow-up interval should be closer when restenosis occurs.

SURGICAL THERAPY

Closed Surgical Commissurotomy

The initial surgical approach for the relief of MS introduced in 1948, was "closed" commissurotomy; i.e., dilation of the stenotic valve via the left atrium, without direct visualization of the valve.[83] This procedure has the advantage that it can be performed using a left thoracotomy approach and does not require cardiopulmonary bypass. Typically, after palpation of the fused commissures with the surgeon's finger, a transventricular dilator is inserted through the left atrial appendage and across the mitral valve. The dilator is opened one or more times to split the fused commissures. The disadvantages of this procedure are the risk of embolic events due to dislodging atrial thrombi, incomplete relief of MS, and induction of excessive MR due to tearing of the leaflets rather than opening of the fused commissures.

Closed mitral commissurotomy results in excellent relief of MS symptoms with an operative mortality averaging 3% to 4%.[83,84] Most patients have significant improvement in symptoms after closed mitral commissurotomy and have an average increase of 1.0 cm² in valve area.[85] Extensive calcification of the valve is associated with a suboptimal hemodynamic result and poor clinical outcome.

Long-term outcome after closed commissurotomy is quite good with 31% to 50% of patients requiring reoperation within 15 years after the initial procedure and 76% at 20 years.[86,87] Recurrent symptoms most often are due to incomplete relief of MS with the initial procedure or a combination of worsened MR and residual MS. Restenosis after an initially successful procedure is the least common indication for reoperation.[88]

Predictors of late death are age, male gender, and the presence of atrial fibrillation. Multivariate predictors of the need for subsequent valve replacement are functional class, mitral valve calcification and subvalvular fusion, and the adequacy of the initial surgical procedure.

This operation is effective and easily accessible, which explains its frequent use until very recently in developing countries.

Open Surgical Commissurotomy

Open mitral commissurotomy is usually performed via a median sternotomy with the patient on full cardiopulmonary bypass. The mitral valve apparatus is directly visualized from the left atrium with careful sharp dissection of the fused commissures under direct vision. In addition, the degree of valve opening can be further improved by release of fused chordae or correction of chordal shortening.[89] If needed, an annuloplasty ring can be used to decrease the severity of coexisting MR.

Compared with closed commissurotomy, the advantages of the open procedure are the ability to visualize the valve structure in detail and to perform a more directed surgical repair. The left atrium also can be evaluated more fully, allowing detection and removal of left atrial thrombus. As with the closed approach, the best hemodynamic results and long-term outcome are seen in patients with little valve calcification, flexible and mobile leaflets, and only minimal MR.

With appropriate patient selection and in experienced hands open commissurotomy is feasible in 80% to 90% of referred subjects with an operative mortality of about 1%.[89-91] The hemodynamic results of open commissurotomy are at least equivalent to those with the closed technique, with valve area increasing by about 1.0 cm² on average. Long-term outcome after open surgical commissurotomy has been excellent with a rate of reoperation for mitral valve replacement of 0% to 16% at 36 to 53 months and 10-year actuarial survival rates of 81% to 90%.[89-92]

Mitral Valve Replacement

In patients with mitral stenosis who require valve replacement, a mechanical valve is usually appropriate because of their better durability in the mitral position and because most patients require long-term anticoagulation for atrial fibrillation.

Most studies reporting the operative mortality for mitral valve replacement include patients with both MS and regurgitation. Operative mortality ranges between 3% and 15% and correlates with age, functional class, pulmonary hypertension, and the presence of coronary artery disease.[92-95]

Long-term outcome after valve replacement for MS depends on the durability and hemodynamics of the prosthetic valve; complications associated with the prosthetic valve; the risks of chronic anticoagulation; any residual anatomic or hemodynamic abnormalities due to MS, such as pulmonary hypertension, left atrial enlargement, atrial fibrillation, or right ventricular enlargement and dysfunction; and involvement of other valves by the rheumatic process.

BALLOON MITRAL COMMISSUROTOMY

BMC is similar to surgical commissurotomy with splitting of the closed commissures.[96] Sometimes the fracturing of calcification may play a role in specific circumstances.

Patient Selection

The application of BMC depends on three major factors: the patient's clinical condition; valve anatomy; and the experience of the medical and surgical teams of the institution concerned.

Evaluation of patient's clinical condition must take into account the degree of functional disability, the presence of contraindications to transseptal catheterization, and the alternative risk of surgery as a function of the underlying cardiac and noncardiac status. Exercise testing is recommended to show symptoms in asymptomatic patients or in those with doubtful symptoms.

Contraindications to transseptal catheterization include suspected left atrial thrombosis, severe hemorrhagic disorder, and severe cardiothoracic deformity. Increased surgical risk could be of cardiac origin (previous surgical commissurotomy or aortic valve replacement) or extracardiac origin (comorbidity such as respiratory insufficiency or older age).

The first step in the evaluation of valve anatomy is to establish the severity of MS. The performance of BMC is usually restricted to patients with moderate to severe MS (valve area <1.5 cm²).[22,23] However, definition of a threshold of valve area above which BMC should not be performed is somewhat arbitrary because, in addition to measuring valve area, one must also take into account body surface area, functional disability, and pulmonary pressures at rest and on exercise.

With the assessment of anatomy the aim is also to establish indications and prognostic considerations. It is critical to ensure that there are no anatomic contraindications to the technique. The first of these is the presence of left atrial thrombosis, which must be excluded by systematic performance of

TEE a few days before the procedure. The second is the degree of MR. The third, the coexistence of another valve disease on the aorta or tricuspid valve, should be looked for.

For prognostic considerations, echocardiographic assessment allows the classification of patients into anatomic groups with a view to predicting the results. Most investigators use the Wilkins score,[42,97] whereas others, such as Iung et al,[98] use a more general assessment of valve anatomy. Controversy exists regarding the most effective echocardiography scoring system in the prediction of results of BMC. In fact, none of the scores available today have been shown to be superior to the others; and all echocardiographic classifications have the same limitations regarding the weight given the estimation of each lesion, their reproducibility, and the lack of assessment of localized changes in specific portions of the valve apparatus (leaflets and commissures), which may increase the risk of severe MR.[41-47] More recent scores that take into account the uneven distribution of the anatomic deformities of the leaflets or the commissural area are promising, but their exact value needs to be validated in large series.[99]

Experience of the Medical and Surgical Teams

The incidence of technical failures and complications, particularly those related to transseptal catheterization, is clearly related to the operator's experience. In addition to improvements in the management of the interventional procedure, experience improves the selection of patients by means of clinical evaluation and echocardiographic assessment.[26,100]

Even though the considerable simplification resulting from the use of the Inoue balloon may lead to a false sense of security when the technique is applied, BMC clearly should be restricted to teams that have extensive experience with transseptal catheterization and are able to perform an adequate number of procedures. The interventionists who perform BMC must also be able to perform emergency pericardiocentesis. Immediate surgical backup does not seem to be compulsory. The exact arrangement for surgical backup varies from institution to institution, according to the severity of the condition being treated and the experience of the cardiologic and surgical teams.

Technique

The transvenous or antegrade approach is the most widely used. Transseptal catheterization, which allows access to the left atrium, is the first step in the procedure and one of the most crucial. The retrograde technique without transseptal catheterization in which the balloon is introduced through the femoral artery is currently seldom used.[101]

The Inoue technique (Figure 14-9), the first to be developed,[96,102] is now used almost exclusively. The Inoue balloon is made of nylon and rubber micromesh and is self-positioning and pressure extensible. The balloon has three distinct parts, each with a specific elasticity, which can be inflated sequentially. The Inoue balloon comes in four sizes, ranging from 24 to 30 mm, and each is pressure dependent, so that its diameter can be varied by up to 4 mm as required by circumstances. Balloon size is usually chosen according to patient characteristics: height and body surface area.[102,103] The use of a stepwise dilatation technique under echocardiographic guidance is recommended (Figure 14-10). The first inflation is performed to the minimum diameter of the balloon chosen. The balloon is then deflated and withdrawn into the left atrium. If MR has not increased and valve area is insufficient, the balloon is readvanced across the mitral valve, and inflation is repeated with the balloon diameter increased by 1 to 2 mm.

Other techniques such as the double-balloon technique and its variant, the multi-track balloons,[104] are very seldom used in developing countries in which economic constraints lead to reuse of the balloons. The metallic commissurotome has been abandoned.

In experienced teams, the use of TEE[105] or intracardiac echocardiography[106,107] is limited to rare patients in whom difficulty is encountered during the transseptal catheterization or particularly high-risk circumstances, such as severe cardiothoracic deformity or pregnancy.

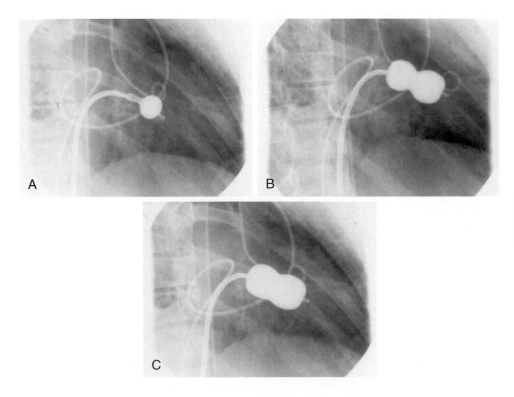

FIGURE 14–9 Fluoroscopic images recorded during a percutaneous balloon commissurotomy using an Inoue balloon. **A,** The distal balloon has been inflated to secure the position at the valvular level. **B,** the proximal segment also has been inflated. **C,** the dilating segment is briefly inflated.

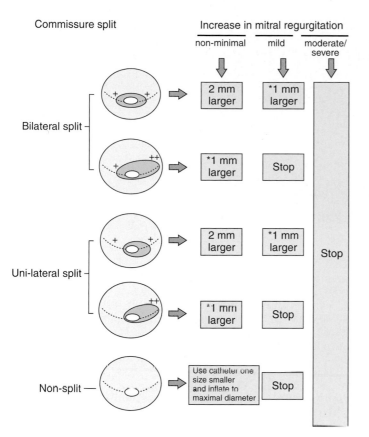

Commissure split

Increase in mitral regurgitation

| non-minimal | mild | moderate/severe |

Bilateral split

2 mm larger | *1 mm larger

*1 mm larger | Stop

Uni-lateral split

2 mm larger | *1 mm larger

*1 mm larger | Stop

Stop

Non-split

Use catheter one size smaller and inflate to maximal diameter | Stop

FIGURE 14–10 Decision making during the stepwise dilation technique using the Inoue balloon, according to echocardiographic findings after each balloon inflation. +, incomplete split; ++, complete split; *, stop in patients with severely diseased valves or those older than 65. (*From Topol E (ed): Textbook of Interventional Cardiology, 5th ed. Philadelphia, WB Saunders, 2008, with permission*).

Monitoring of the Procedure and Assessment of Immediate Results

Two methods are used to assess immediate results in the catheterization laboratory: hemodynamics and echocardiography. Although echocardiography may be difficult to perform in the catheterization laboratory for logistic reasons, it provides essential information on the efficacy of the procedure and also enables early detection of complications. The evaluation of the results necessitates a combined analysis of the following: (1) commissural opening shown by a parasternal short-axis view (this can be done using two-dimensional transthoracic echocardiography or more recently three-dimensional real-time echocardiography); (2) measurement of valve area using planimetry[29] because the pressure half-time measurement is not adequate in the acute setting[33]; (3) measurement of mean gradient; and (4) the presence and degree of MR assessed in several views with a special attention to MR originating in the commissural areas. The following criteria have been proposed for the desired end point of the procedure: (1) mitral valve area greater than 1 cm²/m² of body surface area, (2) complete opening of at least one commissure, or (3) appearance or increment of regurgitation greater than one fourth of classification.[102] Tailoring the strategy to the individual circumstances is important; clinical factors as well as anatomic factors and the cumulative data of periprocedural monitoring should be taken into account. For example, balloon size, increments of size, and expected final valve area are smaller in elderly patients, in patients with very tight MS or extensive valve and subvalvular disease, and in patients with nodular calcification.

Immediately after the procedure, the most accurate evaluation of valve area is provided by planimetry using echocardiography (Figure 14-11).[29] To allow for the slight loss in valve area that occurs during the first 24 hours, echocardiography should be performed 1 or 2 days after BMC, when calculation

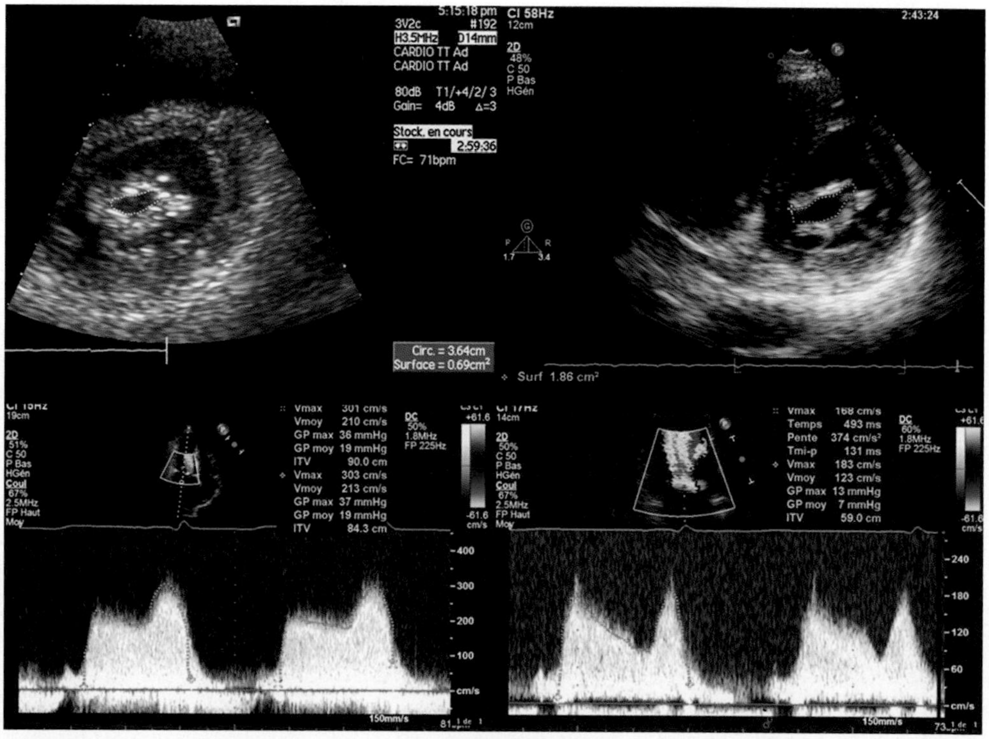

14

Rheumatic Mitral Valve Disease

FIGURE 14–11 Assessment of the immediate result of balloon mitral commissurotomy. *Top,* Two-dimensional echocardiography (parasternal short-axis view) shows opening of both commissures and an increase in valve area from 0.69 to 1.86 cm². *Bottom,* Doppler imaging of transmitral flow shows a decrease of mean mitral gradient from 19 to 7 mmHg.

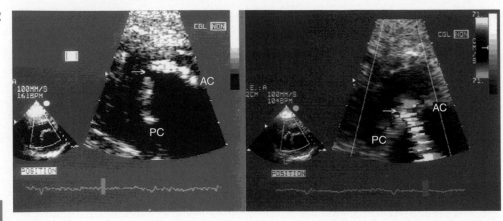

FIGURE 14–12 Severe mitral regurgitation due to an anterior leaflet tear after balloon mitral commissurotomy (transesophageal echocardiography). *Left,* Two-dimensional echocardiography showing the leaflet tear (*arrow*). *Right,* Color Doppler imaging showing severe mitral regurgitation originating from the leaflet tear (*arrow*). AC, anterior commissure; PC, posterior commissure. (*Courtesy of Dr. Cormier*).

of the valve area may be done using planimetry, the pressure half-time method, or the continuity equation. Despite its dependence on flow conditions, mean mitral gradient should be assessed because it has prognostic value. The final assessment of the degree of regurgitation may be made using angiography or Doppler color flow imaging. Transesophageal examination is recommended in patients with severe MR to determine the mechanisms involved (Figure 14-12). The most sensitive method for the assessment of atrial septal shunting is Doppler color flow imaging, which shows the severity of the defect and detects shunting in a more sensitive way than does the assessment of hemodynamics, especially when TEE is used.

Immediate Results

The technique of BMC has now been evaluated in several thousand patients with different clinical conditions and valve anatomy.[26,43,48,98,101,108-118]

Efficacy

The results shown in Table 14-4 demonstrate that BMC usually provides an increase of more than 100% in valve area.

Overall good immediate results, defined by a final valve area greater than 1.5 cm² without MR greater than grade 2/4, are observed in more than 80% of patients.

The improvement in valve function results in an immediate decrease in left atrial pressure and a slight increase in cardiac index. A gradual decrease in pulmonary arterial pressure and pulmonary vascular resistance is seen. High pulmonary vascular resistance continues to decrease over time in the absence of restenosis.[119]

BMC has a beneficial effect on exercise capacity.[120] In addition, studies have shown that this technique improves left atrial and left atrial appendage pump function and decreases left atrial stiffness.

Failures

Failure rates range from 1% to 17%.[26,98,101,109-118,121] Most failures occur in the early part of the investigators' experience. Others are due to unfavorable anatomy.

Risks

Procedural mortality ranges from 0% to 3% (Table 14-5).[26,98,101,109-118,121,122] The main causes of death are left ventricular perforation or the poor general condition of the patient.

TABLE 14–4	Immediate Results of Balloon Mitral Commissurotomy (BMC): Increase in Mitral Valve Area				
			Mitral valve area (cm²)		
Study	**n**	**Age (yr)**	**Before BMC**	**After BMC**	**Technique**
Chen, 1995[109]	4832	37	1.1	2.1	Inoue balloon
Meneveau, 1998[110]	532	54	1.0	1.7	Double-balloon or Inoue balloon
Stefanadis, 1998[111]	441	44	1.0	2.1	Modified single-balloon, double-balloon, or Inoue balloon (retrograde)
Bonhoeffer, 2000[104]	100	31	0.8	2.0	Multi-track balloon
Hernandez, 1999[112]	561	53	1.0	1.8	Inoue balloon
Kang, 2000[113] (randomized comparison)	152 150	42 40	0.9 0.9	1.8 1.9	Inoue balloon
Ben Farhat, 2001[114]	654	33	1.0	2.1	Inoue or double-balloon
Arora, 2002[115]	4850	27	0.7	1.9	Inoue or double-balloon or metallic commissurotome
Palacios, 2002[116]	879	55	0.9	1.9	Inoue or double-balloon
Neumayer, 2002[117]	1123	57	1.1	1.8	Inoue balloon
Iung, 2004[26]	2773	47	1.0	1.9	Inoue balloon, single-balloon, or double-balloon
Fawzy, 2007[118]	520	31	0.9	2.0	Inoue balloon

TABLE 14–5 | **Severe Complications of Balloon Mitral Commissurotomy**

	n	Age (yr)	In-hospital death (%)	Tamponade (%)	Embolic Events (%)	Severe Mitral Regurgitation (%)
National Heart, Lung, Blood Institute Registry[121]* (1987-1989) Center BMC volume	738	54				
n < 25			2	6	4	4
25 ≤ n < 100			1	4	2	3
n ≥ 100			0.3	2	1	3
Chen, 1995[109]* (1985-1994)	4832	37	0.1	0.8	0.5	1.4
Meneveau, 1998[110] (1986-1996)	532	54	0.2	1.1	—	3.9
Stefanadis, 1998[111]* (1988-1996)	441	44	0.2	0	0	3.4
Hernandez, 1999[112] (1989-1995)	620	53	0.5	0.6	—	4.0
Ben Farhat, 2001[114] (1987-1998)	654	33	0.5	0.6	1.5	4.6
Arora, 2002[115] (1987-2000)	4850	27	0.2	0.2	0.1	1.4
Palacios, 2002[116] (1986-2000)	879	55	0.6	1.0	1.8	9.4
Neumayer, 2002[117] (1989-2000)	1123	57	0.4	0.9	0.9	6.0
Iung, 2004[26] (1986-2001)	2773	47	0.4	0.2	0.4	4.1
Fawzy, 2007[118] (1989-2004)	551	31	0	0.7	0.5	1.6

*Multicenter series.

The incidence of hemopericardium varies from 0.5% to 12%. Pericardial hemorrhage may be related to transseptal catheterization or to apex perforation by the guide wire or the balloon itself when the double-balloon technique is used. Embolism is encountered in 0.5% to 5% of patients.

The frequency of severe MR ranges from 2% to 19%. Surgical findings[98,123-127] have shown that it is mostly related to noncommissural leaflet tearing, which could be associated with chordal rupture. The development of severe MR depends more on the distribution of the morphologic changes of the valve than on their severity.[44,51,128] Severe MR may be well tolerated, but more often it is not, and surgery on a scheduled basis is necessary. In most patients, valve replacement is required because of the severity of the underlying valve disease. Conservative surgery has been successfully performed in patients with less severe valve deformity.[126]

The frequency of atrial septal defect reported after BMC varies from 10% to 90%, depending on the technique used for its detection.[129] These shunts are usually small and without clinical consequences.

Although urgent surgery (within 24 hours) is seldom needed for complications, it may be required for massive hemopericardium resulting from left ventricular perforation intractable to treatment by pericardiocentesis or, less frequently, for severe MR with poor hemodynamic tolerance.[97,98,123-125]

Predictors of Immediate Results

The prediction of results is multifactorial.[97,98,130,131] Several studies have shown that, in addition to morphologic factors, preoperative variables such as age, history of surgical commissurotomy, functional class, small mitral valve area, presence of MR before BMC, atrial fibrillation, high pulmonary artery pressure, and the presence of severe tricuspid regurgitation, as well as procedural factors such as balloon type and size, are all independent predictors of the immediate results. The identification of variables linked to outcome enabled the development of predictive models, from which it seems that the sensitivity of prediction is high. Nevertheless, specificity is low, which indicates insufficient prediction of poor immediate results. This latter finding is particularly true with regard to the lack

of accurate prediction of severe MR. This low specificity is related to the intrinsic limitations of the prediction of immediate results, that is, to the possibility of good results in patients who have a high risk for poor results. The possibility of good results in theoretically unsuitable patients has been demonstrated in experimental studies and confirmed clinically.

Long-Term Results

Data from follow-up of up to 17 years can now be analyzed. In clinical terms the overall long-term results of BMC are good (Table 14-6).[110-116,118,132-138] Late outcome after BMC differs

TABLE 14–6 | **Late Results after Balloon Mitral Commissurotomy**

Study	n	Age (yr)	Maximum Follow-up (yr)	Event-Free Survival (%)
Cohen 1992[132]	146	59	5	51*
Dean, 1996. (National Heart, Lung, and Blood Institute registry)[133]	736	54	4	60*
Orrange, 1997[134]	132	44	7	65*
Meneveau, 1998[110]	532	54	7.5	52†
Stefanadis, 1998[111]	441	44	9	75†
Hernandez, 1999[112]	561	53	7	69†
Iung, 1999[135]	1024	49	10	56†
Ben Farhat, 2001[114]	654	34	10	72†
Palacios, 2002[116]	879	55	12	33†
Fawzy, 2007[118]‡	520	31	17	31†

*Survival without intervention.
†Survival without intervention and in New York Heart Association class I or II.
‡Patients with good immediate results.

according to the quality of the immediate results and depends on patient characteristics (Figures 14-13 and 14-14).

When the immediate results are unsatisfactory, patients experience only transient or no functional improvement, and delayed surgery is usually performed when the extracardiac conditions allow. Conversely, if BMC is initially successful, then survival rates are excellent, functional improvement occurs in the majority of patients, and the need for secondary surgery is infrequent. When clinical deterioration occurs in these patients, it is late and mainly related to mitral restenosis. Determining the incidence of restenosis by echocardiography is compromised by the absence of a uniform definition. It has generally been defined as a loss of more than 50% of the

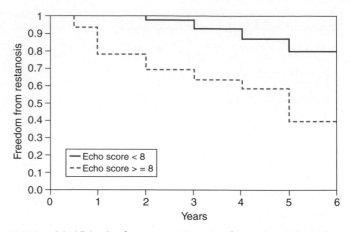

FIGURE 14–15 Freedom from restenosis in a series of 181 patients with initially successful balloon mitral commissurotomy and adequate echocardiographic data in those with an echocardiographic score less than 8 or 8 or greater. Restenosis was defined as a valve area less than 1.5 cm² and a 50% loss of the initial gain in valve area. (*From Wang A, Krasuski RA, Warner JJ, et al: Serial echocardiographic evaluation of restenosis after successful percutaneous mitral commissurotomy. J Am Coll Cardiol 2002;39:328-334, with permission*).

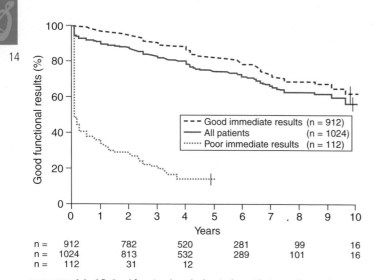

n =	912	782	520	281	99	16
n =	1024	813	532	289	101	16
n =	112	31	12			

FIGURE 14–13 Good functional results (survival considering cardiovascular-related deaths with no need for mitral surgery or repeat dilatation and in NYHA functional class I or II) after balloon mitral commissurotomy in 1024 patients. (*From Iung B, Garbarz E, Michaud P, et al: Late results of percutaneous mitral commissurotomy in a series of 1024 patients: analysis of late clinical deterioration: frequency, anatomical findings, and predictive factors. Circulation 1999;99:3272-3278, with permission*).

initial gain with a valve area becoming less than 1.5 cm². After a successful procedure, the incidence of echocardiographically identified restenosis is usually low, ranging from 2% to 40% at time intervals of 3 to 6 years (Figure 14-15).[112,136,138] The possibility of repeating BMC in patients with recurrent MS is one of the potential advantages of this nonsurgical procedure. Repeated BMC can be proposed if recurrent stenosis leads to symptoms or occurs several years after an initially successful procedure and the predominant mechanism of restenosis is commissural refusion.[139-142] Currently, results of only a small number of series on repeat BMC are available; these show good immediate and midterm outcome in patients with favorable characteristics. Although the results are less favorable in patients presenting with worse characteristics, repeat BMC has a palliative role in patients who are not candidates for surgery.[140,142] These preliminary results are encouraging; however, a definition of the exact role of repeat BMC must await larger series with longer follow-up.

The degree of MR generally remains stable or slightly decreases during follow-up. Atrial septal defects are likely to close over time in the majority of patients because of a reduction in the interatrial pressure gradient. The persistence of shunts is related to their magnitude or to unsatisfactory relief of the valve obstruction. They very seldom require treatment on their own. Finally, clinical series of surgical and balloon commissurotomies suggest that intervention reduces markers of the risk of embolism such as intensity of left atrial echocardiographic contrast, size, and function.[143-148] No direct evidence that BMC reduces the incidence of atrial fibrillation exists, even if its favorable influence on predictors of atrial fibrillation,[149-153] such as atrial size or degree of obstruction, seems to indicate that this is indeed the case. It is recommended that electric shock cardioversion be performed after successful BMC if atrial fibrillation is of recent onset and severe left atrial enlargement is absent.[81]

Surgical commissurotomy has been compared with BMC in several studies, mostly in patients with favorable characteristics. These studies consistently showed that BMC is at least comparable to surgical commissurotomy regarding short-term and midterm follow-up up to 7 years.[154-157]

Predictors of Long-Term Results

Prediction of long-term results is multifactorial[110,116,135,138] and is based on clinical variables such as age; valve anatomy as

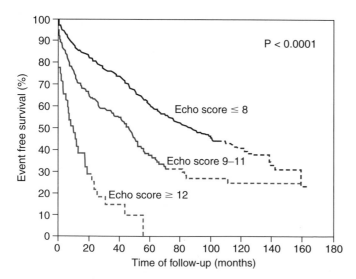

FIGURE 14–14 Event-free survival (alive and free of mitral valve replacement or redoing of balloon mitral commissurotomy) after balloon mitral commissurotomy according to echocardiographic score. (*From Palacios IF, Sanchez PL, Harrell LC, et al: Which patients benefit from percutaneous mitral balloon valvuloplasty? Pre-valvuloplasty and post-valvuloplasty variables that predict long-term outcome. Circulation 2002;105:1465-1471, with permission.*)

assessed by different echocardiographic scores; factors related to the evolutional stage of the disease, i.e., a higher New York Heart Association class before BMC; history of previous commissurotomy; severe tricuspid regurgitation; cardiomegaly; atrial fibrillation; high pulmonary vascular resistances; and the results of the procedure (final valve area, final gradient, and degree of regurgitation). The quality of the late results is generally considered to be independent of the technique used.[113] The identification of these predictors provides important information for patient selection and is relevant to follow-up: patients who have good immediate results but who have a high risk of further events must be carefully followed to detect deterioration and allow for timely intervention.

Applications of Balloon Mitral Commissurotomy in Special Patient Groups

After Surgical Commissurotomy

This category of patients is of interest because in Western countries recurrent MS is becoming more frequent than primary MS, and reoperation in this context is associated with a higher risk of morbidity and mortality and requires valve replacement in most patients.[158-160] BMC is feasible in this setting and significantly improves valve function. On the whole, the results are good, even if slightly less satisfactory than those obtained in patients without previous commissurotomy; this finding probably can be attributed to less favorable characteristics observed in patients who previously underwent operations. These encouraging preliminary data suggest that BMC may postpone reoperation in selected patients with restenosis after commissurotomy. The indications for BMC in this subgroup of patients are similar to those for primary BMC, but echocardiographic examination must exclude any patients in whom restenosis is due mainly to valve rigidity without significant commissural refusion. The latter mechanism could be responsible for the exceptional cases of MS that develop in patients who have undergone mitral ring annuloplasty for correction of MR.

Patients at High Risk for Surgery

Preliminary series have suggested that BMC can be performed safely and effectively in patients with severe pulmonary hypertension.[161-163]

In Western countries many patients with MS have concomitant noncardiac disease, which may also increase the risk of surgery.[4,25] BMC can be performed as a life-saving procedure in critically ill patients,[164,165] as the sole treatment when a patient has an absolute contraindication to surgery, or as a "bridge" to surgery in other patients. In this context, dramatic improvement has been observed in young patients, but, conversely, the outcome is very bad in elderly patients presenting with end-stage disease, for whom conservative treatment often is more appropriate.

In elderly patients, BMC results in moderate, but significant, improvement in valve function at an acceptable risk, although subsequent functional deterioration is frequent.[25,166-169] Therefore, BMC is a valid, if only a palliative, treatment for these patients, particularly when the alternative of surgery carries a high risk because of age, comorbidities, and the evolutive stage of the disease.

During pregnancy, surgery carries a substantial risk of fetal mortality and morbidity, especially if extracorporeal circulation is required. The experience of BMC during pregnancy is still limited[170-175] but suggests the following. From a technical point of view, during the last weeks of pregnancy, which was when BMC was performed in most patients, the procedure may be more difficult because of the enlarged uterus. The procedure is effective, and results in normal delivery in most patients. Regarding radiation exposure, BMC is safe for the fetus, provided protection is given with the use of a shield that completely surrounds the patient's abdomen and if the procedure is performed after the 20th week of gestation. Preliminary series have shown satisfactory development of the infants over 5 to 10 years of follow-up. Nevertheless, it must be borne in mind that, in addition to radiation, BMC carries the potential risk of related hypotension and the ever-present risk of complications that require urgent surgery. In summary, these data, which now represent several hundreds of patients, suggest that BMC can be a useful technique in the treatment of pregnant patients with MS and refractory heart failure despite medical treatment.

TREATMENT STRATEGY

An image of current practice can be derived from the Euro Heart Survey on Valvular Heart Disease,[1] which was performed prospectively in 92 centers throughout Europe during a 4-month period in 2001. It showed that BMC is now used in more than one third of patients with MS, with the other patients being treated by valve replacement mostly using mechanical prostheses. Thus, in current practice, percutaneous intervention has almost replaced surgical commissurotomy.[176] This change is due to the good results of the interventional techniques and also to the fact that most surgeons have lost experience with the conservative techniques for treatment of MS because of the limited number of procedures performed.

Intervention should be done only in patients with significant MS (valve area <1.5 cm²) because beyond this threshold, the risks probably outweigh the benefits, and these patients can usually be managed well with medical treatment.[22,23,177] There may be rare cases for which the procedure may be offered to patients with slightly larger valve areas if they have a large stature, are highly symptomatic, and have favorable presenting characteristics.

Surgery is the only alternative when BMC is contraindicated.

Because the most important contraindication is left atrial thrombosis, the recommendation is self-evident if the thrombus is free-floating or is situated in the left atrial cavity and also applies when the thrombus is located on the interatrial septum. Short series have suggested that BMC can be performed when the thrombus is located in the left atrial appendage[178]; however, it has not been shown to our satisfaction that use of the Inoue technique under transesophageal guidance precludes a risk of embolism. This risk is considered a contraindication for the technique in the current guidelines. If the patient is clinically stable, as is the case for most patients with MS, anticoagulant therapy can be given for 2 to 6 months,[179] and if a new transesophageal examination shows that the thrombus has disappeared, BMC can be attempted.[22,23]

Other contraindications for BMC are as follows (Table 14-7):
1. MR more than mild. BMC can, however, be considered in selected patients with moderate MR if the risk for surgery is high or even prohibitive often is more appropriate.
2. Severe mitral valve calcification
3. Absence of commissural fusion
4. Combined MS and severe aortic disease, for which surgery is obviously indicated in the absence of contraindications. On the other hand, the coexistence of moderate aortic valve disease and severe MS is another situation in which BMC is preferable to postpone the inevitable subsequent surgical treatment of both valves.[180]
5. Combined severe tricuspid stenosis and tricuspid regurgitation with clinical signs of heart failure. This is an indication for surgery on both valves. The existence of tricuspid regurgitation is not a contraindication to the procedure even though it represents a negative prognostic factor.[181]

TABLE 14–7	Contraindications to Percutaneous Mitral Commissurotomy

Mitral valve area >1.5 cm²
Left atrial thrombus
More than mild mitral regurgitation
Severe or bicommissural calcification
Absence of commissural fusion
Severe concomitant aortic valve disease or severe combined tricuspid stenosis and regurgitation
Concomitant coronary artery disease requiring bypass surgery

From Vahanian A, Baumgartner H, Bax J, et al: Guidelines on the management of valvular heart disease. Eur Heart J 2007;28:230-268, with permission.

6. Coronary disease requiring bypass surgery.[22,23] In most of these patients valve replacement is preferred, whereas open commissurotomy may be performed by experienced teams in young patients who are in sinus rhythm with no or mild calcification and have mild to moderate MR.

The therapeutic decision to perform BMC is straightforward in patients with severe mitral stenosis for whom surgery is contraindicated and in patients who are "ideal candidates for the percutaneous approach." BMC also preferable to surgery, at least as a first attempt, in patients with an increased risk for surgery. Surgery may be higher risk because of a cardiac condition as is the case in patients with restenosis after surgical commissurotomy, previous aortic valve replacement, or severe pulmonary hypertension. BMC can be performed as a life-saving procedure in critically ill patients, as the sole treatment in patients with an absolute contraindication to surgery, or as a bridge to surgery in the other patients. It can also be performed in elderly patients as a palliative procedure or in pregnant patients who remain symptomatic despite medical treatment.

In symptomatic patients with favorable characteristics such as young patients with good anatomy (i.e., pliable valves and moderate subvalvular disease [echocardiographic score ≤8]), who are often seen in countries where rheumatic fever is still present, results of BMC are generally excellent (Table 14-8; Figures 14-16 and 14-17).[182-184] In addition, if restenosis occurs, patients treated by BMC could undergo repeat balloon procedures or surgery without the difficulties and inherent risk resulting from pericardial adhesions and chest wall scarring. BMC would thus seem to be the procedure of choice for these patients in whom we may expect to further delay surgery, enabling, for example, pregnancy to occur.

Controversy remains regarding the performance of the procedure in asymptomatic patients and in those with unfavorable anatomy. The level of evidence for performing BMC in asymptomatic patients is low because no randomized comparison exists between the results of BMC and medical therapy for such patients (Table 14-9; Figures 14-17 and 14-18). For these patients, the goal is not to prolong life or to decrease symptoms but rather to prevent thromboembolism. Truly asymptomatic patients, however, are not usually candidates for the procedure because of the small but definite risk inherent in the technique. For patients in the latter group, BMC may be considered in selected patients, i.e., those with a high risk of thromboembolism (previous history of embolism or heavy spontaneous contrast in the left atrium), recurrent atrial arrhythmias, and pulmonary hypertension. BMC can also be performed when systolic pulmonary pressure is greater than 50 mmHg at rest. In the ACC/AHA guidelines the procedure can be recommended if systolic pulmonary pressure is greater than 60 mmHg on

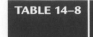

TABLE 14–8	Recommendations for Percutaneous Mitral Commissurotomy in Symptomatic Patients with Mitral Stenosis

ACC/AHA Guidelines[22]	ESC Guidelines[23]
Symptomatic patients (NYHA functional class II, III, or IV), with moderate or severe mitral stenosis* and valve morphology favorable for percutaneous balloon valvotomy in the absence of left atrial thrombus or moderate to severe mitral regurgitation (**IA**)	Patients with mitral stenosis and valve area <1.5 cm²:
Patients with moderate or severe mitral stenosis* who have a nonpliable calcified valve, are in NYHA functional class III-IV, and are either not candidates for surgery or are at high risk for surgery (**IIaC**)	Symptomatic patients with favorable characteristics† for percutaneous mitral commissurotomy (**IB**)
Symptomatic patients (NYHA functional class II, III, or IV), with mitral valve area >1.5 cm² if there is evidence of hemodynamically significant mitral stenosis based on pulmonary artery systolic pressure >60 mmHg, pulmonary artery wedge pressure ≥25 mmHg, or mean mitral valve gradient >15 mmHg during exercise (**IIbC**)	Symptomatic patients with contraindications or high risk for surgery (**IC**)
As an alternative to surgery for patients with moderate or severe mitral stenosis* who have a nonpliable calcified valve and are in NYHA functional class III-IV (**IIbC**)	As initial treatment in symptomatic patients with unfavorable anatomy but otherwise favorable clinical characteristics† (**IIaC**)

*See Table 14-1. Numbers in parentheses indicate level of recommendation (I, IIa or IIb) and level of evidence (A, B or C). See appendix for definitions.

†Favorable characteristics for percutaneous mitral commissurotomy can be defined by the absence of several of the following:

clinical characteristics: old age, history of commissurotomy, NYHA class IV, atrial fibrillation, and severe pulmonary hypertension; and

anatomic characteristics: echocardiography score ≥8, Cormier score 3 (calcification of mitral valve of any extent, as assessed by fluoroscopy), very small mitral valve area, and severe tricuspid regurgitation.

ACC, American College of Cardiology; AHA, American Heart Association; ESC, European Society of Cardiology; NYHA, New York Heart Association.

exercise.[22] However, this latter threshold should be refined by the increasing experience gained in exercise echocardiography. The European guidelines do not fix a threshold for systolic pulmonary pressure on exercise but recommend performing BMC if symptoms appear during exercise.[23] Finally, BMC can be considered for asymptomatic patients requiring major extracardiac surgery or to allow for pregnancy.

In asymptomatic patients, BMC should only be performed by experienced interventionists and when valve anatomy is favorable, in which case a safe and successful procedure can be expected. It could be expected that in the future BMC could be combined with percutaneous closure of the left atrial appendage[185] or catheter ablation of atrial fibrillation[186] to further decrease the embolic risk.

Much remains to be done in refining the indications for BMC in patients with unfavorable anatomy.[187-190] For this group, some favor immediate surgery because of the less satisfying results of BMC, whereas others prefer BMC as an initial treatment for selected candidates and reserve surgery for patients in whom this treatment fails.

Among patients with less favorable valve anatomy the comparison between the results of BMC and of surgery is also difficult. Unfortunately, no randomized study has been performed to examine this issue. Indications in this subgroup of patients must take into account their heterogeneity

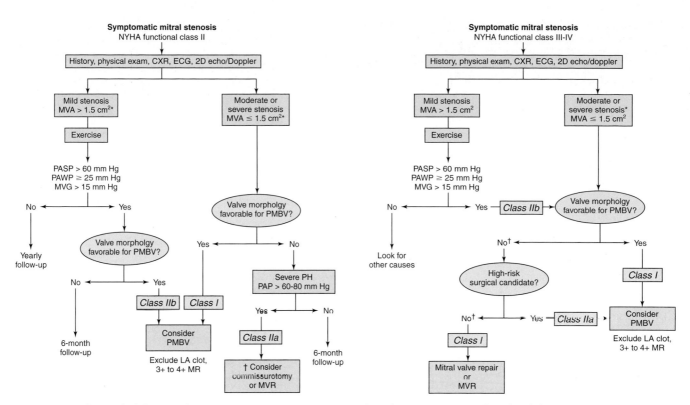

FIGURE 14–16 Indications for balloon mitral commissurotomy in symptomatic patients with mitral stenosis: American College of Cardiology/American Heart Association guidelines. AF, atrial fibrillation; CXR, chest radiograph; 2D, two-dimensional; ECG, electrocardiogram; echo, echocardiography; LA, left atrial; MVA, mitral valve area; MVG, mean mitral valve pressure gradient; MR, mitral regurgitation; MVR, mitral valve replacement; NYHA, New York Heart Association; PASP, pulmonary artery systolic pressure; PAP, pulmonary artery pressure; PH, pulmonary hypertension; PAWP, pulmonary artery wedge pressure; PMBV, percutaneous mitral balloon valvuloplasty. (*From Bonow RO, Carabello BA, Chatterjee K, et al: ACC/AHA 2006 guidelines for the management of patients with valvular heart disease: a report of the American College of Cardiology/American Heart Association Task Force on Practice Guidelines (writing committee to revise the 1998 Guidelines for the Management of Patients with Valvular Heart Disease): developed in collaboration with the Society of Cardiovascular Anesthesiologists: endorsed by the Society for Cardiovascular Angiography and Interventions and the Society of Thoracic Surgeons. J Am Coll Cardiol 2006;48:e1-e148, with permission.*)

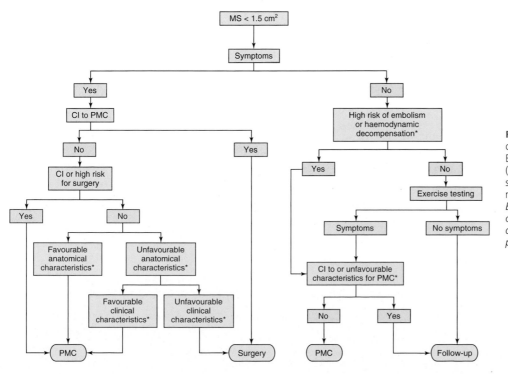

FIGURE 14–17 Indications for balloon mitral commissurotomy in patients with mitral stenosis: European Society of Cardiology guidelines (see Table 14-8 for definitions). MS, mitral stenosis; CI, contra-indication; PMC, percutaneous mitral commissurotomy (*From Vahanian A, Baumgartner H, Bax J, et al: Guidelines on the management of valvular heart disease. Eur Heart J 2007;28:230-268, with permission*).

14

Rheumatic Mitral Valve Disease

TABLE 14–9	Recommendations for Percutaneous Mitral Commissurotomy in Asymptomatic Patients with Mitral Stenosis

ACC/AHA Guidelines[22]	ESC Guidelines[23]
Asymptomatic patients with moderate or severe MS* and valve morphology favorable for BMC who have pulmonary hypertension (pulmonary artery systolic pressure >50 mmHg at rest or >60 mmHg with exercise) in the absence of left atrial thrombus or moderate to severe MR (**IC**) Asymptomatic patients with moderate or severe MS* and valve morphology favorable for BMC who have new onset of atrial fibrillation in the absence of left atrial thrombus or moderate to severe MR (**IIbC**)	Asymptomatic patients with MS with valve area <1.5 cm², favorable characteristics for BMC and high thromboembolic risk or high risk of hemodynamic decompensation: Previous history of embolism (**IIaC**) Dense spontaneous contrast in the left atrium (**IIaC**) Recent or paroxysmal atrial fibrillation (**IIaC**) Systolic pulmonary pressure >50 mmHg at rest (**IIaC**) Need for major noncardiac surgery (**IIaC**) Desire of pregnancy (**IIaC**)

*See Table 14-1.

ACC, American College of Cardiology; AHA, American Heart Association; ESC, European Society of Cardiology.

14

with respect to anatomy and clinical status. An individualized approach is favored that allows for the multifactorial nature of prediction (Figure 14-19). Current opinion is that surgery can be considered to be the treatment of choice in patients with bicommissural or heavy calcification. On the other hand, BMC can be attempted as a first approach in patients with extensive lesions of the subvalvular apparatus or moderate or unicommissural calcification. Clinical status also may argue in favor of BMC, e.g., in young patients the expectation is further delaying valve replacement with its inherent mortality and morbidity. However, surgery should be considered reasonably early after unsatisfactory results or with secondary deterioration.[22,23] Extending our knowledge regarding this group will require evaluation of multifactorial predictive models and consideration of anatomic scores that may be developed using new echocardiographic methods, such as three-dimensional imaging (Figure 14-20).[30,32]

In conclusion, the good results that have been obtained with BMC enable us to say that, currently, this technique has an important place in the treatment of MS and has virtually replaced surgical commissurotomy. In treatment of MS, BMC and valve replacement must be considered not as rivals but complementary techniques, with each applicable at the appropriate stage of the disease.

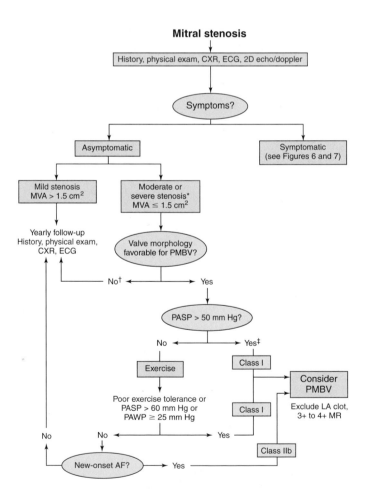

FIGURE 14-18 Indications for balloon mitral commissurotomy in asymptomatic patients with mitral stenosis. American College of Cardiology/American Heart Association guidelines. AF, atrial fibrillation; CXR, chest radiograph; 2D, two-dimensional; ECG, electrocardiogram; LA, left atrial; MR, mitral regurgitation; MVA, mitral valve area; PASP, pulmonary artery systolic pressure; PAWP, pulmonary artery wedge pressure; PMBV, percutaneous mitral balloon valvuloplasty. (*From Bonow RO, Carabello BA, Chatterjee K, et al: ACC/AHA 2006 guidelines for the management of patients with valvular heart disease: a report of the American College of Cardiology/American Heart Association Task Force on Practice Guidelines (writing committee to revise the 1998 Guidelines for the Management of Patients with Valvular Heart Disease): developed in collaboration with the Society of Cardiovascular Anesthesiologists: endorsed by the Society for Cardiovascular Angiography and Interventions and the Society of Thoracic Surgeons. J Am Coll Cardiol 2006;48:e1-e148, with permission*).

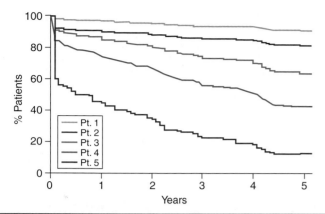

Patient	Age (years)	NYHA class	Rhythm	Calcification	Valve area (cm²)
1	< 50	II	sinus	1	1.25–1.5
2	< 50	II	sinus	2	1–1.25
3	50–70	III	sinus	2	1.25–1.5
4	50–70	III	A. fib	2	1.25–1.5
5	≥ 70	III	A. fib	3	0.75–1

FIGURE 14–19 Predicted probability of good immediate results (valve are ≥1.5 cm² without regurgitation greater than grade 2/4) and good late functional results (survival with no intervention and in New York Heart Association [NYHA] functional class I or II) after balloon mitral commissurotomy in calcified mitral stenosis, according to patient characteristics. The extent of calcification is graded from 1 (small nodule) to 4 (extensive calcification). (*From Iung B, Garbarz E, Doutrelant L, et al: Late results of percutaneous mitral commissurotomy for calcific mitral stenosis. the advantage of an individual assessment for patient selection. Am J Cardiol 2000;85:1308-1314, with permission*).

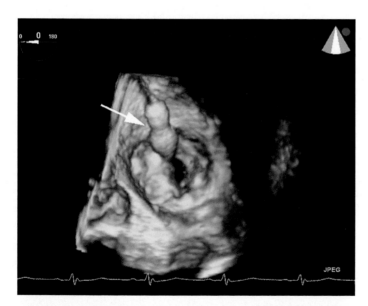

FIGURE 14–20 Monitoring of balloon mitral commissurotomy. Real-time three-dimensional transesophageal echocardiography. Inoue balloon (*arrow*) is inflated just before crossing the mitral valve. (*Courtesy of Dr. Brochet*).

REFERENCES

1. Iung B, Baron G, Butchart EG, et al: A prospective survey of patients with valvular heart disease in Europe: the Euro Heart Survey on valvular heart disease. Eur Heart J 2003;13:1231-1243.
2. Roberts WC, Virmani R: Aschoff bodies at necropsy in valvular heart disease: evidence from an analysis of 543 patients over 14 years of age that rheumatic heart disease, at least anatomically, is a disease of the mitral valve. Circulation 1978;57:803-807.
3. Okay T, Deligonul U, Sancaktar O, Kozan O: Contribution of mitral valve reserve capacity to sustained symptomatic improvement after balloon valvulotomy in mitral stenosis: implications for restenosis. J Am Coll Cardiol 1993;22:1691-1696.
4. Carroll JD, Feldman T: Percutaneous mitral balloon valvotomy and the new demographics of mitral stenosis. JAMA 1993;270:1731-1736.
5. Rizvi SFH, Khan MA, Kundi A, et al: Current status of rheumatic heart diseases in rural Pakistan. Heart 2004;90:394-399.
6. Marijon E, Ou P, Celermajer DS, et al: Prevalence of rheumatic heart disease detected by echocardiographic screening. N Engl J Med 2007;357:470-476.
7. Rahimtoola SH, Durairaj A, Mehra A, et al: Current evaluation and management of patients with mitral stenosis. Circulation 2002;106:1183-1188.
8. Lee MM, Park SW, Kim CH, et al: Relation of pulmonary venous flow to mean left atrial pressure in mitral stenosis with sinus rhythm. Am Heart J 1993;126:1401-1407.
9. Shaw TRD, Northridge DB, Sutaria N: Mitral balloon valvotomy and left atrial thrombus. Heart 2005;91:1088-1089.
10. Peverill RE, Harper RW, Gelman J, et al: Determinants of increased regional left atrial coagulation activity in patients with mitral stenosis. Circulation 1996;94:331-339.
11. Yamamoto K, Ikeda U, Mito H, et al: Endothelin production in pulmonary circulation of patients with mitral stenosis. Circulation 1994;89:2093-2098.
12. Mahoney PD, Loh E, Blitz LR, Herrmann HC: Hemodynamic effects of inhaled nitric oxide in women with mitral stenosis and pulmonary hypertension. Am J Cardiol 2001;87:188-192.
13. Remetz MS, Cleman MW, Cabin HS: Pulmonary and pleural complications of cardiac disease. Clin Chest Med 1989;10:545-592.
14. Otto CM, Davis KB, Reid CL, et al: Relation between pulmonary artery pressure and mitral stenosis severity in patients undergoing balloon mitral commissurotomy. Am J Cardiol 1993;71:874-878.
15. Morrison DA, Lancaster L, Henry R, Goldman S: Right ventricular function at rest and during exercise in aortic and mitral valve disease. J Am Coll Cardiol 1985;5:21-28.
16. Gaasch WH, Folland ED: Left ventricular function in rheumatic mitral stenosis. Eur Heart J 1991;12(Suppl):66-69.
17. Voelker W, Berner A, Regele B, et al: At effects of exercise on valvular resistance in patients with mitral stenosis. J Am Coll Cardiol 1993;22:777-782.
18. Tunick PA, Freedberg RS, Gargiulo A, Kronzon I: Exercise Doppler echocardiography as an aid to clinical decision making in mitral valve disease. J Am Soc Echocardiogr 1992;5:225-230.
19. Dahan M, Paillole C, Martin D, Gourgon R: Determinants of stroke volume response to exercise in patients with mitral stenosis: a Doppler echocardiographic study. J Am Coll Cardiol 1993;21:384-389.
20. Schwammenthal E, Vered Z, Agranat O, et al: Impact of atrioventricular compliance on pulmonary artery pressure in mitral stenosis: a exercise echocardiographic study. Circulation 2001;102:2378-2384.
21. Li M, Dery JP, Dumesnil JG, et al: Usefulness of measuring net atrioventricular compliance by Doppler echocardiography in patients with mitral stenosis. Am J Cardiol 2005;96:432-435.
22. Bonow RO, Carabello BA, Chatterjee K, et al: ACC/AHA 2006 guidelines for the management of patients with valvular heart disease: a report of the American College of Cardiology/American Heart Association Task Force on Practice Guidelines (writing committee to revise the 1998 Guidelines for the Management of Patients with Valvular Heart Disease): developed in collaboration with the Society of Cardiovascular Anesthesiologists: endorsed by the Society for Cardiovascular Angiography and Interventions and the Society of Thoracic Surgeons. J Am Coll Cardiol 2006;48:e1-e148.
23. Vahanian A, Baumgartner H, Bax J, et al: Guidelines on the management of valvular heart disease. Eur Heart J 2007;28:230-268.
24. Wood P: An appreciation of mitral stenosis. I. Clinical features. Br Med J 1954;1:1051-1063.
25. Shaw TRD, Sutaria N, Prendergast B: Clinical and haemodynamic profiles of young, middle aged, and elderly patients with mitral stenosis undergoing mitral balloon valvotomy. Heart 2003;89:1430-1436.
26. Iung B, Nicoud-Houel A, Fondard O, et al: Temporal trends in percutaneous mitral commissurotomy over a 15-year period. Eur Heart J 2004;25:702-708
27. Iung B, Vahanian A: Echocardiography in the patient undergoing catheter balloon mitral valvuloplasty: patient selection, hemodynamic results, complications and long-term outcome. In Otto CM (ed): The Practice of Clinical Echocardiography, 3rd ed. Philadelphia, WB Saunders, 2007:481-501.
28. Faletra F, Pezzano A Jr, Fusco R, et al: Measurement of mitral valve area in mitral stenosis: four echocardiographic methods compared with direct measurement of anatomic orifices. J Am Coll Cardiol 1996;28:1190-1197.
29. Baumgartner H, Hung J, Bermejo J, et al: Echocardiographic assessment of valve stenosis: EAE/ASE recommendations for clinical practice. Eur J Echocardiogr. 2008 Dec 8. [Epub ahead of print].
30. Zamorano J, Cordeiro P, Sugeng L, et al: Real-time three-dimensional echocardiography for rheumatic mitral valve stenosis evaluation: an accurate and novel approach. J Am Coll Cardiol 2004;43:2091-2096.
31. Sebag IA, Morgan JG, Handschumacher MD, et al: Usefulness of three-dimensionally guided assessment of mitral stenosis. Am J Cardiol 2005;96:1151-1156.
32. Messika-Zeitoun D, Brochet E, Holmin C, et al: Three-dimensional evaluation of the mitral valve area and commissural opening before and after percutaneous mitral commissurotomy in patients with mitral stenosis. Eur Heart J 2007;28:72-79.
33. Thomas JD, Wilkins GT, Choong CYP, et al: Inaccuracy of mitral pressure half-time immediately after percutaneous mitral valvotomy: dependence on transmitral gradient and left atrial and ventricular compliance. Circulation 1988;78:980-993.
34. Karp K, Teien D, Bjerle P, Eriksson P: Reassessment of valve area determinations in mitral stenosis by the pressure half-time method: impact of left ventricular stiffness and peak diastolic pressure difference. J Am Coll Cardiol 1989;13:594-599.
35. Chen C, Wang Y, Guo B, Lin Y: Reliability of the Doppler pressure half-time method for assessing effects of percutaneous mitral balloon valvuloplasty. J Am Coll Cardiol 1989;13:1309-1313.
36. Messika-Zeitoun D, Meizels A, Cachier A, et al: Echocardiographic evaluation of the mitral valve area before and after percutaneous mitral commissurotomy; the pressure half-time revisited. J Am Soc Echocardiogr 2005;18:1409-1414.

37. Nakatani S, Masuyama T, Kodama K, et al: Value and limitations of Doppler echocardiography in the quantification of stenotic mitral valve area: comparison of the pressure half-time and the continuity equation methods. Circulation 1988;77:78-85.

38. Messika-Zeitoun D, Yiu SF, Cormier B, et al: Sequential assessment of mitral valve area during diastole using colour M-mode flow convergence analysis: new insights into mitral stenosis physiology. Eur Heart J 2003;24:1244-1253.

39. Otto CM, Davis KB, Holmes DR Jr, et al: Methodologic issues in clinical evaluation of stenosis severity in adults undergoing aortic or mitral balloon valvuloplasty: the NHLBI balloon valvuloplasty registry. Am J Cardiol 1992;69:1607-1616.

40. Izgi C, Ozdemir N, Cevik C, et al: Mitral valve resistance as a determinant of resting and stress pulmonary artery pressure in patients with mitral stenosis: a dobutamine stress study. J Am Soc Echocardiogr 2007;10:1160-1166.

41. Reid CL, Chandraratna PA, Kawanishi DT, et al: Influence of mitral valve morphology on double-balloon catheter balloon valvuloplasty in patients with mitral stenosis: analysis of factors predicting immediate and 3-month results. Circulation 1989;80:515-524.

42. Wilkins GT, Weyman AE, Abascal VM, et al: Percutaneous balloon dilatation of the mitral valve: an analysis of echocardiographic variables related to outcome and the mechanism of dilatation. Br Heart J 1988;60:299-308.

43. Vahanian A, Michel PL, Cormier B, et al: Results of percutaneous mitral commissurotomy in 200 patients. Am J Cardiol 1989;63:847-852.

44. Fatkin D, Roy P, Morgan JJ, Feneley MP: Percutaneous balloon mitral valvotomy with the Inoue single-balloon catheter: commissural morphology as a determinant of outcome. J Am Coll Cardiol 1993;21:390-397.

45. Cannan CR, Nishimura RA, Reeder GS, et al: Echocardiographic assessment of commissural calcium: a simple predictor of outcome after percutaneous mitral balloon valvotomy. J Am Coll Cardiol 1997;29:175-180.

46. Sutaria N, Shaw TRD, Prendergast B, Northridge DB: Transoesophageal echocardiographic assessment of mitral valve commissural morphology predicts outcome after balloon mitral valvotomy. Heart 2006;92:52-57.

47. Turgeman Y, Atar S, Rosenfeld T: The subvalvular apparatus in rheumatic mitral stenosis. methods of assessment and therapeutic implications. Chest 2003;124:1929-1936.

48. Nobuyoshi M, Hamasaki N, Kimura T, et al: Indications, complications, and short-term clinical outcome of percutaneous transvenous mitral commissurotomy. Circulation 1989;80:782-792.

49. Bassand JP, Schiele F, Bernard Y, et al: The double-balloon and Inoue techniques in percutaneous mitral valvuloplasty: comparative results in a series of 232 cases. J Am Coll Cardiol 1991;18:982-989.

50. Miche E, Bogunovic N, Fassbender D, et al: Predictors of unsuccessful outcome after percutaneous mitral valvotomy including a new echocardiographic scoring system. J Heart Valve Dis 1996;5:430-435.

51. Padial LR, Abascal VM, Moreno PR, et al: Echocardiography can predict the development of severe mitral regurgitation after percutaneous mitral valvulotomy by the Inoue technique. Am J Cardiol 1999;83:1210-1213.

52. Vahanian A, Palacios IF: Percutaneous approaches to valvular diseases. Circulation 2004;109:1572-1579.

53. Zoghbi WA, Enriquez-Sarano M, Foster E, et al: Recommendations for evaluation of the severity of native valvular regurgitation with two-dimensional and Doppler echocardiography. J Am Soc Echocardiogr 2003;16:777-802.

54. Dreyfus GD, Corbi PJ, Chan KM, Bahrami T: Secondary tricuspid regurgitation or dilatation: which should be the criteria for surgical repair? Ann Thorac Surg 2005;79:127-132

55. Black IW, Hopkins AP, Lee LC, Walsh WF: Left atrial spontaneous echo contrast: a clinical and echocardiographic analysis. J Am Coll Cardiol 1991;18:398-404.

56. Hecker SL, Zabalgoitia M, Ashline P, et al: Comparison of exercise and dobutamine stress echocardiography in assessing mitral stenosis. Am J Cardiol 1997;80:1374-1377.

57. Reis G, Motta MS, Barbosa MM, et al: Dobutamine stress echocardiography for noninvasive assessment and risk stratification of patients with rheumatic mitral stenosis. J Am Coll Cardiol 2004;43:393-401.

58. Lin SJ, Brown PA, Watkins MP, et al: Quantification of stenotic mitral valve area with magnetic resonance imaging and comparison with Doppler ultrasound. J Am Coll Cardiol 2004;44:133-137.

59. Messika-Zeitoun D, Serfaty JM, Laissy JP, et al: Assessment of the mitral valve area in patients with mitral stenosis by multislice computed tomography. J Am Coll Cardiol 2006;48:411-413.

60. Segal J, Lerner DJ, Miller DC, et al: When should Doppler-determined valve area be better than the Gorlin formula? Variation in hydraulic constants in low flow states. J Am Coll Cardiol 1987;9:1294-1305.

61. Petrossian GA, Tuzcu EM, Ziskind AA, et al: Atrial septal occlusion improves the accuracy of mitral valve area determination following percutaneous mitral balloon valvotomy. Cathet Cardiovasc Diagn 1991;22:21-24.

62. Meira ZMA, Goulart EMA, Colosimo EA, Mota CCC: Long term follow up of rheumatic fever and predictors of severe rheumatic valvar disease in Brazilian children and adolescents. Heart 2005;91:1019-1022.

63. Marcus RH, Sareli P, Pocock WA, Barlow JB: The spectrum of severe rheumatic mitral valve disease in a developing country: correlations among clinical presentation, surgical pathologic findings, and hemodynamic sequelae. Ann Intern Med 1994;120:177-183.

64. Dubin AA, March HW, Cohn K, Selzer A: Longitudinal hemodynamic and clinical study of mitral stenosis. Circulation 1971;44:381-389.

65. Gordon SP, Douglas PS, Come PC, Manning WJ: Two-dimensional and Doppler echocardiographic determinants of the natural history of mitral valve narrowing in patients with rheumatic mitral stenosis: implications for follow-up. J Am Coll Cardiol 1992;19:968-973.

66. Sagie A, Freitas N, Padial LR, et al: Doppler echocardiographic assessment of long-term progression of mitral stenosis in 103 patients: valve area and right heart disease. J Am Coll Cardiol 1996;28:472-479.

67. Rowe JCBE, Sprague H, White P: The course of mitral stenosis without surgery: ten and twenty year perspectives. Ann Intern Med 1960;52:741-749.

68. Olesen KH: The natural history of 271 patients with mitral stenosis under medical treatment. Br Heart J 1962;24:349-357.

69. Horstkotte D, Niehues R, Strauer BE: Pathomorphological aspects, aetiology and natural history of acquired mitral valve stenosis. Eur Heart J 1991;12(Suppl B):55-60.

70. Moreyra AE, Wilson AC, Deac R, et al: Factors associated with atrial fibrillation in patients with mitral stenosis: a cardiac catheterization study. Am Heart J 1998;135:138-145.

71. Ramsdale DR, Arumugan N, Singh SS, et al: Holter monitoring in patients with mitral stenosis and sinus rhythm. Eur Heart J 1987;8:164-170.

72. Triposkiadis F, Trikas A, Tentolouris K, et al: Effect of atrial fibrillation on exercise capacity in mitral stenosis. Am J Cardiol 1995;76:282-286.

73. Wolf PA, Dawber TR, Thomas HE Jr, Kannel WB: Epidemiologic assessment of chronic atrial fibrillation and risk of stroke: the Framingham study. Neurology 1978;28:973-977.

74. Selzer A, Cohn KE: Natural history of mitral stenosis: a review. Circulation 1972;45:878-890.

75. Fatkin D, Feneley M: Stratification of thromboembolic risk of atrial fibrillation by transthoracic echocardiography and transesophageal echocardiography: the relative role of left atrial appendage function, mitral valve disease, and spontaneous echocardiographic contrast. Prog Cardiovasc Dis 1996;39:57-68.

76. Dajani A, Taubert K, Ferrieri P, et al: Treatment of acute streptococcal pharyngitis and prevention of rheumatic fever: a statement for health professionals. Committee on Rheumatic Fever, Endocarditis, and Kawasaki Disease of the Council on Cardiovascular disease in the Young, the American Heart Association. Pediatrics 1995;96:758-764.

77. Wilson W, Taubert KA, Gewitz M, et al: Prevention of infective endocarditis: Guidelines from the American Heart Association. Circulation 2007;116:1736-1754.

78. Al Kasab SM, Sabag T, al Zaibag M, et al: β-Adrenergic receptor blockade in the management of pregnant women with mitral stenosis. Am J Obstet Gynecol 1990;163:137-140.

79. Patel JJ, Dyer RB, Mitha AS: β-Adrenergic blockade does not improve effort tolerance in patients with mitral stenosis in sinus rhythm. Eur Heart J 1995;16:1264-1268.

80. Stoll BC, Ashcom TL, Johns JP, et al: Effects of atenolol on rest and exercise hemodynamics in patients with mitral stenosis. Am J Cardiol 1995;75:482-484.

81. Hu CL, Jiang H, Tang QZ, et al: Comparison of rate control and rhythm control in patients with atrial fibrillation after percutaneous mitral balloon valvotomy: a randomised controlled study. Heart 2006;92:1096-1101.

82. Pérez-Gómez F, Alegrya E, Berjón J, et al: Comparative effects of antiplatelet, anticoagulant, or combined therapy in patients with valvular and nonvalvular atrial fibrillation: a randomized multicenter study. J Am Coll Cardiol 2004;44:1557-1566.

83. Ellis LB, Harken DE: Closed valvuloplasty for mitral stenosis. N Engl J Med 1964;270:643.

84. John S, Bashi VV, Jairaj PS, et al: Closed mitral valvotomy: early results and long-term follow-up of 3724 consecutive patients. Circulation 1983;68:891-896.

85. Feigenbaum H, Linback RE, Nasser WK: Hemodynamic studies before and after instrumental mitral commissurotomy: a reappraisal of the pathophysiology of mitral stenosis and the efficacy of mitral valvotomy. Circulation 1968;38:261-276.

86. Ellis LB, Singh JB, Morales DD, Harken DE: Fifteen-to twenty-year study of one thousand patients undergoing closed mitral valvuloplasty. Circulation 1973;48:357-364.

87. Hickey MS, Blackstone EH, Kirklin JW, Dean LS: Outcome probabilities and life history after surgical mitral commissurotomy: implications for balloon commissurotomy. J Am Coll Cardiol 1991;17:29-42.

88. Higgs LM, Glancy DL, O'Brien KP, et al: Mitral restenosis: an uncommon cause of recurrent symptoms following mitral commissurotomy. Am J Cardiol 1970;26:34-37.

89. Smith WM, Neutze JM, Barratt Boyes BG, Lowe JB: Open mitral valvotomy: effect of preoperative factors on result. J Thorac Cardiovasc Surg 1981;82:738-751.

90. Halseth WL, Elliott DP, Walker EL, Smith EA: Open mitral commissurotomy: a modern re-evaluation. J Thorac Cardiovasc Surg 1980;80:842-848.

91. Antunes MJ, Vieira H, Ferrao de Oliveira J: Open mitral commissurotomy: the 'golden standard.' J Heart Valve Dis 2000;9:472-477.

92. Vahanian A, Iung B, Pierard L, et al: Valvular heart diseases. In Camm J, Luscher T, Serruys P (eds): The ESC Textbook of Cardiovascular Medicine. London, Blackwell Publishing, 2006;21:625-670.

93. Hammermeister K, Sethi GK, Henderson WG, et al: Outcomes 15 years after valve replacement with a mechanical versus a bioprosthetic valve: final report of the Veterans Affairs randomised trial. J Am Coll Cardiol 2000;36:1152-1158.

94. Junod FI, Harlan BJ, Payne J, et al: Preoperative risk assessment in cardiac surgery: comparison of predicted and observed results. Ann Thorac Surg 1987;43:59-64.

95. Arom KV, Nicoloff DM, Kersten TE, et al: Ten years' experience with the St. Jude medical valve prosthesis. Ann Thorac Surg 1989;47:831-837.

96. Inoue K, Owaki T, Nakamura T, et al: Clinical application of transvenous mitral commissurotomy by a new balloon catheter. J Thorac Cardiovasc Surg 1984;87:394-402.

97. Abascal V, Wilkins GT, O'shea JP, et al: Prediction of successful outcome in 130 patients undergoing percutaneous balloon mitral valvotomy. Circulation 1990;82:448-456.

98. Iung B, Cormier B, Ducimetiere P, et al: Immediate results of percutaneous mitral commissurotomy. Circulation 1996;94:2124-2130.

99. Mezilis ME, Salame MY, Oakly DG: Predicting mitral regurgitation following percutaneous mitral valvotomy with the Inoue balloon: comparison of two echocardiographic scoring systems. Clin Cardiol 1999;22:453-458

100. Tuzcu EM, Block PC, Palacios IF, et al: Comparison of early versus late experience with percutaneous mitral balloon valvuloplasty. J Am Coll Cardiol 1991;17:1121-1124.

101. Stefanadis CI, Stratos CG, Lambrou SG, et al: Accomplishments and perspectives with retrograde nontransseptal balloon mitral valvuloplasty. J Interv Cardiol 2000;13:269-280.

102. Vahanian A, Cormier B, Iung B: Percutaneous transvenous mitral commissurotomy using the Inoue balloon: international experience. Cathet Cardiovasc Diagn 1994;2:8-15.

103. Chen C, Wang X, Wang Y, et al: Value of two-dimensional echocardiography in selecting patients and balloon sizes for percutaneous balloon mitral valvuloplasty. J Am Coll Cardiol 1989;14:1651-1658.
104. Bonhoeffer P, Hausse A, Yonga G: Technique and results of percutaneous mitral valvuloplasty with the multi-track system. J Interv Cardiol 2000;13:263-269.
105. Park SH, Kim MA, Hyon MS: The advantages of on-line transesophageal echocardiography guide during percutaneous balloon mitral valvuloplasty. J Am Soc Echocardiogr 2000;13:26-34.
106. Green NE, Hansgen AR, Carroll JD: Initial clinical experience with intracardiac echocardiography in guiding balloon mitral valvuloplasty: technique, safety, utility, and limitations. Catheter Cardiovasc Interv 2004;63:385-394.
107. Liang KW, Fu YC, Lee WL, et al: Intra-cardiac echocardiography guided trans-septal puncture in patients with dilated left atrium undergoing percutaneous transvenous mitral commissurotomy. Int J Cardiol 2007;117:418-421.
108. The National Heart, Lung and Blood Institute Balloon Valvuloplasty Registry participants: Multicenter experience with balloon mitral commissurotomy: NHLBI Balloon Valvuloplasty Registry report on immediate and 30-day follow-up results. Circulation 1992;85:448-461.
109. Chen CR, Cheng TO: Percutaneous balloon mitral valvuloplasty by the Inoue technique: a multicenter study of 4832 patients in China. Am Heart J 1995;129: 1197-1202.
110. Meneveau N, Schiele F, Seronde MF, et al: Predictors of event-free survival after percutaneous mitral commissurotomy. Heart 1998;80:359-364.
111. Stefanadis C, Stratos C, Lambrou S, et al: Retrograde nontransseptal balloon mitral valvuloplasty: immediate results and intermediate long-term outcome in 441 cases—a multi-centre experience. J Am Coll Cardiol 1998;32:1009-1016.
112. Hernandez R, Bañuelos C, Alfonso F, et al: Long-term clinical and echocardiographic follow-up after percutaneous mitral valvuloplasty with the Inoue balloon. Circulation 1999;99:1580-1586.
113. Kang DH, Park SW, Song JK, et al: Long-term clinical and echocardiographic outcome of percutaneous mitral valvuloplasty: randomized comparison of Inoue and double-balloon techniques. J Am Coll Cardiol 2000;35:169-175.
114. Ben Farhat M, Betbout F, Gamra H, et al: Predictors of long-term event-free survival and of freedom from restenosis after percutaneous balloon mitral commissurotomy. Am Heart J 2001;142:1072-1079.
115. Arora R, Kalra GS, Singh S, et al: Percutaneous transvenous mitral commissurotomy: immediate and long-term follow-up results. Cathet Cardiovasc Interv 2002;55: 450-456.
116. Palacios IF, Sanchez PL, Harrell LC, et al: Which patients benefit from percutaneous mitral balloon valvuloplasty? Pre-valvuloplasty and post-valvuloplasty variables that predict long-term outcome. Circulation 2002;105:1465-1471.
117. Neumayer U, Schmidt HK, Fassbender D, et al: Early (three-month) results of percutaneous mitral valvotomy with the Inoue balloon in 1,123 consecutive patients comparing various age groups. Am J Cardiol 2002;90:190-193.
118. Fawzy ME, Shoukri M, Al Buraiki J, et al: Seventeen years' clinical and echocardiographic follow up of mitral balloon valvuloplasty in 520 patients, and predictors of long-term outcome. J Heart Valve Dis 2007;16:454-460.
119. Krishnamoorthy KM, Dash PK, Radhakrishnan S, Shrivastava S: Response of different grades of pulmonary artery hypertension to balloon mitral valvuloplasty. Am J Cardiol 2002;90:1170-1173.
120. Tanabe Y, Oshima M, Suzuki M, et al: Determinants of delayed improvement in exercise capacity after percutaneous transvenous mitral commissurotomy. Am Heart J 2000;139:889-894.
121. The National Heart, Lung, and Blood Institute Balloon Valvuloplasty Registry: Complications and mortality of percutaneous balloon mitral commissurotomy. Circulation 1992;85:2014-2024.
122. Harrison KJ, Wilson JS, Hearne SE, et al: Complications related to percutaneous transvenous mitral commissurotomy. Cathet Cardiovasc Diagn 1994;2:52-60.
123. Varma PK, Theodore S, Neema PK, et al: Emergency surgery after percutaneous transmitral commissurotomy: operative versus echocardiographic findings, mechanisms of complications, and outcomes. J Thorac Cardiovasc Surg 2005;130:772-776.
124. Zimmet AD, Almeida AA, Harper RW, et al: Predictors of surgery after percutaneous mitral valvuloplasty. Ann Thorac Surg 2006;82:828-833.
125. Choudhary SK, Talwar S, Venugopal P: Severe mitral regurgitation after percutaneous transmitral commissurotomy: underestimated subvalvular disease. J Thorac Cardiovasc Surg 2006;131:927.
126. Acar C, Jebara VA, Grare PH, et al: Traumatic mitral insufficiency following percutaneous mitral dilation: anatomic lesions and surgical implications. Eur J Cardiothorac Surg 1992;6:660-664.
127. Hernandez R, Macaya C, Benuelos C, et al: Predictors, mechanisms and outcome of severe mitral regurgitation complicating percutaneous mitral valvotomy with the Inoue balloon. Am J Cardiol 1993;70:1169-1174.
128. Reifart N, Nowak B, Baykut D, et al: Experimental balloon valvuloplasty of fibrotic and calcific mitral valves. Circulation 1990;81:1105-1111.
129. Cequier A, Bonan R, Dyrda I, et al: Atrial shunting after percutaneous mitral valvuloplasty. Circulation 1990;81:1190-1197.
130. Herrmann HC, Ramaswamy K, Isner JM, et al: Factors influencing immediate results, complications, and short-term follow-up status after Inoue balloon mitral valvotomy: a North-American multicenter study. Am Heart J 1992;124:160-166.
131. Feldman T, Carroll JD, Isner JM, et al: Effect of valve deformity on results and mitral regurgitation after Inoue balloon commissurotomy. Circulation 1992;85:180-187.
132. Cohen DJ, Kuntz RE, Gordon SP, et al: Predictors of long-term outcome after percutaneous balloon mitral valvuloplasty. N Engl J Med 1992;327:1329-1335.
133. Dean LS, Mickel M, Bonan R, et al: Four-year follow-up of patients undergoing percutaneous balloon mitral commissurotomy: a report from the National Heart, Lung, and Blood Institute Balloon Valvuloplasty Registry. J Am Coll Cardiol 1996;28: 1452-1457
134. Orrange S, Kawanishi D, Lopez B, et al: Actuarial outcome after catheter balloon commissurotomy in patients with mitral stenosis. Circulation 1997;95:382-389.
135. Iung B, Garbarz E, Michaud P, et al: Late results of percutaneous mitral commissurotomy in a series of 1024 patients: analysis of late clinical deterioration: frequency, anatomic findings, and predictive factors. Circulation 1999;99:3272-3278.
136. Wang A, Krasuski RA, Warner JJ, et al: Serial echocardiographic evaluation of restenosis after successful percutaneous mitral commissurotomy. J Am Coll Cardiol 2002;39:328-334.
137. Chen CR, Cheng T, Chen JY, et al: Long-term results of percutaneous balloon mitral valvuloplasty for mitral stenosis: a follow-up study to 11 years in 202 patients. Cathet Cardiovasc Diagn 1998;43:132-139.
138. Langerveld J, Thijs Plokker HW, Ernst SMPG, et al: Predictors of clinical events or restenosis during follow-up after percutaneous mitral balloon valvotomy. Eur Heart J 1999;20:519-526.
139. Iung B, Garbarz E, Michaud P, et al: Immediate and mid-term results of repeat percutaneous mitral commissurotomy for restenosis following earlier percutaneous mitral commissurotomy. Eur Heart J 2000;21:1683-1690.
140. Pathan AZ, Mahdi NA, Leon MN, et al: Is redo percutaneous mitral balloon valvuloplasty (PMV) indicated in patients with post-PMV mitral restenosis? J Am Coll Cardiol 1999;34:49-54.
141. Turgeman Y, Atar S, Suleiman K, et al: Feasibility, safety, and morphologic predictors of outcome of repeat percutaneous balloon mitral commissurotomy. Am J Cardiol 2005;95:989-991.
142. Kim JB, Ha JW, Kim JS, et al: Comparison of long-term outcome after mitral valve replacement or repeated balloon mitral valvotomy in patients with restenosis after previous balloon valvotomy. Am J Cardiol 2007;99:1571-1574.
143. Stefanadis C, Dernellis J, Stratos C, et al: Effects of balloon mitral valvuloplasty on left atrial function in mitral stenosis as assessed by pressure-area relation. J Am Coll Cardiol 1998;32:159-168.
144. Chiang CW, Lo SK, Ko YS, et al: Predictors of systemic embolism in patients with mitral stenosis: a prospective study. Ann Intern Med 1998;128:885-889.
145. Porte JM, Cormier B, Iung B, et al: Value of transesophageal echocardiography in the follow-up of successful percutaneous mitral valvotomy. Arch Mal Coeur 1994;87: 211-218.
146. Cormier B, Vahanian A, Iung B, et al: Influence of percutaneous mitral commissurotomy on left atrial spontaneous contrast of mitral stenosis. Am J Cardiol 1993;71:842-847.
147. Zaki A, Salama M, El Masry M, et al: Immediate effect of balloon valvuloplasty on hemostatic changes in mitral stenosis. Am J Cardiol 2000;85:370-375.
148. Chen MC, Wu CJ, Chang HW, et al: Mechanism of reducing platelet activity by percutaneous transluminal mitral valvuloplasty in patients with rheumatic mitral stenosis. Chest 2004;125:1629-1634.
149. Krasuski RA, Assar MD, Wang A, et al: Usefulness of percutaneous balloon mitral commissurotomy in preventing the development of atrial fibrillation in patients with mitral stenosis. Am J Cardiol 2004;93:936-939.
150. Leon MN, Harrell LC, Simosa HF, et al: Mitral balloon valvotomy for patients with mitral stenosis in atrial fibrillation: immediate and long-term results. J Am Coll Cardiol 1999;34:1145-1152.
151. Langerveld J, van Hemel NM, Kelder JC, et al: Long-term follow-up of cardiac rhythm after percutaneous mitral balloon valvotomy: does atrial fibrillation persist?. Europace 2003;5:47-53.
152. Fan K, Lee KL, Chow WH, et al: Internal cardioversion of chronic atrial fibrillation during percutaneous mitral commissurotomy: insight into reversal of chronic stretch-induced atrial remodeling. Circulation 2002;105:2746-2752.
153. Krittayaphong R, Chotinaiwatarakul C, Phankingthongkum R, et al: One-year outcome of cardioversion of atrial fibrillation in patients with mitral stenosis after percutaneous balloon mitral valvuloplasty. Am J Cardiol 2006;97:1045-1050.
154. Turi ZG, Reyes VP, Soma Raju B, et al: Percutaneous balloon vs. surgical closed commissurotomy for mitral stenosis. Circulation 1991;83:1179-1185.
155. Reyes VP, Raju BS, Wynne J, et al: Percutaneous balloon valvuloplasty compared with open surgical commissurotomy for mitral stenosis. N Engl J Med 1994;331:961-967.
156. Ben Fahrat M, Ayari M, Maatouk F: Percutaneous balloon versus surgical closed and open mitral commissurotomy: seven-year follow-up results of a randomized trial. Circulation 1998;97:245-250.
157. Cardoso LF, Grinberg M, Pomerantzeff PM, et al: Comparison of open commissurotomy and balloon valvuloplasty in mitral stenosis: a five-year follow-up. Arq Bras Cardiol 2004;83:248-252.
158. Iung B, Garbarz E, Michaud P, et al: Percutaneous mitral commissurotomy for restenosis after surgical commissurotomy: late efficacy and implications for patient selection. J Am Coll Cardiol 2000;35:1295-1302.
159. Jang IK, Block PC, Newell JB, et al: Percutaneous mitral balloon valvotomy for recurrent mitral stenosis after surgical commissurotomy. Am J Cardiol 1995;75:601-605.
160. Fawzy ME, Hassan W, Shoukri M, et al: Immediate and long-term results of mitral balloon valvotomy for restenosis following previous surgical or balloon mitral commissurotomy. Am J Cardiol 2005;96:971-975.
161. Alfonso F, Macaya C, Hernandez R, et al: Percutaneous mitral valvuloplasty with severe pulmonary artery hypertension. Am J Cardiol 1993;72:325-330.
162. Maoqin S, Guoxiang H, Zhiyuan S, et al: The clinical and hemodynamic results of mitral balloon valvuloplasty for patients with mitral stenosis complicated by severe pulmonary hypertension. Eur J Intern Med 2005;16:413-418.
163. Umesan CV, Kapoor A, Sinha N, et al: Effect of Inoue balloon mitral valvotomy on severe pulmonary arterial hypertension in 315 patients with rheumatic mitral stenosis: immediate and long-term results. J Heart Valve Dis 2000;9:609-615.
164. Goldman J, Slade A, Clague J: Cardiogenic shock to mitral stenosis treated by balloon mitral valvuloplasty. Cathet Cardiovasc Diag 1998;43:195-197.
165. Vahanian A, Iung B, Nallet O: Percutaneous valvuloplasty in cardiogenic shock. In Hasdai D, Berger P, Battler A, Holmes D (eds): Cardiogenic Shock: Diagnosis and Treatment. Towota, NJ, Humana, 2002:181-193.

242

166. Hildick-Smith DJR, Taylor GJ, Shapiro LN: Inoue balloon mitral valvuloplasty: long-term clinical and echocardiographic follow-up of a predominantly unfavorable population. Eur Heart J 2000;21:1691-1698.

167. Tuzcu EM, Block PC, Griffin BP, et al: Immediate and long-term outcome of percutaneous mitral valvotomy in patients 65 years and older. Circulation 1992;85:963-971.

168. Iung B, Cormier B, Farah B, et al: Percutaneous mitral commissurotomy in the elderly. Eur Heart J 1995;16:1092-1099.

169. Sutaria N, Elder AT, Shaw TRD: Long term outcome of percutaneous mitral balloon valvotomy in patients aged 70 and over. Heart 2000;83:433-438.

170. Esteves CA, Ramos AIO, Braga SLN, et al: Effectiveness of percutaneous balloon mitral valvotomy during pregnancy. Am J Cardiol 1990;68:930-934.

171. Iung B, Cormier B, Elias J, et al: Usefulness of percutaneous balloon commissurotomy for mitral stenosis during pregnancy. Am J Cardiol 1994;73:398-400.

172. Presbitero P, Prever SB, Brusca A: Interventional cardiology in pregnancy. Eur Heart J 1996;17:182-188.

173. Mangione JA, Lourenco RM, Souza dos Santo E, et al: Long-term follow-up of pregnant women after percutaneous mitral valvuloplasty. Cathet Cardiovasc Interv 2000;50:413-417.

174. de Souza JA, Martinez EE Jr, Ambrose JA, et al: Percutaneous balloon mitral valvuloplasty in comparison with open mitral valve commissurotomy for mitral stenosis during pregnancy. J Am Coll Cardiol 2001;37:900-903.

175. Sivadasanpillai H, Srinivasan A, Sivasubramoniam S, et al: Long-term outcome of patients undergoing balloon mitral valvotomy in pregnancy. Am J Cardiol 2005;95:1504-1506.

176. Palacios IF: Farewell to surgical mitral commissurotomy for many patients. Circulation 1998;97:223-226.

177. Pan M, Medina A, Suarey de Lejo J, et al: Balloon valvuloplasty for mild mitral stenosis. Cathet Cardiovasc Diagn 1991;24:1-5.

178. Chen WJ, Chen MF, Liau CS, et al: Safety of percutaneous transvenous balloon mitral commissurotomy in patients with mitral stenosis and thrombus in the left atrial appendage. Am J Cardiol 1992;70:117-119.

179. Silaruks S, Thinkhamrop B, Kiatchoosakun S, et al: Resolution of left atrial thrombus after 6 months of anticoagulation in candidates for percutaneous transvenous mitral commissurotomy. Ann Intern Med 2004;140:101-105.

180. Chen CR, Cheng TO, Chen JY, et al: Percutaneous balloon mitral valvuloplasty for mitral stenosis with and without associated aortic regurgitation. Am Heart J 1993;125:128-137.

181. Song H, Kang DH, Kim JH, et al: Percutaneous mitral valvuloplasty versus surgical treatment in mitral stenosis with severe tricuspid regurgitation. Circulation 2007;116(Suppl I):I-246-I-250.

182. Gamra H, Betbout F, Ben Hamda K, et al: Balloon mitral commissurotomy in juvenile rheumatic mitral stenosis: a ten-year clinical and echocardiographic actuarial results. Eur Heart J 2003;24:1349-1356.

183. Fawzy ME, Stefadouros MA, Hegazy H, et al: Long term clinical and echocardiographic results of mitral balloon valvotomy in children and adolescents. Heart 2005;91:743-748.

184. Kothari SS, Ramakrishnan S, Kumar CK, et al: Intermediate-term results of percutaneous transvenous mitral commissurotomy in children less than 12 years of age. Catheter Cardiovasc Interv 2005;64:487-490.

185. Sievert H, Lesh MD, Trepels T, et al: Percutaneous left atrial appendage transcatheter occlusion to prevent stroke in high-risk patients with atrial fibrillation: early clinical experience. Circulation 2002;105:1887-1889.

186. Adragao P, Machado FP, Aguiar C, et al: Ablation of atrial fibrillation in mitral valve disease patients: five year follow-up after percutaneous pulmonary vein isolation and mitral balloon valvuloplasty. Rev Port Cardiol 2003;22:1025-1036.

187. Tuzcu ME, Block PC, Griffin B, et al: Percutaneous mitral balloon valvotomy in patients with calcific mitral stenosis: immediate and long-term outcome. J Am Coll Cardiol 1994;23:1604-1609.

188. Ping Zhang H, Allen JW, Lau FYK, et al: Immediate and late outcome of percutaneous balloon mitral valvotomy in patients with significantly calcified valves. Am Heart J 1995;129:501-506.

189. Post JR, Feldman T, Isner J, et al: Inoue balloon mitral valvotomy in patients with severe valvular and subvalvular deformity. J Am Coll Cardiol 1995;25:1129-1136.

190. Iung B, Garbarz E, Doutrelant L, et al: Late results of percutaneous mitral commissurotomy for calcific mitral stenosis. Am J Cardiol 2000;85:1308-1314.

14

CHAPTER 15

Myxomatous Mitral Valve Disease

Brian P. Griffin

Mitral valve prolapse is a common disorder that has been recognized as a specific condition since the 1960s when Barlow and Bosman[1] used cineangiography to delineate the cause of systolic clicks and murmurs. Before this, myxomatous change in mitral valve tissue had been recognized pathologically. However, it was only with the arrival of two-dimensional (2D) echocardiography in the 1970s and subsequently that the natural history and pathophysiology of the condition and its complications became manifest. Mitral valve prolapse (MVP), a term originally coined by Criley et al,[2] is now recognized as the major cause of mitral regurgitation (MR) in developed countries and a cause of premature mortality and considerable morbidity if not diagnosed and appropriately managed.[3,4] In this chapter I will outline the pathogenesis of myxomatous mitral valve disease, its natural history, clinical manifestations, and the current approach to diagnosis and management of the disease and its complications.

DEFINITION

One of the difficulties in diagnosing MVP and managing patients with MVP is the appropriate classification of the patient. Myxomatous mitral valve disease and MVP are conditions that occur together but are not necessarily synonymous (Figure 15-1).[5,6] Understanding the interplay between these entities is essential. Myxomatous mitral valve disease is a pathologic condition in which the mitral valve leaflets and chordae are thickened, where there is hooding of the leaflets, and in which abnormal accumulations of mucopolysaccharides are seen in chordae and leaflets.[3,7] The valve abnormalities and especially the chordal elongation produce prolapse of the leaflets recognized echocardiographically that in some cases leads to MR.[8] A systolic click and murmur are characteristic clinical findings.[9] This condition is associated with complications in a substantial minority of those affected and may eventually lead to the need for valve surgery.[10-12] However, myxomatous mitral valve disease may exist in a preclinical phase without any overt echocardiographic or clinical manifestations.

Superior displacement of part of a mitral valve leaflet in systole on 2D echocardiography is commonly seen even in normal people. Before the refinement of echocardiographic diagnosis, prolapse was diagnosed in a substantial portion of the population.[13] Even with stricter echocardiographic criteria for diagnosis, superior displacement of the mitral valve leaflets is seen in the absence of leaflet thickening or MR in some normal people. This form of prolapse appears to arise in many instances from a disproportion between mitral leaflet size and left ventricular (LV) size. It is seen with a small left ventricle and may disappear with volume loading.[14-16] It is seen in atrial septal defect, for instance, and may disappear on closure of the septal defect.[17,18] This subtle type of prolapse is not a precursor of myxomatous changes in the mitral valve and appears to have a very benign prognosis. Differentiating those with true myxomatous disease from those with valve-ventricle disproportion is not always possible especially on one evaluation. Serial evaluation with echocardiography at yearly or greater intervals will usually allow differentiation to be made. However, it is usually possible to determine high-risk features that substantially increase the likelihood of subsequent adverse events clinically and on the initial echocardiogram.

ANATOMY OF THE NORMAL AND MYXOMATOUS MITRAL VALVE

A basic knowledge of the anatomy of the normal mitral valve is important in understanding and recognizing the variable presentation of myxomatous mitral valve disease.[19,20] The mitral valve consists of anterior and posterior leaflets attached at their base to a fibrous or fibromuscular ring, the mitral annulus (Figure 15-2). The leaflets in turn are attached to papillary muscles by chordae tendineae, one of whose functions is to prevent eversion or prolapse of the leaflets in systole. The anterior leaflet is generally larger than the posterior leaflet and is triangular in shape. The anterior area leaflet has two distinct portions, a thin translucent area at the base and a more

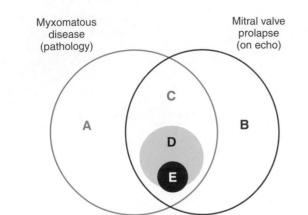

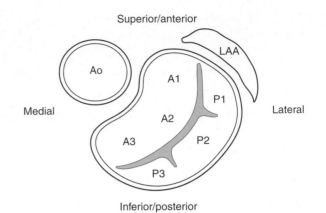

FIGURE 15–1 Interaction of myxomatous disease of the mitral valve, which is diagnosed on pathologic examination, and mitral valve prolapse, which is diagnosed on an echocardiogram. Myxomatous disease can exist in a preclinical state before the onset of prolapse. **A**, Mitral valve prolapse may occur on echocardiography as a benign condition without myxomatous change mainly due to valve-ventricle disproportion. **B**, Myxomatous valve disease is a major cause of mitral valve prolapse. **C**, Some of these patients. **D**, have high-risk clinical and echocardiographic features that make them more prone to the development of complications. **E**, such as severe mitral regurgitation requiring surgery and endocarditis.

FIGURE 15–3 Carpentier system of nomenclature for individual segments of mitral valve. A, anterior leaflet; Ao, aorta; LAA: left atrial appendage; P, posterior leaflet. *(From Foster GP, Isselbacher EM, Rose GA, et al: Accurate localization of mitral regurgitant defects using multiplane transesophageal echocardiography. Ann Thorac Surg 1998;65:1025–1031, with permission.)*

Branching of chordae before insertion is usual but not invariable. At the commissures, a single large chord branches into multiple smaller chordae that then insert at the free edge of each leaflet. The chordae to either half of the leaflets arise from each of the papillary muscles. The chordae to the posterior leaflet are inserted into each of the scallops, explaining why chordal rupture may lead to prolapse or flail of an individual scallop.

The coaptation area of the two leaflets is much greater than that of the mitral orifice and that of the anterior leaflet may be sufficient in itself to cover the entire orifice in systole. In mitral valve repair, this property is advantageous when resection of a prolapsing portion of the posterior leaflet is necessary; the anterior leaflet provides most of the coverage of the mitral orifice without allowing significant leakage. In many instances, the posterior leaflet provides an anchor or keystone against which the anterior leaflet abuts to maintain a stable and competent coaptation surface. Prolapse of the posterior leaflet may cause the anterior leaflet to prolapse because of loss of this keystone function in the absence of any major pathologic change in the anterior leaflet or its chordae.

Myxomatous disease of the mitral valve may affect one or both leaflets and may affect many or only some of the chordae. Prolapse or flail of the posterior leaflet is the most common indication for surgical intervention. In one study of more than 1,000 patients undergoing surgery for myxomatous MR, more than 50% had evidence of chordal rupture to the posterior leaflet.[21] The middle scallop is the most frequent segment affected, followed by the lateral and then the medial scallop. Carpentier has provided a surgical classification of mitral valve anatomy that is widely used. In this classification, the mitral valve has six segments, three in the anterior leaflet (A1, A2, and A3) and three in the posterior leaflet (P1, P2, and P3). The posterior leaflet segments consist of the naturally occurring scallops (P1, medial; P2, middle; and P3, lateral); the anterior segments comprise the areas adjoining each of the three posterior scallops (Figure 15-3).[22,23]

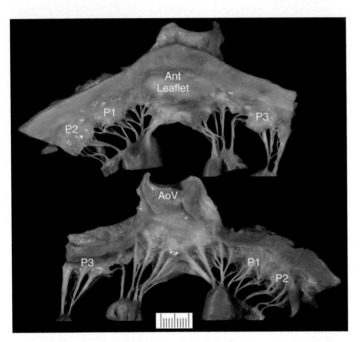

FIGURE 15–2 Normal mitral valve showing thin translucent leaflets and chordae and papillary muscles from atrial side (*top*) and ventricular side (*bottom*). The two leaflets (Ant, anterior) and the three scallops of the posterior leaflet (P1, P2, and P3) are shown. Ao V, aortic valve.

opaque thicker area at the free edge (the rough zone) where coaptation with the posterior leaflet occurs. The posterior leaflet is smaller, has a longer attachment to the annulus, and is generally segmented by clefts at the free edge into three segments or scallops (medial, middle, and lateral). The anterior and posterior leaflets meet at the two commissures (posteromedial and anterolateral) and are fused there by a rim of valve tissue of variable (<1 cm) width.

Normal chordae vary widely in number and appearance and are classified as primary, secondary, and tertiary on the basis of their attachments at the free edge, ventricular surface, and leaflet base, respectively. The normal valve has on average 25 primary chordae of which 9 insert in the anterior leaflet, 14 in the posterior leaflet, and 1 at each of the commissures.

ETIOLOGY AND PATHOLOGY OF MITRAL VALVE PROLAPSE

MVP is a degenerative condition of the mitral valve and is more evident later in life. It occurs in specific connective tissue disorders such as Marfan syndrome, Ehlers-Danlos syndrome, osteogenesis imperfecta, and pseudoxanthoma elasticum, thus suggesting a role for abnormalities of structural proteins in its genesis.[19,24-28] However, the majority of cases are idiopathic in nature, and although characteristic abnormalities on both gross pathologic and histologic examination are evident, the precise mechanism of disease remains to be determined. Pathologically, myxoid degeneration of valve tissue is distinctive.[29] Grossly, there is enlargement and thickening of the leaflets and chords, interchordal hooding of the leaflets, and annular dilatation with elongated and frequently ruptured chordae (Figure 15-4). The tissue has a spongy texture. The redundancy of leaflet tissue is often

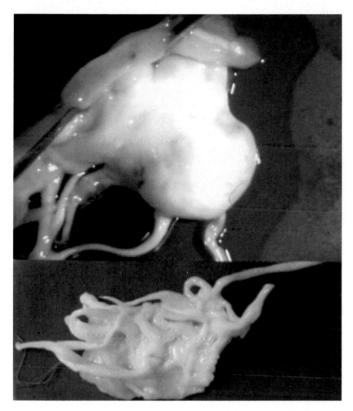

FIGURE 15–4 Gross appearance of myxomatous valve and chordae illustrating the thickening and spongy appearance of leaflets and chordae.

substantial, and fibrin deposits and even microthrombi may be evident in the folds at the base of the leaflets.[30-32] These are postulated to be a source of embolism. Platelet activation at the site of roughened endothelium in the valve has also been postulated.[31] The increased motion of valves and chords often leads to fibrosis of both valve tissue and endocardium at points of contact in the atrium and ventricles. These fibrosed areas have been postulated by some to be a source of increased arrhythmogenicity.[33]

The mitral valve has three layers histologically: the atrialis, a layer of collagen and elastic tissue that forms the atrial aspect of the leaflet; the spongiosa or middle layer that contains structural proteins and proteoglycans; and the fibrosa or ventricularis that consists predominantly of collagen and is on the ventricular side of the leaflet (Figure 15-5).[34] In myxomatous disease, the spongiosa shows an accumulation of proteoglycans and glycosaminoglycans that extends into the chords and the fibrosa and has reduced collagen staining.[35] The increased extracellular matrix gives the tissue a blue color on hematoxylin and eosin staining and was the original basis for the myxomatous label. The increased proteoglycans in the fibrosa are postulated to interfere with tensile strength. An inflammatory infiltrate is not seen in myxomatous tissue, but myofibroblasts are modulated to a more activated format.[36]

The myxomatous mitral valve has been classified into two types on the basis of its surgical appearance by Carpentier.[37] One type is called Barlow disease and is seen in younger patients with marked redundancy of the tissue and prolapse that may involve multiple segments and is more difficult to repair.[30,38] This type is also seen in connective tissue disorders such as Marfan syndrome. Fibroelastic deficiency, the other type, is seen in older patients who have myxomatous changes confined to a single segment, typically the posterior middle scallop. The rest of the valve does not appear myxomatous. There is considerable overlap between these groups and in our and others' experience it has proven difficult to differentiate them reproducibly on either the gross or histologic appearance of the valve.[37]

At a mechanical level considerable abnormality is noted in myxomatous valve disease, which in part explains the pathophysiology. Fragmentation and irregularity of both collagen and elastin have been reported.[39-41] When myxomatous

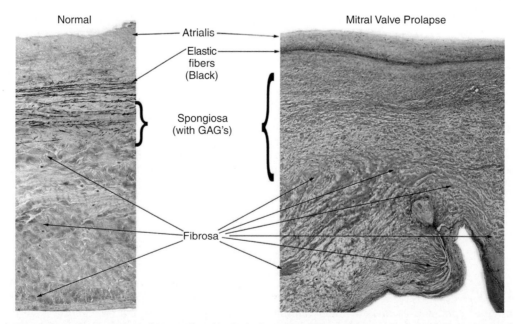

FIGURE 15–5 Histologic appearance of a mitral valve leaflet normally and in mitral valve prolapse. The spongiosa is thicker in mitral valve prolapse with a greater concentration of glycosaminoglycans (GAGs), some of which extend into the fibrosa. *(Courtesy of Rene Rodriguez, MD, Department of Cardiovascular Pathology, Cleveland Clinic.)*

valve tissue obtained at the time of mitral valve surgery is subjected to formal stress/strain analysis, the leaflets are more extensible and less stiff than normal but have relatively minor reductions in tensile strength.[42] Tensile strength is seriously compromised in the chordae despite the increase in thickness and extensibility. Myxomatous chordae fail at 25% of the load that it takes to rupture a normal chord.[43] They exhibit areas of thickening due to glycosaminoglycan deposition and fibrous sheath formation.[44] The poor load-bearing qualities of these chordae suggest that the collagen in the fibrous sheath does not add any tensile strength.[45]

Biochemically, alterations in myxomatous tissue have also been noted. The major abnormalities relate not only to the increased amounts of glycosaminoglycans (GAGs) but also to the types produced. GAGs have multiple roles including imparting specific qualities to connective tissue and modifying the structure of collagen. GAGs are incorporated with proteins as proteoglycans, which have also inherent specific properties.[46] These properties may in turn be further modified by combination with other proteoglycans. In myxomatous chordae, the amount of GAGs is twice that of normal, without any change in cellularity, suggesting that this increase occurs because of either increased production or decreased degradation or a combination.

Similar to the mechanical findings, the degree of biochemical abnormality in myxomatous tissue is more marked in chordal tissue than in the leaflets.[46] Although the individual GAGs in valve and chordal tissue are similar, their proportions differ substantially. These proportions are further altered in myxomatous tissue as is the chain length of the GAGs themselves. In myxomatous chordae, there is an excess of hyaluronan and chondroitin-6-sulfate compared with normal levels. Hyaluronan and chondroitin-6-sulfate are constituents of the proteoglycan versican. Versican is a large proteoglycan that in combination with hyaluronan is thought to increase hydration and sponginess of connective tissue. These properties are ideal to withstand compressive forces such as those that occur at the coaptation surface. In addition, myxomatous chordae have decreased amounts of 4-sulfated GAGs commonly seen in the small proteoglycan decorin. Decorin is important in collagen fibrillogenesis and its reduction may further explain the decrease in the tensile strength encountered in these chordae.[47]

Interestingly, the proportions of GAGs seen in myxomatous chordae more closely resemble those of normal leaflets than normal chordae. It is unclear why this occurs, whether it is genetically determined or whether local environmental factors in the valve itself play a role. The recent finding that GAG production is modulated in a cell culture model of valve tissue by alterations in environmental factors such as tissue strain and location suggests that GAG synthesis or degradation is responsive to local environmental conditions.[48] A neural network that is impaired or damaged in the myxomatous process has also been described in valves.[49] This too, could potentially be involved in aligning appropriate GAG production with a sensed physiologic stimulus such as tension or compression. In addition to changes in GAGs, an increase in matrix-metalloproteinases and other degradative enzymes is reported in myxomatous mitral valve disease.[36] These enzymes appear to be produced by cells within the valve tissue, are capable of structural protein degradation, and may play a role in the structural abnormalities in this disease or may occur in response to the disease alterations.

GENETIC FACTORS

Myxoid degeneration of the mitral valve is often familial although the severity of expression varies considerably within a given family, suggesting that environmental influences are also important.[50,51] The inheritance is considered to be autosomal dominant with variable penetrance that is influenced by both age and gender. It is uncommon in our experience at Cleveland Clinic to perform surgery for myxoid MR on more than one member of an affected family despite the familial nature of the disease. Work from Devereux and colleagues suggested that although MVP occurs with frequency in the families of those affected, the severity of the lesion is very variable within the same kindred.[51,52] In one study, probands with thickened leaflets were more likely to have family members with prolapse (53%) than those without significant leaflet thickening (27%). In multiple studies, heterogeneity of findings in relatives of probands is seen. Thus, leaflet thickening or involvement of one or both leaflets may vary in family members, suggesting that phenotypic expression is affected by multiple other factors rather than a specific genotype.[51]

At least three separate loci for the MVP trait have been identified in extended families with multiple affected members. These include a locus identified in 1999 in France (MMVP1), which was mapped to chromosome 16p11.2-p12.1.[53] A further locus, MMVP2, was identified in 2003 by Freed et al[54] on chromosome 11p15.4. A third locus (MMVP3) on chromosome 13 (13q31.3-q32.1) was reported by Nesta et al[55] in a family of 43 members of whom 9 had conventional diagnostic criteria for MVP. Prolapse configuration was not uniform in those affected and both thickened and nonthickened prolapsing leaflets were seen; prolapse involved the posterior leaflet in some and both leaflets in others. The proteins coded by the three reported MVP loci are unknown as yet as these studies were performed with linkage analysis.[56] However, the locus on chromosome 13 has genes of potential interest that involve cell growth and differentiation.

The occurrence of myxomatous MVP in association with other inherited connective tissue disorders raised the question as to whether proteins involved in these disorders might underlie idiopathic myxomatous degeneration. So far, however, the genes encoding the primary collagens in valve tissue have not been linked to autosomal dominant MVP.[57,58] Multiple single nucleotide polymorphisms are detected at a higher frequency in idiopathic myxoid degeneration compared with a control population, but their significance remains unclear.[59,60] In a rare related condition, X-linked myxomatous valvular dystrophy, in which all of the valves are thickened, mutations in filamin A, a gene that previously was identified only as a cause of neurologic and skeletal disorders, have been implicated.[61]

MVP is not confined to humans. Specific breeds of dog including the King Charles Cavalier Spaniel and the dachshund have a high prevalence of prolapse that may lead to severe MR and congestive heart failure later in life.[62,63] The disease is associated with dysmorphic leaflets and is inherited, suggesting a strong genetic linkage though the specific genetic determinants remain to be elucidated. An experimental murine model of Marfan syndrome–associated MVP has recently been described in which transforming growth factor-β signaling is increased as a result of fibrillin-1 deficiency.[64] Interestingly, the mitral valve changes progressed over time. Abnormal signaling involving the transforming growth factor-β system has also been postulated as a mechanism of abnormality in X-linked valve dystrophy.[65] Although these animal models provide very useful insights into mechanism of disease, the pathophysiological mechanisms operating in human idiopathic MVP appear to differ from those in either Marfan syndrome or the X-linked disorder.[25,66]

EPIDEMIOLOGY AND NATURAL HISTORY

The currently accepted prevalence of MVP in the community is based on the Framingham study.[67] In that population-based study, echocardiograms on 3,491 individuals (1,845 men and

1,646 women) were reviewed. The mean age of the population was 55 years. MVP was determined on long-axis views of the valve and was seen in 84 subjects or 2.4% of the population. Classic prolapse in which leaflet thickness greater than 5 mm and leaflet prolapse are present was seen in 1.3% of those studies and nonclassic prolapse in which leaflet displacement alone was apparent occurred in 1.1%. There was no significant gender difference in prevalence unlike earlier studies without a strict echocardiographic definition in which women predominated. Prevalence was 2% to 3% in each decade of age from 30 to 80. The subjects with MVP had a greater likelihood of MR than those without prolapse, with more regurgitation being evident in the group with classic prolapse who had on average mild regurgitation. Those with nonclassic prolapse had on average trace MR. Other complications such as atrial fibrillation, congestive heart failure, cerebrovascular disease, or syncope were no more common in the MVP group than in the rest of the population studied. MVP has been detected in many population groups of different ethnic and racial backgrounds.[68] In one Canadian study, the prevalence was similar in Caucasian, Indian, and Chinese populations.[69]

Once MVP has been established by echocardiography, long-term follow-up suggests a more complicated course than with community screening as in the Framingham study. Thus, in Olmsted County, site of the Mayo Clinic, a study identified 833 asymptomatic patients with MVP between 1989 and 1998 of whom about two thirds presented with a murmur, and in one third MVP was detected on an echocardiogram for another reason.[70] The mean age of this cohort was 47 years. Those presenting with a murmur tended to have more severe MR and a larger left atrium and were less likely to have atrial fibrillation at the outset. Ten-year mortality for the total cohort was 19% but was not statistically greater than expected. Cardiovascular mortality at 10 years was 9%. Predictors of cardiovascular mortality were moderate or greater MR or LV ejection fraction less than 50%. Site of prolapse, presence of flail, or LV size did not influence mortality. Cardiovascular morbid events in follow-up occurred in 171 patients. These included heart failure in 60, new-onset atrial fibrillation in 51, ischemic neurologic events in 38, peripheral thromboembolism in 11, endocarditis in 4, and mitral valve surgery in 65 patients. Ten-year cardiovascular morbidity was 30% and was predicted by age of 50 or older, left atrial size of 40 mm or greater, MR of any severity but higher odds ratio for more severe MR, flail leaflet, and baseline atrial fibrillation. Gender, location of prolapse, LV size, or valve thickening did not independently predict cardiovascular morbidity.

Prior studies of patients with MVP also suggested high-risk features clinically and on an echocardiogram. In a cohort of 237 asymptomatic or minimally symptomatic patients with MVP studied in the 1980s at Mayo Clinic who were followed for an average of 6 years, the survival at 8 years was predicted to be 88%, no different from that of a control population. Factors indicative of worse outcome included an end-diastolic LV dimension of greater than 6 cm, which was an indicator of a need for mitral valve surgery. Valve redundancy was another strong negative predictor, with sudden death, infective endocarditis, or a cerebral ischemic event occurring in 10% of the 97 patients with this finding, whereas only 1 of 140 patients without redundancy experienced such an event.[12] In another study of 456 patients reported in the late 1980s, the population was classified as having classic MVP on the basis of leaflet thickening and redundancy or nonclassic MVP on the basis of the absence of these features. Complications were more common in the classic group. These included endocarditis in 3.5% of the classic group versus 0% of the nonclassic group, significant MR in 12% and 0%, respectively, and the need for mitral valve surgery in 7% and 1%, respectively. There was a significant incidence of stroke of 6% to 7% that was similar in both groups.

The age of onset of MVP is variable. One study failed to detect MVP in neonates, even in offspring of affected parents.[71] It appears to be relatively uncommon in pediatric populations except in the setting of a primary disorder of connective tissue such as Marfan syndrome.[72] Symptomatic presentation is most common in midlife and surgical intervention for severe MR is most likely in the 6th or 7th decade.[21,73] In one study, the average time from detection of a murmur to symptomatic presentation was 24 years.[74] Once symptoms occurred, surgical intervention was required within 1 year and the mean age at surgery was 60 years. Thus, by inference, it appears that the mean age at which the murmur was detected was 35 years.

Given the asymptomatic nature of MVP for many years, the earliest clinical abnormalities go undetected. Even in those who may be anticipated to have a likelihood of early detection, such as physicians or executives with yearly physical examinations, detection of a murmur or click may occur only in middle age. This fact suggests that, at least in many people, the change in valve function sufficient to be clinically evident does occur relatively late and is not solely due to a failure in detection. Thus, in the Framingham study a systolic murmur was heard only in 23% of patients with classic MVP, in 10% of those with nonclassic prolapse, and in 4% of those without prolapse, whereas a click was heard in 11%, 8%, and 1.5%, respectively, of these groups.

It was estimated in the earlier era of echocardiographic diagnosis of MVP that approximately 4% of men and 1.5% of women in Australia[75] with the condition would eventually require surgery, whereas the estimates for the United States were 5% and 1.5%, respectively.[76] Given the surfeit of diagnosis of MVP in this era, the likelihood is that with a stricter definition of prolapse a greater proportion of these patients will eventually need surgery. Thus, a more recent estimate of the need for mitral valve surgery by age 70 is 11% in men with mitral prolapse and 6% for women.[77]

Despite the risk of complications, MVP appears to have a prognosis that is excellent. When patients with severe MR from MVP undergo repair surgery at an appropriate time, there is considerable evidence that their survival is as good as if not better than that of a control population without MVP.[73,78,79] This is not necessarily true if a mitral valve replacement is performed or if MR has led to LV dysfunction.[80-82] The excellent prognosis in reported series of MVP may reflect a lower than expected rate of coronary artery disease in these series either by design (exclusion of patients with both coronary disease and mitral repair in surgical series) or by chance. In the Framingham study, MVP subjects showed a trend to a lower prevalence of coronary disease. In one surgical series in which patients with coronary artery disease and myxomatous disease were compared with those with ischemic heart disease alone, survival was impaired equally in both groups and was dependent on severity of ischemic heart disease and LV dysfunction.[83] Failure to appropriately intervene surgically in MVP with severe MR does lead to impaired survival, however, illustrating the importance of careful follow-up of these patients at regular intervals.[84] Referral to surgery before the onset of symptoms or of LV dilatation or dysfunction is now indicated by the most recent American College of Cardiology (ACC)/American Heart Association (AHA) guidelines if successful repair has a likelihood of greater than 90%.[85]

DIAGNOSIS AND CLINICAL FEATURES

Symptoms

Most patients presenting with MVP for the first time are asymptomatic, and the diagnosis is made on the basis of the characteristic physical findings or because an echocardiogram is being performed for another reason. Nevertheless, patients with MVP may present with specific symptoms referable to the valve. These include shortness of breath or even heart failure when significant MR is already present. Sudden onset of shortness of breath and heart failure requiring immediate treatment may result from acute chordal rupture or from valve leaflet perforation or valve disruption in endocarditis.[86] Patients with MVP may experience chest pain that is atypical for angina.[87] The mechanism by which this occurs is unknown. Palpitations are common in patients with MVP, even in those with little or no MR.[88] Most frequently these consist of ventricular extrasystoles that may be multifocal or clustered. Atrial extrasystoles are also common.[89] However, in a blinded study of Holter monitor recordings from patients with MVP and control subjects, no difference in frequency or complexity of rhythm disturbance was noted.[90] Nevertheless, once MR is present, arrhythmia is common and is more frequent in women and with advancing age.[89] Atrial fibrillation and atrial flutter are common later in the course of MVP when significant MR has been established for some time and atrial enlargement has ensued.[91] Rarely, MVP is manifested initially by ventricular tachycardia or sudden death.[33,92,93] MVP may also present as subacute bacterial endocarditis[94,95] with fever and systemic illness or with a stroke or transient ischemic attack.[96,97]

Cardiac Physical Findings

MVP is reliably diagnosed by both physical examination and by 2D echocardiography. Classic findings of MVP on examination include a dynamic mid-systolic to late systolic click followed by a high-pitched systolic murmur heard at the cardiac apex. With more advanced MR, the murmur may extend throughout systole, and with severe MR or associated LV dysfunction, a third sound may be heard and the click may be inaudible, but the murmur is usually loud.[98,99] The click is thought to result from stretching of redundant valve and chordal tissue. A click may occur without any murmur when the leaflets are redundant but not regurgitant. In addition, systolic clicks may arise from other pathologic conditions including bicuspid aortic valve, atrial myxoma, or pericarditis. A click, therefore, is sensitive but not very specific for the diagnosis of MVP although a mid-systolic click with late systolic murmur is highly likely to represent myxomatous degeneration of the mitral valve. Provocative maneuvers such as the Valsalva maneuver, squatting, and leg raises may improve the diagnostic likelihood of MVP by illustrating that the click moves within systole in response to volume and loading changes.[100] A reduction in end-diastolic volume such as that occurring with the Valsalva maneuver or standing causes the click to occur earlier, whereas an increase in end-diastolic volume such as that occurring with squatting or decreasing contractility or increasing afterload (hand-grip) will move the click later in systole. The murmur may radiate based on the direction of the regurgitant leak and the leaflet that is prolapsing. Thus, with anterior leaflet prolapse and a posteriorly directed jet, the murmur may be appreciated very well at the back.

Noncardiac Physical Findings

Secondary causes of MVP such as Marfan syndrome have specific skeletal and morphologic findings that aid in their identification. These are not seen routinely in idiopathic MVP, which, in contrast, has no specific features other than the cardiac manifestations that render the diagnosis likely.[101] Those with MVP in the Framingham study were significantly leaner than those without prolapse based on lower body mass index and waist to hip ratio.[67] Lower weight and blood pressure in patients with MVP have been described in other studies.[88] Older studies suggested a higher incidence of skeletal abnormalities associated with MVP such as straight back and asthenic build.[88,102]

Echocardiographic Diagnosis

A 2D echocardiogram is required for precise diagnosis of MVP and to determine the presence of MR and other findings that affect prognosis and risk of complications (Figure 15-6). Usually a transthoracic echocardiogram is adequate for diagnostic purposes although both transesophageal echocardiography (TEE) and three-dimensional (3D) echocardiography may provide specific information that is not available from the transthoracic window. Prolapse was detected initially on echocardiography by M-mode. The characteristic appearance of late systolic hammocking of the mitral leaflets was used to make the diagnosis. However, apart from demonstrative purposes, M-mode has little role in current day diagnosis of prolapse. Stress echocardiography provides powerful additional diagnostic and prognostic information in selected individuals.

On 2D echocardiography, MVP is diagnosed when either or both of the leaflets are displaced 2 mm or more in systole above a line connecting the annular hinge points in the parasternal or apical long-axis view.[103-105] Displacement of the leaflets above this line in other imaging windows and specifically the apical four-chamber window should not be considered abnormal. In an earlier era, prolapse identified in the apical four-chamber view was considered to be diagnostic of true MVP. This led to an epidemic of MVP diagnosis, with it being diagnosed in as many as 38% of teenage girls.[13]

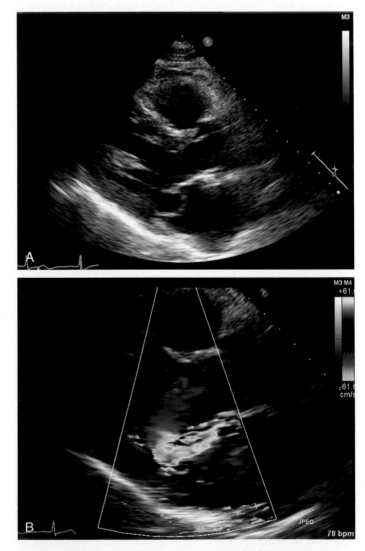

FIGURE 15–6 A, Parasternal long-axis view of prolapse of the posterior mitral leaflet into the left atrium (LA) (*arrow*). **B,** the anteriorly directed regurgitant jet of mitral regurgitation (MR) away from the prolapsing leaflet is demonstrated.

Levine et al[103-105] demonstrated in the late 1980s using 3D echocardiography that the mitral annulus was not planar but rather had a complex saddle-shaped structure in which the anterior and posterior portions of the annulus are higher than those laterally (Figure 15-7). Thus, in the anteroposterior axis, the annulus is concave upward, whereas in the mediolateral axis the annulus is concave downward. The result is that in the apical four-chamber plane, even normal leaflets may appear to break the annular plane. Levine et al[103] went on to show that prolapse identified only in the apical four-chamber view did not exhibit the other features of pathologic MVP, such as chamber enlargement or leaflet thickening, and should not be considered abnormal. Myxomatous changes in the mitral valve leaflets may lead to thickening of leaflets and chordae and to enlargement of the mitral valve annulus.[106] This is especially evident when MR is present. Thickening of the leaflets to 5 mm or greater is considered "classic" MVP and is predictive of subsequent complications (Figure 15-8).[107] Mitral valve thickening is measured in diastole from the leading to the trailing edge of the thickest area of the midportion of the leaflet and not as the dimension of maximal area of focal leaflet thickening.[67] In many instances, the leaflets and chordae are very thick-

ened and redundant.[12,108] It is also common to identify tricuspid valve prolapse in patients with MVP.[109] Tricuspid valve prolapse may occur in up to 40% of all MVP, whereas aortic valve prolapse is much less prevalent and occurs in 1% to 2% of patients with MVP.[85] The thickness of the leaflets changes much more than normally from systole to diastole in MVP on echocardiography.[110] This result has been attributed to inherent increased thickening of the valve structures that has been demonstrated pathologically and also to increased redundancy of the leaflet tissue. Although apical four-chamber views are not useful in detecting mild MVP, once the diagnosis has been made, this imaging window is very helpful in defining the precise leaflet involvement and the severity of MR. In addition, prolapse of the lateral scallop of the posterior leaflet may be evident only in this view.

In a substantial number of patients, there is evidence of chordal disruption on echocardiography.[111,112] In this instance, a portion of one or the other, or rarely both, leaflets may exhibit motion independent of normal leaflet tissue. Chordal rupture in this situation may either be partial or complete and usually leads to impaired coaptation over a substantial portion of the valve surface, giving rise to severe MR. This is not invariably the case, however. Coaptation may be

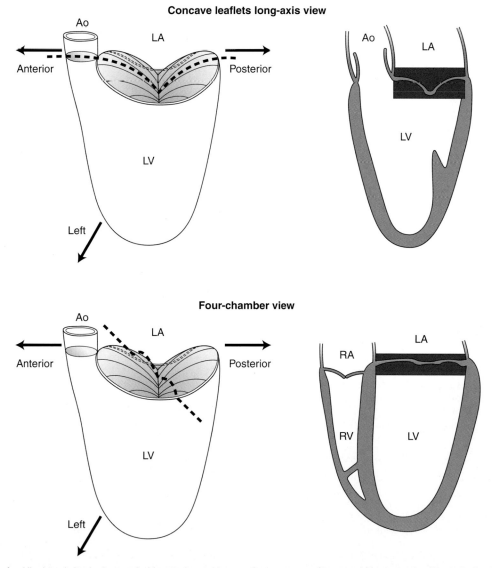

FIGURE 15–7 Model of saddle shaped mitral valve annulus showing how apparent prolapse may occur from an apical cross-sectional image in the absence of any prolapse in a long-axis cross-section. Ao, aorta; LA, left atrium; LV, left ventricle; RA, right atrium; RV, right ventricle. *(From Levine RA, Triulzi MO, Harrigan P, et al: The relationship of mitral annular shape to the diagnosis of mitral valve prolapse. Circulation 1987;75:756–767, with permission.)*

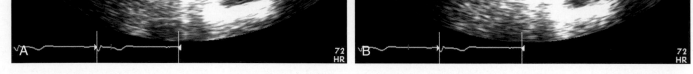

FIGURE 15–8 Parasternal long-axis echocardiogram of bileaflet prolapse in systole (*left*) and diastole (*right*). Significant thickening and redundancy are noted of the leaflets in diastole consistent with "classic" mitral valve prolapse.

maintained despite a flail segment if the other leaflet is large. Prolapsing and flail leaflets are usually reliably identified by transthoracic echocardiography, but TEE has been shown in multiple studies to improve the ability to detect a flail segment.[113-115]

Classification of Prolapse on Echocardiography

MVP is classified on the basis of the leaflet involvement as involving the anterior leaflet, the posterior leaflet, or both. This classification has prognostic value in determining the likelihood of repair and may have some independent value in defining the nature of the disease itself. Unileaflet prolapse especially involving the posterior leaflet is more common than bileaflet prolapse and appears to be more likely to result in flail. Bileaflet prolapse tends to occur at a younger age, is more likely to be associated with myxomatous changes in other valves, and tends to have more dynamic changes in severity of MR.[108] The leaflet involved in prolapse is determined not only by the apparent displacement of the leaflet but also by the direction of the jets or jets when regurgitation is present. Thus, anterior leaflet prolapse is associated with excess motion of the anterior leaflet and a posteriorly directed jet of MR. Posterior leaflet prolapse generally causes an anteriorly directed jet of MR. In bileaflet prolapse, two jets of regurgitation may be identified, or if the prolapse of each leaflet is symmetrical, there may be one central jet. In identifying bileaflet prolapse, jet direction is particularly important. As detailed in the section on anatomy, apparent prolapse of the anterior leaflet can occur with severe posterior leaflet prolapse due to loss of the anchoring effect of the posterior leaflet. Unlike in true bileaflet prolapse where two jets or a central jet is evident, only an anteriorly directed jet is seen and repair is as likely as with isolated posterior leaflet prolapse.[116]

Localization of Prolapse and Flail by Echocardiography

In identifying the site of prolapse by echocardiography, first, the 2D appearances should be assessed and then the origin and direction of the accompanying jet of MR should be analyzed. In the 2D assessment, the long-axis views are paramount when the diagnosis is suspected rather than established. In more severe prolapse when the diagnosis is not in doubt but an assessment of the severity of the lesion is needed, additional views need to be taken into account, including the short-axis view of the valve on which the prolapsing or flail segment or segments may be apparent as a mass-like lesion

and may even simulate an infective vegetation.[117] Off-axis views and the four-chamber view may help determine which leaflet is prolapsing or whether both are prolapsing. Lateral scallop involvement of the posterior leaflet may be particularly challenging to decipher. The regurgitant jet may appear to be directed anteriorly in some views but posteriorly in others, which is understandable as the lateral scallop is quite anteriorly located (see Figure 15-3). A short-axis view of the valve may be particularly helpful in identifying the excess motion of the lateral scallop in this situation and the origin of the regurgitant jet.

TEE is particularly useful in determining the precise site of prolapse and seems to be superior to transthoracic imaging in many instances.[118] The key imaging planes on TEE are the midesophageal view at 40 to 60° on multiplane imaging and the orthogonal view at 130 to 150°. At 40 to 60°, the imaging plane is parallel to a line between the commissures and is helpful in determining whether the prolapse involves the medial (to the left) or lateral (to the right) scallop. The orthogonal view at 130 to 150° is most useful in identifying prolapse of the middle scallop or segment as this imaging plane bisects this scallop. Short-axis views of the mitral valve may also be acquired by TEE in the short-axis transgastric view. When the mitral valve has been examined systematically in a segmental approach and the results are compared with the surgical findings, TEE has been reported to be 96% accurate in one study.[23] In another study of myxomatous mitral valve disease, localization of the abnormality to the posterior leaflet was 78% sensitive and 92% specific with sensitivity being least when the medial scallop was affected.[119] Commissural prolapse is often difficult to detect as it may lead to prolapse of a portion of both leaflets with a large prolapsing mass that may simulate a vegetation. Recognition is enhanced from a short-axis view of the valve on which the commissures are evident and by 3D echocardiography.[120] In addition, the regurgitant jet is often very eccentric in origin in standard views and is seen to originate at the affected commissure in short-axis views.

Assessment of Mitral Regurgitation

MR is one of the major complications of MVP and so it is essential that an echocardiographic evaluation include a full assessment with quantification when feasible of the severity of the lesion. MR assessment is detailed in another chapter, so only important pitfalls in assessment specific to myxomatous mitral valve disease will be summarized here.

1. MR from a prolapsing mitral valve is often eccentric in nature, and the color display may underestimate the true severity.[121] It is important to examine the left atrium in multiple views including off-axis views to fully define the jet. TEE is helpful in this situation to image the jet.

2. In quantifying MR with the proximal isovelocity surface area technique, care must be taken to account for the effects of wall constraint on the proximal isovelocity surface area, which is particularly common with a large flail segment (Figure 15-9).[122] Wall constraint of the proximal convergence area leads to a loss of a true hemispheric proximal convergence zone and a spuriously large radius being measured. These factors lead to a gross overestimation of the regurgitant volume and the regurgitant orifice. Correction factors are available but are somewhat difficult to use as they involve calculating and allowing for the true angle made by the convergence area.[123] Fortunately, when constraint is present, the MR is usually already severe and quantitation, although inaccurate, does not misrepresent the appropriate grading of MR as severe in these patients.

3. The duration of regurgitation is inconstant in myxomatous, MR more so than in MR with other etiologies.[124] Thus, MR may be severe when it occurs but is confined to the latter half of systole rather than holosystolic. In deciding the effects of MR on LV size and function (an important consideration in appropriately timing surgical intervention), not only the severity of the MR but also its duration is important.[125] Color M-mode may be very helpful in determining the true duration of the regurgitation as may the continuous wave Doppler profile of the MR jet (Figure 15-10). Dynamic changes in the apparent severity of the lesion may involve the duration as well as the severity. The severity of MR is especially dynamic in prolapsing mitral valves probably as a result of the effects of loading and geometry on the chordae and leaflets. Patients who are asymptomatic at rest and with apparently moderate MR may exhibit marked symptoms on exercise as a result of both an increase in the severity and the duration of the regurgitation.[126,127] Stress echocardiography is very helpful in situations in which there is a discrepancy between the symptoms and apparent severity of MR at rest in myxomatous disease and an increase in severity of MR on exercise may have predictive value in determining the need for earlier surgical intervention.[128]

Echocardiography in Defining Likelihood of Repair

Myxomatous mitral valve disease is associated with excess tissue, and this usually allows the possibility of repair in centers experienced in the necessary surgical techniques. The current ACC/AHA guidelines stipulate that surgical intervention should be predicated on the likelihood of repair as defined by the valve lesion and the center at which the surgery is to take place.[85] Surgical intervention is indicated earlier when repair appears likely because the short-term and long-term morbidity and mortality associated with repair are much more favorable than those with mitral valve replacement. It is increasingly possible to repair even complex myxomatous disease lesions that a decade ago would have required valve replacement.[129-131] In experienced centers, it is now possible to repair a posterior leaflet prolapse or flail in more than 90% of instances.[21] Extensive calcification of the leaflet that precludes leaflet resection is the usual reason that a posterior leaflet lesion is not repairable. This situation too is usually evident echocardiographically, at least to an experienced reader. Currently bileaflet prolapse lesions can usually be repaired in experienced centers. Anterior leaflet prolapse, anterior leaflet flail, and flail of both leaflets have been the most difficult lesions to repair. It is difficult to resect diseased areas from the anterior leaflet because of its sail-like configuration and the absence of true segmentation. Anterior leaflet repair has therefore required chordal transfer techniques, and durability has not been as good as for repair of posterior leaflet lesions. With the

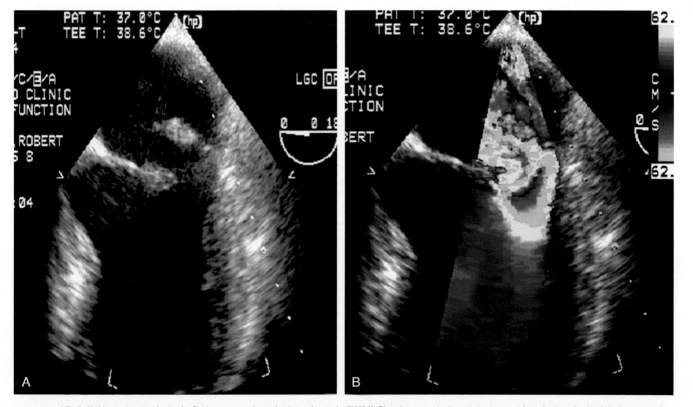

FIGURE 15–9 Flail posterior mitral valve leaflet by transesophageal echocardiography (TEE) (*left*) and severe mitral regurgitation seen by color Doppler (*right*). The proximal convergence area is constrained by the wall and is no longer a true hemisphere. Proximal isovelocity surface area measurement of regurgitant orifice area from this image will overestimate the true area because of the change in the geometry of the convergence area.

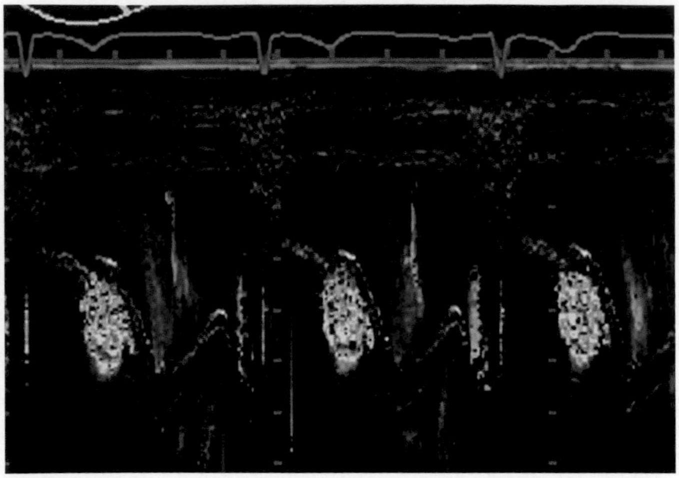

FIGURE 15–10 Color M-mode echocardiography of mitral regurgitation in an asymptomatic patient with bileaflet prolapse and a large regurgitant orifice area but normal left atrial and ventricular size. The regurgitant jet is confined to the second half of systole (between *arrows*) so that the total volume of regurgitation is much lower than would have been anticipated on the basis of the regurgitant orifice area.

advent of more physiologic and user-friendly artificial chordae, the likelihood of durable repair in this situation has also improved substantially.[132] Given the importance of defining the likelihood of repair when one is helping a patient determine the optimal timing for surgical intervention, TEE should be used if the transthoracic images are suboptimal or fail to define adequately the mechanism of MR.

Three-Dimensional Echocardiography

Improvements in real-time 3D echocardiography whether acquired from the transthoracic windows or by the transesophageal approach have led to a rapid evolution of the ability to image complex structures and in particular the myxomatous mitral valve. In a recent study of 112 patients with myxomatous mitral valve disease who were undergoing mitral valve repair, Pepi et al[133] compared 3D TEE, 2D TEE, and both 3D and 2D transthoracic echocardiography in the localization of the site of prolapse using the surgical findings as the gold standard. 3D TEE was significantly more accurate at 96% than the other techniques. 3D transthoracic echocardiography and 2D TEE were similarly accurate at 90% and 87%, respectively, with 2D transthoracic echocardiography being the least accurate at 77%. Multiple areas of prolapse were more likely to be detected by the 3D approach as were commissural lesions. Earlier studies with older technology had suggested no real advantage of 3D over 2D TEE evaluation.[134] It is possible to measure the regurgitant orifice directly in myxomatous mitral valves with 3D TEE. However, this measurement requires considerable off-line processing that makes it of limited feasibility clinically.[135]

Other Diagnostic Techniques

Electrocardiography

Electrocardiographic changes, particularly flattening or inversion of the T wave in the inferior leads have been identified in patients with MVP.[10] QT prolongation is uncommon but has been reported in individual patients with prolapse. Patients MVP may demonstrate abnormal electrocardiographic responses to exercise, and false-positive ST segment depression has been reported in 10% to 60% of patients studied.[10] An imaging study in addition to the electrocardiogram is likely to be more specific when coronary disease is being evaluated in these patients and is a useful screening tool in intermediate-risk patients.[136] An increase in ventricular ectopy with salvoes

of ventricular premature beats may also occur with exercise, particularly in the cool-down phase.[10] Ventricular ectopy is usually worsened by concomitant MR and frequently improves but may not normalize after successful valve surgery. The cause and significance of the electrocardiographic changes and ectopy have been debated for years with autonomic abnormalities being postulated as a cause by some.[137]

Angiography

Although an LV angiogram is no longer used to make the diagnosis of MVP, certain characteristic findings are often evident. The right anterior oblique projection is best for posterior leaflet prolapse, whereas the left anterior oblique projection is optimal for anterior leaflet prolapse. The mitral leaflets are seen to be displaced beyond their point of attachment to the annulus. Other abnormalities may be evident such as MR, annular calcification, and impaired motion of the basal portion of the left ventricle.[138]

Other Imaging Techniques

Nuclear scintigraphy may be of value in excluding coronary artery disease in those patients with chest pain. Although echocardiography is usually adequate to assess LV function, when another assessment of ejection fraction is required, a gated blood pool scan is usually the methodology of choice in these patients. Magnetic resonance imaging and computed tomographic scanning at present have limited value compared with echocardiography in defining valve morphology and hemodynamics and are not routinely used in the evaluation of MVP.

MITRAL VALVE PROLAPSE SYNDROME

MVP has been associated with numerous symptoms such as atypical chest pain, fatigue, orthostatic hypotension, shortness of breath on exertion, palpitations, syncope, panic attack, and anxiety.[137] Findings of asthenic build, low blood pressure, and repolarization abnormalities on the electrocardiogram have all been characterized as the MVP syndrome. In the era before the rationalization of the echocardiographic diagnosis of MVP and in which the apparent prevalence of MVP in the community was high, it is understandable how it appeared that many of these manifestations clustered with the diagnosis of MVP, which in turn gave a convenient and not too grave a diagnosis to account for them. Many studies indicated abnormalities in catecholamines, adrenergic activity, and autonomic function in this patient population.[139-141] Echocardiography was performed in many patients presenting with nonspecific symptoms as a screening tool to identify a possible cause of the symptoms. This selection bias amplified the association of MVP with many other disorders.

Newer studies have suggested that with a more appropriate diagnosis of MVP based on long-axis views there is little, if any, association between true MVP and this cluster of symptoms and clinical findings.[142] Thus, in the Framingham Heart Study, those with MVP did not have an increased risk of developing psychiatric abnormalities or electrocardiographic changes or of experiencing atypical chest pain, panic disorder, or dyspnea compared with that for the general population.[143,144] Furthermore, studies that included asymptomatic patients with MVP failed to detect abnormal autonomic or neuroendocrine function at rest or with tilt-testing.[145] Whether there are subgroups of patients with MVP who have true autonomic abnormalities remains to be determined. A polymorphism at the 1166 position of the angiotensin II receptor has been detected more commonly in patients with MVP than in control subjects and appears to be associated with postural hypotension and enhanced vasomotor response.[146]

Patients with MVP syndrome are managed symptomatically and with counseling on the benign nature of the condition.

If there is concern for a true abnormality at the valve or if this is in doubt, echocardiography should be performed after an interval usually of 1 year. β-Blockade in small doses may be helpful in treating symptomatic palpitations or atypical chest pain. If anxiety disorder or panic disorder appears to be the underlying problem, referral to a specialist clinic is often beneficial.

MANAGEMENT OF THE ASYMPTOMATIC PATIENT

Patients with MVP, mild, or no MR and mild or no symptoms are managed expectantly with the assurance that their prognosis is excellent. Table 15-1 details the current ACC/AHA guidelines for echocardiography in these patients. Those who exhibit high-risk features on an echocardiogram such as leaflet thickening should be followed more closely with a yearly echocardiogram. Those in whom no high-risk features are present may be followed-up more infrequently. Patients with mild prolapse and atypical chest pain should undergo a stress echocardiogram or stress nuclear study if the pretest probability of coronary artery disease is in the intermediate range. Stress electrocardiography in the setting of MVP is associated with a high incidence of false-positive ST depression and is best avoided when the diagnosis of ischemia is required. In those with palpitations, Holter monitoring is useful to detect the precise cause of arrhythmia, although a serious rhythm disturbance is rare.

Good health measures such as avoidance of caffeine or alcohol and an exercise program and reassurance often suffice in reducing or eliminating symptoms. In more refractory instances, symptomatic relief of atypical chest pain and palpitations may be afforded by the empiric use of small doses of β-blockers. Exercise is encouraged in those with MVP. Competitive exercise should be avoided by those with moderate LV enlargement, LV dysfunction, uncontrolled tachyarrhythmias, long-QT interval, unexplained syncope, prior

resuscitation from cardiac arrest, or aortic root enlargement.[147] Heavy weight lifting should also be avoided in those with MVP as this, theoretically at least, may lead to further chordal extension by increasing LV wall stress and thus worsening prolapse and MR. This prohibition generally remains in force even after successful surgical repair, given the residual abnormality of leaflet and chordal tissue. Pregnancy is not contraindicated in MVP on the basis of the diagnosis alone.[85]

Previously, the decision about endocarditis prophylaxis was complicated and somewhat obscure in patients with MVP and was predicated on the presence of MR either clinically or on echocardiography.[148,149] However, the most recent AHA endocarditis prophylaxis guidelines have substantially clarified and simplified this decision. The AHA no longer recommends the use of antibiotic prophylaxis in any form of MVP unless a prior episode of endocarditis has been documented or unless surgical repair or replacement of the valve has taken place.[150]

COMPLICATIONS OF MITRAL VALVE PROLAPSE

Although in many respects a benign condition, MVP is associated with significant complications. These include endocarditis, sudden cardiac death, cerebrovascular events, and MR of a severity to necessitate surgery. Both clinical and echocardiographic parameters are useful in identifying those at increased risk of these complications (Table 15-2). Although MVP is equally prevalent in men and women, men are much more likely to develop significant complications.[151] In most surgical series of patients with myxomatous disease undergoing valve surgery, men outnumber women by a factor of 2 or 3:1.[21] Similarly, men are more prone to endocarditis. The reasons that men are more likely to present with a complicated course are unknown. It has been postulated that men have higher LV wall stress and thus greater tension is exerted on valve tissue and chordae, thus leading to a higher risk of leaflet and chord rupture.[152] Other clinical factors associated with a higher risk of complications include higher blood pressure and higher body mass index.

The echocardiographic findings in multiple studies that have been associated with a complicated course include impaired LV function, more severe MR, and leaflet thickness greater than 5 mm (see Table 15-2). The latter is associated with a greater than a 10-fold increase in risk of sudden death, infective endocarditis, or cerebrovascular event.

Infective Endocarditis

Patients with MVP have a 3- to 8-fold increased risk of developing endocarditis, although the absolute risk at approximately 0.2% per year is relatively low.[151,153,154] Nevertheless, endocarditis is a cause of significant morbidity and mortality when it occurs and may bring forward the time when surgical intervention is required because of an increase in severity of MR. Furthermore, the destruction of the valve tissue in severe cases of endocarditis may preclude successful repair. Risk factors for development of endocarditis include male gender, age older than 45, the presence of a systolic murmur, and thickening and redundancy of the leaflets.[12,95,107,151,154] Vortices produced by the turbulent jet of MR and the redundant thickened valve tissue are thought to increase the likelihood that a bacteremia of a suitable organism will infect the valve. Patients without MR do not appear to have an increased risk of endocarditis. The risk in those with prolapse and a systolic murmur has been estimated to be 0.05% per year.[155] The new guidelines suggest that the risk of bacteremia is as likely with everyday dental hygiene such as flossing or cleaning as with specific

TABLE 15–1	ACC/AHA Guidelines for Echocardiography in Asymptomatic Mitral Valve Prolapse

Class I
Echocardiography is indicated for the diagnosis of MVP and assessment of MR, leaflet morphology, and ventricular compensation in asymptomatic patients with physical signs of MVP. (Level of Evidence: B)

Class IIa
1. Echocardiography can effectively exclude MVP in asymptomatic patients who have been diagnosed without clinical evidence to support the diagnosis. (Level of Evidence: C)

2. Echocardiography can be effective for risk stratification in asymptomatic patients with physical signs of MVP or known MVP. (Level of Evidence: C)

Class III
1. Echocardiography is not indicated to exclude MVP in asymptomatic patients with ill-defined symptoms in the absence of a constellation of clinical symptoms or physical findings suggestive of MVP or a positive family history. (Level of Evidence: B)

2. Routine repetition of echocardiography is not indicated for the asymptomatic patient who has MVP and no MR or MVP and mild MR with no changes in clinical signs or symptoms. (Level of Evidence: C)

ACC, American College of Cardiology; AHA, American Heart Association; MR, mitral regurgitation; MVP, mitral valve prolapse.
From Bonow RO, Carabello B, Chatterjee K, et al: ACC/AHA 2006 guidelines for the management of patients with valvular heart disease: a report of the American College of Cardiology/American Heart Association Task Force on Practice Guidelines. J Am Coll Cardiol. 2006;48:e1-148, with permission.

TABLE 15–2	Use of Echocardiography for Risk Stratification in MV Prolapse			
Study (Year)	N	Features Examined	Outcome	P <
Chandraratna et al. (1984)[184]	86	MV leaflets >5 mm	↑ Cardiovascular abnormalities (60% vs. 6%; Marfan syndrome, TVP, MR, dilated ascending aorta)	0.001
Nishimura et al. (1985)[12]	237	MV leaflet ≥5 mm	↑ Sum of sudden death, endocarditis, and cerebral embolus	0.02
		LVID ≥60 mm	↑ MVR (26% vs. 3.1%)	0.001
Marks et al. (1989)[107]	456	MV leaflet ≥5 mm	↑ Endocarditis (3.5% vs. 0%)	0.02
			↑ Moderate-severe MR (11.9% vs. 0%)	0.001
			↑ MVR (6.6% vs. 0.7%)	0.02
			↑ Stroke (7.5% vs. 5.8%)	NS
Takamoto et al. (1991)[185]	142	MV leaflet 3 mm or greater, redundant, low echo density	↑ Ruptured chordae (48% vs. 5%)	
Babuty et al. (1994)[186]	58	Undefined MV thickening	No relation to complex ventricular arrhythmias	NS
Zuppiroli et al. (1994)[89]	119	MV leaflet greater than 5 mm	↑ Complex ventricular arrhythmias	0.001
Avierinos et al. (2002)[70]	833	Risk factors for:	↑ Cardiovascular mortality	
		Moderate to severe MR	HR 3.0, CI 1.5–5.8	0.002
		EF < 50%	HR 3.8, CI 1.6–8.1	0.003
		Risk factors for:	↑ Cardiovascular morbidity (sum of CHF, new AF, neuro, emb, endocarditis, MVR)	
		LA size ≥ 40 mm	HR 2.7, CI 1.9–3.8	0.001
		Slight MR	HR 3.6, CI 2.0–7.0	0.001
		Moderate to severe MR	HR 9.1, CI 4.9–18.3	0.001
		Flail	HR 2.6, CI 1.5–2.6	0.002

AF, atrial fibrillation; CHF, heart failure; CI, 95% confidence intervals; EF, ejection fraction; emb, peripheral embolic events; HR, hazard ratio; LA, left atrial; LVID, left ventricular internal diameter; MR, mitral regurgitation; MV, mitral valve; MVR, mitral valve surgery; N, number of patients; neuro, ischemic neurological events; NS, not significant; TVP, tricuspid valve prolapse. ↑ indicates increase.

Adapted and expanded from Cheitlin MD, Armstrong WF, Aurigemma GP, et al: ACC/AHA/ASE 2003 Guideline Update for the Clinical Application of Echocardiography: summary article. A report of the American College of Cardiology/American Heart Association Task Force on Practice Guidelines. J Am Soc Echocardiogr. 2003;16:1091-110.

dental procedures and that specific prophylaxis therefore is probably not useful. When endocarditis occurs in MVP, it is treated as for other etiologies, based on the susceptibility of the organism. Surgical repair if feasible is indicated when a hemodynamically severe regurgitant leak ensues, if bacteriologic cure proves impossible with antibiotics alone, or if embolization from a vegetation has occurred or appears to be likely. As discussed earlier, a flail portion of valve in MVP can simulate a vegetation and is a common source of a false-positive diagnosis of endocarditis. Awareness of this possibility and the use of more advanced imaging techniques such as TEE in addition to repeated cultures and the involvement of an infectious disease specialist usually help resolve the clinical problem. Because MR is frequently severe in these patients anyway, surgical intervention is often warranted, and the final diagnosis is made on the basis of the pathologic findings.

Cerebrovascular Ischemic Events

An increased incidence of cerebrovascular events has been reported in MVP, especially in younger patients.[156-158] Multiple potential mechanisms for thromboembolism exist, including platelet and fibrin aggregates on the valve,[30] abnormal platelet aggregation,[159] other detritus such as calcium on the valve in older patients and onset of atrial arrhythmias especially in older patients with more severe MR, and left atrial enlargement. The earlier studies suggesting an increased risk of cerebral thromboembolism in young patients with MVP

have been challenged. In a study of 213 consecutive patients 45 years of age or younger with ischemic stroke or a transient ischemic attack identified over a 10-year period, Gilon et al[160] found that only 1.9% had MVP compared with 2.7% of control subjects. A study from the Mayo Clinic also indicated that the relative risk for stroke in younger patients with uncomplicated MVP was not increased, although the risk in patients with prolapse generally was increased by a factor of 2.[161] In a more recent study from the Mayo Clinic of 777 patients with MVP followed from 1989 to 1998, prolapse doubled the likelihood of a cerebral ischemic event. However, most of the events occurred in patients older than 50 and were predicted by advancing age, leaflet thickening, atrial fibrillation at follow-up, and cardiovascular surgery.[162] Thus, MVP, especially when complicated by other comorbidities, may increase the risk of cerebral embolism, but the risk is low in young people with uncomplicated MVP.

The increased risk imposed by altered platelet aggregation and fibrin or platelet aggregates has also been questioned. Platelet aggregates are uncommon in pathologic studies and platelet activation studies have suggested that the severity of MR may be more important than myxomatous disease itself in causing activation.[159,163] Table 15-3 details the current ACC/AHA guidelines for the management of patients with MVP who have symptoms of transient ischemic attacks or stroke. Aspirin is usually considered the first line of therapy unless there is evidence of or substantial risk of thrombus generation within the heart, in which case full anticoagulation with warfarin is indicated.

TABLE 15–3	ACC/AHA Guidelines for Antithrombotic Therapy in Mitral Valve Prolapse

Class I

1. Aspirin therapy (75-325 mg/day) is recommended for symptomatic patients with MVP who experience cerebral transient ischemic attacks. (Level of Evidence: C)

2. In patients with MVP and atrial fibrillation, warfarin therapy is recommended for patients aged older than 65 or those with hypertension, MR murmur, or a history of heart failure. (Level of Evidence: C)

3. Aspirin therapy (75-325 mg/day) is recommended for patients with MVP and atrial fibrillation who are younger than 65 years old and have no history of MR, hypertension, or heart failure. (Level of Evidence: C)

4. In patients with MVP and a history of stroke, warfarin therapy is recommended for patients with MR, atrial fibrillation, or left atrial thrombus. (Level of Evidence: C)

Class IIa

1. In patients with MVP and a history of stroke, who do not have MR, atrial fibrillation, or left arterial thrombus, warfarin therapy is reasonable for patients with echocardiographic evidence of thickening (≥5 mm) and/or redundancy of the valve leaflets. (Level of Evidence: C)

2. In patients with MVP and a history of stroke, aspirin therapy is reasonable for patients who do not have MR, atrial fibrillation, left atrial thrombus, or echocardiographic evidence of thickening (≥5 mm) or redundancy of the valve leaflets. (Level of Evidence: C)

3. Warfarin therapy is reasonable for patients with MVP with transient ischemic attacks despite aspirin therapy. (Level of Evidence: C)

4. Aspirin therapy (75-325 mg/day) can be beneficial for patients with MVP and a history of stroke who have contraindications to anticoagulants. (Level of Evidence: B)

Class IIb

Aspirin therapy (75-325 mg/day) may be considered for patients in sinus rhythm with echocardiographic evidence of high-risk MVP. (Level of Evidence: C)

ACC, American College of Cardiology; AHA, American Heart Association; MR, mitral regurgitation; MVP, mitral valve prolapse.

From Bonow RO, Carabello B, Chatterjee K, et al: ACC/AHA 2006 guidelines for the management of patients with valvular heart disease: a report of the American College of Cardiology/American Heart Association Task Force on Practice Guidelines. J Am Coll Cardiol. 2006;48:e1-148, with permission.

Sudden Cardiac Death and Ventricular Arrhythmia

Sudden cardiac death occurs at a yearly rate of 40 per 10,000 in those with MVP, a rate that is low but still at least twice as high as that in the general population.[164] The presumed cause of this increased risk is ventricular arrhythmia,[7,33,165] although severe valve disruption due to acute chordal tear has been implicated in case reports.[166] Multiple electrical abnormalities have been reported in MVP including increased QT dispersion and ventricular arrhythmia that may be accentuated by volume loading from MR.[167,168] In fact, MR may be more important in the genesis of ventricular arrhythmia than MVP itself.[168] The true significance of these findings and their relationship to sudden death are unknown.

Risk factors for sudden death include significant MR,[164] redundant valve tissue,[12] and decreased LV systolic function.[169] Autopsy studies of sudden death victims in this population have indicated more severe myxomatous changes in the valve.[170] Other autopsy series suggest an excess of women, particularly in younger age groups.[33,92,171] MVP is a very rare cause of sudden death in competitive athletes.[172] The risk of sudden cardiac death is reported to be increased when the mitral valve is flail, with the mechanism presumably being the addition

of severe MR to the increased susceptibility of myxomatous disease itself.[169,173] Sudden death rates of up to 2% per year have been reported in this setting, which is five times higher than that estimated in those with uncomplicated MVP, but the group studied in that report tended to be older (mean age 67 years). Predictors of risk include atrial fibrillation, worsening functional class, and lower ejection fraction. Early surgical intervention appears to protect from the risk of sudden death in this older patient population with severe MR.[84,174]

In patients with symptomatic ventricular arrhythmia and significant MR in whom the valve is likely to be repaired, surgical intervention will probably improve but not eradicate symptoms completely and is the best initial approach. Implantable cardiac defibrillators are indicated in survivors of a sudden death episode. Patients with impaired LV function, those with frequent episodes of nonsustained ventricular tachycardia, and those with sustained ventricular tachycardia are best referred to an electrophysiologist for assessment with electrophysiologic testing as needed. In those with normal LV ventricular function, symptomatic improvement may result from β-blockade. In the rare patient with very frequent symptomatic unifocal ventricular arrhythmia, electrophysiologic mapping and ablation of the focus may allow improvement in symptoms.

Mitral Regurgitation

MR of a severity to cause severe volume loading of the left ventricle and to necessitate eventual surgical intervention is the most frequent complication of MVP. MR tends to progress over time for a number of reasons. Progressive lengthening of chordae predisposes to more MR. The ventricular and annular remodeling due to MR causes further chordal stretching and ever more MR. Eventually, chordal strength is sufficiently diminished or stress on the chordae exceeds its load-bearing capacity and a chord ruptures, leading to a flail segment and even more severe MR.

Risk factors for development of progressively severe MR include male gender, hypertension, increased body mass index, and increasing age.[74,152] Severe MR is relatively uncommon in patients before the fifth decade.[75] Echocardiographic factors associated with increased risk of severe MR include redundant thickened leaflets, prolapse involving the posterior leaflet, and increased ventricular size.[12,107,175] Conversely, patients who have thin leaflets and little MR at the outset appear to have a relatively low risk of subsequently developing severe MR.[67,107] In a study of 285 patients with MVP and lesser degrees of MR over a 4- to 5-year follow-up, progression of a grade or more of MR developed in 38% and was predicted by age and initial grade of MR. Progression was associated with a greater increase in left atrial and LV size.[176]

The indications for surgery in patients with severe MR and the management of these patients in the operating room by both the echocardiographer and surgeon are addressed in other chapters. Mitral valve repair is highly likely when MVP is the etiology of the MR. Therefore, the threshold to intervene surgically is lowered in these patients when severe MR is present and competent experienced repair surgery is available to the patient. Outcomes are superior for mitral valve repair in this setting compared with that in other etiologies of MR such as ischemic or rheumatic disease, both in terms of the initial success of the repair, its durability over time, and the life expectancy of the patient. Excellent durability of mitral repair out to 20 years has now been reported.[177]

Follow-up after Mitral Valve Repair

Close follow-up is required in patients with MVP after successful valve surgery. Echocardiography is usually performed before discharge to redefine baseline data including any residual MR, the valve gradient, presence of systolic anterior motion of the mitral valve and any resultant outflow obstruction, and LV size and function. As postoperative LV function has been shown to define the subsequent risk of heart failure and survival, it is an important parameter in follow-up.[82] LV ejection fraction may decline with successful eradication of MR based on the changes in loading. An ejection fraction less than 50% is associated with worse outcomes postoperatively, and prophylactic use of angiotensin-converting enzyme inhibitors and β-blockers is appropriate.[178] LV dysfunction may normalize subsequently due to successful remodeling of the ventricle.[179] Systolic anterior motion is less common with current surgical techniques such as sliding annuloplasty.[118,129] Older studies suggest that systolic anterior motion develops more frequently in the presence of an annuloplasty ring and in those with relatively small ventricles preoperatively.[180] Mild systolic anterior motion and outflow obstruction or provocable outflow obstruction often improve with β-blockade and may diminish or disappear over time as remodeling occurs.[181] Rarely, more severe outflow obstruction may require subsequent reoperation for correction. Repair with a sliding annuloplasty is often possible, but when it is not feasible a mechanical valve may need to be implanted to forestall obstruction from bioprosthetic struts. Residual mitral stenosis is exceedingly rare after mitral valve repair in an experienced center, given the excess tissue present in myxomatous disease. Endocarditis is also rare after mitral valve repair although endocarditis prophylaxis is indicated under recent AHA guidelines. When endocarditis occurs, medical management is usually successful if the leaflets alone are involved whereas surgical debridement is required if the annuloplasty is involved.[182] In a study of 1,072 patients, the risk of reoperation in myxomatous mitral valve disease was 7% in the first 10 years after initial surgery.[21] Risk factors for reoperation include more complex anatomy, chordal transfer procedures, and inadequate early results. In approximately 50% of patients requiring reoperation, progression of the degenerative or myxomatous process was the major factor, but these patients only comprised 1.5% of the initial operative cohort. Occasionally these patients may present abruptly with chordal rupture and a flail segment. This may manifest as severe heart failure or rarely as intravascular hemolysis.[183]

CONCLUSIONS AND FUTURE PERSPECTIVES

Myxomatous mitral valve disease with MVP has been recognized as a clinical entity for less than 50 years. Theories about its prevalence, cause, and significance have varied widely over that time period. During the last two decades there has been growing consensus based on considerable data regarding its prevalence, natural history, risk for complications, and effective treatment of MR by valve repair. We still have major knowledge gaps with regard to the pathogenesis of the condition and the molecular basis by which it occurs. We are still unable to detect true myxomatous mitral valve disease in its preclinical state, and patients are not detected until the onset of significant valve changes heralded by clinically manifestations or echocardiography. Hopefully, as our understanding of the molecular and genetic nature of the condition increases, more precise diagnostic tools will become available that will allow early detection in those at risk and more precise stratification of those most likely to develop complications. Furthermore, with knowledge of the aberrant molecular pathways leading to disease, it may then be possible to intervene prophylactically to lessen the likelihood of complications or, in the most attractive scenario, to forestall complications and the need for surgical intervention.

REFERENCES

1. Barlow JB, Bosman CK: Aneurysmal protrusion of the posterior leaflet of the mitral valve: an auscultatory-electrocardiographic syndrome. Am Heart J 1966;71:166-178.
2. Criley JM Lewis KB, Humphries JO, Ross RS: Prolapse of the mitral valve: clinical and cine-angiocardiographic findings. Br Heart J 1966;28:488-496.
3. Olson LJ, Subramanian R, Ackermann DM, et al: Surgical pathology of the mitral valve: a study of 712 cases spanning 21 years. Mayo Clin Proc 1987;62:22-34.
4. Waller BF, Morrow AG, Maron BJ, et al: Etiology of clinically isolated, severe, chronic, pure mitral regurgitation: analysis of 97 patients over 30 years of age having mitral valve replacement. Am Heart J 1982;104:276-288.
5. Hayek E, Gring CN, Griffin BP: Mitral valve prolapse. Lancet 2005;365:507-518.
6. Nishimura RA, McGoon MD: Perspectives on mitral-valve prolapse. N Engl J Med 1999;341:48-50.
7. Davies MJ, Moore BP, Braimbridge MV: The floppy mitral valve: Study of incidence, pathology, and complications in surgical, necropsy, and forensic material. Br Heart J 1978;40:468-481.
8. Jeresaty RM, Edwards JE, Chawla SK: Mitral valve prolapse and ruptured chordae tendineae. Am J Cardiol 1985;55:138-142.
9. Barlow JB: Mitral valve billowing and prolapse—an overview. Aust N Z J Med 1992;22:541-549.
10. Devereux RB, Perloff JK, Reichek N, et al: Mitral valve prolapse. Circulation 1976;54:3-14.
11. Devereux RB, Kramer-Fox R, Kligfield P: Mitral valve prolapse: causes, clinical manifestations, and management. Ann Intern Med 1989;111:305-317.
12. Nishimura RA, McGoon MD, Shub C, et al: Echocardiographically documented mitral-valve prolapse: long-term follow-up of 237 patients. N Engl J Med 1985; 313:1305-1309.
13. Warth DC, King ME, Cohen JM, et al: Prevalence of mitral valve prolapse in normal children. J Am Coll Cardiol 1985;5:1173-1177.
14. Lax D, Eicher M, Goldberg SJ: Mild dehydration induces echocardiographic signs of mitral valve prolapse in healthy females with prior normal cardiac findings. Am Heart J 1992;124:1533-1540.
15. Aufderheide S, Lax D, Goldberg SJ: Gender differences in dehydration-induced mitral valve prolapse. Am Heart J 1995;129:83-86.
16. Lax D, Eicher M, Goldberg SJ: Effects of hydration on mitral valve prolapse. Am Heart J. 1993;126:415-418.
17. Schreiber TL, Feigenbaum H, Weyman AE: Effect of atrial septal defect repair on left ventricular geometry and degree of mitral valve prolapse. Circulation 1980;61:888-896.
18. Suchon E, Podolec P, Plazak W, et al: Mitral valve prolapse associated with ostium secundum atrial septal defect—a functional disorder. Acta Cardiol 2004;59:237-238.
19. Come PC, Fortuin NJ, White RI Jr, et al: Echocardiographic assessment of cardiovascular abnormalities in the Marfan syndrome: comparison with clinical findings and with roentgenographic estimation of aortic root size. Am J Med 1983;74:465-474.
20. Antunes MJ: Mitral Valve Repair. Starnberg, Germany: Verlag R.S. Schultz, 1989.
21. Gillinov AM, Cosgrove DM, Blackstone EH, et al: Durability of mitral valve repair for degenerative disease. J Thorac Cardiovasc Surg 1998;116:734-743.
22. Carpentier A: Cardiac valve surgery—the "French correction." J Thorac Cardiovasc Surg 1983;86:323-337.
23. Foster GP, Isselbacher EM, Rose GA, et al: Accurate localization of mitral regurgitant defects using multiplane transesophageal echocardiography. Ann Thorac Surg 1998;65:1025-1031.
24. Pyeritz RE, Wappel MA: Mitral valve dysfunction in the Marfan syndrome: clinical and echocardiographic study of prevalence and natural history. Am J Med 1983;74: 797-807.
25. Weyman AE, Scherrer-Crosbie M: Marfan syndrome and mitral valve prolapse. J Clin Invest 2004;114:1543-1546.
26. Jaffe AS, Geltman EM, Rodey GE, et al: Mitral valve prolapse: a consistent manifestation of type IV Ehlers-Danlos syndrome. The pathogenetic role of the abnormal production of type III collagen. Circulation 1981;64:121-125.
27. Hortop J, Tsipouras P, Hanley JA, et al: Cardiovascular involvement in osteogenesis imperfecta. Circulation. 1986;73:54-61.
28. Pyeritz RE, Weiss JL, Renie WA, et al: Pseudoxanthoma elasticum and mitral-valve prolapse. N Engl J Med 1982;307:1451-1452.
29. van der Bel-Kahn J, Becker AE: The surgical pathology of rheumatic and floppy mitral valves: distinctive morphologic features upon gross examination. Am J Surg Pathol 1986;10:282-292.
30. Anyanwu AC, Adams DH: Etiologic classification of degenerative mitral valve disease: Barlow's disease and fibroelastic deficiency. Semin Thorac Cardiovasc Surg 2007;19:90-96.
31. Fisher M, Weiner B, Ockene IS, et al: Platelet activation and mitral valve prolapse. Neurology 1983;33:384-386.
32. Virmani R, Atkinson JB, Forman MB: The pathology of mitral valve prolapse. Herz 1988;13:215-226.
33. Chesler E, King RA, Edwards JE: The myxomatous mitral valve and sudden death. Circulation 1983;67:632-639.
34. Olsen EG, Al-Rufaie HK: The floppy mitral valve: study on pathogenesis. Br Heart J 1980;44:674-683.
35. Baker PB, Bansal G, Boudoulas H, et al: Floppy mitral valve chordae tendineae: histopathologic alterations. Hum Pathol 1988;19:507-512.
36. Rabkin E, Aikawa M, Stone JR, et al: Activated interstitial myofibroblasts express catabolic enzymes and mediate matrix remodeling in myxomatous heart valves. Circulation 2001;104:2525-2532.
37. Fornes P, Heudes D, Fuzellier JF, et al: Correlation between clinical and histologic patterns of degenerative mitral valve insufficiency: a histomorphometric study of 130 excised segments. Cardiovasc Pathol 1999;8:81-92.
38. Flameng W, Meuris B, Herijgers P, et al: Durability of mitral valve repair in Barlow disease versus fibroelastic deficiency. J Thorac Cardiovasc Surg 2008;135:274-282.

15

39. Tamura K, Fukuda Y, Ishizaki M, et al: Abnormalities in elastic fibers and other connective-tissue components of floppy mitral valve. Am Heart J 1995;129:1149-1158.

40. King BD, Clark MA, Baba N, et al: "Myxomatous" mitral valves: collagen dissolution as the primary defect. Circulation 1982;66:288-296.

41. Akhtar S, Meek KM, James V: Immunolocalization of elastin, collagen type I and type III, fibronectin, and vitronectin in extracellular matrix components of normal and myxomatous mitral heart valve chordae tendineae. Cardiovasc Pathol 1999;8:203-211.

42. Barber JE, Kasper FK, Ratliff NB, et al: Mechanical properties of myxomatous mitral valves. J Thorac Cardiovasc Surg 2001;122:955-962.

43. Barber JE, Ratliff NB, Cosgrove DM, 3rd, et al: Myxomatous mitral valve chordae. I: Mechanical properties. J Heart Valve Dis 2001;10:320-324.

44. Grande-Allen KJ, Ratliff NB, Griffin BP, et al: Case report: outer sheath rupture may precede complete chordal rupture in fibrotic mitral valve disease. J Heart Valve Dis 2001;10:90-93.

45. Lis Y, Burleigh MC, Parker DJ, et al: Biochemical characterization of individual normal, floppy and rheumatic human mitral valves. Biochem J 1987;244:597-603.

46. Grande-Allen KJ, Griffin BP, Ratliff NB, et al: Glycosaminoglycan profiles of myxomatous mitral leaflets and chordae parallel the severity of mechanical alterations. J Am Coll Cardiol 2003;42:271-277.

47. Nasuti JF, Zhang PJ, Feldman MD, et al: Fibrillin and other matrix proteins in mitral valve prolapse syndrome. Ann Thorac Surg 2004;77:532-536.

48. Gupta V, Werdenberg JA, Mendez JS, et al: Influence of strain on proteoglycan synthesis by valvular interstitial cells in three-dimensional culture. Acta Biomat 2008;4:88-96.

49. Oki T, Fukuda N, Kawano T, et al: Histopathologic studies of innervation of normal and prolapsed human mitral valves. J Heart Valve Dis 1995;4:496-502.

50. Devereux RB, Brown WT, Kramer-Fox R, et al: Inheritance of mitral valve prolapse: effect of age and sex on gene expression. Ann Intern Med 1982;97:826-832.

51. Zuppiroli A, Roman MJ, O'Grady M, et al: A family study of anterior mitral leaflet thickness and mitral valve prolapse. Am J Cardiol 1998;82:823-826.

52. Pini R, Greppi B, Kramer-Fox R, et al: Mitral valve dimensions and motion and familial transmission of mitral valve prolapse with and without mitral leaflet billowing. J Am Coll Cardiol 1988;12:1423-1431.

53. Disse S, Abergel E, Berrebi A, et al: Mapping of a first locus for autosomal dominant myxomatous mitral-valve prolapse to chromosome 16p11.2–p12.1. Am J Hum Genet 1999;65:1242-1251.

54. Freed LA, Acierno JS Jr, Dai D, et al: A locus for autosomal dominant mitral valve prolapse on chromosome 11p15.4. Am J Hum Genet 2003;72:1551-1559.

55. Nesta F, Leyne M, Yosefy C, et al: New locus for autosomal dominant mitral valve prolapse on chromosome 13: clinical insights from genetic studies. Circulation 2005;112:2022-2030.

56. Roberts R: Another chromosomal locus for mitral valve prolapse: close but no cigar. Circulation 2005;112:1924-1926.

57. Henney AM, Tsipouras P, Schwartz RC, et al: Genetic evidence that mutations in the COL1A1, COL1A2, COL3A1, or COL5A2 collagen genes are not responsible for mitral valve prolapse. Br Heart J 1989;61:292-299.

58. Wordsworth P, Ogilvie D, Akhras F, et al: Genetic segregation analysis of familial mitral valve prolapse shows no linkage to fibrillar collagen genes. Br Heart J 1989;61:300-306.

59. Chou HT, Hung JS, Chen YT, et al: Association between angiotensinogen gene M235T polymorphism and mitral valve prolapse syndrome in Taiwan Chinese. J Heart Valve Dis 2002;11:830-836.

60. Chou HT, Chen YT, Shi YR, et al: Association between angiotensin I-converting enzyme gene insertion/deletion polymorphism and mitral valve prolapse syndrome. Am Heart J 2003;145:169-173.

61. Kyndt F, Schott JJ, Trochu JN, et al: Mapping of X-linked myxomatous valvular dystrophy to chromosome Xq28. Am J Hum Genet 1998;62:627-632.

62. Pedersen HD, Kristensen BO, Lorentzen KA, et al: Mitral valve prolapse in 3-year-old healthy Cavalier King Charles Spaniels: an echocardiographic study. Can J Vet Res 1995;59:294-298.

63. Olsen LH, Fredholm M, Pedersen HD: Epidemiology and inheritance of mitral valve prolapse in Dachshunds. J Vet Intern Med 1999;13:448-456.

64. Ng CM, Cheng A, Myers LA, et al: TGF-β-dependent pathogenesis of mitral valve prolapse in a mouse model of Marfan syndrome. J Clin Invest 2004;114:1586-1592.

65. Charitakis K, Basson C: Degenerating heart valves; fill them up with filamin? Circulation 2007;115:2-4.

66. Levine R, Slaugenhaupt S: Molecular genetics of mitral valve prolapse. Curr Opin Cardiol 2007;22:171-175.

67. Freed LA, Levy D, Levine RA, et al: Prevalence and clinical outcome of mitral-valve prolapse. N Engl J Med 1999;341:1-7.

68. Oke DA, Ajuluchukwu JN, Mbakwem A, et al: Clinical and echocardiographic assessment of Nigerian patients seen at the Lagos University Teaching Hospital with features of mitral valve prolapse. West Afr J Med 2000;19:200-205.

69. Theal M, Sleik K, Anand S, et al: Prevalence of mitral valve prolapse in ethnic groups. Can J Cardiol 2004;20:511-515.

70. Avierinos JF, Gersh BJ, Melton LJ 3rd, et al: Natural history of asymptomatic mitral valve prolapse in the community. Circulation 2002;106:1355-1361.

71. Nascimento R, Freitas A, Teixeira F, et al: Is mitral valve prolapse a congenital or acquired disease? Am J Cardiol 1997;79:226-227.

72. Tayel S, Kurczynski TW, Levine M, et al: Marfanoid children: etiologic heterogeneity and cardiac findings. Am J Dis Child 1991;145:90-93.

73. Mohty D, Orszulak TA, Schaff HV, et al: Very long-term survival and durability of mitral valve repair for mitral valve prolapse. Circulation 2001;104(Suppl I):I-1-I-7.

74. Kolibash AJ, Jr., Kilman JW, Bush CA, et al: Evidence for progression from mild to severe mitral regurgitation in mitral valve prolapse. Am J Cardiol 1986;58:762-767.

75. Wilcken DE, Hickey AJ: Lifetime risk for patients with mitral valve prolapse of developing severe valve regurgitation requiring surgery. Circulation 1988;78:10-14.

76. Devereux RB: Mitral valve prolapse and severe mitral regurgitation. Circulation 1988;78:234-236.

77. St John Sutton M, Weyman AE: Mitral valve prolapse prevalence and complications: an ongoing dialogue. Circulation 2002;106:1305-1307.

78. Rosenhek R, Rader F, Klaar U, et al: Outcome of watchful waiting in asymptomatic severe mitral regurgitation. Circulation 2006;113:2238-2244.

79. Enriquez-Sarano M, Schaff HV, Orszulak TA, et al: Valve repair improves the outcome of surgery for mitral regurgitation: a multivariate analysis. Circulation 1995;91:1022-1028.

80. Ling LH, Enriquez-Sarano M, Seward JB, et al: Early surgery in patients with mitral regurgitation due to flail leaflets: a long-term outcome study. Circulation 1997;96:1819-1825.

81. Enriquez-Sarano M, Avierinos JF, Messika-Zeitoun D, et al: Quantitative determinants of the outcome of asymptomatic mitral regurgitation. N Engl J Med 2005;352:875-883.

82. Enriquez-Sarano M, Schaff HV, Orszulak TA, et al: Congestive heart failure after surgical correction of mitral regurgitation: a long-term study. Circulation 1995;92:2496-2503.

83. Gillinov AM, Blackstone EH, Rajeswaran J, et al: Ischemic versus degenerative mitral regurgitation: does etiology affect survival? Ann Thorac Surg 2005;80:811-819.

84. Ling LH, Enriquez-Sarano M, Seward JB, et al: Clinical outcome of mitral regurgitation due to flail leaflet. N Engl J Med 1996;335:1417-1423.

85. Bonow RO, Carabello B, Chatterjee K, et al: ACC/AHA 2006 guidelines for the management of patients with valvular heart disease: a report of the American College of Cardiology/American Heart Association Task Force on Practice Guidelines (writing committee to revise the 1998 Guidelines for the Management of Patients with Valvular Heart Disease). J Am Coll Cardiol 2006;48:e1-148.

86. Roberts WC, Braunwald E, Morrow AG: Acute severe mitral regurgitation secondary to ruptured chordae tendineae: clinical, hemodynamic, and pathologic considerations. Circulation 1966;33:58-70.

87. Alpert MA, Mukerji V, Sabeti M, et al: Mitral valve prolapse, panic disorder, and chest pain. Med Clin North Am 1991;75:1119-1133.

88. Devereux RB: Recent developments in the diagnosis and management of mitral valve prolapse. Curr Opin Cardiol 1995;10:107-116.

89. Zuppiroli A, Mori F, Favilli S, et al: Arrhythmias in mitral valve prolapse: relation to anterior mitral leaflet thickening, clinical variables, and color Doppler echocardiographic parameters. Am Heart J 1994;128:919-927.

90. Kramer HM, Kligfield P, Devereux RB, et al: Arrhythmias in mitral valve prolapse: effect of selection bias. Arch Intern Med 1984;144:2360-2364.

91. Kernis SJ, Nkomo VT, Messika-Zeitoun D, et al: Atrial fibrillation after surgical correction of mitral regurgitation in sinus rhythm: incidence, outcome, and determinants. Circulation 2004;110:2320-2325.

92. Anders S, Said S, Schulz F, et al: Mitral valve prolapse syndrome as cause of sudden death in young adults. Forensic Sci Int 2007;171:127-130.

93. Dollar AL, Roberts WC: Morphologic comparison of patients with mitral valve prolapse who died suddenly with patients who died from severe valvular dysfunction or other conditions. J Am Coll Cardiol 1991;17:921-931.

94. Danchin N, Voiriot P, Briancon S, et al: Mitral valve prolapse as a risk factor for infective endocarditis. Lancet 1989;1:743-745.

95. MacMahon SW, Hickey AJ, Wilcken DE, et al: Risk of infective endocarditis in mitral valve prolapse with and without precordial systolic murmurs. Am J Cardiol 1987;59:105-108.

96. Kelley RE, Pina I, Lee SC: Cerebral ischemia and mitral valve prolapse: case-control study of associated factors. Stroke 1988;19:443-446.

97. Watson RT: TIA, stroke, and mitral valve prolapse. Neurology 1979;29:886-889.

98. Desjardins VA, Enriquez-Sarano M, Tajik AJ, et al: Intensity of murmurs correlates with severity of valvular regurgitation. Am J Med 1996;100:149-156.

99. Tribouilloy CM, Enriquez-Sarano M, Mohty D, et al: Pathophysiologic determinants of third heart sounds: a prospective clinical and Doppler echocardiographic study. Am J Med 2001;111:96-102.

100. Weis AJ, Salcedo EE, Stewart WJ, et al: Anatomic explanation of mobile systolic clicks: implications for the clinical and echocardiographic diagnosis of mitral valve prolapse. Am Heart J 1995;129:314-320.

101. Roman MJ, Devereux RB, Kramer-Fox R, et al: Comparison of cardiovascular and skeletal features of primary mitral valve prolapse and Marfan syndrome. Am J Cardiol 1989;63:317-321.

102. Udoshi MB, Shah A, Fisher VJ, et al: Incidence of mitral valve prolapse in subjects with thoracic skeletal abnormalities—a prospective study. Am Heart J 1979;97:303-311.

103. Levine RA, Stathogiannis E, Newell JB, et al: Reconsideration of echocardiographic standards for mitral valve prolapse: lack of association between leaflet displacement isolated to the apical four chamber view and independent echocardiographic evidence of abnormality. J Am Coll Cardiol 1988;11:1010-1019.

104. Levine RA, Triulzi MO, Harrigan P, et al: The relationship of mitral annular shape to the diagnosis of mitral valve prolapse. Circulation 1987;75:756-767.

105. Levine RA, Handschumacher MD, Sanfilippo AJ, et al: Three-dimensional echocardiographic reconstruction of the mitral valve, with implications for the diagnosis of mitral valve prolapse. Circulation 1989;80:589-598.

106. Weissman NJ, Pini R, Roman MJ, et al: In vivo mitral valve morphology and motion in mitral valve prolapse. Am J Cardiol 1994;73:1080-1088.

107. Marks AR, Choong CY, Sanfilippo AJ, et al: Identification of high-risk and low-risk subgroups of patients with mitral-valve prolapse. N Engl J Med 1989;320:1031-1036.

108. Mills WR, Barber JE, Skiles JA, et al: Clinical, echocardiographic, and biomechanical differences in mitral valve prolapse affecting one or both leaflets. Am J Cardiol 2002;89:1394-1399.

109. Brown AK, Anderson V: Two dimensional echocardiography and the tricuspid valve: leaflet definition and prolapse. Br Heart J 1983;49:495-500.

110. Louie EK, Langholz D, Mackin WJ, et al: Transesophageal echocardiographic assessment of the contribution of intrinsic tissue thickness to the appearance of a thick mitral valve in patients with mitral valve prolapse. J Am Coll Cardiol 1996;28:465-471.

111. Chandraratna PA, Aronow WS: Incidence of ruptured chordae tendineae in the mitral valvular prolapse syndrome: an echocardiographic study. Chest 1979;75:334-339.

112. Grenadier E, Alpan G, Keidar S, et al: The prevalence of ruptured chordae tendineae in the mitral valve prolapse syndrome. Am Heart J 1983;105:603-610.

Ischemic Mitral Regurgitation

Ronen Beeri, Yutaka Otsuji, Ehud Schwammenthal,
and Robert A. Levine

KEY POINTS

- Restricted leaflet motion is the principal mechanism for ischemic mitral regurgitation.
- Increased leaflet tethering caused by papillary muscle displacement and left ventricular dilatation, as opposed to left ventricular dysfunction alone, is the main determinant of ischemic mitral regurgitation.
- The dynamic nature of ischemic mitral regurgitation can often cause underestimation of its severity. Exercise may therefore provide a better evaluation of the true severity and prognosis of ischemic mitral regurgitation.
- Mitral regurgitation is a major contributor to remodeling after a relatively small myocardial infarction.
- Clinical impression suggests that mitral regurgitation remains common despite medical therapy and significantly increases morbidity and mortality.
- Mitral regurgitation relief by revascularization alone in chronic coronary artery disease is problematic.
- Recurrent mitral regurgitation may in principle help explain limitations of annuloplasty to improve outcomes, given the lack of durable effective repair.
- The dynamics of ischemic mitral regurgitation indicate the need for continuing intensive heart failure therapy.

In contrast to fixed organic valvular lesions, ischemic mitral regurgitation (MR) is often overlooked in the face of the primary ventricular dysfunction that causes it. There is a growing body of evidence, however, that ischemic MR itself has a primary adverse influence on myocardial contractility that compounds the ventricular lesion and causes a vicious and downward spiral of heart failure and death. Ischemic MR doubles mortality after myocardial infarction (MI) in patients presenting with chronic heart failure and after surgical or catheter revascularization.[1-10] It occurs in approximately one fifth of patients after acute MI, even in the reperfusion era, and 50% of those with overt congestive heart failure.[3-12] Although MR due to organic lesions primarily affects prognosis when it is moderate to severe, even mild ischemic MR significantly affects survival.[5-8]

The severity of ischemic MR is difficult to gauge clinically, as murmurs are frequently inaudible, so its importance may often be unrecognized.[9] Ischemic MR frequently progresses despite medical and surgical interventions, which are in evolution. It therefore represents a common clinical problem with a primary impact on the patient and the myocardium for which uniformly effective therapeutic strategies are lacking. Understanding its mechanism can lead to more comprehensive therapy for patients with left ventricular (LV) dysfunction.

MECHANISMS

Burch et al[13,14] initially ascribed ischemic MR to papillary muscle (PM) dysfunction. Normally, as the left ventricle shortens longitudinally, systolic PM shortening maintains a relatively constant distance between the PM tips and mitral annulus to prevent prolapse. It was therefore reasoned that PM contractile dysfunction could produce MR via a prolapse mechanism. Matsuzaki et al and others,[15-19] however, have shown that isolated PM ischemic dysfunction fails to produce MR, for which adjacent LV wall dysfunction or dilatation is prerequisite. Clinical echocardiographic observations have further demonstrated that prolapse is uncommon as the sole mechanism of ischemic MR.[20-23]

Burch et al[13,14] alternatively postulated restricted leaflet motion as the basis of ischemic MR. The PMs in their normal orientation balance the forces generated by LV pressure on the leaflet surface by exerting force roughly parallel to the ventricle and perpendicular to the leaflet surface. Infarction and myocardial dysfunction cause the myocardial segments underlying the PMs to bulge outward and displace the PMs, so that they pull the leaflets in posterior and lateral directions and away from their normal coaptation at the annular level (Figure 16-1). Localized inferior or global LV remodeling also increases the tethering distance between the PM tips and the anterior annulus. This draws the leaflets into the ventricle and restricts their motion toward closure, as proposed by White,[24] Levy and Edwards,[25] Silverman and Hurst,[26] and Perloff and Roberts,[27] based on anatomic principles.

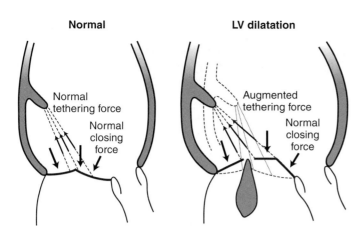

FIGURE 16–1 Basic principles of tethering mechanism for ischemic mitral regurgitation (MR) and balance of opposed closing and tethering forces acting on the leaflets. Augmented tethering force created by papillary muscle displacement apically displaces the leaflets and causes MR.

This apically restricted leaflet motion, termed *incomplete mitral leaflet closure* (IMLC) was first demonstrated with two-dimensional echocardiography (Figure 16-2)[22,23] and associated with increased leaflet tethering by Ogawa et al[22] and Godley et al.[23] Because of his formalin injection studies confirming LV inferior wall damage as prerequisite for ischemic MR, Alain Carpentier renamed *PM dysfunction* to *PM wall dysfunction* [personal communication], referring to tethering caused by displacement of the PMs by changes in the underlying LV wall. For this reason and others discussed below, replacing the term *PM dysfunction* with *PM tethering* lends greater clarity to diagnostic and therapeutic discussions.

Kaul et al[28] elegantly confirmed that reducing PM perfusion failed to cause either prolapse or MR. In contrast, global hypoperfusion with LV dysfunction and dilatation, despite continued PM perfusion and contraction, caused IMLC with MR. This finding led those authors to postulate that MR results not from PM dysfunction but from global LV dysfunction that decreases the leaflet closing force exerted by the left ventricle,[29] as opposed to PM wall tethering per se. Determining whether contractile dysfunction or LV geometry is the dominant cause of ischemic MR, however, has practical therapeutic implications: LV contractile dysfunction demands effective inotropic therapy, revascularization, or transplantation, whereas tethering might respond to modifying LV wall or PM geometry.

New models were therefore required to dissect the effects of LV contractile dysfunction from those of dilatation and geometric change. The engineering flow model is an ideal setting to model independent variation in PM position and transmitral pressure, which generates the leaflet closing force [(LV pressure – left atrial pressure) × annular area].

He et al[30] reproduced MR in excised mitral valves by displacing the PMs apically, posteriorly, and outwardly, based on clinical observations, without changing transmitral pressures. This reproduced IMLC, with MR directly proportional to leaflet tethering. In vivo, He et al pharmacologically created global LV dysfunction but with only limited LV dilatation through combined pericardial restraint and decreased preload. This dissected the effects of LV dysfunction and dilatation: isolated LV contractile dysfunction (ejection fraction <20%) without dilatation failed to cause significant MR; LV dilatation was a prerequisite for IMLC and MR.[29] To quantify tethering geometry, Otsuji et al[31] used three-dimensional (3D) echocardiographic data to standardize the tethering length from the PM tips to the anterior mitral annulus (see Figure 16-1). In the global dysfunction model, Otsuji et al[31] found that tethering length was the only independent predictor of MR, not LV ejection fraction or dP/dt. MR also correlated with LV sphericity, consistent with the key observations of Kono et al[32] and Sabbah et al[33,34] that MR relates not to LV dilatation per se but to increased sphericity that displaces the PMs outward and posteriorly, as verified by 3D echocardiography.[31] Therefore, increased leaflet tethering caused by PM displacement and LV dilatation, as opposed to LV dysfunction alone, is the main determinant of ischemic MR.

The centrality of geometric change in the mechanism of ischemic MR has been demonstrated by a number of other acute and chronic animal studies[35-38] and the clinical investigation of Yiu et al,[39] which strongly correlated PM tethering,

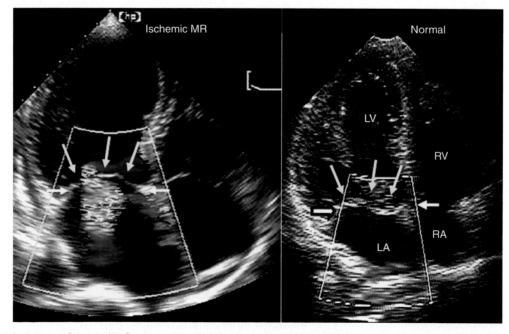

FIGURE 16–2 Apical displacement of the mitral leaflets in a patient with ischemic mitral regurgitation (MR). In contrast with a normal subject in whom the mitral leaflets close at the annular level (*yellow* and *white arrows*) (*right panel*), the patient with ischemic MR has apically displaced leaflet closure (*yellow arrows*) (*left panel*).

16

activation with extracellular matrix degradation,[62] and acceleration of apoptotic cell death,[63] culminating in systolic enlargement, extensive fibrosis, and LV failure, which predicts cardiac events.

MR considerably alters the load on the left ventricle.[64] It increases diastolic wall stress, which can induce eccentric LV hypertrophy and subsequent dilatation and failure,[65] and it thereby increases early systolic wall stress. Although MR permits LV emptying into the lower-pressure left atrium during systole, it actually increases end-systolic wall stress and hence afterload in patients with chronic MR because of induced LV remodeling that decreases contractility and increases end-systolic volume.[66,67] MR induces further LV dilatation by activating neurohumoral and cytokine components of the remodeling cascade.[68-70] As MR is both a cause and a result of LV remodeling, it can potentially exacerbate the vicious cycle spiraling down to cardiac failure unless the remodeling or the MR is reversed (Figure 16-7).[35,38,71] The ability of LV volume overload to potentiate cardiac remodeling is consistent with the reversal of remodeling by LV assist devices in patients with end-stage heart failure.[72]

Knowing whether MR in the MI setting causes more pronounced remodeling than MI alone is important because MR can potentially be eliminated to relieve the volume overload. Separating these two dynamic processes in an experimental model is a challenge because in most existing models they are linked. Beeri et al[73] therefore adapted the LV-to-left atrial (LA) shunt used by Braunwald et al[74-76] and by Rankin et al[77] to create moderate, standardized MR-like flow, independent of a modest anteroapical MI that by itself does not cause MR. In this controlled model, moderate MR worsened post-MI remodeling, increasing both diastolic and systolic LV volumes to reflect volume overload and reduced global function. Reduced contractility was apparent in physiologic measures such as preload-recruitable stroke work, which paralleled decreased single-cell contractility in the noninfarcted myocardium and reduced levels of sarcoplasmic reticulum Ca^{+2}-ATPase, a direct correlate of contractility.[73] As Enriquez-Sarano et al[78] indicated, this controlled model reveals an independent effect of MR on LV remodeling in a way that cannot readily be done in the clinical setting.

In this model, several mediators of the hypertrophic process underwent biphasic changes in the noninfarcted myocardium of animals with MR-type volume overload. These include gp130, a glycoprotein that forms heterodimers to produce different receptors, notably of the interleukin-6/cardiotrophin-1/leukemia inhibitory factor family, linked to cardiomyocyte hypertrophy[79,80]; their reduced abundance, manifested by reduced gp130 levels, has been associated with the transition from hypertrophy to failure.[81,82] Biphasic changes were also observed in Akt (protein kinase B), which is a serine-threonine kinase activated by several pro-survival

and pro-hypertrophic factors, and growth factor receptors activating phosphoinositide-3 kinase.[83] Constitutive activation of Akt in a rat model of ischemia-reperfusion injury reduced cell death and improved function.[84] As for gp130, reduced levels of Akt are related to increased apoptosis and a transition from compensatory hypertrophy to a failure phenotype.[85] In the LV-to-LA shunt ischemic MR model of Beeri et al,[73] although both infarct plus MR and infarct-only sheep had elevated expression of Akt and gp130 after 1 month, the MR sheep demonstrated a notable reduction in these protein levels after 3 months, compared with the animals without MR and with baseline. The pro-hypertrophic process, which begins in both groups at 1 month, continues in the animals without MR but is down-regulated at 3 months in the MR group, in association with continued adverse remodeling and LV dysfunction.[77] Caspase-3 levels, in contrast, remain elevated in MI plus MR sheep, generating an ongoing drive to cell death that further promotes the transition to failure. These findings are consistent with the emerging view of LV remodeling in general as a failed attempt to compensate for initial stresses on the myocardium, in this case exacerbated by the MR volume overload[81,86] and in other settings reflecting the transition from hypertensive hypertrophy to failure.[87,88] In the same model, there was also excessive activation of matrix metalloproteinases in the noninfarcted remote zone of the MI plus MR sheep. This could induce excess extracellular matrix turnover and potentially exacerbate remodeling. Tissue matrix metalloproteinase inhibitors showed a progressive rise from baseline to sacrifice that was significantly greater with MR, suggesting a possible shift from matrix turnover to matrix accumulation and stabilization over time, a response typical of remodeling myocardium.[89] All of these findings suggest strongly that MR is a major contributor to remodeling after a relatively small myocardial infarction, with reduced contractility, decreased hypertrophic drive, increased apoptotic signaling, and altered matrix turnover (see Figure 16-7).

THERAPY

Medical Therapy

The literature regarding medical therapy is limited. Post-MI and heart failure patients commonly present with moderate MR despite treatment with diuretics, angiotensin-converting enzyme (ACE) inhibitors, and β-adrenergic antagonists. Effects of medical therapy can be divided into 1) acute effects of MR per se and 2) chronic effects on LV remodeling.

Regarding the acute effects on MR volume, we need to recall the dynamic balance of tethering and closing forces (see Figure 16-1).[30,51,90] Transmitral pressure, which drives regurgitant flow, also promotes valve closure.[91] Therefore, increased systemic blood pressure might reduce MR by increasing the closing force. However, increased afterload without inotropic stimulation promotes increased LV volume, tethering, and MR (Table 16-1).[92] Inotropic agents, in contrast, can raise LV pressure without increasing tethering, so MR will decrease.[90,93] However, long-term treatment with inotropic agents is not a viable outpatient option, and inotropic agents may ultimately promote LV remodeling and tethering. Reduction in preload by diuretics or vasodilators or a combined preload and afterload reduction can reduce LV size, tethering, and MR.[94,95] Occasionally, however, reducing the closing force by acute afterload reduction may actually increase MR, if the failing ventricle is incapable of decreasing in size in response to the reduction in afterload.[96]

Regarding chronic effects of therapy, acute LV decompression by vasodilators and diuretics is not the same as true reversal of the complex molecular, cellular, and interstitial remodeling process. ACE inhibitors, angiotensin receptor blockers, and β-blockers can attenuate progressive

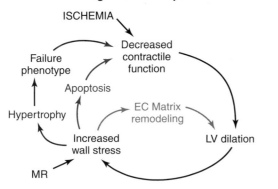

Remodeling: Failed compensation

FIGURE 16-7 Summary of molecular pathways relating mitral regurgitation and left ventricular remodeling. EC, extracellular.

TABLE 16–1	Potential Effects of Medical Therapy on the Forces Determining Mitral Regurgitant Orifice Size		
	Closing Force (Left Ventricular Pressure – Left Atrial Pressure)	Tethering Force (Papillary Muscle Displacement)	Net Effect (Regurgitant Orifice Area)
Noninotropic vasopressor	↑	↑↑↑	↑↑
Inotropic vasopressor	↑	↓	↓↓
Diuretics/ nitrates	↑	↓	↓↓
Pure arterial vasodilators	↓	↓↔	↓↔↑

LV remodeling after acute MI but not necessarily prevent or reverse it.[8,97-100] There are no published data from large trials regarding whether attenuation of remodeling by ACE inhibitors or angiotensin receptor blockers decreases the post-MI incidence of ischemic MR. Clinical impression suggests that MR remains common despite use of these drugs and significantly increases morbidity and mortality. Aggressive medical treatments with the combination of β-blockers and ACE inhibitors have shown beneficial effects on LV remodeling and MR.[101-104] Practically, however, we must deal with the many patients with significant MR in whom current medical therapy appears to have limited effectiveness.

Nonpharmacologic Therapy

Tei et al[105] have reported reduced LV volume and MR in congestive heart failure with vasodilation after thermal treatment (Figure 16-8), mediated by a change in loading conditions and an improvement of impaired vascular function after a hot bath or sauna.[106] Efficacy and periodicity of long-term treatment are being investigated.

Cardiac Resynchronization Therapy

Electrical therapy can also attenuate ischemic MR in patients with heart failure.[107] There are at least three mechanisms. Biventricular pacing, with more effective LV contraction, can reduce end-systolic volume acutely as well as in the chronic phase, reducing tethering. Resynchronization also increases the leaflet closing force in direct correlation with increased *dP/dt*, as shown by Breithardt et al[108] in patients with left bundle branch block. Physiologically, a more rapid rise in LV pressure will prolong the duration of maximal LV forces that promote leaflet closure and oppose tethering and therefore reduce the total volume of MR, based on its dynamic nature (see Figure 16-5, right). Kanzaki et al[109] have also shown that eliminating delayed lateral wall activation with discoordinated PM contraction reduces MR. Electrical therapy will therefore be most useful in those patients with cardiomyopathy whose *dP/dt* rises and lateral wall conduction delay falls with pacing; but there is no evidence of benefit in patients with preserved LV synchronicity or inferior MI. Importantly, although St John Sutton et al[110] have reported significantly decreased MR in the Multicenter InSync Randomized Clinical Evaluation, the extent of the reduction in volume and severity of MR and the increase in ejection fraction were consistently 2- to 3-fold greater in nonischemic patients than in patients with ischemic heart failure despite significantly larger baseline volumes and lower ejection fractions.[111,112]

Percutaneous and Surgical Coronary Revascularization

Emergent revascularization of acute coronary occlusion can reverse ischemic MR. Leor et al[113] and Tenenbaum et al[114] showed that early thrombolysis of first inferior MIs reduces localized LV remodeling and MR. Delayed reperfusion may yield less benefit.[9] Picard et al[115] have shown that MR conveys considerable excess mortality in acute MI with shock for comparable LV function; improved survival is achieved by early revascularization, but MR continues to reduce survival despite early intervention.

In contrast to the clear therapeutic opportunity provided by rapid reperfusion, MR relief by revascularization alone in chronic coronary artery disease is problematic. Aklog et al[56] reported persistent moderate or severe MR in 77% of revascularized patients, without established means to predict improvement.

Surgery of the Valve and Its Apparatus

Mitral Annuloplasty. Annular ring size reduction is the current standard surgical treatment. Bolling introduced the increasingly common practice of implanting rings one or two sizes smaller than predicted by measuring the fibrous intertrigonal annulus, with better surgical outcome compared with

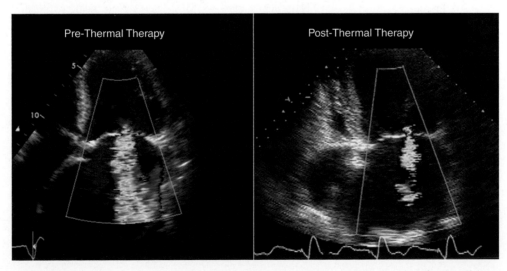

FIGURE 16–8 Both the apical displacement of the mitral leaflets and the degree of mitral regurgitation are markedly diminished after thermal therapy. *(Courtesy of Chuwa Tei et al, Kagoshima University, Japan.)*

that for full-size annuloplasty.[116-120] However, as Carlos Duran has stated (personal communication), this attempts to *compensate* for the fundamental problem, not correct it. Although annular dilatation is a significant facet of ischemic MR and annuloplasty is often effective,[116-120] long-term failures are increasingly recognized. Many experienced centers report the initial disappearance of ischemic MR, but recurrent MR develops, often months postoperatively, in 30% or more of patients, challenging satisfactory early results.[71,121-124] Recurrent MR after annuloplasty is also associated with poorer outcome.[125] In principle, catheter-based techniques to reduce annular size share with surgical annuloplasty the liability of considerable persistence of MR,[126-128] augmented by their limitation in encompassing the entire annulus from the posteriorly located coronary sinus, which bears a variable relation to the annulus itself; this may conceivably allow annular redilatation in the chronic phase. Annuloplasty itself has also been associated with adverse effects on basal ventricular strains.[129] Recurrent MR may in principle help explain limitations of annuloplasty to improve outcomes,[124,130] given the lack of durable effective repair.

Unfavorable results are related to the basic nature of mitral annuloplasty. Annular size reduction does not relieve ventricular tethering but does shift the posterior annulus and leaflet anteriorly in an attempt to restore the lost coaptation zone between the leaflets (Figure 16-9A). Rings shift the posterior annulus anteriorly, but the PM position remains posterior, so posterior leaflet tethering can be enhanced, with its anterior excursion markedly restricted.[131] Excessive tethering of the posterior leaflet is related to persistent/recurrent ischemic MR after surgical ring annuloplasty (see Figure 16-9B).[132-135] Changes in MR jet direction after surgical annuloplasty indicate changing coaptation geometry in the mechanism of recurrent ischemic MR.[136,137] In addition, the left ventricle is a moving target and often continues to remodel and dilate, rendering initial repair ineffective.[71,121-124,129] Recent reports therefore indicate a high incidence of high-grade recurrent MR in 35% of patients 6 months postoperatively.[52,71,121-124]

In trying to predict postoperative MR by preoperative evaluations, the greater the preoperative tethering, for example, measured by restriction of leaflet closure expressed as an angle or depth of coaptation relative to the annulus, the greater the postoperative MR.[121,138-142] Reversibility of LV remodeling will also depend on the impact of concomitant coronary artery bypass grafting, so that prediction of recurrent MR in the individual patient remains challenging.

In an effort to overcome these limitations, modified annular approaches, such as asymmetric annuloplasty with apical displacement of the medial annulus, often at the side of an affected PM, to restore a more normal annular three-dimensional saddle shape, and predominant anteroposterior (septal-lateral) annular reduction to bring the leaflets together most effectively have been used.[143-148] All of these approaches share the limitation that, so long as the LV remodeling is not addressed, MR may persist or recur,[149] and controlled studies are needed.

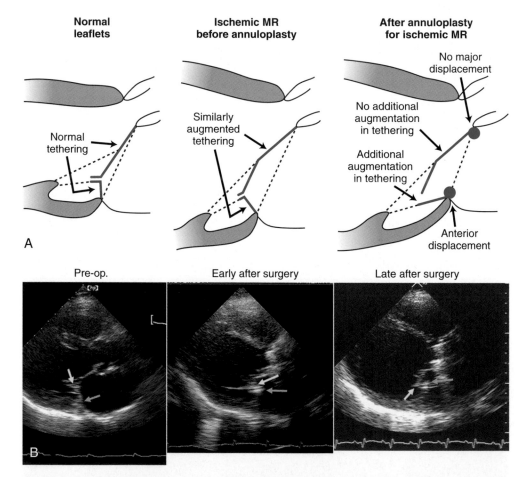

FIGURE 16–9 A, Potential mechanism of persistent or recurrent mitral regurgitation (MR) after annuloplasty for ischemic MR. Left ventricular (LV) remodeling with outward displacement of papillary muscles similarly increases tethering angles between anterior leaflet or posterior leaflet (PML) and the annular line (*middle*). Although surgical annuloplasty may not displace the anterior annulus fixed at the aortic root, this procedure hoists the posterior annulus anteriorly, which may specifically augment posterior leaflet tethering with recurrent MR (*right*). **B**, Serial changes in posterior leaflet tethering in a patient with severe aortic regurgitation, LV dysfunction, and functional MR. Preoperatively, leaflet coaptation (*yellow arrow*) is more anterior than the posterior annulus (*pink arrow*). Early after surgery with aortic valve replacement and mitral annuloplasty, mitral leaflet coaptation is barely more anterior than the posterior annulus; there was no MR then. Late after surgery, the LV dilates and mitral coaptation is more posterior than the posterior annulus, indicating increased tethering as the basis for recurrent MR. (*Diagrams by Yutaka Otsuji of University of Occupational and Environmental Health, Japan.*)

Tethering Reduction Procedures: Left Ventricular Plasty. Subvalvular tethering can be relieved by modifying LV, leaflet, or chordal structures. Early approaches involved scar resection with PM reimplantation.[132] More recent approaches use ventricular reconstruction to restore a less spherical ventricle and reduce MR, as in theSurgical Treatment of Ischemic Heart Failure (STICH) trial.[150-155] The Dor excision and patching of large dysfunctional areas reduces MR, but LV dilatation, tethering, and MR may recur, especially in patients with extensive volume reduction and subsequent LV diastolic dysfunction.[155,156] This procedure has been modified to restore a less spherical left ventricle, for example, septal anterior ventricular exclusion or overlapping plasty to achieve better contraction by reducing short-axis dimension without extensively reducing long-axis dimension and volume to cause a stiff ventricle.[157,158]

Tethering can be reduced by infarct plication to reduce bulging, as reported by Liel-Cohen et al.[38] Plication was inspired by the observation of J. Luis Guerrero, an experienced physiologic surgeon, that manually repositioning the PM-bearing wall inward and anteriorly reduces tethering and MR; plication prolongs this benefit. This infarct plication effect can also be achieved by less invasive methods. Hung et al[159,160] have applied a localized patch containing an epicardial balloon over inferior infarcts. In the beating heart, injecting saline into the buttressed balloon repositions the underlying wall and PM anteriorly, reversing leaflet tenting and MR. Thus, a relatively simple external device can reverse tethering and MR adjustably under echocardiographic guidance in the beating heart. McCarthy's Coapsys device spans the left ventricle with a reinforced suture that hoists a small pad at the posterior base anteriorly toward the right ventricular free wall.[101] The localized LV compression and need for anterior attachment without coronary or right ventricular compromise merit exploration. External constraint can also limit ventricular remodeling,[162] and global constraint devices for congestive heart failure do not appear to cause constriction. The potential for minimally invasive port access implantation has particular value in advanced heart failure.

Alternatively, repopulating damaged myocardium with cells derived from autologous skeletal myoblasts or from embryonic stem cells could reduce MR mechanically if increased wall thickness decreases bulging and reduces wall stress; in a report by Messas et al[163] autologous skeletal myoblast engraftment into a large, scarred sheep infarct blunted the progression of remodeling and MR over 8 weeks.

Direct Procedures for Papillary Muscle Displacement. Langer and Schafers[164] and Kron et al[165] have brought displaced PMs closer to the annulus using sutures. Others have used internal slings or have surgically buckled displaced PMs anteriorly.[166] Direct PM repositioning may also be combined with LV plasty to improve leaflet mobility and coaptation (Figure 16-10).[167]

Procedures to Leaflets. In theory, leaflet elongation can reduce MR[168,169] but is seldom attempted because of concerns regarding durability and complexity. Surgical or percutaneous suturing together of leaflet edges (Alfieri repair) can improve coaptation[170] but with considerable frequency of substantial ischemic MR after this maneuver on the stretched leaflets.[171] Leaflet suturing may have its greatest value when coaptation is asymmetric, with one leaflet overshooting the other, decreasing the coaptational surface and increasing MR (Figure 16-11).[172]

Procedures to Chordae. Fine marginal chordae position the leaflet tips and prevent prolapse; thicker intermediate (basal or strut) chordae insert closer to the leaflet bases. With increased tethering, the basal anterior leaflet near the annulus becomes nearly rigid and tented apically by these basal chordae (see Figure 16-1, right).[173] Messas et al[174] proposed that cutting a limited number of these basal chordae can reduce ischemic MR; eliminating the anterior leaflet bend can make the leaflets less taut and improve coaptation. As an initial approach, the two most central basal chordae to the anterior leaflet were cut at their valvular insertions because they are most stretched by PM displacement away from the LV center.

Relief of MR without prolapse has been confirmed in several settings: 1) Chordal cutting decreases leaflet tension for the same tethering length in an in vitro model[174]; 2) in sheep with acute inferobasal infarction, LV ejection fraction, pressure, and dP/dt are unchanged as MR decreases[175]; 3) with greater inferobasal remodeling 2 months post-MI, the LV ejection fraction is not decreased by chordal cutting[175]; and 4) with chordal cutting at the onset of inferobasal infarcts known to produce progressive MR,[35,36] no MR or post-MI LV ejection fraction decline has been demonstrated after a mean follow-up of 33 weeks (up to 43 weeks).[175] Goetz et al[176] have confirmed that chordal cutting increases leaflet mobility, which could benefit the tethered valve. Alternatively, Gore-Tex chordal elongation is feasible.

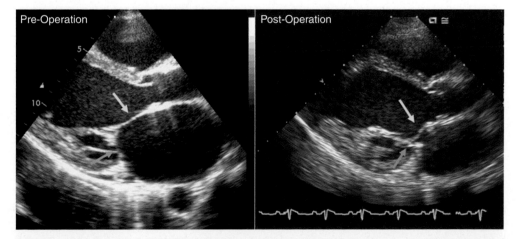

FIGURE 16–10 Improved anterior leaflet mobility after surgical left ventricular plasty (septal anterior ventricular exclusion) with papillary muscle approximation and mitral annuloplasty. Before surgery, both anterior and posterior leaflet closure was restricted (*left panel, yellow* and *pink arrows*). After the surgery, restriction of posterior leaflet closure was augmented because of the annuloplasty (*right panel, pink arrow*). However, restriction of anterior leaflet closure is improved postoperatively (*yellow arrow*), with the leaflet curving to meet the posterior leaflet. *(Courtesy of Ryuzo Sakata, Kagoshima University, Japan.)*

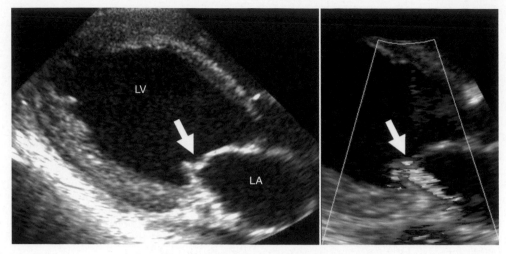

FIGURE 16–11 Relative prolapse of anterior mitral leaflet (AML). Both the AML and posterior leaflet (PML) are tethered and displaced toward left ventricular cavity. However, the tethering is predominant in the PML relative to the AML, resulting in relative prolapse of the distal AML with a posteriorly directed wall jet. LA, left atrium; LV, left ventricle.

Regarding the potential effects of chordal cutting on LV function, a recent series of papers from a single group reported results ranging from no change in LV function to decreases in various segmental or global measures.[177-180] Complete chordal transsection can reduce LV function, particularly in chronically volume-overloaded ventricles, leading to the current practice of chordal-sparing valve replacement.[181] In isolated hearts, however, even severing all basal chordae only slightly decreased shortening of a single myocardial segment. To reduce tethering in treating ischemic MR, only two chords have been cut,[174,175] and although these chords individually bear more stress, Kunzelman and Cochran[182] have suggested that "it may be possible surgically to remove basal chordae without seriously compromising mitral valve function." Basal chordae have been disconnected in routine repair of rheumatic and myxomatous valves for decades without adverse effect.[183,184] Further, reducing MR may predominantly decompress the ventricle and reduce wall stress, thereby increasing contractile function. As the ultimate clinical proof, several surgical groups have begun cutting chords to increase leaflet mobility and coaptation after annuloplasty (Figure 16-12). Borger et al[184] have cut the medial chords to both leaflets in patients with inferior MIs without any decrease in LV

function over at least 1-year of follow-up. Wakiyama et al[185] in Kobe, Japan, have applied chordal cutting in global LV dysfunction. Several approaches have been used, including one through an aortotomy.[186] Chordal elongation or transocation[187] can obviate concerns about disconnection: Komeda and Shimamoto[188] have connected the papillary muscle heads and the anterior annulus after cutting basal chordae, effectively elongating the chordal tethering mechanism without deterioration in cardiac function. Minimally invasive transcatheter approaches are conceivable, because the basal chordae are immobile relative to the heart.[189]

To summarize, ischemic MR is a ventricular disease, distinct from structural leaflet changes. It causes substantial remodeling in addition to that induced by the MI itself. Isolated annuloplasty is often effective but with intrinsic limitations demonstrated by increasing reports of persistent and recurrent ischemic MR. The tethering mechanism provides both annular and subvalvular targets for therapy, including reversing LV geometric changes as well as leaflet or chordal modification. As in the case of prolapse, the likelihood of repair will be enhanced by having a versatile "tool kit" of options, obviating the need for valve replacement.[190] Detailed mapping of geometric substrates should allow us to tailor the ideal combination of annular, ventricular, and chordal approaches to

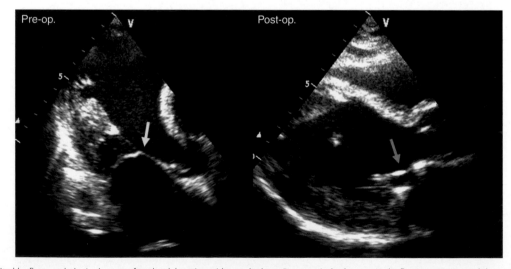

FIGURE 16–12 Mitral leaflet morphologic changes after chordal cutting with annuloplasty. Preoperatively, the anterior leaflet is convex toward the apex, especially at its mid-portion (*yellow arrow*). Postoperatively, the leaflet becomes concave (*pink arrow*), indicating relief of tethering.

achieve the best result in each patient.[191] Finally, the dynamics of ischemic MR indicate the need for continuing intensive heart failure therapy.

REMAINING QUESTIONS

Can we predict patients in whom revascularization alone will reduce MR? To date, only limited studies with low-dose dobutamine or positron emission tomography have explored whether preoperative viability, particularly in PM-bearing segments, can predict MR improvement. Because higher-dose dobutamine may nonspecifically decrease LV volume and MR, prediction of improvement after revascularization is not promising.[92,93] Exercise testing may possibly help predict benefit if exercise-improved inferobasal motion reduces MR.[59]

Do patients with MR undergoing bypass surgery benefit from mitral valve repair? It is controversial whether a concomitant mitral valve procedure has incremental benefit or not, with some reports describing beneficial effects[192-195] and others reporting no significant benefit.[196] The various conclusions can be related to the absence of a standard therapy that can eliminate ischemic MR in the majority of patients over a long period.

Does eliminating ischemic MR reduce LV remodeling? It has now been shown that ischemic MR can itself initiate remodeling.[77] Carabello et al,[197] Zile et al,[67] and Tsutsui et al[198] conclusively established that important MR—nonischemic in that case—causes progressive deterioration of LV contractile function at a cellular and molecular level, with a downward spiral of dilatation, increased wall stress, and decreased contractile function that can be reversed by correcting the MR. The presence of even a moderate amount of MR at the time of coronary artery bypass surgery by itself confers a worse prognosis.[135,199] Numerous clinical series in structural valve disease, most recently from Enriquez-Sarano et al,[200] emphasize reduced survival when mitral valve repair is delayed until the point of LV dysfunction. MR is therefore a potent stimulus for remodeling in the nonischemic heart, and ischemia can further drive that process.

Beeri et al[201] have demonstrated in their animal model that early repair of ischemic-type moderate MR induces reverse remodeling, as manifested by reduced LV volumes, improved load-independent measures of global contractility, and reversal of intracellular activation of pro-hypertrophic and pro-apoptotic pathways. Early MR repair appears to produce even greater activation of compensatory mechanisms than is present with comparable MI alone in the absence of MR, suggesting that MR might induce a "reverse remodeling momentum" that becomes evident when the MR itself is repaired. The pioneering work of Bach and Bolling[116] in patients with dilated cardiomyopathies further proves that reducing MR can reverse LV dilatation and dysfunction, as well as the associated, often counterproductive, neurohumoral cascade.

Does the mitral valve adapt to chronic tethering? Ischemic MR can be viewed as a mismatch between leaflet and annular size. Using a validated method for 3D reconstruction of total leaflet area developed by Handschumacher, Chaput et al,[202] have shown an average of 35% greater leaflet area in patients with LV dysfunction (inferior or global) compared with that in normal control subjects. Although systolic stretch acutely increases leaflet size,[203] Chaput et al[202] measured leaflet area in diastole, independent of any superimposed systolic stretch. Despite these changes in leaflet area, consistent with valve plasticity, the adequacy of leaflet adaptation varies among patients, with a variable ratio of total leaflet area to the tented leaflet closure area required to occlude the orifice based on tethering geometry. A lower total-to-closure leaflet area ratio strongly and independently predicts MR. The underlying adaptive mechanisms merit investigation as potential therapeutic targets.

DIAGNOSIS

Ischemic MR murmurs are frequently faint or inaudible,[9] which may reflect the mid-systolic decrease in flow rate (see Figure 16-5),[50] decreased LV-to-LA pressure gradients and limited acoustic transmission. The absence of intrinsic or organic leaflet lesions or chordal or PM rupture and the presence of apically displaced leaflets in systole confirm ischemic etiology. Jet area may overestimate severity as the jet expands into a dilated atrium.[204] Calculating flow rate from velocity multiplied by surface area proximal to the orifice will underestimate true values if the velocity surface is assumed to be hemispherical; it is generally hemielliptical, paralleling a slit-like orifice.[205,206] The vena contracta dimension in a long-axis view is extremely useful, because the regurgitant orifice scales up or down with the vena contracta dimension perpendicular to the coaptation line.[207] Dynamic MR variation indicates the need to integrate flow throughout systole.[50,208,209] Evaluation at rest may under-represent the burden on the active patient,[57,58] and intraoperative evaluation is heavily influenced by changes in load and tethering.[54-56]

SUMMARY AND PERSPECTIVES

Ischemic MR is a substantial remaining frontier in the successful move from valve replacement to repair and presents a growing opportunity for minimally invasive therapeutic measures. Experience with this condition highlights the lessons of exercise testing in valvular heart disease. Treating ischemic MR is an important element of the broader effort to treat heart failure and limit remodeling by external constraint and cardiac resynchronization.

Understanding the mechanism of ischemic MR is leading to improved therapies that target its primary causes. Providing a range of therapeutic options has the potential to offer a more flexible approach that can be adapted to a wide range of patients with diverse LV and valvular changes. The guiding principle is to achieve a comprehensive repair that addresses tethering at both the annular and ventricular ends of the leaflets. Looking ahead to the near future, we can envision that evaluation of mitral annular and ventricular dimensions will allow us to tailor therapies individually to the patient. Cardiac imaging has been critical to our understanding of ischemic MR and is likely to be an important guide for more effective therapies to realign the mitral valve with its attachments.

Acknowledgments

Drs. Ronen Beeri and Yutaka Otsuji contributed equally to this chapter. We thank Mark D. Handschumacher, BS, for his outstanding contributions to the graphics, 3D conceptualization, and analysis and J. Luis Guerrero, BS, Judy Hung, MD, and Emanuel Messas, MD, for conceptual contributions.

This work was supported in part by the Leducq Foundation Transatlantic Network of Excellence in Mitral Valve Disease (Grant 07 CVD 04), by US-Israel Binational Science Foundation Grants 2001037 and 2005250, and by Grants R01 HL38176, R01 HL72265, and K24 67434 of the National Institutes of Health, Bethesda, MD.

REFERENCES

1. Levine RA, Schwammmenthal E: ischemic mitral regurgitation on the threshold of a solution: from paradoxes to unifying concepts. Circulation 2005;112:745-758.
2. Bursi F, Enriquez-Sarano M, Jacobsen SJ, Roger VL: Mitral regurgitation after myocardial infarction: a review. Am J Med 2006;119:103-112.
3. Koelling TM, Aaronson KD, Cody RJ, et al: Prognostic significance of mitral regurgitation and tricuspid regurgitation in patients with left ventricular systolic dysfunction. Am Heart J 2002;144:524-529.
4. Ellis SG, Whitlow PL, Raymond RE, Schneider JP: Impact of mitral regurgitation on long-term survival after percutaneous coronary intervention. Am J Cardiol 2002;89:315-318.
5. Feinberg MS, Schwammenthal E, Shlizerman L, et al: Prognostic significance of mild mitral regurgitation by color Doppler echocardiography in acute myocardial infarction. Am J Cardiol 2000;86:903-907.
6. Barzilai B, Davis VG, Stone PH, Jaffe AS: Prognostic significance of mitral regurgitation in acute myocardial infarction: the MILIS7 Study Group. Am J Cardiol 1990;65:1169-1175.

7. Grigioni F, Enriquez-Sarano M, Zehr KJ, et al: Ischemic mitral regurgitation: long-term outcome and prognostic implications with quantitative Doppler assessment. Circulation 2001;103:1759-1764.
8. Lamas GA, Mitchell GF, Flaker GC, et al: Clinical significance of mitral regurgitation after acute myocardial infarction. Circulation 1997;96:827-833.
9. Lehmann KG, Francis CK, Dodge HT, the TIMI Study Group: Mitral regurgitation in early myocardial infarction: incidence, clinical detection and prognostic implications. Ann Intern Med 1992;117:10-17.
10. Tcheng JE, Jackman JD Jr, Nelson CL, et al: Outcome of patients sustaining acute ischemic mitral regurgitation during myocardial infarction. Ann Intern Med 1992;117:18-24.
11. Kisanuki A, Otsuji Y, Kuroiwa R, et al: Two-dimensional echocardiographic assessment of papillary muscle contractility in patients with prior myocardial infarction. J Am Coll Cardiol 1993;21:932-938.
12. Trichon BH, Felker GM, Shaw LK, et al: Relation of frequency and severity of mitral regurgitation to survival among patients with left ventricular systolic dysfunction and heart failure. Am J Cardiol 2003;91:538-543.
13. Burch GE, De Pasquale NP, Phillips JH: Clinical manifestations of papillary muscle dysfunction. Arch Intern Med 1963;112:112-117.
14. Burch GE, DePasquale NP, Phillips JH: The syndrome of papillary muscle dysfunction. Am Heart J 1968;75:399-415.
15. Hider CF, Taylor DE, Wade JD: The effect of papillary muscle damage on atrio-ventricular valve function in the left heart. Q J Exp Physiol Cogn Med Sci 1965;50:15-22.
16. Miller GE Jr, Kerth WJ, Gerbode F: Experimental papillary muscle infarction. J Thorac Cardiovasc Surg 1968;56:611-616.
17. Tsakiris AG, Rastelli GC, Amorim Dde S, et al: Effect of experimental papillary muscle damage on mitral valve closure in intact anesthetized dogs. Mayo Clin Proc 1970;45:275-285.
18. Mittal AK, Langston M Jr, Cohn KE, et al: Combined papillary muscle and left ventricular wall dysfunction as a cause of mitral regurgitation: an experimental study. Circulation 1971;44:174-180.
19. Matsuzaki M, Yonezawa F, Toma Y, et al: Experimental mitral regurgitation in ischemia-induced papillary muscle dysfunction. J Cardiol 1988;18(Suppl):121-126.
20. Izumi S, Miyatake K, Beppu S, et al: Mechanism of mitral regurgitation in patients with myocardial infarction: a study using real-time two-dimensional Doppler flow imaging and echocardiography. Circulation 1987;76:777-785.
21. Van Dantzig JM, Delemarre BJ, Koster RW, et al: Pathogenesis of mitral regurgitation in acute myocardial infarction: importance of changes in left ventricular shape and regional function. Am Heart J 1996;131:865-871.
22. Ogawa S, Hubbard FE, Mardelli TJ, Dreifus LS: Cross-sectional echocardiographic spectrum of papillary muscle dysfunction. Am Heart J 1979;97:312-321.
23. Godley RW, Wann LS, Rogers EW, et al: Incomplete mitral leaflet closure in patients with papillary muscle dysfunction. Circulation 1981;63:565-571.
24. White P: Heart Disease, 4th ed. New York, McMillan, 1952:672.
25. Levy MJ, Edwards JE: Anatomy of mitral insufficiency. Prog Cardiovasc Dis 1962;5:119-144.
26. Silverman ME, Hurst JW: The mitral complex: interaction of the anatomy, physiology, and pathology of the mitral annulus, mitral valve leaflets, chordae tendineae, and papillary muscles. Am Heart J 1968;76:399-418.
27. Perloff JK, Roberts WC: The mitral apparatus: functional anatomy of mitral regurgitation. Circulation 1972;46:227-239.
28. Kaul S, Spotnitz WD, Glasheen WP, Touchstone DA: Mechanism of ischemic mitral regurgitation: an experimental evaluation. Circulation 1991;84:2167-2180.
29. Dent JM, Spotnitz WD, Nolan SP, et al: Mechanism of mitral leaflet excursion. Am J Physiol Heart Circ Physiol 1995;269(6 Pt 2):H2100-H2108.
30. He S, Fontaine AA, Schwammenthal E, et al: Integrated mechanism for functional mitral regurgitation: leaflet restriction versus coapting force: in vitro studies. Circulation 1997;96:1826-1834.
31. Otsuji Y, Handshumacher MD, Schwammethal E, et al: Insights from three-dimensional echocardiography into the mechanisms of functional mitral regurgitation: direct in vivo demonstration of altered leaflet geometry. Circulation 1997;96:1999-2008.
32. Kono T, Sabbah HN, Rosman H, et al: Left ventricular shape is the primary determinant of functional mitral regurgitation in heart failure. J Am Coll Cardiol 1992;20:1594-1598.
33. Sabbah HN, Kono T, Stein PD, et al: Left ventricular shape changes during the course of evolving heart failure. Am J Physiol Heart Circ Physiol 1992;263(1 Pt 2):H266-H270.
34. Sabbah HN, Rosman H, Kono T, et al: On the mechanism of functional mitral regurgitation. Am J Cardiol 1993;72:1074-1076.
35. Otsuji Y, Handschumacher MD, Liel-Cohen N, et al: Mechanism of ischemic mitral regurgitation with segmental left ventricular dysfunction: three-dimensional echocardiographic studies in models of acute and chronic progressive regurgitation. J Am Coll Cardiol 2001;37:641-648.
36. Llaneras MR, Nance ML, Streicher JT, et al: Large animal model of ischemic mitral regurgitation. Ann Thorac Surg 1994;57:432-439.
37. Gorman RC, McCaughan JS, Ratcliffe MB, et al: Pathogenesis of acute ischemic mitral regurgitation in three dimensions. J Thorac Cardiovasc Surg 1995;109:684-693.
38. Liel-Cohen N, Guerrero JL, Otsuji Y, et al: Design of a new surgical approach for ventricular remodeling to relieve ischemic mitral regurgitation. Circulation 2000;101:2756-2763.
39. Yiu SF, Enriquez-Sarano M, Tribouilloy C, et al: Determinants of the degree of functional mitral regurgitation in patients with systolic left ventricular dysfunction: a quantitative clinical study. Circulation 2000;102: 1400-6.
40. Kumanohoso T, Otsuji Y, Yoshifuku S, et al: Mechanism of higher incidence of ischemic mitral regurgitation in patients with inferior myocardial infarction: quantitative analysis of left ventricular and mitral valve geometry in 103 patients with prior myocardial infarction. J Thorac Cardiovasc Surg 2003;125:135-143.
41. Kwan J, Shiota T, Agler DA, et al: Geometric differences of the mitral apparatus between ischemic and dilated cardiomyopathy with significant mitral regurgitation: real-time three-dimensional echocardiography study. Circulation 2003;107: 1135-1140.
42. Lai DT, Tibayan FA, Myrmel T, et al: Mechanistic insights into posterior mitral leaflet inter-scallop malcoaptation during acute ischemic mitral regurgitation. Circulation 2002;106(Suppl I):I-40-I-45.
43. Boltwood CM, Tei C, Wong M, Shah PM: Quantitative echocardiography of the mitral complex in dilated cardiomyopathy: the mechanism of functional mitral regurgitation. Circulation 1983;68:498-508.
44. Otsuji Y, Kumanohoso T, Yoshifuku S, et al: Isolated annular dilation does not usually cause important functional mitral regurgitation: comparison between patients with lone atrial fibrillation and those with idiopathic or ischemic cardiomyopathy. J Am Coll Cardiol 2002;39:1651-1656.
45. Otsuji Y, Gilon D, Jiang L, et al: Restricted diastolic opening of the mitral leaflets in patients with left ventricular dysfunction: evidence for increased valve tethering. J Am Coll Cardiol 1998;32:398-404.
46. Messas E, Guerrero JL, Handschumacher MD, et al: Paradoxic decrease in ischemic mitral regurgitation with papillary muscle dysfunction: insights from three-dimensional and contrast echocardiography with strain rate measurement. Circulation 2001;104:1952-1957.
47. Uemura T, Otsuji Y, Nakashiki K, et al: Papillary muscle dysfunction attenuates ischemic mitral regurgitation in patients with localized basal inferior left ventricular remodeling: insights from tissue Doppler strain imaging. J Am Coll Cardiol 2005;46:113-119.
48. Khankirawatana B, Khankirawatana S, Mahrous H, Porter TR: Assessment of papillary muscle function using myocardial velocity gradient derived from tissue Doppler echocardiography. Am J Cardiol 2004;94:45-49.
49. Komeda M, Glasson JR, Bolger AF, et al: Papillary muscle-left ventricular "complex." J Thorac Cardiovasc Surg 1997;113:292-300.
50. Schwammenthal E, Chen C, Benning F, et al: Dynamics of mitral regurgitant flow and orifice area: physiologic application of the proximal flow convergence method: clinical data and experimental testing. Circulation 1994;90:307-322.
51. Schwammenthal E, Popescu AC, Popescu BA, et al: Mechanism of mitral regurgitation in inferior wall acute myocardial infarction. Am J Cardiol 2002;90:306-309.
52. Hung J, Otsuji Y, Handschumacher MD, et al: Mechanism of dynamic regurgitant orifice area variation in functional mitral regurgitation: physiologic insights from the proximal flow convergence technique. J Am Coll Cardiol 1999;33:538-545.
53. Grande-Allen KJ, Barber JE, Klatka KM, et al: Mitral valve stiffening in end-stage heart failure: evidence of an organic contribution to functional mitral regurgitation. J Thorac Cardiovas Surg 2005;130:783-790.
54. Sheikh KH, Bengtson JR, Rankin JS, et al: Intraoperative transesophageal Doppler color flow imaging used to guide patient selection and operative treatment of ischemic mitral regurgitation. Circulation. 1991;84:594-604.
55. Bach DS, Deeb GM, Bolling SF: Accuracy of intraoperative transesophageal echocardiography for estimating the severity of functional mitral regurgitation. Am J Cardiol 1995;76:508-512.
56. Aklog L, Filsoufi F, Flores KQ, et al: Does coronary artery bypass grafting alone correct moderate ischemic mitral regurgitation? Circulation 2001;104(Suppl I):I-68-I-75.
57. Lancellotti P, Lebrun F, Pierard LA: Determinants of exercise-induced changes in mitral regurgitation in patients with coronary artery disease and left ventricular dysfunction. J Am Coll Cardiol 2003;42:1921-1928.
58. Levine RA: Dynamic mitral regurgitation: more than meets the eye. N Engl J Med 2004;351:1681-1684.
59. Lancellotti P, Troisfontaines P, Toussaint AC, Pierard LA: Prognostic importance of exercise-induced changes in mitral regurgitation in patients with chronic ischemic left ventricular dysfunction. Circulation 2003;108:1713-1717.
60. Lapu-Bula R, Robert A, Van Craeynest D, et al: Contribution of exercise-induced mitral regurgitation to exercise stroke volume and exercise capacity in patients with left ventricular systolic dysfunction. Circulation 2002;106:1342-1348.
61. Pierard LA, Lancellotti P: The role of ischemic mitral regurgitation in the pathogenesis of acute pulmonary edema. N Engl J Med 2004;351:1627-1634.
62. Spinale FG, Coker ML, Thomas CV, et al: Time-dependent changes in matrix metalloproteinase activity and expression during the progression of congestive heart failure: relation to ventricular and myocyte function. Circ Res 1998;82:482-495.
63. Cheng W, Kajstura J, Nitahara JA, et al: Programmed myocyte cell death affects the viable myocardium after infarction in rats. Exp Cell Res 1996;226:316-327.
64. Carabello BA: Mitral valve regurgitation. Curr Probl Cardiol 1998;23:202-241.
65. Spinale FG, Ishihra K, Zile MR, et al: Structural basis for changes in left ventricular function and geometry because of chronic mitral regurgitation and after correction of volume overload. J Thorac Cardiovasc Surg 1993;106:1147-1157.
66. Corin WJ, Monrad ES, Murakami T, et al: The relationship of afterload to ejection performance in chronic mitral regurgitation. Circulation 1987;76:59-67.
67. Zile MR, Gaasch WH, Levine HT: Left ventricular stress-dimension-shortening relations before and after correction of chronic aortic and mitral regurgitation. Am J Cardiol 1985;56:99.
68. Dell'Italia LJ, Meng QC, Balcells E, et al: Increased ACE and chymase-like activity in cardiac tissue of dogs with chronic mitral regurgitation. Am J Physiol 1995;269:H2065-H2073.
69. Kapadia SR, Yakoob K, Nader S, et al: Elevated circulating levels of serum tumor necrosis factor- in patients with hemodynamically significant pressure and volume overload. J Am Coll Cardiol 2000;36:208-212.
70. Talwar S, Squire IB, Davies JE, Ng LL: The effect of valvular regurgitation on plasma cardiotrophin-1 in patients with normal left ventricular systolic function. Eur J Heart Failure 2000;2:387-391.
71. Hung J, Papakostas L, Tahta SA, et al: Mechanism of recurrent ischemic mitral regurgitation post-annuloplasty: Continued LV remodeling as a moving target. Circulation 2004;110(Suppl I):85-90.

72. Moazami N, Argenziano M, Kohomoto T, et al: Inflow valve regurgitation during left ventricular assist device support may interfere with reverse ventricular remodeling. Ann Thorac Surg 1998;65:628-31.

73. Beeri R, Yosefy C, Guerrero JL, et al: Mitral regurgitation augments post-myocardial infarction remodeling: failure of hypertrophic compensation. J Am Coll Cardiol 2008;51:476-486.

74. Braunwald E, Welch GH Jr, Sarnoff SJ: Hemodynamic effects of quantitatively varied experimental mitral regurgitation. Circ Res 1957;5:539-545.

75. Braunwald E, Welch GH Jr, Morrow AG: The effects of acutely increased systemic resistance on the left atrial pressure pulse: a method for the clinical detection of mitral insufficiency. J Clin Invest 1958;37:35-40.

76. Braunwald E: Mitral regurgitation: physiologic, clinical and surgical considerations. N Engl J Med 1969;281:425-433.

77. Rankin JS, Nicholas LM, Kouchoukos NT: Experimental mitral regurgitation: effects on left ventricular function before and after elimination of chronic regurgitation in the dog. J Thorac Cardiovasc Surg 1975;70:478-488.

78. Enriquez-Sarano M, Loulmet DF, Burkhoff D: The conundrum of functional mitral regurgitation in chronic heart failure. J Am Coll Cardiol 2008;51:487-489.

79. Hirota H, Yoshida K, Kishimoto T, Taga T: Continuous activation of gp130: a signal-transducing receptor component for interleukin 6-related cytokines, causes myocardial hypertrophy in mice. Proc Natl Acad Sci USA 1995;92:4862-4866.

80. Kunisada K, Tone E, Fujio Y, et al: Activation of gp130 transduces hypertrophic signals via STAT3 in cardiac myocytes. Circulation 1998;98:346-352.

81. Hirota H, Chen J, Betz UAK, et al: Loss of a gp130 cardiac muscle cell survival pathway is a critical event in the onset of heart failure during biomechanical stress. Cell 1999;97:189-198.

82. Zolk O, Ng LL, O'Brien RJ, et al: Augmented expression of cardiotrophin-1 in failing human hearts is accompanied by diminished glycoprotein 130 receptor protein abundance. Circulation 2002;106:1430-1432.

83. Shioi T, Kang PM, Douglas PS, et al: The conserved phosphoinositide 3-kinase pathway determines heart size in mice. EMBO J 2000;19:2537-2548.

84. Matsui T, Tao J, del Monte F, et al: Akt activation preserves cardiac function and prevents injury after transient cardiac ischemia in vivo. Circulation 2001;104:330-335.

85. Haq S, Choukroun G, Lim HW, et al: Differential activation of signal transduction pathways in human hearts with hypertrophy versus advanced heart failure. Circulation 2001;103:670-677.

86. Mann DL, Bristow MR: Mechanisms and models in heart failure. the biomechanical model and beyond. Circulation 2005;111:2837-2849.

87. Rosen BD, Edvardsen T, Lai S, et al: Left ventricular concentric remodeling is associated with decreased global and regional systolic function. The Multi-Ethnic Study of Atherosclerosis. Circulation 2005;112:984-991.

88. Drazner MH: The transition from hypertrophy to failure: how certain are we? Circulation 2005;112:936-938.

89. Spinale FG, Coker ML, Bond BR, Zellner JL: Myocardial matrix degradation and metalloproteinase activation in the failing heart: a potential therapeutic target. Cardiovasc Res 2000;46:225-238.

90. Keren G, Katz S, Strom J, et al: Dynamic mitral regurgitation: an important determinant of the hemodynamic response to load alterations and inotropic therapy in severe heart failure. Circulation 1989;80:306-313.

91. Rodbard S, Williams F: The dynamics of mitral insufficiency. Am Heart J 1954;48:521-539.

92. Keren G, Katz S, Gage J, et al: Effect of isometric exercise on cardiac performance and mitral regurgitation in patients with severe congestive heart failure. Am Heart J 1989;118(5 Pt 1):973-979.

93. Heinle SK, Tice FD, Kisslo J: Effect of dobutamine stress echocardiography on mitral regurgitation. J Am Coll Cardiol 1995;25:122-127.

94. Stevenson LW, Bellil D, Grover-McKay M, et al: Effects of afterload reduction (diuretics and vasodilators) on left ventricular volume and mitral regurgitation in severe congestive heart failure secondary to ischemic or idiopathic dilated cardiomyopathy. Am J Cardiol 1987;60:654-658.

95. Rosario LB, Stevenson LW, Solomon SD, et al: The mechanism of decrease in dynamic mitral regurgitation during heart failure treatment: importance of reduction in the regurgitant orifice size. J Am Coll Cardiol 1998;32:1819-1824.

96. Kizilbash AM, Willett DL, Brickner ME, et al: Effects of afterload reduction on vena contracta width in mitral regurgitation. J Am Coll Cardiol 1998;32:427-431.

97. Pfeffer MA, Lamas GA, Vaughan DE, et al: Effect of captopril on progressive ventricular dilatation after anterior myocardial infarction. N Engl J Med 1988;319:80-86.

98. St John Sutton M, Pfeffer MA, Moye L, et al: Cardiovascular death and left ventricular remodeling two years after myocardial infarction: baseline predictors and impact of long-term use of captopril: information from the Survival and Ventricular Enlargement (SAVE) trial. Circulation 1997;96:3294-3299.

99. Greenberg B, Quinones MA, Koilpillai C, et al: Effects of long-term enalapril therapy on cardiac structure and function in patients with left ventricular dysfunction: results of the SOLVD echocardiography substudy. Circulation 1995;91:2573-2581.

100. Konstam MA, Kronenberg MW, Rousseau MF, et al: Effects of the angiotensin converting enzyme inhibitor enalapril on the long-term progression of left ventricular dilatation in patients with asymptomatic systolic dysfunction. SOLVD (Studies of Left Ventricular Dysfunction) Investigators. Circulation 1993;88(5 Pt 1):2277-2283.

101. Lowes BD, Gill EA, Abraham WT, et al: Effects of carvedilol on left ventricular mass, chamber geometry, and mitral regurgitation in chronic heart failure. Am J Cardiol 1999;83:1201-1205.

102. Capomolla S, Febo O, Gnemmi M, et al: β-Blockade therapy in chronic heart failure: diastolic function and mitral regurgitation improvement by carvedilol. Am Heart J 2000;139:596-608.

103. Remme WJ, Riegger G, Hildebrandt P, et al: The benefits of early combination treatment of carvedilol and an ACE-inhibitor in mild heart failure and left ventricular systolic dysfunction. The Carvedilol and ACE-Inhibitor Remodelling Mild Heart Failure Evaluation Trial (CARMEN). Cardiovasc Drugs Ther 2004;18:57-66.

104. Doughty RN, Whalley GA, Walsh HA, et al: Effects of carvedilol on left ventricular remodeling after acute myocardial infarction: the Capricorn Echo Substudy. Circulation 2004;109:201-206.

105. Tei C, Horikiri Y, Park JC, et al: Acute hemodynamic improvement by thermal vasodilation in congestive heart failure. Circulation 1995;91:2582-2590.

106. Kihara T, Biro S, Imamura M, et al: Repeated sauna treatment improves vascular endothelial and cardiac function in patients with chronic heart failure. J Am Coll Cardiol 2002;39:754-759.

107. Ypenburg C, Lancellotti P, Tops LF, et al: Acute effects of initiation and withdrawal of cardiac resynchronization therapy on papillary muscle dyssynchrony and mitral regurgitation. J Am Coll Cardiol 2007;50:2071-2077.

108. Breithardt OA, Sinha AM, Schwammenthal E, et al: Acute effects of cardiac resynchronization therapy on functional mitral regurgitation in advanced systolic heart failure. J Am Coll Cardiol 2003;41:765-770.

109. Kanzaki H, Bazaz R, Schwartzman D, et al: A mechanism for immediate reduction in mitral regurgitation after cardiac resynchronization therapy: insights from mechanical activation strain mapping. J Am Coll Cardiol 2004;44:1619-1625.

110. St John Sutton MG, Plappert T, Abraham WT, et al: Effect of cardiac resynchronization therapy on left ventricular size and function in chronic heart failure. Circulation 2003;107:1985-1990.

111. Gorcsan J 3rd, Abraham T, Agler DA, et al: Echocardiography for cardiac resynchronization therapy: recommendations for performance and reporting: a report from the American Society of Echocardiography Dyssynchrony Writing Group endorsed by the Heart Rhythm Society. J Am Soc Echocardiogr 2008;21:191-213.

112. St John Sutton MG, Plappert T, Hilpisch KE, et al: Sustained reverse left ventricular structural remodeling with cardiac resynchronization at one year is a function of etiology: quantitative Doppler echocardiographic evidence from the Multicenter InSync Randomized Clinical Evaluation (MIRACLE). Circulation 2006;113:266-272.

113. Leor J, Feinberg MS, Vered Z, et al: Effect of thrombolytic therapy on the evolution of significant mitral regurgitation in patients with a first inferior myocardial infarction. J Am Coll Cardiol 1993;21:1661-1666.

114. Tenenbaum A, Leor J, Motro M, et al: Improved posterobasal segment function after thrombolysis is associated with decreased incidence of significant mitral regurgitation in a first inferior myocardial infarction. J Am Coll Cardiol 1995;25:1558-1563.

115. Picard MH, Davidoff R, Sleeper LA, et al: Echocardiographic predictors of survival and response to early revascularization in cardiogenic shock. Circulation 2003;107:279-284.

116. Bach DS, Bolling SF: Early improvement in congestive heart failure after correction of secondary mitral regurgitation in end-stage cardiomyopathy. Am Heart J 1995;129:1165-1170.

117. Bolling SF, Pagani FD, Deeb GM, Bach DS: Intermediate-term outcome of mitral reconstruction in cardiomyopathy. J Thorac Cardiovasc Surg 1998;115:381-386.

118. Bach DS, Bolling SF: Improvement following correction of secondary mitral regurgitation in end-stage cardiomyopathy with mitral annuloplasty. Am J Cardiol 1996;78:966-969.

119. Bax JJ, Braun J, Somer ST, et al: Restrictive annuloplasty and coronary revascularization in ischemic mitral regurgitation results in reverse left ventricular remodeling. Circulation 2004;110(Suppl II):II-103-II-108.

120. Geidel S, Schneider C, Lass M, et al: Changes of myocardial function after combined coronary revascularization and mitral valve downsizing in patients with ischemic mitral regurgitation and advanced cardiomyopathy. J Thorac Cardiovasc Surg 2007;55:1-6.

121. Calafiore AM, Gallina S, DiMauro M, et al: Mitral valve procedure in dilated cardiomyopathy: repair or replacement. Ann Thorac Surg 2001;71:1146-1152.

122. Tahta SA, Oury JH, Maxwell JM, et al: Outcome after mitral valve repair for functional ischemic mitral regurgitation. J Heart Valve Dis 2002;11:11-14.

123. McGee EC, Gillinov AM, Blackstone EH, et al: Recurrent mitral regurgitation after annuloplasty for functional ischemic mitral regurgitation. J Thorac Cardiovasc Surg 2004;128:916-924.

124. Mihaljevic T, Lam BK, Rajeswaran J, et al: Impact of mitral valve annuloplasty combined with revascularization in patients with functional ischemic mitral regurgitation. J Am Coll Cardiol 2007;49:2191-201.

125. Dahlberg PS, Orszulak TA, Mullany CJ, et al: Late outcome of mitral valve surgery for patients with coronary artery disease. Ann Thorac Surg 2003;76:1539-1547.

126. Daimon M, Gillinov AM, Liddicoat JR, et al: Dynamic change in mitral annular area and motion during percutaneous mitral annuloplasty for ischemic mitral regurgitation: preliminary animal study with real-time 3-dimensional echocardiography. J Am Soc Echocardiogr 2007;20:381-388.

127. Dubreuil O, Basmadjian A, Ducharme A, et al: Percutaneous mitral valve annuloplasty for ischemic mitral regurgitation: first in man experience with a temporary implant. Catheter Cardiovasc Interv 2007;69:1053-1061.

128. Webb JG, Harnek J, Munt BI, et al: Percutaneous transvenous mitral annuloplasty: initial human experience with device implantation in the coronary sinus. Circulation 2006;113:851-855.

129. Cheng A, Nguyen TC, Malinowski M, et al: Effects of undersized mitral annuloplasty on regional transmural left ventricular wall strains and wall thickening mechanisms. Circulation 2006;114(Suppl I):I-600-I-609.

130. Wu AH, Aaronson KD, Bolling SF, et al: Impact of mitral valve annuloplasty on mortality risk in patients with mitral regurgitation and left ventricular systolic dysfunction. J Am Coll Cardiol 2005;45:381-387.

131. Green GR, Dagum P, Glasson JR, et al: Restricted posterior leaflet motion after mitral ring annuloplasty. Ann Thorac Surg 1999;68:2100-2106.
132. Zhu F, Otsuji Y, Yotsumoto G, et al: Mechanism of persistent ischemic mitral regurgitation after annuloplasty: importance of augmented posterior mitral leaflet tethering. Circulation 2005;112(Suppl I):I-396-I-401.
133. Kuwahara E, Otsuji Y, Iguro Y, et al: Mechanism of recurrent/persistent ischemic/functional mitral regurgitation in the chronic phase after surgical annuloplasty: importance of augmented posterior leaflet tethering. Circulation. (2006);114(Suppl I):I-529-34.
134. Marasco SF: Surgical correction of posterior leaflet tethering in ischemic mitral regurgitation. J Cardiovasc Surg (Torino) 2007;48:667-670.
135. Grossi EA, Crooke GA, DiGiorgi PL, et al: Impact of moderate functional mitral insufficiency in patients undergoing surgical revascularization. Circulation 2006;114(Suppl I): I-573-I-576.
136. Senechal M, Magne J, Pibarot P, et al: Direction of persistent ischemic mitral jet after restrictive valve annuloplasty: implication for interpretation of perioperative echocardiography. Can J Cardiol 2007;23(Suppl B):48B-52B.
137. Cheng A, Nguyen TC, Malinowski M, et al: Undersized mitral annuloplasty inhibits left ventricular basal wall thickening but does not affect equatorial wall cardiac strains. J Heart Valve Dis 2007;16:349-358.
138. Kongsaerepong V, Shiota M, Gillinov AM, et al: Echocardiographic predictors of successful versus unsuccessful mitral valve repair in ischemic mitral regurgitation. Am J Cardiol 2006;98:504-508.
139. Agricola E, Oppizzi M, Pisani M, et al: Ischemic mitral regurgitation: mechanisms and echocardiographic classification. Eur J Echocardiogr 2008;9:207-221.
140. Roshanali F, Mandegar MH, Yousefnia MA, et al: A prospective study of predicting factors in ischemic mitral regurgitation recurrence after ring annuloplasty. Ann Thorac Surg 2007;84:745-749.
141. Digiammarco G, Liberi R, Giancane M, et al: Recurrence of functional mitral regurgitation in patients with dilated cardiomyopathy undergoing mitral valve repair: how to predict it. Interact Cardiovasc Thorac Surg 2007;6:340-344.
142. Magne J, Pibarot P, Dagenais F, et al: Preoperative posterior leaflet angle accurately predicts outcome after restrictive mitral valve annuloplasty for ischemic mitral regurgitation. Circulation 2007;115:782-791.
143. David TE: Techniques and results of mitral valve repair for ischemic mitral regurgitation. J Card Surg 1994;9(suppl):274-277.
144. Levine RA, Handschumacher MD, Sanfilippo AJ, et al: Three-dimensional echocardiographic reconstruction of the mitral valve, with implications for the diagnosis of mitral valve prolapse. Circulation 1989;80:589-598.
145. Gorman JH 3rd, Jackson BM, Enomoto Y, Gorman RC: The effect of regional ischemia on mitral valve annular saddle shape. Ann Thorac Surg 2004;77:544-548.
146. Timek TA, Lai DT, Tibayan F, et al: Septal-lateral annular cinching abolishes acute ischemic mitral regurgitation. J Thorac Cardiovasc Surg 2002;123:881-888.
147. Daimon M, Fukuda S, Adams DH, et al: Mitral valve repair with Carpentier-McCarthy-Adams IMR ETLogix annuloplasty ring for ischemic mitral regurgitation: early echocardiographic results from a multi-center study. Circulation 2006;114(Suppl I): I-588-I-593.
148. Filsoufi F, Castillo JG, Rahmanian PB, et al: Remodeling annuloplasty using a prosthetic ring designed for correcting type-iiib ischemic mitral regurgitation. Rev Esp Cardiol 2007;60:1151-1158.
149. Langer F, Rodriguez F, Ortiz S, et al: Subvalvular repair: the key to repairing ischemic mitral regurgitation? Circulation 2005;112(Suppl I):I-383-I-389.
150. Frater RWM, Cornellissen P, Sisto D: Mechanisms of ischemic mitral insufficiency and their surgical correction. In Vetter HO, Hetzer R, Schmutzler H (eds): Ischemic Mitral Incompetence. New York, Springer-Verlag, 1991, pp 117-130.
151. Stanley AW Jr, Athanasuleas CL, Buckberg GD, RESTORE Group: Left ventricular remodeling and functional mitral regurgitation: mechanisms and therapy. Semin Thorac Cardiovasc Surg 2001;13:486-495.
152. Mickleborough LL, Carson S, Ivanov J: Repair of dyskinetic or akinetic left ventricular aneurysm: results obtained with a modified linear closure. J Thorac Cardiovasc Surg 2001;121:675-682.
153. Mickleborough LL: Is mitral valvuloplasty always indicated in patients with poor left ventricular function and ischemic cardiomyopathy? J Thorac Cardiovasc Surg 2001;121:97.
154. Kaza AK, Patel MR, Fiser SM, et al: Ventricular reconstruction results in improved left ventricular function and amelioration of mitral insufficiency. Ann Surg 2002;235:828-832.
155. Di Donato M, Sabatier M, Dor V, et al: Effects of the Dor procedure on left ventricular dimension and shape and geometric correlates of mitral regurgitation one year after surgery. J Thorac Cardiovasc Surg 2001;121:91-96.
156. Otsuji Y, Kuwahara E, Yuge K, et al: Relation of aneurysmectomy in patients with advanced left ventricular remodeling to post-operative left ventricular filling pressure, re-dilatation with ischemic mitral regurgitation. Am J Cardiol 2005;95:517-521.
157. Saga T, Miyamoto T: An alternative technique for the repair of left ventricular aneurysm. Asian Cardiovasc Thorac Ann 1999;7:74-75.
158. Terai H, Tao K, Sakara R: Surgical treatment for ischemic mitral regurgitation: strategy for a tethered valve. Ann Thorac Cardiovasc Surg 2005;11:288-292.
159. Hung J, Chaput M, Guerrero JL, et al: Persistent reduction of ischemic mitral regurgitation by papillary muscle repositioning: structural stabilization of the papillary muscle-ventricular wall complex. Circulation 2007;116(Suppl I):I-259-I-263.
160. Hung J, Guerrero JL, Handschumacher MD, et al: Reverse ventricular remodeling reduces ischemic mitral regurgitation: echo-guided device application in the beating heart. Circulation 2002;106:2594-600.
161. Inoue M, McCarthy PM, Popovic ZB, et al: The Coapsys device to treat functional mitral regurgitation: in vivo long-term canine study. J Thorac Cardiovasc Surg 2004;127:1068-1076;discussion 1076-7.
162. Kelley ST, Malekan R, Gorman JH III, et al: Restraining infarct expansion preserves left ventricular geometry and function after acute anteroapical infarction. Circulation 1999;99:135-142.
163. Messas E, Bel A, Morichetti MC, et al: Autologous myoblast transplantation for chronic ischemic mitral regurgitation. J Am Coll Cardiol 2006;47:2086-2093.
164. Langer F, Schafers HJ: Ring plus string: papillary muscle repositioning as an adjunctive repair technique for ischemic mitral regurgitation. J Thorac Cardiovasc Surg 2007;133:247-249.
165. Kron IL, Green GR, Cope JT: Surgical relocation of the posterior papillary muscle in chronic ischemic mitral regurgitation. Ann Thorac Surg 2002;74:600-601.
166. Hvass U, Tapia M, Baron F, et al: Papillary muscle sling: a new functional approach to mitral repair in patients with ischemic left ventricular dysfunction and functional mitral regurgitation. Ann Thorac Surg 2003;75:809-811.
167. Ueno T, Sakata R, Iguro Y, et al: A new surgical approach to reduce tethering in ischemic mitral regurgitation by relocation of separate heads of the posterior papillary muscle. Ann Thorac Surg 2006;81:2324-2325.
168. Dobre M, Koul B, Rojer A: Anatomic and physiologic correction of the restricted posterior mitral leaflet motion in chronic ischemic mitral regurgitation. J Thorac Cardiovasc Surg 2000;120:409-411.
169. Langer F, Rodriguez F, Cheng A, et al: Posterior mitral leaflet extension: an adjunctive repair option for ischemic mitral regurgitation? J Thorac Cardiovasc Surg 2006;131:868-877.
170. Alfieri O, Maisano F, De Bonis M, et al: The double-orifice technique in mitral valve repair: a simple solution for complex problems. J Thorac Cardiovasc Surg 2001;122:674-681.
171. Bhudia SK, McCarthy PM, Smedira NG, et al: Edge-to-edge (Alfieri) mitral repair: results in diverse clinical settings. Ann Thorac Surg 2004;77:1598-606.
172. Agricola E, Oppizzi M, Maisano F, et al: Echocardiographic classification of chronic ischemic mitral regurgitation caused by restricted motion according to tethering pattern. Eur J Echocardiogr 2004;5:326-334.
173. Nesta F, Otsuji Y, Handschumacher MD, et al: Leaflet concavity: a rapid visual clue to the presence and mechanism of functional mitral regurgitation. J Am Soc Echocardiogr. 2003;16:1301-1308.
174. Messas E, Guerrero JL, Handschumacher MD, et al: Chordal cutting: a new therapeutic approach for ischemic mitral regurgitation. Circulation 2001;104:1958-1963.
175. Messas E, Pouzet B, Touchot B, et al: Efficacy of chordal cutting to relieve chronic persistent ischemic mitral regurgitation. Circulation 2003;108(Suppl II):II-111-II-115.
176. Goetz WA, Lim HS, Pekar F, et al: Anterior mitral leaflet mobility is limited by the basal stay chords. Circulation 2003;107:2969-2974.
177. Messas E, Yosefy C, Chaput M, et al: Chordal cutting does not adversely affect left ventricle contractile function. Circulation. 2006;114(Suppl I):I-524-I-528.
178. Timek TA, Nielsen SL, Green GR, et al: Influence of anterior mitral leaflet second-order chordae on leaflet dynamics and valve competence. Ann Thorac Surg 2001;72:535-541.
179. Nielsen SL, Timek TA, Green GR, et al: Influence of anterior mitral leaflet second-order chordae tendineae on left ventricular systolic function. Circulation 2003;108:486-491.
180. Rodriguez F, Langer F, Harrington KB, et al: Importance of mitral valve second-order chordae for left ventricular geometry, wall thickening mechanics, and global systolic function. Circulation 2004;110(Suppl II):II-115-II-122.
181. David TE, Uden DE, Strauss HD: The importance of the mitral apparatus in left ventricular function after correction of mitral regurgitation. Circulation 1983;68(Suppl II):II-76-II-82.
182. Kunzelman KS, Cochran RP: Mechanical properties of basal and marginal mitral valve chordae tendineae. ASAIO Trans 1990;36:M405-M408.
183. Carpentier A: Cardiac valve surgery: the "French correction." J Thorac Cardiovasc Surg 1983;86:323-337.
184. Borger MA, Murphy PM, Alam A, et al: Initial results of the chordal-cutting operation for ischemic mitral regurgitation. J Thorac Cardiovasc Surg 2007;133:1483-1492.
185. Wakiyama H, Okada Y, Kitamura A, et al: Chordal cutting for the treatment of ischemic mitral regurgitation: two case reports. J Cardiol 2004;44:113-117.
186. Fayad G, Modine T, Azzaoui R, et al: Chordal cutting technique through aortotomy to treat chronic ischemic mitral regurgitation: surgical technique. Int J Surg 2008;6:36-39.
187. Fukuoka M, Nonaka M, Masuyama S, et al: Chordal "translocation" for functional mitral regurgitation with severe valve tenting: an effort to preserve left ventricular structure and function. J Thorac Cardiovasc Surg 2007;133:1004-1011.
188. Komeda M, Shimamoto T: Cutting secondary chordae and placing dual taut stitches between the anterior mitral fibrous annulus and the heads of each papillary muscle to treat ischemic mitral regurgitation without deteriorating left ventricular function. J Thorac Cardiovasc Surg 2008;135:226-227.
189. van Rijk-Zwikker GL, Delemarre BJ, Huysmans HA: Mitral valve anatomy and morphology: relevance to mitral valve replacement and valve reconstruction. J Card Surg 1994;9(Suppl):255-261.
190. Borger MA, Alam A, Murphy PM, et al: Chronic ischemic mitral regurgitation: repair, replace or rethink? Ann Thorac Surg 2006;81:1153-1161.
191. Watanabe N, Ogasawara Y, Yamaura Y, et al: Quantitation of mitral valve tenting in ischemic mitral regurgitation by transthoracic real-time three-dimensional echocardiography. J Am Coll Cardiol 2005;45:763-769.
192. Prifti E, Bonacchi M, Frati G, et al: Should mild-to-moderate and moderate ischemic mitral regurgitation be corrected in patients with impaired left ventricular function undergoing simultaneous coronary revascularization? J Card Surg 2001;16:473-483.
193. Di Donato M, Frigiola A, Menicanti L, et al: Moderate ischemic mitral regurgitation and coronary artery bypass surgery: effect of mitral repair on clinical outcome. J Heart Valve Dis 2003;12:272-279.
194. Grossi EA, Bizekis CS, LaPietra A, et al: Late results of isolated mitral annuloplasty for "functional" ischemic mitral insufficiency. J Card Surg 2001;16:328-332.
195. Akins CW, Hilgenberg AD, Buckley MJ, et al: Mitral valve reconstruction versus replacement for degenerative or ischemic mitral regurgitation. Ann Thorac Surg 1994;58:668-676.

196. Tolis GA Jr, Korkolis DP, Kopf GS, Elefteriades JA: Revascularization alone (without mitral valve repair) suffices in patients with advanced ischemic cardiomyopathy and mild-to-moderate mitral regurgitation. Ann Thorac Surg 2002;74:1476-1481.

197. Carabello BA, Nakano K, Corin W, et al: Left ventricular function in experimental volume overload hypertrophy. Am J Physiol 1989;256:H974-H981.

198. Tsutsui H, Spinale FG, Nagatsu M, et al: Effects of chronic β-adrenergic blockade on the left ventricular and cardiocyte abnormalities of chronic canine mitral regurgitation. J Clin Invest 1994;93:2639-2648.

199. Di Mauro M, Di Giammarco G, Vitolla G, et al: Impact of no-to-moderate mitral regurgitation on late results after isolated coronary artery bypass grafting in patients with ischemic cardiomyopathy. Ann Thorac Surg 2006;81:2128-2134.

200. Enriquez-Sarano M, Avierinos JF, Messika-Zeitoun D, et al: Quantitative determinants of the outcome of asymptomatic mitral regurgitation. N Engl J Med 2005;352:875-883.

201. Beeri R, Yosefy C, Guerrero JL, et al: Early repair of moderate ischemic mitral regurgitation reverses left ventricular remodeling: a functional and molecular study. Circulation 2007;116(Suppl I):I-288-I-293.

202. Chaput M, Handschumacher M, Tournoux F, et al: Mitral leaflet adaptation to ventricular remodeling: occurrence and adequacy in patients with functional mitral regurgitatation. Circulation 2008;118-845-852.

203. Timek TA, Lai DT, Dagum P, et al: Mitral leaflet remodeling in dilated cardiomyopathy. Circulation 2006;114(Suppl I):I-518-I-523.

204. McCully RB, Enriquez-Sarano M, Tajik AJ, Seward JB: Overestimation of severity of ischemic/functional mitral regurgitation by color Doppler jet area. Am J Cardiol 1994;74:790-793.

205. Utsunomiya T, Ogawa T, Doshi R, et al: Doppler color flow "proximal isovelocity surface area" method for estimating volume flow rate: effects of orifice shape and machine factors. J Am Coll Cardiol 1991;17:1103-1111.

206. Yosefy C, Levine RA, Solis J, et al: Proximal flow convergence region as assessed by real-time 3-dimensional echocardiography: challenging the hemispheric assumption. J Am Soc Echocardiogr 2007;20:389-396.

207. Roberts BJ, Grayburn PA: Color flow imaging of the vena contracta in mitral regurgitation: technical considerations. J Am Soc Echocardiogr 2003;16:1002-1006.

208. Buck T, Mucci RA, Guerrero JL, et al: The power-velocity integral at the vena contracta: a new method for direct quantification of regurgitant volume flow. Circulation 2000;102:1053-1061.

209. Buck T, Plicht B, Hunold P, et al: Broad-beam spectral Doppler sonification of the vena contracta using matrix-array technology: a new solution for semi-automated quantification of mitral regurgitant flow volume and orifice area. J Am Coll Cardiol 2005;45:770-779.

CHAPTER 17

Mitral Regurgitation: Timing of Surgery

Rick A. Nishimura and Hartzell V. Schaff

KEY POINTS

- Irreversible left ventricular dysfunction may occur with long-standing volume overload and leads to a poor prognosis.
- The natural history of patients with severe mitral regurgitation is poor, with 90% of patients either dying or undergoing an operation.
- Increasing severity of the degree of mitral regurgitation is related to poor outcome, especially for patients with an effective regurgitant orifice greater than 40mm^2.
- Mitral valve repair is preferred over mitral valve replacement because of lower operative mortality and better long-term outcome.
- The important predictors of late mortality and heart failure after an operation are reduced ejection fraction, older age, elevated serum creatinine, elevated systolic blood pressure, presence of coronary artery disease, and advanced functional class.
- An operation for severe mitral regurgitation should ideally be performed before the onset of ventricular dysfunction, as residual left ventricular dysfunction may occur even with "normal" preoperative systolic function.
- Patients with severe acute mitral regurgitation should undergo an early operation, despite hemodynamic stabilization.
- Patients with severe mitral regurgitation who have already developed severe symptoms (New York Heart Association class III or IV) despite normal left ventricular function will benefit from a mitral valve operation.
- A mitral valve operation is indicated for patients with severe mitral regurgitation due to a primary valvular abnormality when left ventricular dysfunction is present on an echocardiogram (ejection fraction ≤60% or end-systolic dimension ≥40mm).
- In institutions with surgical expertise in mitral valve repair, it is reasonable to proceed with an operation in the asymptomatic patient with severe mitral regurgitation and normal systolic function.

The optimal timing for surgery for severe mitral regurgitation has been controversial.[1-4]

In the symptomatic patient with severe mitral regurgitation, relief of volume overload by mitral valve repair or replacement improves symptoms and functional status.[5,6] Thus, the primary indication for an operation in a patient with severe mitral regurgitation has been the presence of severe symptoms.[7,8] Recent evidence suggests, however, that the natural history of severe mitral valve regurgitation is not benign and that surgical correction of mitral valve regurgitation in asymptomatic patients may improve survival and reduce the risk of complications such as congestive heart failure and atrial fibrillation. In the past, clinicians have been reluctant to subject asymptomatic patients with mitral regurgitation to an operation because of upfront operative mortality and morbidity as well as the potential long-term complications of a valve prosthesis. In current practice, however, severe mitral valve regurgitation due to degenerative disease can be repaired in more than 90% of patients with very low operative risk (<1% to 2%).

It is well known that chronic volume overload may lead to irreversible left ventricular systolic dysfunction, and this can develop before the onset of symptoms.[9-11] Once systolic dysfunction occurs, the outcome becomes poorer, whether or not an operation is performed. Conventional measurements of ventricular function do not reliably predict the onset of left ventricular dysfunction, because of changes in load on the ventricle imposed by the mitral regurgitation.[9,10,12,13] It is important, therefore, to identify and correct severe valve regurgitation before irreversible left ventricular dysfunction occurs.[1,2]

There have been recent advances in our knowledge, diagnosis, and treatment of mitral regurgitation. The pathophysiology of the volume overload on the left ventricle and its eventual outcome on ventricular function is now better understood.[9,12,14] The natural history of severe mitral regurgitation has recently been clarified and elucidated.[15,16] Echocardiography can now be used to accurately assess noninvasively the valve morphology and severity of the regurgitation in most patients and to determine the effect of the volume overload on the left ventricle.[17] Current operative interventions have resulted in a much lower operative mortality and better long-term outcome than was possible several decades ago, with clear benefits of mitral valve repair over valve replacement.[2,3,18,19] All of these advances have provided an incentive to change the indication for timing of operations in patients with mitral regurgitation, setting a new paradigm of an early operation before the onset of ventricular dysfunction. In this chapter we will outline these newer advances and provide recommendations regarding optimal timing of surgery for mitral regurgitation.

RECENT ADVANCES

Pathophysiology

There are several general stages that describe the hemodynamic response to the excessive volume overload of mitral regurgitation in terms of intrinsic left ventricular myocardial as well as circulatory responses (Table 17-1). These stages include 1) an acute volume overload stage, 2) a chronic compensated stage, and 3) a decompensated stage with irreversible left ventricular dysfunction.[1,9,14,20]

Acute Volume Overload Stage

In patients with acute mitral regurgitation, there is an acute volume load placed on the left atrium and an unconditioned left ventricle, resulting in an immediate increase in left atrial pressure that is reflected back to the pulmonary circulation. This volume overload causes symptoms of severe shortness of breath and many times leads to pulmonary congestion. As blood is directed back into the left atrium, there is less forward stroke volume and thus systemic cardiac output falls.

The short-term ventricular response to volume overload is an increase in left ventricular volume from a lengthening of sarcomeres along their normal length tension curve so that total stroke volume increases via the Starling mechanism.[9] Fractional shortening of the left ventricle increases and end-systolic volume decreases as the result of the low resistance runoff into the low pressure left atrium. There is thus a decrease in the integrated systolic wall tension. If forward cardiac output can be maintained by these compensatory mechanisms and if left atrial pressure is lowered by therapy, there will then be an evolution from the acute to the chronic compensated stage of mitral regurgitation.[9,14,20]

Chronic Compensated Stage

The major compensatory mechanism that occurs in this chronic steady state of mitral regurgitation is ventricular enlargement. Ventricular dilatation occurs from rearrangement of sarcomeres, added in series and parallel.[14,21] The individual sarcomeres are not extended beyond their optimal contractile length and, thus, the stretch (or preload) on the individual sarcomere is normalized. The increase in left ventricular cavity size allows a greater left ventricular volume as a result of the valvular regurgitation while normal diastolic pressures are maintained.

Wall stress on the left ventricle is dependent on left ventricular pressure, volume, and wall thickness. The initial unloading of the left ventricle by the low resistance runoff into the left atrium is countered by an increase in left ventricular size during this compensatory stage, returning systolic wall stress to normal levels.[20,22-24] In this chronic compensated stage of mitral regurgitation, there is appropriate ventricular adaptation by ventricular dilatation with adequate forward cardiac output and maintenance of normal filling pressures. Patients remain asymptomatic during this phase, and the normalized preload and wall stress help the left ventricle maintain normal contractility. Patients may remain in this chronic compensated stage for years to decades after the onset of mitral regurgitation.[9,12,14]

Decompensated Stage with Irreversible Left Ventricular Dysfunction

In patients with severe mitral regurgitation, there will eventually be progressive left ventricular enlargement beyond that of a compensated stage.[9,14,20,25,26] This progressive left ventricular enlargement is due to increasing severity of mitral regurgitation, continued compensatory chamber enlargement, or a combination of both. Mitral valve competence is highly dependent on the integrated function of the entire mitral valve apparatus, including the mitral annulus, papillary muscle orientation, chordae, and leaflets. Progressive left ventricular enlargement itself can cause increasing degrees of mitral regurgitation from altered ventricular geometry and annular dilatation; thus, the axiom "mitral regurgitation begets mitral regurgitation." In degenerative mitral regurgitation, disruption of supporting structures such as rupture of chordae may occur, further increasing the severity of mitral regurgitation. As disease progresses, systolic wall stress on the left ventricle is increased because of increased circumferential stress from a larger ventricular minor axis as the left ventricle assumes a more spherical shape.[9,12,13,20,26] An increase in end-diastolic stress occurs from further stretching of the myocytes beyond their normal contractile length, leading to an increase in end-diastolic pressure as the ventricle overfills. The effect of the continued abnormally elevated wall stresses on the ventricle results in a decreased contractile state, with reduced myofiber content and interstitial fibrosis.[27,28] As this process continues, irreversible left ventricular dysfunction occurs, which leads to the decompensated stage of mitral regurgitation. Once irreversible left ventricular dysfunction is present, the prognosis is poor.

Transition Stage

Development of symptoms is an unreliable guide to the transition from the compensated to the uncompensated stage. By the time significant symptoms of dyspnea do occur, there may already be significant irreversible dysfunction. The usual ejection phase indices of ventricular contractility may not reflect deterioration of left ventricular systolic function, because of the dependence of these indices on the load imposed on the left ventricle. Preload, afterload, and wall stress are abnormal and variable in patients with mitral regurgitation and indices such as ejection fraction or fractional shortening may remain normal despite a progressive decrease in the contractile function of the left ventricle. Therefore, other parameters such as preload corrected ejection fraction, end-systolic wall stress normalized for end-systolic volume index, mass normalization of left ventricular elastance, and end-systolic wall stress normalization of ejection fraction have all been proposed as possible indices of a deterioration in intrinsic left ventricular

TABLE 17–1	Stages of Mitral Regurgitation		
	Acute	Chronic Compensated	Chronic Decompensated
Symptoms	↑↑	—	↑↑↑
Left ventricular size	↑	↑↑	↑↑↑
Ejection fraction	>70%	>60%	≤60%
End-systolic dimension	<40 mm	<40 mm	≥40 mm
Wall stress	↓↓	N	↑↑
Preload (myofiber)	↑	N	↑↑↑

17

function.[10,13,20,26,29,30] However, although studies of these indices have been able to identify those patients who have already entered into the decompensated stage, none has been shown to determine when the transition stage begins. Indeed, as discussed below, the outcome of patients with mitral valve regurgitation depends largely on the severity of valve leakage, and, in current practice, criteria for optimal timing of intervention rely mainly on quantitative measurements of the severity of mitral valve leakage rather than on indices of ventricular function, size, or wall stress. The goal of optimal timing is to intervene before the decompensated stage of irreversible left ventricular dysfunction occurs.

Natural History of Mitral Regurgitation

Prior reports on the natural history of mitral regurgitation have been highly variable for a multitude of reasons, including the small population of patients studied, selection bias and multiple etiologies of valve disease, the presence of concomitant other cardiovascular disease, and incomplete hemodynamic data. Also, many of these studies did not compare outcome in patients with mitral valve regurgitation with expected survival of patients without heart disease. In the 1970s, Rapaport[31] reported a relatively good prognosis for patients with mitral regurgitation, with an 80% 5-year survival and 60% 10-year survival in medically treated patients with mitral regurgitation. In the same era, Hammermeister et al[32] reported a much more ominous survival in the medically treated cohort, with a 55% 5-year survival and 20% 10-year survival.[32]

Subsequent studies have helped to reconcile these initial discrepant findings. In the 1980s, Ramanathan et al[33] reported a 5-year survival of 70% in medically treated patients, intermediate between the previous results of Rapaport and Hammermeister et al. The patients were categorized into minimally symptomatic patients, for whom 4-year survival was more than 80% and those with severe symptoms, for whom 4-year survival was 55%. Thus, symptom status was identified as an important predictor of natural history. Reports in the mid-1980s showed that survival in medically treated patients was strongly linked to ventricular function, with short-term survival being poor in patients with subnormal left ventricular or right ventricular function, irrespective of symptoms.[16,34]

Recent data from the 1990s have further clarified the natural history of severe mitral regurgitation.[2,15,19,35] Based on studies of follow-up of patients with a flail posterior leaflet (a surrogate for severe mitral regurgitation), the natural history of isolated mitral regurgitation is now well accepted (Figure 17-1). In these patients who were followed for more than 10 years, there was an excess mortality rate (6.3% yearly) in comparison with the expected survival rate (Figure 17-2). Twenty percent of patients died while under medical management; 69% of the deaths were due to cardiac causes. High morbidity was also noted, with a 10-year incidence of atrial fibrillation of 30% and of heart failure of 63%. Once heart failure developed, the prognosis was worse, with a 5-year survival of less than 20%. At 10 years, 90% of patients with a flail posterior leaflet had either died or had undergone surgical repair because of the development of symptoms.[15]

These recent data also confirmed that the outcome of patients with severe mitral regurgitation was highly dependent on initial symptoms and ventricular function. In patients with New York Heart Association functional class III or IV symptoms, there was considerable mortality (34% yearly) if they did not undergo an operation (Figure 17-3). Even those patients in New York Heart Association functional class I or II had a mortality of 4.1% per year. Those patients with an ejection fraction of less than 60% also had substantial mortality in comparison with those whose ejection fraction was 60% or higher. Ten-year survival was 61% in patients with an ejection fraction higher than 60%

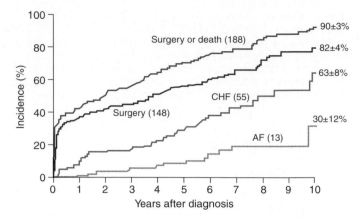

FIGURE 17–1 Incidence of atrial fibrillation (AF), congestive heart failure (CHF), mitral valve operation, and operation or death in 229 patients with isolated mitral regurgitation due to flail mitral valve leaflet between 1980 and 1989. There is a high event rate at the 10-year follow-up. *(From Ling LH, Enriquez-Sarano M, Seward JB, et al: Clinical outcome of mitral regurgitation due to flail leaflet. N Engl J Med 1996;335:1417-1423, with permission.)*

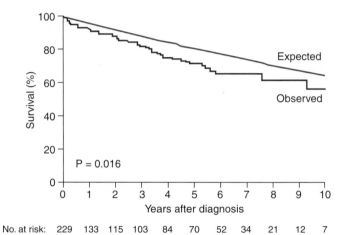

No. at risk: 229 133 115 103 84 70 52 34 21 12 7

FIGURE 17–2 Long-term survival with medical treatment compared with expected survival in 229 patients with mitral regurgitation due to a flail mitral valve leaflet. There was decreased survival in the patients with a flail mitral valve compared with expected survival. *(From Ling LH, Enriquez-Sarano M, Seward JB, et al: Clinical outcome of mitral regurgitation due to flail leaflet. N Engl J Med 1996;335:1417-1423, with permission.)*

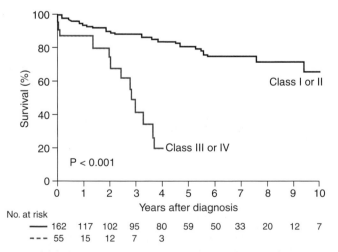

No. at risk
— 162 117 102 95 80 59 50 33 20 12 7
--- 55 15 12 7 3

FIGURE 17–3 Overall long-term survival with medical treatment in 229 patients with flail mitral valve leaflet, according to New York Heart Association class. *(From Ling LH, Enriquez-Sarano M, Seward JB, et al: Clinical outcome of mitral regurgitation due to flail leaflet. N Engl J Med 1996;335:1417-1423, with permission.)*

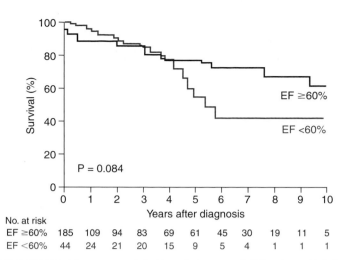

FIGURE 17–4 Long-term survival with medical treatment in 229 patients with flail mitral valve leaflet, according to ejection fraction (EF). *(From Ling LH, Enriquez-Sarano M, Seward JB, et al: Clinical outcome of mitral regurgitation due to flail leaflet. N Engl J Med 1996;335:1417-1423, with permission.)*

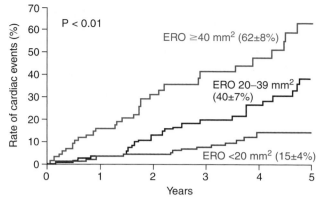

FIGURE 17–5 Kaplan-Meier estimates of the mean (± SE) rates of cardiac events among patients with asymptomatic mitral regurgitation under medical management according to the effective regurgitant orifice (ERO). Cardiac events were defined as death from cardiac causes, congestive heart failure, or new atrial fibrillation. Values in parentheses are event rates at 5 years. *(From Enriquez-Sarano M, Avierinos JF, Messika-Zeitoun D, et al: Quantitative determinants of the outcome of asymptomatic mitral regurgitation. N Engl J Med 2005;352:875-883, with permission.)*

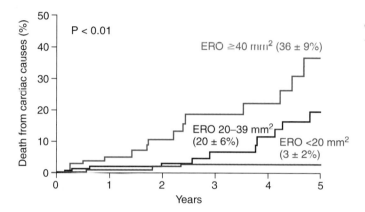

FIGURE 17–6 Kaplan-Meier estimates of the mean (± SE) rates of death from cardiac causes among patients with asymptomatic mitral regurgitation under medical management, according to the effective regurgitant orifice (ERO). Values in parentheses are survival rates at 5 years. *(From Enriquez-Sarano M, Avierinos JF, Messika-Zeitoun D, et al: Quantitative determinants of the outcome of asymptomatic mitral regurgitation. N Engl J Med 2005;352:875-883, with permission.)*

compared with 40% for patients with an ejection fraction less than 60% (Figure 17-4).[15] It was also shown that sudden death is a relatively frequent catastrophic event, responsible for approximately one-fourth of the deaths in patients receiving medical treatment.[36,37] Overall, these data indicate the serious prognostic implication of severe mitral regurgitation, as well as the finding that nearly 90% of these patients will either die or require an operation in 10 years.

The natural history of predominantly asymptomatic patients with moderately severe mitral regurgitation and normal ventricular function has been controversial. Rosen in 1994[16] reported a benign prognosis, with no deaths and no progression to subnormal ventricular function after 5 years of follow-up. However, in that report, there was a 10% average annual risk of development of symptoms, leading to surgery. More data on the natural history of asymptomatic patients with mitral regurgitation have been accumulated based not only on the ability to measure ventricular function but also on the ability to quantify the degree of mitral regurgitation.[38] Stratified by quantitative Doppler echocardiography, 456 patients with asymptomatic organic mitral regurgitation were prospectively followed. Five years after the diagnosis, 22% of patients had died (14% from cardiac causes), and one third of patients had a cardiac event defined as death from a cardiac cause, heart failure, or new atrial fibrillation. Independent determinants of survival were age, the presence of diabetes, and also the effective regurgitant orifice (ERO), which provides a quantitative measure of severity of mitral regurgitation. Those patients with an ERO of at least 40 mm² had a 5-year survival rate lower than expected on the basis of U.S. census data (58% versus 78 %). Compared with patients with a ERO of less than 20 mm², those with an ERO of at least 40 mm² had an increased risk of death from any cause, death from cardiac causes, and sudden death (Figures 17-5 and 17-6).

Overall, the presence of severe mitral regurgitation portends a poor prognosis, even in the asymptomatic patient with a preserved ejection fraction. This insight into the natural history of mitral regurgitation in these patients has important implications regarding timing of surgery. Data show very clearly that patients with a regurgitant volume of at least 60 mL/beat or an ERO of at least 40 mm² have a poor outcome with medical management alone. In addition, close follow-up of patients with intermediate grades of mitral regurgitation (ERO 20 to 39 mm²) is essential. Although these patients with less severe mitral regurgitation have a low risk of death and cardiac events during the first 12 to 18 months after diagnosis, the rates of death and other complications increase substantially thereafter.[38]

Advances in Surgical Intervention

Determination of the optimal timing of a valve operation requires knowledge of the risks and benefits of the operation itself. There have been significant changes in the surgical treatment of mitral regurgitation, with substantial effects on the operative mortality and long-term outcome (Figure 17-7). In North America, the most common cause for mitral regurgitation is degenerative valve disease, and the most common pathophysiologic mechanism is leaflet prolapse.[39,40] More than 95% of patients with leaflet prolapse can have valve repair with low operative risk and with durability that approaches that of prosthetic replacement (Figure 17-8). In our clinic, operative risk for valve repair in patients 75 years or younger is less than 1%. The linearized risk of reoperation after repair of posterior leaflet prolapse is approximately 0.5% per year, and rates of reintervention after repair of anterior or bileaflet prolapse are similarly low (1.6% and 0.9% per year, respectively). Indeed, the durability of mitral valve repair for all subsets of patients with leaflet prolapse in the current era (0.74% per year overall rate of reoperation) is similar to that after mitral valve replacement.[41-43]

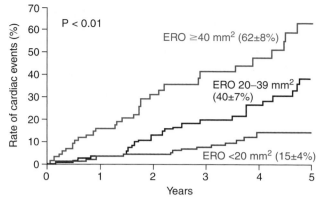

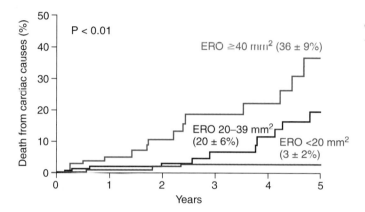

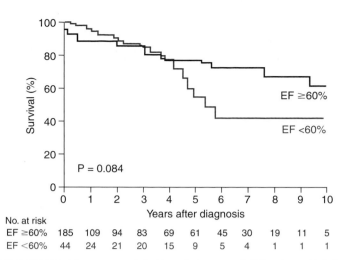

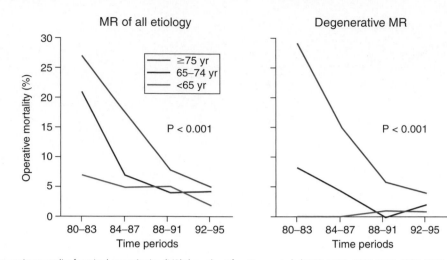

FIGURE 17–7 Trends in operative mortality for mitral regurgitation (MR) throughout four time periods (1980-1983, 1984-1987, 1988-1991, and 1992-1995). The operative mortality is shown for patients 75 years or older (*blue line*), between 65 and 74 years (*red line*), and younger than 65 years (*green line*). *Left,* Trends in operative mortality for all causes of mitral regurgitation, *Right,* Trends in operative mortality for degenerative mitral regurgitation. The probability value applies to the time trends for patients in all age groups. *(From Detaint D, Sundt TM, Nkomoet VT, et al: Surgical correction of mitral regurgitation in the elderly: Outcomes and recent improvements. Circulation 2006;114:265-272, with permission.)*

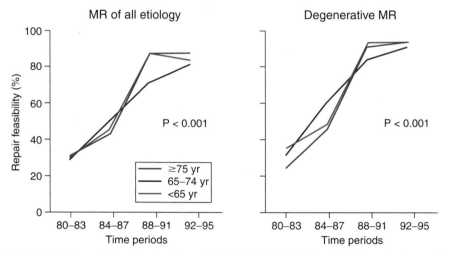

FIGURE 17–8 Trends in feasibility of mitral valve repair throughout four time periods (1980-1983, 1984-1987, 1988-1991, and 1992-1195) for patients 75 years or older (*blue line*), between 65 and 74 years (*red line*), and younger than 65 years (*green line*). *Left,* trends in valve repair for all causes of mitral regurgitation. *Right,* trends in valve repair for degenerative mitral regurgitation. The probability value applies to the time trends for all age group patients. *(From Detaint D, Sundt TM, Nkomoet VT, et al: Surgical correction of mitral regurgitation in the elderly: outcomes and recent improvements. Circulation 2006;114:265-272, with permission.)*

Mitral valve repair is preferred over prosthetic replacement because of low operative mortality and elimination of device-related complications such as ventricular rupture, thrombus formation, and mechanical malfunction.[2,3,18,19,41,44] With valve repair, the chordal apparatus is preserved, and studies in patients having valve replacement show that the preservation of mitral valve attachments preserves ventricular geometry and systolic function.[45,46] Also, valve repair has a much lower rate of late complications than prosthetic replacement. The survival advantage of repair over replacement extends to patients who undergo reoperation for late failure of the initial repair.[42]

There have also been improvements in outcome of patients who cannot undergo mitral valve repair but require mitral valve replacement. Studies have shown that preservation of the chordal apparatus at the time of valve insertion results in a smaller postoperative chamber size, prevents the postoperative increase in systolic stress, and maintains normal ejection performance.[47-50] Thus, the preservation of the chordal apparatus lessens the risk of ventricular dysfunction after a mitral valve operation, compared with the situation in which supporting mitral valve structures were resected.[47-50]

Predictors of Surgical Outcome

Early Mortality

The factors that have been shown to influence early mortality after a mitral valve operation are age and functional class of the patient.[51] Operative mortality continues to improve each decade and is related to surgical expertise.[41,51,52]

Late Outcome

The major cause of death after surgical correction of mitral regurgitation is continued heart failure.[2,12,51,53,54] The important predictors of late mortality and heart failure after an operation are reduced ejection fraction, older age, elevated serum creatinine concentration, elevated systolic blood pressure, presence of coronary artery disease, and advanced functional class (Figure 17-9).[51,53]

As would be expected, postoperative left ventricular dysfunction, as assessed by ejection fraction, remains a major predictor of poor outcome.[2,12,14,51,53,54] A decreased ejection fraction is highly associated with future mortality and the onset of heart failure. Thus, it is essential that one is able to attempt to determine factors associated with postoperative left ventricular dysfunction.

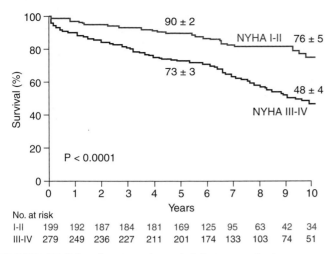

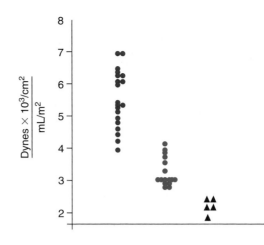

FIGURE 17–9 Overall postoperative survival after an operation for severe mitral regurgitation. Patients in New York Heart Association (NYHA) classes I and II are compared with those for patients in NYHA classes III and IV. Numbers at the bottom indicate patients at risk. *(From Tribouilloy CM, Enriquez-Sarano M, Schaff HV, et al: Impact of preoperative symptoms on survival after surgical correction of organic mitral regurgitation: Rationale for optimizing surgical indications. Circulation 1999;99:400-405, with permission.)*

FIGURE 17–11 End-systolic wall stress/end-systolic volume index ratio (ESWS/ESVI) for normal subjects (*blue circles*) versus two groups of patients who underwent a mitral valve operation. The patients who did well after the operation are shown in *green circles*, and the patients who either died or remained in severe heart failure are shown in *red triangles*. The patients who did poorly had a lower ESWS/ESVI ratio. The *asterisk* denotes a patient who had an ejection fraction of 80% but in whom there was severe left ventricular dysfunction suggested by the ESWS/ESVI. *(From Carabello BA, Nolan SP, McGuire LB: Assessment of preoperative left ventricular function in patients with mitral regurgitation: value of the end-systolic wall stress-end-systolic volume ratio. Circulation 1981;64:1212-1217, with permission.)*

Predictors of Postoperative Left Ventricular Dysfunction

Prediction of residual postoperative left ventricular systolic dysfunction has been attempted in a multitude of studies.[10,13,20,26,29,30] The ejection phase indices of ventricular function (ejection fraction and fractional shortening) were not thought to be of benefit in evaluating intrinsic contractility of the left ventricle because of changes in the load on the ventricle from the severe mitral regurgitation (Figure 17-10). Thus, other parameters had been identified, such as preload corrective ejection fraction, end-systolic volume index normalized to wall stress, and diastolic volume

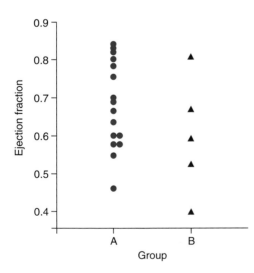

FIGURE 17–10 The preoperative ejection fraction is shown according to patients who did well after an operation (*blue circles*) versus patients who either died or who had severe heart failure after an operation (*red triangles*). Note the very small number of patients in this initial study, which was performed before the use of mitral valve repair. *(From Carabello BA, Nolan SP, McGuire LB: Assessment of preoperative left ventricular function in patients with mitral regurgitation: value of the end-systolic wall stress-end-systolic volume ratio. Circulation 1981;64:1212-1217, with permission.)*

mass normalization of left ventricular elastance. Despite the elegant pathophysiologic theoretical models underlying these parameters, these studies showed that they only demonstrated when it was too late for an operation (Figure 17-11).[10,13,20,26,29,30] The cutoff values from each study predicted when patients had a high risk of severe heart failure or death after an operation but did not predict the optimal timing of surgery. It must be noted that these prior studies may not be applicable to surgical outcomes today, as they included small number of patients, patients with mixed valve disease, conservative selection bias, and the use of valve replacement with or without chordal sparing.[10,13,20,26,29,30]

Recent studies have looked at the determinants of residual postoperative left ventricular dysfunction in the era of mitral valve repair.[2,3,19,51,53-56] Overall, ejection fraction drops by approximately 10% in patients with degenerative mitral regurgitation, on average from 58% to 50%.[53] Despite the limitations of the ejection fraction, this measurement has emerged as the best predictor for determining postoperative left ventricular systolic dysfunction, as well as the onset of heart failure and/or mortality (Figure 17-12)[2,3,19,51,53-56] Patients with a preoperative ejection fraction of less than 60% have a higher incidence of postoperative left ventricular dysfunction as well as an increased incidence of poor outcome.[2,51,53] Even those with ejection fractions between 50 and 60% had a poorer outcome than those patients with an ejection fraction greater than 60%.[51,53]

End-systolic volume (or dimension) has been another useful parameter that has emerged in the predicting of adverse outcome after a mitral valve operation.[10,12,13] The end-systolic dimension incorporates both the increased preload of the heart as well as the intrinsic contractility, as there will be cessation of ejection when the ventricle can no longer contract against its afterload. The end-systolic dimension is also a direct single measurement rather than a calculated value and therefore has excellent reproducibility if properly obtained by echocardiography. Thus, the combination of end-systolic dimension and ejection fraction has been valuable in identifying patients who have already reached the irreversible

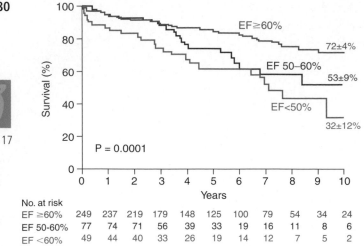

FIGURE 17–12 Late survival of patients undergoing operation for severe mitral regurgitation, according to the preoperative echocardiographic ejection fraction (EF). Numbers at risk for each interval are indicated at the bottom. *(From Enriquez-Sarano M, Tajik AJ, Schaff HV, et al: Echocardiographic prediction of survival after surgical correction of organic mitral regurgitation. Circulation 1994;90:830-837, with permission.)*

stage of left ventricular dysfunction.[12,25,53] In those patients with an ejection fraction of less than 60% or an end-systolic dimension of greater than 40 mm, irreversible left ventricular dysfunction is assumed to be present.[1]

Unexpected Left Ventricular Dysfunction

The criteria of an ejection fraction of less than 60% and end-systolic dimension of greater than 40 mm again determine when the patient has reached the stage of irreversible left ventricular dysfunction.[1,53] However, these criteria do not determine when the transition to left ventricular dysfunction begins to occur. Thus, *unexpected left ventricular dysfunction*, which is defined as a depressed ejection fraction after the correction of mitral regurgitation, may occur even before these parameters are reached (Figure 17-13). It is important to recognize that the cutoff criteria are measurements of when the decompensated stage of left ventricular dysfunction is

reached. Ideally, an operation should be performed before this end stage occurs.[2,3,18,41,53]

Effect of Surgical Correction on Outcome

From the foregoing discussion, it is clear that hemodynamically severe mitral regurgitation does not have a benign course. A strategy of initial medical treatment and delayed surgical intervention for symptomatic patients is accompanied by excess morbidity and mortality (Figure 17-14).[2,3,41,55] Several lines of investigation indicate that earlier referral for correction of severe mitral regurgitation improves the outlook for these patients.

In a further analysis of 221 patients with flail mitral valve leaflets, patients were stratified according to the timing of surgery.[19] Sixty-three patients who had a mitral valve operation within 1 month of diagnosis were categorized as having an early operation. Among the remaining 158 patients designated as the "conservatively" managed group, 80 had a later operation. Because this was an observational, nonrandomized study, some patient characteristics were different in comparing the two groups. Patients having an early operation were younger and more likely to have symptoms and atrial fibrillation, but there was no difference in the ejection fraction between the groups. Patients in the early operation group had improved overall survival rate compared with those managed conservatively (10-year survival 79% versus 65%, P = 0.028) (Figure 17-15). The beneficial effect of an early operation was observed in asymptomatic and minimally symptomatic patients as well as those with more serious heart failure.

A clear weakness among observational studies comparing the outcomes of an early operation versus conservative management is the potential for selection bias. The improved outcome of patients undergoing an early operation might theoretically be attributable to the more favorable risk profile. However, multivariate analysis suggested that an early operation was an independent predictor of improved survival, along with greater freedom from congestive heart failure and new-onset atrial fibrillation.[19]

An analysis of the causes of death also strongly indicated that the beneficial effect of correction of the mitral regurgitation was due to improved postsurgical cardiovascular physiology and not simply patient selection.[19] In the study of patients

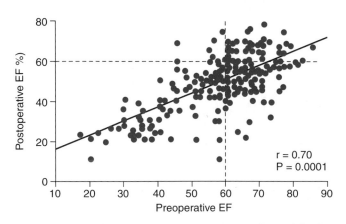

FIGURE 17–13 Correlation between the postoperative ejection fraction (EF) and the preoperative ejection fraction. Although there is a linear correlation between the preoperative and postoperative ejection fractions, there remain a number of patients who have a postoperative ejection fraction less than 60%, despite a preoperative ejection fraction greater than 60%. This represents the group of patients with "unexpected left ventricular dysfunction" after operation. *(From Enriquez-Sarano M, Tajik AJ, Schaff HV, et al: Echocardiographic prediction of left ventricular function after correction of mitral regurgitation: results and clinical implications. J Am Coll Cardiol 1994;24:1536-1543, with permission.)*

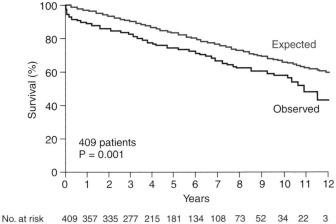

FIGURE 17–14 Postoperative survival of 409 patients after a mitral valve operation compared with expected survival. Survival was 75% at 5 years, 58% at 10 years, and 44% at 12 years. Numbers at the bottom represent the number of patients at risk for each interval and percentage of the expected survival for specific intervals. *(From Enriquez-Sarano M, Tajik AJ, Schaff HV, et al: Echocardiographic prediction of survival after surgical correction of organic mitral regurgitation. Circulation 1994;90:830-837, with permission.)*

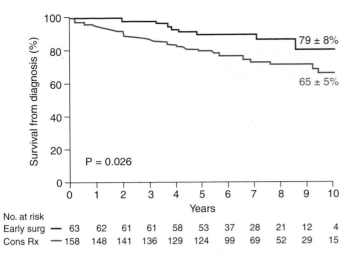

FIGURE 17-15 The outcome of 221 patients with flail leaflets undergoing operation. Early surgery is defined as patients who had a mitral valve operation within 1 month after diagnosis and comprised of 63 patients. Conservative therapy comprised 158 patients initially treated conservatively (80 of whom who operated on later). Overall 10-year survival is shown, with improved long-term survival in patients who underwent the strategy of early surgery. (*From Ling LH, Enriquez-Sarano M, Seward JB, et al: Early surgery in patients with mitral regurgitation due to flail leaflets: a long-term outcome study. Circulation 1997;96:1819-1825, with permission.*)

with flail mitral valve leaflets, a high percentage of all deaths were attributable to cardiovascular causes. However, there were only six cardiovascular deaths during follow-up among patients having an early operation compared with 35 in the conservatively managed group. The 5- and 10-year cardiac death rates were $8 \pm 4\%$ for patients having early correction of mitral regurgitation compared with 16 ± 3 and $29 \pm 5\%$ for conservatively managed patients ($P = 0.025$) and, in multivariate analysis, an early operation was associated with decreased cardiovascular mortality (adjusted risk ratio, 0.18; $P = 0.002$).

ACUTE MITRAL REGURGITATION

Etiology and Presentation

Acute mitral regurgitation is usually due to an acute structural problem of the mitral valve apparatus, either infection causing destruction of the mitral valve leaflets or chordae, spontaneous chordal rupture, or papillary muscle rupture from a myocardial infarction. In acute severe mitral regurgitation, a sudden volume overload is imposed on an unprepared left atrium and left ventricle, with a severe increase in left atrial pressure and a reduction in forward stroke volume and cardiac output.[9,12] Pulmonary edema usually occurs, sometimes even accompanied by cardiogenic shock. If the volume overload is not tolerated, an urgent operation must be performed.

Clinical Evaluation

Acute severe mitral regurgitation must be considered in any patient presenting with hemodynamic compromise. In patients with acute severe mitral regurgitation, the physical examination itself may be misleading. Heart sounds may be difficult to hear because of the respiratory distress. The systolic murmur of mitral regurgitation may be soft, early in systole, and may even be absent as there is rapid equilibration of left atrial and left ventricular pressures. Transthoracic echocardiography is useful for demonstrating a hyperdynamic left ventricle, which rules out a myocardial or pericardial etiology for the hemodynamic compromise. However, because of problems with obtaining high resolution imaging in a critically ill patient, a structural abnormality of the mitral valve

may not be able to be determined by transthoracic echocardiography. Doppler echocardiography may help in identifying a dense continuous wave mitral regurgitation signal with a "V-wave cutoff." Transesophageal echocardiography should be performed to accurately assess the etiology and severity of mitral regurgitation. The structural abnormality causing the mitral regurgitation, such as leaflet perforation, chordal rupture, or rupture of the papillary muscle, should be visualized. The presence of other abnormalities such as vegetations or regional wall motion abnormalities is useful to determine the etiology of the valve regurgitation.

Visualization of an unsupported segment of the mitral apparatus coupled with an eccentric jet of mitral regurgitation on a color flow image in this clinical setting is all that is required for confirmation of acute severe mitral regurgitation. Quantitation of mitral regurgitation severity is not necessary in this acute situation and only adds time to the echocardiographic examination. Cardiac catheterization is no longer required for diagnosis and left ventriculography can be potentially harmful. A limited coronary angiogram should be performed before the operation if the patient is hemodynamically stable.

Treatment

Medical therapy has a limited role in patients with acute severe mitral regurgitation causing hemodynamic compromise and is used mainly to stabilizing the patient in preparation for an operation. Intravenous diuretics are used to decrease pulmonary congestion, and afterload reduction with drugs such as nitroprusside will increase forward cardiac output and reduce filling pressures.[57] Antibiotics should be given if infective endocarditis is suspected. An intra-aortic balloon pump can stabilize hemodynamics to a greater degree than what can be done with medical therapy. If possible an intra-aortic balloon should be placed if the patient is stable enough to be taken to the catheterization laboratory for preoperative coronary angiography. However, the ultimate goal is to proceed as soon as possible with the operation for either mitral valve repair or replacement.[58-60]

There may be a subset of patients who present with lesser degrees of acute mitral regurgitation. These patients will have mild pulmonary congestion that responds initially to medical therapy and may be the subset of patients who have either a rupture of secondary chordae or those who have developed a partial papillary muscle rupture associated with myocardial infarction. In these patients, an early operation is still warranted as there is a high likelihood of acute deterioration during medical observation.[58,59]

CHRONIC MITRAL REGURGITATION

Etiology of Mitral Regurgitation

It is important to determine the etiology of chronic mitral regurgitation (Figure 17-16) when considering timing of surgery. Different surgical techniques are performed based on valve morphology and underlying etiologies, and these different surgical techniques have important implications as to the timing of a particular operation. The competent mitral valve depends on the coordinated function of all the components of the mitral valve apparatus: valve leaflets, annulus, papillary muscles, chordae tendineae, and the left ventricular myocardium. The maintenance of the chordal, annular, and subvalvular continuity and mitral geometric relationships is important in the preservation of overall left ventricular function. Under normal conditions, mitral valve competence is maintained during systole by both passive and active function of the mitral annulus and cusps, subvalvular apparatus, and ventricular wall. The posterior annulus is a muscular

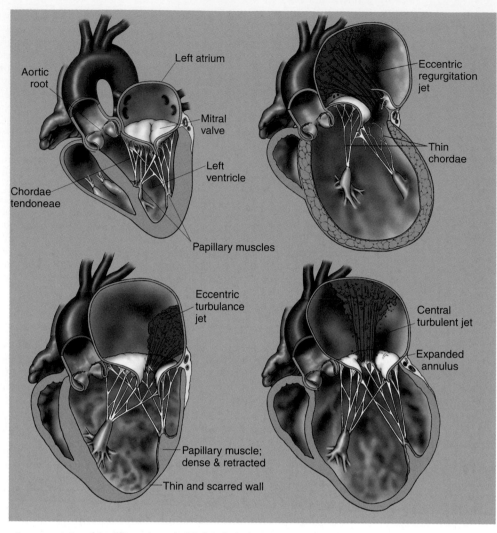

FIGURE 17–16 Schematic representation of the different types of etiologies of mitral regurgitation. *Top left,* normal; *top right,* degenerative mitral regurgitation; *bottom left,* ischemic mitral regurgitation; *bottom right,* functional mitral regurgitation due to left ventricular dilatation.

structure, which shortens at end-systole with a sphincter-like contraction, thus narrowing the annulus and promoting leaflet coaptation. The papillary muscle to annular distance during normal posterolateral left ventricular segmental contraction facilitates the closing motion of normal mitral valve leaflets, permitting their free edges to move centrally. Prolapse into the left atrium is prevented early in systole by papillary muscle contraction and shortening, which produces tension along the chordae and subsequently draws the free edges apically.

Mitral regurgitation occurs when there is an abnormality of the mitral valve leaflets, chordal apparatus, and papillary muscle structures or when there is functional and structural abnormality of the underlying supporting ventricular myocardium. A clinically relevant categorization for the etiology of chronic mitral regurgitation is to divide it into two categories: 1) primary valvular abnormality or 2) abnormality of supporting structures (Table 17-2).

In the United States, the most common cause of primary valvular abnormality resulting in severe mitral regurgitation is degenerative mitral valve disease.[39,40] In degenerative mitral valve disease there is myxomatous degeneration of the mitral valve leaflets and an elongated and redundant chordal apparatus. The thickened redundant leaflets will prolapse back into the left atrium, causing mal-coaptation of leaflet edges and subsequent regurgitation. Rupture of the chor-

dae structures, which causes abrupt increases in the severity of mitral regurgitation due to unsupported segments of the mitral leaflets, is not uncommon in degenerative mitral valve disease, especially in older men.[61,62] Other etiologies for primary valvular mitral regurgitation include rheumatic disease, senile calcific disease, and rare causes such as drug-induced mitral valve disease, healed infective endocarditis, and mitral regurgitation associated with systemic disease. It is important to be able to differentiate between these etiologies, as the likelihood of successful repair is higher for degenerative mitral regurgitation, whereas in primary valvular regurgitation of other etiologies, complete repair is less likely.

TABLE 17–2	Categorization of Etiology of Mitral Regurgitation	
Primary Valvular Causes	**Abnormal Supporting Structures**
Degenerative	Ischemic mitral regurgitation
Rheumatic	Functional mitral regurgitation
Infective	
Other	
Systemic disease	
Drug-induced	
Senile calcific	

Mitral regurgitation can also result from abnormalities of the underlying supporting structures. Ischemic mitral regurgitation occurs when there is myocardial ischemia or infarction interrupting the normal mechanics of contraction of the annulus, posterolateral myocardium, and shortening of the papillary muscle.[63-68] This disruption of the normal contraction sequence results in loss of cusp coaptation. Hypokinesia of the myocardial segments adjacent to the posterior annulus may disrupt annular contraction and early leaflet coaptation and may even result in acute dilatation during systole. Whereas rupture of the head of the papillary muscle produces severe regurgitation in the acute setting, ischemic mitral regurgitation requires a chronically infarcted fibrotic and shortened papillary muscle in conjunction with an akinetic adjacent scar of the left ventricular wall.[63-68] Overall, there is restricted cusp motion resulting in tethering and tenting. The tenting may also occur in combination with annular dilatation from dysfunction of the base of the heart. Because of the influence of cardiac loading conditions on ventricular geometry, the degree of mitral regurgitation is dependent on changes in load imposed on the left ventricle.

Functional mitral regurgitation is due to progressive dilatation of the left ventricle in the presence of a normal mitral valve apparatus.[69,70] The ventricular dilatation leads to a cycle of volume overload within an already dilated left ventricle, progression of annular dilatation, increased left ventricular wall tension, and loss of coaptation of mitral leaflets. Myocardial thinning and dilatation, blunting of the aortomitral angle, widening of the intrapapillary muscle distance, increased leaflet tethering, and decreased leaflet closing forces all will lead to altered forces generated by the papillary muscles. These morphologic changes combine to result in loss of the zone of coaptation and the central jet of mitral regurgitation.

Clinical Evaluation

The clinical evaluation of a patient with chronic mitral regurgitation requires a comprehensive history and physical examination, as well as properly selected noninvasive and invasive testing. The onset of symptoms is one of the major indications for an operation and thus the patient's history is essential. In patients with chronic mitral regurgitation, there may be an insidious onset of symptoms, so that patients may not be cognizant of the extent of effort intolerance. In some patients, the classic symptoms of dyspnea may be absent and manifestations of severe mitral regurgitation could be symptoms of fatigue and tiredness from a reduced forward cardiac output. Some patients do not admit to symptoms, and it is important to obtain other information regarding exercise tolerance, either through a careful detailed history from family and friends or by performing a formal exercise test.

A detailed physical examination of patients with mitral regurgitation is essential in this evaluation. The physical examination is needed to determine whether there are any signs of heart failure (elevated venous pressure or pulmonary rales) but mainly is useful to evaluate the severity of mitral regurgitation. There are several limitations in determining severity of mitral regurgitation by current noninvasive and invasive testing. Thus, the physical examination and these diagnostic modalities need to be correlated to accurately determine the severity of mitral regurgitation.

The typical holosystolic murmur of mitral regurgitation is a key finding, as most patients with severe mitral regurgitation have a clearly audible apical holosystolic murmur. An early diastolic filling sound is a very helpful finding, as this reflects increased antegrade flow across the mitral valve and is a very specific sign for severe mitral regurgitation. Patients with functional mitral regurgitation may have a large color flow jet of central regurgitation on a two-dimensional color

imaging echocardiogram that could be interpreted as severe mitral regurgitation, but a barely audible murmur on examination is evidence that the mitral regurgitation is not of significant severity.[71] Some patients with bileaflet mitral valve prolapse have only a short mid-systolic to late systolic murmur but have been calculated to have a large effective orifice area on quantitative echocardiography. In these patients, the absence of a holosystolic murmur indicates that the mitral valve chordal apparatus is intact, and most will not have mitral regurgitation that is severe enough to benefit from an operation.

Two-dimensional and Doppler echocardiography are used to determine the etiology of mitral regurgitation and the ventricular response to mitral regurgitation as well as to evaluate the severity of mitral regurgitation. Direct visualization of mitral valve leaflets and the chordal structure and papillary muscle can help differentiate patients with a primary valvular abnormality (e.g., degenerative mitral valve disease or rheumatic mitral valve disease) from those with abnormalities of the supporting structures. A critical feature that must be assessed by echocardiography is the feasibility of valve repair, which depends on the etiology of the mitral regurgitation.[72] The determination of whether or not a valve can be repaired versus replaced has significant implications for timing of surgery. The degenerative mitral valve has the highest chance of repair. With diseases that produce calcification, fibrosis, and chordal shortening such as rheumatic disease, calcific senile disease, and mitral valve regurgitation associated with systemic diseases, the likelihood of valve repair is very low. For patients with degenerative mitral valve disease, the overall morphology of the mitral valve leaflets, the primary abnormality causing the regurgitation, and the surrounding structures such as the mitral annulus, determine whether or not a valve can be successfully repaired. Valve repair can be performed with a higher degree of success in patients with posterior leaflet abnormalities, especially a flail unsupported segment in the absence of severe calcification of the annulus. Partial resection of the flail portion and use of a mitral annuloplasty ring are the standards for repair of this abnormality. More complex surgical techniques, such as implantation of neo-chordae, chordal transfer, and other specialized techniques, are required for patients who have an unsupported segment of the anterior leaflet or severe voluminous bileaflet prolapse. Heavy calcification of the mitral annulus will prevent adequate annuloplasty, and the appearance of the annulus should be assessed by echocardiography. In most patients with severe regurgitation due to degenerative mitral valve disease, there will be eccentric jets, the direction of which is determined by the primary leaflet abnormality. With a posterior leaflet abnormality, there will be a large color flow jet directed anteriorly toward the aorta. Conversely, with anterior leaflet abnormalities, there will be color flow jets directed posteriorly.

In ischemic mitral regurgitation, there will be tethering of the posterior leaflet and an akinetic posterolateral segment of the myocardium. This results in "tenting" of the mitral coaptation point, and there will be a posteriorly directed jet. Most cases of ischemic mitral regurgitation are treated by annuloplasty alone, and thus it is important to determine by echocardiography whether there is loss of integrity of the valve apparatus. In functional mitral regurgitation related to left ventricular dilatation, there will usually be a central jet of mitral regurgitation due to asymmetric loss of coaptation of the anterior and posterior leaflets.

It is important to take into consideration left ventricular and left atrial size in the assessment of patients with mitral regurgitation, both of which can be accurately assessed by two-dimensional echocardiography. A two-dimensional directed M-mode for measurement of left ventricular systolic and diastolic dimensions is the most reproducible measurement of left ventricular size in the absence of regional wall motion abnormalities.[1] Prior studies have been based on these simple parameters. However, obtaining these values does require meticulous examination to assure that the measurements are made from a true short axis of the left ventricle. Left atrial dimension or volume is also an important part of the assessment of the patient with mitral regurgitation. If there is severe chronic mitral regurgitation, left atrial enlargement and ventricular dilatation must be present. Despite any quantitative assessment of mitral regurgitation severity, a normal left ventricular size precludes the possibility of surgically significant chronic mitral regurgitation.

The comprehensive two-dimensional and Doppler examinations must also include a systematic approach to determining the severity of mitral regurgitation. As outlined in the American Society of Echocardiography recommendations, a comprehensive evaluation using multiple parameters is needed to fully assess the severity of mitral regurgitation.[17] This includes not only color flow jet parameters but also indirect parameters such as the contour of the transmitral flow velocities, pulmonary vein velocity curves, and secondary pulmonary pressure, as well as continuous wave Doppler intensity and contour. Because decisions for timing of surgery for mitral regurgitation are based on the severity of mitral regurgitation, especially in the asymptomatic patient, it is of value to be able to quantitate the degree of mitral regurgitation. A regurgitant volume and effective orifice area can now be obtained using proximal isovelocity surface area measurements, and these parameters should be a part of all echocardiographic examinations in which mitral regurgitation is a key element.

There may be situations in which a discrepancy is seen between the severity of mitral regurgitation by history and physical examination versus that of echocardiography. Right heart catheterization may be helpful in these instances to determine the pulmonary pressure and left atrial pressure and the absence or presence of a large V wave on the pulmonary artery wedge pressure. A large V wave due to primary diastolic dysfunction of the left ventricle without significant mitral regurgitation can also be seen, and there are patients with a large degree of regurgitant volume into a compliant left atrium who may not have a large V wave.[73] Nonetheless, in symptomatic patients the presence of elevated left atrial pressure and a large V wave are useful findings confirming that mitral regurgitation is causing these symptoms.

Although left ventriculography is still considered a "standard" for determining the severity of mitral regurgitation, there are well-documented limitations to this invasive technique.[74] The density of contrast agent going back into the left atrium is dependent on the size of the left ventricle, function of the left ventricle, size of the left atrium, and filling pressures. The density of the contrast agent going into the left atrium is also dependent on the amount of and speed with which the contrast agent is injected during the left ventriculogram. Premature ventricular contractions or other causes of an irregular heart rhythm may make the severity of mitral regurgitation uninterpretable on a left ventriculogram. However, a reliable indicator of severity of mitral regurgitation can be obtained with a properly performed ventriculogram.

A ventriculogram is not necessary for most patients with mitral regurgitation, especially if the clinical presentation correlates with the echocardiogram. For instance, in a patient with a loud holosystolic murmur, diastolic filling sound, and a flail leaflet on an echocardiogram with a large eccentric jet, a ventriculogram is not required for assessment of the severity of mitral regurgitation. Alternatively, the absence of a loud murmur, normal ventricular size and function, and a central jet of mitral regurgitation on an echocardiogram are all that are needed to determine that mitral regurgitation is not severe enough to warrant an operation. If there is a discrepancy between the noninvasive test results, left ventriculography can be useful in further aiding the decision as to whether the mitral regurgitation is severe enough to warrant intervention.

Exercise testing may be of benefit to evaluate a select subset of patients with mitral regurgitation.[75] This is particularly useful for patients in whom it is unclear whether symptoms are present. Oxygen consumption testing may be performed, as this will determine not only whether there is limited exercise tolerance but also whether the limitation is due to deconditioning or a cardiac etiology. In the latter instance, there should be a plateau of the myocardial oxygen consumption at peak exercise concomitant with symptoms. Whether the ventricular response or pulmonary response to exercise as assessed by exercise echocardiography or radionuclide angiography is of further benefit in determining timing of surgery is still unclear.[76-79]

Primary Valvular Mitral Regurgitation: Indications for Surgery

The optimal timing for surgery in the patient with primary valvular mitral regurgitation depends on multiple factors.[1,2,12,14,41] These include the patient's symptoms, the severity of mitral regurgitation, and the response of the left ventricle to the volume overload. In addition, a major determinant for timing of surgery is the available surgical expertise. The ability to repair a valve rather than replace the valve may have a substantial influence on whether or not an early operation should be considered.[1] Although the number of patients undergoing mitral valve repair for mitral regurgitation has been increasing over the past two decades in the United States and Canada, this technique is still underutilized, as the frequency of repair in the Society of Thoracic Surgeons National Cardiac Database in 2000 was only 35.7% (Figure 17-17).[80] This number is in stark contrast to data from surgical centers that are expert in mitral valve repair, in which the frequency of repair approaches 90% to 95% in patients with severe isolated mitral regurgitation due to degenerative disease.[41] Because repair results in lower operative mortality than replacement (1% to 2% versus 6%), better preservation of left ventricular function, and overall better survival, cardiologists are encouraged to refer candidates for mitral valve repair to these experienced surgical centers.[1]

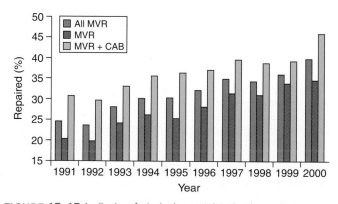

FIGURE 17–17 Application of mitral valve repair (MVR) with or without coronary artery bypass graft (CAB) for all mitral valve procedures both isolated and with associated procedures, is plotted as a percentage of the total number of mitral valve procedures. Application of repair increased overall from 24.6% to 39.8% with associated CAB from 30.8% to 46.0%. Data are from the Society of Thoracic Surgeons National Cardiac Database of 21,741 isolated and combined mitral valve procedures. (*From Savage EB, Ferguson TB Jr, DiSesa VJ: Use of mitral valve repair: analysis of contemporary United States experience reported to the Society of Thoracic Surgeons National Cardiac Database. Ann Thorac Surg 2003;75:820-825, with permission.*)

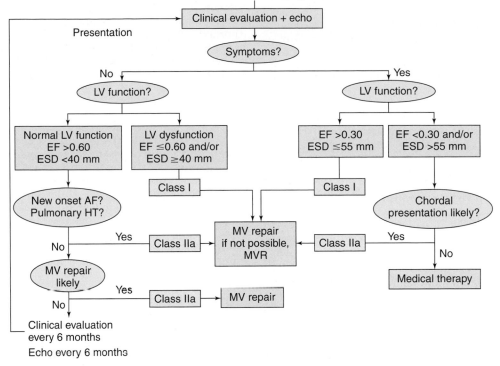

Chronic severe mitral regurgitation

FIGURE 17-18 Management strategy for patients with chronic severe mitral regurgitation. Mitral valve repair may be performed in asymptomatic patients with normal left ventricular function if performed by an experienced surgical team and the likelihood of successful mitral valve repair is greater than 90%. AF, atrial fibrillation; EF, ejection fraction; ESD, end-systolic dimension; HT, hypertension; MV, mitral valve; MVR, mitral valve repair. *(From Bonow RO, Carabello B, Chatterjee K, et al: ACC/AHA 2006 guidelines for the management of patients with valvular heart disease: a report of the American College of Cardiology/American Heart Association Task Force on Practice Guidelines. J Am Coll Cardiol 2006;48:e1-e148, with permission.)*

The following indications for surgery are based on the 2006 American College of Cardiology/American Heart Association Guidelines for Valvular Heart Disease (Figure 17-18).[1]

Symptomatic Patients: Normal Left Ventricular Function

It is well documented that patients with severe mitral regurgitation who have already developed severe symptoms (New York Heart Association class III or IV) despite normal left ventricular function will benefit from a mitral valve operation.[81] Normal left ventricular function is defined as an ejection fraction greater than 60% and end-systolic dimension less than 40 mm on an echocardiogram.[1] The benefit in terms of relief of symptoms and prolongation of life occurs irrespective of whether or not the valve can be repaired or replaced. Severe symptoms indicate an inadequate ability of the left ventricle to respond to the volume overload, and once symptoms occur there is a progressive downhill course with medical treatment alone.

Even patients with mild symptoms (New York Heart Association class II) should be considered for an operation. These patients may have a gradual insidious onset of symptoms but will note a decrease in exercise tolerance with time. The mildly symptomatic patients are most likely entering the transition phase to left ventricular decompensation as even mild symptoms indicate that the left ventricular compensatory mechanisms are becoming overwhelmed with the volume overload. Therefore, patients with any symptoms (New York Heart Association class II, III, and IV), preserved left ventricular function, and severe mitral regurgitation due to a primary valvular abnormality should be considered for an operation.[1]

Symptomatic and Asymptomatic Patients: Left Ventricular Dysfunction

A mitral valve operation is indicated for patients with severe mitral regurgitation due to a primary valvular abnormality when left ventricular dysfunction is present on an echocardiogram (ejection fraction ≤60% or end-systolic dimension ≥40 mm).[1] This recommendation applies to patients who are symptomatic and also asymptomatic. These patients may have already progressed to the stage of irreversible left ventricular dysfunction from the longstanding volume overload. Although it would have been ideal to have patients undergo an operation before they have reached this stage, an operation will probably prevent further deterioration in ventricular function and improve long-term outlook. An operation should be considered irrespective of whether the valve can be repaired or replaced, although valve repair is preferable, given the better effect on ventricular function.

Symptomatic Patients: Severe Left Ventricular Dysfunction

A subset of patients presenting with severe mitral regurgitation are considered to have "end-stage" regurgitation, meaning that ventricular function has significantly deteriorated (ejection fraction less than 30%, end-systolic dimension >55 mm). If a primary valvular abnormality causing the mitral regurgitation is present, there is almost always a concomitant myocardial process contributing to the severe ventricular dysfunction. Nonetheless, careful assessment of valve morphology and quantitation of the severity of regurgitation are important in this distinction, as an operation may still be contemplated. Even though the operative risk is increased and there is a high likelihood of persistent left ventricular dysfunction postoperatively, an operation may be performed to improve symptoms and prevent progressive left ventricular deterioration. In this subset of patients, it is of great importance to assure that the chordal apparatus is preserved to prevent acute ventricular dilatation and, thus, these highest-risk patients are best treated with mitral valve repair.

17

The management of the asymptomatic patient with severe mitral regurgitation due to a primary valvular abnormality who maintains normal systolic function has been controversial.[1,2,4,12,14,24] If these patients are followed until they reach the cutoff values described above (ejection fraction < 60% and/or end-systolic dimension ≥40 mm), they have already entered into the decompensation stage of left ventricular dysfunction.[12,14,24] Postoperative survival is already reduced, and there is a high incidence of postoperative left ventricular systolic dysfunction and eventual recurrent heart failure.[51,53] Thus, there has been impetus to operate before the onset of left ventricular dysfunction to prevent the most serious sequelae of chronic severe mitral regurgitation.

There are no randomized data to use in recommending this approach to all patients. However, in experienced centers, there is a move to operate on patients who maintain normal systolic function if there is a high likelihood of successful valve repair. This change in paradigm for an early operation is based on multiple advances in our understanding of patients with mitral regurgitation, as has been discussed previously. If severe mitral regurgitation is truly present, the natural history studies have uniformly indicated that there is a high likelihood of development of symptoms and/or left ventricular dysfunction over the course of 6 to 10 years.[15,38] Early mitral valve repair can now be performed in experienced centers with <1% mortality and a greater than 90% chance of successful repair. The long-term outcome of the asymptomatic patient who undergoes an early operation is excellent, with an overall survival comparable to that of an age-matched control-matched population (Figure 17-19).[2,3,41,81]

To recommend an operation in these patients, several features must be present. First, it is important to document that there truly is severe mitral regurgitation. Thus, correlation of the physical examination and the diagnostic modalities is essential, and quantitative Doppler assessment is helpful. It is also important to correlate the severity of mitral regurgitation with the effect on the left ventricle and left atrium. Patients with severe mitral regurgitation by necessity must have left ventricular and left atrial enlargement. Finally, the feasibility of mitral valve repair is a combination of the morphology of the mitral valve and the surgical expertise available.

Thus, in institutions with surgical expertise in mitral valve repair, it is reasonable to proceed with an operation in the asymptomatic patient with severe mitral regurgitation and normal systolic function.[1] This decision must be individualized to each patient, however, and the operative risk, patient lifestyle, and patient preference must be taken into consideration. These early operations should be performed only if the operation can be done in a center with a mortality rate of less than 1% and a feasibility of repair greater than 90%.

There is still controversy regarding the optimal approach in this patient population. Not all institutions have surgical expertise in mitral valve repair. If a mitral repair cannot be done with a high degree of success, an early operation in the asymptomatic patient with preserved ventricular function may not be warranted. Several series have shown a good outcome for patients with "watchful waiting," in which patients with mitral regurgitation were followed medically until they reached the criterion of left ventricular dysfunction (ejection fraction <60%).[4,16] Following these guidelines, there were no patients who developed residual left ventricular dysfunction after an operation, but a substantial percentage of patients eventually required an operation. Nearly 50% of all patients developed either symptoms or left ventricular dysfunction or atrial fibrillation by 8 years (Figure 17-20). Adherence to this more conservative approach does require meticulous and continuous follow-up of the patient, which may not be possible for every patient nor care facility. In addition, there is always the unexpected left ventricular dysfunction, which continues to occur even when patients undergo an operation with a normal ejection fraction and a small end-systolic dimension. Thus, if this conservative approach is chosen, the patient and physician must be willing to continue with frequent follow-up visits, with the understanding that the development of irreversible ventricular dysfunction cannot be predicted.

Atrial Fibrillation

Patients with mitral regurgitation due to degenerative disease have a high risk of development of atrial fibrillation, which is independently associated with a high risk of cardiac death or heart failure.[82] Preoperative atrial fibrillation is an independent predictor of reduced long-term survival after a mitral valve operation for chronic severe mitral

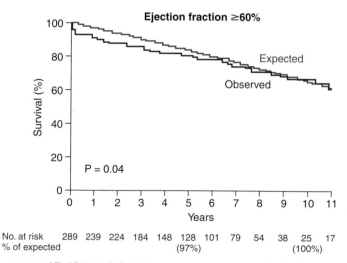

FIGURE 17–19 Survival of patients with a preoperative echocardiographic ejection fraction greater than or equal to 60% compared with expected survival in patients undergoing mitral valve operation for severe mitral regurgitation. The survival was comparable to the reference population. *(From Enriquez-Sarano M, Tajik AJ, Schaff HV, et al: Echocardiographic prediction of survival after surgical correction of organic mitral regurgitation. Circulation 1994;90:830-837, with permission.)*

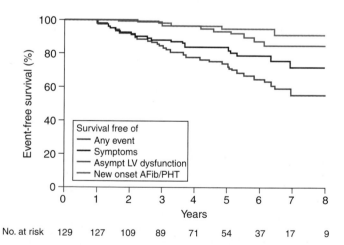

FIGURE 17–20 Kaplan-Meier event-free survival of patients with asymptomatic severe degenerative mitral regurgitation managed according to a watchful waiting strategy. *Solid blue line* shows survival free of any event to indicate an operation. *Red line* shows survival free of symptoms. *Green line* shows survival free of asymptomatic (Asympt) left ventricular (LV) dysfunction. *Purple line* shows survival free of asymptomatic development of atrial fibrillation (AFib) and/or pulmonary hypertension (PHT) to indicate an operation. *(From Rosenhek R, Rader F, Klaar U, et al: Outcome of watchful waiting in asymptomatic severe mitral regurgitation. Circulation 2006;113:2238-2244, with permission.)*

regurgitation.[83-85] Predictors of postoperative atrial fibrillation are an enlarged left atrium and a prolonged duration of preoperative atrial fibrillation; persistent atrial fibrillation after the operation occurs in 80% of patients with preoperative atrial fibrillation with a duration of 3 months or longer but in no patient with preoperative atrial fibrillation of less than 3 months.[83]

To prevent the adverse long-term sequelae of atrial fibrillation, the onset of atrial fibrillation in those patients with severe mitral regurgitation and a valve suitable for repair is an indication for an operation.[1] In patients with chronic atrial fibrillation presenting for a mitral valve operation, a concomitant maze procedure or pulmonary vein isolation should be considered.[86-88]

Ischemic Mitral Regurgitation: Indications for Surgery

Many patients with ischemic heart disease have ischemic mitral regurgitation, and the presence of ischemic mitral regurgitation has subsequently been shown to have a significant impact on prognosis (Figure 17-21).[89-91] There is some degree of ischemic mitral regurgitation detected in as many as 40% of individuals with acute myocardial infarction.[89,90,92] Those who have even mild degrees of ischemic mitral regurgitation after infarction have a cardiovascular risk that is two to four times higher than that of those without ischemic mitral regurgitation, both within the first 2 weeks and long term.[93] Those patients with ischemic mitral regurgitation have greater degrees of heart failure and are more likely to experience recurrent myocardial infarction than those without ischemic mitral regurgitation.[89,90,92] The more severe the mitral regurgitation is, the poorer the survival (Figure 17-22).[89] In patients undergoing coronary artery bypass grafting, one of 10 will have some degree of ischemic mitral regurgitation, and such patients have higher operative mortality and lower long-term survival than those without mitral regurgitation.[94,95]

Revascularization alone can result in improvement of the ischemic mitral regurgitation in selected patients, as mitral regurgitation arises when ischemia or infarction interrupts the normal interaction between the mitral annulus, subvalvular apparatus, and left ventricular wall.[96,97] However, it is difficult to determine whether or not revascularization alone will influence the severity of mitral regurgitation in an individual patient. In addition, changes in load will significantly influence the severity of mitral regurgitation with ischemic

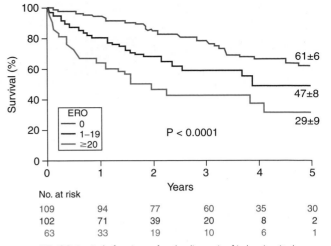

FIGURE 17–22 Survival of patients after the diagnosis of ischemic mitral regurgitation, according to the degree of mitral regurgitation as graded by the effective regurgitant orifice (ERO) = 29 mm² or <20 mm². *(From Grigioni F, Enriquez-Sarano M, Zehr KJ, et al: Ischemic mitral regurgitation: long-term outcome and prognostic implications with quantitative Doppler assessment. Circulation 2001;103:1759-1764, with permission.)*

mitral regurgitation, particularly when the patient is undergoing cardiopulmonary bypass.[98] The late survival after bypass alone in the presence of ischemic mitral regurgitation has been reported to be between 60% and 94% at 3 years and 52% and 81% in 5 years.[97,99-101] In patients with only mild ischemic mitral regurgitation, 3-year survival rates are reported to be 84% and 94%.[102,103] In patients with moderate mitral regurgitation, the 3-year survival varies from 61% to 84% after bypass alone, with only a modest improvement in New York Heart Association functional status and angina severity score.[97,99-101]

In the past, it was felt that the addition of mitral valve repair or replacement to a bypass operation doubled the operative risk. However, more recent series have shown a lower operative mortality.[104] Mitral valve repair has become the preferred method to treat mitral regurgitation with concomitant coronary artery bypass grafting.[99,105,106] The operative mortality associated with valve replacement appears to be twice that of repair using a band or ring annuloplasty. In addition, repair preserves the subvalvular apparatus and prevents potential complications associated with prosthetic valves. Residual regurgitation of a moderate or even mild degree appears to negatively affect late survival.[107] Compared with isolated bypass operations in selected patients, a survival advantage for combined procedures has been reported by some.[104,106,108-111] Others have not shown a survival benefit when mitral repair was added to a bypass operation (Figure 17-23).[112]

The surgical approach to ischemic mitral regurgitation remains controversial.[99,112] Most would agree that severe mitral regurgitation on an echocardiogram or angiogram constitutes the need for mitral intervention at the time of the bypass operation. Patients who have only mild ischemic mitral regurgitation would probably not benefit from any operative intervention. However, there is debate regarding the management of patients with moderate degrees of ischemic mitral regurgitation, not only for optimal treatment but also for when "mild" becomes "moderate." Prior studies evaluating the outcomes of the different approaches to ischemic mitral regurgitation have all been retrospective with significant selection bias. It is hoped that prospective randomized trials currently underway will provide guidance for this subset of patients in the future.

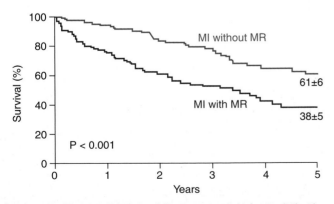

FIGURE 17–21 Survival of patients following myocardial infarction (MI) with ischemic mitral regurgitation (MR) and without ischemic mitral regurgitation. *(From Grigioni F, Enriquez-Sarano M, Zehr KJ, et al: Ischemic mitral regurgitation: long-term outcome and prognostic implications with quantitative Doppler assessment. Circulation 2001;103:1759-1764, with permission.)*

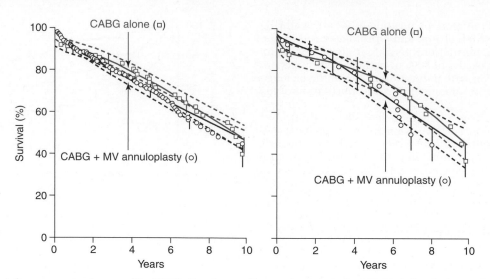

FIGURE 17–23 Survival after coronary artery bypass grafting (CABG) either alone or with concomitant mitral valve (MV) annuloplasty for functional ischemic mitral regurgitation (MR). Symbols represent deaths positioned according to the Kaplan-Meier estimator, vertical bars are 68% confidence limits, and numbers in parentheses are patients still alive. *Solid lines* are parametric estimates enclosed within 68% confidence limits. *Left,* Unadjusted survival based on 37 deaths after CABG alone and 92 after CABG plus MV annuloplasty. *Right,* Propensity matched survival, based on 19 deaths after CABG alone and 19 after CABG plus MV annuloplasty. *(From Mihaljevic T, Lam BK, Rajeswaran J, et al: Impact of mitral valve annuloplasty combined with revascularization in patients with functional ischemic mitral regurgitation. J Am Coll Cardiol 2007;49:2191-2201, with permission.)*

Functional Mitral Regurgitation: Indications for Surgery

Functional mitral regurgitation is due to progressive dilatation of the annular-ventricular apparatus with altered ventricular geometry and a resultant loss of leaflet coaptation. The severity of mitral regurgitation in these patients with severe left ventricular dysfunction is highly dependent on the load on the heart. Thus, with aggressive medical therapy to decrease left ventricular volume and annular dilatation, there can be a significant decrease in dynamic mitral regurgitation. However, some patients will continue to have severe mitral regurgitation despite optimal medical therapy.

In these patients with severe functional mitral regurgitation, there is a significant decrease in the efficiency of left ventricular contraction and work expended by the left ventricle, as the work used to generate regurgitant flow does not contribute to effective forward cardiac output. It is felt by some that eliminating reversal of flow alleviates the excess of work placed on the left ventricle. With use of mitral valve repair to change the detrimental alterations in the annular-ventricular unit, both valve competency and ventricular function may be restored.[69,70,113-115]

Valve repair appears to be relatively safe in this high-risk patient population, which consists of patients with severe functional mitral regurgitation, New York Heart Association functional class II to IV, ejection fraction less than 35%, and a dilated left ventricle.[69,114,115] An overall operative mortality of 1.5% to 5% has been demonstrated. Valve repair has been shown to improve New York Heart Association class for each patient, with an associated improvement in ejection fraction, cardiac output, and end-diastolic volumes along with a reduction in sphericity index and regurgitant fraction, all consistent with reverse remodeling.

However, these data have not been replicated in other centers.[116,117] Thus, the optimal indication and therapy for these patients with functional mitral regurgitation remain unknown. Until more data are available, aggressive medical therapy including the use of biventricular pacing should be considered the first line of care for patients with severe left ventricular dysfunction and functional mitral regurgitation.[116,118,119] We reserve operations for patients with significant functional regurgitation who remain symptomatic despite optimal medical treatment.

REFERENCES

1. Bonow RO, Carabello B, Chatterjee K, et al: ACC/AHA 2006 guidelines for the management of patients with valvular heart disease: a report of the American College of Cardiology/American Heart Association Task Force on Practice Guidelines (writing Committee to Revise the 1998 guidelines for the management of patients with valvular heart disease) developed in collaboration with the Society of Cardiovascular Anesthesiologists endorsed by the Society for Cardiovascular Angiography and Interventions and the Society of Thoracic Surgeons. J Am Coll Cardiol 2006;48:e1-e148.
2. Enriquez-Sarano M, Orszulak TA, Schaff HV, et al: Mitral regurgitation: a new clinical perspective. Mayo Clinic Proc 1997;72:1034-1043.
3. Enriquez-Sarano M, Schaff HV, Frye RL: Early surgery for mitral regurgitation: the advantages of youth. Circulation 1997;96:4121-4123.
4. Rosenhek R, Rader F, Klaar U, et al: Outcome of watchful waiting in asymptomatic severe mitral regurgitation. Circulation 2006;113:2238-2244.
5. Crawford MH, Souchek J, Oprian CA, et al: Determinants of survival and left ventricular performance after mitral valve replacement. Department of Veterans Affairs Cooperative Study on Valvular Heart Disease. Circulation 1990;81:1173-1181.
6. McGoon MD, Fuster V, McGoon DC, et al: Aortic and mitral valve incompetence: long-term follow-up (10 to 19 years) of patients treated with the Starr-Edwards prosthesis. J Am Coll Cardiol 1984;3:930-938.
7. Fowler NO, van der Bel-Kahn JM: Indications for surgical replacement of the mitral valve: with particular reference to common and uncommon causes of mitral regurgitation. Am J Cardiol 1979;44:148-157.
8. Selzer A, Katayama F: Mitral regurgitation: clinical patterns, pathophysiology and natural history. Medicine (Baltimore) 1972;51:337-366.
9. Carabello BA:. Mitral regurgitation: basic pathophysiologic principles. Mod Concepts Cardiovasc Dis 1988;57:53-58.
10. Carabello BA, Nolan SP, McGuire LB: Assessment of preoperative left ventricular function in patients with mitral regurgitation: value of the end-systolic wall stress-end-systolic volume ratio. Circulation 1981;64:1212-1217.
11. Schuler G, Peterson KL, Johnson A, et al: Temporal response of left ventricular performance to mitral valve surgery. Circulation 1979;59:1218-1231.
12. Carabello BA, Crawford FA Jr: Valvular heart disease [see comment] [erratum appears in N Engl J Med 1997;337:507]. N Engl J Med 1997;337:32-41.
13. Carabello BA, Williams H, Gash AK, et al: Hemodynamic predictors of outcome in patients undergoing valve replacement [erratum appears in Circulation 1987 Mar;75:650]. Circulation 1986;74:1309-1316.
14. Gaasch WH, John RM, Aurigemma GP: Managing asymptomatic patients with chronic mitral regurgitation. Chest 1995;108:842-847.
15. Ling LH, Enriquez-Sarano M, Seward JB, et al: Clinical outcome of mitral regurgitation due to flail leaflet. N Engl J Med 1996;335:1417-1423.
16. Rosen SE, Borer JS, Hochreiter C, et al: Natural history of the asymptomatic/minimally symptomatic patient with severe mitral regurgitation secondary to mitral valve prolapse and normal right and left ventricular performance. Am J Cardiol 1994;74:374-380.
17. Zoghbi WA, Enriquez-Sarano M, Foster E, et al: Recommendations for evaluation of the severity of native valvular regurgitation with two-dimensional and Doppler echocardiography. J Am Soc Echocardiogr 2003;16:777-802.
18. Enriquez-Sarano M, Schaff HV, Orszulak TA, et al: Valve repair improves the outcome of surgery for mitral regurgitation. A multivariate analysis. Circulation 1995;91:1022-1028.
19. Ling LH, Enriquez-Sarano M, Seward JB, et al: Early surgery in patients with mitral regurgitation due to flail leaflets: a long-term outcome study. Circulation 1997;96:1819-1825.

20. Gaasch WH, Zile MR: Left ventricular function after surgical correction of chronic mitral regurgitation. Eur Heart J 1991;12(Suppl B):48-51.

21. Ross J Jr, Sonnenblick EH, Taylor RR, et al: Diastolic geometry and sarcomere lengths in the chronically dilated canine left ventricle. Circ Res 1971;28:49-61.

22. Ross J Jr: Adaptations of the left ventricle to chronic volume overload. Circ Res 1974;35(Suppl II):64-70.

23. Ross J Jr: The concept of afterload mismatch and its implications in the clinical assessment of cardiac contractility. Jpn Circ J 1976;40:865-875.

24. Ross J Jr: The timing of surgery for severe mitral regurgitation. N Engl J Med 1996;335:1456-1458.

25. Wisenbaugh T, Skudicky D, Sareli P: Prediction of outcome after valve replacement for rheumatic mitral regurgitation in the era of chordal preservation. Circulation 1994;89:191-197.

26. Zile MR, Gaasch WH, Carroll JD, Levine HJ: Chronic mitral regurgitation: predictive value of preoperative echocardiographic indexes of left ventricular function and wall stress. J Am Coll Cardiol 1984;3(2 Pt 1):235-242.

27. Fuster V, Danielson MA, Robb RA, et al: Quantitation of left ventricular myocardial fiber hypertrophy and interstitial tissue in human hearts with chronically increased volume and pressure overload. Circulation 1977;55:504-508.

28. Spinale FG, Ishihra K, Zile M, et al: Structural basis for changes in left ventricular function and geometry because of chronic mitral regurgitation and after correction of volume overload. J Thorac Cardiovasc Surg 1993;106:1147-1157.

29. Mirsky I, Corin WJ, Murakami T, et al: Correction for preload in assessment of myocardial contractility in aortic and mitral valve disease: application of the concept of systolic myocardial stiffness. Circulation 1988;78:68-80.

30. Wisenbaugh T: Does normal pump function belie muscle dysfunction in patients with chronic severe mitral regurgitation? Circulation 1988;77:515-525.

31. Rapaport E: Natural history of aortic and mitral disease. Am J Cardiol 1975;35:221-227.

32. Hammermeister KE, Fisher L, Kennedy W, et al: Prediction of late survival in patients with mitral valve disease from clinical, hemodynamic, and quantitative angiographic variables. Circulation 1978;57:341-349.

33. Ramanathan KB, Knowles J, Connor MJ, et al: Natural history of chronic mitral insufficiency: relation of peak systolic pressure/end-systolic volume ratio to morbidity and mortality. J Am Coll Cardiol 1984;3:1412-1416.

34. Hochreiter C, Niles N, Devereux RB, et al: Mitral regurgitation: relationship of noninvasive descriptors of right and left ventricular performance to clinical and hemodynamic findings and to prognosis in medically and surgically treated patients. Circulation 1986;73:900-912.

35. Enriquez-Sarano M, Basmadjian AJ, Rossi A, et al: Progression of mitral regurgitation: a prospective Doppler echocardiographic study. J Am Coll Cardiol 1999;34:1137-1144.

36. Ciancamerla F, Paglia I, Catuzzo B, et al: Sudden death in mitral valve prolapse and severe mitral regurgitation: is chordal rupture an indication to early surgery? J Cardiovasc Surg 2003;44:283-286.

37. Grigioni F, Enriquez-Sarano M, Ling LH, et al: Sudden death in mitral regurgitation due to flail leaflet. J Am Coll Cardiol 1999;34:2078-2085.

38. Enriquez-Sarano M, Avierinos JF, Messika-Zeitoun D, et al: Quantitative determinants of the outcome of asymptomatic mitral regurgitation. N Engl J Med 2005;352:875-883.

39. Olson LJ, Subramanian R, Ackermann DM, et al: Surgical pathology of the mitral valve: a study of 712 cases spanning 21 years. Mayo Clin Proc 1987;62:22-34.

40. Waller BF, Morrow AG, Maron BJ, et al: Etiology of clinically isolated, severe, chronic, pure mitral regurgitation: analysis of 97 patients over 30 years of age having mitral valve replacement. Am Heart J 1982;104(2 Pt 1):276-288.

41. Schaff HV, Suri RM, Enriquez-Sarano M: Indications for surgery in degenerative mitral valve disease. Semin Thorac Cardiovasc Surg 2007;19:97-102.

42. Suri RM, Schaff HV, Dearani JA, et al: Recurrent mitral regurgitation after repair: should the mitral valve be re-repaired? J Thorac Cardiovasc Surg 2006;132:1390-1397.

43. Suri RM, Schaff HV, Dearani JA, et al: Survival advantage and improved durability of mitral repair for leaflet prolapse subsets in the current era. Ann Thorac Surg 2006;82:819-826.

44. Duran CM: Surgical techniques for the repair of anterior mitral leaflet prolapse. J Card Surg 1999;14:471-481.

45. Kouris N, Ikonomidis I, Kontogianni D, et al: Mitral valve repair versus replacement for isolated non-ischemic mitral regurgitation in patients with preoperative left ventricular dysfunction: a long-term follow-up echocardiography study. Eur J Echocardiogr 2005;6:435-442.

46. Lillehei CW: New ideas and their acceptance: as it has related to preservation of chordae tendinea and certain other discoveries. J Heart Valve Dis 1995;4(Suppl 2):S106-S114.

47. David TE, Burns RJ, Bacchus CM, Druck MN: Mitral valve replacement for mitral regurgitation with and without preservation of chordae tendineae. J Thorac Cardiovasc Surg 1984;88(5 Pt 1):718-725.

48. Hennein HA, Swain JA, McIntosh CL, et al: Comparative assessment of chordal preservation versus chordal resection during mitral valve replacement. J Thorac Cardiovasc Surg 1990;99:828-837.

49. Horskotte D, Schulte HD, Bircks W, Strauer BE: The effect of chordal preservation on late outcome after mitral valve replacement: a randomized study. J Heart Valve Dis 1993;2:150-158.

50. Rozich JD, Carabello BA, Usher BW, et al: Mitral valve replacement with and without chordal preservation in patients with chronic mitral regurgitation: mechanisms for differences in postoperative ejection performance. Circulation 1992;86:1718-1726.

51. Enriquez-Sarano M, Tajik AJ, Schaff HV, et al: Echocardiographic prediction of survival after surgical correction of organic mitral regurgitation. Circulation 1994;90:830-837.

52. Cohn LH, Couper GS, Kinchla NM, Collins JJ Jr: Decreased operative risk of surgical treatment of mitral regurgitation with or without coronary artery disease. J Am Coll Cardiol 1990;16:1575-1578.

53. Enriquez-Sarano M, Tajik AJ, Schaff HV, et al: Echocardiographic prediction of left ventricular function after correction of mitral regurgitation: results and clinical implications. J Am Coll Cardiol 1994;24:1536-1543.

54. Essop MR: Predictors of left ventricular dysfunction following mitral valve repair for mitral regurgitation. J Am Coll Cardiol 2004;43:1925; author reply -6.

55. Dujardin KS, Seward JB, Orszulak TA, et al: Outcome after surgery for mitral regurgitation. Determinants of postoperative morbidity and mortality. J Heart Valve Dis 1997;6:17-21.

56. Mohty D, Enriquez-Sarano M: The long-term outcome of mitral valve repair for mitral valve prolapse. Curr Cardiol Rep 2002;4:104-110.

57. Yoran C, Yellin EL, Becker RM, et al: Mechanism of reduction of mitral regurgitation with vasodilator therapy. Am J Cardiol 1979;43:773-777.

58. Nishimura RA, Gersh BJ, Schaff HV: The case for an aggressive surgical approach to papillary muscle rupture following myocardial infarction: "From paradise lost to paradise regained." Heart 2000;83:611-613.

59. Nishimura RA, Schaff HV, Shub C, et al: Papillary muscle rupture complicating acute myocardial infarction: analysis of 17 patients. Am J Cardiol 1983;51:373-377.

60. Nishimura RA, Schaff HV, Gersh BJ, et al: Early repair of mechanical complications after acute myocardial infarction. JAMA 1986;256:47-50.

61. Nishimura RA, McGoon MD: Perspectives on mitral-valve prolapse. N Engl J Med 1999;341:48-50.

62. Nishimura RA, Tajik AJ: Follow-up observations in patients with mitral valve prolapse. Herz 1988;13:326-334.

63. Kumanohoso T, Otsuji Y, Yoshifuku S, et al: Mechanism of higher incidence of ischemic mitral regurgitation in patients with inferior myocardial infarction: quantitative analysis of left ventricular and mitral valve geometry in 103 patients with prior myocardial infarction. J Thorac Cardiovasc Surg 2003;125:135-143.

64. Levine RA: Dynamic mitral regurgitation—more than meets the eye. N Engl J Med 2004;351:1681-1684.

65. Levine RA, Schwammenthal E: Ischemic mitral regurgitation on the threshold of a solution: from paradoxes to unifying concepts. Circulation 2005;112:745-758.

66. Otsuji Y, Gilon D, Jiang L, et al: Restricted diastolic opening of the mitral leaflets in patients with left ventricular dysfunction: evidence for increased valve tethering. J Am Coll Cardiol 1998;32:398-404.

67. Otsuji Y, Handschumacher MD, Schwammenthal E, et al: Insights from three-dimensional echocardiography into the mechanism of functional mitral regurgitation: direct in vivo demonstration of altered leaflet tethering geometry. Circulation 1997;96:1999-2008.

68. Yiu SF, Enriquez-Sarano M, Tribouilloy C, et al: Determinants of the degree of functional mitral regurgitation in patients with systolic left ventricular dysfunction: A quantitative clinical study. Circulation 2000;102:1400-1406.

69. Bolling SF: Mitral reconstruction in cardiomyopathy. J Heart Valve Dis 2002;11(Suppl 1):S26-S31.

70. Bolling SF, Pagani FD, Deeb GM, Bach DS: Intermediate-term outcome of mitral reconstruction in cardiomyopathy. J Thorac Cardiovasc Surg 1998;115:381-388.

71. McCully RB, Enriquez-Sarano M, Tajik AJ, Seward JB: Overestimation of severity of ischemic/functional mitral regurgitation by color Doppler jet area. Am J Cardiol 1994;74:790-793.

72. Enriquez-Sarano M, Schaff HV, Frye RL: Mitral regurgitation: what causes the leakage is fundamental to the outcome of valve repair. Circulation 2003;108:253-256.

73. Fuchs RM, Heuser RR, Yin FC, Brinker JA: Limitations of pulmonary wedge V waves in diagnosing mitral regurgitation. Am J Cardiol 1982;49:849-854.

74. Croft CH, Lipscomb K, Mathis K, et al: Limitations of qualitative angiographic grading in aortic or mitral regurgitation. Am J Cardiol 1984;53:1593-1598.

75. Messika-Zeitoun D, Johnson BD, Nkomo V, et al: Cardiopulmonary exercise testing determination of functional capacity in mitral regurgitation: physiologic and outcome implications. J Am Coll Cardiol 2006;47:2521-2527.

76. Armstrong GP, Griffin BP: Exercise echocardiographic assessment in severe mitral regurgitation. Coron Artery Dis 2000;11:23-30.

77. Lee R, Haluska B, Leung DY, et al: Functional and prognostic implications of left ventricular contractile reserve in patients with asymptomatic severe mitral regurgitation. Heart 2005;91:1407-1412.

78. Supino PG, Borer JS, Schuleri K, et al: Prognostic value of exercise tolerance testing in asymptomatic chronic nonischemic mitral regurgitation. Am J Cardiol 2007;100:1274-1281.

79. Wu WC, Aziz GF, Sadaniantz A: The use of stress echocardiography in the assessment of mitral valvular disease. Echocardiography 2004;21:451-458.

80. Savage EB, Ferguson TB Jr, DiSesa VJ: Use of mitral valve repair: analysis of contemporary United States experience reported to the Society of Thoracic Surgeons National Cardiac Database. Ann Thorac Surg 2003;75:820-825.

81. Tribouilloy CM, Enriquez-Sarano M, Schaff HV, et al: Impact of preoperative symptoms on survival after surgical correction of organic mitral regurgitation: rationale for optimizing surgical indications. Circulation 1999;99:400-405.

82. Grigioni F, Avierinos JF, Ling LH, et al: Atrial fibrillation complicating the course of degenerative mitral regurgitation: determinants and long-term outcome. J Am Coll Cardiol 2002;40:84-92.

83. Chua YL, Schaff HV, Orszulak TA, Morris JJ: Outcome of mitral valve repair in patients with preoperative atrial fibrillation: should the maze procedure be combined with mitral valvuloplasty? J Thorac Cardiovasc Surg 1994;107:408-415.

84. Eguchi K, Ohtaki E, Matsumura T, et al: Pre-operative atrial fibrillation as the key determinant of outcome of mitral valve repair for degenerative mitral regurgitation. Eur Heart J 2005;26:1866-1872.

85. Lim E, Barlow CW, Hosseinpour AR, et al: Influence of atrial fibrillation on outcome following mitral valve repair. Circulation 2001;104(12 Suppl 1):I59-I63.

86. Bando K, Kasegawa H, Okada Y, et al: Impact of preoperative and postoperative atrial fibrillation on outcome after mitral valvuloplasty for nonischemic mitral regurgitation. J Thorac Cardiovasc Surg 2005;129:1032-1040.

87. Handa N, Schaff HV, Morris JJ, et al: Outcome of valve repair and the Cox maze procedure for mitral regurgitation and associated atrial fibrillation. J Thor Cardiovasc Surg 1999;118:628-635.

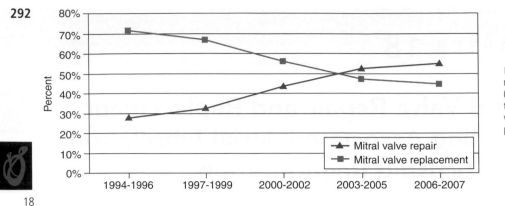

FIGURE 18–1 Mitral valve repair versus mitral valve replacement. Data from the Society of Thoracic Surgery (STS) National Adult Cardiac Surgery Database 2007 show that an increasing percentage of patients undergoing mitral valve surgery are having a mitral valve repair. This includes patients undergiong concomitant procedures.

to patients much earlier in the course of their disease. Initially mitral valve surgery was reserved for patients with advanced symptoms because of the high mortality and morbidity of the procedure and the complications of long-term valve replacement. The situation has changed now, however, with predictable subsets of patients who can expect a successful, durable repair with a very low risk operation. The most recent guidelines suggest that mitral valve repair should be considered in experienced centers for asymptomatic patients with the assumption that the chances for repair are 90% or greater and that the repair would leave little or no residual mitral regurgitation (MR).[6] However, repair still seems to be underutilized in the United States and Europe according to database studies,[7,8] although the trend toward repair is increasing (Figure 18-1). In this chapter we will focus on recent data summarizing techniques and results of mitral valve surgery, and the surgical treatment of two common associated conditions, tricuspid regurgitation (TR) and atrial fibrillation (AF).

MITRAL VALVE ANATOMY AND FUNCTION

Functional Anatomy and Classification of Mitral Regurgitation

In a discussion of surgical treatment, it is important to understand the functional anatomy and different pathophysiologies and the use of a "common language" between cardiologists and surgeons. The functional anatomy of the mitral valve includes the left ventricle, the subvalvular apparatus, the annulus, the valve leaflets, and the left atrium.[9] Carpentier[3] developed a functional classification of mitral regurgitation (Figure 18-2). Type I valve dysfunction is characterized by normal leaflet motion. Lesions that cause type I dysfunction include annular dilatation and leaflet perforation. Type II valve dysfunction is characterized by excessive leaflet motion and leaflet prolapse. Lesions that cause type II dysfunction include chord rupture or elongation and papillary muscle rupture or elongation. Type III valve dysfunction is characterized by restricted leaflet motion. Type IIIA dysfunction occurs when leaflet motion is restricted in diastole. Rheumatic mitral valve disease is the most common etiology of type IIIA dysfunction. Type IIIB dysfunction occurs when leaflet motion is restricted in systole. Ischemic cardiomyopathy is the most common etiology of type IIIB dysfunction. Asymmetric tethering of the posteromedial chords results in restriction of the P3 segment of the posterior leaflet. Anatomically the valve leaflets can be described by segments. The posterior leaflet is divided into three segments or scallops: P1 (lateral), P2 (middle), and P3 (medial). A1, A2, and A3 segments of the anterior leaflet correspond to the opposing posterior leaflet segments (Figure 18-3).

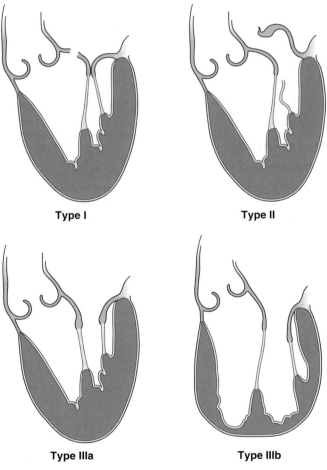

| Type I | Type II |
| Type IIIa | Type IIIb |

FIGURE 18–2 Carpentier functional classification of mitral regurgitation. Type I dysfunction is characterized by normal leaflet motion. Type II dysfunction is characterized by excessive leaflet motion. Type III dysfunction is characterized by restricted leaflet motion with type IIIa occurring during diastole and type IIIb during systole. *(Modified from Adams DH, Anyanwu AC, Rahmanian PB, Filsoufi F: Current concepts in mitral valve repair for degenerative disease. Heart Fail Rev 2006;11: 241-257, with permission.)*

The Mitral Valve Complex and Annulus

The normal mitral valve annulus has a three-dimensional "saddle" shape with both muscular and fibrous portions.[10] The fibrous trigones (left and right), including the central fibrous body, border the aortomitral continuity (subaortic curtain) on each side. The posterior annulus, away from the fibrous skeleton is largely muscular and is most likely to dilate, although the anterior fibrous portion also dilates.[11-13]

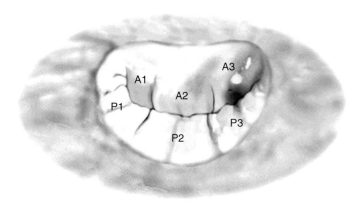

FIGURE 18–3 Anatomy of the normal mitral valve. Looking at the valve from the atrium, the posterior leaflet is divided into P1, P2, and P3 scallops. Similarly, the anterior leaflet is divided into corresponding segments A1, A2, and A3. *(From Fedak PW, McCarthy PM, Bonow RO: Evolving concepts and technologies in mitral valve repair. Circulation 2008;117:963-974, with permission.)*

The mitral valve complex tethers the fibrous skeleton and annulus of the heart to the ventricle and therefore helps maintain left ventricular (LV) shape and function.[14] This function creates "valvular-ventricular interaction" and has become one of the most fundamental concepts underpinning the techniques of valve repair or chord-sparing MVR.[15-21] Lillehei et al,[15] well ahead of other clinicians, recommended that the subvalvular apparatus be preserved during mitral valve surgery to preserve LV function and maintain LV size and shape. These concepts were confirmed by elegant experimental studies demonstrating that removing the chordal apparatus led to LV dilatation, increased wall stress, impaired mechanical function, and decreased LV contractility. Further studies indicated that preservation of chordae facilitated the recovery of both global ventricular and myocyte function after correction of chronic MR, and late survival after MVR was improved. The concept of preserving the valvular-ventricular interaction is now well established and can be applied to the majority of patients. However, the most challenging are those patients with extensive leaflet and annular calcification such as that seen in advanced rheumatic mitral valve disease, in whom resection of leaflets and calcium is required for effective seating of the mitral prosthesis.

MITRAL VALVE REPAIR

Surgical Preparation and Perioperative Care

The majority of mitral valve operations are elective, and therefore there is time for adequate preparation to create an optimal outcome. Coronary angiography is typically performed in all patients 45 years or older and in patients 35 years or older in the presence of chest pain or other objective evidence of myocardial ischemia, LV dysfunction, history of coronary artery disease (CAD), or coronary risk factors such as heredity, tobacco use, hyperlipidemia, hypertension, physical inactivity, obesity, and diabetes.[6] Angiography typically involves only the coronary arteries but may include a left ventriculogram depending on the preoperative echocardiogram findings, especially for patients with ischemic MR and prior myocardial infarction. Right heart catheterization is considered for patients with pulmonary hypertension and LV dysfunction. If the coronary angiogram shows no significant CAD, we typically arrange preoperative autologous blood donation of one or two units before surgery. Because AF is common in patients with mitral valve disease, and there are now effective surgical therapies for AF at the time of mitral valve surgery (as discussed later in this chapter), we carefully

determine any history suggesting AF. If the patient has not had documented AF but has clinical episodes that sound suspicious for AF, then we may obtain preoperative Holter monitoring. We routinely have patients scheduled for valve surgery see a dentist to ensure there is no ongoing periodontal inflammation that may predispose to postoperative endocarditis. Finally, with the increasing prevalence of methicillin-resistant *Staphylococcus aureus*, all patients undergo a nasal swab before surgery, and any patient whose test results are positive for *S. aureus*, whether methicillin-sensitive or -resistant, are treated with nasal mupirocin for 5 days before surgery.

The need for warfarin for anticoagulation after mitral valve repair in patients with sinus rhythm before and after surgery is controversial. Although some centers use only aspirin, others recommend warfarin for approximately 3 months because of a low risk for transient ischemic attacks and other such embolic events that may occur early while endothelial cells are growing onto the prosthetic rings.[22] No randomized trials have been performed to test either strategy.

Surgical Approaches

The standard surgical approach for mitral valve surgery is a full sternotomy. Exposure of the valve is typically through the interatrial groove, which provides excellent exposure. A variety of self-retaining retractors are available to facilitate this exposure. Additional maneuvers to optimize exposure include mobilizing the superior vena cava and mobilizing and retracting the inferior vena cava. We retract the inferior vena cava up and to the left to help expose the posterior medial commissure. Some surgeons prefer a biatrial approach across the atrial septum, especially when performing concomitant tricuspid valve surgery. In rare instances of poor exposure (typically a small left atrium with early severe MR after myocardial infarction) then dividing the superior vena cava to allow reflection of the entire right atrium and a more extended incision along the dome of the left atrium may be useful.

A variety of minimally invasive procedures are now being performed for mitral valve surgery. These include upper or lower hemisternotomies, small right thoracotomies typically using femoral vessel cannulation, and robotic approaches with port access.[23-26] None of the minimally invasive procedures have gone through randomized trials compared with standard sternotomy incisions. Perceived benefits include improved patient acceptance, improved cosmetic results, safety and effectiveness equivalent to that with conventional mitral valve repair and replacement, shorter length of hospital stay, and reduced postoperative disability. Although these claims appear to be valid for some surgeons in some centers, these procedures have not become routine practice for the majority of surgeons because of the perceived difficulty and possibility for inferior outcomes. Robotic operations, especially in their earlier applications, were associated with relatively long cross clamp and cardiopulmonary bypass times, high rates of residual MR after repair, and increased incidence of perioperative stroke.[24,26-29]

Repair Techniques: Myxomatous (Degenerative) Mitral Prolapse

Type II dysfunction is associated with ruptured (flail) or elongated prolapsing chords in the majority of patients. The annulus is also dilated in most patients. A variety of techniques are available to treat leaflet prolapse or flail:
1. Historically the techniques popularized by Carpentier included quadrangular resection of the segment of posterior leaflet that included the prolapsing or ruptured chords.[3,4,30,31] Variations on this technique have included trapezoid or triangular resections that reduce the amount of annular distortion (Figure 18-4).[32-34]

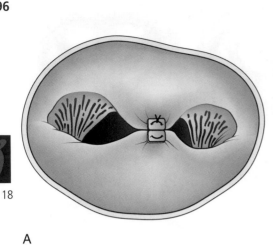

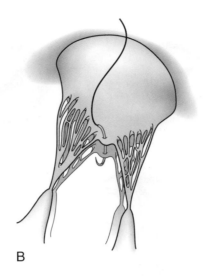

A

B

18

FIGURE 18–8 Edge-to-edge technique (Alfieri technique). The anterior leaflet is approximated to the posterior leaflet creating a double-orifice mitral valve as seen from atrium (**A**) and from the ventricle (**B**).

chord is placed into this "trench" and then the papillary muscle is sutured together to hold the chord at the proper distance. This procedure has largely been supplanted by chord transfer and more recently by use of artificial neo-chords.

After resection of the prolapse or flail segment of the leaflet, the annulus has to be reconstructed if a rectangular or trapezoid resection has been used. The annulus is frequently just sutured together (plicated) at this location.[30,32] Larger resections can also be treated with "compression" sutures that are placed approximately 1 cm apart.[32,65] After tying the compression sutures, the width of resection is usually reduced by half.[32] The remaining annulus can then be plicated. The goal of these techniques is to have the base of the leaflet segments (typically P1 and P3) easily approximated, without any tension, so that when the two edges of the leaflet are sewn back together there is no disruption of the suture line.

Early repairs were performed to the leaflet segments, and the annulus was reconstructed without the routine use of ring annuloplasty. Recurrent MR in that patient population led to more routine use of annuloplasty rings.[66,67] A variety of rings are commercially available and have been recently reviewed but suture plasty is still used by some surgeons.[68] Because the annulus is typically dilated in patients with myxomatous disease, the goal of the rings is to restore the annulus to normal shape or to use the ring to accommodate the pathologic condition of the leaflets.[32] Some rings are based on the normal shape of the annulus and leaflets (Figure 18-9).[69] Use of these rings is considered a "remodeling" annuloplasty that restores the annulus to its normal shape. Other rings are incomplete or C-shaped and rely on anchoring of the ring into the fibrous trigones.[70,71] One ring was designed specifically for the pathologic condition of myxomatous disease to accommodate the elongated leaflets and to move the coaptation point to reduce the risk of SAM.[32,68] Although flexible annuloplasty may have theoretical benefits, in clinical practice and in a randomized trial these have not been demonstrated.[72] Both the complete remodeling rings and the C-shaped rings can be found commercially in soft, flexible materials that attempt to recreate the annular changes during systole and diastole or in more rigid materials that are encased in silicone and Dacron.[68]

Ischemic or Functional Mitral Regurgitation: Indications and Repair Techniques

Occasionally a patient will present with acute severe MR after an acute myocardial infarction with pulmonary edema. Rapid assessment is necessary to determine whether the patient has a ruptured papillary muscle because this group of patients requires an emergency operation with either mitral valve repair

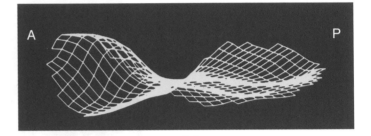

LA

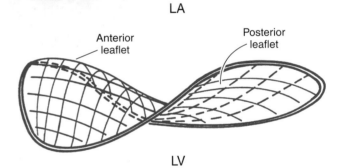

LV

FIGURE 18–9 Normal three-dimensional structure of the mitral valve and annulus. The mitral valve is nonplanar, although the original mitral valve rings were flat and planer. The mitral valve has a saddle shape, with the highest point (toward the left atrium, away from the left ventricle) at the middle of the anterior leaflet adjacent to the aortic valve and at P2. LA, left atrium; LV, left ventricle; A, anterior; P, posterior. *(From Levine RA, Handschumacher MD, Sanfilippo AJ, et al: Three-dimensional echocardiographic reconstruction of the mitral valve, with implications for the diagnosis of mitral valve prolapse. Circulation 1989;80:589-598, with permission.)*

or MVR. Far more commonly, however, the patient develops LV dysfunction with tethering of the leaflets and secondary MR (Figure 18-10). The indications for surgery in this situation may be more controversial. However, in the setting of significant CAD with myocardial viability requiring coronary artery bypass, adding mitral valve surgery would now be considered the standard of care in most circumstances.[6,73] Intraoperative downgrade of MR under general anesthesia at the time of coronary artery bypass should be ignored (Figure 18-11).[74] The controversy now includes what amount of MR warrants mitral valve repair at the time of coronary bypass. Some authors have indicated that adding repair of ischemic MR to coronary artery bypass does not improve survival.[75,76] However, more recent data indicate that even as little as mild to moderate MR when left uncorrected is associated with reduced late survival or an increase in major adverse cardiac events, and it rarely resolves

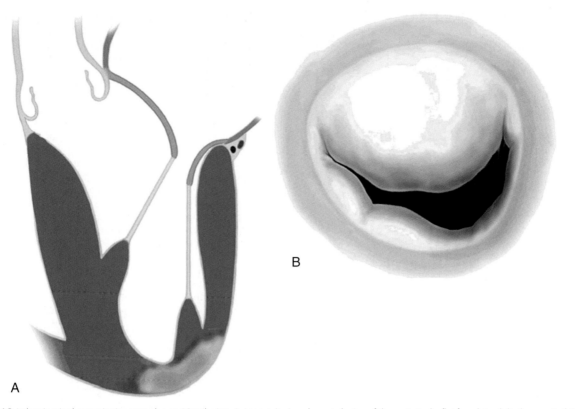

FIGURE 18–10 Ischemic mitral regurgitation secondary to P3 tethering. **A,** Long-axis view shows tethering of the posterior leaflet from lateral displacement of the papillary muscle after myocardial infarction. **B,** Surgeon's view of the mitral valve shows P3 tethering.

FIGURE 18–11 Underestimation of mitral regurgitation (MR) on intraoperative transesophageal echocardiography (TEE). Assessment of MR by intraoperative TEE showed significant intraoperative downgrade with only 11% of patients having 3+ MR. Postoperative echocardiography shows that 40% of these same patients had either 3+ or 4+ MR. *(From Aklog L, Filsoufi F, Flores KQ, et al: Does coronary artery bypass grafting alone correct moderate ischemic mitral regurgitation? Circulation 2001;104:I-68-I-75, with permission.)*

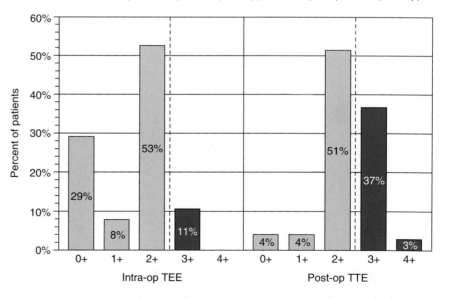

Distribution of MR severity on intraoperative (Intra-op) TEE and postoperative (Post-op) TTE

after coronary bypass alone (Figure 18-12).[74,77-80] Therefore, although the controversy still exists, indications are that coronary artery bypass grafting alone will leave many patients with significant residual MR. Adding mitral valve repair today is not thought to add significantly to operative mortality or morbidity in many patients and may be appropriate, especially in a younger patient.[6,74,77-83]

A multicenter, international, randomized clinical trial (Moderate Mitral Regurgitation In Patients Undergoing CABG [MoMic], personal communication, Per Weirup, Aarhus, Denmark, April 2, 2008) was launched in 2008 to address this controversy. It has been reported that of patients undergoing coronary artery bypass, 20% will have some associated MR.[84]

The majority of these patients will have ischemic MR due to their CAD. The remainder will have mitral valve pathologic lesions unrelated to their CAD. Distinguishing between the two conditions is important for preoperative risk stratification, as patients with ischemic MR generally have impaired LV function and worse CAD.[85,86] Nevertheless, patients with concomitant MR should undergo repair if it is graded at 3+ (moderate-severe) or 4+ (severe)[6] and be considered for repair if it is 2+ (moderate).[77,87] Often a simple restrictive mitral annuloplasty is all that is required to repair the MR.

Whether the valve can be repaired or needs to be replaced is an area that is actively being investigated. Type IIIB MR is characterized by "normal" leaflet morphology with systolic

18

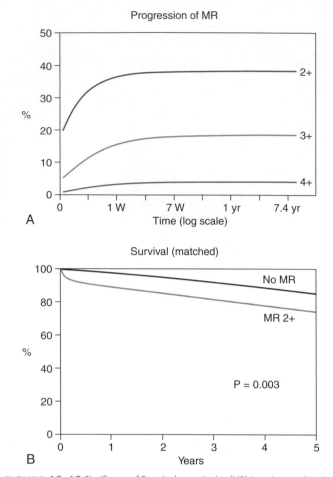

FIGURE 18–12 Significance of 2+ mitral regurgitation (MR) in patients undergoing coronary artery bypass surgery. A, Progression of MR after surgery. B, Patients with 2+ MR had worse survival. *(From Lam BK, Gillinov AM, Blackstone EH, et al: Importance of moderate ischemic mitral regurgitation. Ann Thorac Surg 2005;79:462-470, with permission.)*

restriction of leaflet motion due to ventricular dilatation and tethering of the papillary muscles.[88] Repair has historically been difficult in this group not because the surgical technique is difficult, but the tethering makes it difficult to get the leaflets to coapt adequately (Figure 18-13).[89] Although the leaflets appear normal, they may be "stiffer" because of biochemical changes that may lead to increased fibrosis and theoretically may delay leaflet closure.[90,91]

Whereas a variety of techniques may be used in myxomatous valve repair, for type IIIB MR, the options are more limited and the most prevalent today is the concept of *restrictive mitral annuloplasty*. A small restrictive annuloplasty ring significantly reduces the size of the annulus and leads to better coaptation of the leaflets.[92-95] Clinical experience has indicated that flexible rings may be less effective than rigid rings in accomplishing this goal.[96-99] The main goal is to decrease the septal-lateral dimension. Because the intertrigone distance dilates in this condition, a partial flexible band may not effectively close the septal-lateral dimension, and recurrent MR may develop.[11-13,68,96,100] Therefore, more experience is being gained with small rigid rings, including two designed specifically for functional MR.[68,94,95,101] Additional techniques include subvalvular procedures to cut secondary chords, suture placement to pull the posterior papillary muscles toward the annulus, imbricating the papillary muscles together, and techniques to reshape the ventricle.[102-109] Reshaping the ventricle can be performed directly through surgical reconstruction (such as repairing a posterior aneurysm). Experimentally it has been performed using an inflatable balloon that will move the posterior wall closer to the annulus and restore more normal geometry.[110] Clinically ventricular reshaping has been performed with the Coapsys device (Myocor Inc., Maple Grove, MN), which uses an adjustable transventricular splint to pull the posterior papillary muscle, posterior wall, and therefore leaflets into more normal alignment.[106,111,112] The Coapsys device is still experimental and is undergoing a phase II clinical trial.

MITRAL VALVE RE-REPAIR

Recurrent MR after mitral valve repair should be addressed in a systematic fashion similar to that for primary disease. Failed repairs typically falls into one of two groups: early failures caused by procedure-related factors, and late failures caused by progressive disease.[113,114] Early failures from procedure-related factors such as suture dehiscence, rupture of shortened chordae, SAM, hemolysis, and incomplete repair with residual MR can often be addressed with a re-repair. Conversely, late failures are characterized by new valve pathologic lesions and are less amenable to repair, unless they are caused by progressive annular dilatation due to incorrect ring sizing or failure to use a ring.[115] These cases of recurrent MR often are better addressed with MVR. Overall, of patients with recurrent MR, less than half are able to successfully undergo mitral valve re-repair.[113-115] In these selected patients, mitral valve re-repair can be performed with 93% freedom from another reoperation at 10 years.[113]

MITRAL VALVE REPLACEMENT

Although mitral valve repair is generally the preferred choice for MR, replacement is still sometimes necessary, particularly in patients with rheumatic mitral valve disease with leaflet and

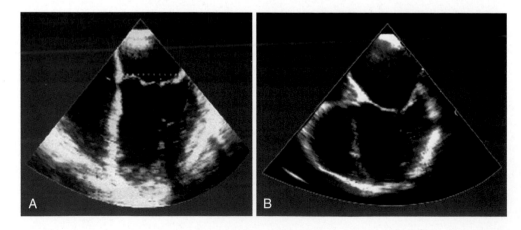

FIGURE 18–13 Mitral valve coaptation depth. **A**, Coaptation depth is illustrated in a healthy patient. **B**, Repair in a patient with ischemic mitral regurgitation is more difficult due to greater coaptation depth. *(From Calafiore AM, Gallina S, Di Mauro M, et al: Mitral valve procedure in dilated cardiomyopathy: repair or replacement? Ann Thorac Surg 2001;71:1146-1152, with permission.)*

subvalvular involvement or degenerative disease with mitral annular and leaflet calcification (frequently older patients), endocarditis with extensive valve destruction, and repair that will leave the patient with residual MR higher than 1+.[6,68,116,117] A fundamental decision must be made about whether a mechanical or tissue valve will be used. The original Starr-Edwards ball-in-cage prosthesis has largely been supplanted by bileaflet or tilting disc mechanical valves. The concern with mechanical valves is the requirement for lifelong warfarin administration. Despite adequate anticoagulation, the risk of thromboembolism with mechanical valves is approximately 2% per year and is on the higher end for valves placed in the mitral position.[6,22,118] The requirement for lifelong use of warfarin also has an attendant risk for significant bleeding episodes, which is approximately 1.5% per year.[22,118] Whereas mechanical valves have excellent durability, in practice the valve may need to be explanted because of obstructive pannus formation, thrombus at the pivots, or bleeding and stroke complications related to warfarin administration, or endocarditis.

Bioprostheses have the advantage of a low thromboembolic risk and, therefore, no requirement for anticoagulation unless indicated for other reasons such as concomitant AF.[6,22] Although first-generation mitral bioprostheses were associated with poor durability, newer-generation bioprostheses have a 10-year actuarial freedom from structural valve deterioration of approximately 64% to 98%.[119-125] Furthermore, many younger patients wish to avoid the risks associated with warfarin administration and face the possibility of a future reoperation. The 2006 American College of Cardiology (ACC)/American Heart Association (AHA) guidelines suggest the use of bioprostheses in patients older than 65 years and also state that a "bioprosthesis is reasonable for MVR in patients under 65 years of age in sinus rhythm who elect to receive this valve for lifestyle considerations after detailed discussions of the risks of anticoagulation versus the likelihood that a second MVR may be necessary in the future."[6] Selected centers now report excellent results for patients undergoing elective reoperation with mitral bioprosthetic re-replacement with mortality as low as 2%.[126,127] Ultimately the choice of prosthesis for mechanical valve replacement is made after discussion between the physician and patient, taking into account the patient's age and overall medical condition, the risk of chronic warfarin administration in relation to the patient's lifestyle, and the risk of future reoperation. There is a distinct trend in the United States away from use of mechanical valves toward use of tissue valves. Data from the Society of Thoracic Surgeons (STS) (Figure 18-14) indicate that the majority of U.S. patients now receive bioprosthetic valves.

The technique for MVR has changed little over the past decades. The Starr-Edwards valve required that the valve leaflets, chords, and subvalvular apparatus be removed to avoid interference with the movement of the poppet within the cage. It was recognized, however, that preserving the valvular-ventricular interactions led to better LV function, and, therefore, the chordal attachments (to the posterior leaflet in particular) were preserved in the majority of patients. It is more difficult to preserve the anterior leaflet because that leaflet tissue may cause LV outflow tract obstruction. Nevertheless, bileaflet chord-sparing replacement can be performed in many patients with a resection of the body of the anterior leaflet and moving the remaining chords away from the outflow tract.[128] In a randomized trial, complete retention of chords resulted in improved ejection fraction and smaller LV chamber size compared with posterior chordal retention only.[128,129] The situations most commonly requiring mitral valve replacement, however, occur in patients with rheumatic valve disease with extensive fibrosis and calcification in whom this may be difficult. Annular calcification is not uncommon and requires debridement to allow safe seating of the prosthesis without the development of perivalvular leaks. The Cavitron ultrasonic surgical aspirator can help pulverize the calcium and facilitate proper placement of the prosthesis. Care must be taken with debridement of the calcium, however, because full-thickness debridement will lead to ventricular disruption, a surgical catastrophe that can be difficult to repair.

Patient-prosthesis mismatch, which has been examined in aortic valve replacement, has also been identified in MVR. Placing too small a mitral prosthesis in relation to the patient's body size has been associated with elevated pulmonary artery pressures, recurrent heart failure, and poor survival.[130-132] Proposed guidelines to avoid patient prosthesis mismatch include using a mitral prosthesis with a projected indexed effective orifice area of no less than $1.2 \, mm^2/m^2$, whenever possible.[133] The frequency of this complication seems to be far less during mitral valve replacement than during aortic valve replacement.

Atrial Fibrillation in Patients Undergoing Mitral Valve Surgery

Preoperative AF is common in many patients undergoing cardiac surgery but is most common in patients undergoing mitral valve surgery.[134,135] Recent data from the STS National Adult Cardiac Surgery Database indicate that 27.3% of patients undergoing mitral valve surgery had a history of AF before surgery, but in single center reports this incidence has been as high as 39%, and for those undergoing mitral valve reoperation it was 54%.[134,135] AF is typically identified in patients with impaired ventricular function, larger left atria, and comorbidities and in older patients.[134,136-138] Recent reports have used statistical methods to account for these baseline differences to examine whether AF itself increases the risk of surgery and impairs late outcomes after surgery. Studies in patients undergoing coronary artery bypass and aortic valve replacement have indicated that patients with preoperative AF have an independent risk for late mortality (and early

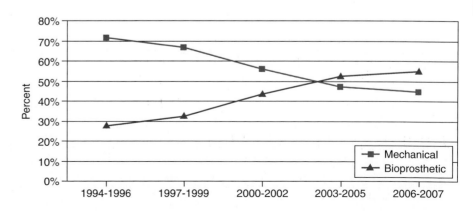

FIGURE 18–14 Bioprosthetic versus mechanical valves in mitral valve replacement. Data from the Society of Thoracic Surgeons (STS) National Adult Cardiac Surgery Database 2007 show that more bioprosthetic than mechanical valves are being used over time. This includes patients undergoing concomitant procedures.

mortality in one study) and are significantly more likely to develop major adverse cardiac events.[138-140] One recent study also indicated that for patients undergoing mitral valve repair, AF increased the risk for mortality and major adverse cardiac events (Figure 18-15).[136]

The Cox maze procedure was first performed with mitral valve repair in 1992,[141] and late results indicate that this strategy has been a very effective surgical treatment of AF.[142-144] The late outcomes for the Cox maze procedure have indicated a

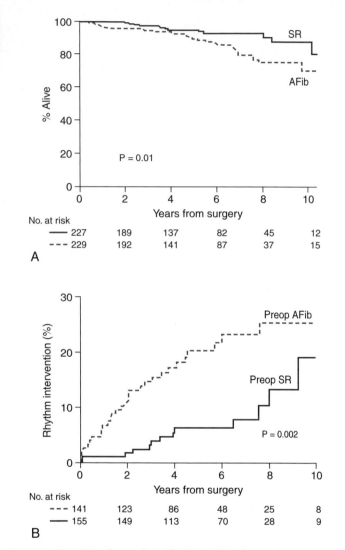

FIGURE 18–15 Significance of atrial fibrillation (AFib) after mitral valve surgery. Survival for patients with atrial fibrillation is worse (**A**) and the rate of rhythm intervention is higher (**B**) than for those in sinus rhythm (SR) after mitral valve surgery. *(From Ngaage DL, Schaff HV, Mullany CJ, et al: Influence of preoperative atrial fibrillation on late results of mitral repair: is concomitant ablation justified? Ann Thorac Surg 2007; 84:434-442, with permission.)*

very low risk for stroke and excellent freedom from symptomatic recurrent AF.[135,142,143,145] Retrospective studies performed in patients with mechanical mitral valves who had AF indicate that the stroke risk is much lower in patients treated with the maze procedure than in patients who are not treated with the maze procedure.[146] However, the classic Cox maze procedure was a complex operation and when added to mitral valve operations was not widely adopted because of the additional cross clamp and cardiopulmonary bypass times.

In the late 1990s, the pulmonary veins were identified as the source of origin of AF in patients with paroxysmal AF and no evidence of structural heart disease (lone AF).[147] Although the pulmonary veins are now accepted to be the site of initiation of AF in many patients, this source has not been well confirmed in patients with structural heart disease such as mitral valve disease. However, electrically isolating the pulmonary veins does provide an excellent anatomic and electrophysiologic procedure to decrease the risk of AF. New technologies were developed to rapidly ablate cardiac tissue to reproduce the lesions created by the Cox maze procedure but without cutting atrial tissue.[148,149] These technologies include unipolar and bipolar radiofrequency, microwave, high-intensity focused ultrasound, cryoablation, and lasers.[148-150] With these new technologies, it became much easier for surgeons to add ablation for AF when the patient was undergoing mitral valve surgery. It is now reported that in patients with a history of AF who are undergoing mitral valve surgery, some type of AF ablation is performed in 52% and as many as 86% in some centers.[134,135] Data from the STS Database indicate that patients with AF ablation have only 9 minute longer cross clamp and bypass times.[134]

Five prospective randomized clinical trials have now been conducted to examine the outcomes of treatment of AF with these new ablation devices during mitral valve surgery in patients with permanent AF (Table 18-1).[151-155] A variety of different energy sources and technologies were used to create ablation lines. These randomized trials confirmed that 1) untreated permanent AF persists in the vast majority of patients after mitral valve surgery (5% to 33% were in normal sinus rhythm at late follow-up), 2) adding ablation using the new technologies was safe and did not add any measurable morbidity or mortality, as found in the STS Database report,[134] and 3) adding the ablation technology significantly increased the rate of return to sinus rhythm compared with that in the control group (range of 44% to 93% in sinus rhythm).

Multicenter and single-center studies have also confirmed the success of ablation with mitral valve surgery for permanent and paroxysmal AF.[135,137,146,150,156-159] Controversy still exists regarding the exact lesion set for ablation, that is, whether the lesions should be just in the left atrium or in the left and right atrium (biatrial) and what is the most effective technology to create transmural lesions (Figure 18-16).[160] A large meta-analysis indicated a benefit of biatrial lesions (92.0% to 87.1% free from AF) versus left side lesions only (86.1% to 73.4%).[161] It has been hard to define "success" after AF ablation by catheter or surgical therapy.[160,162] This complex

TABLE 18–1 | **Prospective Randomized Trials of Permanent Atrial Fibrillation Ablation with Mitral Valve Surgery**

Author, Year	No. Patients	Technology	Control Follow-up NSR	Treated Follow-up NSR
Schuetz et al., 2003[155]	43	Microwave	33.3%	80% ($P = 0.036$)
Abreu Filho et al., 2005[151]	70	Unipolar cooled RF	26.9%	79.4% ($P = 0.001$)
Akpinar et al., 2003[152]	67	Unipolar RF	9.4%	93.6% ($P = 0.0001$)
Doukas et al., 2005[154]	101	Unipolar RF	4.5%	44.4% ($P = 0.001$)
Deneke et al., 2002[153]	30	Unipolar cooled RF	26.7%	81.8% ($P = 0.005$)

NSR, normal sinus rhythm; RF, radiofrequency.

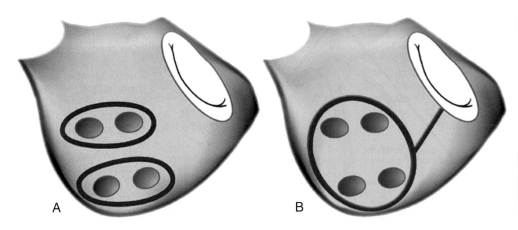

18

Mitral Valve Repair and Replacement, Including Associated Atrial Fibrillation and Tricuspid Regurgitation

FIGURE 18–16 Atrial fibrillation lesion set. Pulmonary vein isolation can be performed without opening the left atrium, and the lesion set is seen from within the left atrium (**A**). More extensive lesion sets require a left atriotomy order to perform the left atrial isthmus lesion connecting the isolated pulmonary veins to the mitral annulus (**B**).

subject was recently addressed in a joint document from the Heart Rhythm Society, European Heart Rhythm Association, and European Cardiac Arrhythmia Society in collaboration with the ACC, AHA, and STS.[160] This is an unusual end point as some patients develop paroxysmal AF, and new ways to indicate freedom from AF are required. In summary, in consideration of the facts that 1) preoperative AF leads to reduced survival and late major adverse cardiac events and 2) five randomized clinical trials, a large registry, and multi-institutional and single-center studies indicate the safety and success of AF ablation using new technologies, the document authors recommended ablation of AF at the time of concomitant surgery: "It is advisable that all patients with documented AF referred for other cardiac surgeries undergo a left or biatrial procedure for AF at an experienced center, unless it...will add significant risk...."[160] It should be noted, however, that the current prospective trials have not had enough patients or long-term follow-up to document that increased return to sinus rhythm reduces major adverse cardiac event rates or improves late survival.

TRICUSPID VALVE SURGERY

Patients with mitral valve disease frequently develop pulmonary hypertension with secondary right ventricular dilatation and "functional" TR. Other patients (rare now in the United States) may also have organic tricuspid valve disease due to rheumatic valve disease. Exact data regarding the frequency of TR in patients undergoing mitral valve surgery are not often reported, but in a recent study from our center, preoperative TR of 2+ or higher (moderate or greater) was present in 32% and tricuspid surgery was performed in 26% of patients undergoing mitral valve surgery.[135] Higher degrees of TR are more common in patients with severe LV dysfunction, elderly patients, and those with long-standing symptomatic MR.[135,163,164]

The threshold for adding tricuspid valve repair to mitral surgery varies considerably and largely relies on "expert opinion." The ACC/AHA guidelines address indications for tricuspid surgery at the time of mitral surgery: class I—severe TR with mitral valve disease (B); class IIA—tricuspid valve replacement with structural nonrepairable disease (C); class IIB—less than or severe TR during MVR with pulmonary hypertension or tricuspid valve dilatation (C).[6] In one report it was noted that for patients with ischemic MR, unrepaired TR progressed and by 3 years after surgery 74% of patients had TR of 2+ or higher (Figure 18-17).[165] Another study indicated that for patients with myxomatous mitral valve disease, those with zero or mild TR with annular dilatation (≥70 mm) when unrepaired had lower functional class and more progression of TR compared with another group of patients

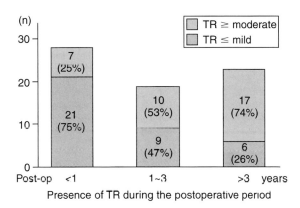

FIGURE 18–17 Progression of tricuspid regurgitation (TR) after surgery for ischemic mitral regurgitation. When TR is left unrepaired, up to 74% of patients will develop moderate TR at 3 years. *(From Matsunaga A, Duran CM: Progression of tricuspid regurgitation after repaired functional ischemic mitral regurgitation. Circulation 2005;112:I-453-I-457, with permission.)*

who had tricuspid annuloplasty.[166] Whereas early mitral surgeons thought TR would resolve after mitral valve surgery,[167] experience has taught us that TR usually persists and may increase after mitral valve surgery.[82,165,168]

There are a variety of techniques that can be used to repair the tricuspid valve including suture techniques (deVega and bicuspidization), repair with flexible rings, and repair with near complete remodeling rings.[135,169-173] Because of the proximity of the atrioventricular node to the septal-anterior leaflet commissure, surgeons avoid placing sutures in this region. Recurrent TR after repair has been high with many similar mechanisms and factors predisposing to ischemic MR.[174-176] Suture repairs have been shown to be less durable than ring repairs in most studies.[172,176-179] Similar to ischemic MR, severe tethering of the leaflets by the distended ventricle appears to be a risk factor for failure (Figure 18-18).[174,175] Pulmonary hypertension has also been shown to be a risk factor for failure.[175,180] Unique to tricuspid valve surgery is the presence of permanent pacing wires that traverse the tricuspid valve that also increase the risk for late failure (Figure 18-19).[176] Although repair is preferable and is possible in the vast majority of patients, occasionally tricuspid replacement may be preferred and was used in 5% in our series of patients with the most severe tethering.[135]

The need for tricuspid surgery indicated a high-risk patient according to the STS Database. Unadjusted mortality for just mitral valve surgery was 7.7% but was 10.8% for mitral with tricuspid surgery and 10.7% for isolated tricuspid surgery.[181] Patients with tricuspid disease frequently present late in the natural history of the disease with poor LV function.[182-184]

29. Robicsek F: Robotic cardiac surgery: time told! J Thorac Cardiovasc Surg 2008;135: 243-246.

30. Adams DH, Anyanwu AC, Rahmanian PB, Filsoufi F: Current concepts in mitral valve repair for degenerative disease. Heart Fail Rev 2006;11:241-257.

31. Deloche A, Jebara VA, Relland JY, et al: Valve repair with Carpentier techniques: the second decade. J Thorac Cardiovasc Surg 1990;99:990-1002.

32. McCarthy PM, McGee EC, Rigolin VH, et al: Initial clinical experience with Myxo-ETlogix mitral valve repair ring. J Thorac Cardiovasc Surg. 2008;136:73-81.

33. Gazoni LM, Fedoruk LM, Kern JA, et al: A simplified approach to degenerative disease: triangular resections of the mitral valve. Ann Thorac Surg 2007;83:1658-1665.

34. Suri RM, Schaff HV, Dearani JA, et al: Survival advantage and improved durability of mitral repair for leaflet prolapse subsets in the current era. Ann Thorac Surg 2006;82:819-826.

35. David TE: Artificial chordae. Semin Thorac Cardiovasc Surg 2004;16:161-168.

36. Dreyfus GD, Corbi P, Rubin S, Aubert S: Posterior leaflet preservation in mitral valve prolapse: a new approach to mitral repair. J Heart Valve Dis 2006;15:528-530.

37. von Oppell UO, Mohr FW: Chordal replacement for both minimally invasive and conventional mitral valve surgery using premeasured Gore-Tex loops. Ann Thorac Surg 2000;70:2166-2168.

38. Lawrie GM, Earle EA, Earle NR: Feasibility and intermediate term outcome of repair of prolapsing anterior mitral leaflets with artificial chordal replacement in 152 patients. Ann Thorac Surg 2006;81:849-856.

39. Perier P: A new paradigm for the repair of posterior leaflet prolapse: respect rather than resect. Operative techniques in thoracic and cardiovascular surgery: a comparative atlas: an official publication of the American Association for Thoracic Surgery. 2005;10:180-193.

40. Gillinov AM, Cosgrove DM: Chordal transfer for repair of anterior leaflet prolapse. Semin Thorac Cardiovasc Surg 2004;16:169-173.

41. Salati M, Moriggia S, Scrofani R, Santoli C: Chordal transposition for anterior mitral prolapse: early and long-term results. Eur J Cardiothorac Surg 1997;11:268-273.

42. Duran CM: Surgical techniques for the repair of anterior mitral leaflet prolapse. J Card Surg 1999;14:471-481.

43. Smedira NG, Selman R, Cosgrove DM, et al: Repair of anterior leaflet prolapse: chordal transfer is superior to chordal shortening. J Thorac Cardiovasc Surg 1996;112:287-292.

44. Perier P, Clausnizer B, Mistarz K: Carpentier "sliding leaflet" technique for repair of the mitral valve: early results. Ann Thorac Surg 1994;57:383-386.

45. Jebara VA, Mihaileanu S, Acar C, et al: Left ventricular outflow tract obstruction after mitral valve repair: results of the sliding leaflet technique. Circulation 1993;88(Suppl II):II-30-II-34.

46. Maslow AD, Regan MM, Haering JM, et al: Echocardiographic predictors of left ventricular outflow tract obstruction and systolic anterior motion of the mitral valve after mitral valve reconstruction for myxomatous valve disease. J Am Coll Cardiol 1999;34: 2096-2104.

47. Adams DH, Anyanwu AC, Rahmanian PB, et al: Large annuloplasty rings facilitate mitral valve repair in Barlow's disease. Ann Thorac Surg 2006;82:2096-2101.

48. Quigley RL: Prevention of systolic anterior motion after repair of the severely myxomatous mitral valve with an anterior leaflet valvuloplasty. Ann Thorac Surg 2005;80: 179-182.

49. Alfieri O, De Bonis M, Lapenna E, et al: "Edge-to-edge" repair for anterior mitral leaflet prolapse. Semin Thorac Cardiovasc Surg 2004;16:182-187.

50. Alfieri O, Maisano F: An effective technique to correct anterior mitral leaflet prolapse. J Card Surg 1999;14:468-470.

51. Bhudia SK, McCarthy PM, Smedira NG, et al: Edge-to-edge (Alfieri) mitral repair: results in diverse clinical settings. Ann Thorac Surg 2004;77:1598-1606.

52. Brinster DR, Unic D, D'Ambra MN, et al: Midterm results of the edge-to-edge technique for complex mitral valve repair. Ann Thorac Surg 2006;81:1612-1617.

53. Feldman T, Wasserman HS, Herrmann HC, et al: Percutaneous mitral valve repair using the edge-to-edge technique: six-month results of the EVEREST Phase I Clinical Trial. J Am Coll Cardiol 2005;46:2134-2140.

54. Frapier JM, Sportouch C, Rauzy V, et al: Mitral valve repair by Alfieri's technique does not limit exercise tolerance more than Carpentier's correction. Eur J Cardiothorac Surg 2006;29:1020-1025.

55. Kherani AR, Cheema FH, Casher J, et al: Edge-to-edge mitral valve repair: the Columbia Presbyterian experience. Ann Thorac Surg 2004;78:73-76.

56. Maisano F, Caldarola A, Blasio A, et al: Midterm results of edge-to-edge mitral valve repair without annuloplasty. J Thorac Cardiovasc Surg 2003;126:1987-1997.

57. Mascagni R, Al Attar N, Lamarra M, et al: Edge-to-edge technique to treat post-mitral valve repair systolic anterior motion and left ventricular outflow tract obstruction. Ann Thorac Surg 2005;79:471-474.

58. Oc M, Doukas G, Alexiou C, et al: Edge-to-edge repair with mitral annuloplasty for Barlow's disease. Ann Thorac Surg 2005;80:1315-1318.

59. Sartipy U, Albage A, Mattsson E, Lindblom D: Edge-to-edge mitral repair without annuloplasty in combination with surgical ventricular restoration. Ann Thorac Surg 2007;83:1303-1309.

60. Croft LR, Jimenez JH, Gorman RC, et al: Efficacy of the edge-to-edge repair in the setting of a dilated ventricle: an in vitro study. Ann Thorac Surg 2007;84:1578-1584.

61. Gillinov AM, Shortt KG, Cosgrove DM 3rd. Commissural closure for repair of mitral commissural prolapse. Ann Thorac Surg 2005;80:1135-1136.

62. Aubert S, Barreda T, Acar C, et al: Mitral valve repair for commissural prolapse: surgical techniques and long term results. Eur J Cardiothorac Surg 2005;28:443-447.

63. Perier P: Surgical repair of the prolapsing anterior leaflet with chordal shortening. Semin Thorac Cardiovasc Surg 2004;16:174-181.

64. Dreyfus GD, Souza Neto O, Aubert S: Papillary muscle repositioning for repair of anterior leaflet prolapse caused by chordal elongation. J Thorac Cardiovasc Surg 2006;132:578-584.

65. Dzemali O, Kleine P, Moritz A: Annular compression stitch for quadrangular resections in mitral valve repair. J Heart Valve Dis 2006;15:132-135.

66. Cohn LH, Couper GS, Aranki SF, et al: Long-term results of mitral valve reconstruction for regurgitation of the myxomatous mitral valve. J Thorac Cardiovasc Surg 1994;107:143-151.

67. Gillinov AM, Cosgrove DM, Blackstone EH, et al: Durability of mitral valve repair for degenerative disease. J Thorac Cardiovasc Surg 1998;116:734-743.

68. Fedak PW, McCarthy PM, Bonow RO: Evolving concepts and technologies in mitral valve repair. Circulation 2008;117:963-974.

69. Carpentier AF, Lessana A, Relland JY, et al: The "physio-ring": an advanced concept in mitral valve annuloplasty. Ann Thorac Surg 1995;60:1177-1186.

70. Gillinov AM, Cosgrove DM 3rd, Shiota T, et al: Cosgrove-Edwards Annuloplasty System: midterm results. Ann Thorac Surg 2000;69:717-721.

71. Fasol R, Meinhart J, Deutsch M, Binder T: Mitral valve repair with the Colvin-Galloway Future Band. Ann Thorac Surg 2004;77:1985-1988.

72. Chang BC, Youn YN, Ha JW, et al: Long-term clinical results of mitral valvuloplasty using flexible and rigid rings: a prospective and randomized study. J Thorac Cardiovasc Surg 2007;133:995-1003.

73. Allman KC, Shaw LJ, Hachamovitch R, Udelson JE: Myocardial viability testing and impact of revascularization on prognosis in patients with coronary artery disease and left ventricular dysfunction: a meta-analysis. J Am Coll Cardiol 2002;39:1151-1158.

74. Aklog L, Filsoufi F, Flores KQ, et al: Does coronary artery bypass grafting alone correct moderate ischemic mitral regurgitation? Circulation 2001;104(Suppl I):I-68-I-75.

75. Diodato MD, Moon MR, Pasque MK, et al: Repair of ischemic mitral regurgitation does not increase mortality or improve long-term survival in patients undergoing coronary artery revascularization: a propensity analysis. Ann Thorac Surg 2004;78:794-799.

76. Tolis GA Jr, Korkolis DP, Kopf GS, Elefteriades JA: Revascularization alone (without mitral valve repair) suffices in patients with advanced ischemic cardiomyopathy and mild-to-moderate mitral regurgitation. Ann Thorac Surg 2002;74:1476-14801.

77. Lam BK, Gillinov AM, Blackstone EH, et al: Importance of moderate ischemic mitral regurgitation. Ann Thorac Surg 2005;79:462-470.

78. Mallidi HR, Pelletier MP, Lamb J, et al: Late outcomes in patients with uncorrected mild to moderate mitral regurgitation at the time of isolated coronary artery bypass grafting. J Thorac Cardiovasc Surg 2004;127:636-644.

79. Paparella D, Mickleborough LL, Carson S, Ivanov J: Mild to moderate mitral regurgitation in patients undergoing coronary bypass grafting: effects on operative mortality and long-term significance. Ann Thorac Surg 2003;76:1094-1100.

80. Prifti E, Bonacchi M, Frati G, et al: Ischemic mitral valve regurgitation grade II-III: correction in patients with impaired left ventricular function undergoing simultaneous coronary revascularization. J Heart Valve Dis 2001;10:754-762.

81. Adams DH, Filsoufi F, Aklog L: Surgical treatment of the ischemic mitral valve. J Heart Valve Dis 2002;11(Suppl 1):S21-S25.

82. McCarthy PM: Valve surgery for patients with left ventricular dysfunction. In McCarthy PM, Young JB (eds): Heart Failure: a Combined Medical and Surgical Approach. Malden, MA, Blackwell Futura, 2007, pp 153-173.

83. Levine RA, Schwammenthal E: Ischemic mitral regurgitation on the threshold of a solution: from paradoxes to unifying concepts. Circulation 2005;112:745-758.

84. Breisblatt WM, Cerqueira M, Francis CK, et al: Left ventricular function in ischemic mitral regurgitation—a precatheterization assessment. Am Heart J 1988;115(suppl 1):77-82.

85. Zeldis SM, Hamby RI, Aintablian A: The clinical and hemodynamic significance of mitral regurgitation in coronary artery disease. Cathet Cardiovasc Diagn 1980;6:225-232.

86. Gahl K, Sutton R, Pearson M, et al: Mitral regurgitation in coronary heart disease. Br Heart J 1977;39:13-18.

87. Schroder JN, Williams ML, Hata JA, et al: Impact of mitral valve regurgitation evaluated by intraoperative transesophageal echocardiography on long-term outcomes after coronary artery bypass grafting. Circulation 2005;112(Suppl I):I-293-I-298.

88. Ryan LP, Jackson BM, Parish LM, et al: Mitral valve tenting index for assessment of subvalvular remodeling. Ann Thorac Surg 2007;84:1243-1249.

89. Calafiore AM, Gallina S, Di Mauro M, et al: Mitral valve procedure in dilated cardiomyopathy: repair or replacement? Ann Thorac Surg 2001;71:1146-1153.

90. Grande-Allen KJ, Borowski AG, Troughton RW, et al: Apparently normal mitral valves in patients with heart failure demonstrate biochemical and structural derangements: an extracellular matrix and echocardiographic study. J Am Coll Cardiol 2005;45:54-61.

91. Grande-Allen KJ, Barber JE, Klatka KM, et al: Mitral valve stiffening in end-stage heart failure: evidence of an organic contribution to functional mitral regurgitation. J Thorac Cardiovasc Surg 2005;130:783-790.

92. Bolling SF, Pagani FD, Deeb GM, Bach DS: Intermediate-term outcome of mitral reconstruction in cardiomyopathy. J Thorac Cardiovasc Surg 1998;115:381-3868.

93. Dion R, Benetis R, Elias B, et al: Mitral valve procedures in ischemic regurgitation. J Heart Valve Dis 1995;4(Suppl 2):S124-S131.

94. Daimon M, Fukuda S, Adams DH, et al: Mitral valve repair with Carpentier-McCarthy-Adams IMR ETlogix annuloplasty ring for ischemic mitral regurgitation: early echocardiographic results from a multi-center study. Circulation 2006;114(Suppl I):I-588-I-593.

95. Braun J, van de Veire NR, Klautz RJ, et al: Restrictive mitral annuloplasty cures ischemic mitral regurgitation and heart failure. Ann Thorac Surg 2008;85:430-437.

96. Miller DC: Ischemic mitral regurgitation redux—to repair or to replace? J Thorac Cardiovasc Surg 2001;122:1059-1062.

97. Spoor MT, Geltz A, Bolling SF: Flexible versus nonflexible mitral valve rings for congestive heart failure: differential durability of repair. Circulation 2006;114 (Suppl I):I-67-I-71.

98. Tahta SA, Oury JH, Maxwell JM, et al: Outcome after mitral valve repair for functional ischemic mitral regurgitation. J Heart Valve Dis 2002;11:11-19.

99. McGee EC, Gillinov AM, Blackstone EH, et al: Recurrent mitral regurgitation after annuloplasty for functional ischemic mitral regurgitation. J Thorac Cardiovasc Surg 2004;128:916-924.

100. Tibayan FA, Rodriguez F, Langer F, et al: Does septal-lateral annular cinching work for chronic ischemic mitral regurgitation? J Thorac Cardiovasc Surg 2004;127:654-663.

101. Votta E, Maisano F, Bolling SF, et al: The Geoform disease-specific annuloplasty system: a finite element study. Ann Thorac Surg 2007;84:92-101.

102. Kron IL, Green GR, Cope JT: Surgical relocation of the posterior papillary muscle in chronic ischemic mitral regurgitation. Ann Thorac Surg 2002;74:600-601.

103. Barletta G, Toso A, Del Bene R, et al: Preoperative and late postoperative mitral regurgitation in ventricular reconstruction: role of local left ventricular deformation. Ann Thorac Surg 2006;82:2102-2109.

104. Borger MA, Murphy PM, Alam A, et al: Initial results of the chordal-cutting operation for ischemic mitral regurgitation. J Thorac Cardiovasc Surg 2007;133:1483-1492.

105. Hvass U, Tapia M, Baron F, et al: Papillary muscle sling: a new functional approach to mitral repair in patients with ischemic left ventricular dysfunction and functional mitral regurgitation. Ann Thorac Surg 2003;75:809-811.

106. Mishra YK, Mittal S, Jaguri P, Trehan N: Coapsys mitral annuloplasty for chronic functional ischemic mitral regurgitation: 1-year results. Ann Thorac Surg 2006;81:42-46.

107. Rama A, Praschker L, Barreda E, Gandjbakhch I: Papillary muscle approximation for functional ischemic mitral regurgitation. Ann Thorac Surg 2007;84:2130-2131.

108. Langer F, Schafers HJ: RING plus STRING: papillary muscle repositioning as an adjunctive repair technique for ischemic mitral regurgitation. J Thorac Cardiovasc Surg 2007;133:247-249.

109. Smerup M, Funder J, Nyboe C, et al: Strut chordal-sparing mitral valve replacement preserves long-term left ventricular shape and function in pigs. J Thorac Cardiovasc Surg 2005;130:1675-1682.

110. Hung J, Guerrero JL, Handschumacher MD, et al: Reverse ventricular remodeling reduces ischemic mitral regurgitation: echo-guided device application in the beating heart. Circulation 2002;106:2594-2600.

111. Fukamachi K, Inoue M, Doi K, et al: Reduction of mitral regurgitation using the Coapsys device: a novel ex vivo method using excised recipients' hearts. ASAIO J 2005;51:82-84.

112. Grossi EA, Saunders PC, Woo YJ, et al: Intraoperative effects of the Coapsys annuloplasty system in a randomized evaluation (RESTOR-MV) of functional ischemic mitral regurgitation. Ann Thorac Surg 2005;80:1706-1711.

113. Dumont E, Gillinov AM, Blackstone EH, et al: Reoperation after mitral valve repair for degenerative disease. Ann Thorac Surg 2007;84:444-450.

114. Suri RM, Schaff HV, Dearani JA, et al: Recurrent mitral regurgitation after repair: should the mitral valve be re-repaired? J Thorac Cardiovasc Surg 2006;132:1390-1397.

115. Shekar PS, Couper GS, Cohn LH: Mitral valve re-repair. J Heart Valve Dis 2005;14:583-587.

116. Jokinen JJ, Hippelainen MJ, Pitkanen OA, Hartikainen JE: Mitral valve replacement versus repair: propensity-adjusted survival and quality-of-life analysis. Ann Thorac Surg 2007;84:451-458.

117. Gillinov AM, Wierup PN, Blackstone EH, et al: Is repair preferable to replacement for ischemic mitral regurgitation? J Thorac Cardiovasc Surg 2001;122:1125-1141.

118. Grunkemeier GL, Li HH, Naftel DC, et al: Long-term performance of heart valve prostheses. Curr Probl Cardiol 2000;25:73-154.

119. Masters RG, Haddad M, Pipe AL, et al: Clinical outcomes with the Hancock II bioprosthetic valve. Ann Thorac Surg 2004;78:832-836.

120. Rizzoli G, Bottio T, Thiene G, et al: Long-term durability of the Hancock II porcine bioprosthesis. J Thorac Cardiovasc Surg 2003;126:66-74.

121. David TE, Ivanov J, Armstrong S, et al: Late results of heart valve replacement with the Hancock II bioprosthesis. J Thorac Cardiovasc Surg 2001;121:268-277.

122. Legarra JJ, Llorens R, Catalan M, et al: Eighteen-year follow-up after Hancock II bioprosthesis insertion. J Heart Valve Dis 1999;8:16-24.

123. Poirer NC, Pelletier LC, Pellerin M, Carrier M: 15-year experience with the Carpentier-Edwards pericardial bioprosthesis. Ann Thorac Surg 1998;66(Suppl):S57-S61.

124. Neville PH, Aupart MR, Diemont FF, et al: Carpentier-Edwards pericardial bioprosthesis in aortic or mitral position: a 12-year experience. Ann Thorac Surg 1998;66 (6 Suppl):S143-S147.

125. Marchand M, Aupart M, Norton R, et al: Twelve-year experience with Carpentier-Edwards PERIMOUNT pericardial valve in the mitral position: a multicenter study. J Heart Valve Dis 1998;7:292-298.

126. Potter DD, Sundt TM 3rd, Zehr KJ, et al: Risk of repeat mitral valve replacement for failed mitral valve prostheses. Ann Thorac Surg 2004;78:67-72.

127. Borger MA, Yau TM, Rao V, et al: Reoperative mitral valve replacement: importance of preservation of the subvalvular apparatus. Ann Thorac Surg 2002;74:1482-1487.

128. Yun KL, Sintek CF, Miller DC, et al: Randomized trial of partial versus complete chordal preservation methods of mitral valve replacement: a preliminary report. Circulation 1999;100(19 Suppl II):II-90-II-94.

129. Yun KL, Sintek CF, Miller DC, et al: Randomized trial comparing partial versus complete chordal-sparing mitral valve replacement: effects on left ventricular volume and function. J Thorac Cardiovasc Surg 2002;123:707-714.

130. Li M, Dumesnil JG, Mathieu P, Pibarot P: Impact of valve prosthesis-patient mismatch on pulmonary arterial pressure after mitral valve replacement. J Am Coll Cardiol 2005;45:1034-1040.

131. Lam BK, Chan V, Hendry P, et al: The impact of patient-prosthesis mismatch on late outcomes after mitral valve replacement. J Thorac Cardiovasc Surg 2007;133:1464-1473.

132. Magne J, Mathieu P, Dumesnil JG, et al: Impact of prosthesis-patient mismatch on survival after mitral valve replacement. Circulation 2007;115:1417-1425.

133. Pibarot P, Dumesnil JG: Prosthesis-patient mismatch in the mitral position: old concept, new evidences. J Thorac Cardiovasc Surg 2007;133:1405-1408.

134. Gammie JS, Haddad M, Milford-Beland S, et al: Atrial fibrillation correction surgery: lessons from the Society of Thoracic Surgeons National Cardiac Database. Ann Thorac Surg 2008;85:909-914.

135. McCarthy PM: Adjunctive procedures in degenerative mitral valve repair: tricuspid valve and atrial fibrillation surgery. Semin Thorac Cardiovasc Surg 2007;19:121-126.

136. Ngaage DL, Schaff HV, Mullany CJ, et al: Influence of preoperative atrial fibrillation on late results of mitral repair: is concomitant ablation justified? Ann Thorac Surg 2007;84:434-443.

137. Lim E, Barlow CW, Hosseinpour AR, et al: Influence of atrial fibrillation on outcome following mitral valve repair. Circulation 2001;104(Suppl I):I-59-I-63.

138. Quader MA, McCarthy PM, Gillinov AM, et al: Does preoperative atrial fibrillation reduce survival after coronary artery bypass grafting? Ann Thorac Surg 2004;77:1514-1524.

139. Ngaage DL, Schaff HV, Mullany CJ, et al: Does preoperative atrial fibrillation influence early and late outcomes of coronary artery bypass grafting? J Thorac Cardiovasc Surg 2007;133:182-189.

140. Ngaage DL, Schaff HV, Barnes SA, et al: Prognostic implications of preoperative atrial fibrillation in patients undergoing aortic valve replacement: is there an argument for concomitant arrhythmia surgery? Ann Thorac Surg 2006;82:1392-1399.

141. McCarthy PM, Cosgrove DM 3rd, Castle LW, et al: Combined treatment of mitral regurgitation and atrial fibrillation with valvuloplasty and the Maze procedure. Am J Cardiol 1993;71:483-486.

142. Prasad SM, Maniar HS, Camillo CJ, et al: The Cox maze III procedure for atrial fibrillation: long-term efficacy in patients undergoing lone versus concomitant procedures. J Thorac Cardiovasc Surg 2003;126:1822-1828.

143. Schaff HV, Dearani JA, Daly RC, et al: Cox-Maze procedure for atrial fibrillation: Mayo Clinic experience. Semin Thorac Cardiovasc Surg 2000;12:30-37.

144. McCarthy PM, Gillinov AM, Castle L, et al: The Cox-Maze procedure: the Cleveland Clinic experience. Semin Thorac Cardiovasc Surg 2000;12:25-29.

145. Cox JL, Ad N, Palazzo T: Impact of the maze procedure on the stroke rate in patients with atrial fibrillation. J Thorac Cardiovasc Surg 1999;118:833-840.

146. Bando K, Kobayashi J, Kosakai Y, et al: Impact of Cox Maze procedure on outcome in patients with atrial fibrillation and mitral valve disease. J Thorac Cardiovasc Surg 2002;124:575-583.

147. Haissaguerre M, Jais P, Shah DC, et al: Spontaneous initiation of atrial fibrillation by ectopic beats originating in the pulmonary veins. N Engl J Med 1998;339:659-666.

148. Gillinov AM, McCarthy PM, Blackstone EH, et al: Bipolar radiofrequency to ablate atrial fibrillation in patients undergoing mitral valve surgery. Heart Surg Forum 2004;7:E147-E152.

149. Damiano RJ, Voeller RK: Surgical and minimally invasive ablation for atrial fibrillation. Curr Treat Options Cardiovasc Med 2006;8:371-376.

150. Ninet J, Roques X, Seitelberger R, et al: Surgical ablation of atrial fibrillation with off-pump, epicardial, high-intensity focused ultrasound: results of a multicenter trial. J Thorac Cardiovasc Surg 2005;130:803-809.

151. Abreu Filho CA, Lisboa LA, Dallan LA, et al: Effectiveness of the maze procedure using cooled-tip radiofrequency ablation in patients with permanent atrial fibrillation and rheumatic mitral valve disease. Circulation 2005;112(Suppl I):I-20-I-25.

152. Akpinar B, Sanisoglu I, Guden M, et al: Combined off-pump coronary artery bypass grafting surgery and ablative therapy for atrial fibrillation: early and mid-term results. Ann Thorac Surg 2006;81:1332-1337.

153. Deneke T, Khargi K, Grewe PH, et al: Efficacy of an additional MAZE procedure using cooled-tip radiofrequency ablation in patients with chronic atrial fibrillation and mitral valve disease: a randomized, prospective trial. Eur Heart J 2002;23:558-566.

154. Doukas G, Samani NJ, Alexiou C, et al: Left atrial radiofrequency ablation during mitral valve surgery for continuous atrial fibrillation: a randomized controlled trial. JAMA 2005;294:2323-2329.

155. Schuetz A, Schulze CJ, Sarvanakis KK, et al: Surgical treatment of permanent atrial fibrillation using microwave energy ablation: a prospective randomized clinical trial. Eur J Cardiothorac Surg 2003;24:475-480.

156. Gillinov AM, Sirak J, Blackstone EH, et al: The Cox maze procedure in mitral valve disease: predictors of recurrent atrial fibrillation. J Thorac Cardiovasc Surg 2005;130:1653-1660.

157. Gillinov AM, Bakaeen F, McCarthy PM, et al: Surgery for paroxysmal atrial fibrillation in the setting of mitral valve disease: a role for pulmonary vein isolation? Ann Thorac Surg 2006;81:19-28.

158. Handa N, Schaff HV, Morris JJ, et al: Outcome of valve repair and the Cox maze procedure for mitral regurgitation and associated atrial fibrillation. J Thorac Cardiovasc Surg 1999;118:628-635.

159. Mokadam NA, McCarthy PM, Gillinov AM, et al: A prospective multicenter trial of bipolar radiofrequency ablation for atrial fibrillation: early results. Ann Thorac Surg 2004;78:1665-1670.

160. Calkins H, Brugada J, Packer DL, et al: HRS/EHRA/ECAS expert Consensus Statement on catheter and surgical ablation of atrial fibrillation: recommendations for personnel, policy, procedures and follow-up. A report of the Heart Rhythm Society (HRS) Task Force on catheter and surgical ablation of atrial fibrillation. Heart Rhythm 2007;4:816-861.

161. Barnett SD, Ad N: Surgical ablation as treatment for the elimination of atrial fibrillation: a meta-analysis. J Thorac Cardiovasc Surg 2006;131:1029-1035.

162. Shemin RJ, Cox JL, Gillinov AM, et al: Guidelines for reporting data and outcomes for the surgical treatment of atrial fibrillation. Ann Thorac Surg 2007;83:1225-1230.

163. Koelling TM, Aaronson KD, Cody RJ, et al: Prognostic significance of mitral regurgitation and tricuspid regurgitation in patients with left ventricular systolic dysfunction. Am Heart J 2002;144:524-529.

164. Nath J, Foster E, Heidenreich PA: Impact of tricuspid regurgitation on long-term survival. J Am Coll Cardiol 2004;43:405-409.

165. Matsunaga A, Duran CM: Progression of tricuspid regurgitation after repaired functional ischemic mitral regurgitation. Circulation 2005;112(Suppl I):I-453-I-457.

166. Dreyfus GD, Corbi PJ, Chan KM, Bahrami T: Secondary tricuspid regurgitation or dilatation: which should be the criteria for surgical repair? Ann Thorac Surg 2005;79:127-132.

167. Braunwald NS, Ross J Jr, Morrow AG: Conservative management of tricuspid regurgitation in patients undergoing mitral valve replacement. Circulation 1967;35(Suppl I): I-63-I-69.

168. Simon R, Oelert H, Borst HG, Lichtlen PR: Influence of mitral valve surgery on tricuspid incompetence concomitant with mitral valve disease. Circulation 1980;62(suppl I): I-152-I-157.

18

169. De Vega NG, De Rabago G, Castillon L, et al: A new tricuspid repair. Short-term clinical results in 23 cases. J Cardiovasc Surg (Torino) 1973;Spec No:384-386.

170. Ghanta RK, Chen R, Narayanasamy N, et al: Suture bicuspidization of the tricuspid valve versus ring annuloplasty for repair of functional tricuspid regurgitation: mid-term results of 237 consecutive patients. J Thorac Cardiovasc Surg 2007;133:117-126.

171. McCarthy JF, Cosgrove DM 3rd: Tricuspid valve repair with the Cosgrove-Edwards Annuloplasty System. Ann Thorac Surg 1997;64:267-268.

172. Matsuyama K, Matsumoto M, Sugita T, et al: De Vega annuloplasty and Carpentier-Edwards ring annuloplasty for secondary tricuspid regurgitation. J Heart Valve Dis 2001;10:520-524.

173. Filsoufi F, Salzberg SP, Coutu M, Adams DH: A three-dimensional ring annuloplasty for the treatment of tricuspid regurgitation. Ann Thorac Surg 2006;81:2273-2277.

174. Fukuda S, Song JM, Gillinov AM, et al: Tricuspid valve tethering predicts residual tricuspid regurgitation after tricuspid annuloplasty. Circulation 2005;111:975-979.

175. Fukuda S, Gillinov AM, McCarthy PM, et al: Determinants of recurrent or residual functional tricuspid regurgitation after tricuspid annuloplasty. Circulation 2006;114(Suppl I):I-582-I-587.

176. McCarthy PM, Bhudia SK, Rajeswaran J, et al: Tricuspid valve repair: durability and risk factors for failure. J Thorac Cardiovasc Surg 2004;127:674-685.

177. Tang GH, David TE, Singh SK, et al: Tricuspid valve repair with an annuloplasty ring results in improved long-term outcomes. Circulation 2006;114(Suppl I):I-577-I-581.

178. Rivera R, Duran E, Ajuria M: Carpentier's flexible ring versus De Vega's annuloplasty. A prospective randomized study. J Thorac Cardiovasc Surg 1985;89:196-203.

179. Yada I, Tani K, Shimono T, et al: Preoperative evaluation and surgical treatment for tricuspid regurgitation associated with acquired valvular heart disease: the Kay-Boyd method vs the Carpentier-Edwards ring method. J Cardiovasc Surg (Torino) 1990;31:771-777.

180. Shah PM, Raney AA: Tricuspid valve disease. Curr Probl Cardiol 2008;33:47-84.

181. Rankin JS, Hammill BG, Ferguson TB Jr, et al: Determinants of operative mortality in valvular heart surgery. J Thorac Cardiovasc Surg 2006;131:547-557.

182. Bernal JM, Gutierrez-Morlote J, Llorca J, et al: Tricuspid valve repair: an old disease, a modern experience. Ann Thorac Surg 2004;78:2069-2075.

183. Kuwaki K, Morishita K, Tsukamoto M, Abe T: Tricuspid valve surgery for functional tricuspid valve regurgitation associated with left-sided valvular disease. Eur J Cardiothorac Surg 2001;20:577-582.

184. Kim HK, Kim YJ, Park JS, et al: Determinants of the severity of functional tricuspid regurgitation. Am J Cardiol 2006;98:236-242.

185. David TE: Outcomes of mitral valve repair for mitral regurgitation due to degenerative disease. Semin Thorac Cardiovasc Surg 2007;19:116-120.

186. El Khoury G, Noirhomme P, Verhelst R, et al: Surgical repair of the prolapsing anterior leaflet in degenerative mitral valve disease. J Heart Valve Dis 2000;9:75-81.

187. Fucci C, Cicco GD, Chiari E, et al: Edge-to-edge mitral valve repair for isolated prolapse of the anterior leaflet caused by degenerative disease. J Cardiovasc Med 2007; 8:354-358.

188. De Bonis M, Lorusso R, Lapenna E, et al: Similar long-term results of mitral valve repair for anterior compared with posterior leaflet prolapse. J Thorac Cardiovasc Surg 2006;131:364-370.

189. Enriquez-Sarano M, Schaff HV, Orszulak TA, et al: Valve repair improves the outcome of surgery for mitral regurgitation: a multivariate analysis. Circulation 1995;91:1022-1028.

190. Thourani VH, Weintraub WS, Guyton RA, et al: Outcomes and long-term survival for patients undergoing mitral valve repair versus replacement: effect of age and concomitant coronary artery bypass grafting. Circulation 2003;108:298-304.

191. Gazoni LM, Kern JA, Swenson BR, et al: A change in perspective: results for ischemic mitral valve repair are similar to mitral valve repair for degenerative disease. Ann Thorac Surg 2007;84:750-758.

192. Kang DH, Kim MJ, Kang SJ, et al: Mitral valve repair versus revascularization alone in the treatment of ischemic mitral regurgitation. Circulation 2006;114(Suppl I):I-499-I-503.

193. Gillinov AM, Blackstone EH, Rajeswaran J, et al: Ischemic versus degenerative mitral regurgitation: does etiology affect survival? Ann Thorac Surg 2005;80:811-819.

194. Acker MA, Bolling S, Shemin R, et al: Mitral valve surgery in heart failure: insights from the Acorn Clinical Trial. J Thorac Cardiovasc Surg 2006;132:568-577, 577.

195. Ling LH, Enriquez-Sarano M, Seward JB, et al: Early surgery in patients with mitral regurgitation due to flail leaflets: a long-term outcome study. Circulation 1997;96:1819-1825.

196. Ling LH, Enriquez-Sarano M, Seward JB, et al: Clinical outcome of mitral regurgitation due to flail leaflet. N Engl J Med 1996;335:1417-1423.

197. Bridgewater B, Hooper T, Munsch C, et al: Mitral repair best practice: proposed standards. Heart 2006;92:939-944.

198. Adams DH, Anyanwu A: Pitfalls and limitations in measuring and interpreting the outcomes of mitral valve repair. J Thorac Cardiovasc Surg 2006;131:523–529.

199. David TE, Ivanov J, Armstrong S, et al: A comparison of outcomes of mitral valve repair for degenerative disease with posterior, anterior, and bileaflet prolapse. J Thorac Cardiovasc Surg 2005;130:1242–1249.

200. Madaric J, Watripont P, Bartunek J, et al: Effect of mitral valve repair on exercise tolerance in asymptomatic patients with organic mitral regurgitation. Am Heart J 2007;154:180-185.

CHAPTER **19**

Percutaneous Transcatheter Treatment for Mitral Regurgitation

Peter C. Block

KEY POINTS

- Mitral regurgitation can be broadly categorized as being either degenerative or functional. Degenerative mitral regurgitation can be managed by surgical correction with a high degree of success. Functional mitral regurgitation is less amenable to surgery regardless of cause.
- Percutaneous repair of mitral regurgitation using the Evalve mitral clip device has been shown to be save and effective. The EVEREST I, a phase I trial, is complete. The EVEREST II trial is a randomized trial comparing standard surgical correction with percutaneous repair and will have core laboratory review of both surgical and percutaneous repair at 1-year follow-up.
- Coronary sinus devices can be placed percutaneously with relative ease. Because of the proximity of the coronary sinus to the posterior mitral annulus, theoretically any device that contracts or constricts the coronary sinus will change the mitral line of coaptation and reduce mitral regurgitation. However, in early trials coronary sinus devices have shown only mild to moderate reduction of mitral regurgitation.
- Functional mitral regurgitation is a secondary phenomenon, usually due to either ischemic myocardial disease or cardiomyopathy and annular dilation. Any percutaneous device that is designed to repair functional mitral regurgitation must address the fact that the etiology is a myocardial, not valvular, abnormality.

In the next decades, treatment of congestive heart failure (CHF) due to ischemic heart disease, structural valve disease, and cardiomyopathy will continue to be a major challenge for cardiologists. The common path that brings patients with CHF to medical attention is the development of left ventricular (LV) failure, frequently associated with mitral regurgitation (MR).[1-3] The presence of MR, whether the primary cause of CHF or a secondary phenomenon, inflicts a further volume load on the already failing left ventricle, causing myocardial dilation, papillary muscle displacement, and thus more MR. MR begets MR (Figure 19-1).

In adults, MR can be broadly characterized as being due to degenerative valvular abnormalities (mitral valve prolapse, mitral cleft, rheumatic disease, and others) or functional abnormalities. The latter include mitral annular dilation due to cardiomyopathic LV dilation or abnormalities of the mitral supporting apparatus (chordal displacement because of papillary muscle scarring, ischemic dysfunction, or LV remodeling due to myocardial infarction in particular).

There are only few medical options for the treatment of MR. The aim of current therapy is symptom relief (diuretics) with unloading to help the failing left ventricle perform more efficiently. Drugs used to increase inotropy, arguably aside from the use of digitalis, have been unsuccessful clinically. There are no long-term studies to show that use of vasodilators reduces the regurgitant fraction in chronic MR. In patients with MR due to ischemia or functional MR due to dilated cardiomyopathy, however, preload reduction may be beneficial[4] and converting enzyme inhibitors, β-blockers, and biventricular pacing may all be helpful.[5-8] The American College of Cardiology/American Heart Association guidelines recommend surgical correction of MR for asymptomatic patients even before LV dilation or systolic dysfunction occur. Intervention for patients after symptoms have developed is also recommended.[9]

Current operative strategies for the multiple etiologies of MR include leaflet repair (reshaping, edge-to-edge approximation, and pericardial patch), leaflet mobilization, chordal repair usually combined with annuloplasty, and valve replacement.[10-24] Surgery is most successful for patients with degenerative valve disease. In such patients surgical valve repair in most instances, accompanied by placement of an annuloplasty device, produces good long-term outcomes,[10-13,25-27] although the reoperation

PERCUTANEOUS REPAIR BEYOND DIRECT VALVULAR INTERVENTION

Even in patients in whom the initial cause of MR is purely valvular, the increased volume load on the left ventricle ultimately leads to both LV hypertrophy and dilation. As the ventricle dilates, secondary changes occur that further increase MR: the mitral annulus enlarges and the papillary muscles and chordae tendineae move outward, thereby changing the relationships of the entire supporting apparatus of the mitral leaflets. Similarly in patients with cardiomyopathy or ischemic disease of the left ventricle who develop MR, LV dilation leads to further remodeling as the ventricle compensates for the increased volume load. Remodeling is associated with profound changes in the LV myocardium.

The central role of LV myocardial changes in MR is demonstrated in a canine model of MR induced by chordal rupture. In studies using that model, MR is associated with infiltration of mast cells, increased activity of matrix metalloproteinases, decreased tissue inhibition of metalloproteinases, and increased chymase activity. These result in a rapid loss of extracellular matrix collagen, increased LV compliance, increased myocyte integrin adhesion, myofiber slippage, myocyte hypertrophy, and decreased LV contraction.[36-41] In experimental and spontaneous MR in dogs, the LV collagen loss allows LV dilation and decreased contractility, in turn leading to further remodeling as time goes on. In the same model, angiotensin-converting enzyme inhibition and angiotensin II receptor blockade have failed to attenuate the collagen loss and myocardial dilation and hypertrophy.[40] These data support the notion that MR is associated with important degenerative changes in the left ventricle. Thus, clinical use of diuretics, converting enzyme inhibitors, or other receptor blockers may improve symptoms because of LV unloading, but the underlying pathophysiologic changes of the LV myocardium are unaffected, and it is not surprising that such therapy has little effect on progression of MR or the development of LV failure. In the final analysis, functional MR is due to underlying LV myocardial dysfunction that may be little affected by a reduction in MR once structural myocardial changes occur. Therefore, the aim of therapy should be to intervene at an early stage of MR before secondary, and perhaps irreversible, myocardial changes can occur.

In an attempt to deal with the complex pathophysiology of MR, most surgical treatment includes more than simply direct valve repair. Surgical experience has shown that the majority of mitral repair procedures should involve placement of some kind of annuloplasty device. Conceptually the reason is that the pathophysiology of MR produces abnormalities of the mitral annulus, changes in alignment of the chordae tendineae and the papillary muscles, and dilation of the LV wall. Because mitral annular distortion or dilation is a common accompaniment of valvular and functional MR, there is resultant displacement of both mitral leaflets and diminution of the depth or even loss of the line of coaptation of the valve. If coaptation of the mitral leaflets does not occur, severe MR results.

Numerous surgical strategies have been developed to reposition the annulus or leaflets. For example, surgical annuloplasty, by shortening the length of the posterior annulus and the attached posterior leaflet, moves the posterior leaflet toward the anterior leaflet, thereby reestablishing a more normal line of mitral coaptation. Direct surgical repair of ruptured chordae tendineae and release of shortened chordae have also been successful strategies.[42]

Just as the percutaneous edge-to-edge procedure is based on surgical principles, several other types of novel percutaneous devices have recently been developed to reestablish mitral valve coaptation. These fall into several broad categories, and all are designed to support or cinch the posterior mitral annulus or support the myocardium. The theoretical result of their deployment is movement of the posterior leaflet toward the anterior leaflet or realignment of the supporting structures of the mitral valve, thereby reestablishing the coaptation line and decreasing MR.

Coronary Sinus Devices

The coronary sinus (CS) runs from the lateral LV wall medially to the right atrium. Its course is roughly parallel to the posterior mitral annulus, and in some patients it lies just posterior to the annulus along most of its course (Figure 19-4).[43-47] A device placed within the CS that could either cinch or compress

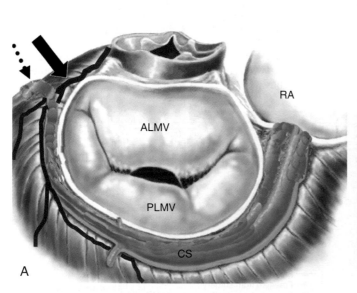
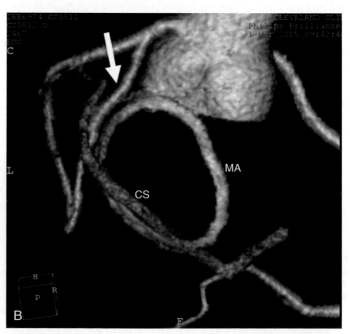

FIGURE 19–4 A, Illustration of the relationship of the coronary sinus to surrounding cardiac structures, including the circumflex coronary artery (*arrow*) and great cardiac vein (*dashed arrow*). **B,** Computed tomographic scan of the aortic root, circumflex coronary artery, (arrow), and mitral annulus. ALMV, anterior leaflet of the mitral valve; CS, coronary sinus; MA, mitral annulus; PLMV, posterior leaflet of the mitral valve; RA, right atrium. *(Courtesy of S. Kapadia, MD, and E. M. Tuzcu, MD, Cleveland Clinic, Cleveland, Ohio.)*

the CS or directly move it forward should also move the posterior leaflet toward the anterior leaflet (see Figure 19-4A). This would reduce MR in patients in whom the line of coaptation was separated. Several such devices have been designed and tested in animal models of MR with success, and some are in early clinical trials. The Viacor PTMA device (Viacor, Wilmington, MA), CARILLON Mitral Contour Device (Cardiac Dimensions, Kirkland, WA), and the MONARC device (Edwards Lifesciences, Irvine, CA) are examples.[45-52]

The Viacor PTMA Device

The Viacor PTMA device consists of a series of shaped nitinol rods which are placed through the proximal access hub of a multi-lumen catheter extending from the CS to the anterior interventricular vein (AIV) (see Figure 19-5). The therapeutic rods vary in length and stiffness, directly moving the posterior annulus toward the anterior leaflet, thereby realigning the mitral line of coaptation and reducing MR (Figure 19-6). The 7-F over-the-wire multi-lumen catheter is introduced through the left or right subclavian vein and advanced through the CS, GCV and AIV. Proximal and distal marker bands assist in aligning the 'working length' of the catheter (the portion of the catheter wound with polyester surgical suture for enhanced stability) with the midpoint of the CS-GCV opposite P2 and the ostium of the CS. Diagnostic rods are then inserted into the lumens of the catheter to determine the amount of movement of the posterior annulus needed to reduce MR. With stiffness and length confirmed for optimized annular push,

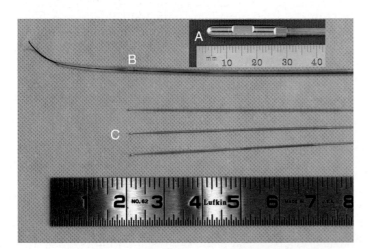

FIGURE 19–5 The Viacor device. **A,** Proximal end of delivery catheter. **B,** 7-F delivery catheter. **C,** Nitinol treatment rods.

the diagnostic rods are replaced with the therapeutic rods. Once the PTMA® device is drawn back to optimal position and reduction in MR is confirmed the CSG sheath is removed in conventional peel-away fashion. The proximal end of the implant is then anchored just outside its subclavian venous entry site, similar to a pacemaker generator.

The system is unique in a number of ways. The implanted therapeutic rods can be exchanged for higher pressure rods in the future should the reduction in MR prove adequate or if MR reappears, even weeks after the initial implantation. Another unique characteristic is that the entire system can be removed if necessary.

The Viacor PTMA device has been shown to be effective in acute and chronic animal models of ischemic MR.[48-52] The device significantly reduced the septal-lateral annular dimensions of the mitral valve with resultant reduction of MR due to realignment of the line of coaptation (Figures 19-6 and 19-7). In a pilot study of four patients with ischemic cardiomyopathy who underwent temporary implantation of the Viacor PTMA device, it was reported that the device could not be successfully implanted in one patient because of tortuous venous anatomy. The remaining three patients had successful device implantation.[53] Effective regurgitant orifice was reduced from 0.25 ± 0.06 to $0.07 \pm 0.03\,cm^2$, the annular anteroposterior diameter was reduced from 40.75 ± 4.3 to $35.2 \pm 1.6\,mm$, and regurgitant volume decreased from 45.5 ± 24.4 to $13.3 \pm 7.3\,mL$.[52,53]

To date, 34 intention-to-treat patients have been evaluated in feasibility studies conducted outside the United States. Whereas previous generations of the PTMA device achieved decreases in the anteroposterior diameter of the mitral annulus somewhat less than those achieved with open surgical procedures, the current generation of the device is showing more promise in is approximating surgical grade corrections. Clinical experience with the progressively improving PTMA device and implantation methods suggest a plausible expectation of clinical efficacy. Correlation of sustained AP reduction with changes in mitral regurgitation, chamber volumes, and clinical measures will benefit from further study, though early human implants suggests a durable reduction in anteroposterior diameter of the annulus. In all cases patients treated with PTMA® tolerated the procedure well and have experienced no procedure or device-related permanent clinical sequelae, and all patients were discharged. There have been no major cardiac adverse events (death, MI, tamponade, emergent cardiac surgery, and stroke) within the study group within 30 days of the procedure. Five patients died within one year of enrollment due to progression of heart failure, determined to be unrelated to the implant or PTMA procedure.

FIGURE 19–6 Result of placement of therapeutic rods into the delivery catheter. **A,** Original position of the coronary sinus before placement of the therapeutic devices (*dotted lines*). **B,** Amount of movement of the CS and posterior mitral annulus resulting from rod placement (*arrow*).

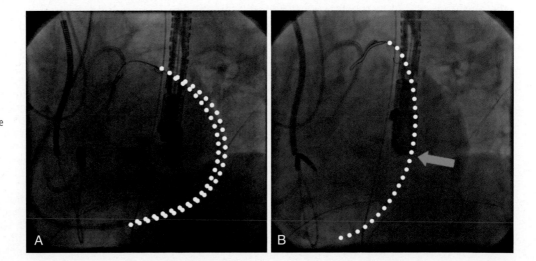

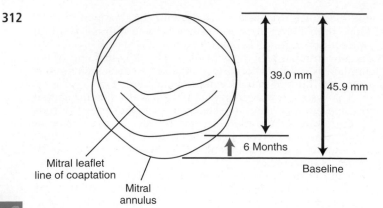

FIGURE 19–7 Three-dimensional echocardiographic tracings of the mitral annulus and mitral valve line of coaptation in end-diastole before and 6 months after placement of the Viacor device. The pretreatment posterior annulus and mitral valve line of coaptation (red) are moved forward.

19

Interestingly, there has been no case of myocardial injury due to impingement of the circumflex coronary artery in the early studies. This result may be due to the outward distribution of forces along the distal and proximal vessel segments. Careful preimplant screening is critical. Cardiac computed tomographic evaluation of the relationships of the CS, the great cardiac vein, and the anterior interventricular vein to the mitral annulus, and identification of unusual circumflex coronary artery crossovers of the CS are invaluable in patient selection.

The Carillon Mitral Contour Device

Cardiac Dimensions has developed the Carillon Mitral Contour System, a percutaneous mitral annuloplasty device intended for patients with heart failure and functional MR. This device comprises two helical nitinol anchors connected by a nitinol ribbon. It is intended to be positioned in the CS or great cardiac vein along the posterior annulus of the mitral valve (Figure 19-8). Jugular venous access is first obtained to facilitate placement of a 9-F delivery catheter to the CS. Coronary arterial and venous angiograms are used to characterize the relevant anatomy and allow for proper device selection, which depends on the length and diameter of the CS or great cardiac vein in the target locations of the vein. After the appropriate device is selected, it is advanced through the delivery catheter, and the distal anchor is deployed and locked into position near the anterior commissure of the mitral valve. The helical wireform anchors are oversized relative to the venous dimensions to ensure proper anchoring. With the proximal anchor still collapsed in the delivery catheter, tension is placed on the delivery system so as to plicate the periannular tissue. The exact degree of tissue plication

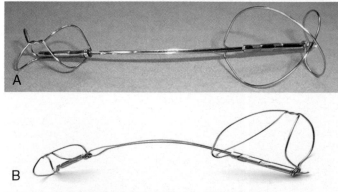

FIGURE 19–8 Top (**A**) and side view (**B**) of the CARILLON device.

is adjustable depending on the underlying anatomy and is determined by real-time assessment of the MR jet evaluated by echocardiography. Once MR reduction has been achieved, the proximal anchor is deployed and locked into position, near the posterior commissure of the mitral valve. While the Carillon device is still connected to the delivery system, safety and efficacy are carefully assessed. Quantitative echocardiographic measures are used to confirm MR reduction. In addition, coronary arteriograms are obtained to ensure no reduction of coronary flow in adjacent coronary arteries. If either insufficient MR reduction is seen or if there is significant reduction of coronary arterial flow, the device may be recaptured by simply advancing the delivery catheter over the anchor wireforms and retracting the device back into the catheter. A second device may be positioned in a new location to optimize efficacy or reduce the impact of the device on coronary flow.

The Carillon device has been tested for short- and long-term safety and efficacy in preclinical animal experiments.[54-56] The studies have shown reductions in septal-lateral mitral annular dimensions, reductions in MR measured by decreased regurgitant volumes, and reduced effective regurgitant orifice areas and improvement in hemodynamics. Interestingly, reductions in neurohormonal responses (norepinephrine and brain natriuretic peptide levels) to congestive heart failure in these models have also been demonstrated.

The device has also been tested in temporary and permanent implants.[57,58] A first-in-man study demonstrated the feasibility and safety of temporary deployment of this device. Of five patients with heart failure and functional MR (mean age 52 ± 9 years) recruited for the study, four had anatomy suitable for deployment of the device. Transthoracic echocardiography and coronary angiography were performed before and after temporary placement and tensioning of the device via the right internal jugular vein. Displacement of the distal anchor occurred in two patients, probably because of undersizing. In one patient the left circumflex coronary artery was initially compromised, and the device was placed more proximally. Despite these technical limitations, temporary deployment produced a significant reduction in the septal-lateral mitral annular dimension from 35.5 ± 4.7 to 32.2 ± 4.6 mm ($P = 0.02$), with evidence of a reduction in the MR color Doppler area from 98.3 ± 43.6 to 83.3 ± 35.1 mm^2 ($P = 0.09$) and reductions in the MR jet area to left atrium area ratio (36 ± 18% to 30 ± 14%). There were no intraprocedural adverse events.[57] The phase I Carillon Mitral Annuloplasty Device European Union Study (AMADEUS) has completed enrollment of the initial 30 patients with functional MR due to congestive heart failure treated with this device. The objective of the study was to evaluate the safety of deploying and implanting the Carillon implant in the CS and secondarily to evaluate the clinical changes associated with device implantation. Inclusion criteria were diagnosis of dilated cardiomyopathy (either ischemic or a nonischemic in etiology) and at least 2+ MR. Patients were excluded if they had any of the following: coronary or venous anatomy that precluded placement of the Carillon implant, previous mitral valve repair or replacement, moderate or severe myxomatous valvular degeneration (with or without mitral leaflet prolapse), rheumatic mitral disease, chordal rupture, severe mitral annular calcification, systolic hypertension greater than 160 mm Hg, or renal dysfunction (serum creatinine >2.5 mg/dL).

Preliminary reports of this trial have been encouraging with an implantation success rate of 70% with more than 75% of patients showing a reduction in MR severity. Commensurate with MR reduction, patients also experienced a one-grade improvement in New York Heart Association (NYHA) functional class. Two patients required recapturing of the device before final deployment because of compromised coronary artery flow from device compression. Importantly, not all coronary arteries that were crossed by the device had compromised flow.[59] The ability to recapture the device after deployment of the distal and proximal anchors allows for the assessment of adequate MR reduction and coronary flow before release of the proximal anchor. Follow-up of all patients continues. The COMPETENT Trial, a pilot safety study of the Carillon Mitral Contour System for the treatment of functional MR is under development. It will be initiated at seven sites in the United States.

The Monarc Device

The Edwards Lifesciences Monarc device has distal and proximal stent-like anchors that are delivered through a 12-F guiding catheter into the CS. A unique metal strip, covered by a biodegradable material connects the two anchors. Once deployed, as a biodegradeable coating disintegrates, the connector shortens, thereby shortening the distance between the two anchors and cinching the CS, moving the posterior leaflet forward (Figure 19-9). Early human experience with the first-generation Edwards CS annuloplasty device, called Viking, was reported by Webb et al.[60] The Viking device has two nitinol stent-like anchors. The distal, smaller anchor lies near the junction of the great cardiac vein/CS junction, and the larger, proximal anchor is placed in the CS near its orifice. The anchors are connected by a unique spring-like segment that shortens over time at body temperature. As the connector shortens over a period of weeks after implantation, it indirectly displaces the posterior annulus anteriorly, which reduces annular diameter and septal-lateral dimensions. Five patients with chronic ischemic MR underwent percutaneous transvenous implantation of the Viking device. Distal injection through an angiographic catheter is used to opacify the CS. Radiopaque markers allow estimation of vessel length and diameter and selection of an appropriately sized implant. A suitable device was selected on the basis of the measured length and diameter of the target segment. A 12-F guiding catheter is advanced over a guide wire well into the CS, and the device delivery catheter is then passed over the wire, through the guiding catheter, and into the CS. The distal anchor is placed, preferably in the great cardiac vein, using radiopaque markers on the delivery catheter, retrograde injections through the guiding catheter, and left coronary arterial injections to monitor precise placement. When the devise is positioned correctly, the distal anchor is released by retracting the outer restraining sheath with the thumb slider mechanism on the delivery catheter handle. Slack is then removed from the bridge element by withdrawing and tensioning the delivery catheter, and the proximal anchor is positioned just within the CS ostium. The restraining

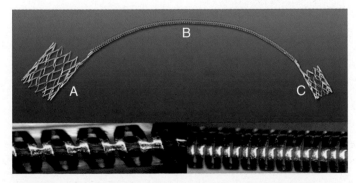

FIGURE 19-9 The MONARC device. *Top,* The distal anchor (C) and proximal anchor (A) are connected by a spring-like segment (B) that shortens over time. *Bottom left,* The spring-like connector at implantation. *Bottom right,* The shortened connector 6 weeks after implantation.

outer sheath is then completely retracted, and the delivery catheter and coaxial wire are removed. Migration of the anchors was not observed. Although there were no adverse clinical events associated with device separation, feasibility study enrollment was discontinued. The mitral annulus diameter at baseline was 36 ± 3 mm and at the 3-month follow-up was 35 ± 1 mm. No significant transmitral gradients were documented at any point during follow-up. LV EF at baseline was 42 ± 11% and at the 3-month follow-up was 50 ± 6%. NYHA functional class at baseline was 2.4 ± 0.5 and at the 3-month follow-up was 2 ± 0.7. Implantation was successful in four patients, although one patient did not have a decrease in MR grade at hospital discharge. Baseline MR in the entire group was grade 3.0 ± 0.7 and was reduced to grade 1.6 ± 1.1 at the last postimplantation visit when the device was intact or at the last postprocedural visit in the patient in whom the device was not successfully implanted. Separation of the bridge section of the device 28 to 81 days after implantation occurred in three of four implanted devices, with a resultant increase in MR. The authors concluded that percutaneous implantation of the Viking device intended to remodel the mitral annulus is feasible, although the favorable effects on MR were minimal.

The Monarc system is a second-generation percutaneous mitral annuloplasty device. Similar to the Viking device, but with a reinforced bridge connector, it is made of nitinol and consists of a larger proximal anchor, a flexible shortening bridge segment, and a smaller distal anchor. The Evolution phase I study is a prospective, multicenter feasibility study using the Monarc system.[61,62] The aim of the study is to evaluate the short-term safety of the Monarc system in treating patients with functional MR and heart failure. Patients must have functional MR 2+ or higher at echocardiography with dilated cardiomyopathy or myocardial infarction/ischemia. The CS must have a target length between 14 and 18 mm and distal target AIV diameter 3 mm or greater. Exclusion criteria include revascularization within the past 3 months, presence of an intracardiac defibrillator or pacing leads in the CS, EF less than 25%, mitral valve prolapse, or significant mitral annular calcification. Procedural success (correct device implantation and absence of in-hospital major cardiac events) and 30-day safety evaluation for the occurrence of death, tamponade, or myocardial infarction are end points. A secondary safety analysis monitored for the 90-day occurrence of device migration from the target area, death, myocardial infarction, device embolization, CS thrombosis, or pulmonary embolus. Enrollment has been completed with 55 patients receiving implants (Figure 19-10). More than 90.9% of patients had NYHA functional class II or III heart failure. Baseline EF was 36.4 ± 9.4% (range 22.7 to 55.2%). MR severity ranged from 2+ (51%) to 4+ (23%). The device was implanted in 49 of 55 patients (89%). Of the six patients who did not receive the device, four had tortuous anatomy and two had inappropriate CS dimensions. The device was implanted at the intended location and without major adverse cardiac events in 42 of the 49 patients (86%). The 30-day event-free survival from death, myocardial infarction, or cardiac tamponade was 90%. At 180 days an interim safety analysis indicated that nine patients had experienced a major adverse cardiac event (five deaths, two myocardial infarctions, and two cardiac tamponades). Three of these events were adjudicated as being device or procedure related. One patient experienced a myocardial infarction due to compression of a first diagonal branch from the distal anchor of the device; two patients had cardiac tamponade probably due to guide wire perforation of the CS.[63] Importantly, there were no bridge separations as occurred with the first-generation Viking device. MR reduction increased one grade or more from 30 to 180 days (48.5% and 92.3% of patients, respectively) as a result of the delayed bridge shortening. The Evolution II

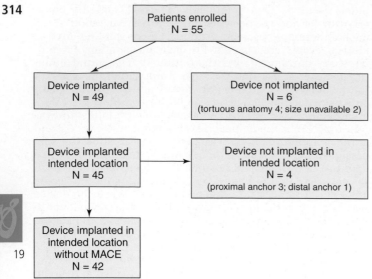

FIGURE 19–10 Ladder diagram of clinical outcome of initial studies of the MONARC device. Of 55 patients enrolled, 42 had the device implanted at the desired location without a major adverse cardiac event (MACE).

placed in the coronary sinus but is also passed through a myocardial path completely around the mitral annulus, exiting once again near the mouth of the coronary sinus. Presumably cinching of this device produces more complete reduction of the annular diameter and greater reduction of MR. Proof of theoretical use will have to await the outcome of animal and ultimately clinical trials.

Anatomic Limitations

Despite the ingenuity of these devices, there are important questions that arise concerning the anatomic relationship of the CS to the posterior annulus of the mitral valve and the coronary vessels. First, the proximal circumflex coronary artery shortly after its bifurcation from the left main coronary runs across the course of the CS. If the circumflex artery lies between the CS and the posterior annulus, any device that cinches the CS and has a distal anchor beyond the circumflex artery crossing will compress the artery and compromise blood flow to the posterolateral myocardium. In patients in whom the circumflex artery lies more lateral than the CS anchor or in whom the circumflex artery does not course between the annulus and CS but instead courses outside the CS, this is not a problem. The circumflex marginal coronary artery branches might present the same dilemma. Second, in many patients the CS does not course parallel to the posterior annulus but instead lies (usually) above it, overlying the left atrial muscle, or below it, over the left ventricle. A device that cinches or moves the left atrial wall forward might also displace the posterior annulus initially, but stretching of the more compliant left atrial muscle over time might result in reappearance of MR. Last, as the annulus of the mitral valve dilates, especially in heart failure due to cardiomyopathy, the CS changes in its relation to the posterior annulus and may elongate, making a CS device less effective. Despite these concerns, initial trials of these devices in humans seem to indicate that they may play a role in the treatment of selected patients with MR. Careful screening of patients using computed tomography and/or magnetic resonance imaging might help select those with the most favorable relationship of the CS to the mitral annulus who will have the highest likelihood of successful MR reduction using these devices.[44]

To more closely mimic the most common surgical strategies for mitral repair (direct valvular repair plus placement of an annuloplasty device), one might envision a combination of percutaneous strategies as well. Thus, direct clipping (or

study will be a nonrandomized multicenter prospective consecutive registry study in 19 clinical sites. End points are 30-day freedom from major adverse cardiovascular events and MR reduction of at least one grade from baseline.

Comparison of Devices

A comparison of clinically tested percutaneous CS annuloplasty devices is shown in Figure 19-11. Other designs using the CS might be also potentially useful. For example, constricting only a portion of the CS with a short device placed near its orifice, which also constricts a portion of the right atrial wall, might be useful in that only the medial portion of the CS is cinched by this device. Such medial cinching might be more effective in patients with ischemic posterior papillary muscle dysfunction, in patients with inferoposterior myocardial scarring in which the posterior medial portion of the posterior leaflet is most affected, or in patients with MR originating from the A3-P3 portion of the mitral valve. A "cerclage" device has been tested in animal models. This device is

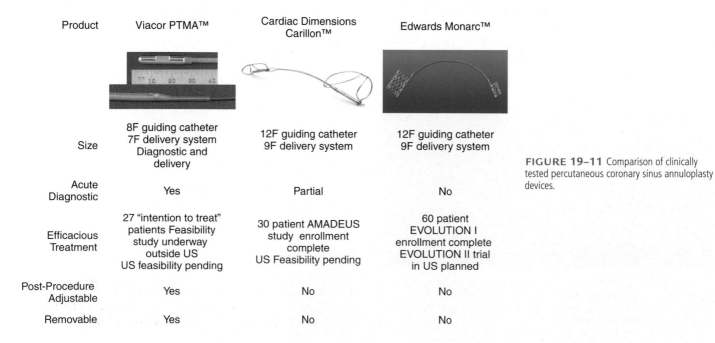

Product	Viacor PTMA™	Cardiac Dimensions Carillon™	Edwards Monarc™
Size	8F guiding catheter 7F delivery system Diagnostic and delivery	12F guiding catheter 9F delivery system	12F guiding catheter 9F delivery system
Acute Diagnostic	Yes	Partial	No
Efficacious Treatment	27 "intention to treat" patients Feasibility study underway outside US US feasibility pending	30 patient AMADEUS study enrollment complete US Feasibility pending	60 patient EVOLUTION I enrollment complete EVOLUTION II trial in US planned
Post-Procedure Adjustable	Yes	No	No
Removable	Yes	No	No

FIGURE 19–11 Comparison of clinically tested percutaneous coronary sinus annuloplasty devices.

other direct repair devices) might in the future be combined with percutaneous placement of a CS or other annuloplasty device. A potential advantage of such combined percutaneous therapy would be that the procedures could be staged. The results of initial direct valve repair could be assessed in the realistic clinical setting of an ambulatory patient. If reduction of MR is inadequate an additional percutaneous annuloplasty procedure could be performed at a later date.

Retrograde Transventricular Mitral Annuloplasty

Mitralign (Tewksbury, MA) has developed a percutaneous transcatheter system based on the concept of surgical suture annuloplasty. Initially the concept included placement of a CS catheter with magnets mounted at the tip behind the P2 segment of the posterior mitral leaflet. A retrograde LV catheter, also with a magnetic tip is advanced from the femoral artery, prolapsed across the aortic valve, and advanced up the posterolateral wall of the left ventricle between the two papillary muscles. The tip of the ventricular catheter lies behind the posterior mitral leaflet and rests against the underside of the mitral annulus at P2. The LV and CS catheters align because of their magnetic tips. Tests with later versions of the device have shown that the placement of a CS catheter and the magnetic tip alignment are not needed, and only a retrograde LV catheter is now used. The retrograde catheter is used for advancement of a special guide wire through the mitral annulus at P2 and into the left atrium. The catheter is removed and replaced with a guiding catheter. The guiding catheter is designed to allow deployment of two to four additional guide wires along the annulus both medial and lateral to the index wire so as to span the P1, P2, and P3 zones. The guiding catheter then serves as a conduit for delivery of specialized anchors into the annular tissue. Once in place, the anchors are cinched together, resulting in a 2- to 3-cm reduction in posterior annular circumference and 0.5- to 1.0-cm reduction in the septal-lateral dimension (Figure 19-12). The results of early studies in humans will determine whether this approach is feasible.

Left Atrial Devices

One device that uses both the CS and the left atrium in its design and function is the PS[3] System, being developed by Ample Medical (Foster City, CA). This system produces septal-lateral shortening of the mitral valve annulus. The system has proven safety and efficacy in animal models.[64] Temporary and permanent human implantations have been performed. The CAFÉ Trial will determine safety and efficacy

of permanent implantations.[65] A T-shaped anchor is first placed in the CS behind the posterior leaflet and a tether is placed across the left atrium and through an atrial septal anchor. The tether is then shortened, thereby pulling the posterior annulus toward the intra-atrial septum and shortening the septal-lateral dimension of the mitral valve and reducing MR (Figures 19-13 and 19-14).

The CS is first wired through a 12-F sheath introduced into the right internal jugular vein. The great cardiac vein (GCV) MagneCath, which has a shaped permanent magnet on its distal tip is then advanced into the great cardiac vein and centered over the mitral valve P2 scallop under fluoroscopic and echocardiographic guidance. With use of standard techniques, a transseptal puncture is then performed, and the tip of a 12-F Mullins catheter is placed into the left atrium. The left atrial (LA) MagneCath, also incorporating a shaped permanent magnet on its distal tip, is then advanced across the left atrium toward the posterior annulus, allowing magnetic linking of the GCV MagneCath and the LA MagneCath tips. A crossing catheter is then advanced from the LA MagneCath into the GCV MagneCath, making a small puncture in the posterior LA wall. A guide wire is passed from the left atrium into the CS and externalized as a continuous loop, and the MagneCaths are removed. The T-bar is then advanced into the CS over the wire, and the bridge is pulled back across the transseptal puncture using the 'loop guide wire and externalized at the right common femoral vein. A septal device similar to the Amplatzer PFO Occluder (AGA Medical, Golden Valley, MN) serves as the interatrial septal anchor. It is deployed over the bridge in a standard fashion, and progressive tension is applied on the bridge to cause septal-lateral shortening. Once the desired degree of shortening is achieved, as assessed by echocardiographic grading of MR reduction, the system is secured (see Figure 19-14).

The primary objective of the first two temporary implants in humans[65] was to evaluate the safety and feasibility of percutaneous septal-lateral shortening by using the PS[3] System. Patients had the PS[3] system implanted immediately before surgical mitral valve repair. Inclusion criteria included grade 2+ to 4+ MR with preserved leaflet anatomy, NYHA functional class II-IV, and LV EF less than 30%. Candidates were excluded if they had a myocardial infarction, coronary artery bypass grafting (CABG), or percutaneous coronary intervention within the last 3 months, calcified mitral annulus or subvalvular apparatus, prior mitral valve surgery, CS pacing leads, left atrial thrombus or left atrial diameter less than 40 mm, and body weight less than 50 kg. The PS[3] System was implanted percutaneously under echocardiographic and fluoroscopic guidance. At the completion of the implant, patients were transferred

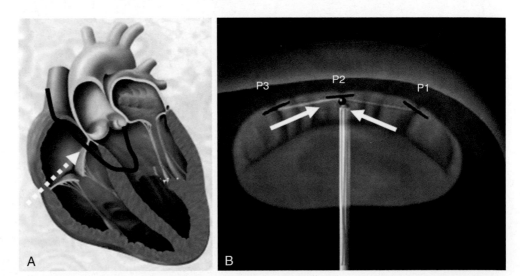

FIGURE 19–12 The Mitralign concept. **A,** A retrograde guiding catheter (*dotted arrow*) is placed with its tip behind the posterior mitral leaflet against the annulus. **B,** Anchors are placed in the mitral annular tissue spanning P1 to P3 through a retrograde catheter system and cinched together, reducing the mitral annulus and septal-lateral dimension (*arrows* indicate cinching of the anchors).

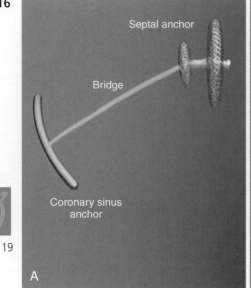
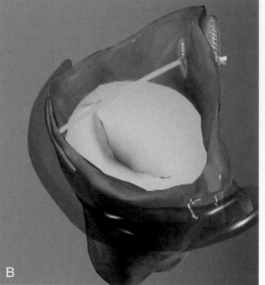

19

FIGURE 19–13 The Ample PS³ system. **A**, Device components consist of a coronary sinus anchor, bridge, and septal anchor. **B**, Schematic representation of the device in place. Reduction of the mitral septal-lateral dimension results from shortening the bridge between the septal wall and great cardiac vein anchors.

Septal anchor

Bridge

Coronary sinus anchor

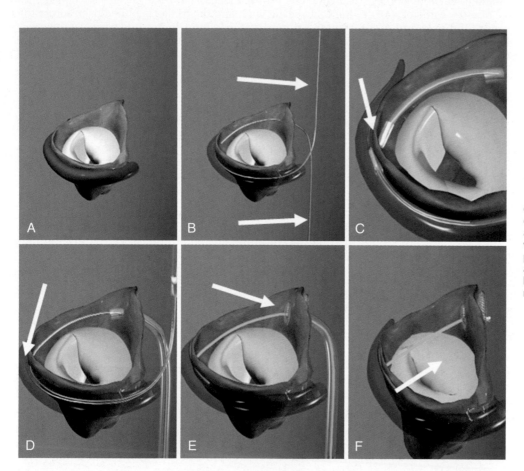

FIGURE 19–14 Sequence of placement of the Ample PS³ system. **A**, Left atrial view of coronary sinus and mitral valve. **B**, Guide wire access (*arrows*) from jugular vein and femoral vein. **C**, MagneCath delivery (*arrow*). **D**, Anchor placed in great cardiac vein (*arrow*). **E**, Septal anchor deployment (*arrow*). **F**, shortening of bridge results in septal-lateral shortening of the mitral valve (*arrow*).

to the cardiac surgical operating room, where cardiopulmonary bypass was initiated, and the right and left atria were examined under direct visualization to assess device implantation. The device was then removed under direct observation, and surgery proceeded as planned. In both cases, the MagneCaths were delivered successfully and the PS³ System was implanted successfully without significant arrhythmia or hemodynamic instability. In both patients, significant stepwise septal-lateral shortening was achieved with septal-lateral

reductions of 29% and 31%, respectively. In both patients MR was reduced (2+ to 1+ in the first patient and 3+ to 1+ in the second patient). Left coronary/great cardiac vein angiography showed no compromise of the left circumflex coronary artery in either patient after device implantation. Strong safety and efficacy have been demonstrated in 6-month animal experiments.[66] The PS3 system has the unique feature that in addition to shortening the septal-lateral dimension of the mitral annulus by direct tension of the bridge the posterior annulus and the upper posterior myocardium are also pulled upward, thereby helping support the posterior myocardium in patients with ventricular scarring or dilation.

Another unique concept for treatment of MR relies on heating the mitral annular collagen to cause the collagen strands to shorten. Collagen shortening in turn shortens the length of the mitral annulus, moves the posterior leaflet forward, and reduces MR. The QuantumCor approach is based on the principle that the mitral valve annulus has a high collagen content. Radiofrequency energy is applied directly to the mitral annular tissue through a catheter system, causing the covalent bonds to break and the collagen to shrink.

The QuantumCor device is a heat probe that can be shaped to conform to the mitral annulus. The unique properties of this approach are that the valve annulus is treated directly, no specific patient anatomy is required for the technology to be effective, and no foreign body is left behind in the circulation.

The QuantumCor technology remodels the native annular collagen. As healing occurs, new collagen forms, infiltrating the areas treated previously. In addition, because small segments of the annulus are treated, some annular tissue is not affected by the initial procedure. If, over time, additional annular remodeling is needed, repeat procedures on untreated segments of tissue as well as newly deposited collagen are feasible. The QuantumCor technology has undergone preclinical testing in acute and chronic animal studies (Figure 19-15). The study objectives were to validate the energy protocol, achieve acute remodeling consistent with clinical expectations, and verify that remodeling was maintained over 180 days. These studies were done via a surgical approach, with direct visualization in a still heart with no blood flow. In acute animal studies the septal-lateral and anteroposterior mitral valve dimensions were measured using intracardiac echocardiography. The posterior annulus was then directly treated with the animal on cardiopulmonary bypass. Direct measurements were done to confirm acute annular shrinkage. Seven animals were followed chronically. Clinically appropriate remodeling of the mitral annulus was achieved in all animals with mean shrinkage of 22% (Figure 19-16). In the four animals that completed the 180-day study, the degree of remodeling was 21.5% immediately after the procedure and 26% at 180 days (personal communication, QuantumCor, December 2007). Early human trials for safety and efficacy are underway.

Theoretically it would seem possible to place a device within the left atrium similar to the annuloplasty rings that are inserted surgically. To completely mimic surgical placement such a device would have to span the posterior annulus from trigone to trigone of the native valve and produce contraction of the annulus by plicating sutures or similar effects. Such a device would have to be easily passed through a transseptal guiding catheter and then be positioned exactly. Although these requirements might pose difficult technical challenges, the result would be a device that constrained the posterior mitral annulus in a manner closely similar to surgical repair.

The normally functioning LV myocardium, papillary muscles, chordae tendineae, and mitral leaflets work together in concert to achieve an adequate line of coaptation of the mitral valve and an absence of MR. To function properly, these supporting structures must lie within a virtual cylinder that has its upper opening above the mitral annulus and its lower opening at the LV apex (Figure 19-17). Any abnormality of the intraventricular supporting structures that results in displacement of the mitral apparatus outside of this virtual cylinder will produce MR. For example, inferoposterior myocardial infarction results in myocardial thinning and expansion. In addition, the posterior papillary muscle may also be affected, with shortening and fibrosis. Because of dilation of the inferoposterior myocardial wall and compensatory remodeling of the remaining myocardium, the papillary muscle with its attached chordae tendineae tether the posterior leaflet so that the line of coaptation is no longer adequate, and MR occurs. Similarly, in cardiomyopathy, MR develops as the left ventricle thins and dilates (see Figure 19-17). As the left ventricle dilates to accommodate the increased volume need, further displacement of the papillary muscles and annular dilation occur, increasing MR.[67,68] Because of these pathophysiologic principles, the strategy of simple placement of an annuloplasty device, with or without direct anatomic repair, is frequently inadequate to decrease MR long term, especially in patients with ischemic cardiomyopathy.[69,70] Thus, unique devices that support and reposition the myocardium as well as the mitral annulus have been developed.

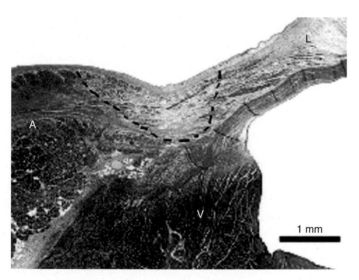

FIGURE 19–15 Histopathologic section of mitral annulus after treatment with the QuantumCor device (Masson's trichrome stain). The *dotted black line* outlines an area of necrosis and fibrosis. L, mitral leaflet, V, left ventricle, A, atrium.

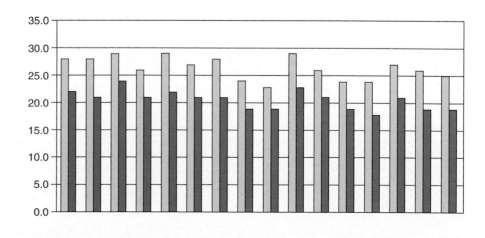

FIGURE 19–16 Mitral valve anteroposterior dimension measurements before (blue bars) and after (red bars) treatment in 16 animals with the QuantumCor device. The mean reduction was 23.8% with a measured mean anteroposterior reduction of 5.75 ± 0.86 mm. *x*-axis, anteroposterior dimension in millimeters.

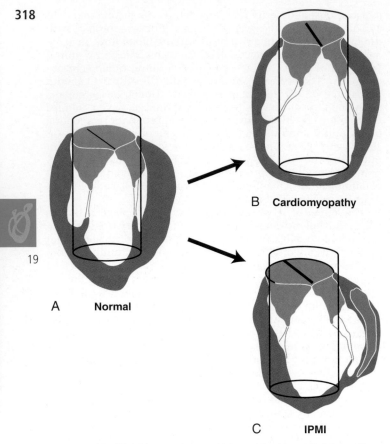

B **Cardiomyopathy**

19

A **Normal**

C **IPMI**

FIGURE 19–17 A, Diagram of a normal left ventricle without MR. A "virtual" cylinder from the mitral annulus to the ventricular apex encompasses the mitral leaflets, chordae tendineae, and papillary muscles. **B**, Diagram of a dilated ventricle in idiopathic cardiomyopathy. Most of the supporting structures of both mitral leaflets lie outside the virtual cylinder. MR is present because of loss of mitral coaptation and annular dilation. **C**, Diagram of the left ventricle after inferoposterior myocardial infarction (IPMI). Note that the virtual cylinder no longer encloses the posterior papillary muscle and chordal tips. Tethering of the posterior leaflet results in MR.

Myocardial/Annular Support Devices

The Coapsys Device

The surgical Coapsys device (Myocor, Maple Grove, MN) was designed to treat both mitral annular dilation and LV geometry changes. It has the advantages of being implanted at the time of CABG surgery on a closed and beating heart without atriotomy or cardiopulmonary bypass and associated aortic cross-clamp and can also be adjusted intraoperatively under echocardiographic guidance. The implant is designed to decrease mitral annular septal-lateral dimensions and reposition and stabilize the papillary muscles, thereby reducing MR by improving leaflet coaptation. It consists of posterior and anterior pads connected by a flexible, subvalvular chord (Figure 19-18). The two pads are placed on the epicardial surface of the heart with the load-bearing subvalvular chord passing across the left ventricle. The posterior pad has superior and inferior heads configured to create shape change at the mitral annular level as well as the LV free wall at the level of the papillary muscles. The relative positioning of the posterior and anterior pads allows the chord to pass through the left ventricle in a subvalvular path between the papillary muscles and below the valve leaflets, ensuring that the implant does not affect the function of these structures. The device is sized by shortening the subvalvular chord that draws the anterior and posterior pads together. The anterior pad is fixed to the subvalvular chord after the device is sized.

Clinical indications for the Coapsys device have focused on patient groups that have essentially normal leaflet pathology and motion, with MR attributable mainly to annular dilation or papillary muscle displacement alone or in combination. The device is not intended to treat MR arising from primary degenerative MR.

Preclinical studies with the Coapsys implant investigated the acute and chronic physiologic effects of ventricular shape change on mitral valve repair in a canine tachycardia-induced dilated cardiomyopathy model. The results of these studies indicated that the Coapsys device was well tolerated, produced no immediate harmful effects, and generated significant improvements in mitral valve function.[71]

The prospective, nonrandomized, single-center feasibility study Treatment of Functional Mitral Regurgitation without Atriotomy or CPB Clinical Evaluation [TRACE]) was designed to evaluate the intraoperative treatment of ischemic functional MR in patients using the Coapsys device. In this trial, patients referred for CABG with preoperative ischemic MR (grade 2 or higher) were included in the study. Patients with structural abnormalities of the mitral apparatus identified by echocardiography were excluded. During surgery and after completion of all grafts, patients were evaluated by TEE for MR status, and the Coapsys device was implanted in those who demonstrated post-CABG intraoperative MR of grade 2 or higher. In a subset of 11 patients completing a 1-year echocardiographic follow-up from the TRACE trial, Mishra et al[72,73] detailed the chronic efficacy of the Coapsys implant for the treatment of ischemic MR. These patients were followed serially at baseline, and at 1, 3, and 12 months after implantation. The MR grade was reduced from 2.9 ± 0.5 at baseline to 1.1 ± 0.6 after 12 months. Clinical assessment of NYHA functional status in these patients demonstrated significant improvement from 2.5 ± 0.5 at baseline to 1.2 ± 0.4 after 12 months. In a subsequent analysis from the same trial, Mittal et al[75] described chronic changes in LV geometry in a set of 24 patients. In this patient cohort, MR was reduced from 3.0 ± 0.6 at baseline to 1.2 ± 1.2 after 12 months. Statistically significant reductions occurred in end-diastolic and end-systolic diameters, as well as in the LV length. In addition, there was a statistically significant improvement of EF 12 months after Coapsys implantation, which implies ongoing reverse remodeling of the myocardium. From baseline to the 1-year follow-up, the effect on MR grade, MR jet area, and NYHA functional class were, respectively, 2.9 ± 0.5 to 1.1 ± 0.8, 7.4 ± 2.9 to $3.0 \pm 1.6 \, cm^2$, and 2.5 ± 0.5 to 1.2 ± 0.4 (all $P < 0.05$ versus baseline). A corresponding reduction in both LV end-diastolic and end-systolic dimensions was also seen, decreasing from approximately 5.5 cm to about 4.8 cm and from 4.7 cm to 4.2 cm, respectively (Figure 19-19). There were no deaths, device failures, reemergence of grade 3+ or 4+ MR, heart failure readmission, or valve reoperations.[72-75]

Although this device showed initial promise, the Coapsys Annuloplasty System is no longer being evaluated.

Percutaneous Approaches

A logical next step stemming from surgical implantation is that intrapericardial positioning of the pads of the Coapsys device can also be performed using percutaneous catheters. The iCoapsys device is such a percutaneous adaptation that is based on the success of the surgically placed Coapsys device.

A large-bore short catheter is first placed just inside the parietal pericardium from a subxiphoid approach. The first catheter to be positioned through the access catheter is the intracardiac echocardiography (ICE) probe delivery catheter. This malleable coaxial catheter with a distal vacuum stabilization cup was loaded with an 8- or 10-F AcuNav (Siemens Medical

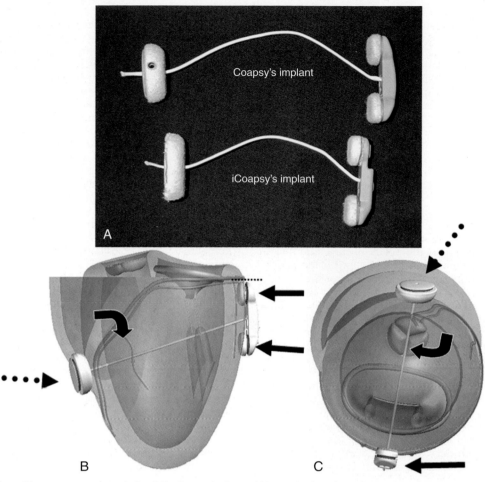

FIGURE 19–18 The Myocor/Coapsys transventricular device. **A**, The Coapsys implant and iCoapsys implant. The implants consist of two epicardial pads connected by a flexible subvalvular chord. Each is constructed of biocompatible implant materials. **B** and **C**, The superior head of the posterior pad is positioned at the mitral annular level; the inferior head at a level just above the papillary muscles (*solid arrows*). The subvalvular chord (*curved arrows*) traverses the left ventricle and passes through the anterior pad (*dotted arrows*) placed just to the right of the interventricular groove.

FIGURE 19–19 Reduction in grade of mitral regurgitation grade (*left*) and left ventricular dimensions (*right*) in 15 patients in the TRACE feasibility trial. Mitral regurgitation (MR) grade measured at baseline, discharge from hospital and 1 month and 12 months after implant. Both left ventricular (LV) end-diastolic dimension (LVEDD) and left ventricular end-systolic dimension (LVESD) are decreased at 1 year compared with baseline.

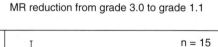

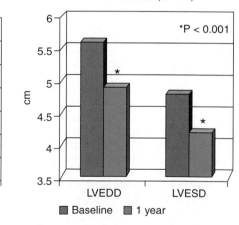

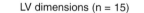

Systems, Malvern, PA) ICE imaging probe for positioning on the anterior surface of the heart. Combined left coronary and right ventriculography is carried out to establish landmarks for the anterior epicardial pad. The catheter containing the ICE transducer is positioned 1 to 2 cm medial to the mid-left anterior descending coronary artery (LAD) and over a septal muscle band that extends from the interventricular septum into the right ventricle and is seen on right ventricular angiography. Additional adjustments in catheter position can be made to

display ICE images from the catheter tip of the left ventricle in short axis, extending from the mid-papillary muscles apically and to the mitral annulus at the base. This catheter tip is then temporarily fixed in place with vacuum.

A posterior sighting catheter is then advanced through the access sheath so its tip lies on the posterior epicardial surface. Its distal vacuum cup is positioned on the mid-posterior LV wall using left coronary angiographic guidance for placement 2 to 3 cm apical to the circumflex coronary artery in the atrioventricular groove. Fine adjustments of the posterior catheter tip are made using epicardial ICE guidance to establish placement of the posterior cup midway between the papillary muscles (see Figure 19-6B). Vacuum is applied for posterior cup fixation. Fluoroscopy in multiple angulated views is used to establish a view that results in precise superimposition of the anterior ICE imaging transducer over the posterior sighting cup. The ICE delivery catheter is then removed and replaced by an anterior sighting catheter and the distal vacuum cup is placed on the anterior epicardial surface. The anterior sighting catheter is adjusted so that it is superimposed over the posterior cup in the "sighting view" and vacuum is applied for fixation. Left coronary angiography is performed while the anterior sighting cup is positioned to confirm placement 1 to 2 cm medial to the mid-LAD segment.

By centering ring markers on the anterior and posterior sighting cups, the anterior sighting catheter is adjusted to precisely aim the anterior cup at the posterior cup, and a snare is deployed in the left ventricle. A needle and leader assembly is then passed through the posterior catheter until the tip of the needle is through the snare. The posterior needle and leader assembly is snared and exteriorized through the anterior LV catheter. Both sighting catheters are removed, leaving the leader behind with both ends exteriorized. The subvalvular chord is attached to the leader and drawn from the posterior ventricular puncture out the anterior puncture, leaving both ends exteriorized.

The posterior pad mounted on its delivery catheter is attached to the posterior side of the subvalvular chord, inserted through the access sheath, and positioned on the posterior epicardial surface under coronary angiographic guidance. A steering lever permits precise longitudinal orientation of the pad segments at the papillary muscle and valve annulus levels. The anterior side of the subvalvular chord is threaded though the anterior pad attached to its delivery catheter and tracked onto the anterior surface of the heart. A similar steering lever on the proximal end of the anterior delivery catheter is used to orient the anterior pad parallel to the LAD with left coronary angiographic guidance. The anterior-posterior pad distance is reduced by tensioning the subvalvular chord using a sizing instrument, until MR is appropriately reduced. A staple is then locked on the subvalvular chord, securing the chord to the pad. It is important to note the implant up to this point can be completely withdrawn or different sized pads can be exchanged and repositioned. The anterior and posterior pad delivery catheters are removed and a cautery device is used to trim the remaining anterior portion of the subvalvular chord.

Only two patients were treated using this device. In the first patient right ventricular perforation occurred before introduction of the therapeutic catheters, and the procedure was abandoned. In the second patient the device was successfully deployed and MR significantly reduced. Although the intrapericardial therapeutic route and the iCoapsys device are novel and have promise, trials evaluating the safety and efficacy of this approach have been suspended for now (personal communication, Myocor, Oct 2008).

PERCUTANEOUS MITRAL VALVE REPLACEMENT

Some mitral valvular pathologic conditions are simply not amenable to repair. Severe rheumatic mitral valve fibrosis and calcification and valvular damage from endocarditis are two extreme examples. Thus, mitral valve replacement (MVR) is still a common surgical approach in many patients with MR. Over the last few years the dream of percutaneous MVR has edged closer to reality. There are many problems to

be overcome. Unlike percutaneous aortic valve replacement, in which rotational position of the device seems unimportant, MVR may have to be more exact. This is true especially if the supporting structures of the replacement valve could cause obstruction of the LV outflow tract. In addition, the native valve leaflets must remain behind. Thus, the support mechanism for the replacement valve might cause direct obstruction due to anterior displacement of the septal leaflet of the native mitral valve or might cause systolic anterior mitral leaflet motion with resulting outflow tract obstruction. In addition, the mitral annulus is not as delineated a structure as the aortic annulus, and exact placement within the mitral annulus as well as anchoring of a percutaneously placed valve will be difficult. Last, transcatheter placement whether via a transseptal or retrograde route will require planar deployment of the replacement valve such that the native leaflets do not interfere with the function of the replacement valve.

Despite all of these issues, unique engineering solutions for percutaneous MVR are being developed and tested in animal models. It is likely that initial attempts of transcatheter mitral valve placements in humans will be made in association with minimally invasive surgery. Thus, a transatrial or transapical approach to replacement will be a reasonable early strategy. Ultimately, because the transseptal route offers the major advantage that the femoral or internal jugular veins are large diameter, compliant vessels, it is likely that deployment will be through those vessels or be done transapically similar to present transapical aortic valve replacement.[76] Early animal feasibility experiments are under way. It seems likely that, just as percutaneous aortic valve replacement has led to multicenter phase II trials we will see the same kind of trials for percutaneous MVR in the future. These are all works in progress, and which technologies will be winners and losers is conjecture. Ultimately clinical trials will furnish the necessary data to make those decisions.

REFERENCES

1. Rosen SE, Borer JS, Hochreiter C, et al: Natural history of the asymptomatic/minimally symptomatic patient with severe mitral regurgitation secondary to mitral valve prolapse and normal right and left ventricular performance. Am J Cardiol 1994;74: 374-380.
2. Ling LH, Enriquez-Sarano M, Seward JB, et al: Clinical outcome of mitral regurgitation due to flail leaflet. N Engl J Med 1996;335:1417-1423.
3. Rosen SE, Borer JS, Hochreiter C, et al: Natural history of the asymptomatic/minimally symptomatic patient with severe mitral regurgitation secondary to mitral valve prolapse and normal right and left ventricular performance. Am J Cardiol 1994;74:374-380.
4. Yoran C, Yellin EI, Becker RM, et al: Mechanism of reduction of mitral regurgitation with vasodilator therapy. Am J Cardiol 1979;43:773-777.
5. Capomullu S, Febo O, Gnemmi M, et al: β-blockade therapy in chronic heart failure: diastolic function and mitral regurgitation improvement by carvedilol. Am Heart J 2000;139:596-608.
6. Linde C, Leclercq C, Rex S, et al: long-term benefits of biventricular pacing in congestive heart failure: results from the MUltisite STimulation in cardiomyopathy (MUST) study. J Am Coll Cardiol 2002;40:111-118.
7. Breithardt OA, Sinha AM, Schwammental E, et al: Acute effects of cardiac resynchronization therapy on functional mitral regurgitation in advanced systolic heart failure. J Am Coll Cardiol 2003;41:765-770.
8. St John Sutton MG, Plappert T, Abraham WT, et al: Effect of cardiac resynchronization therapy on left ventricular size and function in chronic heart failure. Circulation 2003;107:1985-1990.
9. Bonow RO, Carabello B, Chatterjee K, et al: ACC/AHA 2006 Guidelines for the Management of Patients with Valvular Heart Disease: Executive Summary. A report of the American College of Cardiology/American Heart Association Task Force on Practice Guidelines. Circulation 2006;114:450-527.
10. Alfieri O, Maisano F, DeBonis M, et al: The edge-to-edge technique in mitral valve repair: a simple solution for complex problems. J Thorac Cardiovasc Surg 2001;122:674-681.
11. Maisano F. Caldarola A. Blasio A, et al: Midterm results of edge-to-edge mitral valve repair without annuloplasty. J Thorac Cardiovasc Surg 2003;126:1987-1997.
12. Kherani AR, Cheema FH, Casher J, et al: Edge-to-edge mitral valve repair: the Columbia Presbyterian experience. Ann Thorac Surg 2004;78:73-76.
13. Mohty D, Orszulak TA, Schaff HV, et al: Very long-term survival and durability of mitral valve repair for mitral valve prolapse. Circulation 2001;104(Suppl I):I-1-I-17.
14. David TE: Techniques and results of mitral valve repair for ischemic mitral regurgitation. J Card Surg 1994;9:274-277.
15. Kron IL, Green GR, Cope JT: Surgical relocation of the posterior papillary muscle in chronic ischemic mitral regurgitation. Ann Thorac Surg 2002;74:600-601.

16. Hvass U, Tapia M, Baron F, et al: Papillary muscle sling: a new functional approach to mitral repair in patients with ischemic left ventricular dysfunction and functional mitral regurgitation. Ann Thorac Surg 2003;75:809-811.

17. Mickleborough LL: Is mitral valvuloplasty always indicated in patients with poor left ventricular function and ischemic cardiomyopathy? J Thorac Cardiovasc Surg 2001;121:97.

18. Timek TA, Lai DT, Tibayan F, et al: Septal-lateral annular cinching abolishes acute ischemic mitral regurgitation. J Thorac Cardiovasc Surg 2002;123:881-888.

19. Grossi EA, Goldberg JD, LaPietra A, et al: Ischemic mitral valve reconstruction and replacement: comparison of long-term survival and complications. J Thorac Cardiovasc Surg 2001;122:1107-1124.

20. Wu AH, Aaronson KD, Bolling SF, et al: Impact of mitral valve annuloplasty on mortality risk in patients with mitral regurgitation and left ventricular systolic dysfunction. J Am Coll Cardiol 2005;45:381-387.

21. Romano MA. Bolling SF: Update on mitral repair in dilated cardiomyopathy. J Cardiac Surg 2004;19:396-400.

22. Bolling SF: Mitral reconstruction in cardiomyopathy. J Heart Valve Dis 2002;11(Suppl 1): S26-S31.

23. Harris KM, Sundt TM III, Aeppli D, et al: Can late survival of patients with moderate ischemic mitral regurgitation be impacted by intervention on the valve? Ann Thorac Surg 2002;74:1468-1475.

24. Gillinov AM, Cosgrove DM, Lytle BW, et al: Reoperation for failure of mitral valve repair. J Thorac Cardiovasc Surg 1997;113:467-473.

25. Gillinov AM, Cosgrove DM, Blackstone EH, et al: Durability of mitral valve repair for degenerative disease. J Thorac Cardiovasc Surg 1998;116:734-743.

26. Gillinov AM, Cosgrove DM: Mitral valve repair for degenerative disease. J Heart Valve Dis 2002;11(Suppl 1):S15-S20.

27. Mohty D, Enriquez-Sarano M: The long-term outcome of mitral valve repair for mitral valve prolapse. Curr Cardiol Rep 2002;4:104-110.

28. Maisano F, Vigano G, Blasio A, et al: Surgical isolated central Alfieri mitral repair intentionally without annuloplasty: "Clinical proof of principle for an endovascular approach." Eurointervention 2006;2:181-186.

29. Silvestry F, Rodriguez L, Herrmann H, et al: Echocardiographic guidance and assessment of percutaneous repair for mitral regurgitation with the Evalve MitraClip: lessons learned from EVEREST. J Am Soc Echocardiogr 2007;20:1131-1140.

30. Foster E, Wasserman HS, Gray W, et al: Quantitative assessment of severity of mitral regurgitation by serial echocardiography in a multicenter clinical trial of percutaneous mitral valve repair. Am J Cardiol 2007;100:1577-1583.

31. Feldman T, Wasserman HS, Herrmann HC, et al: Percutaneous mitral valve repair using the edge-to-edge technique: six-month results of the EVEREST phase I clinical trial. J Am Coll Cardiol, 2005;46:2134-2140.

32. Feldman T: EVEREST Registry (Endovascular Valve Edge-to-Edge Repair Studies) reduction in mitral regurgitation 12 months following percutaneous mitral valve repair [Abstract]. Clin Cardiol 2007;30:416-417.

33. Herrmann HC, Kar S, Fail P, et al: Stability of mitral valve area and gradient following percutaneous repair of mitral regurgitation with the MitraClip device [Abstract]. J Am Coll Cardiol 2008;51:B79.

34. Bonow RO, Carabello B, de Leon AC, et al: ACC/AHA Guidelines for the Management of Patients with Valvular Heart Disease. A Report of the American College of Cardiology/American Heart Association Task Force on Practice Guidelines (Committee on Management of Patients with Valvular Heart Disease). J Am Coll Cardiol 1998;32: 1486-1582.

35. Carabello BA, Kar S, Rinaldi M, et al: Significant reverse remodeling of the left ventricle one year after percutaneous mitral repair with the MitraClip® device in patients with pre-existing systolic LV Dysfunction [Abstract]. Circulation 2007;116(Suppl II):II-357.

36. Stewart JA, Wei C, Brower GL, et al: Cardiac mast cell- and chymase-mediated matrix metalloproteinase activity and left ventricular remodeling in mitral regurgitation in the dog. J Mol Cell Cardiol 2003;35:311-319.

37. Urabe Y, Mann DL, Kent RL, et al: Cellular and ventricular contractile dysfunction in experimental canine mitral regurgitation. Circ Res 1992;70:131-147.

38. Tallaj J, Wei CC, Hankes GH, et al: β_1-Adrenergic receptor blockade attenuates angiotensin II-mediated catecholamine release into the cardiac interstitium in mitral regurgitation. Circulation 2003;108:225-230.

39. Schultz D, Su X, Wei CC, et al: Downregulation of ANG II receptor is associated with compensated pressure-overload hypertrophy in the young dog. Am J Physiol Heart Circ Physiol 2002;282:H749-H756.

40. Perry GJ, Wei C-C, Hankes GH, et al: Angiotensin II receptor blockade does not improve left ventricular function and remodeling in subacute mitral regurgitation in the dog. J Am Coll Cardiol 2002;39:1374-1379.

41. Beeri R, Yosefy C, Guerrero JL, et al: Early repair of moderate ischemic mitral regurgitation reverses left ventricular remodeling: a functional and molecular study. Circulation 2007;116(Suppl I):I-288-I-293.

42. Wakiyama H, Okada Y, Kitamura A, et al: Chordal cutting for the treatment of ischemic mitral regurgitation: two case reports. J Cardiol 2004;44:113-117.

43. El Maasarany S, Ferrett CG, Firth A, et al: The coronary sinus conduit function: anatomical study (relationship to adjacent structures). Europace 2005;7:475-481.

44. Choure AJ, Garcia MJ, Hesse B, et al: In vivo analysis of the anatomical relationship of coronary sinus to mitral annulus and left circumflex coronary artery using cardiac multidetector computed tomography: implications for percutaneous coronary sinus mitral annuloplasty. J Am Coll Cardiol 2006;48:1938-1945.

45. Maselli D, Guarracino F, Chiaramonti F, et al: Percutaneous mitral annuloplasty: an anatomic study of human coronary sinus and its relation with mitral valve annulus and coronary arteries. Circulation 2006;114:377-380.

46. Tops LF, Van de Veire NR, Schuijf JD, et al: Noninvasive evaluation of coronary sinus anatomy and its relation to the mitral valve annulus: implications for percutaneous mitral annuloplasty. Circulation 2007;115:1426-1432.

47. Shinbane JS, Lesh MD, Stevenson WG, et al: Anatomic and electrophysiologic relation between the coronary sinus and mitral annulus: implications for ablation of left-sided accessory pathways. Am Heart J 1998;135:93-98.

48. Liddicoat JR, MacNeill BD, Gillinov AM, et al: Percutaneous mitral valve repair: a feasibility study in an ovine model of acute ischemic mitral regurgitation. Catheter Cardiovasc Interv 2003;60:410-416.

49. Daimon M, Shiota T, Gillinov M, et al: Percutaneous mitral valve repair for chronic ischemic mitral regurgitation: a real time three-dimensional echocardiographic study in an ovine model. Circulation 2005;11:2183-2189.

50. Feldman T: Percutaneous mitral annuloplasty: not always a cinch. Catheter Cardiovasc Interv 2007;69:1062-1063.

51. Daimon M, Gillinov AM, Liddicoat JR, et al: Dynamic change in mitral annular area and motion during percutaneous mitral annuloplasty for ischemic mitral regurgitation: preliminary animal study with real-time 3-dimensional echocardiography. J Am Soc Echocardiogr 2007;20:381-388.

52. Dubreuil O, Basmadjian A, Ducharme A, et al: Percutaneous mitral valve annuloplasty for ischemic mitral regurgitation: first in man experience with a temporary implant. Catheter Cardiovasc Interv 2007;69:1053-1061.

53. Noble S, Bilodeau L: Traitement percutané des atteintes valvulaires aortiques et mitrales [Percutaneous therapies for aortic and mitral valvular disease]. Rev Méd Suisse 2007;3:1360-1367.

54. Kaye DM, Byrne M, Alferness C, et al: Feasibility and short-term efficacy of percutaneous mitral annular reduction for the therapy of heart failure-induced mitral regurgitation. Circulation 2003;108:1795-1797.

55. Maniu CV, Patel JB, Reuter DG, et al: Acute and chronic reduction of functional mitral regurgitation in experimental heart failure by percutaneous mitral annuloplasty. J Am Coll Cardiol 2004;44:1652-1661.

56. Byrne MJ, Kaye DM, Mathis M, Reuter DG: Percutaneous mitral annular reduction provides continued benefit in an ovine model of dilated cardiomyopathy Circulation 2004;110:3088-3092.

57. Duffy SJ, Federman J, Farrington C, et al: Feasibility and short-term efficacy of percutaneous mitral annular reduction for the therapy of mitral regurgitation in patients with heart failure. Catheter Cardiovasc Interv 2006;68:205-210.

58. Siminiak TL, Jerzykowska O, Kalmucki P, et al: Percutaneous valve repair for mitral regurgitation using the Carillon Mitral Contour System: description of the method and case report. Kardiol Pol 2007;65:272-278.

59. Schofer J: The Carillon experience. Paper presented at EuroPCR, May, 24, 2007, Barcelona, Spain.

60. Webb JG, Harnek J, Munt B, et al: Percutaneous transvenous mitral annuloplasty: initial human experience with device implantation in the coronary sinus. Circulation 2006;113:851-855.

61. Kuck K, Webb J, Harnek J, et al: Percutaneous treatment of functional mitral regurgitation: interim evolution study results with the MONARC system [Abstract]. Am J Cardiol 2007;100:58L.

62. Harnek J: The MONARC Experience. Paper presented at EuroPCR, May 24, 2007, Barcelona, Spain.

63. Piazza N, Bonan R: Transcatheter mitral valve repair for functional mitral regurgitation: coronary sinus approach. J Interv Cardiol 2007;20:495-508.

64. Rogers JH, Macoviak JA, Rahdert DA, et al: Percutaneous septal sinus shortening: a novel procedure for the treatment of functional mitral regurgitation. Circulation 2006;113:2329-2334.

65. Palacios IF, Condado JA, Brandi S, et al: Safety and feasibility of acute percutaneous septal sinus shortening: first-in-human experience. Catheter Cardiovasc Interv 2007;69:513-518.

66. Rogers J, Palacios I, Condado J, et al: Long-term durability of percutaneous septal-sinus shortening [Abstract]. Am J Cardiol 2007;100:58L.

67. Kono T, Sabbah HN, Rosman H, et al: Left ventricular shape is the primary determinant of functional mitral regurgitation in heart failure. J Am Coll Cardiol 1992;7:1594-1598.

68. Boltwood CM, Tei C, Wong M, et al: Quantitative echocardiography of the mitral complex in dilated heart failure: the mechanism of functional mitral regurgitation. Circulation 1983;68:498-508.

69. McGee EC, Gillinov AM, Blackstone EH, et al: Recurrent mitral regurgitation after annuloplasty for functional ischemic mitral regurgitation. J Thorac Cardiovasc Surg 2004;128:916-924.

70. Lachmann J, Shirani J, Plestis KA, et al: Mitral ring annuloplasty: an incomplete correction of functional mitral regurgitation associated with left ventricular remodeling. Curr Cardiol Rep 2001;3:241-246.

71. Inoue M, McCarthy PM, Popovic ZB, et al: Mitral valve repair without cardiopulmonary bypass or atriotomy using the Coapsys device: device design and implantation procedure in canine functional mitral regurgitation model. Heart Surg Forum 2004;7:E117-E121.

72. Trehan N, Mishra YK, Mittal S: Off -pump valve repair using the Coapsys device: a feasibility study in patients with functional mitral regurgitation [Abstract]. Int J Cardiothorac Vasc Surg 2003;19:2.

73. Mishra YK, Mittal S, Jaguri P, et al: Coapsys mitral annuloplasty for chronic functional ischemic mitral regurgitation: 1 year results. Ann Thorac Surg 2006;81:42-46.

74. Mittal S, Mishra Y, Trehan N: Coapsys® leads to global reversal of left ventricular remodeling: expanded TRACE study analysis [Abstract]. Circulation 2007;116(suppl II):II-373.

75. Grossi EA, Saunders PC, Woo YJ, et al: Intraoperative effects of the Coapsys annuloplasty system in a randomized evaluation (RESTOR-MV) of functional ischemic mitral regurgitation. Ann Thorac Surg 2005;80:1706-1711.

76. Lichtenstein SV, Cheung A Ye J, et al: Transapical transcatheter aortic valve implantation in humans: initial clinical experience. Circulation 2006;114:591-596.

Intraoperative Echocardiography for Mitral Valve Disease

Pravin M. Shah

KEY POINTS

- Transesophageal echocardiography provides a roadmap to the surgeon regarding location and severity of mitral valve pathologic lesions.
- Transesophageal echocardiography provides the ability to detect unexpected associated lesions such as patent foramen ovale, atrial septal defect, other valve disease, and aortic atheromatous disease
- Transesophageal echocardiography is used to confirm results of surgical procedures on the mitral valve.
- Results of mitral valve repair are greatly enhanced by a well-functioning echocardiography/surgical team using a common descriptive language.
- An assessment for paravalvular regurgitation after valve replacement could prevent a future need for reoperation.
- Real-time three-dimensional echocardiography using a transesophageal echocardiography probe is now feasible.
- Real-time three-dimensional transesophageal echocardiography has the potential to provide accurate orientation of pathologic valve lesions.

The modern era of mitral valve surgery began about 60 years ago, starting with closed mitral commissurotomy followed by open heart procedures. The major emphasis of surgery was replacement of diseased valves with artificial prostheses. A wide array of mechanical and tissue valves were developed with various results, especially regarding long-term morbidity and mortality. Carpentier[1] is credited with ushering in a new era of mitral valve repair with standardized techniques and consistent, reproducible results. His group, having follow-up lasting nearly 30 years, has reported long-term freedom from reoperation of nearly 90%.[2] Mitral valve repair is now accepted as a preferred surgical procedure with a high rate of early and long-term success for degenerative myxomatous mitral valve disease. The application of appropriate surgical techniques depends on the recognition of underlying pathologic conditions. These are not always evident by direct surgical inspection in a flaccid, arrested heart.

Intraoperative echocardiography was systematically attempted by the Cleveland group on the beating exposed heart using epicardial placement of a high-frequency probe.[3] Thus, high-quality images of anatomy and function were produced. Echocardiography was repeated after attempted surgical repair. Although promising, this procedure was cumbersome because a cardiologist knowledgeable in echocardiography needed to scrub in, the sterile procedures had to be developed, and surgery was delayed during acquisition of the images. The advent of transesophageal echocardiography (TEE) ushered in a new era. First developed and extensively used were single-plane and biplane images. Omoto and his colleagues in Japan are credited with early work.[4,5] Subsequently, multiplane two-dimensional (2D) TEE imaging was introduced and was applied for intraoperative use. Three-dimensional (3D) TEE was initially carried out with reconstruction of multiple 2D imaging planes.[6] The more recent introduction of real-time 3D TEE appears promising.[7,8] However, the current standard of intraoperative TEE imaging remains multiplane 2D imaging, which provides detailed anatomic and functional assessment.

In this chapter I will examine the role of intraoperative TEE in mitral valve disease before cardiopulmonary bypass and subsequently after the surgical procedure when the patient is removed from bypass. The current use of the multiplane 2D TEE approach will be emphasized and the potential for future use of real time 3D TEE will be discussed.

CHAPTER 20

OBJECTIVES OF INTRAOPERATIVE TRANSESOPHAGEAL ECHOCARDIOGRAPHY

Intraoperative TEE in mitral valve disease has three major objectives. These are the following:

1. Provide a surgical roadmap.[9,10] Echocardiography provides accurate and

reliable information regarding anatomy and function of the mitral valve in real time under a physiologic hemodynamic state. This information is extremely useful in all valve-related matters but especially in patients undergoing mitral valve repair.

2. Check the early surgical outcome after mitral valve surgery.[11] Echocardiography is essential to confirm the immediate outcome and provide assessment of the procedure in a beating, filled heart. It is well recognized that there is limited ability to assess valve function in a flaccid, nonbeating heart.

3. Detect associated pathologic lesions. It is not uncommon for patients undergoing mitral valve surgery to have independent and often undiagnosed lesions. These may be diagnosed with a comprehensive examination and appropriately treated.

SURGICAL ROADMAP OF THE DISEASED MITRAL VALVE

A key element of the echocardiographic roadmap is use of a common language that permits easy and accurate communication between the echocardiographer and the surgeon in the operating room setting. To this end, the definition terminologies and classifications must be agreed upon for mutual understanding.

Definition of Mitral Valve Prolapse

There is often a difference between a cardiologist's and a surgeon's use of the term *mitral valve prolapse*. The terms *prolapse, flail wave, billowing valve,* and *Barlow valve* are used without precise definitions. Because a minor degree of leaflet billowing was diagnosed as mitral valve prolapse, the shape of the annulus, whether saddle or ski slope configuration, became relevant. The normal coaptation of the two leaflets is subannular (Figure 20-1). The following definitions are proposed.

The term *prolapse* may be restricted to indicate superior displacement past the annular plane of the free margin or margins of one or both leaflets and may be subclassified as 1) flail mitral valve (Figure 20-2) or 2) billowing valve with free edge prolapse (Figure 20-3). The flail valve is often associated with chordae rupture, although some patients may have extreme chordal elongation without rupture. A less common pathologic lesion resulting in a flail valve prolapse is papillary muscle rupture in the setting of acute myocardial infarction. The billowing valve with prolapse is generally associated with excess tissue, chordal elongation, and free

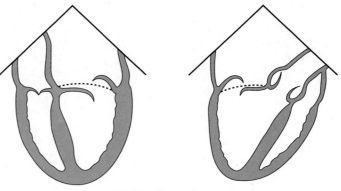

Flail leaflet prolapse

FIGURE 20–2 Schematic diagram of transesophageal echocardiography views showing mitral valve prolapse with chordae rupture with the posterior leaflet going above the annular plane (interrupted lines) in the four-chamber (*left*) and long-axis (*right*) views.

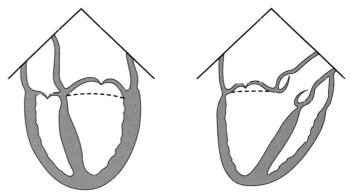

Billowing with prolapse

FIGURE 20–3 Schematic diagram of transesophageal echocardiography views showing bileaflet billowing with mitral valve prolapse in which both leaflets prolapse above the annular plane (interrupted lines).

edge prolapse, which is initially late systolic and later with further chordal elongation becomes holosystolic. Less often, patients with mixed lesions with billowing valve prolapse in one segment may have focal chordae rupture resulting in a localized flail segment. It is important to emphasize that if the term *prolapse* is restricted to indicate superior displacement of free margin of leaflet above the annular plane, the shape of the annulus is irrelevant. The diagnosis of prolapse may be made in either the four-chamber (0°) or long-axis equivalent (120-135°) planes.

The term *billowing valve* should be restricted to describe superior motion of the body near the base of the leaflet. The longer anterior leaflet may often exhibit mild billowing during ventricular systole. The billowing at the base of the leaflet may be considered abnormal when it exceeds 2 mm above the annular plane in a long-axis view (≈130° in the midesophageal plane by TEE) and 5 mm in the four-chamber view (0° in the midesophageal plane). The three scallops of the posterior leaflet have shorter height (length) and do not exhibit billowing. A billowing motion of the posterior leaflet may occur with pathologically increased and redundant tissue and is nearly always abnormal. The abnormal billowing of the anterior and/or posterior leaflets is often associated with myxomatous thickening and excess tissue. The abnormal billowing valve may initially be present without prolapse (i.e., superior displacement of the free edge) (Figure 20-4). As the marginal chordae elongate, there is initially a late systolic prolapse with late systolic regurgitation, and in late stages as chordal elongation proceeds, a holosystolic

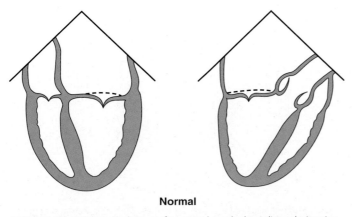

Normal

FIGURE 20–1 Schematic diagram of transesophageal echocardiography imaging planes shows normal coaptation of valve leaflets below the level of the mitral annulus (interrupted line). *Left,* four-chamber (0°) plane; right, long-axis (~135°) plane.

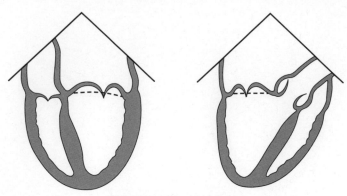

Billowing without prolapse

FIGURE 20–4 Schematic diagram of transesophageal echocardiography views showing abnormal leaflet billowing with the body of both leaflets protruding above the annular plane but with coaptation remaining at or below the annular plane (interrupted lines).

prolapse with holosystolic regurgitation develops. In this setting the chordae elongation often involves both the leaflets, with resulting regurgitation being central.

TERMINOLOGY FOR LEAFLET ANATOMY

Two major terminology classifications to designate components of each leaflet are in use, the Carpentier classification and the Duran classification.

Carpentier Classification

This terminology proposed by Carpentier and widely used refers to the three scallops of the posterior leaflets as P1 (anterolateral), P2 (middle), and P3 (posteromedial) (Figure 20-5). The corresponding segments of the anterior leaflet are labeled A1, A2, and A3. The anterior leaflet having a smoother surface lacks distinctive separation between A1 and A2 and A2 and A3.

Duran Classification

Kumar et al[12] proposed a classification based on chordal insertions from the two groups of papillary muscles. In this approach the lateral half of both leaflets is designated with 1 and the medial half with 2. Thus, the anterior leaflets are divided into A1 with chordae crossing from the anterolateral papillary muscle and A2 with chordae from the posteromedial papillary muscle (Figure 20-6). The posterior leaflet scallops are designated as P1 (anterolateral) and

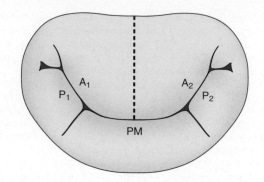

FIGURE 20–6 Duran classification of mitral valve leaflet structure. A, anterior; P, posterior; PM, posterior middle.

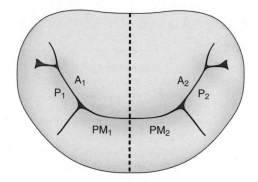

FIGURE 20–7 Modified Duran classification. A, anterior; P, posterior; PM, posterior middle.

P2 (posteromedial) and the larger middle scallop as PM. The PM being a larger scallop, it was subsequently suggested that it be subdivided as PM1 and PM2 based on chordal origins (Figure 20-7).[9]

Although this classification is anatomically more appealing and relevant, it is less widely used. We therefore offer a modified Carpentier classification to incorporate some of the relevant anatomic concepts of the Duran approach.

Modified Carpentier Classification

In an attempt to make the commonly used Carpentier classification more anatomically relevant, we propose division of A2 and P2, two of the larger segments in halves, namely lateral and medial (Figure 20-8). Thus, A2l and P2l are lateral halves with chordal attachments to the anterolateral papillary muscle and A2m and P2m are medial halves with chordal attachments to the posteromedial papillary muscle.

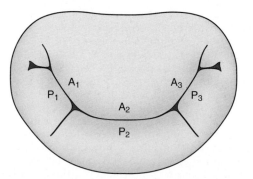

FIGURE 20–5 Carpentier classification of mitral valve leaflet structure. The mitral valve is viewed from the left atrium as seen from the surgeon's perspective. A, anterior; P, posterior.

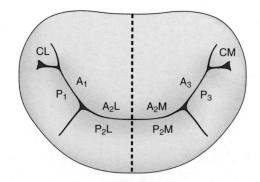

FIGURE 20–8 Modified Carpentier classification. The middle scallops of both anterior (A2) and posterior (P2) leaflets are divided into lateral (L) and medial (M) halves. In addition the lateral and medial commissural scallops are also included (CL and CM, respectively)

The A1, P1, A2l, and P2l are leaflet components with chordae arising from anterolateral papillary muscle, and A3, P3, A2m, and P2m have chordae from the posteromedial papillary muscle. This approach maintains the simplicity of the Carpentier classification without ignoring the important anatomic connections. The commissural scallops are similarly labeled lateral (Cl) and medial (Cm).

DETERMINATION OF PATHOPHYSIOLOGY OF MITRAL REGURGITATION

Diverse disorders affecting different components of the mitral valve apparatus may result in mitral valve regurgitation. The cascade of valve dysfunction may be seen as

Etiology→Structural change→Functional change→ Mitral regurgitation

Intraoperative echocardiography provides 1) assessment of mitral regurgitation, 2) evaluation of functional changes in the valve, and 3) evaluation and localization of structural changes and may further provide 4) clues to determine etiology.

Assessment of Mitral Regurgitation

In general, mitral regurgitation is best quantitated before the patient is brought to the operating room, where general anesthesia may preclude accurate assessment of severity.[13,14] Attention should be directed more to localizing the pathologic lesion and the origin of regurgitant jets. In rare circumstances, when the surgical plan is primarily a coronary artery bypass graft or an aortic valve replacement, one may be called upon to provide quantitation of concomitant mitral regurgitation if the latter was not adequately defined previously. General anesthesia has the tendency to lower systemic vascular resistance, resulting in the potential underestimation of regurgitation severity.[15] The regurgitation severity in an anesthetized patient should be tested both in the basal state and after augmentation of loading conditions. A combination of increased preload and afterload may be used to assess a possible need for mitral valve surgery in patients with coronary artery disease undergoing bypass surgery.

Three major approaches are used for quantitation of mitral regurgitation:

1. Size of the turbulent jet. This is first established visually. It tends to be less reliable, especially for eccentric jets.
2. Flow acceleration using the proximal isovelocity surface area radius. This approach permits quantitation of the effective regurgitation orifice area and of regurgitant volume. Although this is an accepted method for accurate quantitation, there are some limitations.
3. Vena contracta. The zone of vena contracta seen as a narrow "waist" of the jet just above the regurgitant orifice has been purported to provide accurate quantitation. This approach, too, has limitations.

It is probably best to integrate all of the above approaches in the operating room to make a recommendation regarding the need for mitral valve surgery.

Evaluation of Valve Functional Pathology

Carpentier's approach to the functional pathology of mitral regurgitation is commonly used and is shown in Table 20-1.[1] It is simple and provides an accurate description by echocardiography and surgical inspection[16,17]:

Type 1. The leaflet motion is normal, and regurgitation may be caused by leaflet perforation or a cleft valve (Figure 20-9A-D).

TABLE 20–1	Carpentier Classification of Mitral Regurgitation
Type 1: Normal leaflet motion	
Type 2: Leaflet prolapse	
Type 3: Restricted leaflet	
3A. Systolic and diastolic restriction	
3B. Systolic restriction	

From Carpentier A: Cardiac valve surgery—the "French correction." J Thorac Cardiovasc Surg 1983;86:323-337.

Type 2. The leaflets exhibit excessive motion, resulting in valve prolapse of a portion of one or both leaflets. A flail mitral valve is a form of prolapse associated with chordal rupture (Figure 20-10 and Figure 20-11), whereas a billowing valve with prolapse is associated with elongated chords and excess redundant leaflet tissue. This latter condition is also referred to as a *Barlow valve* (Figure 20-12A-F).

Type 3A. Leaflet restriction in systole and diastole is observed in chronic rheumatic mitral valve disease and in other inflammatory or toxic conditions such as valvulopathy resulting from carcinoid heart disease and exposure to ergot or the appetite suppressants phentermine-fenfluramine (phen-fen). There is often considerable scarring and fibrosis of the leaflets with involvement of subvalve structures.

Type 3B. Leaflet restriction observed mainly in systole as seen in dilated or chronic ischemic cardiomyopathy. Leaflet tethering is present with coaptation commonly displaced more apically into the left ventricular cavity. The annulus is dilated along with left ventricular enlargement and outward displacement of the two papillary muscle groups.

Evaluation of Structural Changes in the Valve

Echocardiography permits analysis of all components of the mitral valve apparatus, namely the annulus, the leaflets, the chordae, the papillary muscles, the left ventricle, and the left atrium.[10,17,18,19]

Mitral Annulus

Evaluation of the annulus should include assessment of size and calcification. Annular size is expressed on the basis of diameters in the four-chamber (0°) view and long-axis (130°) view. Although normally elliptical, a dilated annulus assumes a more circular shape. The annular diameter in normal adults is generally less than 3.2 cm. The annular dilatation is multifactorial. Degenerative myxomatous mitral valve disease is commonly associated with annular dilatation as a component of the underlying pathologic lesion. The annulus also dilates as a result of left ventricular and left atrial enlargement. Thus, mitral regurgitation in and of itself results in annular dilatation, which in turn exacerbates the degree of regurgitation. Hence the statement that mitral regurgitation begets more mitral regurgitation. The mitral annulus is typically not dilated in chronic rheumatic disease. The degree of calcification involving the annulus should be examined in multiple views and has great bearing on surgical techniques and operability.

Mitral Leaflets

Structural changes may include thickening, calcification, tears, perforations, clefts, or attached vegetations. The location and extent of changes in different components of the leaflets can be determined by examining multiple cross-sectional views. A knowledge of the precise anatomic display using multiple midesophageal and transgastric echocardiography planes is

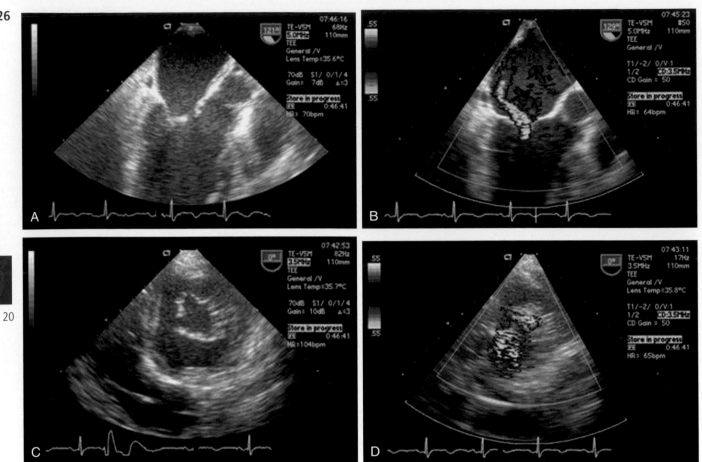

FIGURE 20–9 Mitral regurgitation caused by a cleft anterior mitral leaflet. **A**, normal leaflet coaptation. **B**, regurgitation through the anterior leaflet (A2) cleft. **C**, transgastric short-axis view demonstrating absence of tissue in anterior leaflet (A2) **D**, regurgitant flow through the leaflet gap.

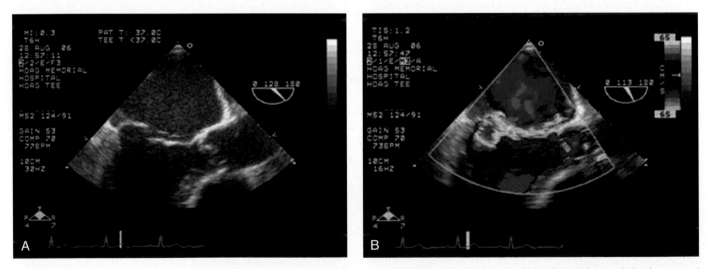

FIGURE 20–10 Transesophageal echocardiographic long-axis view showing a flail posterior leaflet involving the middle scallop (P2) with chordal rupture (**A**) with an eccentric jet directed anteriorly (**B**).

essential for accurate localization of leaflet pathologic lesions (Figure 20-13A).

Chordae Tendineae

The structural abnormalities associated with chordae include elongation, rupture, calcification, shortening, and fusion. These changes may be observed in several echocardiographic planes.

However, direct visualization is achieved best in transgastric views (≈80%) on which both papillary muscle groups and the chordae inserting into the leaflets may be displayed.

Papillary Muscles

The changes in papillary muscle morphology include fibrotic scarring, rupture, or congenital malformations. These are

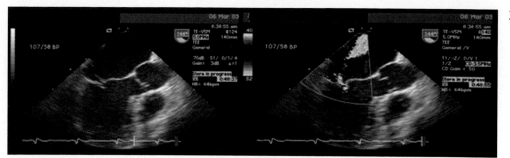

FIGURE 20–11 Transesophageal echocardiographic long-axis view showing a flail anterior leaflet involving the middle scallop (A2) with ruptured chordae (**A**) with a posteriorly directed eccentric jet (**B**).

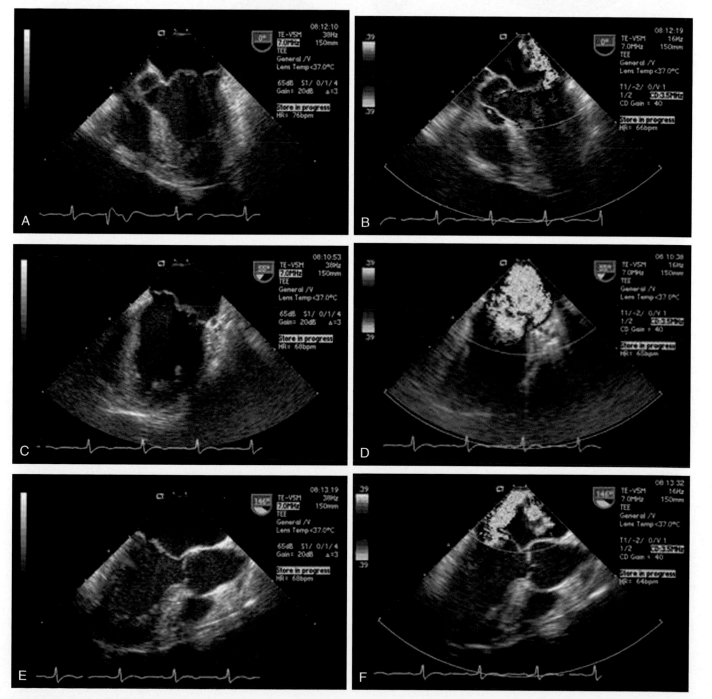

FIGURE 20–12 Transesophageal echocardiographic long-axis view shows bileaflet billowing prolapse (**A**) with a central jet of mitral regurgitation (**B**). In **C**, there is prolapse of all leaflet segments associated with multiple sites of regurgitation (**D**). In **E**, there is bileaflet prolapse of different segments, with associated central regurgitation (**F**).

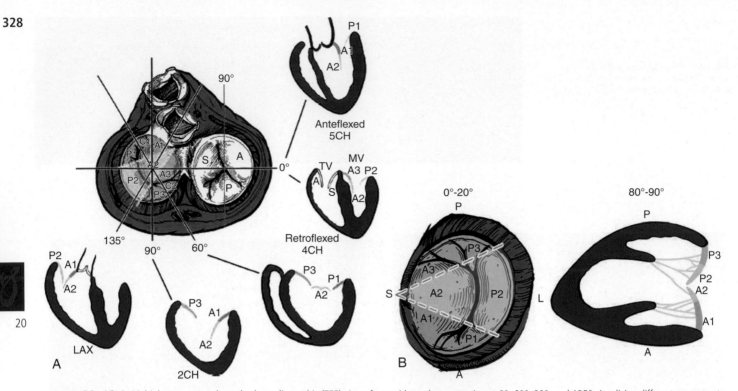

FIGURE 20–13 A, Multiplane transesophageal echocardiographic (TEE) views from mid-esophagus starting at 0°, 60°, 90°, and 135° visualizing different components of the mitral valve anatomy. **B**, TEE views from transgastric planes. The *left panel* at 0° to 20° shows the mitral valves in the short-axis view with leaflet designations based on the original Carpentier classification. The *right panel* shows the papillary muscles and chordae attaching to different components of the valve leaflets. 2CH, two-chamber view; 4CH, four-chamber view; 5CH, five-chamber view; A, anterior, L, lateral, LAX, long axis; MV, mitral valve; P, posterior, S, septal; TV, tricuspid valve. (*Adapted from Carpentier classification.*)

best observed on transgastric short-axis (0°) and longitudinal (80°) views (see Figure 20-13B). A ruptured papillary muscle with a resulting flail valve is readily visualized in the midesophageal views. Several midesophageal planes also provide evaluation of wall motion of segments adjacent to the base of the papillary muscle that have an impact on its function.

Left Ventricle

Size and function of the left ventricle may be comprehensively assessed by examining multiple mid-esophageal and gastric planes. Eccentric displacement of the papillary muscles in a dilated ventricle results in incomplete coaptation of leaflets. Both global and regional ventricular functions influence mitral valve function.

Left Atrium

Intraoperative TEE does not provide accurate assessment of left atrial size and volume. It does provide assessment of the atrial appendage and interatrial septum.

Etiology of Mitral Regurgitation

Echocardiography often provides clues to the etiology of mitral valve disease.

Rheumatic Disease

Thickened and/or calcified leaflets, shortened fused chords, commissural fusion, and a type 3A movement abnormality with doming of the anterior leaflet and fixed posterior leaflet are commonly observed with chronic rheumatic valve disease.

Myxomatous Degenerative Mitral Valve Disease

Thickened, redundant enlarged leaflets, dilated annulus, prolapse with or without billowing, chordae rupture, and chordae elongation, with type 2 leaflet motion are diagnostic features.

Infective Endocarditis

Focal vegetations, chordal rupture, annular abscess, leaflet disruption, and perforation may be observed based on severity of infection and infective agent.

Dilated Cardiomyopathy

Outward displacement of papillary muscles, tethering of leaflets, and apically displaced and incomplete coaptation results in central regurgitation; its severity is highly load dependent (Figure 20-14).

Ischemic Heart Disease

Three distinct types may be identified. The type associated with chronic ischemic left ventricular dysfunction and dilatation is indistinguishable from the changes described for dilated cardiomyopathy. The second type consists of postero-inferior wall akinesia or hypokinesia with restriction of part of the posterior leaflets and an override of the opposing segment of the anterior leaflet. This may be mistaken for mitral valve prolapse, because it results in an eccentric jet of regurgitation (Figure 20-15). However, unlike the mal-coaptation of mitral prolapse, the coaptation and leaflets are subannular. The third type consists of flail mitral valve associated with acute rupture of a papillary muscle head in the setting of acute myocardial infarction (Figure 20-16).

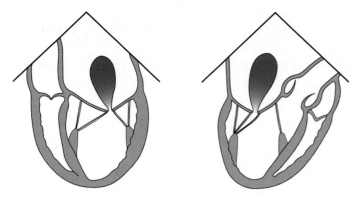

FIGURE 20–14 Schematic diagram of transesophageal echocardiographic views showing tethering of the mitral leaflets caused by left ventricular dilatation and papillary muscle displacement, as would be seen in patients with dilated cardiomyopathy or chronic ischemic heart disease. *Left*, four-chamber view (0°). *Right*, long-axis view (≈135°).

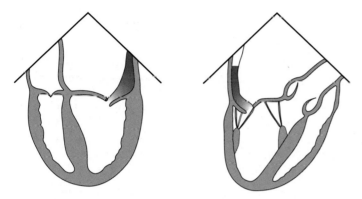

FIGURE 20–15 Schematic diagram of the transesophageal echocardiographic four-chamber (*left*) and long-axis (*right*) views illustrating ischemic dysfunction of the posterior papillary muscle, resulting in anterior leaflet (A2) override and an eccentric jet of mitral regurgitation.

Congenital Cleft Mitral Valve

Although generally associated with an atrioventricular cushion defect, this may occur as an isolated pathologic lesion. Apart from thickening of leaflet edges, no other structural abnormalities are seen. A discontinuity of the leaflet tissue may be seen (see Figure 20-9).

Leaflet Perforation

This is generally a result of infective endocarditis, often involving the aortic valve with secondary seeding of the mitral valve. Minor structural discontinuity along the leaflet at the site of perforation may be observed.

Chronic Inflammatory Processes

Chronic inflammatory causes of mitral regurgitation include 1) exposure to phen-fen, 2) exposure to ergot derivatives, 3) atypical nonbacterial infection, and 4) carcinoid disease. The structural changes include thickening and fibrotic changes that may affect the leaflets and subannular tissues with variable involvement of the chordal structures. The result is restricted leaflet motion.

Fibroelastic Degeneration

This condition is uncommon but may be observed in elderly subjects with a flail mitral valve segment and chordae rupture.

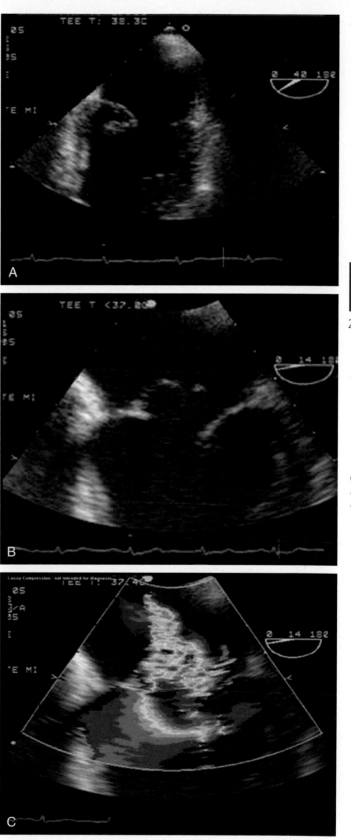

FIGURE 20–16 Acute rupture of a papillary muscle resulting in severe mitral regurgitation. **A**, mitral valve leaflets in diastole. Note the detached tip of the papillary muscle, which results in severe valve prolapse in systole (**B**) and massive mitral regurgitation (**C**).

Typically the leaflets are thin and translucent, unlike for myxomatous disease in which they are thick, redundant, and opaque.

ECHOCARDIOGRAPHY-GUIDED SURGICAL APPROACH

Intraoperative echocardiography provides reliable delineation of pathophysiology as well as localization of abnormalities and may be used to plan appropriate surgical approaches to correct mitral valve diseases.[20,21] A planned surgical approach is subject to change if the findings during the operation vary from those seen with echocardiography. A well-functioning echocardiography-surgery collaborative team would learn from these variances to improve their echocardiographic skills. The following descriptions of commonly observed echocardiographic findings provide a lesion-specific surgical approach.

Dilated Annulus with Normal Leaflet Tissue, Incomplete Tip Coaptation, and Central Regurgitation

This may be seen in chronic ischemic or dilated cardiomyopathy (type 3B), and the mitral regurgitation jet is generally central. The appropriate surgical solution is placement of an annular reduction annuloplasty ring, providing a greater coaptation surface at the free margins. In some patients with ischemic cardiomyopathy, if the predominant regurgitation site is from the A3-P3 region, a Carpentier-McCarthy-Adams ring may be preferred.[22] The design of this asymmetric ring permits better coaptation along the A3, P3, and Cm areas.

Dilated Annulus with Excess Leaflet Tissue and Central Regurgitation

This is observed in billowing mitral valve prolapse (type 2) involving both leaflets. The surgical approach may include 1) resection of excess tissue involving the posterior leaflet, 2) implantation of artificial chords (Gore-Tex chords) or chordal reduction procedures, and 3) placement of an annuloplasty band or ring, the size being determined by the amount of leaflet tissue after surgical resection or reduction.[23] Selection of an inappropriately small annuloplasty band may result in postrepair systolic anterior motion (SAM).[24] In some cases a Myxo ring may be appropriate because the design of this ring displaces the leaflet coaptation posteriorly, thus avoiding leaflet SAM.[25]

Flail Posterior Leaflet Scallop (Type 2) with Chordal Rupture or Elongation and Excess Leaflet Height Associated with Eccentric Regurgitation Jet

The most common site is P2. The surgical approach consists of leaflet resection, with an artificial chord to P2 implanted to the appropriate side of the papillary muscle. The artificial chord placed on P2l would be implanted to the anterolateral papillary muscle and on P2m to the posteromedial papillary muscle. The repair is supported by an annuloplasty band, the size being determined by size of leaflet tissue after repair.

Flail Anterior Leaflet (Commonly at A2) with Chordal Rupture and Eccentric Regurgitation Jet

The surgical approach differs from a flail posterior leaflet pathologic lesion only in that the leaflet resection is limited in extent. Also the artificial chord implantation from A2l or from A2m will go to the corresponding papillary muscle.

Combination of Restricted Posterior Leaflet (Type 3b) and Flail Anterior Leaflet (Type 2)

This offers a special surgical challenge. Resection of secondary chords may free the posterior leaflet and result in restored mobility. The anterior leaflet flail correction is as described above.

Leaflet Perforation

Perforations commonly involve the anterior leaflet at its base and are caused by infective endocarditis affecting the aortic valve with a jet lesion on the mitral valve. The bacterial seeding may result in localized perforation. This may be readily corrected by simple plication or with use of a pericardial patch.

Cleft Mitral Valve

Clefts generally involve A2 as a congenital defect and may occur in association with an atrioventricular cushion defect or may occur in isolation. The correction involves plication for a narrow cleft and a pericardial patch for a larger one.

Mixed Rheumatic Mitral Stenosis and Regurgitation

Rheumatic disease with subvalve pathologic changes may be considered for repair, especially in the absence of marked scarring and shortening of leaflet tissues or extensive calcification. The surgical approach includes commissurotomy, chordotomy, papillotomy, and, in some cases, leaflet extension with pericardial tissue. The annuloplasty ring is a smaller size to permit improved tip coaptation.

Infective Endocarditis

Infections of the mitral valve with vegetations and without extensive tissue destruction and without abscess formation may be suitable for mitral valve repair. The surgical approach consists of vegetectomy, repair of flail segments and ring annuloplasty.

Commissural Prolapse

Commissural prolapse with regurgitation is often difficult to repair, and the surgical approach commonly used consists of a commissural Alfieri stitch, which comprises edge-to-edge plication.[26]

Decisions for Mitral Valve Replacement

Conditions that are likely to require mitral valve replacement based on echocardiographic anatomy include extensive calcification of the mitral annulus, leaflets, and chordate; marked fibrosis and shortening of mitral leaflets; extensive tissue necrosis of leaflets due to infection; extensive subvalvular pathologic changes consisting of marked shortening of the chords with the papillary muscles attached to the leaflets; large annular abscesses; and severely restricted leaflets.

INTRAOPERATIVE ECHOCARDIOGRAPHIC ASSESSMENT OF SURGERY

Mitral Valve Repair

It is essential to assess the anatomic as well as functional aspects of the repaired valve. Anatomically, the tip coaptation should be subannular and should have surface coaptation near the free edge of about 5 to 10 mm. Functionally, the absence of any regurgitation is a desired outcome, but it is not uncommon to see trivial or mild regurgitation after a successful repair. The assessment must be made with a sufficiently filled ventricle and with systolic blood pressure of 110 to 140 mm Hg. If the regurgitation is moderate or greater, localization by careful echocardiographic assessment may be helpful in revision of the repair on a second pump run. In our experience, the second pump run is successful for adequate repair in 75% of patients.

Multiple echocardiographic cross sections should be obtained to look for paravalvular mitral regurgitation. Low-velocity small jets are often related to stitch regurgitation, and these are eliminated after administration of protamine. A turbulent paravalvular jet, even if small, should not be ignored because it may exhibit progression or may be associated with clinical hemolysis.

Postrepair SAM has been known to occur in 5% to 10% of patients with degenerative myxomatous mitral valve prolapse. When SAM is observed, it is important to establish proper ventricular filling, a slower heart rate, and normal blood pressures. If SAM is persistent and is associated with valve regurgitation, a corrective action should be undertaken. This may consist of a reduction of the amount of leaflet tissue, implantation of a larger annuloplasty band or ring, or use of a Myxo ring (Figure 20-17). It is important that leaflet SAM with outflow turbulence and mitral regurgitation not be ignored.

It is also important to assess the mean gradient across the mitral valve. A very small annuloplasty ring may result in mitral stenosis with transvalvular gradients.

Mitral Valve Replacement

After mitral valve replacement, it is important to determine the presence and severity of paravalvular regurgitation and to measure transvalvular gradients. TEE identifies excess leaflet chordal tissue capable of left ventricular outflow obstruction and provides assurance of normal prosthetic valve function, with unobstructed opening of bileaflet discs and normal flow characteristics without central regurgitation of bioprosthetic valves.

IMPACT OF INTRAOPERATIVE ECHOCARDIOGRAPHY ON SURGICAL OUTCOME

It is difficult, if not unethical, to carry out a prospective randomized trial to assess the utility of information provided from intraoperative echocardiography. Because the nature of the anatomic and pathophysiologic information is robust, it would not be appropriate to blind the surgeon. The question of impact on surgical outcome has been approached from two angles. There are reports on the impact of intraoperative echocardiography on predictability of valve repair and on surgical approach.[27,28] We have reported the frequency of valve repair attempted and successful by the same surgeon 3 consecutive years before and after institution of a dedicated echocardiography-surgery team providing detailed echocardiographic analysis before and after valve repair.[29]

The Cleveland Clinic data showed that in approximately 14% of patients, the surgeons altered their surgical technique on basis of the echocardiographic information.[27] The data at this institution showed that the percentage of successful repairs jumped from around 50% to 55% to 85% to 90% after institution of an echocardiography-surgery collaborative team.[29]

These observations support the American College of Cardiology/American Heart Association practice guidelines for the management of patients with valvular heart disease[30] statement that the use of intraoperative echocardiography in mitral valve repair is a class I indication (Table 20-2). Similarly, it also merits a class I indication in surgical management of infective endocarditis. Indeed it is recommended that intraoperative echocardiography for all other valve surgery be considered as a class IIa indication. The overall utility of using intraoperative echocardiography will ultimately depend on the expertise and dedication of the echocardiographer and a collaborative relationship with the

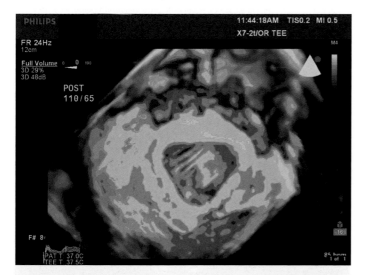

FIGURE 20-17 A three-dimensional transesophageal echocardiographic image of a Myxo annuloplasty ring as seen from the left atrium. The somewhat triangular shape results in posterior displacement of leaflet coaptation, which protects against the development of systolic anterior motion.

TABLE 20-2	American College of Cardiology/American Heart Association Practice Guidelines for Intraoperative Echocardiography in Relevance to Mitral Valve Disease

Class I
1. Intraoperative TEE is recommended for valve repair surgery
2. Intraoperative TEE is recommended for valve surgery for infective endocarditis

Class II A
Intraoperative TEE is reasonable for all patients undergoing cardiac valve surgery

TEE, transesophageal echocardiography.

Bonow RO, Carabello BA, Chatterjee KC, et al: ACC/AHA 2006 guidelines for the management of patients with valvular heart disease; a report of the American College of cardiology/American Heart Association Task Force on Practice Guidelines (writing committee to revise the 1998 Guidelines for the management of patients With Valvular Heart Disease): developed in collaboration with the Society of Cardiovascular Anesthesiologists: endorsed by the Society for Cardiovascular Angiography and Interventions and the Society of Thoracic Surgeons. Circulation 2006;114:e84-e231.

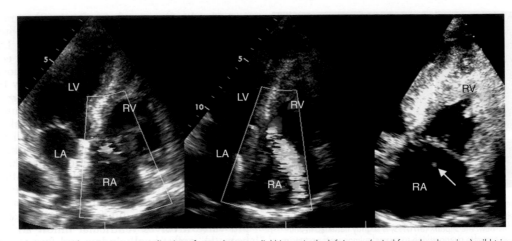

FIGURE 21–3 This composite image demonstrates a complication of an endomyocardial biopsy. In the left image (apical four-chamber view) mild tricuspid regurgitation is seen with color flow Doppler. In the center image, obtained from the same view, an eccentric laterally directed jet of severe tricuspid regurgitation is seen. In the right image a zoomed view of the tricuspid valve is seen. In addition, the severed tricuspid chordae is seen (*arrow*). LA, left atrium; LA, left ventricle; RA, right atrium; RV, right ventricle.

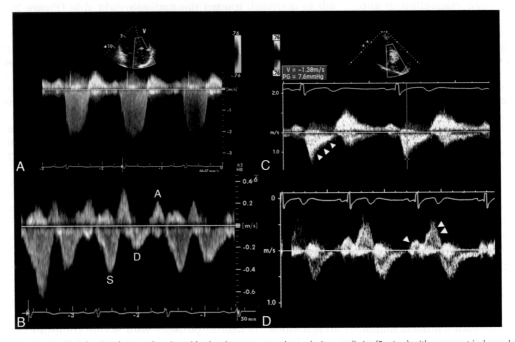

FIGURE 21–4 A, Continuous wave Doppler signal across the tricuspid valve demonstrates a low-velocity systolic jet (2 m/sec) with a symmetrical rounded appearance consistent with mild tricuspid valve regurgitation. Measurement of the peak systolic velocity provides an indirect assessment of right ventricular systolic pressure using the modified Bernoulli equation. **B**, Hepatic vein pulsed-wave Doppler signal with accompanying electrocardiogram tracing demonstrating normal hepatic vein flow in the patient with mild tricuspid regurgitation in **A**. Systolic flow (S) and diastolic flow (D) are seen emanating from the hepatic veins into the inferior vena cava (flow seen displayed below the baseline) and atrial reversal flow (**A**) representing normal flow refluxing into the hepatic veins resulting from atrial contraction. **C**, A dense systolic continuous wave Doppler signal is demonstrated in a patient with severe tricuspid valve regurgitation. Severe tricuspid regurgitation results in a triangular or "dagger-shaped" (*arrowheads*) early peaking tricuspid regurgitant jet profile due to early equilibration of pressures between the right atrium and right ventricle. **D**, Hepatic vein pulsed-wave Doppler signal demonstrating both atrial (*single arrowhead*) and systolic reversed flow (*double arrowhead*), indicating elevation in right atrial pressure and severe tricuspid valve regurgitation in a patient in sinus rhythm. These systolic reversals reflect retrograde flow in the hepatic veins that can be recognized clinically as a pulsatile liver. Hepatic vein systolic reversals may not be specific for severe tricuspid regurgitation when atrial fibrillation is present.

Evaluation of the degree of tricuspid stenosis includes calculation of 1) the mean pressure gradient throughout both phases of respiration and 2) the pressure half-time valve area (the proposed constant to determine tricuspid valve area is 190).[13,21] Unlike the evaluation of mitral stenosis, short-axis 2D imaging of the valve orifice is rarely feasible.

The diagnosis of pulmonic valve disease is often made initially by echocardiography. Two-dimensional imaging of the right ventricular outflow tract may exhibit features of abnormal pulmonic valve motion, doming, prolapse, and partial or complete valve absence. In some patients, the pulmonic valve also can be imaged in an anteriorly angulated apical four-chamber view or in a subcostal short-axis or long-axis view (Figure 21-5A). Two-dimensional echocardiographic images are also used to evaluate right ventricular size and systolic function and right ventricular wall thickness in patients with pulmonic valve disease.

Transesophageal imaging of the pulmonic valve may also be challenging, as the valve is in the far field of the imaging plane. The pulmonic valve is best visualized with the multiplane probe rotated to about 90°, resulting in a long-axis view of the right ventricular outflow tract and pulmonic valve with the aortic valve in an oblique short-axis orientation. Alternatively, the pulmonic valve can be visualized in a transverse plane (0° rotation) with the probe withdrawn to the level of the pulmonary artery bifurcation to obtain an

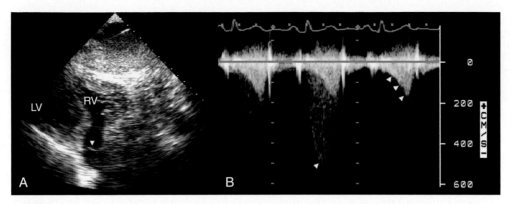

FIGURE 21–5 A, Two-dimensional echocardiogram from a patient with severe pulmonic valve stenosis. The best alignment between the Doppler beam and the pulmonic flow signal was from a subcostal long-axis window with the transducer angled anteriorly. Marked right ventricular hypertrophy was noted and there was systolic doming of the pulmonic valve (*arrowhead*). **B,** From the same patient, the peak velocity recorded with continuous wave Doppler ultrasound for calculation of the transvalvular pressure gradient (*single arrowhead*) suggests a peak gradient over 100 mmHg. Note the late peaking infundibular gradient (*three arrowheads*) from dynamic right ventricular outflow tract obstruction. LV, left ventricle; RV, right ventricle.

image looking straight down the pulmonary artery from the bifurcation to the valve. This view provides a parallel intercept angle for Doppler recordings.

Even from the transesophageal approach, the valve may not be well seen because of interposition of the bronchus between the transducer and the pulmonic valve. When pulmonic stenosis is suspected, it is particularly important to evaluate for subvalvular or supravalvular obstruction, in addition to valvular stenosis, because right ventricular outflow obstruction may take any one of these forms, which have similar clinical manifestations. Rarely, cardiac catheterization is needed to define the exact level of obstruction when the echocardiogram is nondiagnostic.

Evaluation of pulmonic stenosis relies predominantly on measurement of maximal and mean pressure gradients. In theory, valve area can be calculated using the continuity equation, but this calculation is rarely performed clinically because of the difficulty of measuring the transpulmonary volume flow rate (see Figure 21-5B).

Pulmonic regurgitation is graded on a 1 to 4+ scale using color Doppler flow imaging. Severe pulmonic regurgitation is associated with holodiastolic flow reversal in the pulmonary artery. Color flow imaging shows a broad diastolic jet in the right ventricular outflow tract that continues throughout diastole (Figure 21-6A and B). The characteristics of the color flow jet are affected by the regurgitant volume and pressure and also by right ventricular pressures. The pulmonic regurgitant flow may appear laminar and brief because of the low velocity of pulmonic regurgitation when pulmonary pressures are normal. Planimetered color flow jet areas have been demonstrated to correlate well with pulmonic regurgitation severity noted by angiography; however, a high degree of variability and overlap among different grades of regurgitation was observed.[22] The vena contracta width has been used

for assessment of pulmonic regurgitation but this use has not been validated.

Continuous wave Doppler in pulmonic regurgitation is characterized by equal intensities of antegrade and retrograde flow across the pulmonic valve with the signal rapidly reaching baseline (see Figure 21-6C). The density of the continuous wave Doppler signal is a qualitative method of assessing pulmonic regurgitation severity. The deceleration pressure half-time corresponds to the degree of regurgitation and the right ventricular pressures. Rapid equalization or "to and fro" flow with a pressure half-time of less than 100 milliseconds is suggestive but not specific for severe pulmonic regurgitation, with a sensitivity of 76% and specificity of 94%.[23] Early and rapid equilibration of diastolic pressures also occurs in patients with low pulmonary artery end-diastolic pressure and/or increased right ventricular diastolic pressure. Two-dimensional imaging may demonstrate progressive ventricular dilation and dysfunction, suggesting significant regurgitation in the absence of other causes for this observation.[17]

Right Ventricular Size and Function

Although 2D echocardiography can provide a morphologic assessment of right ventricular dimensions and function,[24] accurate measurement of right ventricular dimensions, volumes, and function are difficult because of the complex three-dimensional anatomy of the right ventricular chamber. Right ventricular size and systolic function are evaluated qualitatively in comparison with left ventricular size and function. On transthoracic imaging the right ventricle is seen well in apical and subcostal four-chamber views. Parasternal right ventricular inflow and short-axis views are also helpful. On transesophageal imaging, right ventricular function is best evaluated using the four-chamber view. Three-dimensional echocardiographic imaging offers the possibility of feasible

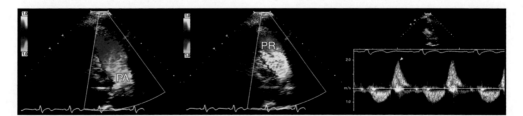

FIGURE 21–6 Transthoracic echocardiographic images of the right ventricular outflow tract from a patient with severe pulmonic valve regurgitation related to prior repair of tetralogy of Fallot. **A,** Color-flow Doppler features demonstrate laminar flow during systole into the pulmonary artery (PA). **B,** Broad laminar regurgitation jet of pulmonic regurgitation (PR) that fills the right ventricular outflow tract during diastole. **C,** Continuous wave Doppler shows an intense holodiastolic flow signal (*arrowhead*) across the pulmonary valve that decelerates rapidly to baseline. There is no pulmonic stenosis (antegrade velocity of 1.0 m/sec) and the low-velocity diastolic flow indicates normal pulmonary diastolic pressures.

clinical measures of right ventricular size and systolic function in the future.[25]

Echocardiography can also provide Doppler-derived surrogate measures of right ventricular function that have been shown to have prognostic value in patients with pulmonary hypertension. These measures include the right-sided index of myocardial performance (Tei index)[26] and measurements of the peak systolic velocity and displacement of the tricuspid annulus using tissue Doppler imaging.[27-29]

The extent of right ventricular hypertrophy can be assessed qualitatively based on the thickness of the right ventricular free wall.[24] The timing of ventricular septal motion also provides insight into right ventricular function as previously discussed. Although patterns of abnormal septal motion may be recognized on 2D imaging, the timing and extent of septal motion are best evaluated using M-mode echocardiography. When right ventricular enlargement and abnormal septal motion are present, the echocardiographer must ensure that these abnormalities are caused by valvular disease rather than by an intracardiac shunt because of the impact on management. An atrial septal defect or anomalous pulmonary veins will result in right-sided chamber enlargement, often with secondary tricuspid regurgitation due to a dilated annulus. Delineation of the atrial septum and pulmonary veins is best performed using transesophageal echocardiography and is indicated in unexplained right-sided chamber enlargement.

Cardiac magnetic resonance (CMR) imaging is an accurate method for the assessment of right ventricular size and function.[30,31] CMR imaging–derived right ventricular dimensions used as predictors of late contractile dysfunction have been defined in several groups of patients with pulmonary regurgitation after repair of tetralogy of Fallot.[32-34] Currently, it is not known whether these parameters correlate with persistent abnormal right ventricular function in patients with primary tricuspid valve regurgitation or pulmonary regurgitation from causes other than postoperative tetralogy of Fallot repair. Unfortunately, although CMR is considered the test of choice to assess right heart volume and systolic function,[35] the availability of this complementary technology is still limited, the data analysis is time consuming, and CMR cannot be performed in patients with defibrillators or pacemakers.[36] Recent data also indicate a detrimental effect of gadolinium in patients with advanced renal disease.[37]

Pulmonary Artery Pressures

Estimation of pulmonary pressures is an essential component of the examination in patients with right-sided valve disease. Pulmonary pressures can be estimated noninvasively from the velocity of the tricuspid regurgitant jet and the appearance of the inferior vena cava. Most patients have some degree of tricuspid regurgitation that permits estimation of right ventricular pressure. The velocity of the regurgitant signal is related to the right ventricular to right atrial systolic pressure difference (P_{RV-RA}) as stated in the simplified Bernoulli equation:

$$P_{RV-RA} = 4(V_{TR})^2$$

where P is pressure, RV is right ventricle, RA is right atrium, V velocity, and TR is tricuspid regurgitation.

To estimate right ventricular systolic pressure, this derived pressure gradient is added to an estimate of right atrial pressure, which is based on the size and respiratory variation of the inferior vena cava caliber (see Chapter 5).

TRICUSPID VALVE ANATOMY

The normal tricuspid valve is characterized by three sail-like leaflets: anterior, posterior, and septal (see Figure 21-2). The anterior leaflet is the most anatomically constant of the three, with the other leaflets varying more often in size and position. The leaflets are attached to the tricuspid valve annulus.

Similar to the mitral valve leaflets, the tricuspid valve leaflets are restrained by chordae tendinea attached to the papillary muscles, which are in turn inserted into the right ventricular wall. Tricuspid valve chordae may also insert directly into the right ventricular free wall, a feature distinguishing the right and left ventricles.

TRICUSPID REGURGITATION

Etiology

Tricuspid regurgitation that is at least moderate or greater in severity is often "functional" in nature. Functional tricuspid regurgitation by definition is not related to primary tricuspid leaflet pathologic lesions but rather is due to another disease process causing right ventricular dilatation, distortion of the subvalvular apparatus, tricuspid annular dilatation, or a combination of these. Causes of clinically significant tricuspid regurgitation are outlined in Table 21-1. Furthermore, a moderate or greater degree of tricuspid regurgitation, regardless of the primary etiology, usually engenders additional tricuspid regurgitation because of the adverse hemodynamic consequence of right ventricular volume overload, resulting in a slow and inexorable clinical and hemodynamic deterioration.

Functional tricuspid regurgitation due to pulmonary hypertension is seen in patients with significant left-sided heart disease, commonly rheumatic in origin, those with primary pulmonary hypertension, and those with pulmonary disease leading to cor pulmonale.[38] As a general rule, when systolic pulmonary artery pressures increase beyond 55 mmHg, tricuspid regurgitation can occur despite anatomically normal tricuspid leaflets, whereas more than mild tricuspid regurgitation occurring in the setting of lower systolic pulmonary pressures (<40 mmHg) probably reflects a structural abnormality of the valve leaflets or the subvalvular apparatus.[16,39] Functional tricuspid regurgitation also results from tricuspid annular dilatation in patients with right ventricular dilation due to right ventricular infarction, dilated cardiomyopathy, or an atrial septal defect or anomalous pulmonary venous drainage.[40-42]

TABLE 21–1	Causes of Tricuspid Valve Regurgitation
Congenital	
Ebstein anomaly	
Tricuspid valve dysplasia	
Tricuspid valve hypoplasia	
Tricuspid valve cleft	
Double orifice tricuspid valve	
Unguarded tricuspid valve orifice	
Right ventricular disease	
Right ventricular dysplasia	
Endomyocardial fibrosis	
Increased right heart pressure	
Acquired	
Annular dilatation	
Left-sided valvular heart disease	
Endocarditis	
Trauma	
Carcinoid heart disease	
Rheumatic heart disease	
Tricuspid valve prolapse	
Iatrogenic (radiation, drugs, biopsy, pacemaker, implantable cardiac defibrillator)	
Right ventricular dilation	
Pulmonary hypertension	
Primary pulmonary hypertension	
Secondary to left-sided heart disease (valvular heart disease; cardiomyopathy, and others)	
Right ventricular volume overload	
Atrial septal defect	
Anomalous pulmonary venous drainage	

Primary tricuspid valve pathologic lesions leading to tricuspid regurgitation may result from blunt trauma or iatrogenic injury or from direct leaflet involvement by specific diseases. When caused by permanent pacemaker or internal cardiac defibrillator leads, the mechanism of valve injury is variable, related to lead entrapment in the tricuspid apparatus, direct leaflet perforation at the time of lead insertion, fibrotic adhesion of the lead to the leaflet, or avulsion or laceration of the tricuspid valve leaflets upon lead removal.[43] Because leaflet injury may be under-recognized in patients who have undergone prior lead implants, a high clinical index of suspicion is warranted, particularly when these patients present with worsening right heart failure.

Direct trauma from transvenous endomyocardial biopsy may occur, particularly in cardiac transplantation patients who undergo repeated biopsies for rejection surveillance (see Figure 21-3).[44] Echocardiographic guidance during the biopsy may avert damage to the tricuspid valve or subvalvular apparatus.

The tricuspid leaflets and supporting structures may also be damaged indirectly by blunt chest trauma, most often after a motor vehicle accident resulting in papillary muscle, valve, or chordal rupture. Associated conduction abnormalities including right and left bundle branch block and left anterior hemiblock are common, occurring in more than 90% of patients with traumatic tricuspid regurgitation. The tricuspid regurgitation murmur is often not initially recognized on physical examination. Moreover, the patient may be asymptomatic and remain so for years after the trauma.[45] Routine use of echocardiography to evaluate victims of blunt chest trauma enhances detection of traumatic tricuspid regurgitation, overcoming the limitations of the history and physical examination. Recent data suggest that severe tricuspid regurgitation due to a flail leaflet is associated with adverse outcomes, favoring early surgical repair (see natural history section).[44]

Direct damage to the tricuspid valve may also occur as a result of infective and marantic endocarditis.[44,46] Right-sided infective endocarditis is usually a manifestation of intravenous drug abuse.[16,47] It is also increasingly seen in patients with indwelling venous catheters used for dialysis or chemotherapy and with infected pacemaker or defibrillator devices. *Staphylococcus aureus* is responsible for 80% of these tricuspid valve infections.[16] Infrequently, marantic (noninfective) endocarditis may occur in the setting of connective tissue diseases such as systemic lupus erythematosus, rheumatoid arthritis, or antiphospholipid antibody syndrome.[48] The tricuspid valve may also be damaged directly in up to 30% to 50% of patients with rheumatic mitral valve disease.[49]

Serotonin (5-HT)-active drugs may also induce tricuspid regurgitation by directly damaging the valve leaflets. This association was first described with the ergot alkaloids, ergotamine and methysergide, used for migraine therapy.[50] The anorectic drugs fenfluramine and dexfenfluramine were subsequently implicated and have since been withdrawn from the market.[51] Pergolide and cabergoline are both dopamine agonists used in the treatment of Parkinson disease and restless leg syndrome. These agents may also induce tricuspid regurgitation by a mechanism similar to that of fenfluramine and dexfenfluramine and also have been voluntarily withdrawn recently.[52-54] The drug-related histopathologic changes seen in these valves include a fibroproliferative response that appears to be mediated by the $5-HT_{2B}$ receptor.[55] These pathologic features are similar to those seen in carcinoid heart disease.

Carcinoid heart disease is a rare but distinctive form of valve disease affecting primarily the right-sided cardiac valves. Carcinoid is a rare tumor arising from argentaffin cells. The primary tumor is usually located in the small bowel and metastasizes to the liver. The primary tumor and metastases produce active substances, including serotonin. Serotonin is recognized as an agent involved in the development and progression of valve disease in patients with carcinoid syndrome.[56] Carcinoid heart disease involves a combination of tricuspid valve regurgitation (Figure 21-7) with rare stenosis as well as pulmonic valve stenosis and regurgitation. Left-sided valvular abnormalities occur in approximately 10% of patients with carcinoid valve disease characteristically due to shunting of blood from the right to left atrium through a patent foramen ovale or atrial septal defect and less commonly due to a bronchial carcinoid or very active carcinoid disease with high levels of circulating serotonin.[57] Rarely, carcinoid valve disease occurs in patients without hepatic metastases; an ovarian carcinoid tumor should be sought in this setting.[58]

Mediastinal radiation can directly damage the tricuspid leaflets. The associated postinflammatory fibrosis and calcification usually manifest 5 or more years after the radiation insult, results in distortion of the leaflets causing tricuspid regurgitation.[16,59,60] Assessment and treatment of tricuspid regurgitation in this setting may be complicated by concomitant dysfunction of other cardiac valves as well as pericardial, myocardial, and coronary artery involvement.

Endomyocardial fibrosis, which is prevalent in tropical Africa, causes fibrosis of the papillary muscle tip and thickening and shortening of the leaflets and chordae leading to regurgitation. This process may affect both mitral and tricuspid valves.

Congenital causes of tricuspid regurgitation are rare and include congenital tricuspid valve prolapse, which may occur as an isolated abnormality or be associated with mitral valve prolapse and other connective tissue disorders.[61,62] The most common congenital cause of tricuspid regurgitation is Ebstein anomaly (Figure 21-8).[63] In Ebstein anomaly there is apical displacement of the septal and posterior tricuspid valve leaflets

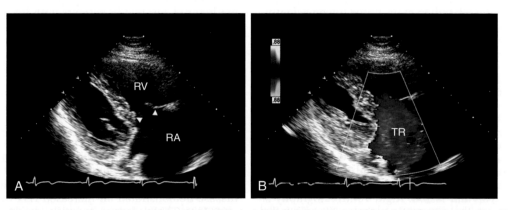

FIGURE 21-7 A, Two-dimensional echocardiographic systolic image (right ventricular inflow view) demonstrates thickened septal and anterior tricuspid valve leaflets (*arrowheads*) and enlargement of the right ventricle (RV) and right atrium (RA) in a patient with carcinoid heart disease. **B,** Color flow Doppler image demonstrates severe tricuspid regurgitation (TR) in the same patient. Note laminar color flow (blue) filling an enlarged right atrium.

21

and annular dilatation is absent, improvement in tricuspid regurgitation can be expected after relief of mitral stenosis alone. However, if severe tricuspid regurgitation is present, the valve is deformed, or there is dilatation of the tricuspid annulus, tricuspid valve surgery is necessary.[16] When patients with multivalvular disease have severe tricuspid regurgitation, tricuspid annuloplasty or replacement is often performed. It is also reasonable to consider tricuspid annuloplasty in patients with more than mild tricuspid regurgitation who are undergoing mitral valve surgery for mitral regurgitation when there is pulmonary hypertension or tricuspid annular dilatation.[16]

Adult patients with an atrial septal defect or other shunt lesion causing tricuspid annular dilatation and more than moderate tricuspid regurgitation should be considered for operative intervention rather than device closure. When these patients with an atrial septal defect are referred for surgery, the operation should include abolition of the cardiac shunt and tricuspid valve repair to decrease the degree of right heart enlargement given the unpredictable reduction in regurgitation after surgical atrial septal defect closure alone. A maze procedure is suggested if there is a history of atrial arrhythmias.[73]

TRICUSPID STENOSIS

Etiology

In developed countries, tricuspid valve stenosis is an exceptionally rare clinical condition, particularly because rheumatic heart disease accounts for about 90% of cases. Moreover, in patients with rheumatic mitral valve disease, only 3% to 5% have concurrent tricuspid stenosis.[88,89] Unusual causes of tricuspid stenosis include carcinoid heart disease,[90] congenital anomalies, infective endocarditis due to large (often fungal) vegetations, and Whipple disease.[91] A right atrial myxoma might present with signs and symptoms mimicking obstruction at the tricuspid valve level (Table 21-4).

Diagnosis

Because patients with rheumatic tricuspid stenosis invariably have coexisting mitral valve disease, it is difficult to separate symptoms specific to tricuspid valve obstruction from those of mitral valve stenosis and/or regurgitation. Reported symptoms include fatigue, dyspnea, and peripheral edema.[89,92,93]

On physical examination, venous pressure is elevated with a prominent "a" wave and characteristically an opening snap, followed by a diastolic rumbling murmur at the right sternal border that varies with respiration.[94] As with tricuspid regurgitation, physical examination findings may be subtle, and the murmur is often inaudible.

Electrocardiography shows atrial fibrillation in 50% of patients, but right atrial enlargement may be evident in those in sinus rhythm.[89,92-94] Chest radiography shows an enlarged right atrium but normal size pulmonary artery and clear lung fields. Tricuspid stenosis can be evaluated at catheterization with measurement of the transvalvular pressure gradient and calculation of valve area. However, because of the ease and accuracy of an echocardiographic assessment, cardiac catheterization is seldom necessary.

TABLE 21–4	Etiology of Tricuspid Stenosis
Rheumatic heart disease	
Congenital tricuspid stenosis	
Right atrial tumors	
Carcinoid heart disease	
Endomyocardial fibrosis	
Valvular vegetations	
Extracardiac tumors	

Echocardiography enables a definitive diagnosis of the etiology and severity of tricuspid stenosis. Rheumatic involvement parallels the changes seen with rheumatic mitral valve disease including commissural fusion and diastolic doming with thickened and shortened chordae. Even on echocardiography, findings can be subtle so that tricuspid valve involvement may be overlooked unless specific attention is directed to tricuspid valve anatomy and motion in patients with rheumatic mitral valve disease. Doppler evaluation of tricuspid stenosis severity has replaced the need for catheterization in these patients.[95-97] Tricuspid stenosis is considered severe when the mean gradient is 7 mmHg or greater and the pressure half-time is 190 milliseconds or longer.[13] According to the ACC/AHA guidelines, severe tricuspid stenosis is defined as a valve area less than 1.0 cm^2.[16]

Natural History

Few data are available on the natural history of isolated tricuspid stenosis because it typically accompanies rheumatic mitral valve disease. In a retrospective study of 13 patients with severe rheumatic tricuspid stenosis, 12 patients underwent surgery for mitral and/or aortic valve involvement and 6 of these had concurrent tricuspid valve surgery.[98] As for mitral stenosis, tricuspid valve obstruction is the result of a chronic, slowly progressive disease process correlating with a gradual increase in stenosis severity and gradual symptom onset.

Medical and Surgical Treatment

Medical therapy for significant tricuspid stenosis usually is ineffective because diuresis to improve systemic venous congestion further reduces cardiac output and thus, surgery should strongly be considered. If atrial fibrillation is present, ventricular rate control is important to promote diastolic filling. Tricuspid stenosis that requires surgery is most commonly due to rheumatic heart disease and is best treated by valve replacement (see Table 21-3).[16,18]

Tricuspid balloon valvotomy has been advocated for tricuspid stenosis of various causes. However, severe TR is a common consequence of this procedure, and results are poor when severe TR develops.[16,99,100]

PULMONIC STENOSIS

Etiology

Pulmonic valve stenosis is related to a congenital or genetic disorder in 95% of patients. Although pulmonic stenosis may be a feature of complex congenital cardiac lesions, such as tetralogy of Fallot, 80% of cases occur in isolation. Rarely carcinoid syndrome or rheumatic valve disease may cause pulmonic stenosis, but these lesions always occur in conjunction with other valve disease.[91]

The abnormal pulmonic valve may be classified as *acommissural* with prominent systolic doming of the valve cusps and an eccentric orifice, *unicommissural* with a single asymmetric commissure, *bicuspid* with fused commissures, or *dysplastic* with severely thickened and deformed valve cusps (Figure 21-13). Evaluation of valve morphology is important as dysplastic valves respond poorly to balloon dilation. The pulmonary annulus and outflow tract may also be narrowed; this type of valve morphology is common in patients with Noonan syndrome.

Pulmonary artery aneurysms may be associated with pulmonic stenosis and are generally benign. Most patients with pulmonary artery enlargement and congenital pulmonic stenosis do not require operative intervention in the absence of symptomatic compression of adjacent structures or pulmonary regurgitation with associated right heart enlargement. Rarely rupture or dissection may occur when severe pulmonary artery dilatation occurs in the setting of severe pulmonary hypertension.[101,102]

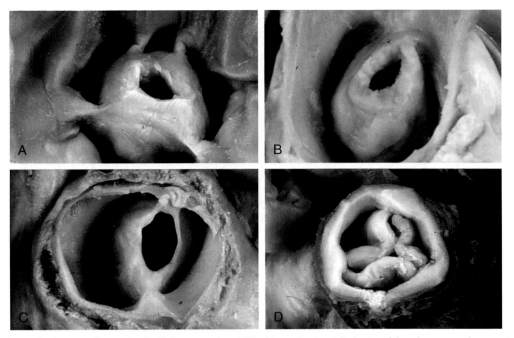

FIGURE 21-13 The abnormal pulmonary valve may be classified as acommissural (**A**) with prominent systolic doming of the valve cusps and an eccentric orifice, unicommissural (**B**), bicuspid with fused commissures (**C**), or dysplastic (**D**) with severely thickened and deformed valve cusps. *(Courtesy of Dr. William D. Edwards, Department of Laboratory Medicine and Pathology, Mayo Clinic College of Medicine.)*

Diagnosis

Most patients with mild or moderate pulmonic stenosis are asymptomatic, and even those with severe obstruction may have no symptoms. Typical symptoms associated with pulmonic stenosis include fatigue and dyspnea due to reduced cardiac output. Some patients delay symptom onset by adjusting their lifestyle and level of activity. Exertional lightheadedness or syncope may occur in adults with pulmonic stenosis associated with systemic or suprasystemic right ventricular pressures. With long-standing severe pulmonic stenosis, right heart failure may occur. Sudden death is uncommon.

Most adults with pulmonic stenosis have a normal appearance. In Noonan syndrome characteristic features include short stature, webbed neck, hypertelorism, low-set ears and hairline, chest wall deformities, and lymphedema. This diagnosis is important to recognize because this is an autosomal dominant condition that has a high frequency of associated cardiac anomalies (reported in 85%), most commonly pulmonic stenosis in 60%.[103] The typically dysplastic pulmonic valve in patients with Noonan syndrome is less amenable to balloon intervention, and surgical treatment should be considered.

Clinical findings depend on the severity of pulmonic stenosis, and other associated cardiac lesions. In mild pulmonic stenosis, the physical examination is characterized by a normal jugular venous pulse, no right ventricular lift, and a pulmonic ejection sound that tends to decrease with inspiration. A pulmonic ejection murmur is usually heard, ending in mid-systole; this murmur increases in intensity with inspiration.

In severe pulmonic stenosis, the jugular venous pressure demonstrates a prominent a wave, and a right ventricular lift is common. A palpable systolic murmur may be noted at the upper left sternal border. A loud and long crescendo-decrescendo pulmonic ejection systolic murmur is present, which is loudest at the upper left sternal border, radiating to the suprasternal notch and left side of the neck. Although an ejection click is common in mild pulmonic stenosis, with increasing severity the click moves closer to the first heart sound and may even

be absent when severe stenosis is present. As pulmonic stenosis progresses, the second heart sound becomes widely split as a result of delayed pulmonic valve closure due to prolongation of the right ventricular ejection time. Eventually, as the severity increases further, pulmonic valve closure is no longer audible. As a consequence of right ventricular hypertrophy, a right-sided fourth heart sound may also be heard.

An electrocardiogram is generally recommended for the initial and serial evaluation of patients with pulmonic stenosis.[16] The electrocardiogram is usually normal in patients with pulmonic stenosis, however when the right ventricular pressure is greater than 60 mmHg, features of right atrial enlargement, right axis deviation, and right ventricular hypertrophy may be present. Depending on the severity of pulmonic stenosis, a right ventricular strain pattern may be present (Figure 21-14A).

The chest radiograph may be normal or may demonstrate features of right heart enlargement and dilatation of the pulmonary artery (see Figure 21-14B). In severe pulmonic stenosis, the vascular markings may be diminished.

Transthoracic Doppler echocardiography is recommended for the initial and serial follow-up evaluation of pulmonic stenosis.[16] The diagnosis of pulmonic stenosis is usually best confirmed by transthoracic echocardiography. Two-dimensional echocardiography demonstrates the thickened pulmonic valve cusps with characteristic doming in systole as the cusps reach their limit of excursion. The severity of pulmonic stenosis is determined by the peak transpulmonary velocity using continuous wave Doppler to calculate the transvalvular pressure gradient (see Figure 21-5). The 2006 ACC/AHA guidelines on the management of valvular heart disease define severe pulmonic stenosis as a peak gradient greater than 60 mmHg, moderate pulmonic stenosis as a peak gradient 36 to 60 mmHg, and mild pulmonic stenosis as a peak gradient less than 36 mmHg.[16] The right ventricular systolic pressure can be confirmed from the tricuspid regurgitant jet velocity using the modified Bernoulli equation. In addition, right ventricular hypertrophy is seen with severe pulmonic stenosis. The degree of coexisting pulmonic regurgitation is evaluated using color-flow Doppler imaging and

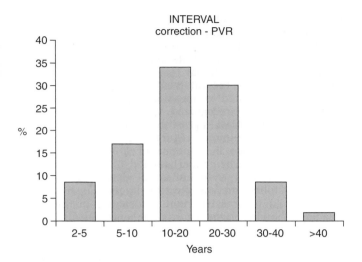

INTERVAL
correction - PVR

FIGURE 21–20 The interval between initial tetralogy of Fallot repair and reoperation for severe pulmonic regurgitation in 51 patients undergoing reoperation. PVR, pulmonic valve replacement. *(From Hazekamp M, Kurvers MM, Schoof PH, et al: Pulmonary valve insertion late after repair of Fallot's tetralogy. Eur J Cardiothorac Surg 2001;19:667-670, with permission.)*

for surgical right ventricular outflow tract reduction, higher preoperative right ventricular volumes were independently associated with a larger decrease of right ventricular volumes. A cutoff value of $160\,mL/m^2$ for normalization of right ventricular end-diastolic volume or $82\,mL/m^2$ for right ventricular end-systolic volume was noted. In this series, a threshold above which right ventricular volumes did not decrease after surgery was not identified (Figure 21-21).[34]

The type of pulmonic valve prosthesis should be individualized, and the operation should be performed by a cardiac surgeon experienced in the management of congenital cardiac disease (see pulmonary stenosis section). An annual echocardiogram is appropriate for patient monitoring, ideally beginning soon after the initial surgery so that residual right ventricular dilation can be distinguished from progressive disease.

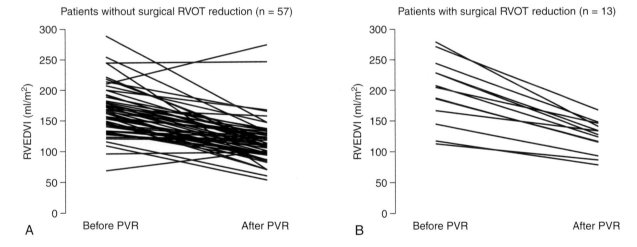

FIGURE 21–21 Impact of pulmonic valve replacement on right ventricular size. The decrease in right ventricular end-diastolic volume index (RVEDVI) is depicted for patients with tetralogy of Fallot, treated with pulmonic valve replacement. *Left*, Patients who did not undergo a surgical right ventricular (RV) outflow tract (RVOT) reduction (*n* = 58). *Right*, patients with a surgical RVOT reduction (*n* = 13). In four patients without surgical RVOT reduction, right ventricular size did not decrease after surgery. Three of these patients developed postoperative pulmonic regurgitation greater that 20%. Note that in patients without surgical RVOT reduction and high RVEDVI, right ventricular size could decrease substantially. Furthermore, two patients were operated on with normal preoperative RVEDVI. Both patients became symptomatic with severe pulmonic regurgitation and a right ventricle that was larger than the left ventricle. *(From Oosterhof T, van Straten A, Vliegen HW, et al: Preoperative thresholds for pulmonary valve replacement in patients with corrected tetralogy of Fallot using cardiovascular magnetic resonance. Circulation 2007;116:545-551, with permission.)*

REFERENCES

1. Bommer W, Weinert L, Neumann A, et al: Determination of right atrial and right ventricular size by two dimensional echocardiography. Circulation 1979;60:91-100.
2. Watanabe T, Katsume H, Matsukubo H, et al: Estimation of right ventricular volume with two dimensional echocardiography. Am J Cardiol 1982;49:1946-1953.
3. Dell'Italia L, Walsh R: Right ventricular diastolic pressure-volume relations and regional dimensions during acute alterations in loading conditions. Circulation 1988;77:1276-1282.
4. Feneley M, Gavaghan T: Paradoxical and pseudoparadoxical interventricular septal motion in patients with right ventricular volume overload. Circulation 1986;74:230-238.

5. Pearlman AS, Clark CE, Henry WL, et al: Determinants of ventricular septal motion: influence of relative right and left ventricular size. Circulation 1976;54:83-91.
6. Louie EK, Rich S, Levitsky S, Brundage BH: Doppler echocardiographic demonstration of the differential effects of right ventricular pressure and volume overload on left ventricular geometry and filling. J Am Coll Cardiol 1992;19:84-90.
7. Dell'Italia L: The right ventricle: anatomy, physiology, and clinical importance. Curr Probl Cardiol 1991;16:653-720.
8. Lee F: Hemodynamics of the right ventricle in normal and disease states. Cardiol Clin 1992;10:59-67.
9. Spann JF Jr, Buccino RA, Sonnenblick EH, Braunwald E: Contractile state of cardiac muscle obtained from cats with experimentally produced ventricular hypertrophy and heart failure. Circ Res 1967;21:341-354.

10. Kramer M, Valantine HA, Marshall SE, et al: Recovery of the right ventricle after single-lung transplantation in pulmonary hypertension. Am J Cardiol 1994;73:494-500.
11. Scuderi LJ, Bailey SR, Calhoon JH, et al: Echocardiographic assessment of right and left ventricular function after single-lung transplantation. Am Heart J 1994;127:636-642.
12. Jardin F, Dubourg O, Guéret P, et al: Quantitative two-dimensional echocardiography in massive pulmonary embolism: emphasis on ventricular interdependence and leftward septal displacement. J Am Coll Cardiol 1987;10:1201-1206.
13. Oh JK, Seward JB, Tajik AJ: The Echo Manual, 3rd ed. Baltimore, Lippincott Williams & Wilkins, 2006.
14. Klein A, Burstow DJ, Tajik AJ, et al: Age-related prevalence of valvular regurgitation in normal subjects: a comprehensive color flow examination of 118 volunteers. J Am Soc Echocardiogr 1990;3:54-63.
15. Baumgartner FJ, Milliken JC, Robertson JM, et al: Clinical patterns of surgical endocarditis. J Card Surg 2007;22:32-38.
16. Bonow RO, Carabello BA, Chatterjee KC, et al: ACC/AHA 2006 guidelines for the management of patients with valvular heart disease: a report of the American College of Cardiology/American Heart Association Task Force on Practice Guidelines. Circulation 2006;114:e84-e231.
17. Zoghbi WA, Enriquez-Sarano M, Foster E, et al: Recommendations for evaluation of the severity of native valvular regurgitation with two-dimensional and Doppler echocardiography. J Am Soc Echocardiogr 2003;16:777-802.
18. Vahanian A, Baumgartner H, Bax J, et al: Guidelines on the management of valvular heart disease: the Task Force on the Management of Valvular Heart Disease of the European Society of Cardiology. Eur Heart J 2007;28:230-268.
19. Pennestrí F, Loperfido F, Salvatori MP, et al: Assessment of tricuspid regurgitation by pulsed Doppler ultrasonography of the hepatic veins. Am J Cardiol 1984;54:363-368.
20. Sakai K, Nakamura K, Satomi G, et al: Evaluation of tricuspid regurgitation by blood flow pattern in the hepatic vein using pulsed Doppler technique. Am Heart J 1984;108(3 Pt 1):516-523.
21. Fawzy ME, Mercer EN, Dunn B, et al: Doppler echocardiography in the evaluation of tricuspid stenosis. Eur Heart J 1989;10:985-990.
22. Kobayashi J, Nakano S, Matsuda H, et al: Quantitative evaluation of pulmonary regurgitation after repair of tetralogy of Fallot using real time flow imaging system. Jpn Circ J 1989;53:721-727.
23. Silversides C, Veldtman GR, Crossin J, et al: Pressure half-time predicts hemodynamically significant pulmonary regurgitation in adult patients with repaired tetralogy of Fallot. J Am Soc Echocardiogr 2003;16:1057-1062.
24. Lang RM, Bierig M, Devereux RB, et al: Recommendations for chamber quantification: a report from the American Society of Echocardiography's Guidelines and Standards Committee and the Chamber Quantification Writing Group, developed in conjunction with the European Association of Echocardiography, a branch of the European Society of Cardiology. J Am Soc Echocardiogr 2005;18:1440-1463.
25. Lang RM, Mor-Avi V, Sugong L, et al: Three-dimensional echocardiography: the benefits of the additional dimension. J Am Coll Cardiol 2006;48:2053-2069.
26. Tei C, Dujardin KS, Hodge DO, et al: Doppler echocardiographic index for assessment of global right ventricular function. J Am Soc Echocardiogr 1996;9:838-847.
27. LaCorte JC, Cabreriza SE, Rabkin DG, et al: Correlation of the Tei index with invasive measurements of ventricular function in a porcine model. J Am Soc Echocardiogr 2003;16:442-447.
28. Meluzin J, Spinarová L, Bakala J, et al: Pulsed Doppler tissue imaging of the velocity of tricuspid annular systolic motion; a new, rapid, and non-invasive method of evaluating right ventricular systolic function. Eur Heart J 2001;22:340-348.
29. Miller D, Farah MG, Liner A, et al: The relation between quantitative right ventricular ejection fraction and indices of tricuspid annular motion and myocardial performance. J Am Soc Echocardiogr 2004;17:443-447.
30. Grothues F, Moon JC, Bellenger NG, et al: Interstudy reproducibility of right ventricular volumes, function, and mass with cardiovascular magnetic resonance. Am Heart J 2004;147:218-223.
31. Møgelvang J, Stubgaard M, Thomsen C, Henriksen O: Evaluation of right ventricular volumes measured by magnetic resonance imaging. Eur Heart J 1988;9:529-533.
32. Buechel ER, Dave HH, Kellenberger CJ, et al: Remodelling of the right ventricle after early pulmonary valve replacement in children with repaired tetralogy of Fallot: assessment by cardiovascular magnetic resonance. Eur Heart J 2005;26:2721-2727.
33. Therrien J, Provost Y, Merchant N, et al: Optimal timing for pulmonary valve replacement in adults after tetralogy of Fallot repair. Am J Cardiol 2005;95:779-782.
34. Oosterhof T, van Straten A, Vliegen HW, et al: Preoperative thresholds for pulmonary valve replacement in patients with corrected tetralogy of Fallot using cardiovascular magnetic resonance. Circulation 2007;116:545-551.
35. Beygui F, Furber A, Delépine S, et al: Routine breath-hold gradient echo MRI-derived right ventricular mass, volumes and function: accuracy, reproducibility and coherence study. Int J Cardiovasc Imaging 2004;20:509-516.
36. Bleeker GB, Steendijk P, Holman ER, et al: Assessing right ventricular function: the role of echocardiography and complementary technologies. Heart 2006;92(Suppl 1):i19-i26.
37. Clorius S, Technau K, Watter T, et al: Nephrogenic systemic fibrosis following exposure to gadolinium-containing contrast agent. Clin Nephrol 2007;68:249-252.
38. Cohen S, Sell JE, McIntosh CL, Clark RE: Tricuspid regurgitation in patients with acquired, chronic, pure mitral regurgitation. II. Nonoperative management, tricuspid valve annuloplasty, and tricuspid valve replacement. J Thorac Cardiovasc Surg 1987;94:488-497.
39. Waller BF, Moriarty AT, Eble JN, et al: Etiology of pure tricuspid regurgitation based on anular circumference and leaflet area: analysis of 45 necropsy patients with clinical and morphologic evidence of pure tricuspid regurgitation. J Am Coll Cardiol 1986;7:1063-1074.
40. Muller O, Shillingford J: Tricuspid incompetence. Br Heart J 1954;16:195.
41. Salazar E, Levine H: Rheumatic tricuspid regurgitation. Am J Med 1962;33:111-129.
42. Sepulveda G, Lukas D: The diagnosis of tricuspid insufficiency—clinical features in 60 cases with associated mitral valve disease Circulation 1955;11:552-562.
43. Lin G, Nishimura RA, Connolly HM, et al: Severe symptomatic tricuspid valve regurgitation due to permanent pacemaker or implantable cardioverter-defibrillator leads. J Am Coll Cardiol 2005;45:1672-1675.
44. Messika-Zeitoun D, Thomson H, Bellamy M, et al: Medical and surgical outcome of tricuspid regurgitation caused by flail leaflets. J Thorac Cardiovasc Surg 2004;128:296-302.
45. Marvin R, Schrank J, Nolan S: Traumatic tricuspid insufficiency. Am J Cardiol 1973;32:723-726.
46. van Son JA, Danielson GK, Schaff HV, Miller FA Jr: Traumatic tricuspid valve insufficiency: experience in thirteen patients. J Thorac Cardiovasc Surg 1994;108:893-898.
47. Chan P, Ogilby JD, Segal B: Tricuspid valve endocarditis. Am Heart J 1989;117:1140-1146.
48. Waller BF, Knapp WS, Edwards JE: Marantic valvular vegetations. Circulation 1973;48:644-650.
49. Duran C: Tricuspid valve surgery revisited. J Card Surg 1994;9(2 Suppl):242-247.
50. Redfield MM, Nicholson WJ, Edwards WD, Tajik AJ: Valve disease associated with ergot alkaloid use: echocardiographic and pathologic correlations. Ann Intern Med 1992;117:50-52.
51. Connolly HM, Crary JL, McGoon MD, et al: Valvular heart disease associated with fenfluramine-phentermine. N Engl J Med 1997;337:581-588.
52. Pritchett AM, Morrison JF, Edwards WD, et al: Valvular heart disease in patients taking pergolide. Mayo Clin Proc 2002;77:1280-1286.
53. Schade R, Andersohn F, Suissa S, et al: Dopamine agonists and the risk of cardiac-valve regurgitation. N Engl J Med 2007;356:29-38.
54. Zanettini R, Antonini A, Gatto G, et al: Valvular heart disease and the use of dopamine agonists for Parkinson's disease. N Engl J Med 2007;356:39-46.
55. Rothman RB, Baumann MH, Savage JE, et al: Evidence for possible involvement of 5-HT(2B) receptors in the cardiac valvulopathy associated with fenfluramine and other serotonergic medications. Circulation 2000;102:2836-2841.
56. Møller JE, Pellikka PA, Bernheim AM, et al: Prognosis of carcinoid heart disease: analysis of 200 cases over two decades. Circulation 2005;112:3320-7.
57. Connolly HM, Schaff HV, Mullany CJ, et al: Surgical management of left-sided carcinoid heart disease. Circulation 2001;104(12 Suppl 1):I36-I40.
58. Chaowalit N, Connolly HM, Schaff HV, et al: Carcinoid heart disease associated with primary ovarian carcinoid tumor. Am J Cardiol 2004;93:1314-1315.
59. Adams MJ, Lipshultz SE, Schwartz C, et al: Radiation-associated cardiovascular disease. Crit Rev Oncol Hematol 2003;45:55-75.
60. Crestanello JA, McGregor CG, Danielson GK, et al: Mitral and tricuspid valve repair in patients with previous mediastinal radiation therapy. Ann Thorac Surg 2004;78:826-831.
61. Chandraratna P, Lopez JM, Fernandez JJ, Cohen LS: Echocardiographic detection of tricuspid valve prolapse Circulation 1975;51:823-826.
62. Weinreich D, Burke JF, Bharati S, Lev M: Isolated prolapse of the tricuspid valve. J Am Coll Cardiol 1985;6:475-481.
63. Attenhofer Jost CH, Connolly HM, Dearani JA, et al: Ebstein's anomaly. Circulation 2007;115:277-285.
64. Celermajer DS, Bull C, Till JA, et al: Ebstein's anomaly: presentation and outcome from fetus to adult. J Am Coll Cardiol 1994;23:170-176.
65. Hansing C, Rowe G: Tricuspid insufficiency: a study of hemodynamics and pathogenesis. Circulation 1972;45:793-799.
66. DePace N, Ross J, Iskandrian AS, et al: Tricuspid regurgitation: noninvasive techniques for determining causes and severity. J Am Coll Cardiol 1984;3:1540-1550.
67. Groves P, Lewis NP, Ikram S, et al: Reduced exercise capacity in patients with tricuspid regurgitation after successful mitral valve replacement for rheumatic mitral valve disease. Br Heart J 1991; 66:295-301.
68. Sagie A, Schwammenthal E, Newell JB, et al: Significant tricuspid regurgitation is a marker for adverse outcome in patients undergoing percutaneous balloon mitral valvuloplasty. J Am Coll Cardiol 1994;24:696-702.
69. Tang GH, David TE, Singh SK, et al: Tricuspid valve repair with an annuloplasty ring results in improved long-term outcomes. Circulation 2006;114(1 Suppl):I577-I581.
70. Fukuda S, Song JM, Gillinov AM, et al: Tricuspid valve tethering predicts residual tricuspid regurgitation after tricuspid annuloplasty. Circulation 2005;111:975-979.
71. Singh SK, Tang GH, Maganti MD, et al: Midterm outcomes of tricuspid valve repair versus replacement for organic tricuspid disease. Ann Thorac Surg 2006;82:1735-1741.
72. Ohata T, Kigawa I, Tohda E, Wanibuchi Y: Comparison of durability of bioprostheses in tricuspid and mitral positions. Ann Thorac Surg 2001;71(5 Suppl):S240-S243.
73. Stulak JM, Dearani JA, Puga FJ, et al: Right-sided maze procedure for atrial tachyarrhythmias in congenital heart disease. Ann Thorac Surg 2006;81:1780-1785.
74. Ratnatunga C, Edwards MB, Dore CJ, Taylor KM: Tricuspid valve replacement: UK Heart Valve Registry mid-term results comparing mechanical and biological prostheses. Ann Thorac Surg 1998;1998:1940-1947.
75. Rizzoli G, Vendramin I, Nesseris G, et al: Biological or mechanical prostheses in tricuspid position? A meta-analysis of intra-institutional results. Ann Thorac Surg 2004;77:1607-1614.
76. Bove E, Kavey RE, Byrum CJ, et al: Improved right ventricular function following late pulmonary valve replacement for residual pulmonary insufficiency or stenosis. J Thorac Cardiovasc Surg 1985;90:50-55.
77. Sadeghi HM, Kimura BJ, Raisinghani A, et al: Does lowering pulmonary arterial pressure eliminate severe functional tricuspid regurgitation? Insights from pulmonary thromboendarterectomy. J Am Coll Cardiol 2004;44:126-132.
78. Hannoush H, Fawzy ME, Stefadouros M, et al: Regression of significant tricuspid regurgitation after mitral balloon valvotomy for severe mitral stenosis. Am Heart J 2004;148:865-70.
79. Song JM, Kang DH, Song JK, et al: Outcome of significant functional tricuspid regurgitation after percutaneous mitral valvuloplasty. Am Heart J 2003;145:371-376.

Infective Endocarditis

Thomas M. Bashore

KEY POINTS

- Infective endocarditis remains a deadly disease with death in one of four patients despite advances in antimicrobial therapy.
- In the past, infective endocarditis was a disease that most commonly involved *Streptococcus viridans* species in younger patients who had rheumatic valvular disease. Now endocarditis is mainly caused by staphylococcal infections, and most patients are elderly, are injection drug users, or have an implanted medical device (prosthetic valve, pacemaker, or defibrillator). Only three fourths of patients with infective endocarditis have known underlying heart disease.
- Endocarditis begins with platelet and fibrin deposition in an area of endothelial damage, with formation of a nonbacterial thrombotic lesion. Bacteria adherence to this lesion occurs, particularly with organisms such as staphylococcal species that have adhesion molecules on their surfaces. Bacterial growth leads to recruitment of inflammatory cells and valvular damage ensues.
- Many of the classic features of infective endocarditis are not seen anymore because of early diagnosis. The modified Duke criteria are important in establishing a diagnosis and rely on the determination of a likely organism and on evidence for valvular vegetations or leaflet destruction. Epiphenomena, such as fever, evidence for inflammatory markers, or signs of peripheral emboli, contribute to the criteria.
- About 15% of patients with infective endocarditis have negative blood cultures. An aggressive approach to uncovering the infective source is necessary including novel culture methods, antibody titers, and molecular and immunologic methods.
- Echocardiography is the key diagnostic tool and provides major diagnostic Duke criteria. Use of an algorithm reduces unnecessary use of echocardiography. In many patients transesophageal echocardiography is critical for diagnosis and evaluation of vegetation size, abscess formation, fistula formation, leaflet perforation, or prosthetic valve dehiscence.
- The prognosis of infective endocarditis is worse in patients with congestive heart failure, altered mental state, general debility, poor left ventricular function, and/or diabetes. Patients undergoing hemodialysis also do poorly as do those with significant emboli. Injection drug users tend to do better than others because of their young age and higher likelihood of tricuspid endocarditis (rather than left-sided disease). Concurrent human immunodeficiency virus infection in injection drug users does not contribute added risk unless their CD4 counts are low.
- Prosthetic valve endocarditis early (<60 days) after surgery tends to be nosocomial, whereas late infections are more similar to native valve infective endocarditis.
- Cardiac device infections are a major source of new cases of infective endocarditis because device use is growing. In most patients device removal, in addition to antibiotics, is needed to cure the infection.
- Patients undergoing surgery tend to do better than those receiving medical treatment, although medical cure rates continue to improve. Congestive heart failure remains the primary reason for surgical intervention. Other indications for surgery are extensive valvular destruction and large vegetations, a paravalvular abscess, ineffective antimicrobial therapy, recurrent emboli, or the presence of a highly resistant organism.
- The type of organism determines the type and duration of therapy. For most native valve endocarditis, 4 weeks of therapy are warranted, whereas prosthetic valve endocarditis generally requires 6 weeks. In select situations with right heart involvement, 2 weeks of therapy may be adequate. More resistant organisms require 8 weeks of treatment, and some unusual organisms may require months or years.

The earliest description of the vegetative lesions of endocarditis has been attributed to Lazarus Riverius (1589-1655),[1] and later Giovanni Lancisi (1654-1720)[2] provided a more complete description of these pathologic lesions of the heart in *De Subitaneis Mortibus* written in 1709. Throughout the 18th and early 19th centuries there were many descriptions of endocarditis by investigators such as Morgagni and Corvisart, yet it was not until the mid to late 19th century that a link was made between the lesions, the associated inflammation, and the sequelae of the disease. In 1841, Bouillard (1796-1881) made the important connection between the inflamed endocardium, a "typhoid" state, and "gangrenous endocarditis." This was followed by observations of Virchow (1821-1902) in 1847 and Kirkes (1823-1864) in 1852 related to the link between vegetative lesions and embolic events.[1]

In his famous 1885 Gulstonian lectures Osler summarized the knowledge at that time and in addition made several important observations. First he described the acute and fulminating forms of the disease and was able to articulate specific characteristics of a more chronic and insidious form. He then improved the nomenclature of the disease and suggested calling the clinical course of the disease either "simple" or "malignant."[3,4] In addition, he described both the classic presentation of a typical case and noted the diagnostic uncertainty in many cases. Finally, Osler believed that endocarditis would turn out to be a "mycotic" process, stating "…in all its forms, an essentially mycotic process; the local and constitutional effects being produced by the growth of valves, and the transference to distant parts of microbes, which vary in character with the disease in which it develops."

Since the days of Osler there have been many advances in our understanding of infective endocarditis (IE) from pathophysiology to diagnosis, prognosis, and treatment, yet our knowledge remains incomplete. What is clear is that this is a serious and dynamic disease process.

EPIDEMIOLOGY

Cardiac Risk Factors

The true incidence of endocarditis is difficult to ascertain. Over the past 10 years, several epidemiologic studies have provided data on both the incidence of endocarditis and insight into populations at risk. In a Swedish urban setting, Hogevik et al[5] found an incidence of 5.9 episodes per 100,000 person-years from 1984 to 1988. During a similar time period, in a Philadelphia metropolitan study the total incidence was calculated to be 9.29 episodes per 100,000 person-years.[6] When intravenous drug abusers were excluded, this incidence fell to 5.02 episodes per 100,000 person-years. In both urban and rural settings in France, the incidence was estimated to be around 2.43 episodes per 100,000 person-years[7] in 1991 and increased to 3.1 episodes per 100,000 person-years in 1999[8] with a peak incidence of 14.5 episodes per 100,000 person-years in the elderly. The growing incidence in elderly individuals has been confirmed in the Medicare population in the United States, with 20.4 episodes per 100,000 person-years in 1998 (a 13.7% increase from 1986).[9] In fact, more than half of all cases of IE in the United States and Europe now occur in patients older than age 60, and the median age of patients has increased steadily during the past 40 years.[10] Endocarditis is therefore now occurring less in patients with poor dentition and rheumatic disease and more in elderly patients and those who undergo procedures to implant devices such as prosthetic valves, pacemakers, and defibrillators.[8,11]

Table 22-1 summarizes cardiac conditions and their estimated incidence of IE per 100,000 patient-years.[12] Sex and

TABLE 22–1	Incidence of Endocarditis
	Per 100,000 Patient-Years
General population	5-7
Underlying cardiac conditions	
Mitral valve prolapse with no murmur	4.6
Mitral valve prolapse with mitral regurgitation	52
Ventricular septal defect	145 (½ risk if closed)
Aortic stenosis	271
Rheumatic heart disease	380-440
Prosthetic heart valve	308-383
Cardiac surgery for native infective endocarditis	630
Prior native endocarditis	740
Surgery for prosthetic infective endocarditis	2160

age also influence the incidence of IE with males predominating. Male to female ratios have been noted to range from 3.2:1 to 9:1.[10,13,14] Of interest, 50% to 70 % of children younger than 2 years who develop IE have no underlying heart disease, whereas older children usually have a congenital heart condition.[15] Endocarditis in injection drug users (IDUs) also may occur when there is no apparent underlying valvular pathologic lesions.

Around 75% of all patients do have underlying structural heart disease at the time of their endocarditis[16,17] with a wide variability from 42% to 98% in different series.[18] Earlier reports before 1967 showed that rheumatic heart disease was the most common cardiac abnormality, being present in 39% of patients.[19] In contrast, a later series from Tennessee showed that rheumatic heart disease was present in only 6% of patients with IE.[17]

In 1999, we estimated that 38% of all cases of endocarditis involve the aortic valve with 34% involving the mitral valve, 8% involving both the aortic and mitral valves, and 4% involving the tricuspid valve. Congenital heart disease represents the underlying disorder in about 3.5% of all cases.[18] Specific valvular lesion involvement is summarized in Table 22-2.[20] Mitral valve lesions, specifically mitral prolapse and mitral regurgitation, are the most common single underlying pathologic lesions now. These are followed by aortic regurgitation, aortic stenosis, prosthetic valves, and finally congenital heart disease (particularly cyanotic heart disease). Endocarditis is unusual in patients with isolated pulmonary stenosis, atrial septal defect, mitral stenosis, or hypertrophic cardiomyopathy.

TABLE 22–2	Specific Predisposing Valvular Lesions in Patients with Endocarditis
	% Endocarditis Cases
Native valve disease	
Mitral regurgitation	21-33
Aortic regurgitation	17-30
Aortic stenosis	10-18
Congenital heart disease	4-18
Cyanotic heart disease	8
Tetralogy of Fallot	2
Ventricular septal defect	1.5
Patent ductus arteriosus	1.5
Eisenmenger syndrome	1.2
Atrial septal defect, coarctation of aorta	<1
Prosthetic valve	12-30

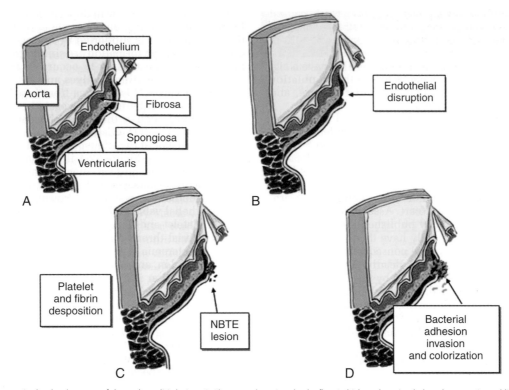

FIGURE 22-2 The steps in the development of the endocarditis lesion. **A,** The normal aortic valve leaflet. A thickened portion below the commissural line is the area where the leaflets coapt and trauma most likely to occur. Endothelium covers the valve and is an extension of aortic and ventricular endothelium. The fibrosa provides major support for the leaflet. The ventricularis underlies the free edge, and the spongiosa lies between the two in the central portion. **B,** The initial insult with endothelial injury and exposure of valve collagen. **C,** Platelet and fibrin deposition with the formation of the nonbacterial thrombotic endocardial lesion (NBTE). **D,** Adhesion of microorganisms and then invasion into the NBTE lesion and colonization. Inflammatory cells become evident and elastin and collagen disruption occurs, and the valve destruction begins.

An important component in the formation of the infected vegetation is adherence of the organisms to the endothelium or to the NBTE lesion. This adherence is by adhesive surface matrix molecules on the microorganism. Certain organisms appear to produce these surface molecules more than others, which may explain their particular attraction for the NBTE lesion. For instance, streptococci that produce surface glucans and dextran appear to be more likely to cause endocarditis than those that do not.[40] Other proteins may also be involved, depending on the organism.[21]

In up to 30% of patients, a preexisting cardiac abnormality may not be evident.[41] Several organisms appear capable of infecting apparently normal valves, including *S. aureus*, some streptococci, *Salmonella, Rickettsia, Borrelia,* and *Candida*.[41] In these patients, endothelial infection may occur via interaction of specific glycoproteins or by endothelial phagocytosis. It has even been postulated that the endothelial cells may contain metabolically latent organisms that eventually damage the endothelium.[42]

The endothelial cells, fibroblasts, and platelets also produce fibronectin that binds to the subendothelial collagen, fibrin, and certain microorganisms, thus facilitating the adherence of the infectious agent. Receptors for fibronectin and adhesive molecules have been found on the surface of *S. aureus, Streptococcus viridans, Streptococcus pneumoniae* and group A, C, and G streptococci, and *Candida albicans*.[40] The adherence mechanism involves both the host extracellular matrix and the adherence surface proteins of the infecting agents. Streptococci may express more than a dozen different microbial surface components that recognize adherence receptors that attach to fibronectin or collagen. One of them, protein F1/SfbI, binds fibronectin and mediates adherence of the streptococci to host cells. Bound fibronectin acts as a bridging molecule toward host cell integrins, which in turn initialize the uptake process that leads to streptococci internalization. Once safely inside the cells, the bacteria can survive, protected from antibiotics and host defense,[43] which may explain why certain organisms, such as staphylococcal species or streptococci, that bind to platelets and incite the clotting mechanism may be more virulent than those organisms that readily shed into the bloodstream. A clumping factor (fibrinogen-binding surface protein) may also help certain organisms, such as *S. aureus*, bind to platelet thrombi.[40]

The fact that *S. aureus* may also induce endothelial cells to produce tissue factor could, at least partially, explain why *S. aureus* adheres to relatively normal valves. Particulate material that may be injected by intravenous drug abusers may also promote *S. aureus* adherence by stimulating adhesive binding molecules on normal heart valves.[40] This concept has been postulated to explain the distinct predilection for the tricuspid valve to be involved in intravenous drug abusers, with one report suggesting that involvement occurs in 78% of cases of endocarditis in this population, followed by involvement of the mitral in 24% and the aortic valve in 8%.[44]

A potential therapeutic approach to prevent this binding was tried with the St. Jude Silzone prosthetic valve ring, a silver-coated polyester ring. Unfortunately, concerns regarding increased paravalvular regurgitation and emboli led to its early withdrawal from clinical trials.[45]

All of these processes eventually lead to the infecting organism proliferating within the vegetation. The cycle of adherence, organism growth, and platelet-fibrin deposition then is repeated again and again as the vegetation develops. After treatment, capillaries and fibroblasts may appear in the lesion, but untreated lesions tend to be avascular. Necrosis, with various stages of healing may occur along with vasculitic components in the healed lesion. Even after successful antimicrobial therapy, many sterile vegetations will persist indefinitely.[46]

DIAGNOSIS

Clinical Manifestations

The prevalence of the clinical features observed in patients with IE is summarized in Table 22-6. Many of the features espoused by Osler in the Gulstonian lectures[4,47] are rarely seen today as therapy for IE is now available, and fewer patients have a prolonged course. Most patients who develop IE have an indolent course from 2 weeks to many months with the presence of vague symptoms. Symptoms include fever, chills, anorexia, weight loss, night sweats, and malaise.

Fever is the most common symptom, occurring in from 64% to 93% of patients with native valve endocarditis, 85% with PVE, and 75% to 88% of IDU patients with IE. It is less common in elderly patients, those with congestive heart failure (CHF), renal failure, severe debility, or previous antibiotic therapy.[48] Persistent fever more than 1 week after therapy requires further investigation into whether there is a persistent cause (e.g., an abscess somewhere), a nosocomial infection, drug fever, or inadequate IE therapy.

A murmur is apparent in 80% to 85% of patients,[21] although auscultation is a dying art in cardiology, and a murmur may not be recognized even when present. The murmur of acute and fulminant aortic regurgitation may be particularly difficult to hear as there is little diastolic gradient. Whereas tricuspid regurgitation should be evident from examination of the jugular venous pulse, the murmur is often quite soft if right ventricular systolic pressure is normal.

A variety of peripheral cutaneous manifestations provide for the classic endocarditis examination (Figure 22-3). Unfortunately, the incidence of many of these events is not high. Emboli can be observed in many areas such as the mouth or conjunctival petechiae, nail bed splinters, skin Janeway lesions or Osler nodes, or funduscopic Roth spots. Splinter hemorrhages tend to occur in the proximal half of the nail bed as opposed to splinters due to trauma that occur in the outer half. Janeway lesions are painless, erythematous skin lesions that often appear in crops on the hands or feet. Biopsies reveal that they are microabscesses without arteritis, and organisms can often be cultured from them.

Osler nodes are painful lesions that present as nodules on the pads of the toes or fingertips and may persist for days. The cause for Osler nodes is unclear, but the fact that they may be seen in nonendocarditis settings, such as in those systemic lupus erythematosus, and the histologic evidence for perivasculitis on biopsy leads many to consider these to be immunologic

TABLE 22–6	Clinical Manifestations of Infective Endocarditis
Symptom or Physical Finding	**%**
Fever	58-90
Weight loss	25-35
Headache	15-40
Musculoskeletal pain	15-40
Altered mentation	10-20
Murmur	80-85
Peripheral stigmata	
Petechiae	10-40
Janeway lesions	6-10
Osler nodes	7-23
Splinter hemorrhages	5-15
Clubbing	10-15
Neurologic manifestations	30-40
Roth spots	4-10
Splenomegaly or infarct	15-50

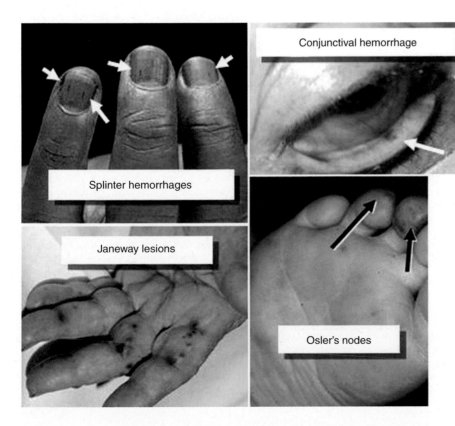

FIGURE 22–3 Peripheral manifestations of infective endocarditis.

phenomena. Rarely, organisms have been cultured from Osler nodes, suggesting that they are simply another manifestation of cutaneous emboli.[49]

Roth spots are retinal hemorrhages with a white center. They most likely represent septic emboli, but like Osler nodes, they have been described in other clinical settings, especially as a manifestation of systemic lupus erythematosus, anemia, diabetes, multiple myeloma, and HIV infection.[50] Frank retinal artery occlusion may also occur.

Musculoskeletal aches and pains are common in IE and often occur early in the course.[51] Any joints can be involved, but back and shoulder pain are most frequently cited.[52] Septic emboli may result in osteomyelitis or bone abscess formation (especially in the spine). Musculoskeletal pain must be taken seriously if it persists during the course of therapy.

Neurologic symptoms are common and are seen in as many as 30% to 50% of patients with IE. Symptoms appear to be more common in IDU patients and those with staphylococcal IE.[53] Embolic stroke is the most common and primary manifestation. Intracranial hemorrhage may occur due to a ruptured arterial vessel, a ruptured mycotic aneurysm, or bleeding into a thrombotic stroke distribution.[54] In addition, neurologic symptoms may be related to cerebritis or meningitis or to toxic or immune-mediated injury. Brain abscess is rare, but microabscesses from virulent organisms, such as *S. aureus*, occur. Meningitis may be a major feature in IE caused by *S. pneumoniae*.

Splenic emboli are probably underreported. In the preantibiotic era, splenomegaly was common. Now about 25% to 50% of patients may have evidence for an enlarged spleen. Autopsy series suggest that splenic infarcts are often present without clinical symptoms.[55]

Evolution of the Duke Criteria

IE has traditionally been defined as an infection of the valves and chordae within the cardiac chambers. This definition has now been expanded to include infection on any structure within the heart including normal endothelial surfaces (e.g., myocardium and valvular structures), prosthetic heart valves (e.g., mechanical, bioprosthetic, homografts, and autografts), and implanted devices (e.g., pacemakers, implantable defibrillators, and ventricular assist devices). Much of the infection noted over the last decade has been on implanted medical devices.

The diagnosis of IE hinges on clinical suspicion and the demonstration of continuous bacteremia. It was not until the late 1970s that Pelletier and Petersdorf[56] developed a case definition based on a 30-year experience of caring for patients with IE in Seattle. Although this case definition was highly specific, it lacked sufficient sensitivity. In 1981, von Reyn et al[57] published an analysis that provided four diagnostic categories in cases of suspected IE (rejected, possible, probable, and definite) and improved both the sensitivity and the specificity of the previous case definition but did not incorporate imaging information from the burgeoning field of echocardiographic imaging.

In 1994, Durack et al[58] from Duke University Medical Center incorporated echocardiography into the criteria for the first time, and these have come to be known as the Duke criteria. These criteria have been validated subsequently by many other studies,[59-61] including the most recent modifications (Table 22-7).[62-64] *Definite* endocarditis is considered to be present if there is *pathologic* evidence (surgical pathologic histology or culture or vegetation histology or culture) *or* if there is *clinical* evidence as demonstrated by two major criteria *or* one major criterion and three minor criteria *or* five minor criteria. *Possible* endocarditis is defined as having one major criterion and one minor criterion *or* three minor criteria. *Rejected* is defined as having a firm alternative diagnosis *or* sustained resolution of the suspected endocarditis evidence

TABLE 22-7 | The Modified Duke Criteria*

I. Major criteria
A. Microbiologic
Typical microorganisms isolated or identified from a pathologic specimen *or* found in positive blood cultures (all 3 or 3 of 4 drawn over 1 hour or 2 positive cultures separated by >12 hours), *or* a single positive blood culture for *Coxiella burnetii* (*or* phase I IgG antibody titer to *C. burnetii* >1:800).
B. Evidence of endocardial involvement
New valvular regurgitation murmur *or* positive echocardiogram results (intracardiac or device mass, *or* para-annular abscess, *or* new dehiscence of prosthetic valve)

II. Minor criteria
A. Predisposition to infective endocarditis
1. Previous infective endocarditis
2. Injection drug use
3. Prosthetic heart valve
4. Mitral valve prolapse
5. Cyanotic congenital heart disease
6. Other cardiac lesions creating turbulent flow within the intracardiac chambers
B. Fever >38° C (100.4° F)
C. Vascular phenomena (e.g., embolic event, mycotic aneurysm, Janeway lesion)
D. Immunologic phenomena (e.g., presence of serologic markers, glomerulonephritis, Osler nodes, or Roth spots)
E. Microbiologic findings not meeting major criteria *or* serologic evidence for an active infection with typical organism

*Definite infective endocarditis = 2 major criteria *or* 1 major criterion and 3 minor *or* 5 minor criteria. *Possible infective endocarditis* = 1 major criterion and 1 minor criterion *or* 3 minor criteria.

after 4 or fewer days of antibiotic therapy *or* no pathologic evidence for endocarditis at surgery or autopsy after 4 or fewer days of therapy.

Major criteria focus on identifying an organism and providing evidence that there is valvular, cardiac, or device infection from that organism. Positive blood culture results play an important role, and when two separate blood cultures show a typical organism, such as *S. aureus, S. viridans* species, *Streptococcus bovis*, HACEK group (*Haemophilus, Actinobacillus, Cardiobacterium, Eikenella*, and *Kingella*), or enterococci in the absence of a primary focus *or* persistently positive blood cultures (≥2 cultures >12 hours apart *or* all 3 blood cultures or 3 of 4 blood cultures drawn within an hour period), then this qualifies as a major criterion. Because of the difficulty in diagnosing Q fever, a single blood culture or an IgG antibody titer greater than 1:800 for *Coxiella burnetii* also qualifies. The other major criteria include clear-cut evidence for cardiac or device vegetation or valve destruction as demonstrated by echocardiographic evidence of a vegetation, abscess, or dehiscence of a prosthetic valve *or* the clinical presence of a new (not changing) regurgitant valve lesion on examination.

Minor criteria focus on the epiphenomena that are part of the endocarditis complex of clinical findings. These include having a predisposition (known heart condition or injection drug use), fever, vascular phenomena (major arterial emboli, septic pulmonary infarction, mycotic aneurysm, intracranial hemorrhage, conjunctival hemorrhage, or Janeway lesions), immunologic phenomena (glomerulonephritis, Osler nodes, Roth spots, rheumatoid factor, or C-reactive protein [CRP]), and soft microbiologic evidence (positive blood culture results that do not meet the criteria outlined as major criteria) or serologic evidence for an active infection with an organism consistent with IE.

There is growing interest in the use of CRP and procalcitonin. A CRP level that is elevated at baseline and normalizes with therapy has been associated with good outcomes,[65] whereas a persistently elevated CRP level despite therapy has been associated with poor outcomes.[66] Procalcitonin, a marker of systemic bacterial infection, has also been shown to be elevated in IE and may be an early marker of the disease.[67,68]

There is also now growing evidence that molecular diagnostic techniques may eventually help refine the Duke criteria, especially regarding culture-negative endocarditis. Molecular and immunologic diagnostic techniques may have a role in discovering infection from fastidious agents such as *C. burnetii*, *Legionella pneumophila*, *Tropheryma whipplei*, *Bartonella* species, HACEK organisms, and fungi. The most readily applicable techniques amplify trace amounts of a given nucleic acid target of microbial DNA in host tissues. In the form of the broad range or the universal 16S RNA gene polymerase chain reaction (PCR), most etiologic agents involved in IE have been identified. The bacterial 16S ribosomal RNA gene has both highly conserved and variable regions, and PCR is able to detect all know bacteria at the genus level and provide identification.[69] Fungal organisms can also be identified. PCR, however, is costly and requires meticulous technique to avoid contaminants and false-positive results. PCR has improved the sensitivity and specificity of diagnosis in excised heart valves though,[70,71] and the advantage will come when real-time, effective PCR methods can be applied to blood samples.

Transthoracic and Transesophageal Echocardiography

Echocardiographic Features

The modified Duke criteria depend on identifying the infected lesion, and echocardiography is the key imaging tool. With the use of echocardiography, there are several findings that provide evidence consistent with IE including vegetations, evidence of annular tissue destruction (abscess), aneurysm, fistula, leaflet perforation, and valvular dehiscence. Echocardiography also provides data regarding ventricular function, evidence for pulmonary hypertension, and an assessment of the hemodynamic consequences of the infection.

Vegetations. On an echocardiogram a vegetation appears as an irregularly shaped, discrete echogenic mass that is adherent to yet distinct from the endothelial cardiac surface. Oscillation of the mass with high-frequency movement independent from that of intrinsic structures is supportive but not mandatory for the echocardiographic diagnosis of a vegetation. Vegetations have the consistency of mid-myocardium (Figure 22-4) but may also have areas of both echolucency and echodensity. Their locations were described earlier (see Figure 22-1). Vegetations may also appear on nonvalvular intravascular structures, such as pacemaker leads (Figure 22-5). Vegetations on prosthetic material may be a particular challenge and transesophageal echocardiography (TEE) imaging is usually required for confirmation. Over time vegetations tend to decrease in size with therapy, although their presence may persist as a less mobile and more echogenic mass.

Not all intracardiac mass lesions represent vegetations from IE. For instance, in systemic lupus erythematosus, inflammatory mass lesions (Libman-Sacks) related to the lupus usually have a broad base and are small. Other sterile vegetations, such as marantic endocarditis, may also occur in patients with advanced malignancies. A mass effect may be seen in patients with myxomatous valves, ruptured chordae unrelated to infection, cardiac tumors, and degenerative valvular changes, especially when there is considerable calcium. Moreover, normal variants such as prominent Lambl excrescences[72] (small filiform processes on the medial tips of the aortic valve), a Chiari network, or a Eustachian valve in the right atrium may mimic IE vegetations on an echocardiogram.

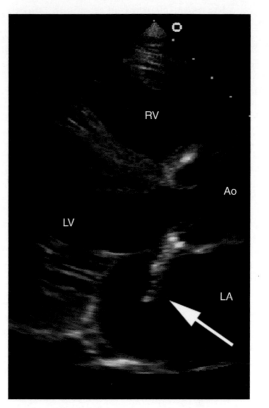

FIGURE 22-4 Typical endocarditis vegetative lesion on the native mitral valve. Echocardiographic consistency of vegetation is similar to the myocardium. Ao, aorta; LA, left atrium; LV, left ventricle; RV, right ventricle. *(From Bashore TM, Cabell C, Fowler V Jr: Update on infective endocarditis. Curr Probl Cardiol 2006;31:274-352, with permission.)*

Since the early 1990s multiple studies have shown a strong association between vegetation size and subsequent thromboembolic risk. Some have found that the risk of embolization was directly related to vegetation size.[73] Tischler and Vaitkus[74] conducted a meta-analysis that incorporated 10 studies involving 738 patients with IE. They found that

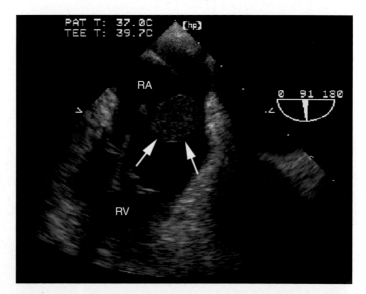

FIGURE 22-5 Endocarditis on a pacemaker or defibrillator lead. Ball-like vegetation on pacemaker lead (vertical echoes seen in right atrium [RA]). Horizontal echoes between RA and right ventricle (RV) represent the tricuspid valve. *(From Bashore TM, Cabell C, Fowler V Jr: Update on infective endocarditis. Curr Probl Cardiol 2006;31:274-352, with permission.)*

the pooled odds ratio (OR) for risk of embolization was three times higher in patients with large vegetations (>10mm) than in patients with no detectable or small vegetations (OR, 2.90; 95% confidence interval [95% CI], 1.95-4.02). Di Salvo et al[75] found that both size and mobility were predictive of embolic events. Unfortunately, there is a relatively high degree of interobserver variability in recording the specific characteristics of vegetations,[76] and this has led some to be skeptical of using a definitive cutoff size measurement to define risk.

Para-Valvular Extension of Infection (Myocardial Abscess Formation). Para-valvular extension of infection, or abscess formation, is one of the most serious complications of IE, signaling an indication for surgical therapy. A myocardial abscess can be defined as a thickened area or mass in the myocardium or annular region with an appearance that is generally nonhomogeneous. There is usually evidence of flow within the cavity, but flow is not mandatory for the diagnosis. An echo-free space suggests that complete liquefaction of the myocardium or aortic wall has occurred. An example of an annular abscess is shown in Figure 22-6.

Abscess formation is associated with substantial morbidity and mortality. The abscess can extend and rupture, creating a fistulous tract. Extension into the septum may affect the conduction system, leading to heart block. Abscess formation is more commonly associated with aortic valve IE, particularly aortic prosthetic valve IE. The mortality rate associated with abscess formation is 1.5 to 2.0 times higher than that for similar patients without abscess formation. Although transthoracic echocardiography (TTE) imaging can establish the diagnosis of abscess formation, overall the resolution associated with typical TTE imaging in adults is insufficient for the full characterization of most intracardiac abscess cavities, and TEE is preferred.

Fistula Formation. Spread of infection from valvular structures to the surrounding paravalvular tissue may place the patient at increased risk of adverse outcomes including heart failure and death. This risk is particularly seen with aortic valve IE, in which aortic abscesses and mycotic pseudoaneurysms involving the sinuses of Valsalva may rupture, leading to the development of aortocavitary or aortopericardial fistulas. Aortocavitary communications, especially to right heart structures, create intracardiac shunts, which may result in further clinical deterioration and hemodynamic instability (Figure 22-7).

Perforation and Valvular regurgitation. There is little information available about valvular perforation, but it is generally accepted that this is either associated with a virulent microorganism, such as *S. aureus* or occurs when the infection process continues for a substantial amount of time without detection. Once a perforation occurs, a significant amount of valvular regurgitation may develop.

Dehiscence of Prosthetic Valve. Dehiscence of a prosthetic valve due to IE is a serious complication. Dehiscence is generally defined as a rocking motion of the prosthetic valve more than 15° in any one plane. This complication may lead to a gross separation of the prosthetic annulus from the native tissue. Invariably, prosthetic valve dehiscence is associated with significant paravalvular regurgitation and usually is associated with hemodynamic compromise. Figure 22-8 shows aortic valve prosthesis dehiscence. Dehiscence represents a relative urgent indication for surgical therapy.

Use and Overuse of Echocardiography

Although echocardiography is the imaging technology of choice for the diagnosis of IE and can detect cardiac involvement in a significant proportion of patients with clinically occult IE,[77] its optimal use is predicated on the appropriate pretest probability of disease.[78] Kuruppu et al[79] have shown that 53% of echocardiograms could be avoided without loss of diagnostic accuracy by using a simple algorithm in patients with a low pretest probability of disease. In addition, Greaves et al[80] have shown that the collective absence of five simple clinical criteria indicated a zero probability of a TTE showing evidence of endocarditis. These clinical criteria included vasculitic/embolic phenomena, the presence of central venous access, a recent history of injection drug use, the presence of a prosthetic valve, and positive blood cultures. Note that in about 15% of patients the sound transmission from the chest wall may be attenuated by a variety of factors (e.g., obesity or lung hyperinflation), obviating a diagnostic image. In these situations, TEE may be preferred as the primary imaging modality.

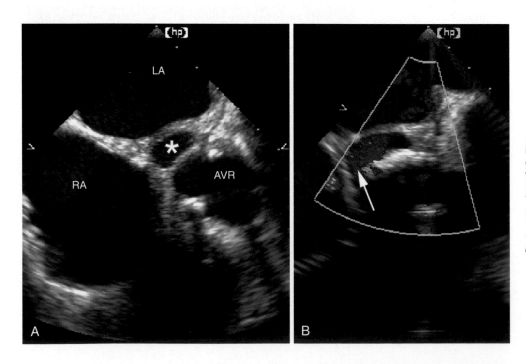

FIGURE 22–6 Annular abscess formation in endocarditis. **A**, asterisk denotes the area of the paravalvular abscess between the aortic valve replacement (AVR) and the left atrium (LA). **B**, The color flow Doppler echocardiogram shows the presence of flow in and out of the abscess. *(From Bashore TM, Cabell C, Fowler V Jr: Update on infective endocarditis. Curr Probl Cardiol 2006;31:274-352, with permission.)*

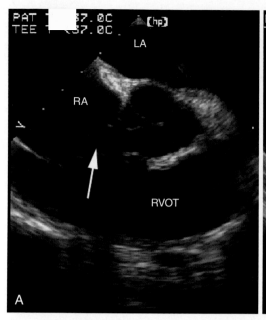

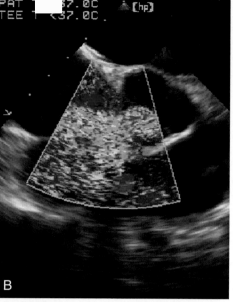

FIGURE 22–7 Fistula formation during infective endocarditis. **A,** An infected sinus of Valsalva aneurysm that has ruptured into the right ventricle (RV) outflow tract (RVOT) and right atrium (RA). **B,** Color-flow Doppler imaging shows a pattern of high velocity flow from the high pressure aorta into the lower pressure right atrium and ventricle. *(From Bashore TM, Cabell C, Fowler V Jr: Update on infective endocarditis. Curr Probl Cardiol 2006;31:274-352, with permission.)*

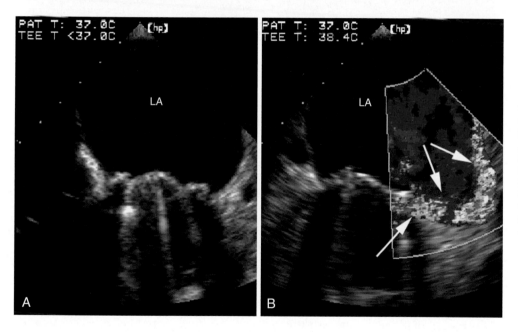

FIGURE 22–8 Prosthetic valve endocarditis with valvular dehiscence. **A,** Transesophageal two-dimensional echocardiogram of a St. Jude mitral valve. **B,** Color-flow Doppler echocardiogram shows severe para-valvular mitral regurgitation (arrows) into the left atrium (LA) due to dehiscence of the mitral valve replacement. *(From Bashore TM, Cabell C, Fowler V Jr: Update on infective endocarditis. Curr Probl Cardiol 2006;31:274-352, with permission.)*

Both TTE and TEE have a significant role in the diagnosis and management of patients with suspected IE. TTE is widely available and can provide rapid important diagnostic information. Under ideal conditions, TTE can reliably identify structures as small as 5 mm in diameter, and TEE can depict structures as small as 1 mm. It is widely accepted that the sensitivity/specificity is superior for TEE compared with TTE (93%/96% versus 46%/95%). As a generality, TEE should be obtained whenever TTE is likely to produce a low yield, such as in the definition of a paravalvular abscess or in patients with a prosthetic valve or a suspected lead or dwelling catheter infection. TEE may be particularly helpful in culture-negative IE. However, TEE may underestimate the presence of a paravalvular abscess.[81]

Figure 22-9 outlines the current guidelines for use of TTE and TEE in the diagnosis and follow-up of patients with IE.[82] This algorithm reflects studies showing that an initial strategy of TEE imaging is the most cost-effective in many clinical situations. For instance, Heidenreich[78] and colleagues have shown that in suspected endocarditis a diagnostic strategy that focuses on TEE as the initial imaging modality is more cost-effective than a staged procedure with TTE and is a better strategy than empiric antibiotic therapy alone. In a similar study, Rosen et al[83] determined the cost-effectiveness of TEE in establishing the duration of therapy for catheter-associated bacteremia.[83] Three management strategies were compared: 1) empirical treatment with 4 weeks of antibiotics (long course); 2) empirical treatment with 2 weeks of antibiotic therapy (short course); and 3) TEE-guided therapy. In the case of the TEE strategy, positive TEE results dictated long-course therapy and negative TEE results dictated short-course therapy. The effectiveness of an empiric long-course strategy and a TEE-guided strategy were both superior to empiric short-course therapy. When costs were accounted for, the TEE-guided strategy was superior to the empiric long-course strategy, which cost more than $1,500,000 per quality-adjusted life year saved.

The algorithm suggests that multiple echocardiographic evaluations may be useful in determining the prognosis of

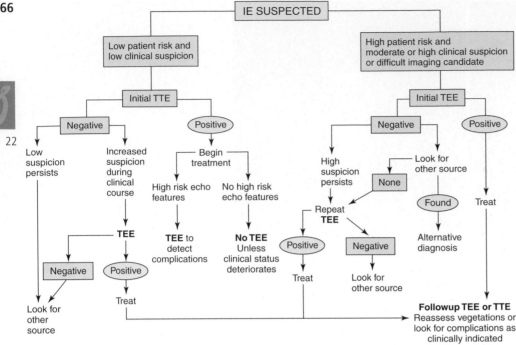

FIGURE 22–9 Algorithm for the effective use of transthoracic (TTE) and transesophageal (TEE) echocardiography. IE, infective endocarditis. *(Modified from Bayer AS, Bolger AF, Taubert KA, et al: Diagnosis and management of infective endocarditis and its complications. Circulation 1998;98:2936-2948, with permission.)*

patients with IE. For instance, if a vegetation stays static or enlarges prognosis is worse than if the vegetation shrinks during therapy.[84]

Serial examinations can be taken to extreme, however. In a recent review of 262 patients with 266 episodes of suspected IE, TTEs were repeated at least once in 192 (72.2%) patients, whereas TEEs were repeated in 49 (18.4%) of patients. The average number of TTE examinations was 2.4, but 6 patients had at least six TTEs. In a similar fashion, the mean number of TEE examinations was 1.7, although four patients had at least four TEEs and one patient had five TEEs. The authors found that although repeated echocardiograms were occasionally helpful, no additional diagnostic information was provided after the second or third echocardiogram (TTE or TEE).[85]

Other Imaging Modalities in Infective Endocarditis

Other imaging modalities may support the diagnosis of IE and/or be used to evaluate the potential for complications. Chest radiography can be used to provide supporting evidence of IE such as nodular pulmonary infiltrates in a febrile injection drug user, suggesting right-sided IE with septic pulmonary emboli.

Computed tomography and magnetic resonance imaging are useful to assess for evidence of thromboembolic complications, such as stroke or visceral embolic events, in patients with IE, but their role in imaging cardiac pathologic lesions is uncertain. There have been times when magnetic resonance or computed tomography has been useful to diagnose abscess formation, especially when TEE is not feasible. Coronary computed tomographic angiography is also useful for excluding coronary artery disease and avoiding the need for cardiac catheterization in middle-aged patients.

COMPLICATIONS

Endocarditis vegetations on native valves may mechanically interfere with valve motion and result in valvular regurgitation. Vegetation growth can result in leaflet perforation and

may cause chordal rupture. Infection may also extend outside the valve leaflets into surrounding structures such as the sinotubular junction, the annulus, the myocardium, the conduction system, or the intravalvular fibrosa. Cavitation in the aortic wall may result in an aortic annular abscess that usually remains in communication with the lumen. Rarely these abscesses can erode to the pericardium or to another cardiac chamber, such as the left atrium or right ventricle.

Endocarditis on prosthetic valves usually begins on the valvular cuff and often extends outside the valvular apparatus, resulting in valvular dehiscence, abscess formation, and myocardial involvement. Vegetations can be large enough to interfere directly with mechanical prosthetic leaflet function and result in both regurgitation and obstruction. Mechanical prosthetic valves appear to have a greater risk for endocarditis in the early period after surgery and bioprosthetic valves later on.[21,86] Implantable rings (as part of valve repair) have the least risk for endocarditis.[87] By 5 years there is probably no real difference in the incidence of endocarditis between mechanical and bioprosthetic valves.[23,88]

Despite improvements in our diagnostic tests and antibiotics, the incidence of complications in patients with endocarditis has not changed much over the last few decades.[89] Table 22-8 provides estimates of the incidence of clinical complications in the modern era.[86] Despite advances in the diagnosis and management of IE, endocarditis remains a disease with unacceptably high morbidity and mortality. More than 50% of patients with IE have some type of serious complication including heart failure, stroke, and paravalvular extension, whereas the in-hospital mortality rates (15% to 20%) and 1-year mortality rates (30% to 40%) have changed little over the past 20 years.[8,90,91] Death is still common and usually relates to cardiogenic shock, multiorgan failure, or stroke.

Cardiac Complications

The most frequent complication from IE is congestive heart failure. Heart failure in endocarditis is usually the result of acute or semiacute valvular regurgitation and not myocardial failure. It is most common with aortic valve

TABLE 22–8	Complications from Infective Endocarditis: Estimates of the Incidence of Complications in the Modern Era

Complication	%
Death	12-45 (24% average)
Congestive heart failure (aortic regurgitation > mitral regurgitation > tricuspid regurgitation)	50-60
Embolization (mitral > aortic valve)	20-25
cardiovascular accident	15
Other major emboli	
Limb	2-3
Mesenteric	2
Splenic	2-3
Glomerulonephritis	15-25
Annular abscess	10-15
Mycotic aneurysm	10-15
Conduction system involvement	5-10
Central nervous system abscess	3-4
Other less common complications (pericarditis, myocarditis, myocardial infarction, intracardiac fistula, metastatic abscess)	1-2

involvement followed by mitral and then tricuspid valve infection.[92] The ability of the heart to withstand the volume overload–related valvular regurgitation is dependent on several factors: the severity of the regurgitation, which valve is involved, the rapidity of the volume overload, and both the size and function of the chamber receiving the volume overload. Mitral regurgitation, for instance, presents both a volume overload and an afterload decrease to the left ventricle, and this may explain why it is better tolerated than acute aortic regurgitation, in which the lesion results in both a volume overload and an afterload increase.[93] The rapid increase in left ventricular diastolic pressures in acute aortic regurgitation may even prematurely close the mitral valve before ventricular systole is initiated. This pre-closure is readily observed by M-mode echocardiography and has been used as an indication that surgical correction is indicated.[94]

Embolization

The second most frequent complication is embolization. Stroke is the most commonly observed major clinical consequence of embolization, and the risk of such embolization appears much greater for mitral than for aortic valve endocarditis.[95,96] Indeed, cerebral infarction due to either emboli or mycotic aneurysm may be the presenting sign of endocarditis in up to 14% of patients.[97] The rate of embolic events declines rapidly after the initiation of effective antibiotics, dropping from an initial 13 events per 1000 patient-days in the first week to less than 1.2 events per 1000 patient-days after 2 weeks of therapy.[98] Pulmonary emboli, usually septic in nature, occur in 66 to 75% of intravenous drug users who have tricuspid valve endocarditis.[99] Emboli may involve virtually any systemic organ, including the liver, spleen, kidney, and abdominal mesenteric vessels. Renal emboli can cause hematuria and flank pain. Splenic infarction may lead to abscess development and cause prolonged fevers or left shoulder pain from diaphragmatic irritation. Coronary emboli can result in myocardial infarction. Distal emboli can produce peripheral metastatic abscesses, especially of the spine or other bony structures. Muscular and joint pains are not uncommon in IE, but severe osteoarticular pain may indicate a bony embolus.[100]

Mycotic Aneurysms

Mycotic aneurysms result from septic embolization to an arterial intraluminal space or to the vasa vasorum of the cerebral vessels. Branch point vessels are the most common sites of presentation. Mycotic aneurysms are uncommon but may be responsible for up to 15% of neurologic complications. The clinical syndrome that results may vary considerably from a slow leak that produces only mild headache and meningeal irritation to sudden intracranial hemorrhage and a major stroke.[101]

Renal Dysfunction

Renal dysfunction is common in patients with endocarditis. Although often attributed to immune complex glomerulonephritis (GN), a recent necropsy and biopsy study[102] revealed that localized infarction was present in 31% and acute GN in 26%. The most common type of GN was vasculitic, without deposition of immunoproteins in glomeruli. Of the renal infarcts, more than half were related to septic emboli, primarily in patients infected with *S. aureus*. Acute interstitial nephritis was found in 10%, presumably due to antibiotic usage. Renal cortical necrosis was also found in 10%. Azotemia due to immune complex–mediated GN generally improves with effective antibiotic therapy. The cause of renal dysfunction in many patients is multifactorial, especially when baseline renal function is abnormal or CHF is present.

Valvular and Paravalvular Abscess Formation

Extension of the infection outside the valve annulus is a serious development and usually requires surgical intervention for cure. These extensions can occur in the myocardium, involve the conduction system, and develop into a true abscess. An annular abscess may initially not communicate with the lumen of the aorta or the cardiac chamber, but as it progresses, it usually breaks through to such areas and is notable for the presence of flow in and out of the pocket as shown by color flow Doppler electrocardiography. Abscesses can form directly on the valve leaflets themselves, a finding that is particularly evident in mitral endocarditis.

Less Common Complications

Other less common complications include the development of pericarditis (either from direct extension of the infection or possibly from embolization to the pericardial vessels) and myocarditis. Invasion of the sinus of Valsalva may result in not only aortic regurgitation but also pericarditis, hemopericardium, and fistula formation into right heart structures.

CLINICAL APPROACH

Common Features

Once treatment for IE is started, fever should resolve within days, the exception being some patients with *S. aureus* infections, in whom it may persist for up to 2 weeks. Recurrent fevers should raise concern that the antibiotics are ineffective, that there is an abscess or other infection somewhere that is not being resolved, or that there is drug fever. All patients should have surveillance blood cultures obtained after 3 to 4 days of intravenous drug therapy. Patients should be monitored daily for new embolic phenomena or signs of worsening hemodynamics.

When therapy begins, most patients should have a percutaneous inserted central catheter or similar long-term access line placed early for antibiotic administration. Patients should have a cardiac examination performed daily and follow-up echocardiography at any sign of a complication from endocarditis.

Although the sedimentation rate is almost universally elevated, its level does not correlate with the effectiveness of therapy. The CRP level, if obtained, should decline with effective therapy. Periodic measures of renal function and complete blood counts and initial hepatic function tests should be obtained and a surveillance blood culture should be obtained 72 hours into therapy. For most patients, minimum inhibitory concentration (MIC) levels of the antibiotics used should be obtained to help guide therapy. The patient should be monitored with telemetry while hospitalized to observe for any arrhythmia and any change in the P-R interval. Any prolongation of the P-R interval should be assumed to be related to abscess formation unless a secondary cause is clearly evident. Infectious disease specialists should be involved to help with the antibiotic decision making, and it is prudent to have input from a cardiothoracic surgeon early in the course to help with the decision making. Consultation with a surgeon is particularly important if there is any hemodynamic instability or evidence of abscess formation and in PVE.

Warfarin presents a particular problem. If the patient is receiving chronic warfarin therapy, the drug should initially be stopped, and the international normalized ratio should be allowed to drift down until it is less than 2.0. At that point unfractionated or low-molecular-weight heparin should be initiated. When it is determined that surgical intervention is not going to be needed, warfarin may be resumed, usually after about 7 days of antimicrobial therapy.

In patients with mechanical prosthetic valves already in place, the average rate of major thromboembolism is about 8% per year,[103] so a brief stoppage of warfarin is warranted. The lowest risk prosthetic valve is the bileaflet aortic valve. Caged ball valves, mitral mechanical valves, the presence of congestive heart failure or atrial fibrillation, a prior history of venous thromboembolism within the last 3 months, or a hypercoagulable state all increase the risk of withholding warfarin.[104] If unfractionated heparin is used, the activated partial thromboplastin time should be kept at around 50 to 65 seconds.

A central nervous system event in a patient receiving warfarin is a potentially devastating occurrence, and it is important to immediately document whether there is bleeding by use of either a head computed tomographic scan or magnetic resonance imaging. If head or gastrointestinal bleeding is present, then the individual clinical scenario must be taken into account to determine how long it is safe to withhold anticoagulation therapy. In general, the effects of warfarin should be reversed with vitamin K, and no anticoagulant should be given for 72 hours. At that time unfractionated heparin or low-molecular-weight heparin can be started. Warfarin can usually be started at the same time, and the heparin can be discontinued when an international normalized ratio of 2.0 has been documented.

Almost all patients who do not undergo surgical intervention for IE can now be treated with an initial 1- to 2-week hospitalization and then home therapy for the remainder of the antibiotic course. Patients should be seen in the outpatient setting at the conclusion of therapy and repeat laboratory results and an echocardiogram are normally obtained.

Determining Prognosis

The clinical examination, the organism involved and its response to therapy, and the echocardiographic information can establish the prognosis and guide future decision making in treatment of IE. A number of studies have examined other factors in an effort to understand prognosis in patients with IE. Chu et al[105] examined 267 consecutive patients with acute IE to determine factors early in the course of IE that were independently associated with mortality. Controlling for severity of illness with APACHE II scoring, they found that the independent predictors of early mortality were the presence of diabetes mellitus (OR, 2.48; 95% CI, 1.24-4.96), S. aureus infection (OR, 2.06; 95% CI, 1.01-4.20), and an embolic event (OR, 2.79; 95% CI, 1.15-6.80).[105] In a similar fashion, Hasbun et al[106] found that five baseline features were independently associated with mortality and developed a scoring system that included the following: mental status: lethargy or disorientation (4 points); Charlson comorbidity scale: 2 or greater (3 points); CHF: moderate to severe (3 points); microbiology: S. aureus (6 points), other nonviridans infection (8 points); and therapy: medical therapy only (5 points). On the basis of this point system, patients with a score of 6 points or less only had 6% mortality at 6 months, whereas patients with a score of more than 15 points had 63% mortality.[106] In other studies, the need for hemodialysis has also been found to portend a poor outcome[107] as has the presence of poor ventricular function.[108] Another recent study suggested that the poorest prognosis is seen in patients with an altered mental state, those with mobile vegetations, and those undergoing hemodialysis.[109]

The Injection Drug User

In IDU patients 75% to 93% of cases of IE develop on an apparently normal tricuspid valve.[21] The incidence of IE in IDU patients ranges from 1% to 5% per year, whereas in patients with IE the concomitant rate of IDU ranges from 5% to 20%.[110] Earlier studies all suggested that endocarditis in IDU patients occurs on the tricuspid valve in 46% to 78% of cases followed by the mitral valve (24% to 32%) then the aortic valve (8% to 19%), with as many as 16% having multiple valves infected.[21] Recently, however, left-sided disease has been increasing in drug users. In one series left-sided involvement occurred in 57% of IDU patients compared with 40% with right-sided disease.[28] Regardless of the site, the most common infecting organism in IDU patients is overwhelmingly S. aureus, which has been reported in up to 82%.[29]

Prognosis in IDU patients with IE is generally better than that in patients with IE but no history of IDU. This paradox can be explained by the fact that IE in IDU patients is often right-sided in nature, which has a much better prognosis (i.e., mortality <5%)[110] than left-sided IE.[111] The IDU patients generally are much younger as well. Of importance, the presence of HIV infection does not appear to alter the diagnostic use of the Duke criteria or the course of the disease,[112] although patients with a very low CD4 count may have a greater risk.[8] Serologic tests for the specific strain of Staphylococcus do not seem to be useful in identifying IE in those with staphylococcal sepsis.[113]

IDU patients with isolated right-sided IE may be eligible for short-course therapy that generally would not be considered in patients with left-sided disease.[114] Because these patients are often medically noncompliant, surgery should be offered with great thought. Several studies have shown that surgical management of IDU patients with IE can be done safely with acceptable outcomes.[115,116] In general, the main indications for surgery in IDU patients are IE caused by microorganisms difficult to eradicate, such as fungi, persistent/recurrent bacteremia despite optimal antimicrobial therapy, and tricuspid valve vegetations greater than 2 cm with a dilated right heart and recurrent pulmonary emboli or right heart failure.[117]

Prosthetic Valve Endocarditis

It is estimated that endocarditis occurs in from 1.4% to 3.1% of patients with a prosthetic valve at 12 months and from 3.0% to 5.7% at 5 years.[21,22,88,118] PVE represents around 10% to 30% of all IE.[119,120] Traditionally two risk periods are defined for the development of PVE: an early (5- to 6-week period) and a late period. However, Karchmer[21] argues that PVE is a continuum, and separates the disease into less than 2 months, 2 to 12 months, and longer than 12 months categories. Early PVE is generally defined as endocarditis that develops in the first 2 months after heart surgery, with most organisms involved considered to be nosocomial, as opposed to late PVE, in which the organisms more likely resemble those causing native valve endocarditis. A transition occurs from 2 to 12 months (Table 22-9). There is a suggestion that mechanical valves are more likely than bioprosthetic valves to get infected in the first year,[118] although by 5 years the risk of infection is similar between the two types of valves.

The signs of IE may be difficult to sort out from those of other postoperative infectious complications during the early period of PVE. Peripheral stigmata and emboli appear less often in early compared with later PVE and the Duke criteria may be more difficult to apply.[121]

PVE is a special case in the decision to perform TEE versus TTE. In almost all instances, TEE provides information that is not observable with TTE. A full evaluation of the infected area should be performed including the annulus of the valve infected, the function of the valve, abscess formation, presence of a fistula tract, assessment for dehiscence, assessment for paravalvular regurgitation, and full assessment of overall regurgitation.

Infected Intracardiac Devices

Intracardiac devices (e.g., pacemakers and implantable defibrillators) have become more commonplace with an aging population. Information from the Medicare database indicates that the device implantation rate showed a relative increase of 42% in the 1990s but that there was a 124% relative increase in patients with documented device infections during the same time period.[122]

Imaging is particularly difficult in patients with device infection, because it is difficult to determine whether a mass on a lead wire is a sterile or an infected thrombus. It is important to image the device throughout its course in the cardiac chambers. Special attention should be directed to the point where the device crosses the tricuspid valve, as trauma may cause endothelial trauma and development of a vegetation. In addition, devices that are placed in the superior vena cava should be imaged as far as possible. Figure 22-10 illustrates a large vegetation on a pacemaker lead.

Gram-positive cocci are the overwhelming cause of an infected intracardiac device. Patients with S. aureus bacteremia and a probable catheter-related infection may have obscure valvular endocarditis and a TEE is generally indicated.[123,124] When there is documented valvular IE in these patients, in almost all instances these devices should be replaced at the time of valvular surgery.[125]

WHEN TO OPERATE IN INFECTIVE ENDOCARDITIS

Medical therapy alone for IE have been reported to be associated with an increase in mortality at 6 months compared with surgery,[106,126,127] although most of the surgical benefit is seen in patients who have moderate to severe heart failure (Figure 22-11). The mortality at 6 months in the medical group was nearly 50%, whereas the mortality in the surgical group was only 15%.[128] In patients without moderate or severe heart failure there was no difference in the medical and surgical groups with 6-month mortality for both at 15%.[106] It is evident that patients with at least moderate heart failure do better with surgery. In all other patients, it is less clear whether surgery has any survival benefit.

Table 22-10 outlines the generally accepted criteria for cardiac surgical procedures in patients with native and prosthetic valve endocarditis. CHF is the major reason to proceed with surgical intervention in IE. This concern is especially important in patients with aortic regurgitation, in whom emergency

TABLE 22–9	Microorganisms Causing Infective Endocarditis in Native Valves, Injection Drug Users, and the Early, Mid, and Late Prosthetic Valve Syndromes					
				Prosthetic Valves (%)		
Organism	Native Valve (%)	IDU (%)	2 mo	2-12 mo	>12 mo
Staphylococci						
Staphylococcus aureus	20-48	50-60	22	12	18
Staphylococcus epidermidis	3-5	—	33	32	11
Streptococci						
Viridans spp.	25-65	1-12	1	9	31
Enterococci	5-17	8-9	8	12	11
Streptococcus bovis	7-10	—	—	—	
β-Hemolytic streptococcus	4-5	10-25	—	—	
Pneumococci	1-3	—	—	—	
Gram-negative bacilli	4-9	5-7	13	3	6
Culture-negative	3-15	3-5	5	2	8
HACEK (including fastidious gram-negative)	2-5	—	0	0	6
Fungi	1-5	0-4	8	12	3
Polymicrobial	1-2	5-7	3	6	5

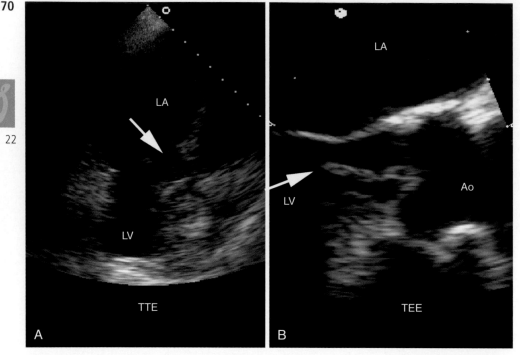

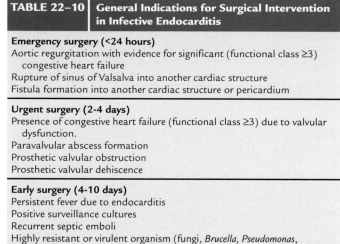

FIGURE 22–10 Transthoracic echocardiogram (TTE) versus transesophageal echocardiogram (TEE) in a patient with aortic valve endocarditis. **A**, In this two-chamber transthoracic echocardiographic view, the vegetation (arrow) is difficult to distinguish on the aortic valve. **B**, Transesophageal view in the same patient readily shows the vegetation (arrow). Ao, aorta; LA, left atrium; LV, left ventricle. *(From Bashore TM, Cabell C, Fowler V Jr: Update on infective endocarditis. Curr Probl Cardiol 2006;31:274-352, with permission.)*

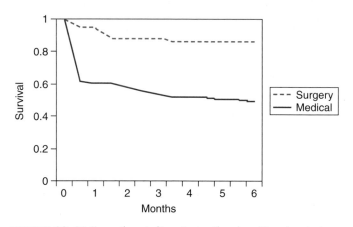

FIGURE 22–11 Six-month survival in patients with endocarditis and moderate-severe heart failure. *(Adapted from Vikram HR, Buenconsejo J, Hasbun R, Quagliarello VJ: Impact of valve surgery on 6-month mortality in adults with complicated, left-sided native valve endocarditis. JAMA 2003;290:3207-3214, with permission.)*

TABLE 22–10	General Indications for Surgical Intervention in Infective Endocarditis

Emergency surgery (<24 hours)
Aortic regurgitation with evidence for significant (functional class ≥3) congestive heart failure
Rupture of sinus of Valsalva into another cardiac structure
Fistula formation into another cardiac structure or pericardium

Urgent surgery (2-4 days)
Presence of congestive heart failure (functional class ≥3) due to valvular dysfunction.
Paravalvular abscess formation
Prosthetic valvular obstruction
Prosthetic valvular dehiscence

Early surgery (4-10 days)
Persistent fever due to endocarditis
Positive surveillance cultures
Recurrent septic emboli
Highly resistant or virulent organism (fungi, *Brucella, Pseudomonas,* antibiotic-resistant enterococci, poorly responsive *Staphylococcus aureus*)
Large (>10 mm) mobile vegetations, especially on the mitral valve
Immediate relapse after completion of prior endocarditis treatment

From Bashore TM, Cabell C, Fowler V Jr: Update on infective endocarditis. Curr Probl Cardiol 2006;31:274-352, with permission.

surgery (within 24 hours) should be performed once CHF is present. The rapid rise in the left ventricular diastolic pressure with acute aortic regurgitation may prematurely close the mitral valve (preclosure demonstrated by M-mode echocardiography) and is an indication for surgery.[94] Emergency surgical intervention should also be performed if there is hemodynamic instability owing to rupture of a sinus of Valsalva into another heart structure or into the pericardium. Urgent surgical intervention (within 2 to 4 days) is indicated if there is any evidence for prosthetic valvular obstruction, paravalvular abscess, prosthetic valve dehiscence, or more than New York Heart Association functional class 2 heart failure. Early surgical intervention (within 4 to 10 days) is indicated if there is evidence for even moderate (functional class 2 CHF), ineffective antimicrobial therapy (persistent fevers, positive surveillance blood cultures, or a highly virulent organism), large (>10 mm) mobile vegetations, recurrence of an embolic event, or endocarditis due to a highly resistant organism or to one for

which therapy is not available (fungi, *Brucella, Pseudomonas,* or antibiotic resistant enterococci).

Embolic neurologic complications result in a significant increase in mortality, and this has led to many to consider early surgery in such patients. The risk of open-heart surgery is also increased. In one retrospective study, 44% had further neurologic deterioration if a nonhemorrhagic cerebral event had occurred with 7 days or less before surgery[129] compared with 16.7% who had neurologic deterioration if surgery was delayed to 8 to 14 days, with only 2.3% experiencing deterioration if surgery was delayed 4 weeks. In hemorrhagic stroke, though, the risk persists for up to 4 weeks. As a general guideline, in most settings, one would advocate delaying valve replacement for 2 to 3 weeks after a nonhemorrhagic central nervous system event and for a month after an intercerebral bleeding episode.

Surgical approaches to valvular endocarditis vary widely. An implantable device, such as a pacemaker or implantable defibrillator, almost always needs to be replaced, and this fact should be taken into consideration when surgery is planned (especially if the patient is dependent on the pacemaker). Surgical valve repair rather than replacement has been growing in popularity[130] as an alternative to valve replacement and should be considered if feasible. Homografts and autografts can often be used now, especially when there is extensive involvement of the valve annular apparatus, and these have become the prosthetic materials of choice in these situations. Paravalvular abscess formation and erosion destroy heart tissue, but the myocardium can be reconstructed using pericardium. Tricuspid valve excision without replacement continues to be advocated in IDUs who are likely to have recurrent tricuspid valve endocarditis,[131] but severe heart failure invariably develops eventually, and this approach is not recommended over valve repair or replacement even in this group of patients for whom treatment is difficult.

MICROBIOLOGY

A huge variety of microorganisms have been implicated in IE, but staphylococci and streptococci account for the majority of all cases. The International Collaboration on Endocarditis-Prospective Cohort Study recently identified the microbiologic agent in 1779 patients from 39 medical centers in 16 countries with definite endocarditis and found that staphylococci were the etiologic agents in 42% and streptococci in 40%.[132] Table 22-9 outlines the prevalence of microorganisms for IDU patients with native valve IE and for those with the early and late infections after prosthetic valves.[18,20,21,99,121,133,134] The following is meant to provide an overview and not a comprehensive discussion of the principles of antibiotic therapy for IE.

Gram-Positive Cocci

Streptococci

Streptococci and staphylococci account for 80% to 90% of cases of IE in which an organism is identified. Streptococci have traditionally been the most common cause of IE,[135] and many community hospitals still report viridans streptococci as the most common isolates among patients with IE.[136] However, staphylococci have assumed increasing importance among isolates in community hospitals in recent years.[137] Viridans streptococci remain the major cause of IE in children and young women with isolated mitral valve involvement. With modern medical and surgical management, the cure rate should exceed 90% in nonenterococcal streptococcal endocarditis.[82]

The most common streptococci isolated from patients with endocarditis are *Streptococcus sanguis*, *Streptococcus bovis*, *Streptococcus mutans*, and *Streptococcus mitior*.[138] Group D organisms included the enterococci and *S. bovis*. There appears to be no correlation, however, between the clinical outcome and the species involved,[139] with the exception of nutritionally deficient strains. *S. bovis* is a normal inhabitant of the gastrointestinal tract, and its association with gastrointestinal lesions is well established.[140]

Enterococci are also normal inhabitants of the gastrointestinal tract and occasionally the anterior urethra. The *Enterococcus* group is responsible for 5% to 18% of the cases of IE, and incidence appears to be rising.[141] Cure is difficult because of intrinsic resistance of the organism to many antibiotics, and a high mortality persists in this disease. Most enterococcal bacteremias are nosocomial in origin and are often polymicrobial (42% in one large series)[142] and associated with serious underlying disorders.

Before 1945, *S. pneumoniae* was the causative agent in approximately 10% of the cases of IE, but this incidence has decreased to approximately 1% to 3% currently.[143] The course is usually fulminant and is often (in approximately one third of patients) associated with paravalvular abscess formation or pericarditis or both. Patients with pneumococcal endocarditis are frequently alcoholic (≈40%) and concurrent meningitis is present in about 70% of patients.[144] Mortality remains at approximately 50% with similar rates in children.[145] Death is usually due to rapid valvular destruction and hemodynamic compromise.[146]

Nutritionally variant streptococci such as *Abiotrophia* species may be difficult to isolate and are implicated in about 5% of the cases of streptococcal endocarditis. IE due to nutritionally deficient streptococci is virtually always indolent in onset and associated with preexisting heart disease.[147] Therapy remains difficult, and prognosis is poor. The closely related organism, *Streptococcus mitis*, has also emerged as an important causative agent of IE among drug users.

Group B streptococci (*Streptococcus agalactiae*) colonize the mouth, vagina, and anterior urethra and are a major cause of invasive infections in neonates and adults. Risk factors for group B streptococcal sepsis and IE in adults include diabetes mellitus, colon carcinoma, alcoholism, hepatic failure, elective abortion, and intravenous drug use.[148] Underlying heart disease is common, and the overall mortality rate is nearly 50%. The organism has large, friable vegetations and frequently major systemic emboli are present. Group A streptococci remain a very rare cause of IE associated with a high complication rate.[149] IE due to *Gemella haemolysans* has also been reported.[150]

Staphylococci

Staphylococci cause at least 30% to 40% of all cases of IE, and 80% to 90% of these are due to coagulase-positive *S. aureus*. Conversely, only a minority of patients (10% 12%) with *S. aureus* bacteremia will have IE.[124] The organism may attack normal heart valves in approximately one third of the patients. The course is often fulminant, and results in death in approximately 25% to 30% of the patients. The proportion of cases of IE attributable to *S. aureus* is increasing due in part to increasing use of dialysis and pacemaker/defibrillator implantation.

Complications, such as myocardial abscesses (with conduction disturbances), purulent pericarditis, and peripheral foci of suppuration are more common in staphylococcal endocarditis than in other forms of IE[151] with mortality rates often exceeding 50% in patients older than 50 years, especially when the infection is acquired nosocomially.[152]

Whereas *Staphylococcus epidermidis* is an important agent in early PVE, it is increasingly being recognized as a cause of native valve endocarditis as well.[153] Rare cases of IE due to other coagulase-negative staphylococci (e.g., *Staphylococcus saprophyticus* or *Staphylococcus capitis*)[154,155] and *Staphylococcus lugdunensis*[156] have been reported. This latter organism tends to cause a substantially more virulent form of IE than that due to other coagulase-negative staphylococci, with high morbidity rates. These strains are frequently misidentified as *S. aureus*.

Gram-Negative Bacilli

IE due to gram-negative aerobic bacilli is uncommon. Narcotic drug users, early prosthetic valve recipients, and patients with cirrhosis[157] appear to have an increased risk for the development of gram-negative bacillary endocarditis. Among members of Enterobacteriaceae, *Salmonella* species are major causes of endocarditis and aortitis.[158] These organisms have an affinity for abnormal cardiac valves. Most (95%) of the patients with *Pseudomonas* endocarditis are IDU patients,[159] and this organism affects normal valves in this situation. Major embolic phenomena, an inability to sterilize valves, neurologic complications (53%), ring and annular abscesses, splenic abscesses, bacteremic relapses, and rapidly progressive CHF are all common. Early surgery is recommended by many authorities for left-sided *Pseudomonas* endocarditis.[160] In contrast, high-dose regimens of antipseudomonal penicillins combined with aminoglycosides have been effective in a majority of patients with isolated right-sided pseudomonal IE.

HACEK and Other Unusual Gram-Negative Bacteria

The organisms within the HACEK group are all fastidious and require 2 to 3 weeks for primary isolation. The clinical syndromes produced by organisms in this group are similar: large friable vegetations, frequent emboli, and the development of CHF and often the eventual need for valve replacement.[161]

The organisms include *Haemophilus* species, predominantly *Haemophilus paraphrophilus*, *Haemophilus parainfluenzae*, and *Haemophilus aphrophilus*, which account for 0.8% to 1.3% of all cases of IE.[162] Emboli to major peripheral arteries may occur, and major central nervous system complications are frequent.[162] A closely related organism, *Actinobacillus actinomycetemcomitans*, is a rare cause of IE.[163] IE due to *Cardiobacterium hominis*[164] resembles the disease caused by *Haemophilus* species. At least 28 cases of *Kingella* endocarditis have been reported[165] with approximately 50% of patients developing complications. Rarer still is IE due to *Eikenella corrodens* for which intravenous drug use has been implicated.[166]

Neisseria gonorrhoeae was responsible for at least 5% to 10% of the cases of IE before the introduction of penicillin but is now rarely seen. Most cases of gonococcal endocarditis now follow an indolent course, in contrast to the often fulminant progression in the preantibiotic era. A high frequency of late complement component deficiencies has been noted in patients with gonococcal endocarditis, and sudden hemodynamic deterioration may occur despite appropriate therapy.[167]

Gram-Positive Bacilli

IE due to corynebacteria (diphtheroids) is uncommon and usually occurs on damaged or prosthetic valves. A recent report[168] emphasized the aggressive nature of these infections, including major vascular complications, the frequent occurrence of septic arthritis, and involvement of native valves. Intravenous drug use is also a predisposing factor. *Listeria monocytogenes*,[169] lactobacilli,[170] and *Erysipelothrix rhusiopathiae*[171] have all been reported to cause IE. These organisms may take several weeks for isolation on blood culture.

Anaerobic Bacteria

Bacteroides fragilis is the most common pathogen associated with this rare form of IE.[172] Approximately 25% of these cases of IE are polymicrobial, usually with mixed with anaerobic or microaerophilic streptococci. The portal of entry for *B. fragilis* is probably the gastrointestinal tract. Thromboembolic episodes are especially common in IE due to *B. fragilis*, possibly attributable to the heparinase produced by this organism. The mortality rate in patients with anaerobic endocarditis has ranged from 21% to 46%.[172] Isolation of these organisms may be improved by the newer anaerobic culture techniques currently in use.

Fungi

Patients with fungal endocarditis include intravenous drug users, patients who have undergone reconstructive cardiovascular surgery, and patients who have received prolonged intravenous antibiotic therapy. Recent evidence suggests a shift in the epidemiology of fungal IE toward patients receiving intensive medical care. The incidence of fungal sepsis increased 270% from 1980 to 2000.[173] In a review of 23 addicts, *Candida parapsilosis* was responsible in 12 patients (52%), and other *Candida* species. (*Candida guilliermondii*, *Candida stellatoidea*, *Candida krusei*, and *Candida tropicalis*) caused most of the remaining cases. *C. albicans* was isolated in only 1 of the 23 IDU patients. In contrast, in 82 patients who developed fungal endocarditis after cardiac surgery, the causative organisms included *C. albicans* and *Aspergillus* species with each accounting for approximately one third of the isolates. *C. parapsilosis* was found in fewer than 10%. Fungal endocarditis has been observed in patients after prolonged intravenous therapy, of whom 50% were infected with *C. albicans*.

The overall cure rate in patients with fungal endocarditis is poor (14.5%) because of poor penetration of antifungal agents into the vegetation,[174] the low toxic-therapeutic ratio of the available antifungal agents, and the usual lack of fungicidal activity with these compounds. A cure is virtually impossible without surgical intervention.[175] The role of promising antifungal agents, including caspofungin[176] and voriconazole,[177] in the management of fungal IE remains to be defined. In a review of *Aspergillus* IE[178] only 15% of 34 patients had positive blood cultures, and only 1 patient survived. Other fungi that have caused IE include *Histoplasma*, *Blastomyces*, *Coccidioides*, *Cryptococcus*, *Hansenula*, *Fonsecaea* (*Hormodendrum*), *Scedosporium prolificans*, *Mucor*, *Paecilomyces*, *Trichosporon beigelii*, *Pseudallescheria boydii*, and *Phialophora*.

Other Microorganisms

Five cases of IE due to *Spirillum minor*, a spirochete, have been reported.[179] This organism is widely distributed in nature, especially in fresh or salt water with organic debris. *S. minor* is the etiologic agent of "rat-bite fever" (sodoku), but rodent to man transmission has not documented in the cases of endocarditis.

IE due to *Coxiella burnetii* (Q fever) is well documented.[180] Risk factors may include exposure to cats, cattle, or rabbits, as well as a previous valvulopathy or pregnancy. The aortic valve is involved in more than 80% of cases. Vegetations are small or absent.[181] The diagnosis is best made serologically; a positive titer of antibody to the phase I antigen as measured by complement fixation or enzyme-linked immunosorbent assay is indicative of chronic infection, whereas a fourfold rise in the titer of antibody to the phase II antigen is associated with active current infection. A phase I antibody titer (generally IgG and/or IgA) greater than 1:1200 is considered diagnostic of Q fever endocarditis and may be useful to follow the response to therapy.[182] PCR probes are under development. The prognosis with medical therapy alone is poor, and valve replacement is usually necessary for a cure. This agent may also cause endarteritis. A single case of IE due to the causative agent of murine typhus has been reported.[183]

Chlamydia psittaci, the agent of psittacosis, has been implicated in at least 10 well-documented cases of IE.[184] Most of the cases have been associated with psittacine bird exposure. *T. whippelii*, the causative agent of Whipple disease, is an occasional cause of IE and has recently been cultivated from human valvular tissue.[185]

The role of viruses in IE is unknown. Experimentally, coxsackie B virus has been shown to produce valvular and mural endocarditis in animals.[186] Although the enteroviruses are commonly implicated in cases of myocarditis or pericarditis in humans, there is no proof that viral infections produce IE in humans. Adenoviruses are capable of producing IE in mice.

"Culture-Negative" Endocarditis

Sterile blood cultures have been noted in 2.5% to 31% of patients with IE.[187,188] However, blood cultures are negative in only approximately 5% of patients with IE confirmed by strict diagnostic criteria.[189,190] The most commonly attributed causes include right-sided endocarditis; cultures taken toward the end of a chronic course (longer than 3 months); uremia supervening in a chronic course; mural endocarditis as in ventricular septal defects, thrombi after myocardial infarction, or infection related to pacemaker wires; slow growth of fastidious organisms such as anaerobes, *Haemophilus* species, *Actinobacillus* species, *Cardiobacterium* species, nutritionally variant streptococci, or *Brucella* species; the prior administration of antibiotics[188]; fungal endocarditis; endocarditis caused by obligate intracellular parasites such as rickettsiae, chlamydiae, *T. whippelii*,[191] and perhaps viruses; or noninfective endocarditis or an incorrect diagnosis. Attention to the proper collection of blood culture specimens, care in the performance of serologic tests, and the use of newer diagnostic techniques may reduce the proportion of culture-negative cases. The use of PCR to assist in the diagnosis has been described earlier. Some clues as to the cause based on the clinical scenario may be found by reviewing Table 22-3.

Polymicrobial Endocarditis

The proportion of cases of IE due to more than one pathogen appears to be rising,[192] particularly in older patients and in the IDU population. Left-sided involvement, two organisms (versus three or more), and an older age were associated with a higher mortality rate as well.

ANTIMICROBIAL TREATMENT

Certain general therapeutic principles provide the framework for the current recommendations for treatment of endocarditis. These include the facts that complete eradication of infection takes weeks to achieve, the infection exists in a sequestered area of impaired host defense, the bacteria in the vegetations may exist in a state of reduced metabolic activity and cell division[193] rendering them less susceptible to the bactericidal action, and parenteral antibiotics are recommended over oral drugs because of the importance of sustained antibacterial activity. Bacteriostatic antibiotics are generally ineffective in the treatment of bacterial endocarditis. In addition, the selection of antibiotics should be based on antimicrobial susceptibility tests, and the treatment should be monitored clinically and with determination of antimicrobial blood levels when indicated.

Recently, the guidelines for the diagnosis, antimicrobial therapy, and management of IE have been revised as an American Heart Association Scientific Statement.[194] The following recommendations for antimicrobial therapy are patterned after these new guidelines and the reader is referred to that document for more details.

Viridans Group Streptococci

Most strains of viridans streptococci, "other" streptococci (including *Streptococcus pyogenes*), and nonenterococcal group D streptococci (primarily *S. bovis*) are sensitive to penicillins (MIC ≤0.12 μg/mL). However, 15% to 20% of viridans streptococci are resistant to this arbitrary concentration of penicillin.[195] In addition,[196] approximately 15% of the strains of *S. mutans* demonstrate a high MIC for penicillin. These organisms should probably be considered penicillin-tolerant, and studies now suggest that tolerance to penicillin among viridans streptococci is more prevalent than reported previously. Nearly all strains of nutritionally dependent streptococci are tolerant to penicillin.[197] The influence of the tolerance phenomenon on the response to penicillin therapy in experimental endocarditis is not known; two studies yielded conflicting results.[198,199]

Highly Penicillin-Susceptible Viridans Group Streptococci and *Streptococcus bovis*

Cure rates of 98% or greater have been reported in patients who complete 4 weeks of therapy with parenteral penicillin/ampicillin or ceftriaxone for endocarditis caused by highly penicillin-susceptible viridans group streptococci or *S. bovis*[200] (MIC ≤0.12 μg/mL)[194] (Table 22-11). The addition of gentamicin sulfate to penicillin may result in synergistic killing and is recommended. In uncomplicated and especially in right-sided endocarditis, treatment with a 2-week regimen of either penicillin or ceftriaxone combined with an aminoglycoside results in cure rates similar to those after monotherapy with penicillin or ceftriaxone administered for 4 weeks.[201] Once-a-day ceftriaxone along with a once-a-day aminoglycoside (netilmicin or gentamicin) works as well as 2 weeks of therapy with penicillin together with an aminoglycoside administered in daily divided dosages.[202] Patients with known extracardiac infection or those with a reduced creatinine clearance of less than 20 mL/min are not candidates for 2-week regimens. Four weeks of penicillin or ceftriaxone monotherapy results in similar outcomes and avoids the use of gentamicin. Compared with penicillin, the advantage of once-daily ceftriaxone is its simplicity for use in therapy administered to outpatients.[203] For patients in whom penicillin or ceftriaxone therapy is contraindicated, vancomycin is considered the most effective alternative. Patients with endocarditis complicating prosthetic valves or other prosthetic material should receive 6 weeks of therapy with penicillin or ceftriaxone with or without gentamicin for the first 2 weeks.[194]

Viridans Group Streptococci and *Streptococcus bovis* with Penicillin Tolerance

Penicillin-resistant viridans group streptococci or *S. bovis* rarely cause IE. The recommended therapy for native valve endocarditis caused by penicillin-resistant strains (MIC >0.12 to ≤0.5 μg/mL) of viridans group streptococci and *S. bovis* includes 4 weeks of penicillin/ampicillin or ceftriaxone plus gentamicin for the first 2 weeks of treatment (see Table 22-11). Experience with the use of vancomycin with or without aminoglycosides is limited.

Viridans Group Streptococci with Penicillin Resistance, Nutritionally Variant Streptococci, and *Gemella* Species

IE due to nutritionally variant streptococci (*Abiotrophia* and *Granulicatella* species), *Gemella* species, and viridans streptococci (MIC for penicillin >0.5 μg/mL) should be treated with the same regimen recommended for penicillin-resistant enterococci (6 weeks of vancomycin combined with

TABLE 22–11 | **Overview of Therapy for Endocarditis Caused by Viridans Group Streptococci or *Streptococcus bovis***

Regimen	Dosage and Route	Duration (per type of valve)
Highly Penicillin-Sensitive Organisms		
Penicillin G	12-18 million U/24 hr either continuous or in 4-6 doses	4 wk for native valve 6 wk for prosthetic
OR		
Ceftriaxone sodium	2 g/24 h IV/IM in one dose	4 wk for native valve 6 wk for prosthetic
OR		
Penicillin G plus gentamicin		2 wk for native valve 6 wk for prosthetic 2 wk for either
Penicillin G	12-18 million U/24 hr either continuous or in 6 divided doses	
Gentamicin	3 mg/kg per 24 hr IV/IM in 1 dose	
OR		
Ceftriaxone sodium plus gentamicin		
Ceftriaxone	2 g/24 h IV/IM in 1 dose	2 wk for native valve 6 wk for prosthetic 2 wk for either
Gentamicin	3 mg/kg per 24 h IV/IM in 1 dose	
OR		
Vancomycin	30 mg/kg per 24 h in 2 equal doses to maximum of 2 g/24 hr	4 wk for native valve 6 wk for prosthetic
Relatively penicillin-resistant organisms		
(Penicillin or ceftriaxone) plus gentamicin		
Penicillin G	24 million U/24 hr either continuously or in 4-6 equally divided dose	4 wk for native valve 6 wk for prosthetic
OR		
Ceftriaxone	2 g/24 h IV/IM in 1 dose	4 wk for native valve 6 wk for prosthetic
PLUS		
Gentamicin	3 mg/kg per 24 h IV/IM in 1 dose	2 wk for native valve 6 wk for prosthetic
OR		
Vancomycin	30 mg/kg per 24 h in 2 equal doses to maximum of 2 g/24 hr	4 wk for native valve 6 wk for prosthetic

IM, intramuscularly; IV, intravenously; prosthetic, prosthetic valve or other prosthetic material.

Modified from Baddour LM, Wilson WR, Bayer AS, et al: Infective endocarditis: diagnosis, antimicrobial therapy, and management of complications. Circulation 2005;111:e394-e434.

gentamicin). Nephrotoxicity is a particular concern with this regimen, though. Therapy is similar to that for enterococcal IE.[194] Patients with prosthetic valve IE should receive 6 weeks of therapy with a combination of penicillin or ceftriaxone together with gentamicin. Vancomycin therapy is suggested only for patients who are unable to tolerate either penicillin or ceftriaxone.

Streptococcus pneumoniae

Patients with endocarditis caused by highly penicillin-susceptible *S. pneumoniae* should receive 4 weeks of antimicrobial therapy with penicillin, cefazolin, or ceftriaxone. Vancomycin should be administered only to patients who are unable to tolerate β-lactam therapy.

Increasingly, however, *S. pneumoniae* organisms with intermediate penicillin resistance (MIC >0.1 to 1.0 μg/mL) or high penicillin resistance (MIC ≥2.0 μg/mL) are being recovered from patients with bacteremia, and penicillin-resistant

S. pneumoniae IE (MIC of penicillin >0.5 μg/mL) has been described.[204] In the majority of these patients, penicillin-resistant *S. pneumoniae* should be treated with a third-generation cephalosporin or a vancomycin-based regimen. A 6-week course of cefotaxime, ceftriaxone, or vancomycin (for cephalosporin-resistant strains) is recommended. Treatment with both vancomycin and ceftriaxone has also been proposed. For those patients with IE who have concomitant meningitis, third-generation cephalosporins are recommended. Before the advent of penicillin resistance, the mortality was approximately 60% for patients with pneumococcal IE treated with antibiotic therapy alone compared with 32% for patients treated with antibiotics plus surgery. Therefore, valve replacement surgery should be considered in many patients with pneumococcal IE.

Enterococcal Endocarditis

Enterococci should be routinely tested in vitro for susceptibility to penicillin and vancomycin (MIC), for β-lactamase production (nitrocephin disk testing), and for high-level resistance to gentamicin and streptomycin (Table 22-12).

The treatment of enterococcal IE is complicated by high rates of antimicrobial resistance among clinical isolates. Because of a defective bacterial autolytic enzyme system, cell wall–active antimicrobial agents are mostly bacteriostatic against enterococci.[205] Improved outcomes can be expected with the synergistic combination of a cell wall–active agent and an aminoglycoside. Penicillin G and ampicillin, in combination with gentamicin or streptomycin, facilitate the intracellular uptake of the aminoglycoside, resulting in a subsequent bactericidal effect. Care must be taken to avoid nephrotoxicity and ototoxicity. Recently, gentamicin has been increasingly substituted for streptomycin.[141]

Enterococcal IE may be treated with 4 weeks of combination therapy.[206] Exceptions include patients with mitral valve involvement, duration of symptomatic illness exceeding 3 months, enterococcal PVE, and relapse(s) of enterococcal endocarditis. In those instances, current guidelines[82,141] suggest ampicillin/penicillin plus an aminoglycoside for 4 to 6 weeks. Vancomycin therapy should be used only if patients are unable to tolerate penicillin or ampicillin. Gentamicin should be used with caution, following drug levels in impaired renal function. Increasing the dosage of gentamicin does not enhance efficacy but increases the risk of nephrotoxicity. A recent study by Olaison et al[207] showed that patients treated with combination therapy, in whom duration of the aminoglycoside was reduced to a median of 15 days, had an overall cure rate of 81% (75 of 93).

The optimal therapy for enterococcal IE with an organism resistant to penicillin but sensitive to vancomycin and gentamicin is unclear because none of the currently available regimens are bactericidal against such strains. Vancomycin is bacteriostatic against enterococci but displays synergy with aminoglycosides. Nephrotoxicity and ototoxicity are always a concern with this regimen. Nevertheless, vancomycin plus gentamicin is usually indicated for enterococcal strains with intrinsic high-level resistance to penicillin (MIC >16 μg/mL). The addition of rifampin to vancomycin is not recommended.

When high levels of resistance to aminoglycosides (MIC >2000 μg/mL for streptomycin and 500-2000 μg/mL for gentamicin) are present, the addition of these agents to cell wall–active agents is no longer synergistic and is not recommended. In these cases, a prolonged course of a cell wall–active agent (8 to 12 weeks) at high dose (20 to 40 million units of penicillin intravenous daily in divided doses or 2 to 3 g of ampicillin intravenously every 4 hours or by continuous infusion) is suggested. Surgical therapy is often necessary for cure. Recent studies also suggest that combining a third-generation

TABLE 22–12 | Overview of Therapy for Native or Prosthetic Endocarditis Caused by *Enterococcus*

Regimen	Dosage and Route	Duration
Susceptible to penicillin, gentamicin and vancomycin		
Ampicillin sodium	12 g/24 h IV in 6 doses	4-6 wk
OR		
Penicillin G	18-30 million U/24 h either continuously or in 6 doses	4-6 wk
PLUS		
Gentamicin	3 mg/kg per 24 h IV/IM in 3 equal doses	4-6 wk
OR		
Vancomycin	30 mg/kg per 24 h IV in 2 equally divided doses	6 wk
PLUS		
Gentamicin	3 mg/kg per 24 h IV/IM in 3 equal doses	6 wk
Susceptible to penicillin, streptomycin, and vancomycin, but resistant to gentamicin		
Ampicillin sodium	12 g/24 h IV in 6 doses	4- 6 wk
OR		
Penicillin G	18-30 million U/24 h either continuously or 6 doses	4-6 wk
PLUS		
Streptomycin sulfate	15 mg/kg per 24 h IV/IM in 2 equal doses	4-6 wk
OR		
Vancomycin	30 mg/kg per 24 h IV in 2 equally divided doses	6 wk
PLUS		
Streptomycin sulfate	15 mg/kg per 24 h IV/IM in 2 equal doses	6 wk
Susceptible to aminoglycosides and vancomycin but resistant to penicillin		
β-*Lactamase—producing strain*		
Ampicillin-sulbactam	12 g/24 h IV in 4 doses	6 wk
PLUS		
Gentamicin	3 mg/kg per 24 h IV/IM in 3 equal doses	6 wk
OR		
Vancomycin	30 mg/kg per 24 h IV in 2 equally divided doses	6 wk
PLUS		
Gentamicin	3 mg/kg per 24 h IV/IM in 3 equal doses	6 wk
Intrinsic penicillin resistance		
Vancomycin	30 mg/kg per 24 h IV in 2 equally divided doses	6 wk
PLUS		
Gentamicin	3 mg/kg per 24 h IV/IM in 3 equal doses	6 wk
Resistant to Penicillin, Aminoglycosides and Vancomycin		
Enterococcus faecium		
Linezolid	1200 mg/24 h IV/PO in 2 equal doses	≥8 wk
OR		
Quinupristin-dalfopristin	22.5 mg/kg per 24 h IV in 3 equal doses	≥8 wk
Enterococcus faecalis		
Imipenem/cilastatin	2 g/24 h IV in 4 doses	≥8 wk
PLUS		
Ampicillin sodium	12 g/24 h in 6 equal doses	≥8 wk
OR		
Ceftriaxone sodium	2 g/24 h IV/IM in 1 dose	≥8 wk
PLUS		
Ampicillin sodium	12 g/24 h IV in 6 doses	≥8 wk

IM, intramuscularly; IV, intravenously; PO, orally.

Modified from Baddour LM, Wilson WR, Bayer AS, et al: Infective endocarditis: Diagnosis, antimicrobial therapy, and management of complications. Circulation 2005;111:e394-e434.

cephalosporin (ceftriaxone or cefotaxime) with ampicillin may be effective.[208] The rationale for these combinations is based on the ability to saturate different penicillin-binding proteins to achieve synergy. High doses of ceftriaxone (e.g., 4 g/day) are used.

IE caused by vancomycin-resistant enterococci (VRE) is difficult to treat at best. In vitro susceptibilities are crucial to guide antibiotic therapy. Most vancomycin-resistant strains of *Enterococcus faecalis* and some of *Enterococcus faecium* are susceptible to ampicillin (MIC <16 μg/mL). For susceptible strains, a regimen of ampicillin or penicillin combined with gentamicin or streptomycin is recommended. For enterococci resistant to ampicillin (MIC ≥16 μg/mL), higher doses of ampicillin can be used. The streptogramin, quinupristin-dalfopristin (QD), is active against gram-positive cocci including VRE and is bacteriostatic against *E. faecium* and uniformly ineffective against all strains of *E. faecalis*; monotherapy with this agent is unlikely to be curative in VRE endocarditis. Some animal model data suggest that the combination of QD and ampicillin may be beneficial, but clinical data supporting this treatment option are lacking.[209]

Linezolid has been used successfully in the treatment of complicated VRE (*E. faecium*) and intravascular infections, including prolonged bacteremia and IE.[210] However, linezolid also is bacteriostatic against VRE (*E. faecalis* or *E. faecium*) and is not recommended as a first-line therapy. There is anecdotal clinical experience with the combination of chloramphenicol plus minocycline.[211] Daptomycin, a novel lipopeptide antibiotic, displays in vitro efficacy against *E. faecium* in pharmacodynamic models with simulated endocardial vegetations, but clinical treatment failures have been reported recently.[212] Neither daptomycin nor another novel agent, tigecycline, have been proven to be effective bacteriocidal agents at this time.[213]

Coagulase-Negative Staphylococci

Coagulase-negative staphylococci (CoNS) are a common cause of early PVE. Often the infection is locally invasive, with prosthetic invasion and destruction occurring in more than half of the patients. The mortality rate is reported to be as high as 63% to 74%.[214] S. epidermidis predominates as a cause of IE. Resistance to β-lactams is found in 80% of CoNS isolates in PVE.[214] Some studies have shown that patients treated with vancomycin and rifampin, with or without gentamicin, have higher cure rates than those treated with vancomycin alone.[215] Current guidelines suggest the use of vancomycin and rifampin (Table 22-13). If the strain is gentamicin susceptible, then gentamicin should be added for the first 2 weeks of therapy both for synergy and to prevent the development of rifampin resistance.[216]

Native valve IE caused by CoNS is uncommon. It is associated with a high rate of heart failure and mortality comparable with those for native valve IE caused by S. aureus.[217] Many patients with native valve IE due to CoNS are susceptible to β-lactams; however, β-lactams should only be used on the basis of susceptibility testing. Most studies suggest a higher cure rate for combination therapy (β-lactam or vancomycin, based on susceptibility testing, plus gentamicin) compared with monotherapy.[218]

Staphylococcus aureus

Staphylococcus aureus is an increasingly important cause of IE and is now the most common cause of IE in some centers.[219] Unfortunately, antimicrobial resistance is also increasing.

Regardless of whether the infection is community- or hospital-acquired, the majority of S. aureus organisms produce β-lactamase and therefore are highly resistant to penicillin G. In these patients the drugs of choice for methicillin-susceptible S. aureus (MSSA) are the semisynthetic, penicillinase-resistant penicillins such as nafcillin or oxacillin sodium. In the unusual patient with S. aureus susceptible to penicillin, penicillin may be used in high doses.[215]

Aminoglycoside use is controversial. Anecdotal case reports in non-IDU patients suggest that gentamicin-nafcillin therapy may be effective in patients who fail to respond to monotherapy with nafcillin.[220] However, a study[221] suggested that the combination does not reduce mortality or the frequency of cardiac complications and increases the frequency of gentamicin-associated nephrotoxicity. There appears to be little evidence that adjunctive gentamicin therapy beyond 3 to 5 days confers additional clinical benefit.

When penicillin agents are not appropriate, first-generation cephalosporins such as cefazolin are indicated, although cefazolin was shown to be less effective in experimental models of MSSA endocarditis.[222] Cefazolin remains a standard therapy for staphylococcal infections, despite case reports suggesting treatment failures that may be explained by the production of type A β-lactamase in patients with MSSA IE.[223]

In MRSA IE and in patients with MSSA IE who have allergies to β-lactams, vancomycin is the drug of choice,[215] although it may be somewhat inferior because of its slow bactericidal activity as well as poor tissue penetration. If the MRSA strain is aminoglycoside-susceptible, gentamicin may be added to vancomycin; however, it should be limited to no more than the initial 3 to 5 days of therapy.

In patients with MRSA IE and serious adverse reactions associated with vancomycin, linezolid is the next-line therapy. It has an excellent pharmacokinetic profile but is bacteriostatic and failures in the treatment of MRSA IE have already been reported.[224] Quinupristin-dalfopristin (QD) has a bactericidal effect against some, but not all, staphylococci[225] and its role is unclear.[226] Adverse characteristics of QD include arthralgias and myalgias and a requirement for central catheter administration. Daptomycin was shown to be effective in animal models of MRSA endocarditis, and some recent data suggest it may be valuable in the clinical setting.[227] Rifampin is not recommended for first-line treatment of staphylococcal native valve IE.[228] Nevertheless, it may play a role in those patients with an inadequate response to conventional therapy.

Right-sided IE commonly occurs in the setting of injection drug use. Although standard treatment consists of 4 weeks of monotherapy, shorter courses of antibiotic therapy have been proposed and use semisynthetic penicillin along with an aminoglycoside at a low dose for 2 weeks. The cure rates

TABLE 22–13	Overview of Therapy for Endocarditis Caused by *Staphylococcus* species	
Regimen	**Dosage and Route**	**Duration**
Methicillin-susceptible organisms (native valves)		
Nafcillin or oxacillin with option of gentamicin	12 g/24 h IV in 4-6 doses	6 wk
Gentamicin in 2 or 3 doses	3 mg/kg per 24 h IV/IM	3-5 days
OR		
Cefazolin with option of gentamicin	6 gm/24 h in 3 divided doses	6 wk
Gentamicin in 2 or 3 doses	3 mg/kg per 24 h IV/IM	3-5 days
Methicillin-resistant organisms (native valves)		
Vancomycin	30 mg/kg per 24 h in 2 equally divided doses	6 wk
Methicillin-susceptible organisms (prosthetic material)		
Nafcillin or oxacillin	12 g/24 h IV in 6 doses	≥6 wk
PLUS		
Rifampin	900 mg/24 h IV/PO in 3 doses	≥6 wk
PLUS		
Gentamicin	3 mg/kg per 24 h IV/IM in 2 or 3 equal doses	2 wk
Methicillin-resistant organisms (prosthetic material)		
Vancomycin	30 mg/kg per 24 h in 2 equal doses to maximum of 2 g/24 hr	≥6 wk
PLUS		
Rifampin	900 mg / 24 h IV/PO in 3 doses	≥6 wk
PLUS		
Gentamicin	3 mg/kg per 24 h IV/IM 2 or 3 equal doses	2 wk

IM, intramuscularly; IV, intravenously; PO, orally.

Modified from Baddour LM, Wilson WR, Bayer AS, et al: Infective endocarditis: diagnosis, antimicrobial therapy, and management of complications. Circulation 2005;111:e394-e434.

(>90% to 95%) obtained with this strategy are comparable to those obtained with 4 weeks of monotherapy.[229] For patients with MSSA infection and complicated right-sided IE, fever lasting longer than 7 days, HIV infection, or large (>1 cm) vegetations, a full 4-week course of therapy is indicated.[101] In all patients with MRSA IE, 4 weeks of intravenous therapy with vancomycin are preferable.

In IDU patients who will not comply with a course of parenteral antibiotic therapy, oral treatment may be an option. Two studies have evaluated the use of predominantly oral 4- week antibiotic regimens (ciprofloxacin plus rifampin) for the therapy of uncomplicated right-sided *S. aureus* endocarditis in IDUs.[230,231] In each study, including one in which more than 70% of patients were HIV-seropositive, cure rates exceeded 90%.

For staphylococcal PVE, combination antibiotic therapy is based on experience with coagulase-negative staphylococcal PVE. For MSSA PVE the recommendation is to use nafcillin or oxacillin in combination with rifampin for 6 to 8 weeks and low-dose gentamicin during the first 2 weeks.[215] For MRSA PVE, vancomycin is substituted for nafcillin or oxacillin. Susceptibility testing of all organisms to each antibiotic must be performed. In animal models, rifampin has been shown to kill staphylococci adherent to prosthetic materials, but resistant strains are common. To minimize resistance to rifampin, it should be added only after antibiotics active against staphylococci have been started. For strains resistant to gentamicin or other aminoglycosides, a fluoroquinolone may be used if the strain is susceptible.[232]

Endocarditis Due to Enterobacteriaceae or Pseudomonas Species

IE due to these organisms is rare and mortality is extremely high. Surgery is generally required for survival. The prognosis is especially poor with left-sided cardiac involvement. Certain combinations of penicillins or cephalosporins and aminoglycosides have been shown to be synergistic against many of these strains and are usually recommended. For IE due to most strains of *Escherichia coli* or *Proteus mirabilis*, a combination of either ampicillin or penicillin with an aminoglycoside, usually gentamicin, or a broad-spectrum cephalosporin is recommended. Third-generation cephalosporins are extremely active against *E. coli* in vitro, and some (e.g., ceftriaxone) have proved effective in animal models of *E. coli* endocarditis.[233]

For *Klebsiella* endocarditis a combination of a third-generation cephalosporin and an aminoglycoside (either gentamicin or amikacin) is recommended. Certain β-lactam/β-lactamase inhibitor combinations (e.g., piperacillin-tazobactam,[234] but not ceftriaxone-sulbactam)[235] are active in experimental models of *Klebsiella* endocarditis. The specific aminoglycoside used is a critical variable and cannot be totally predicted from MIC data alone, as pharmacodynamic characteristics differ markedly in animal models of IE due to gram-negative aerobic bacilli.[236] Endovascular *Salmonella* infections, including IE, may also respond to third-generation cephalosporins.[237] Left-sided IE due to *Serratia marcescens* is refractory to medical therapy alone; valve replacement is invariably required for cure.

Pseudomonas aeruginosa IE is generally associated with IDUs. Medical therapy may be successful in right-heart IE in up to 50% to 75% of patients.[194] If the disease is refractory to antibiotics, tricuspid valve excision or "vegectomy"[238] without valve replacement is indicated, at least over the short haul. Valve replacement is often necessary for a cure of left-sided IE due to *P. aeruginosa* although some medical cures are possible.[44]

The optimal antimicrobial regimen for *P. aeruginosa* IE is unclear. Problems have emerged with all potential regimens in animal models of this disease.[239] Treatment failures of *Pseudomonas* endocarditis in humans have also been due to the selection of isolates with an enhanced production of type Id β-lactamase.[240] Based mostly on clinical experience,[159] the preferred regimen is high-dose tobramycin (8 mg/kg/day intravenously or intramuscularly in divided doses every 8 hours) with maintenance of peak and trough concentrations of 15 to 20 and 2 μg/mL or less, respectively, in combination with either an extended-spectrum penicillin (e.g., ticarcillin, piperacillin, or azlocillin) or ceftazidime or cefepime in full doses. The toxicity associated with this regimen is surprisingly low; combination treatment should be given for a minimum of 6 weeks. The use of quinolones (in combination with an aminoglycoside) appears to be promising in animal models,[239] but the development of resistance during therapy is a concern. With limited experimental data,[241] ceftazidime-tobramycin is preferred over aztreonam-tobramycin. Occasional patients have been successfully treated with imipenem plus an aminoglycoside.[242]

IE due to *Haemophilus* species (and other members of the HACEK group) is generally responsive to 3 weeks of ampicillin alone.[215] β-Lactamase–producing strains have been well documented, though. Because of difficulty in cultivating HACEK organisms in the laboratory, particularly for newer, automated susceptibility testing systems, such strains should be considered as ampicillin-resistant. The third-generation cephalosporins should be regarded as the drugs of choice for treatment of HACEK IE.[241] The place for quinolones (if any) in the therapy of these infections is not known. Duration of treatment for HACEK IE should be 3 to 4 weeks for native valve infections and 6 weeks for prosthetic valve infections.[203,215] See Table 22-14 for details.

Fungal Endocarditis

The incidence of fungal IE has increased impressively in the past decade. Whereas the survival rate in patients treated before 1974 was less than 20%,[174] survival in the current era has increased to approximately 40%, coincident with improved diagnostic techniques.[243]

The optimal therapy has not been determined, though. Antifungal agents alone have been generally unsuccessful in achieving a cure of this disease. When fungal IE is diagnosed, a combined medical-surgical approach is usually recommended.[244]

The mainstay of antifungal drug therapy is amphotericin B. This agent is toxic and produces multiple side effects, including fever, chills, phlebitis, headache, anorexia, anemia, hypokalemia, renal tubular acidosis, nephrotoxic-

TABLE 22–14	Overview of Therapy for Native or Prosthetic Endocarditis Caused by HACEK Organisms	
Regimen	Dosage and Route	Duration
Ceftriaxone sodium	2 g/24 h IV/IM in 1 dose	4 wk
OR		
Ampicillin-sulbactam	12 g per 24 h IV in 4 equally divided doses	4 wk
OR		
Ciprofloxacin	1000 mg/ 24 h PO or 800 mg/24 hr IV in 2 equal doses	4 wk for native valve 6 wk for prosthetic

IM, intramuscularly; IV, intravenously; PO, orally; prosthetic, prosthetic valve or other prosthetic material.

Modified from Baddour LM, Wilson WR, Bayer AS, et al: Infective endocarditis: diagnosis, antimicrobial therapy, and management of complications. Circulation 2005;111:e394-e434.

primary valve repair when anatomically appropriate are now the standard in the majority of experienced surgical centers. Nevertheless, more than 40,000 aortic or mitral valve replacement operations were reported to the Society of Thoracic Surgeons National Adult Cardiac Database in calendar year 2007.[1] Patients who had undergone previous heart valve surgery represented more than 25% of the subjects with valvular heart disease in the 2003 Euro Heart Survey.[2] Familiarity with the specific attributes, durability, and inherent limitations of the currently available heart valve substitutes, as well as their potential for long-term complications, is critical to appropriate clinical decision making for patients in whom repair is not appropriate or feasible. The choice of valve prosthesis is inherently a tradeoff between durability and thrombogenicity, with the associated hazards of anticoagulation. The ideal heart valve substitute remains an elusive goal.[3-5] Most surgical centers use a specific type of mechanical or tissue valve for the majority of their patients. Although standards have been formulated for reporting outcomes after valve surgery,[6] comparisons of prosthetic valve performance are influenced by patient-, surgeon-, and institutional-related factors.[7]

MECHANICAL VALVES

There are three basic types of mechanical prosthetic valves: bileaflet, tilting disk, and ball-cage (Figure 23-1). The St. Jude bileaflet valve is the most widely used mechanical prosthesis worldwide and consists of two pyrolytic semicircular "leaflets" or disks attached by hinges to a rigid valve ring. The open valve has three orifices: a small, tunnel-like central opening between the two disks and two larger semicircular orifices laterally. Its hemodynamic characteristics compare favorably to those of a tilting-disk valve (Table 23-1). Performance indices (the ratio of effective orifice area to the area of the sewing ring) range from 0.40 to 0.70, depending on valve size. Effective orifice areas range from 0.7 cm² for a 19-mm valve to 4.2 cm² for a 31-mm prosthesis. Average peak velocities are 3.0 ± 0.8 m/s in the aortic position and 1.6 ± 0.3 m/s in the mitral position.[8,9] Peak instantaneous gradients can be estimated using the modified Bernoulli equation, but mean gradient calculations are the more useful clinical parameter. The phenomenon of pressure recovery across bileaflet and cage-ball aortic valves magnifies the estimate of the difference between left ventricular (LV) and aortic pressures (i.e., the systolic gradient), especially when the latter is derived from measurements obtained close to the valve, compared with more distally in the ascending aorta.[10,11] There is additional confounding by the contribution of flow acceleration through the narrow central orifice

of a bileaflet valve.[12] Doppler velocity determinations tend to overestimate the transvalvular gradient across bileaflet valves. Published reference tables of expected velocities for the various valve sizes should be consulted and comparison with baseline postoperative studies made to avoid misdiagnosis of prosthetic valve stenosis.[13] The CarboMedics valve is a variation of the St. Jude prosthesis that can be rotated to prevent limitation of leaflet excursion by subvalvular tissue. Both types of bileaflet valves have a small amount of normal regurgitation designed in part to decrease the risk of thrombosis. A small central jet and two converging jets emanating from the hinge points of the disks can be visualized on color Doppler flow imaging.[14-16]

There are two principal tilting disk valves in clinical use. The Medtronic Hall valve has a thin, circular disk of tungsten-impregnated graphite with pyrolytic coating, secured at its center by a curved, central guide strut, within titanium housing. The sewing ring is made of Teflon. The disk opens to 75° in the aortic model and 70° in the mitral model. The Omniscience valve disk is made of pyrolytic carbon and has a seamless polyester knit sewing ring. The disk opens to 80° and closes at an angle of 12° to the annular plane. For both valve types, the major orifice is semicircular in cross-section. Because the disk does not open to 90°, there is slight resistance to flow with estimated pressure gradients of 5 to 25mm Hg in the aortic position and 5 to 10mm Hg in the mitral position (see Table 23-1).[17] Effective orifice areas depend on valve size and range from 1.6 to 3.7 cm², with performance indices of 0.40 to 0.65, similar to those reported for bileaflet mechanical valves.[18] Tilting disk valves also have a small amount of regurgitation, arising from small gaps at the perimeter of the valve.[14,19] With Medtronic Hall valves, there is also a small amount of regurgitation around the central guide strut.[17]

The bulky Starr-Edwards ball-cage valve, the oldest commercially available prosthetic heart valve, is now rarely implanted. Because of its sheer size, it is not suitable for use in the mitral position in patients with small LV cavities, in the aortic position in patients with small aortic root sizes, or for composite aortic valve root reconstruction. The poppet is made of silicone rubber, the cage of Stellite alloy, and the sewing ring of Teflon/polypropylene cloth. The aortic cage is formed by 3 arches located at 120° intervals around the sewing ring. The ball-cage valve is more thrombogenic and has less favorable hemodynamic performance characteristics than either bileaflet or tilting disk valves (see Table 23-1). Antegrade flow occurs around the ball and through the struts of the cage. There is a small amount of regurgitant back flow before the ball seats after ejection.[17]

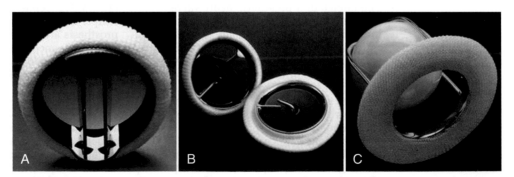

FIGURE 23–1 Mechanical heart valves. **A,** St. Jude bileaflet valve. The occluding mechanism consists of two semicircular leaflets that pivot apart during systole, creating three separate orifices as shown. **B,** Medtronic-Hall tilting disk valve. The disk opens to 75° in the aortic model and 70° in the mitral model. It is retained by an S-shaped center guide strut. **C,** Starr-Edwards ball-cage valve. The poppet is made of siliconized rubber. The sewing ring is more generous than those with bileaflet or tilting disk valves. *(From Antunes MJ, Burke AP, Carabello B et al: In Rahimtoola SH [ed]: Valvular Heart Disease. Philadelphia, Current Medicine, 2005, p 296–297. Braunwald E (series ed): Essential Atlas of Heart Diseases, 3rd ed.)*

TABLE 23–1	Hemodynamic Characteristics of Prosthetic Valves				
	Peak Velocity (m/s) Mean ± SD	Gradient (mmHg) Mean ± SD (Range)	Area (cm²) Mean (Range)	Performance Index* Mean (Range)	Regurgitant Volume* (ml) Mean (Range)
Aortic					
Mechanical					
Bi-leaflet					
St. Jude	3.0±0.8	11±6		0.57 (0.43–0.71)	8.5 (6.8–10.8)
CarboMedics				0.54 (0.40–0.65)	7.9 (6.2–9.6)
Tilting Disk					
Bjork-Shiley	2.5±0.6	14±5		0.48 (0.38–0.58)	7.0 (5.5–9.2)
Medtronic-Hall	2.6±0.3	12±3		0.58 (0.51–0.64)	5.3 (3.0–7.5)
Ball-Cage					
Starr-Edwards	3.1±0.5	24±4		0.33 (0.30–0.36)	4.1 (2.5–5.5)
Tissue					
Stented					
Hancock	2.4±0.4	11±2	1.8 (1.4–2.3)	0.43 (0.41–0.44)	<2
CE Porcine	2.4±0.5	14±6	1.8 (1.2–3.1)	0.44 (0.40–0.48)	<2
CE Pericardial	2.4±1.2	14+4	1.04±0.2 cm²/m²		
Stentless					
SPV-Toronto	2.2±0.4	3 (2–20)	1.8–2.3		Trace
Homograft	1.8±0.4	7±3	2.2 (1.7–3.1)		trace
Mitral					
Mechanical					
Bi-leaflet					
St. Jude	1.6±0.3	5±2	2.9 (1.8–4.4)	0.49 (0.48–0.51)	11.0 (9.7–13.1)
Tilting Disk					
Bjork-Shiley	1.6±0.3	5±2	2.4 (1.6–3.7)	0.44 (0.42–0.45)	6.7
Medtronic-Hall	1.7±0.3	3±1	2.4 (1.5–3.9)	0.48 (0.45–0.53)	9.0 (7.2–10.0)
Ball-Cage					
Starr-Edwards	1.8±0.4	5±2	2.1 (1.2–2.5)	0.28 (0.27–0.29)	–
Tissue					
Hancock	1.5±0.3	4±2	1.7 (1.3–2.7)	0.28 (0.25–0.30)	<2
CE Porcine	1.8±0.2	7±2	2.5 (1.6–3.5)	0.40 (0.35–0.47)	<2
CE Pericardial		4±2	2.6±0.6		

Data are mean ± SD or mean (range).

* =in vitro data

CE = Carpentier Edwards

From Alam M, Rosman HS, Lakier JB, Kemp S, Khaja F, Hautamaki K et al. Doppler and echocardiographic features of normal and dysfunctioning bioprosthetic valves. J Am Coll Cardiol 1987;10:851-858; Reisner SA, Meltzer RS: Normal values of prosthetic valve Doppler echocardiographic parameters: a review. J Am Soc Echocardiogr 1988;1:201-210; Jaffe WM, Coverdale HA, Roche AH, Brandt PW, Ormiston JA, Barratt Boyes BG. Doppler echocardiography in the assessment of the homograft aortic valve. Am J Cardiol 1989;63:1466-1470; Mohr FW, Walther T, Baryalei M, et al. The Toronto SPV bioprosthesis: one-year results in 100 patients. Ann Thorac Surg 1995;60:171-175; Firstenberg MS, Morehead AJ, Thomas JD, et al. Short-term hemodynamic performance of the mitral Carpentier-Edwards PERIMOUNT pericardial valve. Ann Thorac Surg 2001;71(5 Suppl):S285-S288; Milano AD, Blanzola C, Mecozzi G, et al. Hemodynamic performance of stented and stentless aortic bioprostheses. Ann Thorac Surg 2001;72:33-38. Zabalgoitia M. Echocardiographic recognition and quantitation of prosthetic valve dysfunction. In: Otto CM, editor. *The Practice of Clinical Echocardiography*. Philadelphia: W.B. Saunders, 2002; Yoganathan AP, Heinrich RS, Fontaine AA: Fluid dynamics of prosthetic valves. In: Otto CM, editor. *The Practice of Clinical Echocardiography*. Philadelphia: W.B. Saunders, 2002

Durability and Long-Term Outcomes

Currently available mechanical valves have excellent, long-term durability, with up to 40 years for the Starr-Edwards valve and more than 25 years for the St. Jude valve. Structural deterioration, exemplified by some older-generation Bjork-Shiley (strut fracture with disk embolization) and Starr-Edwards (ball variance) prostheses, is now extremely rare. Ten-year freedom from valve-related death exceeds 90% for both St. Jude and CarboMedics bilealfet valves. The Medtronic Hall prosthesis has shown comparable longevity. Actuarial survival rates, which also depend significantly on several patient factors such as age, gender, ventricular function, coronary artery disease, functional status, and major comorbidities, range from 94 ± 2% at 10 years for St. Jude valves to 85 ± 3% at 9 years for Omniscience valves and 60% to 70% at 10 years for Starr-Edwards valves (Table 23-2).[20-26] Long-term issues associated with mechanical valves include infective endocarditis, paravalvular leaks, thromboembolism/valve thrombosis, hemorrhagic complications related to anticoagulation with vitamin K antagonists (VKAs), and pannus ingrowth. All patients with mechanical valves require life-long anticoagulation, the intensity of which varies as a function of prosthesis

TABLE 23–2 | Long-Term Outcome after Mechanical Valve Replacement: Selected Series

Valve Type	Reference	Years Implanted	n	Mean Age (yr)	Actuarial Survival	Complications (% patient-years)			
						Thromboembolism	Bleeding	PVE	Valve Thrombosis
Bileaflet									
St. Jude	27	1977-1987	1298	62 ± 13	Event-free survival 67 ± 8% at 9 yr	1.5	0.56	0.16	0.09
St. Jude	22	1978-1991	91	39 (range 15–50)	94 ± 2% at 10 yr	0.6	0.8	0.4	—
St. Jude AVR	26	1977-1997	1419	63 ± 14	Actuarial survival 82% at 5 yr 51% at 15 yr 45% at 19 yr				
St. Jude AVR + CABG	26	1977-1997	971	70 ± 10	Actuarial survival 72% at 5 yr 45% at 10 yr 15% at 19 yr				
CarboMedics	25	1989-1997	1019	61 ± 10	Event-free survival 82% at 7 yr Mortality rate 2.9%/yr	1.0	1.7	0.1	0.1
Tilting disk									
Medtronic Hall	21	1977-1987	1104	56	Actuarial survival AVR 46 ± 2 % at 15 yr MVR 42 ± 4 % at 15 yr DVR 28 ± 5 % at 15 yr	1.8 1.9 1.9	1.2		0.05 0.19 0.13
Ball-cage									
Starr-Edwards	23	1963-1977	362	40 ± 10	Event-free survival AVR 66.4% at 10 yr MVR 73.4%	AVR 1.36 MVR 1.25	1.06 0.56	—	—
Starr-Edwards	24	1969-1991	1100	57	Survival 59.6 % at 10 yr 31.2% at 20 yr	1.26	0.18	0.39	0.02

AVR, aortic valve replacement; CABG, coronary artery bypass graft; DVR, double valve replacement; MVR, mitral valve replacement; PVE, prosthetic valve endocarditis.

type, position, and number. Thrombogenicity is significantly less for bileaflet and current generation tilting disk valves than for the ball-cage valve. Higher intensity anticoagulation is required for mechanical valves in the mitral versus aortic position, for patients with multiple mechanical prostheses and often for patients with additional risk factors for thromboembolism, such as atrial fibrillation (AF). Tissue valve substitutes are preferred for tricuspid valve replacement because of higher rates (up to 20%) of thrombosis with mechanical valves in this position. Even with appropriately targeted anticoagulation, reported rates of thromboembolism range from 0.6 to 3.3 per 100 patient-years for patients with bileaflet or tilting disk valves. Complications related to anticoagulation in this population occur at rates of 0.9 to 2.3 per 100 patient-years.[28] A 1.4 per 100 patient-years rate of thromboembolism has been reported for the Starr-Edwards 1260 model valve.[24]

TISSUE VALVES

Tissue valves, or bioprostheses, include stented and stentless heterografts (porcine and bovine), also referred to as xenografts, homografts (or allografts) from human cadaveric sources, and autografts of pericardial or pulmonic valve origin. They provide an alternative, less thrombogenic heart valve substitute for which long-term anticoagulation in the absence of additional risk factors is not required.

Stented Heterograft Valves

The stented heterograft valve is a tri-leaflet valve with a circular opening in systole (Figure 23-2). Porcine valves (e.g., Carpentier-Edwards and Hancock) are constructed of glutaraldehyde-fixed porcine aortic leaflets mounted on semisynthetic rigid or flexible stents and the sewing ring. One of the three leaflets of the porcine aortic valve is muscular and is typically replaced during construction with a fibrous leaflet from a second valve.[29,30] There have been several iterative design improvements over time, including glutaraldehyde fixation at low or zero pressure, reconfiguration of the sewing ring, and treatments to retard calcification and reduce leaflet stiffness. The newer bovine pericardial valves (Carpentier-Edwards, see Figure 23-2) offer improved hemodynamic performance compared with earlier-generation porcine bioprostheses (see Table 23-1). In the aortic position, the antegrade velocity approximates 2.4 m/s, mean gradient 14 mm Hg, and indexed valve area 1.04 cm^2/m^2.[31] The pericardial aortic valve has a larger effective orifice area at any given

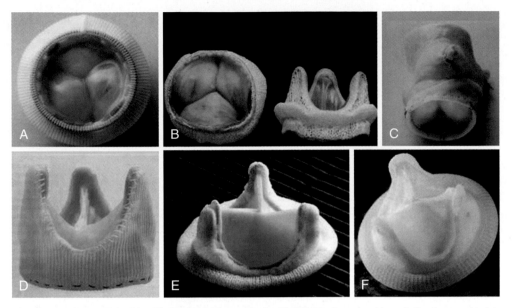

FIGURE 23-2 Bioprosthetic heart valves. **A,** Hancock Modified Orifice (MO) stented valve. The MO valve is produced by replacing the muscular right coronary cusp with the noncoronary cusp from another porcine valve. **B,** Carpentier-Edwards stented porcine valve. The annulus is purposefully asymmetric to obliterate the muscular septal ridge of the porcine right coronary cusp. **C,** Medtronic Freestyle stentless valve. **D,** St. Jude Medical Toronto SPV stentless valve. **E,** Carpentier-Edwards pericardial valve. **F,** Autologous pericardial valve. *(From Grunkemeier GL, Rahimtoola SH, Starr A: Prosthetic heart valves. In Rahimtoola SH (ed): Valvular Heart Disease. Philadelphia, Current Medicine, 1997, pp 13.9-13.11. Braunwald E (series ed): Atlas of Heart Diseases, vol XI.)*

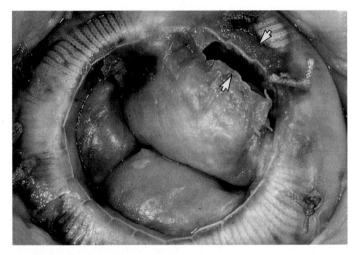

FIGURE 23-3 Bioprosthetic structural valve deterioration of a 5-year-old mitral Hancock porcine valve. There is a linear tear at the base of one of the three cusps (*white arrows*). *(From Antunes MJ, Burke AP, Carabello B, et al: In Rahimtoola SH (ed): Valvular Heart Disease. Philadelphia, Current Medicine, 2005, p 298. Braunwald E (series ed): Essential Atlas of Heart Diseases, 3rd ed.*

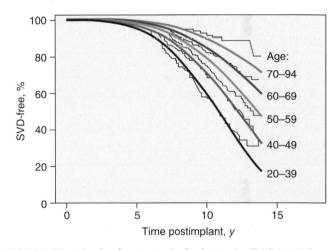

FIGURE 23-4 Freedom from structural valve deterioration (SVD). Actuarial freedom from SVD for 4910 operative survivors of isolated aortic or mitral valve replacement with Hancock or Carpentier-Edwards porcine valves. The curves are stratified by age group and show a significantly lower rate of SVD for older versus younger patients. A Weibull regression model based on patient age and valve position (smooth lines) was used to fit the actuarial Kaplan-Meier curves (jagged lines). *(Adapted from Grunkemeier GL, Jamieson WRE, Miller DC, Starr A: Actual vs. actuarial risk of structural valve deterioration. J Thorac Cardiovasc Surg 1994;108:709-718.)*

valve size between 19 and 29. The average peak gradient in the mitral position is 9 ± 3 mm Hg and the effective orifice area 2.5 ± 0.6 cm².[32] A small degree of regurgitation can be detected by color Doppler flow imaging in 10% of normally functioning bioprostheses. The major drawback with stented porcine valves is their limited durability, typically beginning within 5 to 7 years of implantation, with tissue changes characterized by calcification, fibrosis, tears, and perforations (Figure 23-3). Structural valve deterioration (SVD) occurs earlier for mitral than for aortic bioprosthetic valves, perhaps due to exposure of the mitral prosthesis to relatively higher closing pressures (Table 23-3). The process of SVD is accelerated in younger patients, in those with disordered calcium metabolism (end-stage renal disease), and, possibly, in pregnant women independent of younger age (Figure 23-4). In several older series, the estimated rate of SVD of porcine valves was 3.3% per patient year, with freedom from valve failure at 10 years of 78 ± 2% for aortic valves and 69 ± 2% per patient year for mitral valves.[33,34,43] The rate of valve failure accelerates further after 10 years, such that the actuarial freedom from porcine bioprosthetic SVD is 49 ± 4% at 15 years for aortic valves and 32 ± 4% for mitral valves.[32] By comparison, the rate of freedom from primary tissue failure with pericardial aortic valves is 86% at 12 years[35] (see Table 23-3 and Figure 23-5).

Stentless Heterograft Valves

The rigid sewing ring and stent-based construction of certain bioprostheses allow for easier implantation and maintenance of the three-dimensional relationships of the leaflets. However,

TABLE 23–3 | Long-Term Outcome after Tissue Valve Replacement: Selected Series

Valve Type	Reference	Years Implanted	n	Age (yr ± SD)	Actuarial Survival	Freedom from or (Annual Rate of) Thromboembolism	Freedom from or (Annual rate of) Structural Valve Deterioration
Stented heterografts							
Porcine (Hancock and Carpentier-Edwards)	33	1971-1990	2879	AVR 60 ± 15	77 ± 1% at 5 yr 54 ± 2% at 10 yr 32 ± 3% at 15 yr	92 ± 1% at 10 yr	78 ± 2% at 10 yr 49 ± 4% at 15 yr
				MVR 58 ± 13	70 ± 1% at 5 yr 50 ± 2% at 10 yr 32 ± 3% at 15 yr	86 ± 1% at 10 yr	69 ± 2% at 10 yr 32 ± 4% at 15 yr
Carpentier-Edwards	34	1975-1986	1,195	57.3	57.4 ± 1.5% at 10 yr	(1.6%/patient-year)	(3.3%/patient-year)
Carpentier-Edwards pericardial	35	1984-1995	254	71 (range 25–87)	80 ± 3% at 5 yr 50 ± 8 at 10 yr 36 ± 9 at 12 yr	67 ± 13% at 12 yr	86 ± 9% at 12 yr
Stentless heterografts							
Toronto SPV	36	1987-93	123	61 ± 12	91 ± 4% at 6 yr	87 ± 7% at 6y	(0%)
Medtronic Freestyle	37	1993-1997	95	75	80 ± 6% at 5 yr	(9% at 4 yr)	(0%)
PRIMA Edwards	38	1991-93	200	68.5 ± 8	95% at 1 yr	(3% at 1 yr)	(AV block requiring pacer 7% at 1 yr, mild AR 27% at 1yr)
Homografts							
Cryopreserved	39	1981-91	18	46	85% at 8 yr		85% at 8 yr
Antibiotic sterilized, subcoronary	40	1973-1983	200	50	81 ± 3% at 10 yr 58 ± 4 % at 20 yr	81 ± 3% at 10 yr 31 ± 5% at 20 yr	
Pulmonic autografts							
Pulmonic autografts	41	1986-95	195	8 mo-62 yr			95 ± 2% at 2 yr 81 ± 5% at 8 yr
Pulmonic autografts	42	1991-1997	80	31	98 ± 1% at 5 yr		(0%)

AR, atrial regurgitation; AV, atrioventricular; AVR, aortic valve replacement; MVR, mitral valve replacement.

these features also contribute to impaired hemodynamic performance and accelerated SVD. Stentless porcine valves (Toronto SPV, Edwards, and Medtronic Freestyle) (Figure 23-2) were developed in part to address these issues. Their use has been restricted to the aortic position. Implantation is technically more challenging, whether they are deployed in a subcoronary position or as part of a mini-root, and hence they are preferred by only a minority of surgeons. Early postoperative mean gradients can be less than 15 mm Hg with further improvement in valve performance over time due to aortic root remodeling, lower peak exercise transvalvular gradients, and more rapid reduction in LV mass.[44-51] There is a low incidence of significant aortic regurgitation, although results will vary as a function of technical expertise and appropriate valve sizing at the time of implant. Rates of SVD are low and 6-year actuarial survival rates are as high as 91 ± 4%.[36-38,50] There are few data on patient outcomes after 10 to 15 years.

Homografts

Aortic valve homografts are harvested from human cadavers within 24 hours of death as blocks of tissue comprising the ascending aorta, aortic valve, a portion of the interventricular septum, and the anterior mitral valve leaflet. They are treated with antibiotics and cryopreserved at −196° C.[52] They are now most commonly implanted in the form of a total root

replacement with reimplantation of the coronary arteries and trimming of any excess tissue not required for primary valve replacement. Sizing is based on echocardiographic measurement of the dimensions of the aortic annulus and sinotubular junction. Homograft valves seem to be resistant to infection and are preferred for management of aortic valve and root endocarditis in the acute phase. Neither immunosuppression nor routine anticoagulation is required. Despite earlier expectations, long-term durability beyond 10 years is not superior to that for current-generation pericardial valves. In an echocardiographic follow-up study of 570 patients with aortic valve homografts, 72% had signs of valve dysfunction at 6.8 ± 4.1 years after implantation, with moderate to severe aortic regurgitation in 15.4%, moderate aortic stenosis in 10%, and severe aortic stenosis in 2.5%.[53] Rates of homograft reoperation at 15 years for SVD, which do not account for all cases of SVD, are approximately 20% for patients 41 to 60 years of age and 16% for those older than 60 years at time of implantation.[54] Excessive leaflet and root calcification render reoperations particularly challenging. Mitral homograft valve replacement, a complex technical feat, is not advocated.

Autografts

In the Ross procedure, the patient's own pulmonic valve or autograft is harvested as a small tissue block containing the

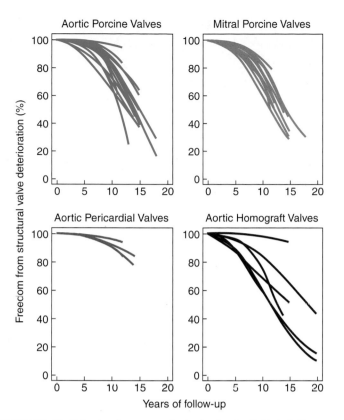

FIGURE 23-5 Freedom from structural valve deterioration (SVD). Weibull distribution curves for freedom from SVD for four types of tissue valves. Note the more gradual rate of SVD for aortic pericardial valves. *(Adapted from Grunkemeier GL, Li H-H, Naftel DC, et al: Long-term performance of heart valve prostheses. Curr Probl Cardiol 2000;25:73-156.)*

pulmonic valve, annulus, and proximal pulmonary artery, and inserted in the aortic position usually as a complete root replacement with reimplantation of the coronary arteries.[55-64] The pulmonic valve and right ventricular outflow tract are then replaced with either an aortic or pulmonic homograft. Thus, the procedure requires two separate valve operations and a longer pump run and has a steep learning curve. With appropriate patient selection at experienced centers of excellence, operative mortality rates are less than 1% and freedom from valve-related death is as high as 84 ± 6% at 14 years.[42,65-67] Advantages of the autograft include the ability to increase in size during childhood growth, excellent hemodynamic performance characteristics, inherent lack of thrombogenicity, and resistance to infection. The hemodynamic performance characteristics of the pulmonary autograft are similar to those of a normal, native aortic valve both at rest and with exercise. However, the homograft in the pulmonic position has a higher mean gradient at rest (9 ± 7 mm Hg) and with exercise (21 ± 14 mm Hg), compared with a normal, native pulmonic valve.[68-70] Early homograft stenosis occurs in 10% to 20% of patients and is due to extrinsic compression from inflammation and adventitial fibrosis.[71,72] The procedure is usually reserved for children and young adults but should be avoided in those with dilated roots given the unacceptably high incidence of accelerated degeneration and pulmonary autograft dilatation with significant regurgitation. The Ross procedure is not practiced widely and surgical opinions differ regarding the best approach to the child or young adult with aortic valve disease. Approximately 15% to 29% of hospital survivors require reoperation over 20 years.[59,65-67,73,74] The use of pericardial autograft valves for either aortic or mitral replacement, in which the patient's own pericardium is fashioned onto a frame in the operating room, has had very limited support,

despite excellent hemodynamic performance characteristics and durability in small patient subsets.[75]

Comparison of Mechanical versus Tissue Valves

Obvious differences between valve types include the enhanced durability and need for anticoagulation with mechanical prostheses versus the significantly more limited durability with tissue valves. Short- to intermediate-term hemodynamic performance characteristics with low-profile mechanical prostheses (e.g., St. Jude) are comparable to those with stented tissue valves of similar size. There are no significant differences in rates of prosthetic valve endocarditis (PVE), although some series have suggested a higher incidence of early (<1 year) infection with mechanical valves versus tissue heterografts.[76] Two earlier randomized trials compared long-term outcomes with a spherical tilting disk valve (Bjork-Shiley) versus those with a stented porcine valve (Hancock or Carpentier-Edwards). In the Veterans Affairs Trial, 575 men were randomly assigned between 1977 and 1982; 394 underwent aortic valve replacement (AVR) and 181 had mitral valve replacement (MVR).[77] Among those undergoing AVR, survival at 15 years was better with mechanical AVR (34% ± 3% versus 21 ± 3%, *P* = 0.02) (Figure 23-6), whereas there was no difference in survival with mechanical versus tissue MVR (81% versus 79%). With AVR, the increased mortality among patients allocated a tissue prosthesis was largely driven by the higher rate of SVD and the risks associated with reoperation. SVD occurred predominantly in patients younger than 65 years, beginning at 5 to 6 years after MVR and 7 to 8 years after AVR. The cumulative incidence of SVD was 23 ± 5% for tissue AVR versus 0 ± 0% for mechanical AVR and 44 ± 8% for tissue MVR versus 5 ± 4% for mechanical MVR.[77] There was an increased risk of bleeding with mechanical valve replacement, but no significant differences were observed for other valve-related complications such as thromboembolism and PVE.

In the Edinburgh Heart Valve Trial, 541 men and women were randomly assigned between 1975 and 1979 and followed for a mean of 12 years after AVR (*n* = 211), MVR (*n* = 261), or AVR plus MVR (*n* = 61).[78] There was a trend for improved survival with mechanical valve replacement (*P* = 0.08), and higher rates of reoperation with tissue valve

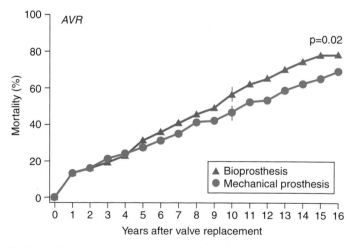

FIGURE 23-6 Mortality after aortic valve replacement (AVR) with a mechanical (Bjork-Shiley) versus stented porcine (Hancock) prosthesis in the Veteran Affairs Randomized Trial. At 15 years, mortality was 66 ± 3% for patients receiving mechanical valves compared with 79 ± 3% for those receiving porcine valves (*P* = 0.02). *(From Hammermeister K, Sethi GK, Henderson WG, et al: Outcomes 15 years after valve replacement with a mechanical versus a bioprosthetic valve: Final report of the Veteran Affairs randomized trial. J Am Coll Cardiol 2000;36:1152-1158.)*

replacement (AVR 22.6 ± 5.7% versus 4.2 ± 2.1%, $P < 0.01$; MVR 43.1 ± 6.0% versus 9.9 ± 3.2%, $P < 0.001$). Bleeding rates were higher with mechanical AVR, but there were no differences in rates of thromboembolism or PVE. A more recent meta-analysis showed no differences in survival between mechanical and tissue valves when patient age and risk factors were included in the model.[79] Although the results from the two randomized trials with valves implanted 20 to 30 years ago are not directly comparable to current outcomes after valve replacement surgery, they are directionally consistent and form the basis of the integrated approach to patient management.

23   CHOICE OF PROSTHETIC HEART VALVE

The need for heart valve replacement surgery marks a major milestone in the natural history of the underlying disease and mandates that clinical indications for the procedure are convincingly met and that valve repair by an experienced surgeon is not an option. Because there is no perfect heart valve substitute, judgment and compromise are required. Important factors to consider include patient age, the desire for pregnancy, the anatomic nature of the valve lesion, the presence of infection, the experience of the surgeon, the risks of anticoagulation, the willingness and ability to take anticoagulant medications reliably, the likelihood of reoperation for SVD over 10 to 15 years, and patient preferences. Recently, there has been a clear trend favoring the use of tissue valves, related to improved durability with current-generation pericardial prostheses, lower rates of mortality and major morbidity with reoperation, and strong patient preferences to avoid the life-style limitations and hazards of anticoagulation therapy.

The balanced recommendations set forth by both American College of Cardiology (ACC)/American Heart Association (AHA)[80] and European Society of Cardiology (ESC)[81] guideline writing committees for patients with valvular heart disease are a useful reference for clinical decision making. Mechanical AVR is recommended when there is a mechanical valve already in place in either the mitral or tricuspid position or both (class I). Bioprothetic AVR is recommended for patients who cannot or will not take VKAs (class I). Mechanical AVR is reasonable for patients younger than 65 years without a contraindication to anticoagulation and for patients already treated with anticoagulation for another indication, such as AF or chronic venous thromboembolic disease (class IIa). Bioprosthetic AVR is reasonable for patients 65 years or older (class IIa) and for patients younger than 65 years, provided the younger patient is fully informed of the tradeoffs between anticoagulation and the likelihood of reoperation (class IIa). In this latter scenario, the predicted risks associated with reoperation should be acceptable. Bioprosthetic AVR might be considered for a young woman contemplating pregnancy (class IIb), so that the hazards of anticoagulation therapy can be avoided in this setting. Homograft AVR is a reasonable choice for patients with active infective endocarditis (class IIa). For MVR, a tissue valve is recommended for any patient unwilling or unable to take VKAs (class I). Mechanical MVR is reasonable for patients in whom there is an independent indication for anticoagulation, especially AF (class IIa). Bioprosthetic MVR is reasonable for patients 65 years or older in sinus rhythm, and for patients younger than 65 years in sinus rhythm who understand the high likelihood of reoperation during their lifetime (class IIa). Isolated tricuspid valve replacement is usually performed with a tissue valve because of the high rates of mechanical valve thrombosis in this position. Mechanical tricuspid valve replacement is recommended when there is a mechanical prosthesis in either or both the mitral or aortic position.

MEDICAL MANAGEMENT AND SURVEILLANCE AFTER VALVE REPLACEMENT

Anticoagulation

There is general agreement among the ACC/AHA,[80] ESC,[81] and American College of Chest Physician (ACCP) guidelines[82] for antithrombotic management of patients with prosthetic heart valves, except for the divergent recommendations discussed below. These differences are due to the lack of a robust evidence base. The guidelines are in agreement that all patients with mechanical heart valves require life-long anticoagulation and that the intensity of anticoagulation varies as a function of valve type, position, and number. Further, more intense anticoagulation is recommended in the presence of additional risk factors for thromboembolism, such as AF, LV systolic dysfunction, a history of thromboembolism, or a hypercoagulable state.

The risk of thromboembolism is highest in the first postoperative month. Anticoagulation should be initiated after surgery as soon as it is deemed safe, preferably within the first 2 days, beginning with heparin and transitioning to a VKA.

For patients at low risk defined as those with either a St. Jude bileaflet or Medtronic Hall tilting disk AVR in sinus rhythm with normal LV systolic function and no other risk factors, a target international normalized ratio (INR) of 2.5 (range, 2.0 to 3.0) is recommended. A higher target INR (3.0; range, 2.5 to 3.5) is recommended if additional risk factors for thromboembolism are present or if the mechanical aortic valve is more thrombogenic (Bjork-Shiley, Omniscience, and Starr-Edwards). Patients with a mechanical MVR are managed to a target INR of 3.0 (range, 2.5 to 3.5), irrespective of valve type.

Patients with a bioprosthetic MVR and risk factors for thromboembolism are managed to a target INR of 2.5 (range, 2.0 to 3.0). There is general agreement that patients with bioprosthetic MVRs without risk factors should be treated with VKAs for the first 3 postoperative months to a target INR of 2.5 (range, 2.0 to 3.0), but lack of consensus regarding the need for VKA therapy in this time frame for patients with bioprosthetic AVRs without risk factors. These specific patients are most often managed with aspirin alone. Long-term treatment of low-risk patients with bioprosthetic AVRs and MVRs consists of low-dose aspirin, although there are no data to support this practice.

The development of thromboembolism at therapeutic levels of anticoagulation in high-risk patients with mechanical and bioprosthetic valves is managed by the addition of low-dose aspirin and/or an increase in the target INR and range. The routine addition of low-dose aspirin to therapeutic anticoagulation is recommended for all patients with mechanical heart valves by the ACC/AHA guideline writing committee (Table 23-4) but reserved for patients with other indications, chiefly atherosclerotic vascular disease, by the ESC and ACCP writing groups, and only if the increased risk of bleeding with dual antithrombotic therapy is considered manageable.

Interruption of Anticoagulation

In the planned interruption of VKA therapy for noncardiac surgery, the following must be taken into account: the nature of the procedure; the magnitude of risk of thromboembolism based on valve type, position, and number; underlying patient risk factors; and the competing risk of periprocedural hemorrhage.[83] Low-risk patients with low-profile bileaflet or tilting disk valves in the aortic position can usually stop VKA therapy 3 to 5 days before noncardiac surgery and then resume it postoperatively as soon as it is considered safe, without the need for a heparin "bridge." In all other patients

TABLE 23–4	Antithrombotic Therapy in Patients with Prosthetic Heart Valves			
	Aspirin (75-100 mg)	Warfarin (INR 2.0-3.0)	Warfarin (INR 2.5–3.5)	No Warfarin
Mechanical prosthetic valves				
A. AVR—Low risk				
<3 mo	Class I	Class I	Class IIa	
>3 mo	Class I	Class I		
B. AVR—High risk				
	Class I		Class I	
C. MVR	Class I		Class I	
Biological prosthetic valves				
A. AVR—Low Risk				
<3 mo	Class I	Class IIa		Class IIb
>3 mo	Class I			Class IIa
B. AVR—High risk				
	Class I	Class I		
C. MVR—Low risk				
<3 mo	Class I	Class IIa		
>3 mo	Class I			Class IIa
D. MVR—High risk				
	Class I	Class I		

Risk factors: atrial fibrillation, left ventricular dysfunction, previous thromboembolism, and hypercoagulable condition. International normalized ratio (INR) should be maintained between 2.5 and 3.5 for aortic tilting disk valves and Starr-Edwards valves. AVR, aortic valve replacement; MVR, mitral valve replacement.

Modified from McAnulty JH and Rahimtolola SH. Anti-thrombotic therapy in valvular heart disease. In Schlant R, Alexander RW [eds]. Hurst's The Heart. New York, NY, McGraw-Hill, 1988, and from Bonow RO, Carabello BA, de Leon A et al. ACC/AHA 2006 Guidelines for the Management of Patients with Valvular Heart Disease. Available at http://www.acc.org/clinical/guidelines/valvular/index.pdf, with permission.

either low-molecular-weight heparin (LMWH) or intravenous unfractionated heparin should be used as a bridge both before and after surgery, as directed by the surgeon. The use of LMWH avoids the need for preoperative hospitalization and has been validated in some settings.[84,85] Randomized trials are lacking, however.

Excessive Anticoagulation

Correction of a supratherapeutic[86] INR should be considered when the INR exceeds 5.0, especially with active bleeding. Rapid correction of a therapeutic INR may also be necessary because of bleeding or the need for emergency noncardiac surgery. Any INR value greater than 4.0 obtained with a finger-stick device should be verified with a laboratory assay performed on a phlebotomized blood specimen. For patients with minimally elevated INRs (4.0 to 5.0) and no active bleeding, the VKA is held for one or two doses, and the INR is repeated. Patients with INRs of 5.0 or greater but less than 9.0 who are not actively bleeding can be managed with oral vitamin K in doses of 1.0 to 2.5 mg. High doses of vitamin K may drive the INR into a subtherapeutic range and lead to a state of relative VKA resistance for up to 1 week. When the INR is 9.0 or greater, a higher dose of oral vitamin K is recommended (2.5 to 5.0 mg). The bioavailability of oral vitamin K exceeds that of subcutaneously administered vitamin K and the INR should correct toward normal over 24 to 48 hours. With serious or life-threatening bleeding at any INR, 10 mg of vitamin K should be given by slow intravenous infusion, supplemented with fresh frozen plasma, prothrombin complex concentrate, or recombinant factor VIIa. Vitamin K administration can be repeated at 12-hour intervals for persistent INR elevation. Intravenous administration of vitamin K may be associated with anaphylactic reactions, although they have also occurred with vitamin K given by alternate routes.

Anticoagulation in Pregnant Women

Management of anticoagulation in the pregnant patient is fraught with hazards for both the mother and fetus. Many consider a mechanical heart valve with the obligate need for anticoagulation to be a contraindication to pregnancy. All choices are associated with an increased risk of spontaneous abortion, and the first principle of management is to engage the mother, her partner, and family in a discussion of the pitfalls of any approach. Warfarin therapy may be relatively safer for the mother, although there is a risk of fetal embryopathy, the incidence of which has been estimated to be 6%.[87] Exposure during the 6th to 12th week of gestation may be most harmful. There are observational data to suggest that the risk of embryopathy may be dose related and that fetal abnormalities are less common with maternal doses of warfarin less than 5 mg/day.[88] Opinions regarding the relative safety of warfarin during pregnancy differ sharply between the United States and Europe.

Unfractionated heparin may be advantageous for the fetus, particularly because it does not cross the placenta, yet older studies in patients with relatively thrombogenic valves suggest that it may be less effective than warfarin for the prevention of thromboembolism or prosthetic valve thrombosis in the mother. The initial experience with LMWH was characterized by unacceptable rates of maternal complications, possibly related to the lack of dose adjustment to maintain therapeutic anti-Xa levels throughout pregnancy.[89]

In the United States, one approach that is often used is dose-adjusted LMWH throughout pregnancy, aiming for anti-Xa levels between 0.7 and 1.2 IU/mL, assessed 4 hours after a subcutaneous dose.[88,90] Importantly, LMWH is not advised if anti-Xa levels cannot be monitored. Testing should be performed at a minimum of every 2 weeks. If unfractionated heparin is used, the activated partial thromboplastin time should be twice control or the anti-Xa level should be 0.5 to 1.0 IU/mL.

For women who choose to use warfarin before 6 and after 12 weeks of gestation, the INR target is 3.0 (range, 2.5 to 3.5). Warfarin should be discontinued at week 36 or 2 to 3 weeks before anticipated delivery, to avoid traumatic bleeding complications in a fully anticoagulated infant. Heparin is given in the weeks leading up to delivery and can be resumed 6 hours post-partum as deemed safe. Warfarin is not excreted in breast milk and is begun the evening after delivery. For high-risk women (MVR or older age, thrombogenic prosthesis, AF, and history of thromboembolism), low-dose aspirin can be added to anticoagulant therapy in the second and third trimesters.[90]

Antiplatelet Therapy

The addition of low-dose aspirin to therapeutic VKA therapy in selected patient subsets has been discussed previously. Dual antiplatelet therapy with aspirin and clopidogrel or with aspirin and dipyridamole is not a substitute for VKA therapy in patients with mechanical heart valves. Clopidogrel is an appropriate choice when antiplatelet therapy is indicated for patients who are allergic to aspirin.

Infective Endocarditis Prophylaxis

There is agreement that patients with prosthetic heart valves constitute one of several groups at high risk for serious complications from infective endocarditis and that antibiotic prophylaxis is reasonable (class IIa) before all dental procedures that involve manipulation of gingival tissue or the periapical region of teeth or perforation of the oral mucosa.[91] Prophylaxis is not recommended before gastrointestinal or genitourinary procedures in the absence of suspected infection. The regimens for dental procedures are provided in Chapter 8.

Morbidity and mortality rates with PVE are higher than those associated with native valve endocarditis, especially when the offending organism is *Staphylococcus aureus*, and an aggressive, multidisciplinary approach to diagnosis and treatment is essential.

Clinical Assessment

Postoperative visits should begin approximately 3 to 4 weeks after valve implantation. The first visit is focused on ensuring a smooth transition from hospital/rehabilitation facility to home, reconciling medications, and assessing neurocognitive function, wound healing, volume status, heart rhythm, and the auscultatory characteristics of prosthetic valve function (Figure 23-7). A grade 1 to 3 midsystolic murmur is audible at the base in all patients after AVR. The intensity varies as a function of valve size, cardiac output, and gradient. The closing sound of a mechanical AVR (A2) is often palpable and distinctly loud, even to the extent that it is a nuisance to the patient. Patients who have undergone conduit replacement of the ascending aorta with valve-sparing reconstruction have a grade 2 to 3 systolic murmur below the suprasternal notch radiating into the carotid arteries and along the course of the clavicles. An aortic diastolic murmur under any circumstances is pathologic. Patients with stented tissue valves in the mitral position have grade 2 or 3 midsystolic murmurs, which are loudest at the left sternal border and indicative of accelerated flow past the stents that extend into the LV outflow tract. With a low-profile mechanical MVR, an outflow murmur of this type is not present. S1 is loud and crisp. A soft, grade 1, low-pitched diastolic murmur can sometimes be heard in the left lateral decubitus position with either a tissue or mechanical MVR, depending on the cardiac output and magnitude of the transvalvular diastolic pressure gradient; it need not indicate valve dysfunction.

The history at subsequent visits is tailored to detect symptoms suggestive of heart failure or reduced functional capacity, arrhythmia, thromboembolism, or infection. Adherence to the recommended schedule of INR determinations and the relative time spent in the therapeutic range should be assessed in all patients receiving anticoagulation. Problems with bleeding should be identified. The interview should include questions regarding other cardiovascular and general health issues, as well as a review of medication adherence, drug interactions, and adverse side effects. A focused cardiovascular examination is repeated at each visit. Instructions regarding antibiotic prophylaxis are repeated. After the 6-month mark, follow-up visits can be conducted annually unless interim problems arise.

A chest radiograph is obtained by the surgeon at the first visit to assess for residual pleural fluid, pneumothorax, lung aeration, and heart size. An electrocardiogram is routinely performed and should be reviewed for rhythm, conduction, and dynamic repolarization changes. Postoperative baseline values for hemoglobin, hematocrit, lactate dehydrogenase, and bilirubin should be established for patients with mechanical heart valves, allowing future comparisons in patients with suspected hemolysis. It is less useful to follow the serum haptoglobin. Other laboratory studies are performed as clinically relevant.

Echocardiography

A complete, postoperative baseline transthoracic echocardiogram (TTE) with color Doppler flow imaging should be performed in all patients after heart valve replacement, typically at the first postoperative outpatient visit or at 3 months after surgery to allow for reequilibration of volume status and early LV remodeling. Correlation with the operative note is critical to an integrated understanding of the TTE findings. Published tables of transvalvular velocities and prosthetic valve areas, as a function of valve type and size, should be consulted to determine whether valve function is acceptable. The phenomenon of pressure recovery, especially with mechanical bileaflet valves, must be considered in interpretation, as previously reviewed. The

Type of Valve	Aortic Prosthesis		Mitral Prosthesis	
	Normal Findings	Abnormal Findings	Normal Findings	Abnormal Findings
Caged-Ball (Starr-Edwards)	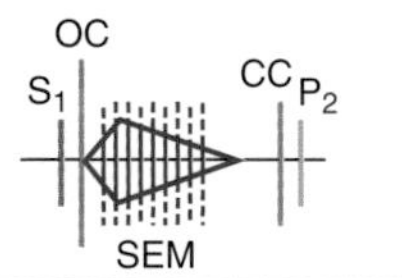 OC, S₁, CC, P₂, SEM	Aortic diastolic murmur; Decreased intensity of opening or closing click	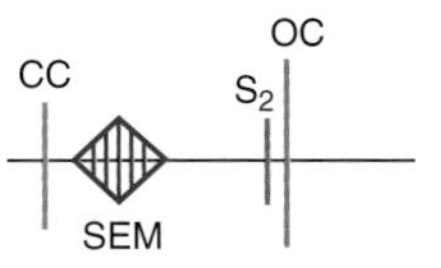 CC, OC, S₂, SEM	Low-frequency apical diastolic murmur; High-frequency holosystolic murmur
Single-Tilting-Disk (Bjork-Shiley or Medtronic-Hall)	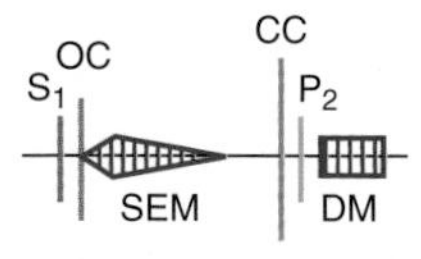 OC, S₁, CC, P₂, SEM, DM	Decreased intensity of closing click	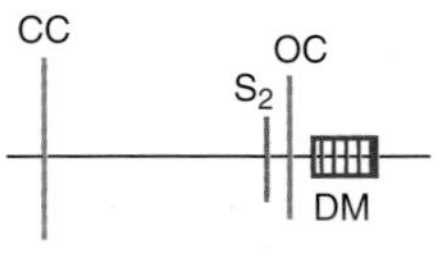 CC, OC, S₂, DM	High-frequency holosystolic murmur; Decreased intensity of closing click
Bileaflet-Tilting-Disk (St. Jude Medical)	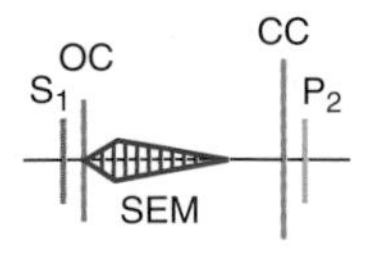 OC, S₁, CC, P₂, SEM	Aortic diastolic murmur; Decreased intensity of closing click	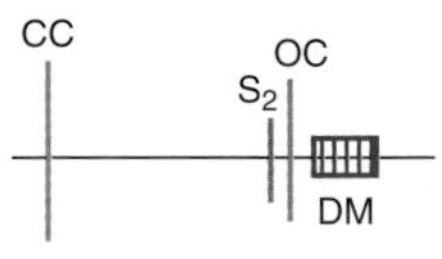 CC, OC, S₂, DM	High-frequency holosystolic murmur; Decreased intensity of closing click
Heterograft Bioprosthesis (Hancock or Carpentier-Edwards)	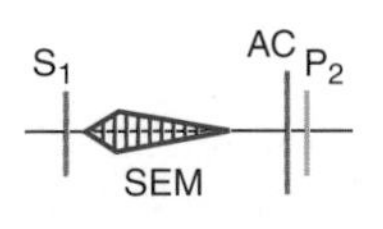 S₁, AC, P₂, SEM	Aortic diastolic murmur	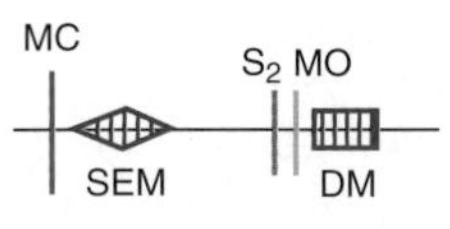 MC, S₂, MO, SEM, DM	High-frequency holosystolic murmur

FIGURE 23–7 Auscultatory characteristics of prosthetic heart valves. Findings are stratified according to valve type and position. AC, aortic closure; CC, closing click; DM, diastolic murmur; MC, mitral valve closure; MO, mitral opening; OC, opening click; SEM, systolic ejection murmur. *(From Vongpatanasin W, Hillis D, Lange RA: Prosthetic heart valves. N Engl J Med 1996;335:407-416.)*

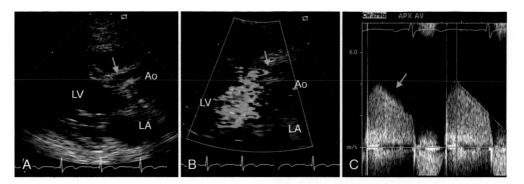

FIGURE 23–8 Transthoracic echocardiograms in a patient with prosthetic valve endocarditis and paravalvular regurgitation. **A,** Parasternal long-axis view shows an echo-free space anterior to a mechanical aortic valve replacement. **B,** Color Doppler imaging shows a diastolic flow disturbance originating in this space with flow into the left ventricular (LV) chamber. **C,** Continuous wave Doppler confirms that this flow is aortic regurgitation, showing the typical timing and velocity curve with a density and slope consistent with severe regurgitation. Ao, aorta; LA, left atrium. *(From Otto CM: Textbook of Echocardiography, 4th Ed, 2009, Philadelphia: Elsevier Saunders.)*

standard TTE examination includes imaging of the valve, measurement of the transvalvular velocity, calculation of instantaneous and mean pressure gradients and valve orifice area, qualitative assessment of the degree of regurgitation, evaluation of LV size and systolic function, and estimation of pulmonary artery systolic pressure. Mean pressure gradients are more useful clinically than instantaneous or maximum pressure gradients because prosthetic valves have very high velocities at the time of valve opening with rapid equilibration thereafter. The baseline expected degree of regurgitation through a mechanical bileaflet or tilting disk valve should be noted. When clinically indicated in patients with suspected valve dysfunction, thrombosis, or infection, transesophageal echocardiography (TEE) can be performed to obtain higher quality images with improved spatial resolution (Figure 23-8 and 23-9). The frequency with which routine, surveillance TTE should be performed in the longitudinal follow-up of patients after prosthetic heart valve replacement has not been established. Small changes in prosthetic valve function are not likely to alter clinical management and may only heighten patient anxiety. Most authorities agree that yearly evaluations are not appropriate in the absence of any clinical change. A repeat TTE can be considered at 5 years for a tissue prosthesis (class IIb), with more frequent evaluations over the next 5 to 10 years, given the expected rate of structural deterioration (20% to 30% failure rates at 10 years and 50% by 15 years).[92-94] It is not clear that repeat, routine TTE is predictably necessary at any future time point after the baseline evaluation for a normally functioning mechanical prosthesis (class III).[80]

The leaflets of a bioprosthesis should appear thin and mobile. The struts of a stented valve are easily identified. The sewing ring/annular interface is thickened and echogenic. Stentless bioprosthetic valves, homografts, and autografts appear very similar to normal, native aortic valves, except for the expected degree of postoperative annular thickening. With time, the homograft root will calcify; the pulmonary autograft may dilate, especially in older patients. The appearance and movement of mechanical bileaflet and tilting-disk valves are very difficult to assess with TTE imaging because of the acoustical shadowing and reverberations inherent to these valves. These limitations can be overcome with multiplane TEE imaging when indicated (Figure 23-10). The pattern and degree of valvular regurgitation can be assessed with color Doppler flow imaging. Because of left atrial shadowing from the prosthesis on TTE imaging, evaluation with TEE is essential in patients with suspected mitral prosthetic valve regurgitation, particularly when it is paravalvular in location. Indirect TTE signs of mitral prosthetic valve

regurgitation include an increased early diastolic transmitral flow velocity, elevated pulmonary artery pressures, and hyperdynamic LV systolic function. TEE is less useful for the assessment of suspected aortic prosthetic valve regurgitation.

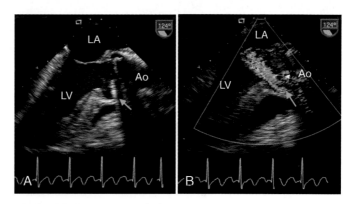

FIGURE 23–9 Transesophageal echocardiography (TEE) in the same patient as Figure 23-8. **A,** TEE provides better definition of the area of valve dehiscence adjacent to the septum (*arrow*). The TEE probe has been positioned so the shadows from the valve prosthesis do not obscure the area of interest. **B,** Color Doppler image shows aortic regurgitation originating from this site. Ao, aorta; LA, left atrium; LV, left ventricle. *(From Otto CM: Textbook of Echocardiography, 4th Ed, 2009, Philadelphia: Elsevier Saunders.)*

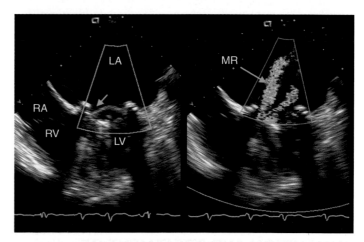

FIGURE 23–10 Prosthetic mitral regurgitation (MR) due to inadequate leaflet closure evaluated by transesophageal echocardiography. The two-dimensional images (*left*) show incomplete closure of the medial valve disk (*arrow*) and color flow imaging (*right*) demonstrates severe prosthetic mitral regurgitation with a wide vena contracta. LA, left atrium; LV, left ventricle; RA, right atrium; RV, right ventricle. *(From Otto CM: Textbook of Echocardiography, 4th Ed, 2009, Philadelphia: Elsevier Saunders.)*

TABLE 24–1 | **Criteria for Sports Participation**

Mitral Stenosis	Sports Participation
Mild (pulmonary systolic pressure <50 mm Hg during exercise, sinus rhythm)	All competitive sports
Moderate (sinus rhythm or atrial fibrillation, pulmonary systolic pressure ≤50 mm Hg)	Low and moderate static and low and moderate dynamic competitive sports
Severe (sinus rhythm or atrial fibrillation, pulmonary artery pressure >50 mm Hg)	Should not participate in any competitive sports
Any severity in atrial fibrillation or with a history of atrial fibrillation or with a mechanical prosthetic valve and must receive long-standing anticoagulation	Should not participate in sports with a risk of bodily contact
After valve repair or transcatheter balloon valvotomy	Based on the residual severity of the mitral stenosis or mitral regurgitation and left ventricular dysfunction as recommended in patients without the procedure

Mitral regurgitation	
Mild to moderate (with sinus rhythm, normal heart size and function, normal pulmonary artery pressures)	All competitive sports
Mild to moderate (sinus rhythm, mild left ventricular enlargement, normal left ventricular systolic function at rest)	Low and moderate static and low, moderate, and high dynamic competitive sports
Severe (left ventricular enlargement, pulmonary hypertension, and any degree of left ventricular dysfunction at rest)	Should not participate in any competitive sports
Any severity and in atrial fibrillation or a history of atrial fibrillation or a mechanical prosthetic valve who must receive long-standing anticoagulation	Should not participate in sports with a risk of bodily contact
After valve repair or transcatheter balloon valvotomy	Low intensity
	Should not participate in sports with a risk of bodily contact or possible trauma
	Selected athletes can participate in low and moderate static and low and moderate dynamic competitive sports

Valvular, subvalvular, and supravalvular aortic stenosis	
Mild (mean gradient <25 mm Hg, normal electrocardiogram, asymptomatic, no aortic dilatation)	All competitive sports with at least annual evaluation of severity
Moderate (mean gradient 25–40 mmHg)	Low-intensity competitive sports
	Selected athletes whose exercise tolerance testing at least to the level of the competition activity demonstrates adequate exercise capacity without symptoms, ST segment changes, or supraventricular or ventricular tachyarrhythmias and with a normal blood pressure response can participate in low and moderate static and low and moderate dynamic competitive sports
	Should not participate in any competitive sports
Severe (mean gradient >40 mmHg) or symptomatic patients with moderate aortic stenosis	

Aortic regurgitation	
Mild or moderate (normal or only mildly increased left ventricular size, asymptomatic, no arrhythmias)	All competitive sports
Moderate (left ventricular enlargement but no aortic root dilatation and asymptomatic and no ventricular arrhythmias on exercise testing)	Low and moderate static and low, moderate, and high dynamic competitive sports
Severe (left ventricular enlargement, marked aortic root dilation, symptoms)	Should not participate in any competitive sports

Tricuspid stenosis	
Combined with mitral stenosis, follow recommendations for mitral stenosis	Isolated—exercise testing to the level of the intensity of the sport

Tricuspid regurgitation	
Mild, moderate, severe (right atrial pressure <20 mmHg, normal right ventricular function, and systolic pressure)	All competitive sports

Pulmonic stenosis	
Mild (peak systolic gradient <40 mmHg, asymptomatic, normal right ventricular function)	All competitive sports
Moderate to severe (peak systolic gradient >40 mm Hg, asymptomatic, normal right ventricular function)	Low-intensity competitive sports

Pulmonic regurgitation	
Severe with marked right ventricular enlargement	Low-intensity competitive sports

Marfan syndrome	
No aortic dilatation, moderate/severe mitral regurgitation, family history of dissection or sudden death in a Marfan relative	Low and moderate static/low dynamic competitive sports
Aortic root dilatation, postoperative aortic root reconstruction, chronic dissection of any artery, moderate/severe mitral regurgitation, or family history of dissection or sudden death in a relative with Marfan syndrome, bicuspid aortic valve	Low-intensity competitive sports only
	Should not participate in sports that have the potential for bodily contact

TABLE 24–2	Etiologies of Mitral Valve Lesions in Children

Congenital

Leaflet hypoplasia
Parachute mitral valve
Isolated cleft mitral valve
Annular hypoplasia
Mitral arcade
Double orifice mitral valve
Mitral valve prolapse
Supravalvular mitral ring
Hammock mitral valve
Chordal elongation or rupture
Papillary muscle hypoplasia
Papillary muscle fusion

Acquired

Anomalous left coronary artery
Myocarditis
Cardiomyopathies
Connective tissue disorders
Endocarditis
Rheumatic fever
Kawasaki disease
Collagen vascular disease
Glycogen storage disease

TABLE 24–3	Defects Associated with Mitral Stenosis

Coarctation of the aorta
Hypoplastic left heart syndrome
Atrioventricular septal defect
Ventricular septal defect
Atrial septal defect
Aortic stenosis
  Valvular
  Subvalvular
Double outlet right ventricle
Single ventricle
Transposition of the great vessels
Tetralogy of Fallot

commissures, chordae, papillary muscles, annular ring, and supramitral area (Figure 24-1).[6] Although mitral stenosis may be acquired from rheumatic fever or after cardiac surgery, the pediatric patient is more likely to have regurgitation. Therefore, rheumatic lesions will be discussed in the regurgitation section and only congenital mitral stenosis will be considered here.

Clinical Presentation

The clinical presentation of mitral stenosis depends on several factors: 1) severity of the obstruction, 2) size of the left ventricle, and 3) presence and severity of associated defects. Left heart size varies, ranging from normal to severely hypoplastic with atresia of the left heart valves. Determination of the degree of left heart hypoplasia may be difficult because the dilated, hypertensive right ventricle distorts the shape of the left ventricle and can make it appear small even though it is normal in size. Similarly, when blood flows through an atrial septal defect rather than into the left ventricle, a potentially adequate left ventricle may be underfilled and appear deceptively small. Several investigators have suggested parameters to aid in determining whether a biventricular repair can be attempted or whether single ventricle palliation must be considered,[7,8] but none of their reports deal with isolated mitral stenosis or provide absolute cutoff values. These studies do provide guidelines, however, and stress the importance of making multiple measurements using standard imaging planes and reference sites.

When mitral stenosis is hemodynamically significant, the left ventricle is underfilled with increased volume in the left atrium. As the left atrial volume continues to increase, pressure within this chamber eventually rises, leading to an increase in pulmonary venous pressure, constriction of arterioles, and an increase in pulmonary artery pressure. As a result, pulmonary blood flow is restricted. Initially, these compensatory changes reduce pulmonary capillary pressure and protect the lungs from pulmonary edema. With time, however, unless there is a shunt lesion, cardiac output drops, and the compensatory mechanisms fail. Symptoms of dyspnea and fatigue develop in older children and tachypnea and poor growth are seen in infants.[4]

The clinical findings of the associated defects are often prominent and may actually obscure the findings of mitral stenosis. Regardless, the child with hemodynamically significant stenosis usually has a diastolic murmur and loud first heart sound. If pulmonary hypertension is present, the second heart sound is narrowly split, and the second component is loud. An opening snap is unusual in congenital mitral stenosis.[5] When the stenosis is severe, infants and younger children will have the classic findings of congestive heart failure—tachypnea, tachycardia, hepatomegaly, and cardiomegaly.

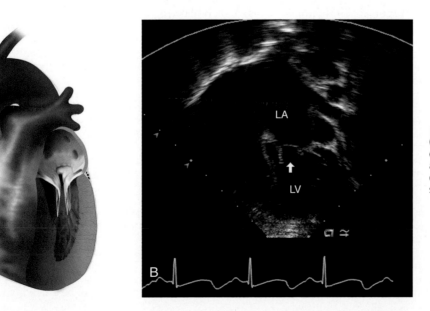

FIGURE 24–1 Schematic diagram (**A**) and comparable apical four-chamber echocardiographic view (**B**) of a fibrous ring above the mitral valve (*arrow* between the opening leaflets) causing congenital mitral stenosis. LA, left atrium; LV, left ventricle.

Electrocardiograms usually reflect the degree of stenosis, and tracings may be normal or show biatrial enlargement. Similarly, depending on the severity of the stenosis, the cardiac silhouette on a chest radiograph ranges from normal to markedly enlarged. If the obstruction is long-standing or severe, left atrial enlargement and the characteristic flow redistribution of pulmonary edema may be seen.[4]

Echocardiography allows detailed imaging of mitral valve anatomy and associated defects as well as assessment of the secondary changes related to hemodynamic alterations.[9] A complete two-dimensional and Doppler examination using standard planes and all imaging windows is needed to adequately evaluate the mitral apparatus, the presence and severity of any associated defects, and the absolute and relative sizes of the cardiac valves and ventricles. Doppler measurements should include mitral peak and mean inflow gradients and assessments of mitral valve area as described in previous chapters. It is important to note, however, that in the presence of a large atrial septal defect or low cardiac output, flow across the valve decreases, and Doppler estimates of valve stenosis are unreliable. When flow decreases, two-dimensional planimetry may be a better indicator of mitral valve area because it is independent of transvalvular flow, especially in older children.[9]

The techniques for obtaining the measurements needed to calculate valve area have been discussed, but their application to younger children and infants has been less reliable for several reasons. First, the value of 220 msec used as a constant in the equation for the pressure half-time was selected because it correlated with a critical mitral valve area of $1.0\,cm^2$ in adults and, thus, is not applicable in small children who normally have very small mitral valve areas. Second, the mitral E and A ratios are age-dependent and may be influenced by changes in atrial or ventricular compliance that occur with growth and maturity. Because pressure half-time depends on left atrial compliance, left ventricular compliance, and peak transmitral pressure gradient as well as mitral valve area, changes in compliance may affect the accuracy of this technique. Third, the Gorlin formula used to calculate mitral valve area is unreliable at rapid heart rates such as those seen in children.[9,10] Mitral annular diameters should routinely be measured and z-scores should be calculated. It should be emphasized that care must be taken to obtain the true annular dimension, rather than the dimension of the stenotic orifice, to avoid underestimating valve size. Finally, estimation of the pulmonary artery pressure obtained from the tricuspid and/or pulmonary regurgitant jets is also an important indicator of stenosis severity.

Cardiac catheterization in younger children and infants with mitral stenosis is deferred until intervention is being considered. In older children, hemodynamic data including left atrial pressure (via a transseptal approach, if needed) and left ventricular end-diastolic pressure are routinely obtained. The severity of the stenosis is estimated by calculating the difference between these two measurements. If the left atrium cannot be entered, the difference between the pulmonary capillary wedge pressure and left ventricular end-diastolic pressure may be used. Because they herald the onset of pulmonary edema or low cardiac output, mean gradients of 12 to 15 mmHg[11] with the typical secondary changes warrant intervention. Pulmonary artery pressures and cardiac outputs are useful for evaluating the overall hemodynamic effects of the stenosis. If an atrial septal defect is present, it may need to be transiently occluded to obtain meaningful measurements.

Mitral stenosis presenting in infancy is uniquely challenging. Because of the wide spectrum of mitral valve malformations, high prevalence of associated defects, and limited experience at any one institution, the optimal management remains controversial.[12]

Treatment

Medical management includes digoxin to slow the heart rate and allow increased filling time, diuretics to reduce pulmonary edema, and enteric feeding with a high caloric formula. Because medical therapy seldom results in a sustained benefit, however, most infants ultimately develop intractable pulmonary edema or low cardiac output. If congenital mitral stenosis is left untreated, the mean survival is 3 years.[5]

A transcatheter mitral valvuloplasty is usually attempted before surgery because of the difficulties in selecting a suitable mechanical prosthesis for an infant. The results from balloon dilation for congenital mitral stenosis appear to be improving with an adequate reduction in the pressure gradient maintained in as many as 62% of patients. Technical adjustments of dilating the valve with gradually increasing balloon sizes and pressures may contribute to the improved short-term outcomes. Younger age and higher predilation left atrial pressure predict a worse survival. In some infants an acceptable gradient reduction is not sustained because of stretching rather than tearing of the valve with a gradual reconfiguration of the apparatus to the original shape or from scarring of a torn valve leaflet, leading to restenosis. Mitral regurgitation from a tear in the valve, disruption of the chordal structures, and/or a partially flail leaflet is the most frequent complication of balloon valvuloplasty. Moderate to severe mitral regurgitation develops in about 28% of patients, and nearly all require valve replacement.[13] It is interesting to note that balloon angioplasty in older children and adolescents for rheumatic mitral stenosis has a safety record and restenosis rate that is comparable to that in adults, suggesting that valve morphology may also play a role in determining success.[14]

Surgical valvuloplasty may be a better solution in some infants, but (with the exception of surgical resection of a supravalvular fibrous ring, with which successful long-term relief is expected),[13,15] acceptable results are far more difficult to achieve for mitral stenosis than for mitral regurgitation. Outcomes are poorer in those with complex associated defects,[16] in those younger than 2 years, and when replacement is required at the initial operation.[13] The repair should only be attempted after an exhaustive preoperative echocardiographic investigation of the mitral valve apparatus. Even then, modifications may be needed as more information is obtained using intraoperative transesophageal echocardiography.[17] Some centers use three-dimensional intraoperative echocardiography to aid the surgeon in tailoring the repair, but there are few data regarding use of this procedure to date. Despite even the most meticulous preparation, the surgical mortality for young children is relatively high at 15% to 26%, and 14% to 34% of the survivors require reoperation within 1 year.[18] Independent risk factors for poor overall freedom from reoperation and midterm survival include age younger than 12 months, cardiothoracic ratio greater than 0.6, and associated cardiac anomalies.[19] When the mitral valve cannot be repaired, a prosthesis must be used. Because bioprosthetic valves thicken, shrink, and calcify early in children, mechanical valves are usually implanted.[20] Management of mechanical valves in growing children differs from that for adults. First, mitral valve replacement may be associated with high early mortality: 21% for children younger than 5 years[21] and 42% for those younger than 2 years.[22] Second, mechanical valves in this setting are palliative at best and will ultimately need replacement with a larger valve, usually within 10 years of the first operation.[23] Third, even the smallest mechanical valve may be difficult to insert in an infant without causing left ventricular outflow obstruction or cardiac distortion. Resection of the subvalvular apparatus or implantation of the valve entirely within the left atrium has been advocated in this group.[24] Fourth, despite apparently successful relief of the stenosis, pulmonary artery hypertension does not always resolve.[24] Last, the logistics of providing anticoagulation for a mechanical valve placed in the mitral position can be challenging in children. Although various treatment regimens have been evaluated, our practice is to anticoagulate with warfarin, maintaining the international normalized ratio at 3 to 4. Maintenance of anticoagulation is often difficult in infants and children and requires careful attention to diet, concurrent medications, growth, and other factors. Thrombus formation has been successfully treated with thrombolytic agents even in young infants.[25]

Mitral Regurgitation

Mitral regurgitation may occur in combination with mitral stenosis but will be discussed here as an isolated lesion. Congenital mitral regurgitation occurs even less often than congenital mitral stenosis.[5] Congenital lesions that result in poor left ventricular function leading to mitral regurgitation despite a normal mitral valve apparatus include cardiomyopathies, myocarditis, or anomalous left coronary artery. Primary treatment is focused on the underlying cause rather than on the regurgitation itself. Therefore, only the common pediatric causes of regurgitation from an abnormal mitral valve will be considered here.

Clinical Presentation

Atrioventricular septal defects are a widely diverse group of anomalies characterized by a unique five-leaflet atrioventricular valve. The valve can have one or two orifices, depending on the presence or absence of a bridging tongue of tissue connecting the anterior and posterior leaflets. A modified subcostal view to visualize the valve en face (Figure 24-2) allows determination of the number of orifices, site of regurgitation, and degree of commitment of the valve to each ventricle.[26-28] Although the most common site of regurgitation is between the left halves of the anterior and posterior bridging leaflets or so-called "cleft," regurgitation may also result from deficient leaflet tissue, poorly coapted commissures involving the left lateral leaflet, abnormal papillary muscles, and chordal anomalies.[29]

Mitral regurgitation may be associated with Marfan syndrome, an inheritable connective tissue disorder caused by defects in fibrillin 1 and affecting the cardiovascular, skeletal, and ocular systems. Fibromyxomatous changes occur in the mitral valve, resulting in leaflet prolapse, chordal elongation, annular dilatation, and ultimately regurgitation.[30] Mitral valve prolapse is the most frequent abnormality seen at the time of presentation (80% to 100%) and mitral regurgitation occurs in 48% to 64% of children with Marfan syndrome. Morbidity and mortality associated with Marfan syndrome presenting in the first year of life are attributed predominantly to mitral valve dysfunction and regurgitation. Otherwise, the mitral valve is usually involved by a mean age of 9.7 years with more than 80% of cases presenting as "silent mitral valve prolapse." The disease is degenerative, and 54% of patients develop regurgitation that subsequently progresses in 84% within 8 years of follow-up.[30,31]

Rheumatic valve disease is discussed in Chapter 14. The mitral valve is involved in 95% of children with rheumatic carditis. Mitral regurgitation results from annular dilatation, chordal elongation, and leaflet prolapse. Typically, mitral regurgitation is seen acutely and may subsequently improve or even resolve, and then, for some, stenosis develops over time.[32] The progression of rheumatic mitral disease from regurgitation to stenosis occurs more rapidly in developing countries where treatment for severe stenosis is routinely needed during childhood. In contrast, surgical or catheter treatment for mitral valve disease can usually be delayed until adulthood in patients in the United States.

Diagnostic Tests

Regardless of etiology, mitral regurgitation can be diagnosed on the basis of the patient's history combined with the presence of a high-frequency, holosystolic murmur located at the apex and radiating to the axilla. If mitral valve prolapse is present, there is a midsystolic click and late systolic murmur that is accentuated with Valsalva maneuvers. Although the chest radiograph and electrocardiogram may show evidence of left atrial and left ventricular enlargement, echocardiography is the mainstay of diagnosis. All available windows must be used to evaluate the entire mitral valve apparatus. Even the complex anatomy of the left atrioventricular valve of an atrioventricular septal defect can be extensively characterized if unique imaging planes are used.[28] The commissure between the anterior and posterior bridging leaflet or

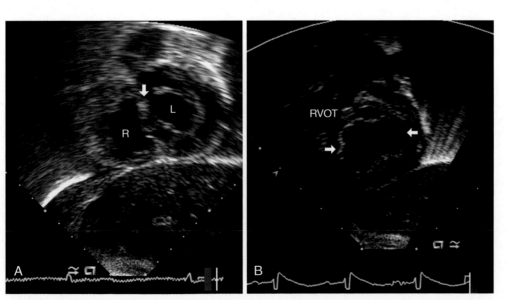

FIGURE 24–2 By rotating the transducer 45° clockwise from the standard subcostal coronal view, the right and left sides of the common atrioventricular valve of an atrioventricular septal defect are seen. **A,** bridging tongue of tissue (*arrow*) dividing the valve into two orifices. **B,** shows a single orifice valve between the arrows. L, left; R, right; RVOT, right ventricular outflow tract.

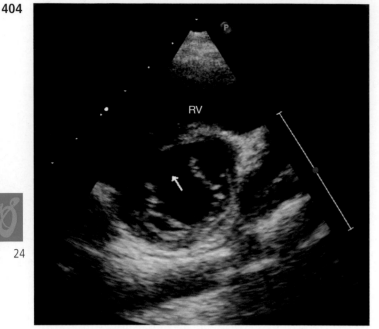

FIGURE 24–3 Two-dimensional parasternal short-axis view demonstrating the commissure between the anterior and posterior bridging (cleft shown by the *arrow*) of a patient with an atrioventricular septal defect. RV, right ventricle.

left atrial area with color Doppler imaging is also used to distinguish mild (<30%), moderate (30%-50%), and severe (>50%) mitral regurgitation.[36]

Although echocardiographic parameters have been identified to predict the need for valve repair in adults, there are few comparable studies focused on outcome data in children. Retrospective studies of children undergoing surgery for mitral regurgitation from a variety of causes have conflicting results regarding the recovery of ventricular function. Whereas early investigators suggested that even with preoperative symptoms, there was recovery of function,[37] more recent studies suggest that late postoperative dysfunction persists if the preoperative left ventricular end-systolic dimension z-score is 6 or greater.[38] Thus, despite concerns of ventricular dilation and impaired function, surgery often is delayed as long as possible due to considerations of patient size, continued growth, and the need for anticoagulation after valve replacement. To date, symptoms remain the most common indication for intervention in the pediatric age group.

Disease Progression

Similar to mitral regurgitation in adult patients, chronic left ventricular volume overload results in compensatory dilation of the left ventricle.[39] Likewise, regurgitation into the left atrium may result in increased left atrial and pulmonary pressures and an increased risk of atrial fibrillation. Patients may be medically managed for a time with digoxin and diuretics. The role of angiotensin-converting enzyme inhibitors remains unclear because there are no large, randomized trials in children.[40] Delaying intervention in children may have some advantages. The likelihood of valvuloplasty success may be greater in the larger child and, if repair fails, a larger prosthesis can be placed. Unfortunately, children with significant regurgitation seem to develop symptoms faster than adults. With severe mitral regurgitation, some investigators report about 16 years from diagnosis to symptoms in the adult,[39] whereas the time span in children has been reported to be less than 3 years.[41] The advantages of delaying surgery in the presence of symptoms must be weighed against the risks of developing arrhythmias, however. Children with long-standing mitral regurgitation develop progressive left atrial enlargement and an increased risk for late atrial arrhythmias that are associated with a poor outcome.[37]

Treatment

The wide spectrum of anatomic abnormalities that lead to mitral regurgitation demands the use of a variety of surgical techniques for repair. The suitability of certain techniques may depend on the etiology of the mitral regurgitation, associated

cleft can be seen from the parasternal short-axis view as it opens toward the interventricular septum (Figure 24-3). Real-time three-dimensional echocardiography (Figure 24-4) has proven to be valuable to characterize the valve leaflets, localize the sites of regurgitation and define the valve anatomy, especially in repaired atrioventricular septal defects with residual lesions or in the unbalanced forms.[33]

Quantification of mitral regurgitation in the adult patient has been well described. These methods have been validated in only a small number of pediatric studies, however, and modifications are recommended. For example, the proximal isovelocity surface area method in children requires color M-mode echocardiography to obtain accurate measurements of the very small radii of the flow convergence zones when heart rates are rapid.[34,35] In addition, the Nyquist limit should be adjusted to about 24 to 31 cm/sec when the proximal isovelocity surface area technique is used in children.[34] Calculation of the ratio of the regurgitant jet area to

FIGURE 24–4 Three-dimensional views of the cleft from a patient with an atrioventricular septal defect from the typical parasternal short-axis (**A**) and then rotated into the "surgeon's" view (**B**). RV, right ventricle. *(Courtesy of Girish Shirali, MD, Medical College of South Carolina, Charleston, SC.)*

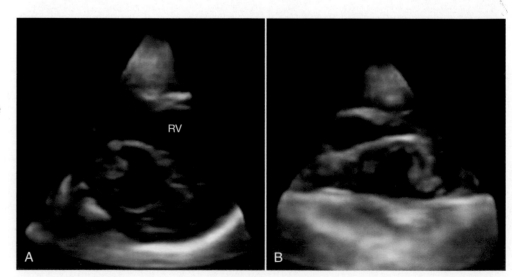

defects, and the surgeon's skill and preference. For example, repair of atrioventricular septal defects can be accomplished with a one- or two-patch technique with a similar incidence of residual regurgitation.[42] In addition, although much is made of making the left atrioventricular valve bileaflet versus trileaflet, successful repairs have been performed with both techniques.[43,44] Success of the repair is strongly dependent on the adequacy of the preoperative evaluation of the entire heart with special attention to the valve and all of its components. After atrioventricular septal defect repair in particular, mild regurgitation is common, moderate regurgitation occurs in about 15% to 30%, and severe regurgitation requiring reoperation occurs in 5% to 19% of patients.[45,46] Although controversial, reported risk factors for postoperative left atrioventricular valve regurgitation include low body weight, relatively small size of the left atrioventricular valve, transitional type of atrioventricular septal defect,[47] severe preoperative atrioventricular valve regurgitation,[46] severe immediate postoperative regurgitation, severe congestive heart failure with progressive annular dilation, and the presence of accessory atrioventricular valve orifices (Figure 24-5).[48] When surgical valvuloplasty is successful, the freedom from reoperation is 97% at 1 year, 93% at 5 years, and 93% at 10 years.[49] Failure to achieve a competent left atrioventricular valve remains the most frequent cause of reoperation and both early and late deaths.[45,48] Despite surgical skill and use of all known operative techniques, about 2% to 5% of valves in this lesion cannot be repaired.[44]

Valve repair techniques must be adapted to the individual child regardless of the etiology of mitral regurgitation.[23] When atrioventricular septal defects and l-transposition are removed from the indications for surgery, the causes of congenital mitral regurgitation include chordal anomalies, annular dilatation, papillary muscle anomalies, leaflet prolapse, posterior leaflet hypoplasia, and a true cleft in the anterior leaflet.[50,51] Because of this diversity, one approach cannot be generalized to all children, and multiple techniques must be individualized for the best results. Intraoperative two-dimensional transesophageal echocardiography is routinely used to provide additional information regarding the valve

architecture, direct the specific details of repair, assess ventricular function, determine whether the valve area is adequate, and assess the technical adequacy of repair. Although it is not yet widely used, three-dimensional transesophageal echocardiography may become routine to determine the degree, mechanisms, and sites of regurgitation including coaptation failure, clefts, and commissural abnormalities.[52] It is important to note, however, that some investigators have reported that the intraoperative transesophageal assessment of the grade of regurgitation does not predict the grade of regurgitation at follow-up.[53] The overall mortality rates for mitral valvuloplasty regardless of etiology range from 0% to 22%.[54] Freedom from reoperation for mitral valvuloplasty in childhood is 83% at 8 years, 68% at 15 years, and 86% at 17 years.[55]

Mitral regurgitation leads to surgical intervention in 24% to 38% of children with Marfan syndrome. It may be the sole indication for repair or may be combined with aortic root dilation requiring concomitant procedures and increasing surgical risk. Nearly all valves (97%) can be repaired in the child who requires surgical intervention; however, because the disease is degenerative, the freedom from reoperation is lower in children than in adults at a 10-year follow-up (41% versus 87%).[56]

Mitral valve repair is also the procedure of choice in children with rheumatic heart disease. In cases of acute rheumatic fever, the disease is characterized by regurgitation that may improve with time, and surgery is rarely needed during this phase. In India, 27% of reconstructions of stenotic and/or regurgitant rheumatic mitral valves were performed in children younger than 15 years. The repair was more difficult, and 5-year reoperation rates were higher at 5% to 27% for children compared with 8% to 10% for adults.[57] Of the 366 children with rheumatic carditis seen at our institution between 1985 and 2003, only 22 (6%) required mitral valve surgery at younger than 21 years of age. Repair was successful in 19 patients, but 3 required valve replacement. Actuarial freedom from reoperation was 78% at 5 years, 65% at 10 years, and 49% at 15 years, indicating the need for long-term surveillance for the possible need for late valve reoperation.[58]

If mitral valve repair fails or when the leaflets are so dysplastic as to preclude repair, mechanical valves are still the best alternative in children.[59] Most investigators report a higher mortality rate for children undergoing mitral valve replacement (30%) compared with those undergoing valvuloplasty.[19] Complete heart block has been reported in as many as 38% of survivors.[49] When the child outgrows the prosthesis, a larger valve can be placed as the mitral annulus will grow even when sewn to a prosthetic valve.[60] Fibrous tissue resection at the atrioventricular junction and translocation maneuvers may facilitate up-sizing of the valve without impairing ventricular function.[25]

AORTIC VALVE

Aortic Valvular Stenosis

The most common form of left ventricular outflow tract obstruction in children,[61] valvular aortic stenosis, occurs in 2% to 8% of infants with congenital heart disease.[62-64] Male infants are three to four times more frequently affected than female infants.[65-67] In children, the stenotic aortic valve is usually bicuspid with commissural fusion (most often adjacent to the right coronary cusp) and thickened valve leaflets that may be of unequal size. A bicuspid aortic valve occurs in as many as 1% to 2% of all individuals, making it the most common form of congenital heart disease.[68,69] Only approximately 2% of children born with an abnormal aortic valve will have significant obstruction or regurgitation by adolescence.[70]

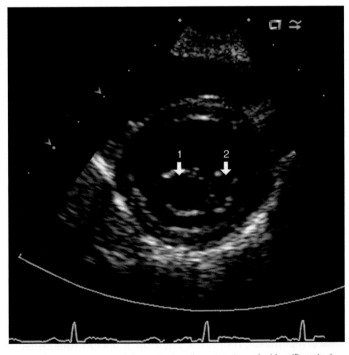

FIGURE 24–5 Parasternal short-axis view demonstrating a double orifice mitral valve (arrows).

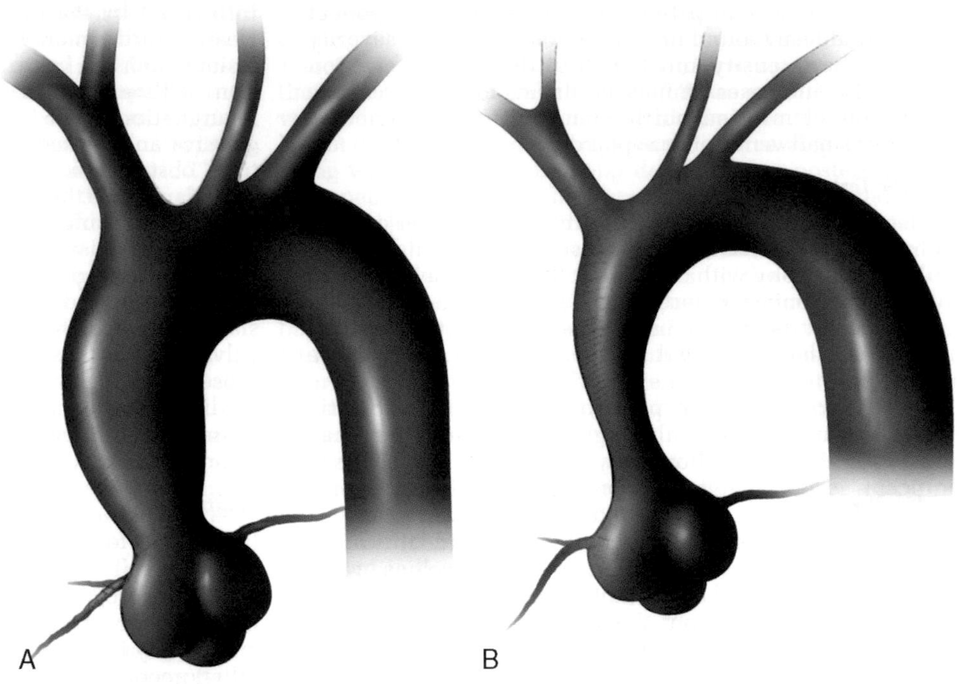

FIGURE 24–9 Drawings illustrating the two main types of supravalvular aortic stenosis: localized, hourglass narrowing (**A**) and diffuse narrowing of the ascending aorta (**B**).

TABLE 24–5	Cardiovascular Anomalies Associated with Supravalvular Aortic Stenosis

Branch and peripheral pulmonary artery stenosis
Aortic valve abnormalities (including bicuspid valve)
Coarctation of the aorta
Stenoses of head and neck vessels
Renal artery stenosis
Abdominal coarctation
Mitral valve abnormalities

reported in up to two thirds of patients (Table 24-5).[142,144,149,150] The free edges of the aortic valve leaflets may be adherent to the supravalvar aortic ridge, sometimes obstructing coronary orifices. Additional narrowing at the origins of the coronary arteries may occur due to intimal hyperplasia, medial hypertrophy, and fibrosis.[142] In the absence of coronary flow obstruction, the coronary arteries are exposed to high pressure and may be dilated or tortuous.[142] Associated stenoses of the branch and peripheral pulmonary arteries are common[148] and may be severe enough to result in right ventricular hypertension. When affected, the pulmonary arteries are usually diffusely hypoplastic, but discrete narrowing may occur.[142] Other associated cardiac anomalies include stenoses of head and neck vessels and/or stenosis of the renal and mesenteric arteries, coarctation of the aorta, and mitral valve abnormalities.[151,152]

Excluding coronary artery changes (and higher pressure to which the coronary arteries are often exposed), the physiology of supravalvular aortic stenosis is similar to that of valvular aortic stenosis. A unique feature of the jet resulting from the supravalvular aortic narrowing is its tendency to hug the aortic wall, resulting in a transfer of kinetic energy to the innominate artery (Coanda effect) and a right arm pressure higher than the left arm pressure.[153]

Clinical Presentation

Most patients are asymptomatic, but children with severe obstruction may exhibit easy fatigability, dyspnea on exertion, angina, dizziness, or syncope.[149] On physical examination, there is a systolic ejection murmur similar in quality and location to that of aortic valve stenosis, but an associated ejection click is uncommon. The aortic component to the second heart sound may be increased because of the high pressure distal to the aortic valve. The Coanda effect may result in a right arm systolic blood pressure that is 5 to 10 mmHg higher than that in the left arm. Transmission of the murmur to the head and neck vessels may be more prominent than with aortic valve stenosis, especially if there is associated narrowing of the brachiocephalic arteries. Associated branch pulmonary stenosis may result in long systolic murmurs that may extend into diastole heard in both lung fields.

Diagnostic Tests

The electrocardiogram is often normal with mild obstruction. Left ventricular hypertrophy is common with more severe aortic obstruction, whereas right ventricular hypertrophy may be seen if there is significant branch or peripheral pulmonary artery stenosis.[154] Similarly, the chest radiograph is usually normal. In contrast with aortic valve stenosis, the ascending aorta is not dilated.[149]

Echocardiography is the optimal modality to confirm a suspected diagnosis, evaluate the degree of obstruction, and identify associated abnormalities. The narrowing at the sinotubular junction and ascending aorta can be identified by two-dimensional imaging from the parasternal long-axis view. The ratio of the diameter of the aorta at the sinotubular junction to the aortic annulus is less than 1.0 in patients with supravalvar aortic stenosis.[155] Doppler imaging shows increased velocity and turbulence at the site of ascending aortic narrowing. However, because of a variety of factors including pressure recovery and the difference between peak-to-peak and peak instantaneous gradients, the Doppler gradient is usually significantly higher than the peak-to-peak gradient obtained at catheterization. A peak Doppler gradient greater than 85 mmHg has been shown to be predictive of a catheter-measured gradient greater than 50 mmHg, the cutoff value often used as an indication for intervention.[156] Echocardiography also allows assessment of the remainder of the ascending aorta, proximal head and neck vessels, aortic arch, aortic valve, and proximal branch pulmonary arteries.

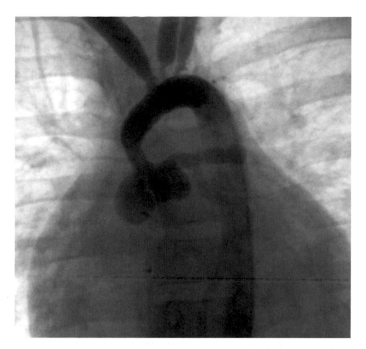

FIGURE 24–10 Aortogram demonstrating diffuse supravalvular narrowing and hypoplasia of the ascending aorta. Note the prominent left coronary artery, minimal filling of the right coronary artery, and narrowing of the origins of head and neck vessels.

Magnetic resonance imaging is used with increasing frequency to evaluate the branch and peripheral pulmonary arteries as well as the supravalvar aortic narrowing.[157]

Cardiac catheterization and angiography are often performed before intervention because of the high incidence of associated abnormalities, including coronary involvement and/or distal pulmonary artery stenoses that may be difficult to assess using echocardiography (Figure 24-10). If the right ventricular pressure is elevated, right ventricular or pulmonary artery angiography should be performed to assess the extent of branch and peripheral pulmonary artery narrowing.

Disease Progression

Supravalvular aortic stenosis tends to be progressive, at least in part due to subnormal growth of the ascending aorta. In contrast, peripheral pulmonary artery stenoses may be stable or actually decrease in severity over time.[158] There is a risk of sudden death, probably related to coronary artery obstruction and the severity of aortic obstruction.[146,158-160] Deaths have also been reported in association with catheterization or surgical procedures.[147,159,161] Long-term survival is influenced by the severity of the obstruction and associated lesions. The overall survival for patients with supravalvular aortic stenosis is reported to be 71% at 17 years after presentation but is influenced by severity. The 30-year survival has been reported to be 95% for those with mild, 73% for those with moderate, and 12% for those with severe stenosis.[145] Approximately 30% of patients with Williams syndrome will eventually require repair of their supravalvular aortic stenosis.[161,162] Systemic hypertension is common and may be related to abnormal vascular compliance, associated coarctation, or renal artery stenosis.[161]

Treatment

Management of supravalvular aortic stenosis depends on severity and symptoms. Patients with mild stenosis may be followed conservatively without intervention. Patients with more severe obstruction and symptoms should be referred for surgical intervention. Some recommend intervention for a left ventricular strain pattern on an electrocardiogram or a catheter-measured peak gradient greater than 50 mmHg in the absence of

symptoms.[147,156] Surgery usually consists of a patch aortoplasty and, if necessary, addressing coronary arteries and any proximal pulmonary artery narrowing. Because the aortic valve is commonly involved, in some patients a concomitant aortic valvotomy or, less commonly, aortic valve replacement, may be necessary.[147,149,163] Small residual gradients are common and may be related to associated valvular abnormalities. Approximately 20% to 25% of patients have aortic regurgitation after surgery.[164] The diffuse type of supravalvular aortic narrowing is more difficult to repair and is associated with a greater likelihood of residual narrowing postoperatively.[164] Preoperative New York Heart Association class 3 to 4 symptoms, the diffuse type of supravalvular aortic stenosis, and the presence and severity of associated lesions influence outcome and the need for reintervention.[149]

Although in general the intervention should be surgical, balloon dilation and/or stenting of supravalvular aortic narrowing have been reported.[165]

Aortic Regurgitation

Aortic regurgitation almost always occurs with associated congenital cardiac abnormalities and is uncommon as a primary lesion. Although most commonly associated with primary abnormalities of the aortic valve, a dilated aortic root and/or annulus, or lesions adjacent to the aortic valve, it may also be acquired from an infectious process such as endocarditis or rheumatic fever or postoperatively when the native pulmonary valve is used as a neo-aortic valve (Table 24-6).[5,166]

The pathophysiology and physical examination of aortic regurgitation are described in Chapter 10.

Clinical Presentation

Most children with mild to moderate aortic regurgitation are asymptomatic. When present, symptoms are more likely to be due to associated abnormalities. With more severe regurgitation, however, symptoms such as dyspnea or chest pain on exertion, palpitations, and even dizziness, syncope, and sudden death may occur.[167]

Diagnostic Tests

The electrocardiogram is often normal in children with mild to moderate aortic regurgitation but may show left ventricular hypertrophy with or without ST and T wave

TABLE 24–6	Cardiovascular Abnormalities Associated with Aortic Regurgitation
Primary abnormality of the aortic valve	
Bicuspid aortic valve	
Stenotic aortic valve before or after intervention	
Dilated aortic root and annulus	
Marfan syndrome	
Tetralogy of Fallot	
Adjacent lesions	
Ventricular septal defect (supracristal or membranous)	
Subaortic stenosis	
Supravalvular aortic stenosis	
Surgical procedures resulting in neo-aortic valve	
Norwood aortic reconstruction procedure	
Arterial switch	
Damus (proximal pulmonary to ascending aorta) anastomosis	
Related to infectious processes	
Endocarditis	
Rheumatic fever (rheumatic heart disease)	
Other congenital abnormalities	
Aortico-left ventricular tunnel	
Ruptured sinus of Valsalva aneurysm	

associated lesions. Adolescents and young adults with rheumatic tricuspid stenosis remain asymptomatic for long periods of time.[220]

Treatment

Medical therapy is generally ineffective in patients with severe tricuspid stenosis and symptoms of congestive heart failure, so these patients should be referred for surgical or catheter-based intervention similar to that used for mitral stenosis.[223]

PULMONARY VALVE

Obstruction of the right ventricular outflow tract can be classified as subvalvular, valvular, or supravalvular and can occur at multiple levels. In this chapter we focus on valvular pulmonary stenosis and pulmonary regurgitation as a result of interventions on the right ventricular outflow tract.

Pulmonary Stenosis

Pulmonary valve stenosis as an isolated lesion accounts for approximately 10% of cardiac malformations.[224] A familial tendency[91] and an association with syndromes, including Noonan syndrome,[225] suggest a genetic cause in some patients. The most common type of pulmonary stenosis involves fusion of the commissures, resulting in doming of the valve into the main pulmonary artery (Figure 24-16).[226] Other forms include dysplastic valves and combined annulus and valvar hypoplasia. Pulmonary stenosis is often associated with other conditions (Table 24-10).

Clinical Presentation

Excluding neonates with critical pulmonary stenosis, the majority of patients are asymptomatic. As the severity of the stenosis increases, right ventricular pressure increases and hypertrophy develops. The increased afterload results in decreased

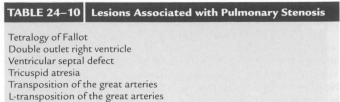

TABLE 24–10	Lesions Associated with Pulmonary Stenosis

Tetralogy of Fallot
Double outlet right ventricle
Ventricular septal defect
Tricuspid atresia
Transposition of the great arteries
L-transposition of the great arteries
Truncus arteriosus

muscle shortening and decreased stroke volume. The volume of blood being ejected decreases and the residual right ventricular volume increases (Frank-Starling relationship). As right ventricular compliance decreases, the increased pressure is transmitted to the right atrium. Cyanosis may occur if an atrial communication is present, allowing right-to-left shunting. If pulmonary stenosis is untreated, the hypertrophied right ventricle will maintain stroke volume for a time, but if long-standing, elevated pressure causes the right heart to dilate and fail.[227] Symptoms of cyanosis, dyspnea, and exertional fatigue develop in patients with severe pulmonary stenosis. Neonates with critical pulmonary stenosis have systemic or suprasystemic right ventricular pressures and will present with severe cyanosis or even die if the ductus arteriosus closes. The right ventricle may have varying degrees of hypoplasia related to the amount of forward flow through the pulmonary valve in early gestation.[228] An in-depth discussion of the physiology in these patients has been provided in the textbook by Rudolph.[229]

Asymptomatic infants and children, who comprise the majority of patients, typically present with a systolic ejection murmur that can radiate throughout the precordium and to the back. The length and frequency of the murmur increase with increasing severity.[230] An ejection click and a thrill in the left second or third intercostal space often accompanies the murmur. The chest radiograph may have a prominent main pulmonary artery segment from poststenotic dilatation. The heart size is normal unless there are associated lesions, heart failure from critical pulmonary stenosis in the newborn, or long-standing, untreated severe disease in the older child. The electrocardiogram reflects the degree of stenosis[231] but is not specific enough to use alone for following progression.[232] In mild pulmonary stenosis, the ECG is often normal but may have mild right axis deviation. In moderate pulmonary stenosis, the ECG is abnormal 90% of the time with an rR or RS complex present in V_1. In severe pulmonary stenosis, the mean frontal axis varies from 100 to 170° and a pure R wave or RS or QR pattern is often present in lead V_1. The T wave in V_1 may be upright in severe stenosis.[224]

Diagnostic Tests

Echocardiography can effectively assess the anatomy and function of the pulmonary valve leaflets by two-dimensional imaging and Doppler interrogation (Figure 24-17). Commissural fusion, dysplastic leaflets, annulus size, associated subvalvular and supravalvular stenoses, and additional anomalies can be identified. Color Doppler imaging shows direction and aliasing of flow through the valve, allowing parallel alignment of the continuous wave Doppler beam for assessment of the stenosis as described in Chapter 21. When serial obstruction occurs at the subvalvular, valvular, and/or supravalvular levels, the simplified Bernoulli equation will be inaccurate as it fails to account for pressure recovery, type, or length of stenoses.[233] Because the Doppler peak instantaneous gradient frequently overestimates the peak-to-peak gradient obtained at cardiac catheterization, many laboratories advocate the use of mean gradients to determine the timing of balloon valvuloplasty.[234] The diameter of the right ventricular anterior wall has been used to assess right ventricular hypertrophy; however, it is not a sensitive indicator of the severity of pulmonary stenosis and must be used in association with other indicators.[235]

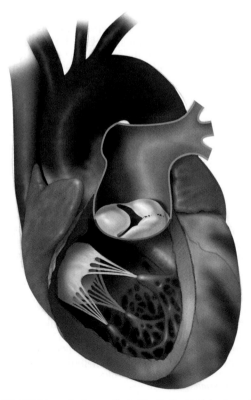

FIGURE 24–16 Schematic diagram illustrating an abnormal doming pulmonary valve and dilated main pulmonary artery.

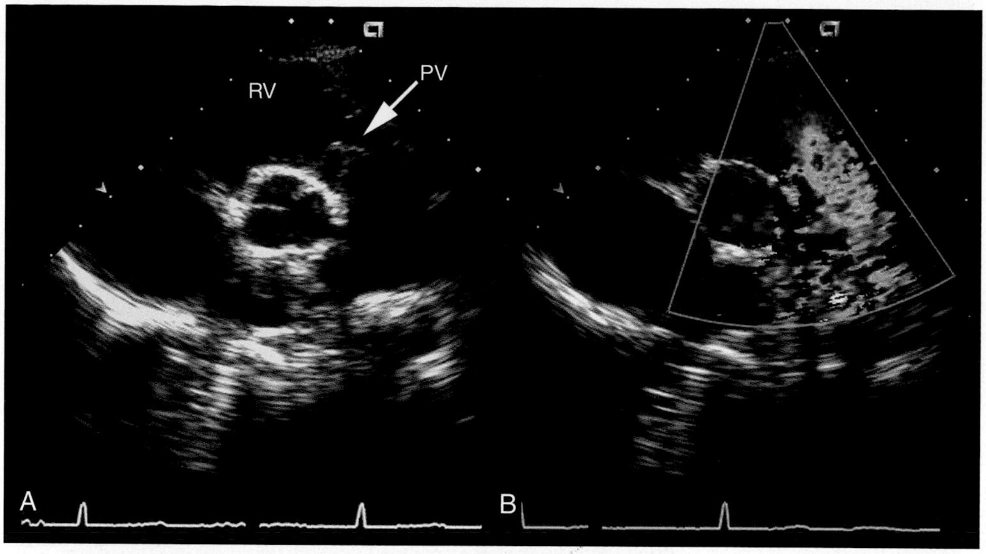

FIGURE 24–17 A, Parasternal short-axis view of a dysplastic and doming pulmonary valve (*arrow*) with poststenotic dilatation of the main pulmonary artery. **B,** Same image with color Doppler added showing flow acceleration at the valve level. PV, pulmonary valve; RV, right ventricle.

Echocardiographic assessment of ventricular size and function is difficult because of the complex shape of the right ventricle and the abnormal motion of the ventricular septum during systole. As a result, there has been a reliance on the "eyeball" method for the right ventricle that has many limitations.[178] Quantification of diastolic function can be derived from Doppler recordings of tricuspid valve inflow as discussed in the adult section. Children with pulmonary stenosis have higher peak A velocities compared with those for normal children, yielding a lower peak E to peak A velocity ratio.[236] This relative shift in right ventricular filling to late diastole is an early finding suggesting diastolic dysfunction. Because old methods for quantification of systolic function were cumbersome and fraught with errors, new techniques independent of ventricular geometry (myocardial performance index, Doppler tissue imaging, and magnetic resonance imaging) have been developed.

Magnetic resonance imaging has emerged as an excellent way to overcome the problem of evaluating the complex-shaped right ventricle. It provides accurate anatomic and functional data. Tracing of the endocardial borders at end-systole and end-diastole allows volumes to be obtained by multiplying the measured areas by the slice thickness and summing the result. Stroke volume and ejection fraction, therefore, can be calculated without any geometric assumption. Magnetic resonance imaging is now considered the standard for RV function assessment.[237]

Cardiac catheterization is restricted to those patients requiring intervention with balloon valvuloplasty. Historically, the gradient used to determine treatment was based on cardiac catheterization. Newer guidelines use a Doppler peak instantaneous gradient for determining mild, moderate, and severe grades. Many children will undergo balloon valvuloplasty for gradients greater than 40 mmHg to avoid being restricted to only low-intensity competitive sports (see Table 24-1).[238] Serial clinical follow-up is recommended for patients with mild valvar pulmonary stenosis as the gradient may gradually change over time (−12 to +3 mmHg/year).[239]

Neonates with severe stenosis that is ductal-dependent require semiemergency treatment to decrease their mortality. Prostaglandin administration is essential before intervention to provide pulmonary blood flow and often remains necessary after intervention until the cyanosis resolves. With right ventricular growth and improved compliance, the cyanosis generally resolves. However, in rare patients, a surgical shunt is required to provide additional pulmonary blood flow and allow discontinuation of the prostaglandins.[240]

Percutaneous balloon valvuloplasty provides immediate relief of the right ventricular outflow obstruction with success rates approaching 95% and mortality rates less than 8%,[241] making it the procedure of choice for the treatment of valvar pulmonic stenosis. The size of the dilation balloon in relation to the valve annulus diameter is the most important technical consideration affecting acute results. Recently, experts have recommended that the balloon/annulus ratio be decreased from a range of 1.2 to 1.4 to a range of 1.2 to 1.25 as this ratio still provides adequate relief of the obstruction and may prevent significant pulmonary regurgitation at late follow-up.[238] Restenosis of the pulmonary valve, defined as a gradient greater than 36 mmHg, continues to be a problem in 8% to 10% of patients.[242] Multiple risk factors for restenosis have been identified: a balloon/pulmonary valve annulus ratio less than 1.2, immediate postvalvuloplasty gradient of 30 mmHg or greater, and smaller pulmonary annulus diameter. Long-term outcome of balloon pulmonary valvuloplasty is excellent with an intervention-free rate of 84% at 10 years and a rate in the high 70% at 15 years.[238] Surgery is currently reserved for patients in whom associated defects require an operative approach or the pulmonary valve annulus is hypoplastic.

Pulmonary Regurgitation

In contrast with pulmonary stenosis, pulmonary regurgitation is more frequently acquired than congenital. A rare exception is absent pulmonary valve (usually associated with tetralogy of Fallot) that presents at birth with a systolic and diastolic (to and fro) murmur from combined stenosis and regurgitation. The branch pulmonary arteries may be massive, compressing airways and resulting in respiratory compromise. The treatment of these infants must be individualized, and details can be obtained from several sources.[243,244] In this section we will focus on pulmonary regurgitation as a result of intervention for right ventricular outflow tract obstruction.

The most frequent cause of pulmonary regurgitation is palliation of right ventricular outflow tract obstruction in patients with tetralogy of Fallot. These patients have anterior deviation of the infundibular septum causing various degrees of right ventricular outflow tract narrowing (Figure 24-18). In addition, the pulmonary valve is often thick and stenotic, and the annulus may be hypoplastic. Repair of this defect in the best-case scenario involves resection of the infundibular muscle and closure of the ventricular septal defect. If the valve annulus is too small, either a patch is placed across the annular ring (transannular patch) or a conduit is placed between the right ventricle and the main pulmonary artery. Although

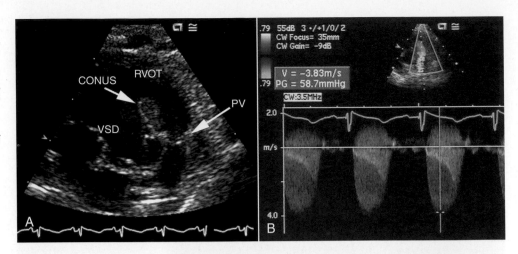

FIGURE 24–18 **A,** Parasternal short-axis view showing a large perimembranous ventricular septal defect with anterior deviation of the conal septum (*arrow*) and a small pulmonary valve annulus (*long arrow*). **B,** Continuous wave Doppler in the same patient showing infundibular and valvar pulmonary stenosis with a peak gradient of 3.8 m/sec. PV, pulmonary valve; RVOT, right ventricular outflow tract; VSD, ventricular septal defect.

TABLE 24–11	Uses for Allograft Material

Tetralogy of Fallot
Pulmonary stenosis
Pulmonary atresia with ventricular septal defect
Double outlet right ventricle with malposed great arteries
Supravalvular pulmonary stenosis
Isolated pulmonary arteries
Supravalvular aortic stenosis
Transposition of the great arteries with ventricular septal defect and
    pulmonary stenosis
Truncus arteriosus
Ross procedure
Aortic root replacement in Marfan syndrome

the mechanisms differ, both may result in hemodynamically significant pulmonary regurgitation. The transannular patch disrupts the integrity of the pulmonary valve and prevents normal coaptation of the leaflets. The cryopreserved human allograft, which is the most commonly used conduit, allows for a competent valve in the outflow but rapidly degenerates in children. This limited durability of the allograft (Table 24-11) has led to a search for alternative valved conduits, including the bovine jugular venous valved conduit, porcine heterograft, or decellularized allograft. Each of these has advantages and disadvantages. The bovine jugular venous valved conduit is easily implantable, comes in a variety of sizes, and has results comparable to those with the allograft but maximal follow-up is 4 years or less.[245,246] Porcine heterografts are more readily available but have lesser long-term durability than cryopreserved allografts.[247] Use of a decellularized allograft minimizes the immune response, but it is unknown whether this will translate into improved long-term durability.[248]

Although previously it was accepted that pulmonary regurgitation might be well tolerated for many years or even a lifetime, this view no longer appears to be true. Recent studies have implicated pulmonary regurgitation in the development of right ventricular dysfunction, impaired exercise performance, and increased incidence of severe arrhythmias and sudden death.[249,250] Thus, careful follow-up is needed and should include a detailed history, physical examination, chest x-ray, electrocardiogram, and echocardiogram. When symptoms are equivocal, an exercise test may be warranted.

In the setting of significant pulmonary regurgitation, the physical examination reveals a long diastolic murmur at the left mid-sternal border and a right ventricular heave if there is significant right ventricular volume overload. Serial chest radiography can often be used to assess progressive cardiomegaly and dilation of the main and branch pulmonary arteries. The electrocardiogram is not useful for assessing right ventricular hypertrophy as nearly all patients with tetralogy of Fallot

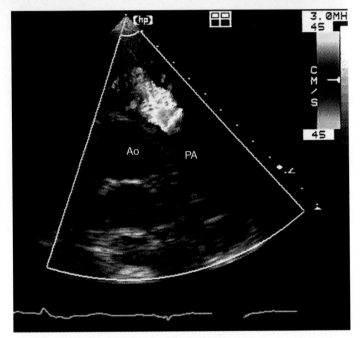

FIGURE 24–19 Color Doppler imaging in the parasternal short-axis view showing severe pulmonary regurgitation with the regurgitant jet encompassing the entire pulmonary annulus. Ao, aorta; PA, pulmonary artery.

have a right bundle branch block postoperatively. Measuring the QRS duration is important, however, because it appears to be a surrogate for right ventricular size. A QRS duration of 180 msec or greater has proven to be sensitive and specific for predicting life-threatening ventricular arrhythmias.[251]

An echocardiogram is useful for estimating right ventricular pressures, pulmonary regurgitation, and right ventricular size and function and for identification of residual lesions. Pulmonary regurgitation may be semiquantitated using color Doppler echocardiography (Figure 24-19). A ratio of the diameter of the regurgitant jet to the diameter of the pulmonary valve annulus of less than 0.4 indicates 1+ pulmonary regurgitation, whereas a ratio greater than 0.7 indicates 3+ regurgitation.[252] Diastolic flow reversal in the branch pulmonary arteries indicates greater than 2+ pulmonary regurgitation. Despite its ready availability and widespread use for serial examinations, echocardiography has limitations in two main areas. First, postoperative scars, chest wall deformities, overlying lung tissue, and occasionally body size impair imaging, especially of the branch pulmonary arteries.[253] Second, the unusual geometry of the right ventricle makes assessment of right ventricular size and function cumbersome.

Because it does not rely on acoustic windows or geometric assumptions, magnetic resonance imaging has emerged as an excellent way to assess the entire right ventricular outflow tract, the main and branch pulmonary arteries and their relationship to the airways, to quantitate the amount of regurgitation, and to evaluate the effect of increased volume on the right ventricle.[254-256] In addition, this technique provides functional data, allowing accurate determination of right ventricular stroke volume and cardiac output.[257] Cine phase-contrast magnetic resonance imaging sequences allow quantification of forward and regurgitant flow in the pulmonary artery to accurately measure regurgitant fraction.[258] Magnetic resonance imaging typically provides sufficient anatomic and functional data so that cardiac catheterization is limited to those requiring an intervention, an electrophysiology study, or evaluation of coronary artery anatomy.

Exercise testing in patients who have undergone surgical repair of tetralogy of Fallot may demonstrate impaired exercise capacity and decreased maximal oxygen consumption that are associated with right ventricular systolic dysfunction.[259]

Medical management in patients with severe pulmonary regurgitation is limited because right ventricular pressures are usually low and the right heart size and function can only be improved by decreasing end-systolic volume. Despite this limitation, the decision to place a new allograft is often delayed as long as possible because of the likelihood of reoperation as the conduit ultimately fails in the growing child. The failure rate is most impressive in children younger than 2 years, with nearly 58% of conduits requiring intervention and 30% being explanted within 3 years.[260] Delays in allograft placement, however, may prove detrimental as evidence suggests that excessive delay is associated with right ventricular dysfunction and exercise intolerance that may persist even after repair in adults. Similar outcome data are not available for children[261] and objective measurements for the correct timing of intervention still need to be defined.

The current guidelines commonly used for pulmonary valve replacement are summarized in Table 24-12.[262] Surgical placement of a cryopreserved human allograft, porcine, or bioprosthetic valve or valved conduit is the standard of care. Conduit sizes are chosen with z-scores of 1 to 3 to maximize both durability and function. Timely placement of an appropriately sized, competent valve that reduces the regurgitant load

on the right ventricle may have several benefits. Typically, right ventricular ejection fraction[263] and exercise performance improve.[264-266] The QRS complex also appears to stabilize, decreasing the risk of atrial and ventricular arrhythmias. Intraoperative cryoablation may further decrease this risk.[261]

The newest field in interventional cardiology is the percutaneous implantation of valves. Percutaneous stent-mounted bovine jugular venous valves have been implanted in the right ventricular outflow tract with good clinical and hemodynamic results. This exciting new technique, although not applicable to patients with severe regurgitation and a dilated right ventricular outflow tract, may provide an earlier alternative to surgery in select patients.[267]

REFERENCES

1. Wilson W, Taubert KA, Gewitz Met al, et al: Prevention of infective endocarditis: guidelines from the American Heart Association: a guideline from the American Heart Association Rheumatic Fever, Endocarditis and Kawasaki Disease Committee, Council on Cardiovascular Disease in the Young, and the Council on Clinical Cardiology, Council on Cardiovascular Surgery and Anesthesia, and the Quality of Care and Outcomes Research Interdisciplinary Working Group. J Am Dent Assoc 2007;138:739-745, 747-760.
2. Maron BJ, Douglas PS, Graham TP, et al: Task Force 1: preparticipation screening and diagnosis of cardiovascular disease in athletes. J Am Coll Cardiol 2005;45:1322-1326.
3. Maron BJ, Ackerman MJ, Nishimura RA, et al: Task Force 4: HCM and other cardiomyopathies, mitral valve prolapse, myocarditis, and Marfan syndrome. J Am Coll Cardiol 2005;45:1340-1345.
4. Baylen BG, Atkinson DE: Mitral inflow obstruction. In Allen HD, Driscoll DJ, Shaddy RE, Feltes TF (eds): Heart Disease in Infants, Children, and Adolescents. Philadelphia, Lippincott Williams & Wilkins, 2008, pp 922-937.
5. Fyler D: Nadas' Pediatric Cardiology. St. Louis, Mosby-Yearbook, 1992.
6. Moore P, Adatia I, Spevak PJ, et al: Severe congenital mitral stenosis in infants. Circulation 1994;89:2099-2106.
7. Colan SD, McElhinney DB, Crawford EC, et al: Validation and re-evaluation of a discriminant model predicting anatomic suitability for biventricular repair in neonates with aortic stenosis. J Am Coll Cardiol 2006;47:1858-1865.
8. Cohen MS, Jacobs ML, Weinberg PM, Rychik J: Morphometric analysis of unbalanced common atrioventricular canal using two-dimensional echocardiography. J Am Coll Cardiol 1996;28:1017-1023.
9. Snider AR: Abnormalities of ventricular inflow. In Snider AR, Serwer GA, Ritter SB (eds): Echocardiography in Pediatric Heart Disease, 2nd ed. St. Louis, Mosby-Year-Book, 1997, pp 385-407.
10. Banerjee A, Kohl T, Silverman NH: Echocardiographic evaluation of congenital mitral valve anomalies in children. Am J Cardiol 1995;76:1284-1291.
11. Lock JE: Hemodynamic evaluation of congenital heart disease. In Lock JE, Fellows KE (eds): Diagnostic and interventional catheterization in congenital heart disease. Boston, Martinus Nijhoff Publishing, 1988, pp 43-44.
12. Serraf A, Zoghbi J, Belli E, et al: Congenital mitral stenosis with or without associated defects: an evolving surgical strategy. Circulation 2000;102(19 Suppl 3):III166-III171.
13. McElhinney DB, Sherwood MC, Keane JF, et al: Current management of severe congenital mitral stenosis: outcomes of transcatheter and surgical therapy in 108 infants and children. Circulation 2005;112:707-714.
14. Fawzy ME, Stefadouros MA, Hegazy H, et al: Long term clinical and echocardiographic results of mitral balloon valvotomy in children and adolescents. Heart 2005;91:743-748.
15. Collison SP, Kaushal SK, Dagar KS, et al: Supramitral ring: good prognosis in a subset of patients with congenital mitral stenosis. Ann Thorac Surg 2006;81:997-1001.
16. Schaverien MV, Freedom RM, McCrindle BW: Independent factors associated with outcomes of parachute mitral valve in 84 patients. Circulation 2004;109:2309-2313.
17. Stellin G, Padalino M, Milanesi O, et al: Repair of congenital mitral valve dysplasia in infants and children: is it always possible? Eur J Cardiothorac Surg 2000;18:74-82.
18. Wood AE, Healy DG, Nolke L, et al. Mitral valve reconstruction in a pediatric population: late clinical results and predictors of long-term outcome. J Thorac Cardiovasc Surg 2005;130:66-73.
19. Prifti E, Vanini V, Bonacchi M, et al: Repair of congenital malformations of the mitral valve: early and midterm results. Ann Thorac Surg 2002;73:614-621.
20. Chauvaud S, Waldmann T, d'Attellis N, et al: Homograft replacement of the mitral valve in young recipients: mid-term results. Eur J Cardiothorac Surg 2003;23:560-566.
21. Vohra HA, Laker S, Stumper O, et al: Predicting the performance of mitral prostheses implanted in children under 5 years of age. Eur J Cardiothorac Surg 2006;29:688-92.
22. Beierlein W, Becker V, Yates R, et al: Long-term follow-up after mitral valve replacement in childhood: poor event-free survival in the young child. Eur J Cardiothorac Surg 2007;31:860-865.
23. Alpagut U, Dayioglu E: Surgery for mitral valvar disease in childhood: should we choose reconstruction or repair? Cardiol Young 2003;13:337-340.
24. Adatia I, Moore PM, Jonas RA, et al: Clinical course and hemodynamic observations after supraannular mitral valve replacement in infants and children. J Am Coll Cardiol 1997;29:1089-1094.
25. Yoshimura N, Yamaguchi M, Oshima Y, et al: Surgery for mitral valve disease in the pediatric age group. J Thorac Cardiovasc Surg 1999;118:99-106.
26. van Son JA, Phoon CK, Silverman NH, Haas GS: Predicting feasibility of biventricular repair of right-dominant unbalanced atrioventricular canal. Ann Thorac Surg 1997;63:1657-1663.

TABLE 24-12	Guidelines for Pulmonary Valve Replacement in Repaired Tetralogy of Fallot with Significant Pulmonary Regurgitation*	
Compelling	Subjective ↓ in exercise ability
	Sustained objective ↓ in exercise capacity
	Symptomatic VT/syncope
	Sustained VT on 24-h ECG monitoring
	Serial RV dilation/↓ in RV ejection fraction
	Increasing RV end-systolic volume
	Onset tricuspid regurgitation with RV dilatation or atrial arrhythmias
Strong	QRS >180 msec or serial increase in QRS duration
	Surgery indicated for other reason (e.g., residual VSD)
	Pregnancy contemplated
Equivocal	RV volume >170 mL/m^2
	150 mL/m^2
	Patient preference

*Pulmonary regurgitation fraction >30%.
ECG, electrocardiogram; RV, right ventricle; VSD, ventricular septal defect; VT, ventricular tachycardia.

169. Day RW, Tani LY: Pulmonary intravascular ultrasound in infants and children with congenital heart disease. Cathet Cardiovasc Diagn 1997;41:395-398.
170. Keane JF, Plauth WH Jr, Nadas AS: Ventricular septal defect with aortic regurgitation. Circulation 1977;56(1 Suppl):I72-I77.
171. Karpawich PP, Duff DF, Mullins CE, et al: Ventricular septal defect with associated aortic valve insufficiency: progression of insufficiency and operative results in young children. J Thorac Cardiovasc Surg 1981;82:182-189.
172. Hisatomi K, Kosuga K, Isomura T, et al: Ventricular septal defect associated with aortic regurgitation. Ann Thorac Surg 1987;43:363-367.
173. Corin WJ, Monrad ES, Murakami T, et al: The relationship of afterload to ejection performance in chronic mitral regurgitation. Circulation 1987;76:59-67.
174. Agozzino L, de Vivo F, Falco A, et al: Non-inflammatory aortic root disease and floppy aortic valve as cause of isolated regurgitation: a clinico-morphologic study. Int J Cardiol 1994;45:129-134.
175. Laudito A, Brook MM, Suleman S, et al: The Ross procedure in children and young adults: a word of caution. J Thorac Cardiovasc Surg 2001;122:147-153.
176. von Bernuth G: 25 years after the first arterial switch procedure: mid-term results. Thor Cardiovasc Surg 2000;48:228-232.
177. Bland EF, Jones TD: Rheumatic fever and rheumatic heart disease: a twenty year report on 1000 patients followed since childhood. Circulation 1951;4:836-843.
178. Askovich B, Hawkins JA, Sower CT, et al: Right ventricle-to-pulmonary artery conduit longevity: is it related to allograft size? Ann Thorac Surg 2007;84:907-12.
179. Tweddell JS, Pelech AN, Frommelt PC, et al: Complex aortic valve repair as a durable and effective alternative to valve replacement in children with aortic valve disease. J Thorac Cardiovasc Surg 2005;129:551-558.
180. Grinda JM, Latremouille C, Berrebi AJ, et al: Aortic cusp extension valvuloplasty for rheumatic aortic valve disease: midterm results. Ann Thorac Surg 2002;74:438-443.
181. Becker AE, Becker MJ, Edwards JE: Pathologic spectrum of dysplasia of the tricuspid valve: features in common with Ebstein's malformation. Arch Pathol 1971;91:167-178.
182. Aaron BL, Mills M, Lower RR:. Congenital tricuspid insufficiency: definition and review. Chest 1976;69:637-641.
183. Donnelly WH, Bucciarelli RL, Nelson RM: Ischemic papillary muscle necrosis in stressed newborn infants. J Pediatr 1980;96:295-300.
184. Bucciarelli RL, Nelson RM, Egan EA, et al: Transient tricuspid insufficiency of the newborn: a form of myocardial dysfunction in stressed newborns. Pediatrics 1977;59: 330-337.
185. Reller MD, Rice MJ, McDonald RW: Tricuspid regurgitation in newborn infants with respiratory distress: echo-Doppler study. J Pediatr 1987;110:760-764.
186. Eichhorn P, Ritter M, Suetsch G, et al: Congenital cleft of the anterior tricuspid leaflet with severe tricuspid regurgitation in adults. J Am Coll Cardiol 1992;20:1175-1179.
187. Hagler DJ, Squarcia U, Cabalka AK, et al: Mechanism of tricuspid regurgitation in paramembranous ventricular septal defect. J Am Soc Echocardiogr 2002;15:364-368.
188. Anderson RH, Silverman NH, Zuberbuhler JR: Congenitally unguarded tricuspid orifice: its differentiation from Ebstein's malformation in association with pulmonary atresia and intact ventricular septum. Pediatr Cardiol 1990;11:86-90.
189. Kobayashi T, Inoue Y, Takeuchi K, et al: Prediction of intravenous immunoglobulin unresponsiveness in patients with Kawasaki disease. Circulation 2006;113:2606-2612.
190. Celermajer DS, Bull C, Till JA, et al: Ebstein's anomaly: presentation and outcome from fetus to adult. J Am Coll Cardiol 1994;23:170-176.
191. Giuliani ER, Fuster V, Brandenburg RO, Mair DD: Ebstein's anomaly: the clinical features and natural history of Ebstein's anomaly of the tricuspid valve. Mayo Clin Proc 1979;54:163-173.
192. Roberson DA, Silverman NH: Ebstein's anomaly: echocardiographic and clinical features in the fetus and neonate. J Am Coll Cardiol 1989;14:1300-1307.
193. Hornberger LK, Sahn DJ, Kleinman CS, et al: Tricuspid valve disease with significant tricuspid insufficiency in the fetus: diagnosis and outcome. J Am Coll Cardiol 1991;17:167-173.
194. Simcha A, Bonham-Carter RE: Ebstein's anomaly: clinical study of 32 patients in childhood. Br Heart J 1971;33:46-49.
195. Celermajer DS, Dodd SM, Greenwald SE, et al: Morbid anatomy in neonates with Ebstein's anomaly of the tricuspid valve: pathophysiologic and clinical implications. J Am Coll Cardiol 1992;19:1049-1053.
196. Yetman AT, Freedom RM, McCrindle BW: Outcome in cyanotic neonates with Ebstein's anomaly. Am J Cardiol 1998;81:749-754.
197. Smallhorn JF, Izukawa T, Benson L, Freedom RM: Noninvasive recognition of functional pulmonary atresia by echocardiography. Am J Cardiol 1984;54:925-926.
198. Vettukattil JJ, Bharucha T, Anderson RH: Defining Ebstein's malformation using three-dimensional echocardiography. Interact Cardiovasc Thorac Surg 2007;6:685-690.
199. Acar P, Abadir S, Roux D, et al: Ebstein's anomaly assessed by real-time 3-D echocardiography. Ann Thorac Surg 2006;82:731-733.
200. Velayudhan DE, Brown TM, Nanda NC, et al: Quantification of tricuspid regurgitation by live three-dimensional transthoracic echocardiographic measurements of vena contracta area. Echocardiography 2006;23:793-800.
201. Wald RM, Adatia I, Van Arsdell GS, Hornberger LK: Relation of limiting ductal patency to survival in neonatal Ebstein's anomaly. Am J Cardiol 2005;96:851-856.
202. Plowden JS, Kimball TR, Bensky A, et al: The use of extracorporeal membrane oxygenation in critically ill neonates with Ebstein's anomaly. Am Heart J 1991;121 (2 Pt 1):619-622.
203. Marsh TD, Shelton LW Jr: Neonatal tricuspid insufficiency with abnormal tricuspid valve treated with extracorporeal membrane oxygenation (ECMO): possible extension of ECMO use. Am J Perinatol 1993;10:36-38.
204. Reemtsen BL, Fagan BT, Wells WJ, Starnes VA: Current surgical therapy for Ebstein anomaly in neonates. J Thorac Cardiovasc Surg 2006;132:1285-1290.
205. Knott-Craig CJ, Goldberg SP, Overholt ED, et al: Repair of neonates and young infants with Ebstein's anomaly and related disorders. Ann Thorac Surg 2007;84:587-593.
206. Gentles TL, Calder AL, Clarkson PM, Neutze JM: Predictors of long-term survival with Ebstein's anomaly of the tricuspid valve. Am J Cardiol 1992;69:377-381.
207. Rossi L, Thiene G: Mild Ebstein's anomaly associated with supraventricular tachycardia and sudden death: clinicomorphologic features in 3 patients. Am J Cardiol 1984;53:332-334.
208. Oechslin EN, Harrison DA, Harris L, et al: Reoperation in adults with repair of tetralogy of Fallot: indications and outcomes. J Thorac Cardiovasc Surg 1999;118:245-251.
209. Pome G, Rossi C, Colucci V, et al: Late reoperations after repair of tetralogy of Fallot. Eur J Cardiothorac Surg 1992;6:31-35.
210. Reddy VM, McElhinney DB, Brook MM, et al: Repair of congenital tricuspid valve abnormalities with artificial chordae tendineae. Ann Thorac Surg 1998;66:172-176.
211. Kawahira Y, Yagihara T, Uemura H, et al: Replacement of the tricuspid valve in children with congenital cardiac malformations. J Heart Valve Dis 2000;9:636-640.
212. Pasque M, Williams WG, Coles JG, et al: Tricuspid valve replacement in children. Ann Thorac Surg 1987;44:164-168.
213. Kaplan M, Kut MS, Demirtas MM, et al: Prosthetic replacement of tricuspid valve: bioprosthetic or mechanical. Ann Thorac Surg 2002;73:467-473.
214. Kawano H, Oda T, Fukunaga S, et al: Tricuspid valve replacement with the St. Jude Medical valve: 19 years of experience. Eur J Cardiothorac Surg 2000;18:565-569.
215. Nakano K, Ishibashi-Ueda H, Kobayashi J, et al: Tricuspid valve replacement with bioprostheses: long-term results and causes of valve dysfunction. Ann Thorac Surg 2001;71:105-109.
216. Dalrymple-Hay MJ, Leung Y, Ohri SK, et al: Tricuspid valve replacement: bioprostheses are preferable. J Heart Valve Dis 1999;8:644-648.
217. Kiziltan HT, Theodoro DA, Warnes CA, et al: Late results of bioprosthetic tricuspid valve replacement in Ebstein's anomaly. Ann Thorac Surg 1998;66:1539-1545.
218. Bartlett HL, Atkins DL, Burns TL, et al: Early outcomes of tricuspid valve replacement in young children. Circulation 2007;115:319-325.
219. Goswami KC, Rao MB, Dev V, Shrivastava S: Juvenile tricuspid stenosis and rheumatic tricuspid valve disease: an echocardiographic study. Int J Cardiol 1999;72:83-86.
220. Roguin A, Rinkevich D, Milo S, et al: Long-term follow-up of patients with severe rheumatic tricuspid stenosis. Am Heart J 1998;136:103-108.
221. Wooley CF, Fontana ME, Kilman JW, Ryan JM: Tricuspid stenosis: atrial systolic murmur, tricuspid opening snap, and right atrial pressure pulse. Am J Med 1985;78:375-384.
222. Minich LL, Tani LY, Ritter S, et al: Usefulness of the preoperative tricuspid/mitral valve ratio for predicting outcome in pulmonary atresia with intact ventricular septum. Am J Cardiol 2000;85:1325-1328.
223. Smith MD, Sagar KB, Mauck HP, et al: Surgical correction of congenital tricuspid stenosis. Ann Thorac Surg 1982;34:329-332.
224. Blieden L, Berant M, Zeevi B: In Moller J, Hoffman J (eds): "Pulmonic stenosis" Pediatric Cardiovascular Medicine, 1st ed. London, Churchill Livingstone, 2000, pp 552-564.
225. Rodriguez-Fernandez HL, Kelly DT, Collado A, et al: Hemodynamic data and angiographic findings after Mustard repair for complete transposition of the great arteries. Circulation 1972;46:799-808.
226. Edwards J: Congenital malformations of the heart and great vessels. In Gould S (ed): Pathology of the Heart. Springfield, IL, Charles C Thomas, 1960, pp 391-397.
227. Rocchini A, Emmanouilides, G: Pulmonary stenosis. In Emmanouilides G, Riemenschneider T, Allen H, Gutgesell H (ed): Heart Disease in Infants, Children, and Adolescents Including the Fetus and Young Adult, 5th ed. Williams & Wilkins, 1995, pp 930-957.
228. Sommer RJ, Rhodes JF, Parness IA: Physiology of critical pulmonary valve obstruction in the neonate. Catheter Cardiovasc Interv 2000;50:473-479.
229. Rudolph AM: Congenital Diseases of the Heart, 2nd ed. Armonk, NY, Futura Publishing, 2001.
230. Vogelpoel L, Schrire V: Auscultatory and phonocardiographic assessment of pulmonary stenosis with intact ventricular septum. Circulation 1960;22:55-72.
231. Bassingthwaighte J, Parkin T, Dushane J: The electrocardiographic and hemodynamic findings in pulmonary stenosis with intact ventricular septum. Circulation 1963;28:893-905.
232. Puchalski MD, Lozier JS, Bradley DJ, et al: Electrocardiography in the diagnosis of right ventricular hypertrophy in children. Pediatrics 2006;118:1052-1055.
233. Simpson IA, Valdes-Cruz LM, Yoganathan AP, et al: Spatial velocity distribution and acceleration in serial subvalve tunnel and valvular obstructions: an in vitro study using Doppler color flow mapping. J Am Coll Cardiol 1989;13:241-248.
234. Silvilairat S, Cabalka AK, Cetta F, et al: Echocardiographic assessment of isolated pulmonary valve stenosis: which outpatient Doppler gradient has the most clinical validity? J Am Soc Echocardiogr 2005;18:1137-1142.
235. Snider AR, Server GA, Ritter SB (eds): Echocardiography in Pediatric Heart Disease, 2nd ed. St. Louis, Mosby-Year Book, 1997.
236. Vermilion RP, Snider AR, Meliones JN, et al: Pulsed Doppler evaluation of right ventricular diastolic filling in children with pulmonary valve stenosis before and after balloon valvuloplasty. Am J Cardiol 1990;66:79-84.
237. Schwerzmann M, Samman AM, Salehian O, et al: Comparison of echocardiographic and cardiac magnetic resonance imaging for assessing right ventricular function in adults with repaired tetralogy of Fallot. Am J Cardiol 2007;99:1593-1597.
238. Rao PS: Percutaneous balloon pulmonary valvuloplasty: state of the art. Catheter Cardiovasc Interv 2007;69:747-763.
239. Gielen H, Daniels O, van Lier H: Natural history of congenital pulmonary valvar stenosis: an echo and Doppler cardiographic study. Cardiol Young1999;9:129-135.
240. Latson LA: Critical pulmonary stenosis. J Interv Cardiol 2001;14:345-350.
241. Tabatabaei H, Boutin C, Nykanen DG, et al: Morphologic and hemodynamic consequences after percutaneous balloon valvotomy for neonatal pulmonary stenosis: medium-term follow-up. J Am Coll Cardiol 1996;27:473-478.
242. McCrindle BW: Independent predictors of long-term results after balloon pulmonary valvuloplasty. Valvuloplasty and Angioplasty of Congenital Anomalies (VACA) Registry Investigators. Circulation 1994;89:1751-1759.
243. Alsoufi B, Williams WG, Hua Z, et al: Surgical outcomes in the treatment of patients with tetralogy of Fallot and absent pulmonary valve. Eur J Cardiothorac Surg 2007;31:354-359.

244. Norgaard MA, Alphonso N, Newcomb AE, et al: Absent pulmonary valve syndrome: surgical and clinical outcome with long-term follow-up. Eur J Cardiothorac Surg 2006;29:682-687.

245. Morales DL, Braud BE, Gunter KS, et al: Encouraging results for the Contegra conduit in the problematic right ventricle-to-pulmonary artery connection. J Thorac Cardiovasc Surg 2006;132:665-671.

246. Boethig D, Breymann T: Contegra pulmonary valved conduits cause no relevant hemolysis. J Card Surg 2004;19:420-425.

247. Homann M, Haehnel JC, Mendler N, et al: Reconstruction of the RVOT with valved biological conduits: 25 years experience with allografts and xenografts. Eur J Cardiothorac Surg 2000;17:624-630.

248. Hawkins JA, Hillman ND, Lambert LM, et al: Immunogenicity of decellularized cryopreserved allografts in pediatric cardiac surgery: comparison with standard cryopreserved allografts. J Thorac Cardiovasc Surg 2003;126:247-253.

249. Abd El Rahman MY, Abdul-Khaliq H, Vogel M, et al: Relation between right ventricular enlargement, QRS duration, and right ventricular function in patients with tetralogy of Fallot and pulmonary regurgitation after surgical repair. Heart 2000;84:416-420.

250. Gatzoulis MA, Till JA, Somerville J, Redington AN: Mechanoelectrical interaction in tetralogy of Fallot: QRS prolongation relates to right ventricular size and predicts malignant ventricular arrhythmias and sudden death. Circulation 1995;92:231-237.

251. Balaji S, Lau YR, Case CL, Gillette PC: QRS prolongation is associated with inducible ventricular tachycardia after repair of tetralogy of Fallot. Am J Cardiol 1997;80:160-163.

252. Williams RV, Minich LL, Shaddy RE, et al: Comparison of Doppler echocardiography with angiography for determining the severity of pulmonary regurgitation. Am J Cardiol 2002;89:1438-1441.

253. Marx GR, GevaT: MRI and echocardiography in children: how do they compare? Semin Roentgenol 1998;33:281-292.

254. Beekman RP, Beek FJ, Meijboom EJ: Usefulness of MRI for the pre-operative evaluation of the pulmonary arteries in tetralogy of Fallot. Magn Reson Imaging 1997;15:1005-1015.

255. Geva T, Greil GF, Marshall AC, et al: Gadolinium-enhanced 3-dimensional magnetic resonance angiography of pulmonary blood supply in patients with complex pulmonary stenosis or atresia: comparison with x-ray angiography. Circulation 2002;106:473-478.

256. Powell AJ, Chung T, Landzberg MJ, Geva T: Accuracy of MRI evaluation of pulmonary blood supply in patients with complex pulmonary stenosis or atresia. Int J Card Imaging 2000;16:169-174.

257. Helbing WA, de Roos A: Clinical applications of cardiac magnetic resonance imaging after repair of tetralogy of Fallot. Pediatr Cardiol 2000;21:70-79.

258. Rebergen SA, Chin JG, Ottenkamp J, et al: Pulmonary regurgitation in the late postoperative follow-up of tetralogy of Fallot: volumetric quantitation by nuclear magnetic resonance velocity mapping. Circulation 1993;88(5 Pt 1):2257-2266.

259. Meadows J, Powell AJ, Geva T, et al: Cardiac magnetic resonance imaging correlates of exercise capacity in patients with surgically repaired tetralogy of Fallot. Am J Cardiol 2007;100:1446-1450.

260. Karamlou T, Blackstone EH, Hawkins JA, et al: Can pulmonary conduit dysfunction and failure be reduced in infants and children less than age 2 years at initial implantation? J Thorac Cardiovasc Surg 2006;132:829-838.

261. Therrien J, Siu SC, McLaughlin PR, et al: Pulmonary valve replacement in adults late after repair of tetralogy of Fallot: are we operating too late? J Am Coll Cardiol 2000;36:1670-1675.

262. Shinebourne EA, Babu-Narayan SV, Carvalho JS: Tetralogy of Fallot: from fetus to adult. Heart 2006;92:1353-1359.

263. Vliegen HW, van Straten A, de Roos A, et al: Magnetic resonance imaging to assess the hemodynamic effects of pulmonary valve replacement in adults late after repair of tetralogy of Fallot. Circulation 2002;106:1703-1707.

264. Discigil B, Dearani JA, Puga FJ, et al: Late pulmonary valve replacement after repair of tetralogy of Fallot. J Thorac Cardiovasc Surg 2001;121:344-351.

265. Eyskens B, Reybrouck T, Bogaert J, et al: Homograft insertion for pulmonary regurgitation after repair of tetralogy of Fallot improves cardiorespiratory exercise performance. Am J Cardiol 2000;85:221-225.

266. Hazekamp MG, Kurvers MM, Schoof PH, et al: Pulmonary valve insertion late after repair of Fallot's tetralogy. Eur J Cardiothorac Surg 2001;19:667-670.

267. Khambadkone S, Coats L, Taylor A, et al: Percutaneous pulmonary valve implantation in humans: results in 59 consecutive patients. Circulation 2005;112:1189-1197.

Valvular Heart Disease in Pregnancy

Karen Stout

KEY POINTS

- Valvular disease may carry a high risk for the mother and fetus in some circumstances, but many women with valvular disease can successfully deliver healthy children.
- Global risk assessment includes assessment of the specific lesion as well as functional status.
- Specific valvular lesions are associated with different risks.
- Severe aortic stenosis has a high complication rate during pregnancy.
- Both moderate and severe mitral stenosis have high complications rates during pregnancy.
- Anticoagulation during pregnancy is a difficult clinical management issue and recommendations must be individualized.
- Women at increased risk for adverse maternal or fetal outcomes should be referred to experienced centers.

Valvular heart disease in pregnant women may present in a variety of different scenarios. Women with known valvular heart disease may present to the physician prior to pregnancy for evaluation of potential maternal and fetal risk. They may also present during pregnancy without preconception counseling. Other women have no previous cardiac history but are diagnosed with valve disease during pregnancy. In each situation, the normal physiologic changes of pregnancy may exacerbate the hemodynamics of the valve lesion, such that women who are asymptomatic in the nongravid state may decompensate during pregnancy. In addition to maternal risk, clinical management is complicated by the potential effects of medications, radiation or surgery on the fetus. However, despite the increased maternal and fetal risks, most women with valvular heart disease can undergo a successful pregnancy when carefully monitored at an experienced center. Optimal management of the pregnant woman with valvular heart disease depends on a team approach by an obstetrician, a cardiologist, and an anesthesiologist experienced in management of these patients.

PHYSIOLOGIC CHANGES OF PREGNANCY

Normal Hemodynamic Changes

Pregnancy

A substantial increase in plasma volume, erythrocyte volume, and cardiac output occurs during pregnancy (Figure 25-1).[1-4] Cardiac output increases by as much as 45% over baseline values, with most of the increase due to a heart rate 20% to 30% higher than baseline, with a smaller incremental increase in stroke volume.[5-8] The increase in cardiac output primarily occurs in the first trimester, beginning as early as 10 weeks of gestation, with the maximal cardiac output achieved by 24 weeks in some studies. Other studies show a continued slow rise in cardiac output in the last two trimesters (Figure 25-2).[7,9,10] Cardiac output is more dependent on heart rate near term. Pulmonary pressures remain normal during pregnancy, which suggests a decrease in pulmonary vascular resistance to compensate for the increased cardiac output.[11] Left ventricular diastolic filling pressures remain normal.[12]

The exact mechanism that initiates the increase in cardiac output during pregnancy is not clear, although hormonal effects are presumed to be important. At the physiologic level, an increase in venous tone leads to preload augmentation,[13] while a decrease in aortic stiffness and alterations in the microcirculation reduce afterload.[5] The decrease in systemic resistance offsets the increase in cardiac output such that blood pressure decreases slightly during pregnancy. Based on echocardiographic data, left ventricular wall stress decreases by about 30%, which decreases the oxygen demands of the myocardium.[4,14] Paradoxically, based on echocardiographic measurements of afterload adjusted velocity of circumferential fiber shortening, several studies suggest that left ventricular contractility may be depressed. The magnitude of this change is unlikely to be clinically significant.[4,14,15] Stroke volume is maintained in the setting of decreased contractility due to the altered loading conditions of pregnancy. At term, the relationship between left ventricular filling pressure and stroke-work index is comparable to the nonpregnant state.[16]

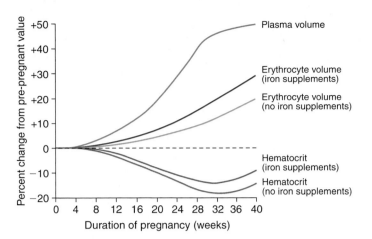

FIGURE 25–1 Plasma and erythrocyte increase during pregnancy. *(From Pitkin RM: Nutritional support in obstetrics and gynecology. Clin Obstet Gynecol 1976;19:489-513, with permission.)*

Positional Changes

Patients with valvular heart disease need to be aware of the effects of positional change on cardiovascular hemodynamics in pregnancy. Orthostatic changes are similar to the nonpregnant state.[17] However, the supine position is associated with compression of the inferior vena cava by the gravid uterus. This results in decreased venous return to the right atrium with a consequent decline in stroke volume and cardiac output. Compression of the inferior vena cava can be prevented by having the patient use a left lateral decubitus position instead of the supine position.[18] Appropriate patient positioning is particularly important at the time of procedures such as surgery or catheterization because the fetus will tolerate hypotension due to caval compression very poorly. Some patients may also need to labor in the left lateral decubitus position.

Peripartum and Postpartum Changes

Peripartum hemodynamics are affected by uterine contractions, the pain of labor and delivery, and immediate blood loss (Figure 25-3). When valve disease is present, these hemodynamic stresses may result in decompensation. The hemodynamic effects of pain include an increased heart rate and stroke volume. During labor, uterine contractions force blood into the circulating blood pool. The increase in intravascular volume with each contraction is accompanied by an increase in heart rate such that cardiac output is augmented by about 20% with each contraction (Figure 25-4).[19,20] Labor and delivery are associated with mild increases in pulmonary and left ventricular diastolic pressures, which may be accentuated in patients with decreased left ventricular compliance. For example, a patient with decreased left ventricular compliance due to aortic stenosis may have substantial increases in left ventricular end-diastolic pressures in the peripartum period, which, if not monitored and treated, may lead to pulmonary edema. Uterine contractions will have large effects on pulmonary pressures in the context of obstruction to left ventricular outflow.

The blood loss with vaginal delivery to some extent compensates for the increased blood volume of pregnancy but may not be well tolerated in women with valvular heart disease. This is particularly true when the left ventricular pressure-volume relationship is very steep, such as in women with severe aortic stenosis. A small loss of volume and preload may result in a large decrease in cardiac output. However, the volume changes with cesarean section are even greater than those with vaginal delivery.[21] Therefore, cesarean section is rarely indicated for cardiac reasons.

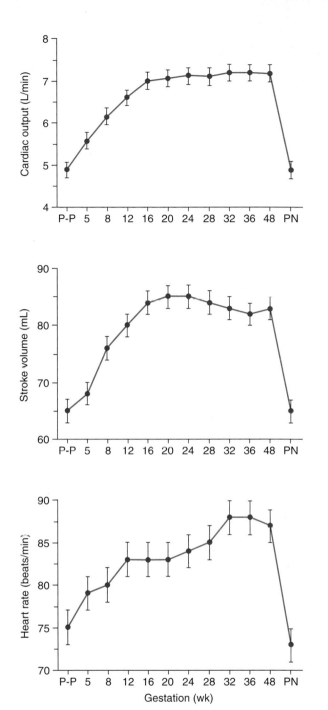

FIGURE 25–2 Increase in cardiac output from the nonpregnant state throughout pregnancy. P-P, prepregnancy; PN, postnatal. *(From Hunter S, Robson SC: Adaptation of the maternal heart in pregnancy. Br Heart J 1992;68: 540-543, with permission.)*

After delivery of the placenta, stroke volume and cardiac output rise by about 10% and remain elevated for about 24 hours. Over the next 2 weeks, cardiac output declines by 25% to 30% due to a decrease in heart rate and intravascular volume.[22,23] In some patients, symptoms occur postpartum due to intra- and extravascular volume shifts that result in spontaneous volume loading.[16,24] Although hemodynamics return toward baseline 6 to 12 weeks after delivery, the new postpartum baseline may be different than prepartum hemodynamics. For example, both left ventricular and aortic dimensions may remain slightly larger than the prepregnancy baseline.[6,23]

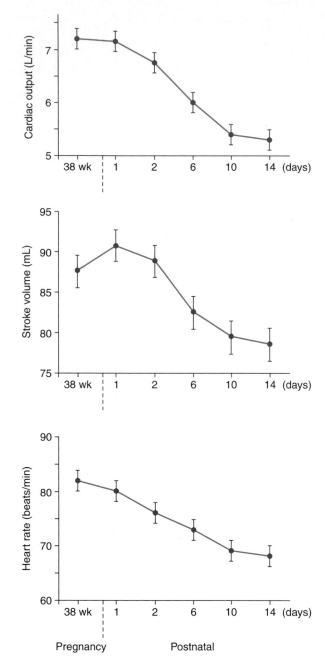

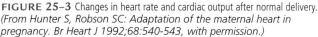

Pregnancy   Postnatal

FIGURE 25-3 Changes in heart rate and cardiac output after normal delivery. *(From Hunter S, Robson SC: Adaptation of the maternal heart in pregnancy. Br Heart J 1992;68:540-543, with permission.)*

Evaluation by Echocardiography

Cardiac Output

Echocardiography is used both to evaluate the presence and severity of valvular heart disease and to monitor the hemodynamic effects of pregnancy.

Cardiac output can be accurately measured by Doppler echocardiography in pregnant women with and without valvular heart disease with a high degree of reproducibility.[9,25,26] In women without aortic valve disease, cardiac output can be measured based on continuous wave Doppler recordings of the ascending aorta in combination with an A-mode measurement of the smallest aortic diameter.[9] When aortic diameters are used, repeat measurement is necessary at each time point because aortic root diameter increases slightly during pregnancy.[27,28]

Cardiac output can also be measured using the left ventricular outflow tract diameter and pulsed Doppler flow velocity

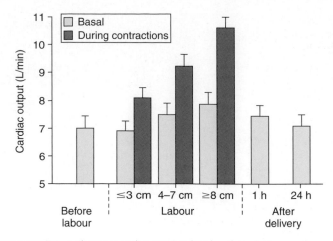

FIGURE 25-4 Changes in cardiac output and stroke volume during normal labor. *(From Hunter S, Robson SC: Adaptation of the maternal heart in pregnancy. Br Heart J 1992;68:540-543, with permission.)*

curve. This method is accurate even in women with aortic valve disease.[10,18,29,30]

Normal Anatomic Changes

Echocardiographic findings reflect the normal physiologic changes of pregnancy. These normal changes need to be taken into account in evaluation of women with valve disease. Left ventricular end-diastolic dimension increases by 2 to 3 mm, with no change in end-systolic dimension, such that both fractional shortening and ejection fraction are increased compared with baseline.[17,28,29,33-34] In addition, both aortic root and left ventricular outflow tract diameters increase by 1 to 2 mm; this increase often persists long term after pregnancy.[27,35] Left atrial size increases by about 4 mm,[28] which is associated with an increase in serum atrial natriuretic peptide levels.[36,37] A small increase in mitral annulus diameter and a larger increase in tricuspid annulus diameter occur.[28]

A small pericardial effusion is seen in 25% of healthy women during pregnancy.[37]

Doppler Changes

The increased cardiac output of pregnancy leads to increased transvalvular flow velocities. Aortic and left ventricular outflow velocities increase by about 0.3 m/sec. The transmitral E-velocity increases by 0 to 0.1 m/sec, with an increase in A-velocity of 0.1 to 0.2 m/sec.[7,28] The greater increase in A-velocity compared with E-velocity results in a shift from the normal E/A ratio seen in young adults (>1.5) to an equalized or reversed E/A ratio. The pulmonary venous flow pattern shows an increase in the velocity, but not duration, of the pulmonary venous A wave.[5]

Mild tricuspid and pulmonic regurgitation are usually seen during pregnancy. Physiologic mitral regurgitation is also common, likely due to annular dilation related to left ventricular dilation.[38]

EPIDEMIOLOGY

The incidence of rheumatic heart disease has declined in industrialized nations during the last 40 years.[39,40] During that same time, successes in diagnostic and therapeutic approaches to congenital heart disease have led to an increase in the number of adults with congenital heart disease. Additionally, other causes of valve disease, including connective tissue disorders such as Marfan syndrome, are increasingly common. Consequently, although rheumatic heart disease remains the more common form of valve disease in pregnancy in developing countries, the profile of valve disease during pregnancy is different in industrialized nations. The nature of congenital heart disease and systemic disease add further complexity to the management of pregnancy and valvular disease, as these patients frequently have a constellation of associated cardiovascular abnormalities beyond the valve disease itself. Some patients may have a systemic right ventricle or aortic pathology that poses additive risk. The spectrum of valve disease in pregnancy makes risk assessment somewhat difficult, but general risk factors have been identified, as well as risks based upon the specific valvular lesion.

RISK FACTORS FOR ADVERSE OUTCOMES

The maternal and fetal risks in women with valvular heart disease are difficult to evaluate because the specific hemodynamics, functional status, previous interventions, and other clinical factors vary substantially from patient to patient. Given the relative infrequency of valve disease in pregnant women, much of our initial understanding is based on case reports and small observational clinical series.

More recently, several multicenter prospective studies have assessed risks for adverse outcomes across large groups of women with diverse cardiac diseases. A prospective multicenter Canadian study evaluated the risk of adverse outcomes in pregnant women with cardiac disease with enrollment of 599 consecutive pregnancies in women with all types of heart disease.[41] This study included 143 women with congenital valve disease and 81 women with acquired valve disease. On multivariate analysis, predictors of adverse maternal events were a history of cardiac events prior to pregnancy, a New York Heart Association (NYHA) functional class greater than II, cyanosis, left heart obstruction, or systemic ventricular dysfunction. These four predictors allow prediction of the risk of maternal events as shown in Table 25-1 and in Figure 25-5.

In this series of 599 consecutive pregnancies, the live birth rate was 98% with fetal death in 1% and neonatal death in 1%. The risk of fetal or neonatal death was predicted by NYHA class greater than II or cyanosis, left heart obstruction, smoking, multiple gestations, and use of anticoagulants throughout pregnancy, as shown in Table 25-2. Neonatal events occurred in 20% of pregnancies, including premature birth in 18% and small-for-gestational-age birthweight in 4% of pregnancies. In women with congenital heart disease but without a recognized genetic syndrome, 7% of the 432 infants had congenital heart disease.

In a second publication from this study, 302 pregnancies in women with heart disease were compared with 575 pregnancies in women without heart disease, matched for clinical, socioeconomic, and obstetric risk factors. Even when matched for these other factors, there was an increased risk of both maternal and fetal complications in women with heart disease. The rate of maternal cardiac complications was 17% versus 0% in the control group. Heart failure and arrhythmias accounted for most of the cardiac complications (94%), with two postpartum deaths due to heart failure or pulmonary hypertension. In addition, the risk of neonatal complications was 2.3 times normal (Figure 25-6). The authors conclude that maternal cardiac and obstetric risk factors have additive effects. Those patients with risk factors for adverse outcomes should be referred to high-risk obstetric clinics (Figure 25-7).[42]

As the number of adults with congenital heart disease increases, the number of women of reproductive age with valve disease in the context of other cardiac abnormalities also increases. Consequently, in patients with a constellation of cardiac abnormalities, identifying the relevant underlying hemodynamic lesion can be difficult. Additionally, the effect

TABLE 25–1	Predictors of Primary Adverse Events* in Pregnant Women with Cardiac Disease
Predictors	**Definition**
Cardiac event before pregnancy	Heart failure Transient ischemic attack Stroke
Functional status	Baseline NYHA class > II Cyanosis
Left heart obstruction	MVA < 2 cm², AVA < 1.5 cm², LVOT gradient > 30 mmHg
Systemic ventricular systolic dysfunction	EF < 40%
Risk Index	
Number of Predictors	**Rate of Cardiac Events**
0	5%
1	27%
>1	75%

*Primary adverse events were defined as pulmonary edema, sustained symptomatic arrhythmia requiring treatment, stroke, cardiac arrest, or cardiac death.
AVA, aortic valve area; EF, ejection fraction; LVOT, left ventricular outflow tract; MVA, mitral valve area; NYHA, New York Heart Association.
From Siu SC, Sermer M, Colman JM, et al: Prospective multicenter study of pregnancy outcomes in women with heart disease. Circulation 2001;104:515-521, with permission.

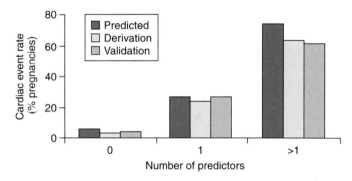

FIGURE 25–5 Frequency of maternal primary cardiac events as predicted by the risk index in Table 25-1. Frequencies are shown for derivation and validation groups, expressed as a function of the number of cardiac predictors. *(From Siu SC, Sermer M, Colman JM, et al: Prospective multicenter study of pregnancy outcomes in women with heart disease. Circulation 2001;104:515-521, with permission.)*

TABLE 25–2	Predictors of Neonatal Events in Women with Cardiac Disease
Predictors of Neonatal Events	
NYHA class > II or cyanosis at the baseline prenatal visit	
Maternal left heart obstruction	
Smoking during pregnancy	
Multiple gestations	
Use of anticoagulants throughout pregnancy	
Risk Index	
Number of Predictors	**Rate of Fetal or Neonatal Death**
0	2%
1 or more	4%

NYHA, New York Heart Association.
From Siu SC, Sermer M, Colman JM, et al: Prospective multicenter study of pregnancy outcomes in women with heart disease. Circulation 2001;104:515-521, with permission.

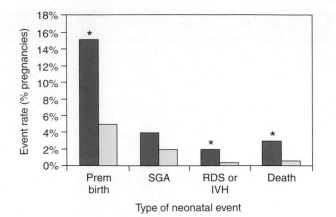

FIGURE 25–6 Event rates in 302 pregnancies in women with heart disease (purple bars) and in 572 pregnancies in women without heart disease (blue bars) subdivided into specific type of neonatal complications. Prem birth, delivery at less than 37 weeks of gestations; SGA, small for gestational age birth weight; RDS or IVH, respiratory distress syndrome or intraventricular hemorrhage; death, fetal or neonatal death. *P < 0.005, heart disease versus controls. *(From Siu SC, Colman JM, Sorensen S, et al: Adverse neonatal and cardiac outcomes are more common in pregnant women with cardiac disease. Circulation 2002;105:2179-2184, with permission.)*

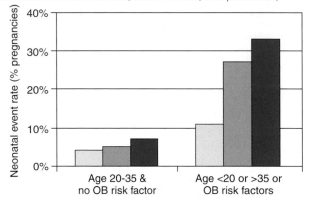

FIGURE 25–7 Frequency of neonatal complications when patients are divided into two groups by the presence or absence of maternal noncardiac risk factors (obstetric high-risk characteristics including smoking, use of anticoagulation, multiple gestation, maternal age). *Light blue bars* represent control group. *Medium blue bars* represent the heart disease group without left heart obstruction or poor functional class/cyanosis. *Dark blue bars* represent the high-risk cardiac patients, with left heart obstruction or poor functional class/cyanosis. *(From Siu SC, Colman JM, Sorensen S, et al: Adverse neonatal and cardiac outcomes are more common in pregnant women with cardiac disease. Circulation 2002;105:2179-2184, with permission.)*

of valve disease in the setting of other congenital defects may have a different impact than valve disease in isolation. Several studies have sought to assess the risks of pregnancy in patients with congenital heart disease, which includes patients with congenital valve abnormalities.

Khairy and colleagues reported 90 pregnancies in 54 women with varied types of congenital heart disease.[43] This study also identified NYHA class 2, prior history of heart failure, and smoking as risk factors for maternal cardiac events. This series had a large number of patients with right-sided lesions and fewer with significant left ventricular outflow obstruction. The right-sided abnormalities were either obstructive lesions (5.7%) or repaired tetralogy of Fallot (28.3%) with pulmonic regurgitation as the dominant abnormality. Significant left ventricular outflow obstruction was present in 17%. They identified severe pulmonic regurgitation or subpulmonic ventricular dysfunction as risks for adverse maternal outcomes (Table 25-3). Multivariate analysis of risks for adverse fetal outcomes also included left ventricular outflow tract obstruction as a risk factor (Table 25-4). As with the Siu study, these authors developed a risk score (Figure 25-8). Notably different in this study is the impact of pulmonic regurgitation and right ventricular dysfunction.

These studies emphasize the importance of placing the valvular disease in the context of a patient's other cardiac lesions, as risk factors for adverse outcomes may be additive. Additionally, functional class is important in risk assessment, independent of the underlying hemodynamic abnormality. Table 25-3 compares identified risk factors from the Valvular Heart Disease Guidelines of the American College of Cardiology (ACC)/American Heart Association (AHA) and the studies by Siu and Khairy.[41,43]

An additional risk consideration is that of aortic pathology, which is associated with many different disease processes. In addition to patients with connective tissue disorders such as Marfan, Ehler-Danlos, or Loeys-Dietz syndromes, aortic dilation can also be seen in patients with congenital heart disease. Congenital abnormalities such as bicuspid aortic valve, tetralogy of Fallot, transposition of the great vessels, and truncus arteriosus all may have associated aortic dilation. Some surgical repairs of congenital heart disease are associated with the development of aortic dilation, including the Ross repair of aortic stenosis or arterial switch repairs for transposition of the great vessels. The risk of dissection in congenital abnormalities does not appear to be as high as the risk in connective tissue disorders,

TABLE 25–3	Comparison of Risks for Adverse Maternal Outcomes		
	ACC/AHA Guidelines[44]	Siu (2001)[41]	Khairy (2006)[43]
Study group*		599 pregnancies, 224 women with heart disease	90 pregnancies, 54 women with congenital heart disease
History		Prior cardiac event or arrhythmia	Prior history of heart failure Smoking history Weight
NYHA class	AR, MS, MR with class III-IV symptoms	NYHA > II or cyanosis	NYHA ≥ 2
Valve lesion	AS with or without symptoms Mechanical prosthesis	Left heart obstruction	Severe pulmonic regurgitation
Ejection fraction	AV or MV disease with EF < 40%	Systemic ventricular dysfunction (EF < 40%)	Decreased subpulmonic ventricular EF Decreased morphologic right ventricular EF
Pulmonary pressures	AV or MV disease with > 75% systemic pulmonary pressures		
Other	Marfan syndrome with or without AR		

*The American College of Cardiology (ACC)/American Heart Association (AHA) guidelines are based on synthesis of data from multiple publications.

AR, aortic regurgitation; AS, aortic stenosis; AV, aortic valve; EF, ejection fraction; MR, mitral regurgitation; MS, mitral stenosis; MV, mitral valve; NYHA, New York Heart Association.

TABLE 25–4	Comparison of Risk Factors for Fetal Complications

Siu (2001)[41]
Cyanosis
NYHA class > II
Left heart obstruction
Smoking
Anticoagulation
Multiple gestation

Khairy (2006)[43]
Decreased saturation
Symptomatic arrhythmia
Subaortic obstruction > 30 mmHg*
Smoking

*The only risk factor remaining in multivariate analysis.

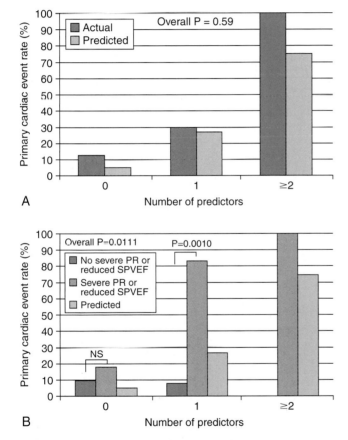

FIGURE 25–8 Risk score for adverse cardiac events during pregnancy. **A,** The actual versus the predicted event rates with 0, 1, and = 2 risk factors. **B,** Further risk stratification based on the presence of severe pulmonic regurgitation (PR) and/or reduction in subpulmonary ventricular ejection fraction (SPVEF). *(From Khairy P, Ouyang DW, Fernandes SM, et al: Pregnancy outcomes in women with congenital heart disease. Circulation 2006;113:517-524, with permission.)*

but as yet this is not well understood. Although the ACC/AHA guidelines recommend consideration of aortic surgery to repair the aorta in patients with bicuspid valves and an aortic diameter greater than 5.0 cm,[44] the aortic diameter that poses increased risk during pregnancy in such patients is not known. In patients with Marfan syndrome, the risk appears highest for those individuals with an aortic diameter greater than 4.0 cm.[45-47]

Pregnancy increases the risk of dissection through several mechanisms, including estrogen interference with collagen deposition, accelerated destruction of the elastic lamellae due to elastase, and decrease in collagen synthesis due to relaxin.[48,49] Although there are few specific data regarding the risk of dissection, aortic pathology may be an important concomitant risk factor during pregnancy.

BASIC CLINICAL APPROACH

Evaluation of Disease Severity

The first step in evaluation of the pregnant woman with possible valve disease is to establish a specific diagnosis and determine the severity of disease. History and physical exam are important in the identification of abnormal cardiac symptoms or abnormal cardiac exam findings.

Pregnant women frequently have symptoms or exam findings that may be suggestive of heart disease (Table 25-5). On exam, a systolic murmur is present in 80% of pregnant women and typically represents a benign flow murmur.[50]

In 103 women without a previous cardiac history who were referred for echocardiography for a murmur appreciated during pregnancy, about 80% had a physical examination consistent with a flow murmur; all these women had a normal echocardiogram.[50] In the 7% with a pansystolic, late systolic, or diastolic murmur, all had abnormal echocardiograms, including three ventricular septal defects, one large atrial septal defect, one atrial septal defect with rheumatic mitral regurgitation, and one nonobstructive hypertrophic cardiomyopathy.

Echocardiography is necessary in pregnant women with a murmur if there is a previous history of cardiac disease, definite cardiac symptoms, arterial oxygen desaturation, a grade 3/6 or louder systolic murmur, or any diastolic murmur. In these patients, echocardiography allows accurate diagnosis of the location and severity of valve disease, associated hemodynamic abnormalities (e.g., pulmonary hypertension), and assessment of left and right ventricular systolic and diastolic dysfunction.

Functional status plays an important role in risk stratification. As evidenced by several studies, poor functional class is a significant risk for maternal and fetal complications with pregnancy. In addition to a careful symptom history, exercise testing may have a role in preconception counseling. If there is a significant valvular lesion and impaired functional status, consideration of valve replacement prior to pregnancy may be indicated.

Management during Pregnancy

Clinical Monitoring

Once the diagnosis of valve disease is made in a pregnant woman, the cardiologist should work with the high-risk obstetrician to determine the optimal intervals for evaluation,

TABLE 25–5	Cardiac Findings During a Normal Pregnancy

Symptoms
Fatigue
Orthopnea
Decreased exercise tolerance
Palpitations
Lower-extremity edema

Physical Examination
Mid-systolic murmur at left sternal border (pulmonic flow murmur)
Split S1
Continuous murmur (mammary souffle or venous hum)
Lower-extremity edema
S3

the potential need for medical therapy, discussion of issues related to labor and delivery, and plans for therapy should the patient decompensate during pregnancy.

These women benefit from very close monitoring during pregnancy by a high-risk obstetrics clinic to prevent maternal and fetal complications. After an initial evaluation, subsequent evaluations are based on the patient's disease severity and clinical course. At each visit a structured review of symptoms is performed, with specific questions to elicit early evidence of orthopnea, paroxysmal nocturnal dyspnea, a decrease in exercise tolerance chest pain, dyspnea, or palpitations. Any change in exercise tolerance, or even subtle symptoms, should prompt reevaluation for cardiac decompensation. In addition, long-range planning for interventions postpartum and plans for future pregnancies should be initiated early to ensure that appropriate postpartum cardiac evaluation is not delayed.

Medical Therapy

Medications need to be carefully reviewed prior to pregnancy so that the patient can avoid medications with adverse fetal effects. New medical therapies are used only as needed for symptoms or prevention of adverse events. Another example is the patients with mechanical prosthetic valves require anticoagulation despite the risks of this therapy. However, when medical therapy is not essential and may not be safe in pregnancy, it should be discontinued during pregnancy. Another example is the woman on an angiotensin-converting enzyme inhibitor for asymptomatic aortic regurgitation who should discontinue this medication before becoming pregnant. On the other hand, medications that are critical to maintaining clinical stability may need to be continued or changed prior to pregnancy. For those patients in whom teratogenic medications are necessary to maintain stability, pregnancy is likely ill advised. For example, women on angiotensin-converting enzyme inhibitors for impaired ventricular function may not tolerate discontinuation or an alternative medication during pregnancy.

Many patients can be managed with few or no medications, even when decompensation occurs. Simple measures such as bedrest, oxygen supplementation, avoidance of the supine position, and patient education can be very effective. When medication is needed, consultation with the pharmacist and obstetrician is needed to determine safety during pregnancy. In a series of 66 pregnancies in women with native valve disease, medications were utilized in 52%, including diuretics in 42%, β-blockers in 34%, calcium channel blockers in 20%, digoxin in 14%, heparin in 6%, hydralazine in 2%, and aspirin in 2%.[51]

Effects of Intercurrent Illness

Women with valve disease who are initially well compensated during pregnancy may abruptly decompensate with superimposition of another hemodynamic stress. Intercurrent febrile events are commonly associated with decompensation.[52] For example, a viral or bacterial infection may lead to cardiac symptoms of angina or heart failure due to the increased metabolic demands associated with fever and tachycardia. Factors that may contribute to decompensation, such as anemia, pulmonary embolus, or infection, should be diligently sought in pregnant women with heart disease when decompensation occurs. Vaccination against influenza and pneumococcus is appropriate.

Medical therapy focuses on treatment of the underlying disease process and measures to decrease hemodynamic stress, such as fever reduction and supplemental oxygen. Some patients may need admission to the intensive care unit, sometime with intubation and mechanical ventilation, as well as invasive hemodynamic monitoring to optimize preload and afterload. In extreme cases, valvuloplasty or surgery may be needed during pregnancy.

Inheritability

Women with congenital heart disease, including congenital valve disease, are more likely to have children with congenital heart disease.[53] Fetal echocardiography has advanced substantially during the last 20 years, allowing diagnosis and hemodynamic assessment of fetal congenital heart disease.[54] Fetal echocardiography is appropriate in those women at higher risk, allowing the opportunity to identify significant cardiac defects and plan appropriately for the care of the fetus after delivery. If a significant cardiac abnormality is identified, there is opportunity prior to delivery to meet with the pediatric cardiologists, perinatologists, and cardiac surgeons to discuss management.

Management in the Peripartum Period

Endocarditis prophylaxis guidelines do not recommend antibiotic prophylaxis for vaginal deliveries in women with valvular heart disease; this recommendation has not changed in the 2007 guidelines.[55]

Peripartum Hemodynamic Monitoring

In patients with severe valve disease, particularly those with left-sided obstructive lesions, a planned delivery with invasive hemodynamic monitoring should be considered. Placement of a Swan-Ganz catheter and arterial line allows continuous monitoring of pulmonary pressures, pulmonary wedge pressure, cardiac output and systemic vascular resistance. These parameters allow optimization of preload and afterload during labor and delivery and in the early postpartum period. In high-risk patients, monitoring may be continued for 24 to 48 hours postpartum to avoid decompensation due to the intravascular fluid shifts during this time period. Patients at highest risk are those with mitral stenosis and aortic stenosis, with the degree of risk increasing in proportion to the severity of valve obstruction. Left ventricular systolic dysfunction in association with valve disease also confers a high risk.

Type of Delivery

There is no difference in peripartum complication rates between vaginal delivery and cesarean section in women with heart disease.[42] In 599 consecutive pregnancies in women with heart disease, 27% were by cesarean section, with 96% of those for obstetric indications. Maternal cardiac status was the indication for cesarean section in only 4% of these patients.

In another series of 66 women with valvular heart disease, the mode of delivery was vaginal in 92%, although only 58% were spontaneous, with forceps or vacuum assistance needed in the remainder. Indications for cesarean section were obstetric in three cases and cardiac in two cases (i.e., heart failure, acute coronary syndrome).[51]

Many high-risk obstetric centers recommend induction of labor to ensure the availability of an experienced cardiac and obstetric team for patient management and to allow placement of pulmonary artery and arterial catheters for hemodynamic monitoring (if needed). The optimal timing of induction is near term, with a favorable cervix. Prolonged inductions should be avoided. Pain control is especially important in women with heart disease to minimize the surges in catecholamines and changes in heart rate and systemic vascular resistance associated with pain. Induction of labor allows early pain control. In addition, if the fetus has a cardiac abnormality, a planned delivery allows prompt care of the newborn infant.

Timing of Surgical Intervention

In women with valvular heart disease who present for evaluation prior to pregnancy, risk assessment can assist in deciding whether surgical intervention before pregnancy is optimal. Most women with mild to moderate valve disease tolerate pregnancy well, such that valve surgery can be deferred. With severe regurgitation or stenosis, decision making is more difficult. If normal hemodynamics can be restored with retention of the native valve, such as mitral valve repair for mitral regurgitation or balloon valvuloplasty for mitral stenosis, intervention for correction of the valve lesion prior to pregnancy usually is indicated. If correction requires valve replacement, the advantages of correcting the hemodynamic abnormality must be weighed against the risks of a prosthetic valve during pregnancy. When valve replacement is needed, the decision of whether to use a mechanical valve or tissue valve is difficult. The issues of anticoagulation are significant during pregnancy in patients with mechanical valves. On the other hand, tissue valves have limited durability, although the impact of pregnancy on durability is debated. Some studies suggest that pregnancy hastens valve degeneration, whereas others suggest the rate of degeneration is related to the young age of the patients, not pregnancy. Individualized recommendations are needed, balancing the risk of anticoagulation against the risk of reoperation.[56-58] In all young women undergoing valve replacement surgery, the possibility of a subsequent pregnancy should be also taken into account when deciding on the type of valve prosthesis.

In women with valvular heart disease who are first seen during pregnancy, surgical intervention usually can be deferred until the postpartum period, even when valve disease is severe. However, surgical intervention may rarely be needed in women with valvular heart disease and hemodynamic compromise during pregnancy that does not respond to medical management. Valve surgery during pregnancy has been performed with a maternal mortality of 3%, similar to nonpregnant women, but with a fetal loss rate between 12% and 20%.[59-61] Risk factors for adverse maternal or fetal outcomes include NYHA class III or higher, left ventricular dysfunction, and emergent procedures. Surgical procedures should be performed by the most experienced surgeon available so to minimize cardiopulmonary bypass time, as risks to the fetus increase with increasing bypass time.[62] Percutaneous mitral valvuloplasty can be performed during pregnancy, if needed, with shielding of the abdomen to limit radiation exposure to the fetus. However, complications at the time of valvuloplasty that require urgent surgical intervention would be expected to have adverse outcomes for the fetus.

Women with severe valve disease who are managed medically during pregnancy should be referred for surgical intervention postpartum using the same criteria as for valve disease in nonpregnant patients (Figure 25-9). However, a postpartum improvement in well-being combined with infant care may result in poor compliance with follow-up visits. Thus, a reasonable approach is to evaluate the valve disease carefully during pregnancy, discuss the options with the patient, and, if intervention is indicated, proceed with valve surgery or balloon valvuloplasty early postpartum, possibly during the same hospital admission.

SPECIFIC VALVULAR LESIONS AND OUTCOMES

Aortic Stenosis

The etiology of aortic stenosis in pregnant women usually is congenital, often a unicuspid valve.[41,63] A substantial number of patients have undergone previous surgical commissurotomy as a child; in 20% restenosis requires reoperation at a mean of 13 (range 3 to 26) years after the initial surgery, at the age when pregnancy is most likely.[64] In women with aortic stenosis, the increased stroke volume of pregnancy is associated with an increase in transaortic velocity and pressure gradient. Valve area calculations are accurate, allowing decision making regarding postpartum management. Many previously asymptomatic women with aortic stenosis have symptom onset during pregnancy due to increased systemic metabolic demands and a limited ability to increase stroke volume.[63,65] Congestive heart failure symptoms also may be due to decreased left ventricular compliance. The relative tachycardia of pregnancy limits the time for diastolic coronary blood flow, sometimes leading to anginal symptoms. Even if pregnancy itself is well tolerated, any superimposed hemodynamic stress, such as infection or anemia, can lead to clinical decompensation.

Aortic stenosis is associated with an increased maternal and fetal risk, with the level of risk related to the severity of left ventricular outflow obstruction.[63,65-67] Symptoms typically increase by one NYHA functional class in about half of patients. Congestive heart failure is the most common complication, reported to occur in as many as 40% of cases.[41,65,68] The risk of neonatal complication is high, affecting as many as 25% of pregnancies in women with aortic stenosis.[41] In a study of 39 patients with aortic stenosis who underwent 49 pregnancies, women with mild and moderate stenosis had no events during pregnancy. Conversely, 40% of those with severe stenosis had events, even when asymptomatic prior to pregnancy.[69]

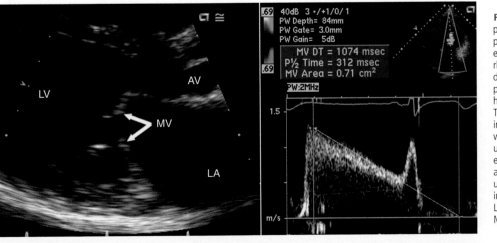

FIGURE 25–9 This 39-year-old woman presented in the third trimester of her fifth pregnancy with dyspnea and crackles on examination. Echocardiography (left) shows rheumatic mitral stenosis with characteristic doming of the mitral leaflets in diastole in a parasternal long axis view. Doppler Pressure half-time (right) shows a valve area of 0.74 cm². The patient was diuresed and symptomatically improved. The remainder of her pregnancy was spent at bedrest, and she underwent an uncomplicated delivery. Dyspnea and pulmonary edema developed in the first 2 days postpartum and responded to diuretics. The woman then underwent balloon valvuloplasty with a significant improvement in her valve area. LV, left ventricle; LA, left atrium; RV, right ventricle; AV, aortic valve; MV, mitral valve.

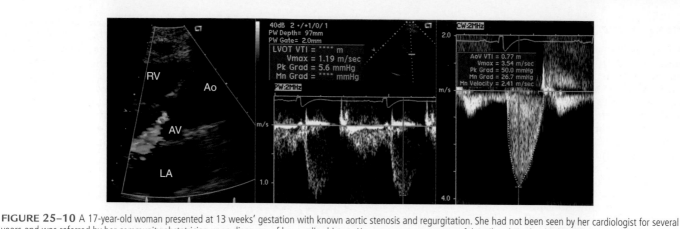

FIGURE 25–10 A 17-year-old woman presented at 13 weeks' gestation with known aortic stenosis and regurgitation. She had not been seen by her cardiologist for several years and was referred by her community obstetrician upon discovery of her cardiac history. Her pregnancy was uneventful until early in the third trimester, when she had palpitations and a near-syncopal event. *Left,* Transthoracic echocardiography of aortic valve in long axis, shows moderate aortic regurgitation and dilated ascending aorta. *Center,* Doppler evaluation of the LV outflow tract (LVOT) for calculation of valve area. *Right,* Doppler evaluation of the aortic valve shows moderate stenosis, with a valve area of 1.1 cm². She was placed on bedrest and underwent an uncomplicated vaginal delivery and subsequent placement of an intrauterine device, as she did not desire more children for at least 5 years. Her peripartum course was complicated by dizziness with ambulation, and exercise testing showed a marked decrease in blood pressure with exercise. Due to significant combined aortic stenosis and regurgitation, she was referred for aortic valve replacement and consideration for aortic root repair. LV, left ventricle; LA, left atrium; RV, right ventricle; AV, aortic valve; Ao, aorta.

Echocardiography allows quantitative evaluation of the severity of aortic stenosis and any associated abnormalities (Figure 25-10). Although aortic stenosis increases the maternal risk, many patients can be managed medically, even when stenosis is severe.[65,70] Patient education and frequent maternal monitoring are used in asymptomatic patients. If symptoms occur, treatment options include bedrest, oxygen supplement, and use of β-blockers to increase left ventricular and coronary diastolic filling times. Intercurrent febrile events are commonly associated with decompensation and often can be managed with fever reduction, β-blockers, supplemental oxygen, and bedrest. With severe decompensation, hemodynamic monitoring in the intensive care unit with optimization of preload and afterload may be needed. Balloon aortic valvuloplasty and aortic valve replacement have been described in patients with severe aortic stenosis who failed medical therapy.[71-73]

Mitral Stenosis

Mitral valve stenosis is most often due to rheumatic valve disease, although congenital mitral stenosis can also be encountered.[40] There is no evidence that pregnancy changes the natural history of rheumatic mitral stenosis.[74] The murmur of mitral stenosis is difficult to appreciate in the pregnant patient. Echocardiography allows accurate evaluation of the severity of stenosis, associated regurgitation, and estimation of pulmonary systolic pressure.

Previously asymptomatic patients with mitral stenosis may first experience symptoms during pregnancy due to the hemodynamic changes of pregnancy.[41] A mild decrease in functional status is experienced by 43% of patients, with 30% experiencing a more severe reduction in functional status, although it should be noted that even normal women have a decrease in functional status with pregnancy.[51] The increased transmitral volume flow rate and the shortened diastolic filling time lead to an increase in left atrial pressure, which may result in congestive heart failure. Symptoms most often begin in the second trimester, with 43% developing heart failure, 20% developing arrhythmias, 50% having a change in medication, and 43% requiring hospitalization during pregnancy.[51]

Beta blockers may be helpful in pregnant women with mitral stenosis by increasing the diastolic filling time, resulting in both a decrease in left atrial pressure and an increase in forward stroke volume.[75] Diuretics may be used judiciously for volume overload if necessary. Diuresis may impair uteroplacental blood flow; therefore, they must be used cautiously. With rheumatic mitral valve disease, it also is important to continue antibiotic prophylaxis to prevent recurrent rheumatic fever during pregnancy.

Admission to the intensive care unit with placement of a pulmonary artery catheter may be needed to guide medical therapy in severely decompensated patients. In patients who are unresponsive to medical therapy, balloon mitral valvuloplasty can be performed during pregnancy, using abdominal shielding to prevent radiation exposure or using transesophageal echocardiography to guide the procedure.[76-81] Immediate and long-term results of balloon valvuloplasty are good even when performed in pregnancy. In a study of 71 NYHA class III-IV patients who underwent valvuloplasty, 98% were NYHA class I-II at the end of pregnancy. Event-free survival at 44 months was 54%. The majority of events were initiation of medical therapy, with some patients undergoing repeat valvuloplasty or mitral valve surgery. The neonates born following valvuloplasty had no clinical abnormalities and had normal growth and development at a mean of 44 months follow-up. This and other data suggest that in patients in whom medical therapy fails, valvuloplasty is an acceptable option.[82,83]

Patients at highest risk for significant decompensation are those with moderate to severe mitral stenosis and cardiac events prior to pregnancy.[51,84-86]

Aortic Regurgitation

Aortic regurgitation is uncommon in pregnant women. Causes include a bicuspid aortic valve, endocarditis, rheumatic valve disease, or aortic root dilation. When aortic root disease is present, such as Marfan syndrome, the risk of pregnancy is more closely linked to the risk of the aortic dissection than to the aortic regurgitation per se. In theory, the decrease in systemic vascular resistance and shortened diastole of pregnancy might decrease aortic regurgitant severity. In reality, aortic regurgitation severity is unchanged, as the decrease in systemic vascular resistance is counterbalanced by the increased intravascular volume and slight increase in aortic root dimension associated with pregnancy. Typically, patients with aortic regurgitation tolerate pregnancy well. If symptoms occur, a careful evaluation to distinguish worsening of valve disease form other causes of symptoms is warranted.

Mitral Regurgitation

Mitral regurgitation in pregnancy may be due to mitral valve prolapse, endocarditis, or rheumatic disease. Mild to moderate mitral regurgitation is well tolerated. Mitral valve prolapse is not associated with increased maternal risk unless severe mitral regurgitation is present.[87,88] Even severe mitral regurgitation may be well tolerated unless atrial fibrillation or pulmonary hypertension complicates the presentation. There also have been case reports of clinical deterioration during pregnancy due to acute severe mitral regurgitation secondary to chordal rupture from endocarditis or myxomatous mitral valve disease.

Management of mitral regurgitation during pregnancy is directed toward careful monitoring during pregnancy and at the time of labor and delivery (Figure 25-11). There are no data to support the use of vasodilators for mitral regurgitation in pregnancy. Pregnancy itself is a powerful afterload reducer. In patients with severe mitral regurgitation who meet ACC/AHA guidelines for surgical intervention, valve repair should be considered in the postpartum period.

Right-Sided Valve Disease

The etiology of pulmonic stenosis in pregnancy is congenital. Thus, severe pulmonic stenosis is rare, having been treated in infancy or childhood. Cases of severe pulmonic stenosis during pregnancy usually are due to restenosis in patients with complex congenital heart disease. Mild to moderate pulmonic stenosis is well tolerated in pregnancy.[51]

Pulmonic stenosis accounted for about 10% of all patients in a series of 599 pregnancies in women with heart disease.[41] There were no adverse cardiac events in these 58 pregnancies and only 1 patient had worsening cardiac symptoms. However, neonatal complications occurred in 17% of these pregnancies.[41] Another study of 17 women with pulmonic stenosis demonstrated no significant maternal and fetal complications during pregnancy.[89] Drenthen and colleagues performed a systematic review of the available literature on pregnancy and women with congenital heart disease.[90] They included 2491 pregnancies, and pulmonic stenosis was present in 123. There were no maternal cardiovascular events during pregnancy. A separate study by the same group evaluating non-cardiac complications of pulmonic stenosis during pregnancy reported a higher than expected rate of pregnancy-induced hypertension and fetal complications including prematurity, small-for-gestational-age status, and intrauterine growth retardation.[91] This has not been seen in other studies, however, and the mechanism for increased pregnancy-induced hypertension is not evident.

Tricuspid stenosis in pregnancy is rare, but treatment with percutaneous balloon valvuloplasty has been reported.

Right-sided valve regurgitation is generally well tolerated in pregnancy. Pulmonic regurgitation also is due to congenital heart disease and is most often a sequelae of a previous surgical procedure, such as repair of tetralogy of Fallot, in pregnant women. In patients with repaired tetralogy of Fallot, maternal and fetal complication rates are generally low, but severe pulmonic regurgitation with impaired right ventricular function, left ventricular dysfunction, and severe pulmonary hypertension are risk factors for maternal cardiac events.[92,93] Tricuspid regurgitation may be due to Ebstein's anomaly or previous endocarditis.[41,94]

Prosthetic Valves

In patients with heart valve prostheses, the hemodynamic changes of pregnancy result in increased transvalvular velocities, even with no change in valve function. However, as for native valves, echocardiographic measures of valve area remain accurate during pregnancy. A baseline echocardiographic study early in pregnancy is useful for comparison, should a change in symptoms occur later in pregnancy.

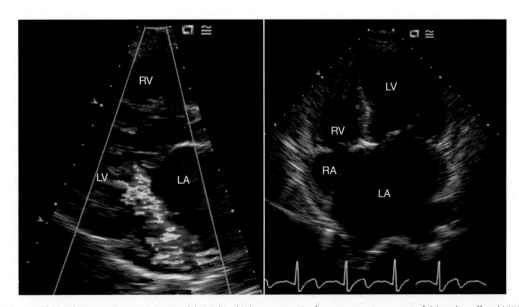

FIGURE 25–11 A 25-year-old gravida 3, para 2 woman presented during her third pregnancy. Her first pregnancy was uneventful, but she suffered NYHA class IV symptoms during the last week of her second pregnancy. At that time she was found to have mitral regurgitation due to rheumatic valve disease. Pulmonary pressures were ≈70 mmHg systolic at that time. She was diuresed and delivered urgently. It was recommended that she undergo valve replacement after delivery, but she did not return for follow-up appointments. She then presented in the second trimester of the current pregnancy with dyspnea. Echocardiographic findings included a parasternal long axis view showing severe mitral regurgitation (Left) and an apical view showing marked left atrial enlargement (Right). Left ventricular size was increased and systolic function mildly decreased. She was diuresed and initially did well, but presented in NYHA class IV symptoms unresponsive to medical therapy. She was again delivered urgently, and had a difficult post-partum course in regard to pulmonary edema, but eventually she improved to her baseline. Valve replacement was again recommended but the patient declined surgical intervention. LV, left ventricle; LA, left atrium; RV, right ventricle; RA, right atrium.

25

The major issues in management of women with heart valve prostheses are anticoagulation for mechanical valves and the risk of valve degeneration with tissue valves.

Women with either tissue or mechanical heart valves have significantly worse outcomes with pregnancy than women without valvular disease.[95-97] Older-generation mechanical valves appear to have higher complication rates[96-99] than newer-generation valves, but little data are available that directly compare the types of valves, and the literature largely reports the experience with older-generation valves.[100]

Women with bioprosthetic valves have fewer thromboembolic or bleeding complications; however, the incidence of maternal death still ranges from 0% to 5%. Data regarding the outcome of bioprosthetic valves during pregnancy are conflicting. Some series suggest a rapid deterioration during or after pregnancy,[56,96-98] whereas others suggest no impact of pregnancy on valve durability.[56-58,101,102] Women with bioprosthetic valves often become pregnant at a time interval after valve replacement when degeneration is likely. Therefore, it remains controversial whether pregnancy itself accelerates valve degeneration or whether the degeneration seen in pregnant women is reflective of the relatively rapid valve degeneration seen in younger patients as a group. Pregnancy with a pulmonic autograft (Ross procedure) has been reported, but the experience with pregnancy after this procedure is limited.[103,104]

Medical Therapy

The basic principles of medical therapy in the pregnant woman with a prosthetic valve are similar to those for the woman with native valve disease. The key elements are quantitative evaluation of valve and cardiac function, careful and frequent antepartum monitoring, judicious use of appropriate medications to relieve symptoms, a planned labor and delivery with optimal pain control, and, in some cases, invasive hemodynamic monitoring.

Anticoagulation

Although the importance of maintaining adequate anticoagulation during pregnancy in women with prosthetic valves is clear,[98,105] the specific approach to management of anticoagulation remains controversial.[97,106] Each option for anticoagulation during pregnancy carries risks for the mother and fetus. Heparin is safe for the fetus, does not cross the placenta, and provides appropriate anticoagulation for the valve when used in therapeutic doses.[107,108] A disadvantage of heparin therapy is development of osteoporosis with a small risk (<2%) of symptomatic fractures but a higher risk of a detectable decrease in bone density (in one third of women).[109-112] In addition, heparin offers significant challenges in optimal methods of drug administration and monitoring of the anticoagulation effect.[99]

Warfarin provides the lowest risk of thromboembolic complications during pregnancy and is easier to administer, although monitoring is similar to that needed with heparin.[100] The major risks of warfarin during pregnancy are the risk of embryopathy and fetal bleeding. Warfarin therapy during pregnancy is associated with first-trimester teratogenicity, particularly between the 6th and 12th weeks of gestation.[113-115] There also may be an increased risk of central nervous system abnormalities with exposure to warfarin at any time in pregnancy.[113] In addition, there is a substantial risk of bleeding in the anticoagulated fetus, especially at the time of delivery.[116] The incidence of warfarin embryopathy is reported to be anywhere from less than 5% to more than 10%.[52,96,100,117,118] In an attempt to consolidate disparate data, many authors have performed literature reviews of the topic. One detailed review found a rate of warfarin embryopathy of 6.4%,[100] whereas another review that emphasized the embryopathy rate in live births found a rate of 7.4% of live births.[58] A reasonable estimate based upon currently available literature is likely 4% to 10%. This adverse effect of warfarin may be dose dependent; in 25 women with a warfarin dose greater than 5 mg/day, fetal complications occurred in 88% and embryopathy in 8%, compared with 33 women on a lower warfarin dose with complications in 15% and embryopathy in 0%.[117]

At this time, there are conflicting data on the use of low-molecular-weight heparin for anticoagulation in pregnant women with mechanical valves.[119-124] In 2002 the Food and Drug Administration issued a recommendation against using enoxaparin for anticoagulation of mechanical heart valves, including during pregnancy.[125]

Unfortunately, there are no randomized controlled trials that compare options for anticoagulation of mechanical heart valves in pregnancy. Available data are cohort studies, small case series, or case reports. Therefore, the literature is rife with reviews and opinion, but little contemporary, quality data on which to make recommendations. Accordingly, the AHA/ACC recommendations emphasize the importance of *continuous effective anticoagulation with frequent monitoring throughout pregnancy.* The guidelines then discuss several options for achieving continuous effective anticoagulation. Class I recommendations for anticoagulation during pregnancy in women with mechanical heart valves are listed in Table 25-6. Options include unfractionated heparin given intravenously or subcutaneously, low-molecular-weight heparin, and warfarin, with the previously discussed caveats regarding risks and benefits of each agent. It should be noted that the guidelines specifically state that if anti-factor Xa levels cannot be monitored, low-molecular-weight heparin should not be used.[44]

With any approach to anticoagulation, close control and monitoring are essential to maintain a therapeutic level and to avoid bleeding or thrombotic complications. In the absence of a meticulous approach to management of anticoagulation, the rate of complications is high.[96] It is likely that many of the hemorrhagic and thromboembolic complications associated with anticoagulation and prosthetic valves during pregnancy could be avoided by a rigorous approach to management and monitoring of anticoagulation.

TABLE 25–6　| ACC/AHA Guidelines Regarding Anticoagulation During Pregnancy

1. Women who stop warfarin from weeks 6 to 12 gestation should be anticoagulated with continuous IV unfractionated heparin, dose-adjusted subcutaneous UFH, or dose-adjusted LMWH.
2. Up to 36 weeks' gestation, the choice of warfarin, continuous IV unfractionated heparin, dose-adjusted subcutaneous UFH, or dose-adjusted LMWH should be discussed fully with the patient. In patients who receive dose-adjusted LMWH, it is administered twice daily, with goal anti-factor Xa levels of 0.7 to 1.2 four hours after administration.
   The target for dose-adjusted UFH should be twice control.
   Warfarin should be dosed to a goal INR of 3 (range 2.5 to 3.0).
3. Warfarin should be stopped 2 weeks prior to planned delivery and replaced with continuous IV UFH.

ACC, American College of Cardiology; AHA, American Heart Association; IV, intravenous; INR, international normalized ratio; LMWH, low-molecular-weight heparin; UFH, unfractionated heparin.

Adapted from Bonow RO, Carabello B, Chatterjee K, et al: ACC/AHA 2006 guidelines for the management of patients with valvular heart disease: a report of the American College of Cardiology/American Heart Association Task Force on Practice Guidelines. J Am Coll Cardiol 2006;48:e1-e148, with permission.

REFERENCES

1. Cole P, St. John Sutton M: Cardiovascular physiology in pregnancy. In Douglas PS (ed): Cardiovascular Health and Disease in Women. Philadelphia, WB Saunders, 1993, pp 305-328.

2. Katz VL: Physiologic changes during normal pregnancy. Curr Opin Obstet Gynecol 1991;3:750-758.

3. Capeless EL, Clapp JF: Cardiovascular changes in early phase of pregnancy. Am J Obstet Gynecol 1989;161:1449-1453.

4. Gilson GJ, Samaan S, Crawford MH, et al: Changes in hemodynamics, ventricular remodeling, and ventricular contractility during normal pregnancy: a longitudinal study. Obstet Gynecol 1997;89:957-962.

5. Mesa A, Jessurun C, Hernandez A, et al: Left ventricular diastolic function in normal human pregnancy. Circulation 1999;99:511-517.

6. Robson SC, Dunlop W: When do cardiovascular parameters return to their preconception values? Am J Obstet Gynecol 1992;167:1479.

7. Mabie WC, DiSessa TG, Crocker LG, et al: A longitudinal study of cardiac output in normal human pregnancy. Am J Obstet Gynecol 1994;170:849-856.

8. Easterling TR, Benedetti TJ: Measurement of cardiac output by impedance technique. Am J Obstet Gynecol 1990;163:1104-1106.

9. Easterling TR, Benedetti TJ, Schmucker BC, et al: Maternal hemodynamics in normal and preeclamptic pregnancies: a longitudinal study. Obstet Gynecol 1990;76:1061-1069.

10. Hunter S, Robson SC: Adaptation of the maternal heart in pregnancy. Br Heart J 1992;68:540-543.

11. Robson SC, Hunter S, Boys RJ, et al: Serial changes in pulmonary haemodynamics during human pregnancy: a non-invasive study using Doppler echocardiography. Clin Sci (Lond) 1991;80:113-117.

12. Clark SL, Cotton DB, Lee W, et al: Central hemodynamic assessment of normal term pregnancy. Am J Obstet Gynecol 1989;161:1439-1442.

13. Edouard DA, Pannier BM, London GM, et al: Venous and arterial behavior during normal pregnancy. Am J Physiol 1998;274:H1605-H1612.

14. Geva T, Mauer MB, Striker L, et al: Effects of physiologic load of pregnancy on left ventricular contractility and remodeling. Am Heart J 1997;133:53-59.

15. Mone SM, Sanders SP, Colan SD. Control mechanisms for physiological hypertrophy of pregnancy. Circulation 1996;94:667-672.

16. Clark SL. Cardiac disease in pregnancy. Crit Care Clin 1991;7:777-797.

17. Easterling TR, Schmucker BC, Benedetti TJ: The hemodynamic effects of orthostatic stress during pregnancy. Obstet Gynecol 1988;72:550-552.

18. McLennan FM, Haites NE, Rawles JM: Stroke and minute distance in pregnancy: a longitudinal study using Doppler ultrasound. Br J Obstet Gynaecol 1987;94:499-506.

19. Robson SC, Dunlop W, Boys RJ, et al: Cardiac output during labour. Br Med J (Clin Res Ed) 1987;295:1169-1172.

20. Lee W, Rokey R, Miller J, et al: Maternal hemodynamic effects of uterine contractions by M-mode and pulsed-Doppler echocardiography. Am J Obstet Gynecol 1989;161:974-977.

21. Strickland RA, Oliver WC Jr, Chantigian RC, et al: Anesthesia, cardiopulmonary bypass, and the pregnant patient. Mayo Clin Proc 1991;66:411-429.

22. Robson SC, Dunlop W, Hunter S: Haemodynamic changes during the early puerperium. Br Med J (Clin Res Ed) 1987;294:1065.

23. Robson SC, Hunter S, Boys RJ, et al: Hemodynamic changes during twin pregnancy. A Doppler and M-mode echocardiographic study. Am J Obstet Gynecol 1989;161:1273-1278.

24. Clark SL, Horenstein JM, Phelan JP, et al: Experience with the pulmonary artery catheter in obstetrics and gynecology. Am J Obstet Gynecol 1985;152:374-378.

25. Robson SC, Boys RJ, Hunter S: Doppler echocardiographic estimation of cardiac output: analysis of temporal variability. Eur Heart J 1988;9:313-318.

26. Robson SC, Murray A, Peart I, et al: Reproducibility of cardiac output measurement by cross sectional and Doppler echocardiography. Br Heart J 1988;59:680-684.

27. Easterling TR, Benedetti TJ, Schmucker BC, et al: Maternal hemodynamics and aortic diameter in normal and hypertensive pregnancies. Obstet Gynecol 1991;78:1073-1077.

28. Sadaniantz A, Kocheril AG, Emaus SP, et al: Cardiovascular changes in pregnancy evaluated by two-dimensional and Doppler echocardiography. J Am Soc Echocardiogr 1992;5:253-258.

29. Robson SC, Hunter S, Moore M, et al: Haemodynamic changes during the puerperium: a Doppler and M-mode echocardiographic study. Br J Obstet Gynaecol 1987;94:1028-1039.

30. Lee W, Rokey R, Cotton DB: Noninvasive maternal stroke volume and cardiac output determinations by pulsed Doppler echocardiography. Am J Obstet Gynecol 1988;158:505-510.

31. Robson SC, Hunter S, Boys RJ, et al: Serial study of factors influencing changes in cardiac output during human pregnancy. Am J Physiol 1989;256:H1060-H1065.

32. Rubler S, Damani PM, Pinto ER: Cardiac size and performance during pregnancy estimated with echocardiography. Am J Cardiol 1977;40:534-540.

33. Vered Z, Poler SM, Gibson P, et al: Noninvasive detection of the morphologic and hemodynamic changes during normal pregnancy. Clin Cardiol 1991;14:327-334.

34. Laird-Meeter K, van de Ley G, Bom TH, et al: Cardiocirculatory adjustments during pregnancy—an echocardiographic study. Clin Cardiol 1979;2:328-332.

35. Hart MV, Morton MJ, Hosenpud JD, et al: Aortic function during normal human pregnancy. Am J Obstet Gynecol 1986;154:887-891.

36. Bradley TD, Logan AG, Kimoff RJ, et al: Continuous positive airway pressure for central sleep apnea and heart failure. N Engl J Med 2005;353:2025-2033.

37. Pouta AM, Rasanen JP, Airaksinen KE, et al: Changes in maternal heart dimensions and plasma atrial natriuretic peptide levels in the early puerperium of normal and pre-eclamptic pregnancies. Br J Obstet Gynaecol 1996;103:988-992.

38. Campos O, Andrade JL, Bocanegra J, et al: Physiologic multivalvular regurgitation during pregnancy: a longitudinal Doppler echocardiographic study. Int J Cardiol 1993;40:265-272.

39. Boudoulas H: Etiology of valvular heart disease. Expert Rev Cardiovasc Ther 2003;1:523-532.

40. Soler-Soler J, Galve E: Worldwide perspective of valve disease. Heart 2000;83:721-725.

41. Siu SC, Sermer M, Colman JM, et al: Prospective multicenter study of pregnancy outcomes in women with heart disease. Circulation 2001;104:515-521.

42. Siu SC, Colman JM, Sorensen S, et al: Adverse neonatal and cardiac outcomes are more common in pregnant women with cardiac disease. Circulation 2002;105:2179-2184.

43. Khairy P, Ouyang DW, Fernandes SM, et al: Pregnancy outcomes in women with congenital heart disease. Circulation 2006;113:517-524.

44. Bonow RO, Carabello BA, Kanu C, et al: ACC/AHA 2006 guidelines for the management of patients with valvular heart disease: a report of the American College of Cardiology/American Heart Association Task Force on Practice Guidelines (writing committee to revise the 1998 Guidelines for the Management of Patients With Valvular Heart Disease): developed in collaboration with the Society of Cardiovascular Anesthesiologists: endorsed by the Society for Cardiovascular Angiography and Interventions and the Society of Thoracic Surgeons. Circulation 2006;114:e84-3231.

45. Milewicz DM, Dietz HC, Miller DC: Treatment of aortic disease in patients with Marfan syndrome. Circulation 2005;111:e150-e157.

46. Lind J, Wallenburg HCS: The Marfan syndrome and pregnancy: a retrospective study in a Dutch population. Eur J Obstetr Gynecol Reprod Biol 2001;98:28-35.

47. Meijboom LJ, Vos FE, Timmermans J, et al: Pregnancy and aortic root growth in the Marfan syndrome: a prospective study. Eur Heart J 2005;26:914-920.

48. Immer FF, Bansi AG, Immer-Bansi AS, et al: Aortic dissection in pregnancy: analysis of risk factors and outcome. Ann Thorac Surg 2003;76:309-314.

49. Bryant-Greenwood GD, Schwabe C. Human relaxins: chemistry and biology. Endocr Rev 1994;15:5-26.

50. Mishra M, Chambers JB, Jackson G: Murmurs in pregnancy: an audit of echocardiography. Br Med J 1992;304:1413-1414.

51. Hameed A, Karaalp IS, Tummala PP, et al: The effect of valvular heart disease on maternal and fetal outcome of pregnancy. J Am Coll Cardiol 2001;37:893-899.

52. Elkayam U, Gleicher N: Cardiac Problems in Pregnancy: Diagnosis and Management of Maternal and Fetal Disease. 3rd ed. New York, Wiley-Liss, 1998.

53. Siu SC, Colman JM: Heart disease and pregnancy. Heart 2001;85:710-715.

54. Gardiner HM: Fetal echocardiography: 20 years of progress. Heart 2001;86:II12-II22.

55. Wilson W, Taubert KA, Gewitz M, et al: Prevention of infective endocarditis: guidelines from the American Heart Association. a guideline from the American Heart Association Rheumatic Fever, Endocarditis, and Kawasaki Disease Committee, Council on Cardiovascular Disease in the Young, and the Council on Clinical Cardiology, Council on Cardiovascular Surgery and Anesthesia, and the Quality of Care and Outcomes Research Interdisciplinary Working Group. Circulation 2007;116:1736-1754.

56. Badduke BR, Jamieson WR, Miyagishima RT, et al: Pregnancy and childbearing in a population with biologic valvular prostheses. J Thorac Cardiovasc Surg 1991;102:179-186.

57. Jamieson WR, Miller DC, Akins CW, et al: Pregnancy and bioprostheses: influence on structural valve deterioration. Ann Thorac Surg 1995;60:S282-S286; discussion S7.

58. Hung L, Rahimtoola SH: Prosthetic heart valves and pregnancy. Circulation 2003;107:1240-1246.

59. Mahli A, Izdes S, Coskun D: Cardiac operations during pregnancy: review of factors influencing fetal outcome. Ann Thorac Surg 2000;69:1622-1626.

60. Pomini F, Mercogliano D, Cavalletti C, et al: Cardiopulmonary bypass in pregnancy. Ann Thorac Surg 1996;61:259-268.

61. Parry AJ, Westaby S: Cardiopulmonary bypass during pregnancy. Ann Thorac Surg 1996;61:1865-1869.

62. Arnoni RT, Arnoni AS, Bonini RC, et al: Risk factors associated with cardiac surgery during pregnancy. Ann Thorac Surg 2003;76:1605-1608.

63. Lao TT, Sermer M, MaGee L, et al: Congenital aortic stenosis and pregnancy—a reappraisal. Am J Obstet Gynecol 1993;169:540-545.

64. Horstkotte D, Loogen F: The natural history of aortic valve stenosis. Eur Heart J 1988;9:57-64.

65. Easterling TR, Chadwick HS, Otto CM, et al: Aortic stenosis in pregnancy. Obstet Gynecol 1988;72:113-118.

66. Arias F, Pineda J: Aortic stenosis and pregnancy. J Reprod Med 1978;20:229-232.

67. Shime J, Mocarski EJ, Hastings D, et al: Congenital heart disease in pregnancy: short-and long-term implications. Am J Obstet Gynecol 1987;156:313-322.

68. Hameed A, Karaalp IS, Tummala PP, et al: The effect of valvular heart disease on maternal and fetal outcome of pregnancy. J Am Coll Cardiol 2001;37:893-899.

69. Silversides CK, Colman JM, Sermer M, et al: Early and intermediate-term outcomes of pregnancy with congenital aortic stenosis. Am J Cardiol 2003;91:1386-1389.

70. Brian JE Jr, Seifen AB, Clark RB, et al: Aortic stenosis, cesarean delivery, and epidural anesthesia. J Clin Anesth 1993;5:154-157.

71. Lao TT, Adelman AG, Sermer M, et al: Balloon valvuloplasty for congenital aortic stenosis in pregnancy. Br J Obstet Gynaecol 1993;100:1141-1142.

72. Sreeram N, Kitchiner D, Williams D, et al: Balloon dilatation of the aortic valve after previous surgical valvotomy: immediate and follow up results. Br Heart J 1994;71:558-560.

73. Banning AP, Pearson JF, Hall RJ: Role of balloon dilatation of the aortic valve in pregnant patients with severe aortic stenosis. Br Heart J 1993;70:544-545.

74. Chesley LC: Severe rheumatic cardiac disease and pregnancy: the ultimate prognosis. Am J Obstet Gynecol 1980;136:552-558.

75. al Kasab SM, Sabag T, al Zaibag M, et al: Beta-adrenergic receptor blockade in the management of pregnant women with mitral stenosis. Am J Obstet Gynecol 1990;163:37-40.

76. Ben Farhat M, Gamra H, Betbout F, et al: Percutaneous balloon mitral commissurotomy during pregnancy. Heart 1997;77:564-567.

77. Gupta A, Lokhandwala YY, Satoskar PR, et al: Balloon mitral valvotomy in pregnancy: maternal and fetal outcomes. J Am Coll Surg 1998;187:409-415.

78. Patel JJ, Mitha AS, Hassen F, et al: Percutaneous balloon mitral valvotomy in pregnant patients with tight pliable mitral stenosis. Am Heart J 1993;125:1106-1109.

79. Ribeiro PA, Fawzy ME, Awad M, et al: Balloon valvotomy for pregnant patients with severe pliable mitral stenosis using the Inoue technique with total abdominal and pelvic shielding. Am Heart J 1992;124:1558-1562.

80. Ruzyllo W, Dabrowski M, Woroszylska M, et al: Percutaneous mitral commissurotomy with the Inoue balloon for severe mitral stenosis during pregnancy. J Heart Valve Dis 1992;1:209-212.

81. Stoddard MF, Longaker RA, Vuocolo LM, et al: Transesophageal echocardiography in the pregnant patient. Am Heart J 1992;124:785-787.

82. Esteves CA, Munoz JS, Braga S, et al: Immediate and long-term follow-up of percutaneous balloon mitral valvuloplasty in pregnant patients with rheumatic mitral stenosis. Am J Cardiol 2006;98:812-816.

83. Mangione JA, Lourenco RM, dos Santos ES, et al: Long-term follow-up of pregnant women after percutaneous mitral valvuloplasty. Catheter Cardiovasc Interv 2000;50:413-417.

84. Silversides CK, Colman JM, Sermer M, et al: Cardiac risk in pregnant women with rheumatic mitral stenosis. Am J Cardiol 2003;91:1382-1385.

85. Reimold SC, Rutherford JD: Clinical practice. Valvular heart disease in pregnancy. N Engl J Med 2003;349:52-59.

86. Elkayam U, Bitar FL Valvular heart disease and pregnancy. Part I: native valves. J Am Coll Cardiol 2005;46:223-230.

87. Jana N, Vasishta K, Khunnu B, et al: Pregnancy in association with mitral valve prolapse. Asia Oceania J Obstet Gynaecol 1993;19:61-65.

88. Tang LC, Chan SY, Wong VC, et al: Pregnancy in patients with mitral valve prolapse. Int J Gynaecol Obstet 1985;23:217-221.

89. Hameed AB, Goodwin TM, Elkayam U: Effect of pulmonary stenosis on pregnancy outcomes—a case-control study. Am Heart J 2007;154:852-854.

90. Drenthen W, Pieper PG, Roos-Hesselink JW, et al: Outcome of pregnancy in women with congenital heart disease: a literature review. J Am Coll Cardiol 2007;49:2303-2311.

91. Drenthen W, Pieper PG, Roos-Hesselink JW, et al: Non-cardiac complications during pregnancy in women with isolated congenital pulmonary valvar stenosis. Heart 2006;92:1838-1843.

92. Veldtman GR, Connolly HM, Grogan M, et al: Outcomes of pregnancy in women with tetralogy of fallot. J Am Coll Cardiol 2004;44:174-180.

93. Meijer JM, Pieper PG, Drenthen W, et al: Pregnancy, fertility, and recurrence risk in corrected tetralogy of Fallot. Heart 2005;91:801-805.

94. Connolly HM, Warnes CA: Ebstein's anomaly: outcome of pregnancy. J Am Coll Cardiol 1994;23:1194-1198.

95. Pavankumar P, Venugopal P, Kaul U, et al: Pregnancy in patients with prosthetic cardiac valve. A 10-year experience. Scand J Thorac Cardiovasc Surg 1988;22:19-22.

96. Sbarouni E, Oakley CM. Outcome of pregnancy in women with valve prostheses. Br Heart J 1994;71:196-201.

97. Born D, Martinez EE, Almeida PA, et al: Pregnancy in patients with prosthetic heart valves: the effects of anticoagulation on mother, fetus, and neonate. Am Heart J 1992;124:413-417.

98. Hanania G, Thomas D, Michel PL, et al: Pregnancy and prosthetic heart valves: a French cooperative retrospective study of 155 cases. Eur Heart J 1994;15:1651-1658.

99. Salazar E, Izaguirre R, Verdejo J, et al: Failure of adjusted doses of subcutaneous heparin to prevent thromboembolic phenomena in pregnant patients with mechanical cardiac valve prostheses. J Am Coll Cardiol 1996;27:1698-1703.

100. Chan WS, Anand S, Ginsberg JS: Anticoagulation of pregnant women with mechanical heart valves: a systematic review of the literature. Arch Intern Med 2000;160:191-196.

101. El SF, Hassan W, Latroche B, et al: Pregnancy has no effect on the rate of structural deterioration of bioprosthetic valves: long-term 18-year follow up results. J Heart Valve Dis 2005;14:481-485.

102. Avila WS, Rossi EG, Grinberg M, et al: Influence of pregnancy after bioprosthetic valve replacement in young women: a prospective five-year study. J Heart Valve Dis 2002;11:864-869.

103. Dore A, Somerville J: Pregnancy in patients with pulmonary autograft valve replacement. Eur Heart J 1997;18:1659-1662.

104. Yap SC, Drenthen W, Pieper PG, et al: Outcome of pregnancy in women after pulmonary autograft valve replacement for congenital aortic valve disease. J Heart Valve Dis 2007;16:398-403.

105. Sareli P, England MJ, Berk MR, et al: Maternal and fetal sequelae of anticoagulation during pregnancy in patients with mechanical heart valve prostheses. Am J Cardiol 1989;63:1462-1465.

106. Vongpatanasin W, Hillis LD, Lange RA: Prosthetic heart valves. N Engl J Med 1996;335:407-416.

107. Ginsberg JS, Hirsh J, Turner DC, et al: Risks to the fetus of anticoagulant therapy during pregnancy. Thromb Haemost 1989;61:197-203.

108. Ginsberg JS, Kowalchuk G, Hirsh J, et al: Heparin therapy during pregnancy. Risks to the fetus and mother. Arch Intern Med 1989;149:2233-2236.

109. Ginsberg JS, Kowalchuk G, Hirsh J, et al: Heparin effect on bone density. Thromb Haemost 1990;64:286-289.

110. Dahlman T, Lindvall N, Hellgren M: Osteopenia in pregnancy during long-term heparin treatment: a radiological study post partum. Br J Obstet Gynaecol 1990;97:221-228.

111. Barbour LA, Kick SD, Steiner JF, et al: A prospective study of heparin-induced osteoporosis in pregnancy using bone densitometry. Am J Obstet Gynecol 1994;170:862-869.

112. Dahlman TC: Osteoporotic fractures and the recurrence of thromboembolism during pregnancy and the puerperium in 184 women undergoing thromboprophylaxis with heparin. Am J Obstet Gynecol 1993;168:1265-1270.

113. Hall JG, Pauli RM, Wilson KM: Maternal and fetal sequelae of anticoagulation during pregnancy. Am J Med 1980;68:122-140.

114. Becker MH, Genieser NB, Finegold M, et al: Chondrodysplasis punctata: is maternal warfarin therapy a factor? Am J Dis Child 1975;129:356-359.

115. Iturbe-Alessio I, Fonseca MC, Mutchinik O, et al: Risks of anticoagulant therapy in pregnant women with artificial heart valves. N Engl J Med 1986;315:1390-1393.

116. Ville Y, Jenkins E, Shearer MJ, et al: Fetal intraventricular haemorrhage and maternal warfarin. Lancet 1993;341:1211.

117. Vitale N, De Feo M, De Santo LS, et al: Dose-dependent fetal complications of warfarin in pregnant women with mechanical heart valves. J Am Coll Cardiol 1999;33:1637-1641.

118. Cotrufo M, De Feo M, De Santo LS, et al: Risk of warfarin during pregnancy with mechanical valve prostheses. Obstet Gynecol 2002;99:35-40.

119. Dulitzki M, Pauzner R, Langevitz P, et al: Low-molecular-weight heparin during pregnancy and delivery: preliminary experience with 41 pregnancies. Obstet Gynecol 1996;87:380-383.

120. Montalescot G, Polle V, Collet JP, et al: Low molecular weight heparin after mechanical heart valve replacement. Circulation 2000;101:1083-1086.

121. Casele HL, Laifer SA, Woelkers DA, et al: Changes in the pharmacokinetics of the low-molecular-weight heparin enoxaparin sodium during pregnancy. Am J Obstet Gynecol 1999;181:1113-1117.

122. Rowan JA, McCowan LM, Raudkivi PJ, et al: Enoxaparin treatment in women with mechanical heart valves during pregnancy. Am J Obstet Gynecol 2001;185:633-637.

123. Leyh RG, Fischer S, Ruhparwar A, et al: Anticoagulation for prosthetic heart valves during pregnancy: is low-molecular-weight heparin an alternative? Eur J Cardiothorac Surg 2002;21:577-579.

124. Ginsberg JS, Chan WS, Bates SM, et al: Anticoagulation of pregnant women with mechanical heart valves. Arch Intern Med 2003;163:694-698.

125. http://www.fda.gov/medwatch/SAFETY/2002/lovenox.htm (accessed February 17, 2009)

APPENDIX 1. ACC/AHA GUIDELINES CLASSIFICATION AND LEVELS OF EVIDENCE

"SIZE OF TREATMENT EFFECT"

<table>
<tr><th></th><th>Class I

Benefit >>> Risk

Procedure/Treatment SHOULD be performed/administered</th><th>Class IIa

Benefit >> Risk

Additional studies with focused objectives needed

IT IS REASONABLE to perform procedure/ administer treatment</th><th>Class IIb

Benefit ≥ Risk

Additional studies with broad objectives needed; additional registry data would be helpful

Procedure/treatment MAY BE CONSIDERED</th><th>Class III

Risk ≥ Benefit

No additional studies needed

Procedure/treatment SHOULD NOT be performed/administered since it is NOT HELPFUL and MAY BE HARMFUL</th></tr>
<tr><td>Level A

*Multiple (3-5) population risk strata evaluated**

General consistency of direction and magnitude of effect</td><td>Recommendation that procedure or treatment is useful/effective

Sufficient evidence from multiple randomized trials or meta-analyses</td><td>Recommendation in favor of treatment or procedure being useful/effective

Some conflicting evidence from multiple randomized trials or meta-analyses</td><td>Recommendation's usefulness/efficacy less well established

Greater conflicting evidence from multiple randomized trials or meta-analyses</td><td>Recommendation that procedure or treatment not useful/effective and may be harmful

Sufficient evidence from multiple randomized trials or meta-analyses</td></tr>
<tr><td>Level B

*Limited (2-3) population risk strata evaluated**</td><td>Recommendation that procedure or treatment is useful/effective

Limited evidence from single randomized trial or non-randomized studies</td><td>Recommendation in favor of treatment or procedure being useful/effective

Some conflicting evidence from single randomized trial or non-randomized studies</td><td>Recommendation's usefulness/efficacy less well established

Greater conflicting evidence from single randomized trial or non-randomized studies</td><td>Recommendation that procedure or treatment not useful/effective and may be harmful

Limited evidence from single randomized trial or non-randomized studies</td></tr>
<tr><td>Level C

*Very limited (1-2) population risk strata evaluated**</td><td>Recommendation that procedure or treatment is useful/effective

Only expert opinion, case studies, or standard-of-care</td><td>Recommendation in favor of treatment or procedure being useful/effective

Only diverging expert opinion, case studies, or standard-of-care</td><td>Recommendation's usefulness/efficacy less well established

Only diverging expert opinion, case studies, or standard-of-care</td><td>Recommendation that procedure or treatment not useful/effective and may be harmful

Only expert opinion, case studies, or standard-of-care</td></tr>
<tr><td>Suggested phrases for writing recomemndations[†]</td><td>should
is recommended
is indicated
is useful/effective/ beneficial</td><td>is reasonable
can be is useful/ effective/beneficial
is probably recommended or indicated</td><td>may/might be considered
may/might be reasonable
usefulness/effectiveness is unknown/unclear/ uncertain or not well established</td><td>is not recommended
is not indicated
should not
is not useful/effective/ beneficial
may be harmful</td></tr>
</table>

(Left vertical axis label: "ESTIMATE OF CERTAINTY (PRECISION) OF TREATMENT EFFECT")

Applying classification of recommendations and level of evidence.

*Data available from clinical trials or registries about the usefulness/efficacy in different subpopulations, such as gender, age, history of diabetes, history of prior myocardial infarction, history of heart failure, and prior aspirin use. A recommendation with Level of Evidence B or C does not imply that the recommendation is weak. Many important clinical questions addressed in the guidelines do not lend themselves to clinical trials. Even though randomized trials are not available, there may be a very clear clinical consensus that a particular test or therapy is useful or effective.

†In 2003 the ACC/AHA Task Force on Practice Guidelines recently provided a list of suggested phrases to use when writing recommendations. All recommendations in this guideline have been written in full sentences that express a complete thought, such that a recommendation, even if separated and presented apart from the rest of the document (including headings above sets of recommendations), would still convey the full intent of the recommendation. It is hoped that this will increase readers' comprehension of the guidelines and will allow queries at the individual recommendation level.

APPENDIX 2. ESC GUIDELINES CLASSIFICATION AND LEVELS OF EVIDENCE

Class I	Class IIa	Class IIb
Evidence and/or general agreement that a given treatment or procedure is beneficial, useful, and effective	Conflicting evidence and/or a divergence of opinion about the usefulness/efficacy of a given treatment or procedure	Conflicting evidence and/or a divergence of opinion about the usefulness/efficacy of a given treatment or procedure
	Weight of evidence/opinion is in favor of usefulness/efficacy	*Usefulness/efficacy is less well established by evidence/opinion*

Level of Evidence A	Level of Evidence B	Level of Evidence C
Data derived from multiple randomized clinical trials or meta-analyses	Data derived from a single randomized clinical trial or large non-randomized studies	Consensus of opinion of the experts and/or small studies, retrospective studies, registries

Note: Page numbers followed by *f* indicates figure and *t* indicates table.